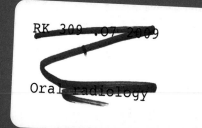

# Oral Radiology

## PRINCIPLES
## and INTERPRETATION

# Oral Radiology
## PRINCIPLES
## and INTERPRETATION

### Sixth Edition

**STUART C. WHITE, DDS, PhD**
Distinguished Professor
Section of Oral and Maxillofacial Radiology
School of Dentistry
University of California, Los Angeles
Los Angeles, California

**MICHAEL J. PHAROAH, DDS, MSc, FRCD(C)**
Professor, Department of Radiology
Faculty of Dentistry
University of Toronto
Toronto, Ontario
Canada

MOSBY

ELSEVIER

11830 Westline Industrial Drive
St. Louis, Missouri 63146

ORAL RADIOLOGY: PRINCIPLES AND INTERPRETATION        ISBN: 978-0-323-04983-2

**Library of Congress Cataloging-in-Publication Data**

Oral radiology : principles and interpretation / [edited by] Stuart C. White, Michael J. Pharoah.—6th ed.
    p. ; cm.
  Includes bibliographical references and index.
  ISBN 978-0-323-04983-2 (pbk. : alk. paper)   1. Teeth—Radiography.   2. Jaws—Radiography.
3. Mouth—Radiography.   I. White, Stuart C.   II. Pharoah, M. J.
  [DNLM:   1. Radiography, Dental. WN 230 O63 2009]
  RK309.O7 2009
  617.6′07572—dc22

                                                                    2008016461

*Vice President and Publisher:* Linda Duncan
*Senior Editor:* John Dolan
*Managing Editor:* Jaime Pendill
*Publishing Services Manager:* Patricia Tannian
*Project Manager:* Claire Kramer
*Design Direction:* Kimberly Denando

Printed in China
Last digit is the print number:   9  8  7  6  5  4  3  2

## TO OUR FAMILIES

Liza

Heather, Kelly, Ingrid, Xander, and Zeke

Linda

Jayson, Edward, and Lian

# CONTRIBUTORS

**Byron W. Benson, DDS, MS**
Professor and Vice Chair
Department of Diagnostic Sciences
Texas A&M Health Science Center
Baylor College of Dentistry
Dallas, Texas

**Sharon L. Brooks, DDS, MS**
Professor
Department of Periodontics and Oral Medicine
University of Michigan
School of Dentistry
Ann Arbor, Michigan

**Laurie C. Carter, DDS, PhD**
Professor and Director
Oral and Maxillofacial Radiology
Director of Advanced Dental Education
Virginia Commonwealth University
School of Dentistry
Richmond, Virginia

**Allan G. Farman, BDS, PhD (odont), DSc (odont)**
Professor, Division of Radiology and Imaging Science
Department of Surgical and Hospital Dentistry
Clinical Professor, Department of Diagnostic Radiology School of
    Medicine
Adjunct Professor, Department of Anatomical Sciences and
    Neurobiology
University of Louisville
Louisville, Kentucky

**Mel L. Kantor, DDS, MPH, PhD**
Professor
Division of Oral and Maxillofacial Radiology
Department of Diagnostic Sciences
UMDNJ New Jersey Dental School
Newark, New Jersey

**Ernest W.N. Lam, DMD, PhD, FRCD(C)**
Associate Professor
Oral and Maxillofacial Radiology
University of Toronto
Toronto, Ontario, Canada

**Linda Lee, DDS, MSc, Dipl ABOP, FRCD(C)**
Dental Oncology
Princess Margaret Hospital
University Health Network
University of Toronto
Toronto, Ontario, Canada

**John B. Ludlow, DDS, MS, FDS, RCSEd**
Professor of Oral and Maxillofacial Radiology
University of North Carolina at Chapel Hill
School of Dentistry
Chapel Hill, North Carolina

**Alan G. Lurie, DDS, PhD**
Professor and Chair
Oral and Maxillofacial Radiology
University of Connecticut
School of Dentistry
Farmington, Connecticut

**André Mol, DDS, MS, PhD**
Assistant Professor
Department of Diagnostic Sciences and General Dentistry
University of North Carolina at Chapel Hill
School of Dentistry
Chapel Hill, North Carolina

**Carol Anne Murdoch-Kinch, DDS, PhD**
Associate Professor
Department of Oral and Maxillofacial Surgery/Hospital Dentistry
University of Michigan
Ann Arbor, Michigan

**Susanne Perschbacher, DDS, MSc, FRCD(C)**
Assistant Professor
Oral and Maxillofacial Radiology
University of Toronto
Toronto, Ontario, Canada

**C. Grace Petrikowski, DDS, MSc, FRCD(C)**
Associate Professor
Faculty of Dentistry, University of Toronto
Toronto, Ontario, Canada

**Axel Ruprecht, DDS, MScD, FRCD(C)**
Gilbert E. Lilly Professor of Diagnostic Sciences
Professor and Director of Oral and Maxillofacial Radiology
Professor of Radiology
Professor of Anatomy and Cell Biology
The University of Iowa
Iowa City, Iowa

**William C. Scarfe, BDS, MS, FRACDS**
Professor
Radiology and Imaging Sciences
University of Louisville
School of Dentistry
Louisville, Kentucky

**Vivek Shetty, DDS, Dr Med Dent**
Professor
Section of Oral and Maxillofacial Surgery
UCLA
School of Dentistry
Los Angeles, California

**Sotirios Tetradis, DDS, PhD**
Professor
Section of Oral and Maxillofacial Radiology
UCLA
School of Dentistry
Los Angeles, California

**Ann Wenzel, PhD, Dr Odont**
Professor and Head
Department of Oral Radiology
School of Dentistry
University of Aarhus
Aarhus, Denmark

**Robert E. Wood, DDS, PhD, FRCD(C), DABFO**
Head, Department of Dental Oncology
Princess Margaret Hospital
Associate Professor, University of Toronto
Toronto, Ontario, Canada

# PREFACE

Each new edition of this textbook provides the opportunity to include recent progress in our rapidly changing field of diagnostic imaging. Every chapter has been revised in light of new knowledge, technology, and techniques. It is the continuing goal of our textbook to present the underlying science of diagnostic imaging, including the core principles of image production and interpretation for the dental student.

For the first time, we are able to offer supplemental resources to both instructors and students. We will have a companion Evolve website (http://evolve.elsevier.com/White/oralradiology) for the sixth edition. For instructors, a test bank and image collection will save time in preparing for lectures and examinations. Students have access to a fully searchable bibliography with MedLine links to assist in research.

We are sincerely appreciative of the contributions of all authors for sharing their expertise with the reader and acknowledge the superb contributions of previous contributors, Kathryn Atchison and Neil Frederiksen.

This edition welcomes three new authors. Dr. William C. Scarfe and Dr. Allan G. Farman, colleagues at the University of Louisville, prepared an excellent new chapter on cone-beam imaging. This imaging modality is rapidly evolving and making substantive superb contributions to diagnostic challenges involving placement of dental implants, detection and interpretation of dental and osseous disease, and cephalometric analysis. Their chapter describes the underlying principles and clinical applications of this technology. Dr. Susanne Perschbacher at the University of Toronto rewrote the chapter on periodontal diseases, a critical subject in oral health that dentists manage daily.

The chapters on radiographic manifestations of disease in the orofacial region have been updated with an effort to keep a balance between the amount of detailed information and the depth of knowledge required for the dental student. The additions include the latest information on etiology and diagnosis and more examples of advanced imaging, including cone-beam computed tomography images. New concepts on the classification of oral and maxillofacial diseases published by the World Health Organization have been introduced. Also, the clinical and radiologic aspects of new entities have been included, such as bisphosphonate-related osteonecrosis in the chapter on inflammatory lesions of the jaws. The chapter on orofacial implants has been expanded and updated to include the application of new imaging modalities and new software programs to keep students and instructors abreast of this rapidly changing field.

**Stuart C. White**
**Michael J. Pharoah**

# ACKNOWLEDGMENTS

We have drawn on the special talents of many of our colleagues as authors of chapters, some for the first time and others for return visits. We thank all for sharing their knowledge and skills. We are also most grateful for the generous support from the staff at Elsevier for their energy and creativity in the presentation of the content of this book.

Finally, we particularly thank our students whose sharp eyes and minds constantly discover new ways for us to improve each edition.

**Stuart C. White**
**Michael J. Pharoah**

# CONTENTS

# PART
# ONE

# Physics of Ionizing Radiation

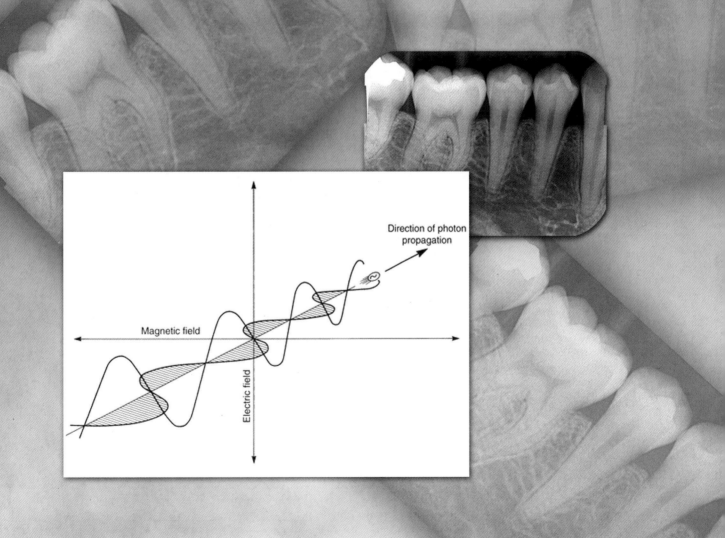

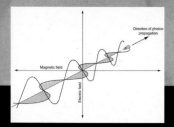

# CHAPTER 1

# Radiation Physics

*One atom says to a friend, "I think I lost an electron." The friends replies, "Are you sure?" "Yes," says the first atom, "I'm positive."*

## Composition of Matter

Matter is anything that has mass and occupies space. Matter occurs in three states: solid, liquid, and gas. Atoms, the fundamental units of matter, cannot be subdivided by chemical methods although they may be composed of many smaller (subatomic) particles. Bohr viewed the atom as a miniature solar system with a nucleus at the center and revolving electrons (Fig. 1-1). Although this classical view of the atom has the virtue of being easily understood, it has been replaced in recent decades by the Standard Model, which describes fundamental particles, and the Quantum Mechanical Model, which describes the arrangement of electrons in an atom.

According to the Standard Model, there are 12 types of fundamental matter particles plus their corresponding antiparticles (Table 1-1). These particles are considered to be fundamental because current experiments show that they have no inner structure and cannot be divided. These fundamental particles consist of six types of quarks and six types of leptons and their antiparticles (particles having an opposite charge but otherwise identical to quarks and leptons). Quarks only exist in association with other quarks, never as solitary particles. Neutrons and protons are made of quarks. Unlike quarks, leptons exist only as solitary particles. The stable leptons are electrons and neutrinos. All visible matter in the universe (that is, all stable matter) is made of up quarks, down quarks, and electrons. Antimatter particles are rare and highly unstable because when they interact with matter, they mutually annihilate into pure energy. The universe is made of 24% matter and 76% dark energy. Only 5% of the matter is in the form of atoms and neutrinos. The nature of the rest of the matter, and of dark energy, is unknown.

In addition to matter particles, the Standard Model describes force carrier particles—particles that mediate interactions between matter particles. They are the means by which matter (quarks and leptons) interacts without touching, such as through magnetism, light, and electrostatic attraction and repulsion. Photons mediate the electromagnetic force, W and Z bosons mediate the weak nuclear force (associated with beta decay), and gluons mediate the strong nuclear force that binds nuclei together. Gravity is speculated to be mediated by gravitons, a fourth type of force particle (but not part of the Standard Model).

## ATOMIC STRUCTURE

### Nucleus

In all atoms except hydrogen, the nucleus consists of positively charged protons and neutral neutrons. A hydrogen nucleus contains a single proton. Protons and neutrons in turn are made of quarks (Fig. 1-2).

Protons (with a charge of 1) consist of two up quarks (charge $\frac{2}{3}$ each) and one down quark (charge $-\frac{1}{3}$). Neutrons are made of one up quark and two down quarks and thus are neutral. Although the positively charged protons repel each other, the nucleus does not fly apart because it is held together by the strong nuclear force, the rapid exchange of gluons. The strong nuclear force overwhelms the repulsive electromagnetic effect at the incredibly short distances inside an atomic nucleus.

The number of protons in the nucleus determines the identity of an element. This is its atomic number ($Z$), the nuclear charge. Each of the more than 100 elements has a specific atomic number, a corresponding number of orbital electrons in the ground state, and unique chemical and physical properties. Nearly the entire mass of the atom consists of the protons and neutrons in the nucleus. The total number of protons and neutrons in the nucleus of an atom is its atomic mass ($A$).

### Electron Orbitals

The *Quantum Mechanical Model* describes contemporary understanding of the arrangement of electrons in an atom. Beginning with the work of Schrödinger, physicists saw electrons as being small particles that exhibit particle-like properties (e.g., they have mass) and wavelike properties (e.g., they generate interference patterns). The previous concept of electrons circling around nuclei in two-dimensional orbits has been replaced by the concept of electrons existing in three-dimensional volumes called *orbitals*. Orbitals represent the probability locations of the electron in space at any instant in time, the regions in which the electron is most likely to exist. Each kind of orbital is characterized by a set of quantum numbers $n$, $l$, and $m$. The principal quantum number ($n$) describes the size of the orbital, the average distance of the electron from the nucleus. The angular momentum quantum number ($l$) describes the shape of the orbital ($l$ can never be greater than $n - 1$). The letters s, p, d, f, g, and h are used to describe orbital shapes and correspond with angular momentum values of 0, 1, 2, 3, 4, and 5, respectively. The s-type orbital is spherical (Fig. 1-3). The s-type orbitals are the first to be filled in every element. Next are the p-type orbitals, which are bilobed and centered on the nucleus. Boron is the first element to contain an electron in a p orbital. Next are the d-type orbitals, which consist of four lobes arranged around the nucleus or they are bilobed with a ring. Scandium is the first element to contain an electron in a d orbital. The magnetic quantum number ($m$) describes the orientation of an orbital in space. In an atom with many electrons the electron clouds of one orbital are superimposed with those of other orbitals. No known atom has more than seven orbitals. Only two electrons may occupy an orbital. Electrons occupy the lowest energy available orbitals first (lowest principal quantum number then the lowest angular momentum). Finally, for the first 18 elements, the orbitals fill up first each of the available orientations (*m*) one at a time so that their spins are unpaired.

In all atoms there is an electrostatic attraction between the positively charged nucleus and its surrounding negatively charged electrons. The amount of energy required to remove an electron from a given orbital must exceed the electrostatic force of attraction between it and the nucleus. This is called the *electron binding energy* of the electron (or *ionization energy*) and is specific for each orbital of each element. Electrons in the 1s orbital of a given element have the greatest binding energy because they are closest to the nucleus. The binding energy of the electrons in each successively larger orbital decreases. For an electron to move from a specific orbital to another orbital farther from the nucleus, energy must be supplied in an amount equal to the difference in binding energies between the two orbitals. In contrast, in moving an electron from an outer orbital to one closer to the nucleus, energy is lost and given up in the form of electromagnetic radiation (see "Characteristic Radiation," p. 10).

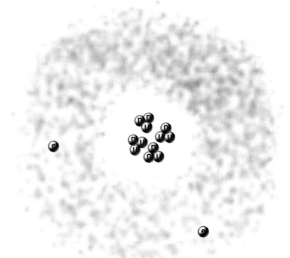

FIG. **1-2** Modern view of helium atom showing nucleus with two protons, each composed of two up quarks (U) and one down quark (D), two neutrons, each made of one up quark and two down quarks, and two surrounding electrons within a spherical orbital.

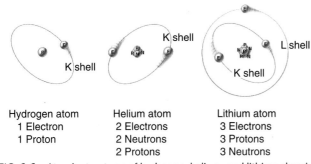

Hydrogen atom
1 Electron
1 Proton

Helium atom
2 Electrons
2 Neutrons
2 Protons

Lithium atom
3 Electrons
3 Protons
3 Neutrons

FIG. **1-1** Atomic structures of hydrogen, helium, and lithium showing electrons orbiting nuclei containing neutrons and protons as described by Bohr in the early twentieth century.

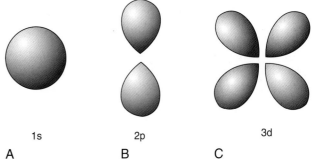

1s　　2p　　3d
A　　B　　C

FIG. **1-3** Electron orbitals look like clouds of varying density, probability plots of the location of the electron. **A,** The s-type electron orbital is spherical and centered around the nucleus. **B,** p-type electron orbitals are bilobed and centered around the nucleus. **C,** Four of the five d-type electron orbitals are made up of four lobes, centered on the nucleus, the other is bilobed with an encircling ring.

TABLE **1-1**
*Fundamental Particles*

| | FAMILIES OF MATTER | | | FORCE CARRIER PARTICLES |
|---|---|---|---|---|
| | I | II | III | |
| Quarks | u up | c charm | t top | γ photon |
| | d down | s strange | b bottom | g gluon |
| Leptons | e electron | μ muon | τ tau | W W boson |
| | $\nu_e$ electron neutrino | $\nu_\mu$ muon neutrino | $\nu_\tau$ tau neutrino | Z Z boson |

## IONIZATION

When the number of electrons in an atom is equal to the number of protons in its nucleus, the atom is electrically neutral. If such an atom loses an electron, the nucleus becomes a positive ion and the free electron a negative ion. This process of forming an ion pair is termed *ionization*. To ionize an atom requires sufficient energy to overcome the electrostatic force binding the electrons to the nucleus. The binding energy of an electron is related to the atomic number of the atom and the orbital type. Large atomic number elements (high *Z*) have more protons in their nucleus and thus bind electrons in any give orbital more tightly than do smaller-*Z* elements. Within a given atom, electrons in the inner orbitals are more tightly bound than the more distant outer orbitals. Tightly bound electrons require the energy of x rays or high-energy particles to remove them, whereas loosely bound electrons can be displaced by ultraviolet radiation. However, *nonionizing radiations*, such as visible light, infrared, and microwave radiation, and radio waves do not have sufficient energy to remove bound electrons from their orbitals.

## Nature of Radiation

Radiation is the transmission of energy through space and matter. It may occur in two forms: particulate and electromagnetic.

## RADIOACTIVITY

Small atoms have roughly equal numbers of protons and neutrons, whereas larger atoms tend to have more neutrons than protons. This makes them unstable and they may break up, releasing α or β particles or γ rays. This process is called *radioactivity*. When a radioactive atom releases an α or β particle, the atom is transmuted into another element. α Particles are helium nuclei consisting of two protons and two neutrons. They result from the radioactive decay of many large atomic number elements. Because of their double positive charge and heavy mass, α particles densely ionize matter through which they pass. Accordingly, they quickly give up their energy and penetrate only a few micrometers of body tissue. (An ordinary sheet of paper absorbs them.) After stopping, α particles acquire two electrons and become neutral helium atoms.

When a neutron in a radioactive nucleus decays, it produces a proton, a β particle, and a neutrino. β Particles are otherwise identical to electrons. High-speed β particles are not densely ionizing; thus, they are able to penetrate matter to a greater depth than α particles

can, up to a maximum of 1.5 cm in tissue. This deeper penetration occurs because β particles are smaller and lighter and carry a single negative charge; therefore they have a much lower probability of interacting with matter than do α particles. β Particles are used in radiation therapy for treatment of some skin cancers.

The capacity of particulate radiation to ionize atoms depends on its mass, velocity, and charge. The rate of loss of energy from a particle as it moves along its track through matter (tissue) is its *linear energy transfer* (LET). A particle loses kinetic energy each time it ionizes adjacent matter. The greater its physical size and charge and the lower its velocity, the greater is its LET. For example, α particles, with their high charge and low velocity, are densely ionizing, lose their kinetic energy rapidly, and thus have a high LET. β Particles are much less densely ionizing because of their lighter mass and lower charge; thus they have a lower LET. High LET radiations concentrate their ionization along a short path, whereas low LET radiations produce ion pairs much more sparsely over a longer path length.

The third type of radioactivity is γ decay. γ Rays are photons, a form of electromagnetic radiation (see later). They result as part of a decay chain where a massive nucleus produced by fission converts from an excited state to a lower-level ground state.

## ELECTROMAGNETIC RADIATION

Electromagnetic radiation is the movement of energy through space as a combination of electric and magnetic fields. It is generated when the velocity of an electrically charged particle is altered. γ, x rays, ultraviolet rays, visible light, infrared radiation (heat), microwaves, and radio waves are all examples of electromagnetic radiation (Fig. 1-4). γ originate in the nuclei of radioactive atoms. They typically have greater energy than do x rays. X rays, in contrast, are produced extranuclearly from the interaction of electrons with large atomic nuclei in x-ray machines. The types of radiation in the electromagnetic spectrum may be ionizing or nonionizing, depending on their energy.

Quantum theory considers electromagnetic radiation as small bundles of energy called *photons*. Each photon travels at the speed of light and contains a specific amount of energy. The unit of photon energy is the *electron volt* (eV), the amount of energy acquired by one electron accelerating through a potential difference of 1 volt ($1.602 \times 10^{-19}$ joules). The relationship between wavelength and photon energy is as follows:

$$E = h \times c / \lambda$$

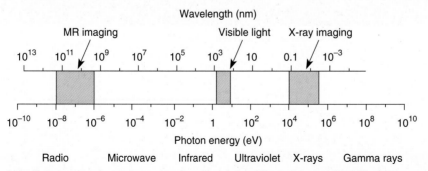

FIG. **1-4** Electromagnetic spectrum showing the relationship among wavelength, photon energy, and physical properties of various portions of the spectrum. Photons with shorter wavelengths have higher energy. Photons used in dental radiography have a wavelength of 0.1 to 0.001 nanometers.

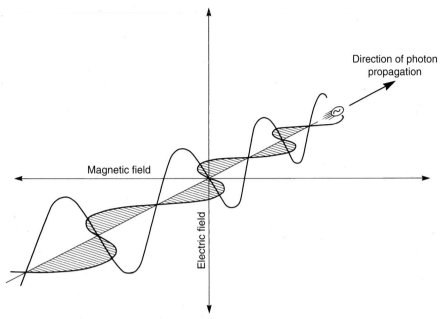

FIG. **1-5**  The electric and magnetic fields associated with a photon.

where $E$ is energy in kiloelectron volts (keV), $h$ is Planck's constant $(6.626 \times 10^{-34}$ joule-seconds or $4.3 \times 10^{-18}$ keV), $c$ is the velocity of light, and $\lambda$ is wavelength in nanometers. This expression may be simplified to the following:

$$E = 1.24 / \lambda$$

Some properties of electromagnetic radiation are best expressed by quantum theory, whereas others are most successfully described by wave theory. The quantum theory of radiation has been successful in correlating experimental data on the interaction of radiation with atoms, the photoelectric effect, and the production of x rays. The wave theory of electromagnetic radiation maintains that radiation is propagated in the form of waves, not unlike the waves resulting from a disturbance in water. Such waves consist of electric and magnetic fields oriented in planes at right angles to one another that oscillate perpendicular to the direction of motion (Fig. 1-5). All electromagnetic waves travel at the velocity of light ($c = 3.0 \times 10^8$ m/sec) in a vacuum. Waves of all kinds exhibit the properties of wavelength ($\lambda$) and frequency ($\nu$) and are related as follows:

$$\lambda \times \nu = c = 3 \times 10^8 \, m/sec$$

where $\lambda$ is in meters and $\nu$ is in cycles per second (hertz). Wave theory is more useful for considering radiation in bulk when millions of quanta are being examined, as in experiments dealing with refraction, reflection, diffraction, interference, and polarization.

High-energy photons such as x rays and $\gamma$ rays are typically characterized by their energy (electron volts), medium-energy photons (e.g., visible light and ultraviolet waves) by their wavelength (nanometers), and low-energy photons (e.g., AM and FM radio waves) by their frequency (KHz and MHz).

## X-Ray Machine

The primary components of an x-ray machine are the x-ray tube and its power supply. The x-ray tube is positioned within the tube head, along with some components of the power supply (Fig. 1-6). Often

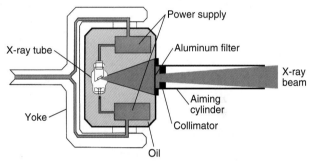

FIG. **1-6**  Tube head (including the recessed x-ray tube), components of the power supply, and the oil that conducts heat away from the x-ray tube. Path of useful x-ray beam from anode through filter and collimator to end of aiming cylinder shown in blue.

the tube is recessed within the tube head to improve the quality of the radiographic image (see Chapter 4). The tube head is supported by an arm that is usually mounted on a wall. A control panel allows the operator to adjust the time of exposure and often the energy and exposure rate of the x-ray beam.

## X-RAY TUBE

An x-ray tube is composed of a cathode and an anode situated within an evacuated glass envelope or tube (Fig. 1-7). Electrons stream from a filament in the cathode to a target in the anode, where they produce x rays. For the x-ray tube to function, a power supply is necessary to (1) heat the cathode filament to generate electrons and (2) establish a high-voltage potential between the anode and cathode to accelerate the electrons toward the anode.

### Cathode

The cathode (see Fig. 1-7) in an x-ray tube consists of a filament and a focusing cup. The *filament* is the source of electrons within the x-ray tube. It is a coil of tungsten wire about 2 mm in diameter and 1 cm or less in length. It is mounted on two stiff wires that support it and carry the electric current. These two mounting wires lead through the glass envelope and connect to both the high- and low-voltage electrical sources. The filament is heated to incandescence by the flow of current from the low-voltage source and emits electrons at a rate proportional to the temperature of the filament.

The filament lies in a *focusing cup* (Fig. 1-8, *A*; see also Fig. 1-7), a negatively charged concave reflector made of molybdenum. The parabolic shape of the focusing cup electrostatically focuses the electrons emitted by the filament into a narrow beam directed at a small rectangular area on the anode called the *focal spot* (Fig. 1-8, *B*; see also Fig. 1-7). The electrons move in this direction because they are both repelled by the negatively charged cathode and attracted to the positively charged anode. The x-ray tube is evacuated to prevent collision of the fast-moving electrons with gas molecules, which would significantly reduce their speed. The vacuum also prevents oxidation, "burnout," of the filament.

### Anode

The anode consists of a tungsten target embedded in a copper stem (see Fig. 1-7). The purpose of the *target* in an x-ray tube is to convert the kinetic energy of the colliding electrons into x-ray photons. The target is made of tungsten, an element that has several characteristics of an ideal target material. It has a high atomic number (74), a high melting point, high thermal conductivity, and low vapor pressure at the working temperatures of an x-ray tube. The conversion of the kinetic energy of the electrons into x-ray photons is an inefficient process with more than 99% of the electron kinetic energy converted to heat. A target made of a high atomic number material is most efficient in producing x rays. Because heat is generated at the anode, the requirement for a target with a *high melting point* is clear. Tungsten also has *high thermal conductivity,* thus readily dissipating its heat into the copper stem. Finally, the *low vapor pressure* of tungsten at high temperatures helps maintain the vacuum in the tube at high operating temperatures. The tungsten target is typically embedded in a large block of copper. Copper, also a good *thermal conductor,* removes heat from the tungsten, thus reducing the risk of the target melting. Additionally, insulating oil between the glass envelope and the housing of the tube head carries heat away from the copper stem. This type of anode is a *stationary anode* because it has no moving parts.

The *focal spot* is the area on the target to which the focusing cup directs the electrons and from which x rays are produced. The sharpness of a radiographic image increases as the size of the focal spot decreases (see Chapter 4). The heat generated per unit target area, however, becomes greater as the focal spot decreases in size. To take advantage of a small focal spot while distributing the electrons over a larger area of the target, the target is placed at an angle to the electron beam (Fig. 1-9). The apparent size of the focal spot seen from a position perpendicular to the electron beam (the *effective focal spot*) is smaller than the actual focal spot size. Typically, the target is inclined about 20 degrees to the central ray of the x-ray beam. This causes the effective focal spot to be approximately 1 × 1 mm, as opposed to the actual focal spot, which is about 1 × 3 mm. This results in a small apparent source of x rays and thus an increase in the sharpness of the image (see Fig. 4-2), with a larger actual focal spot size to improve heat dissipation.

Another method of dissipating the heat from a small focal spot is to use a *rotating anode.* In this case the tungsten target is in the form of a beveled disk that rotates when the tube is in operation (Fig. 1-10). As a result, the electrons strike successive areas of the target, widening the focal spot by an amount corresponding to the circumference of the beveled disk, thus distributing the heat over this extended area.

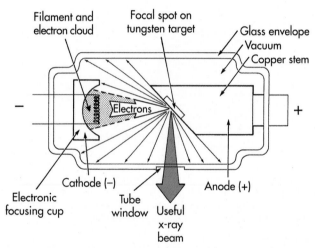

FIG. **1-7** X-ray tube with the major components labeled.

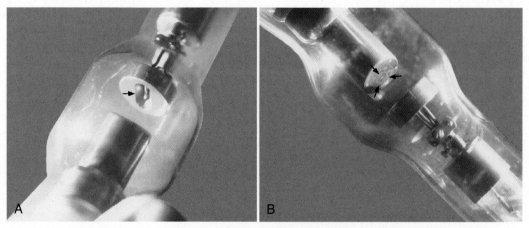

FIG. **1-8** **A,** Focusing cup *(arrow)* containing a filament in the cathode of the tube from a dental x-ray machine. **B,** Focal ipot area *(arrows)* on the target of the tube.

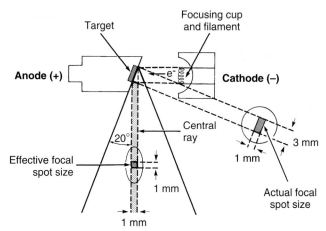

FIG. **1-9** The angle of the target to the central ray of the x-ray beam has a strong influence on the apparent size of the focal spot. The projected effective focal spot is much smaller than the actual focal spot size.

The focal spot of a stationary tube is now a focal track in rotating anode machines. Narrow focal tracks in rotating anode tubes can be used with tube currents of 100 to 500 milliamperes (mA), 10 to 50 times that possible with stationary targets. The target and rotor (armature) of the motor lie within the x-ray tube, and the stator coils (which drive the rotor at about 3000 revolutions per minute) lie outside the tube. Such rotating anodes are not used in intraoral dental x-ray machines but may be used in tomographic or cephalometric units and are always used in medical computed tomography x-ray machines, which require high radiation output.

## POWER SUPPLY

The primary functions of the power supply of an x-ray machine are to (1) provide a low-voltage current to heat the x-ray tube filament and (2) generate a high potential difference between the anode and cathode. The x-ray tube and two transformers lie within an electrically grounded metal housing called the *head* of the x-ray machine. An electrical insulating material, usually oil, surrounds the tube and transformers.

### Tube Current

The *tube current* is the flow of electrons through the tube; that is, from the cathode filament, across the tube to the anode, and then back to the filament. The *filament transformer* (Fig. 1-11) reduces the voltage of the incoming alternating current (AC) to about 10 volts in the filament circuit. This voltage is regulated by the filament current control (mA selector), which adjusts the resistance and thus the current flow through the filament. This in turn regulates the filament temperature and thus the number of electrons emitted. The mA setting on the filament current control actually refers to the tube current, typically about 10 mA, which is measured by the milliammeter. This is not the same as the current in the filament circuit.

Notice also that the tube current is dependent on the tube voltage; as the voltage increases between the anode and cathode, so does the current flow. The hot filament releases electrons, creating a negative space charge around the filament. When the filament wire is positive, the released electrons stay near the filament. The increasingly negative space charge impedes the further release of electrons. When the anode

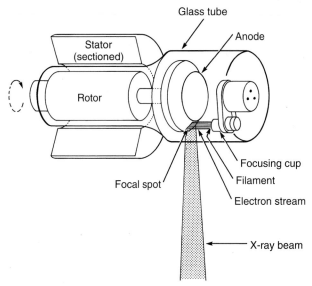

FIG. **1-10** X-ray tube with a rotating anode, which allows heat at the focal spot to spread out over a large surface area.

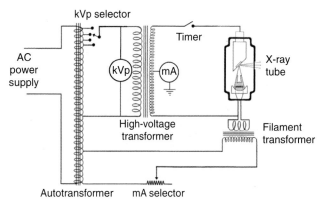

FIG. **1-11** Schematic of dental x-ray machine circuitry and x-ray tube with the major components labeled.

becomes positive, it attracts electrons from the filament, the space charge is reduced, and increasing numbers of electrons are released from the filament, thereby increasing the tube current. The higher the voltage, the greater this effect.

### Tube Voltage

A high voltage is required between the anode and cathode to give electrons sufficient energy to generate x rays. The actual voltage used on an x-ray machine is adjusted with the *autotransformer* (see Fig. 1-11). By using the kilovolt peak (kVp) selector, the operator adjusts the autotransformer and converts the primary voltage from the input source into the desired secondary voltage. The selected secondary voltage is applied to the primary winding of the *high-voltage transformer,* which boosts the peak voltage of the incoming line current (110 V) up to 60,000 to 100,000 V (60 to 100 kV). This boosts the peak energy of the electrons passing through the tube to as high as 60 to 100 keV and provides them sufficient energy to generate x rays. The kVp dial thus selects the peak operating voltage between the anode and cathode.

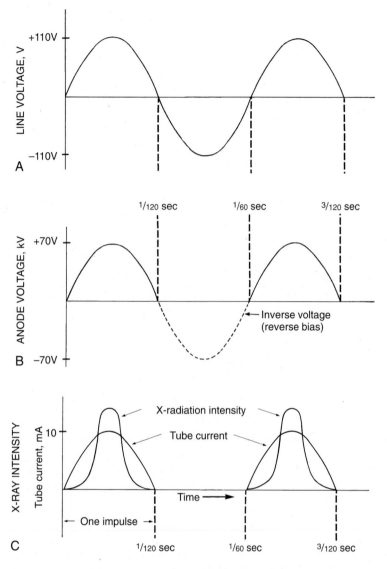

FIG. **1-12** **A**, A 60-cycle AC line voltage at autotransformer. **B**, Voltage at the anode varies up to the kVp setting (70 in this case). **C**, The intensity of radiation produced at the anode increases as the anode voltage increases. (Modified from Johns HE, Cunningham JR: *The physics of radiology,* ed 3, Springfield, Ill, 1969, Charles C Thomas.)

Because the polarity of the line current alternates (60 cycles per second), the polarity of the x-ray tube alternates at the same frequency (Fig. 1-12, *A*). When the polarity of the voltage applied across the tube causes the target anode to be positive and the filament to be negative, the electrons around the filament accelerate toward the positive target and current flows through the tube (Fig. 1-12, *B*). Because the line voltage varies continuously, so does the voltage potential between the anode and cathode.

The operating voltage of an x-ray machine is stated as the kVp. As the tube voltage is increased, the speed of the electrons moving toward the anode increases. When the electrons strike the focal spot of the target, some of their energy converts to x-ray photons. X rays are produced at the target with greatest efficiency when the voltage applied across the tube is high. Therefore the intensity of x-ray pulses tends to be sharply peaked at the center of each cycle (Fig. 1-12, *C*). During the following half (or negative half) of each cycle, the filament becomes positive and the target negative (see Fig. 1-12, *B*). At these times the electrons do not flow across the gap between the two elements of the tube. This half of the cycle is called *inverse voltage* or *reverse bias* (see Fig. 1-12, *B*). No x rays are generated during this half of the voltage cycle (see Fig. 1-12, *C*). Therefore when an x-ray tube

is powered with 60-cycle AC, 60 pulses of x rays are generated each second, each having a duration of $\frac{1}{120}$ second. This type of power supply circuitry, in which the alternating high voltage is applied directly across the x-ray tube, limits x-ray production to half the AC cycle and is called *self-rectified* or *half-wave rectified*. Almost all conventional dental x-ray machines are self-rectified.

Some dental x-ray manufacturers produce machines that replace the conventional 60-cycle AC, half-wave rectified power supply with a full-wave rectified, high-frequency power supply. This results in an essentially constant potential between the anode and cathode. The result is that the mean energy of the x-ray beam produced by these x-ray machines is higher than that from a conventional half-wave rectified machine operated at the same voltage. For a given voltage setting and radiographic density, the images resulting from these constant-potential machines have a longer contrast scale and the patient receives a lower dose compared with conventional x-ray machines.

## TIMER

A timer is built into the high-voltage circuit to control the duration of the x-ray exposure (see Fig. 1-11). The electronic timer controls the length of time that high voltage is applied to the tube and therefore the time during which tube current flows and x rays are produced. Before the high voltage is applied across the tube, however, the filament must be brought to operating temperature to ensure an adequate rate of electron emission. Subjecting the filament to continuous heating at normal operating current shortens its life. To minimize filament damage, the timing circuit first sends a current through the filament for about half a second to bring it to the proper operating temperature and then applies power to the high-voltage circuit. In some circuit designs, a continuous low-level current passing through the filament maintains it at a safe low temperature, thereby further shortening the delay to preheat the filament. For these reasons an x-ray machine may be left on continuously during working hours.

Some x-ray machine timers are calibrated in fractions of a second, whereas others are expressed as number of impulses in an exposure (e.g., 3, 6, 9, 15). The number of impulses divided by 60 (the frequency of the power source) gives the exposure time in seconds. Thus a setting of 30 impulses means that there will be 30 impulses of radiation equivalent to a half-second exposure.

## TUBE RATING AND DUTY CYCLE

X-ray tubes produce heat at the target while in operation. The heat buildup at the anode is measured in heat units (HU), where HU = kVp × mA × seconds. The heat storage capacity for anodes of dental diagnostic tubes is approximately 20 kHU. Heat is removed from the target by conduction to the copper anode and then to the surrounding oil and tube housing and by convection to the atmosphere.

Each x-ray machine comes with a *tube rating* chart that describe the longest exposure time the tube can be energized for a range of voltages (kVp) and tube current (mA) values without risk of damage to the target from overheating. These tube ratings generally do not impose any restrictions on tube use for intraoral radiography. If a dental x-ray unit is used for extraoral exposures, however, it is wise to mount the tube-rating chart by the machine for easy reference. *Duty cycle* relates to the frequency with which successive exposures can be made. The interval between successive exposures must be long enough for heat dissipation. This characteristic is a function of the size of the anode and the method used to cool it.

## Production of X Rays

Most high-speed electrons traveling from the filament to the target interact with target electrons and release their energy as heat. Occasionally, however, electrons convert their kinetic energy into x-ray photons by the formation of *bremsstrahlung* and *characteristic radiation*.

### BREMSSTRAHLUNG RADIATION

The sudden stopping or slowing of high-speed electrons by tungsten nuclei in the target produces bremsstrahlung photons, the primary source of radiation from an x-ray tube. (*Bremsstrahlung* means "braking radiation" in German.) Occasionally electrons from the filament directly hit the nucleus of a target atom. When this happens, all the kinetic energy of the electron is transformed into a single x-ray photon (Fig. 1-13, *A*). The energy of the resultant photon (in keV) is thus numerically equal to the energy of the electron, that is, the voltage applied across the x-ray tube at that instant.

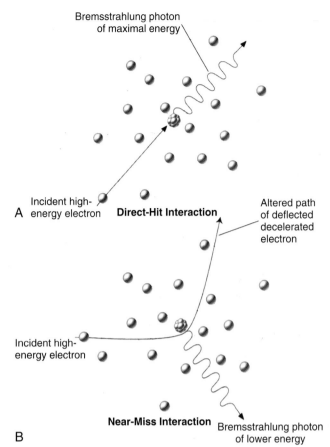

FIG. **1-13** Bremsstrahlung radiation is produced by the direct hit of an electron on a nucleus in the target **(A)** or more frequently, by the passage of an electron near a nucleus, which results in electrons being deflected and decelerated **(B)**.

More frequently, high-speed electrons have near or wide misses with atomic nuclei (see Fig. 1-13, *B*). In these interactions, the electron is attracted toward the positively charged nuclei, its path is altered towards the nucleus, and it loses some of its velocity. This deceleration causes the electron to lose kinetic energy that is given off in the form of many new photons. The closer the high-speed electron approaches the nuclei, the greater is the electrostatic attraction between the nucleus and the electron, braking effect, and energy of the resulting bremsstrahlung photons.

Bremsstrahlung interactions generate x-ray photons with a continuous spectrum of energy. The energy of an x-ray beam is usually described by identifying the peak operating voltage (in kVp). A dental x-ray machine operating at a peak voltage of 70 kVp, for example, applies a fluctuating voltage of up to 70 kVp across the tube. This tube therefore produces a continuous spectrum of x-ray photons with energies ranging to a maximum of 70 keV (Fig. 1-14). The reasons for this continuous spectrum are as follows:

1. The continuously varying voltage difference between the target and filament, which is characteristic of half-wave rectification, causes the electrons striking the target to have varying levels of kinetic energy.
2. The bombarding electrons pass at varying distances around tungsten nuclei and are thus deflected to varying extents. As a

result, they give up varying amounts of energy in the form of bremsstrahlung photons.

3. Many electrons participate in many bremsstrahlung interactions in the target before losing all their kinetic energy. As a consequence, an electron carries differing amounts of energy at the time of each interaction with a tungsten nucleus that results in the generation of an x-ray photon.

## CHARACTERISTIC RADIATION

Characteristic radiation contributes only a small fraction of the photons in an x-ray beam. It occurs when an incident electron ejects an inner electron from the tungsten target. When this happens, an electron from an outer orbital is quickly attracted to the void in the deficient inner orbital (Fig. 1-15). When the outer-orbital electron replaces the displaced electron, a photon is emitted with an energy equivalent to the difference in the two orbital binding energies. The energies of characteristic photons are discrete because they represent the difference of the energy levels of electron orbital levels and hence are characteristic of the target atoms.

## Factors Controlling the X-Ray Beam

An x-ray beam may be modified by altering the beam exposure duration (timer), exposure rate (mA), energy (kVp and filtration), shape (collimation), and intensity (target-patient distance).

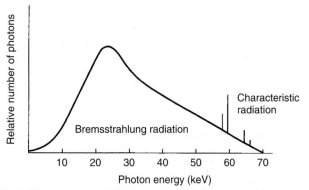

FIG. **1-14**   Spectrum of photons emitted from an x-ray beam generated at 70 kVp. The vast preponderance of radiation is bremsstrahlung, with a minor addition of characteristic radiation.

## EXPOSURE TIME

Changing the time controls the duration of the exposure and thus the number of photons generated (Fig. 1-16). When the exposure time is doubled, the number of photons generated at all energies in the x-ray emission spectrum is doubled, but the range of photon energies is unchanged.

## TUBE CURRENT (mA)

The quantity of radiation produced by an x-ray tube (i.e., the number of photons that reach the patient and film) is directly proportional to the tube current (mA) and the time the tube is operated (Fig. 1-17). As the mA setting is increased, more power is applied to the filament, which heats up and releases more electrons that collide with the target to produce radiation. The quantity of radiation produced is expressed as the product of time and tube current. The quantity of radiation remains constant regardless of variations in mA and time as long as the product remains constant. For instance, a machine operating at 10 mA for 1 second (10 mA) produces the same quantity of radiation when operated at 20 mA for 0.5 second (10 mA). In practice some dental x-ray machines fall slightly short of this ideal constancy. The term *beam quantity* or *beam intensity* refers to the number of photons an x-ray beam.

## TUBE VOLTAGE (kVp)

Increasing the kVp increases the potential difference between the cathode and the anode, thus increasing the energy of each electron when it strikes the target. This results in an increased efficiency of conversion of electron energy into x-ray photons and thus an increase in (1) the number of photons generated, (2) their mean energy, and (3) their maximal energy (Fig. 1-18).

The ability of x-ray photons to penetrate matter depends on their energy. High-energy x-ray photons have a greater probability of penetrating matter, whereas lower-energy photons have a greater probability of being absorbed. Therefore the higher the kVp and mean energy of the x-ray beam, the greater the penetrability of the beam through matter. A useful way to characterize the penetrating quality of an x-ray beam (its energy) is by its half-value layer (HVL). The HVL is the thickness of an absorber, such as aluminum, required to reduce by one half the number of x-ray photons passing through it.

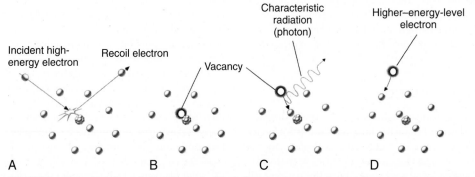

FIG. **1-15**   Characteristic radiation. **A,** An incident electron ejects an electron from in an inner orbital creating a photoelectron and a vacancy. **B,** An electron from an outer orbital fills this vacancy. **C,** A photon is emitted with energy equal to the difference in energy levels between the two orbitals. **D,** Electrons from various orbitals may be involved, giving rise to other photons. The energies of the photons thus created are characteristic of the target atom.

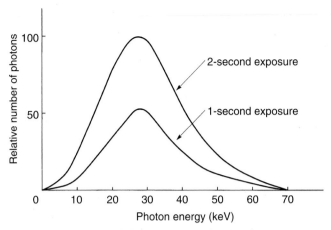

FIG. **1-16** Spectrum of photon energies showing that, as exposure time increases (kVp and tube voltage held constant), so does the total number of photons. The mean energy and maximal energies of the beams are unchanged.

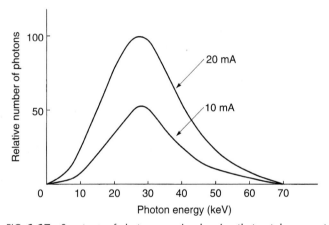

FIG. **1-17** Spectrum of photon energies showing that as tube current (mA) increases (kVp and exposure time held constant), so does the total number of photons. The mean energy and maximal energies of the beams are unchanged. Compare with Figure 1-16.

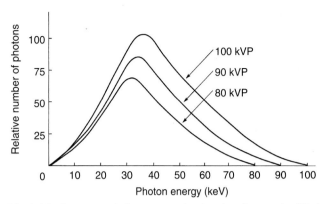

FIG. **1-18** Spectrum of photon energies showing that, as the kVp is increased (tube current and exposure time held constant), there is a corresponding increase in the mean energy of the beam, the total number of photons emitted, and the maximal energy of the photons.

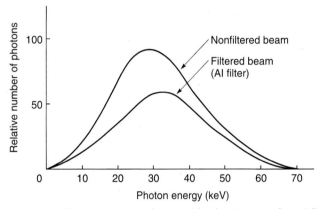

FIG. **1-19** Filtering an x-ray beam with aluminum preferentially removes low-energy photons, thereby reducing the beam intensity while increasing the mean energy of the residual beam.

As the average energy of an x-ray beam increases, so does its HVL. The term *beam quality* refers to the mean energy of an x-ray beam.

Exposure time, tube current (mA), and tube voltage are the three variables found on many x-ray machines. In some machines the setting of the tube current, the setting of the tube voltage, or both are fixed. It is recommended that if the tube current is variable that the operator select the highest mA value available and always operate the machine at this setting. This will result in the lowest exposure time for a given exposure and thus minimize the chance of patient movement. Similarly, if tube voltage can be adjusted, it is recommended that the operator select a desired voltage, perhaps 70 kVp, and leave the machine at this setting. This protocol simplifies selecting the proper patient exposure by using just exposure time as the means to adjust for anatomic location within the mouth and patient size.

## FILTRATION

Although an x-ray beam consists of a spectrum of x-ray photons of different energies, only photons with sufficient energy to penetrate through anatomic structures and reach the image receptor (film or digital) are useful for diagnostic radiology. Photons that are of such low energy that they cannot reach the receptor contribute to patient exposure (risk) but do not offer any benefit. Consequently, to reduce patient dose, such low-energy photons should be removed from the beam. This can be accomplished, in part, by placing an aluminum filter in the path of the beam. An aluminum filter preferentially removes many of the lower-energy photons with lesser effect on the higher-energy photons that are able to contribute to making an image (Fig. 1-19).

*Inherent filtration* consists of the materials that x-ray photons encounter as they travel from the focal spot on the target to form the usable beam outside the tube enclosure. These materials include the glass wall of the x-ray tube, the insulating oil that surrounds many dental tubes, and the barrier material that prevents the oil from escaping through the x-ray port. The inherent filtration of most x-ray machines ranges from the equivalent of 0.5 to 2 mm of aluminum. *Total filtration* is the sum of the inherent filtration plus any added *external filtration* supplied in the form of aluminum disks placed over the port in the head of the x-ray machine. Governmental regulations require the total filtration in the path of a dental

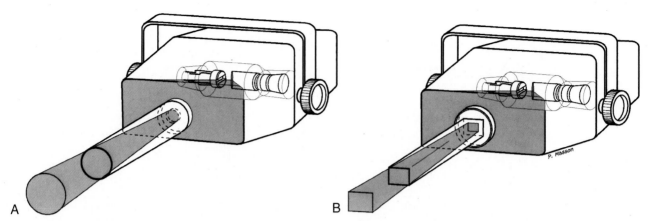

FIG. **1-20** Collimation of an x-ray beam *(blue)* is achieved by restricting its useful size. **A,** Circular collimator. **B,** Rectangular collimator restricts area of exposure to just larger than the detector size.

x-ray beam to be equal to the equivalent of 1.5 mm of aluminum up to 70 kVp and 2.5 mm of aluminum for all higher voltages (see Chapter 3).

## COLLIMATION

A collimator is a metallic barrier with an aperture in the middle used to reduce the size of the x-ray beam and thereby the volume of irradiated tissue (Fig. 1-20). Round and rectangular collimators are most frequently used in dentistry. Dental x-ray beams are usually collimated to a circle 2¾ inches (7 cm) in diameter. A round collimator (see Fig. 1-20, *A*) is a thick plate of radiopaque material (usually lead) with a circular opening centered over the port in the x-ray head through which the x-ray beam emerges. Typically, round collimators are built into open-ended aiming cylinders. Rectangular collimators (see Fig. 1-20, *B*) further limit the size of the beam to just larger than the x-ray film, thereby further reducing patient exposure. Some types of film-holding instruments also provide rectangular collimation of the x-ray beam (see Chapters 3 and 9).

Use of collimation also improves image quality. When an x-ray beam is directed at a patient, the hard and soft tissues absorb about 90% of the photons and about 10% pass through the patient and reach the film. Many of the absorbed photons generate scattered radiation within the exposed tissues by a process called *Compton scattering* (see later). These scattered photons travel in all directions, and some reach the film and degrade image quality. Collimating the x-ray beam thus reduces the exposure area and thus the number of scattered photons reaching the film.

## INVERSE SQUARE LAW

The intensity of an x-ray beam (the number of photons per cross-sectional area per unit of exposure time) depends on the distance of the measuring device from the focal spot. For a given beam the intensity is inversely proportional to the square of the distance from the source (Fig. 1-21). The reason for this decrease in intensity is that an x-ray beam spreads out as it moves from its source. The relationship is as follows:

$$\frac{I_1}{I_2} = \frac{(D_2)^2}{(D_1)^2}$$

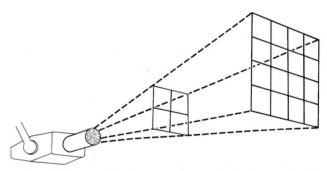

FIG. **1-21** The intensity of an x-ray beam is inversely proportional to the square of the distance between the source and the point of measure.

where *I* is intensity and *D* is distance. Therefore if a dose of 1 Gy is measured at a distance of 2 m, a dose of 4 Gy will be found at 1 m and 0.25 Gy at 4 m.

Therefore changing the distance between the x-ray tube and patient has a marked effect on skin exposure. Such a change requires a corresponding modification of the kVp or mA to keep constant the exposure to the film or digital sensor.

## Interactions of X-Rays with Matter

In dental imaging the x-ray beam enters the face of a patient, interacts with hard and soft tissues, and then strikes a digital sensor or film. The incident beam contains photons of many energies but is spatially heterogeneous. That is, the intensity of the beam is essentially uniform from the center of the beam outward. As the beam goes through the patient, it is attenuated, that is, reduced in intensity. This attenuation results from interactions of individual photons in the beam with atoms in the absorber. The x-ray photons are either absorbed or scattered out of the beam. In absorption interactions, photons ionize absorber atoms, convert their energy into kinetic energy of the ejected electron, and cease to exist. In scattering interactions, photons also interact with absorber atoms but then move off in another direction. The frequency of these interactions depends on the type of tissue exposed. Thus although the incident beam striking the patient is spatially homogenous, the remnant beam, the beam that exits the patient, is spatially heterogeneous. It is this differential exposure of the film that allows a radiograph to reveal the morphologic features of enamel, dentin, bone, and soft tissues through which it has passed.

In a dental x-ray beam there are three means of beam attenuation: (1) coherent scattering, (2) photoelectric absorption, and (3) Compton scattering. In addition, about 9% of the primary photons pass through the patient without interaction (Fig. 1-22 and Table 1-2).

## COHERENT SCATTERING

Coherent scattering (also known as *classical, elastic,* or *Thompson scattering*) may occur when a low-energy incident photon (less than 10 keV) passes near an outer electron of an atom. The incident photon interacts with the electron by causing it to become momentarily excited at the same frequency as the incoming photon (Fig. 1-23). The incident photon ceases to exist. The excited electron then returns to the ground state and generates another x-ray photon with the same frequency (energy) as in the incident beam. Usually the secondary photon is emitted at an angle to the path of the incident photon. The net effect is that the direction of the incident x-ray photon is altered. Coherent scattering accounts for only about 7% of the total number

of interactions in a dental exposure (see Table 1-1). Coherent scattering contributes little to film fog because the number of scattered photons is small and their energy is too low for many of them to reach the film or sensor.

## PHOTOELECTRIC ABSORPTION

Photoelectric absorption is critical in diagnostic imaging. This process occurs when an incident photon interacts with an electron in an inner orbital of an atom of the absorbing medium. The photon ejects the electron from its orbital and it becomes a recoil electron (photoelectron) (Fig. 1-24). At this point the incident photon ceases to exist. The kinetic energy imparted to the recoil electron is equal to the energy of the incident photon minus the binding energy of the electron. In the case of atoms with low atomic numbers (e.g., those in most biologic molecules), the binding energy is small and the recoil electron acquires most of the energy of the incident photon. Most photoelectric interactions occur in the 1s orbital because the density of the

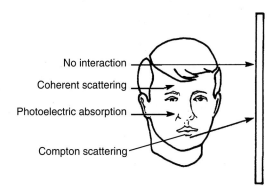

FIG. **1-22** Photons in an x-ray beam interact with the object primarily by Compton scattering, in which case the scattered photon may strike the film and degrade the radiographic image by causing film fog, or photoelectric absorption, in which case they cease to exist. Relatively few photons undergo coherent scattering within the object or pass through the object without interacting and expose the film.

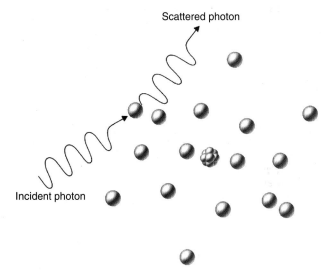

FIG. **1-23** Coherent scattering resulting from the interaction of a low-energy incident photon with an outer electron, causing the outer electron to vibrate momentarily. After this, a scattered photon of the same energy is emitted at a different angle from the path of the incident photon.

---

TABLE **1-2**
## *Fate of 1,000,000 Incident Photons in Bitewing Projection*

| INTERACTION | FATE OF INCIDENT PHOTON | PRIMARY PHOTONS | SCATTERED PHOTONS* | TOTAL† |
|---|---|---|---|---|
| Coherent scattering | Scatters from outer electron | 74,453 | 78,117 | 152,570 |
| Photoelectric absorption | Ejects inner electron and ceases to exist; releases characteristic photon | 268,104 | 261,041 | 529,145 |
| Compton scattering | Ejects outer electron, both scatter | 565,939 | 549,360 | 1,115,300 |
| No interaction | Passes through patient | 91,504 | 379,350 | 470,855 |
| | Total | 1,000,000 | 1,267,868 | 2,267,869 |

From Gibbs SJ: Personal communication, 1986.
*Scattered photons result from primary, Compton, and coherent interactions.
†Note that the sum of the total number of photoelectric interactions and photons that exit the patient equals the total number of incident photons.

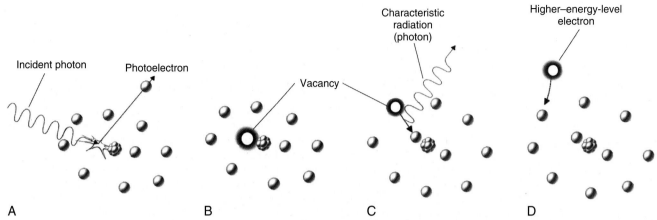

FIG. **1-24** Photoelectric absorption. **A,** Photoelectric absorption occurs when an incident photon gives up all its energy to an inner electron ejected from the atom (a photoelectron). **B,** An electron vacancy in the inner orbital results in ionization of the atom. **C,** An electron from a higher energy level fills the vacancy and emits characteristic radiation. **D,** All orbitals are subsequently filled, completing the energy exchange.

electron cloud is greatest in this region and thus there is a higher probability of interaction. About 23% of interactions in a dental x-ray beam exposure involve photoelectric absorption.

An atom that has participated in a photoelectric interaction is ionized as a result of the loss of an electron. This electron deficiency (usually in the 1s orbital) is instantly filled, usually by a 2s or 2p orbital electron, with the release of characteristic radiation (see Fig. 1-15). Whatever the orbital of the replacement electron, the characteristic photons generated are of such low energy that they are absorbed within the patient and do not fog the film. Recoil electrons ejected during photoelectric absorption travel only short distances in the absorber before they give up their energy through secondary ionizations.

The clinical significance of photoelectric absorption depends on the fact that the frequency of photoelectric interaction varies directly with the *third power of the atomic number* of the absorber. For example, because the effective atomic number of compact bone (Z = 13.8) is greater than that of soft tissue (Z = 7.4), the probability that a photon will be absorbed by a photoelectric interaction in bone is approximately 6.5 times ($13.8^3/7.4^3 = 6.5$) greater than in an equal thickness of soft tissue. This difference is readily seen on dental radiographs as a difference in optical density of the image. It is this difference in the absorption that makes the production of a radiographic image possible.

## COMPTON SCATTERING

Compton scattering occurs when a photon interacts with an outer orbital electron (Fig. 1-25). About 49% of interactions in a dental x-ray beam exposure involve Compton scattering. In this interaction the incident photon collides with an outer electron, which receives kinetic energy and recoils from the point of impact. The path of the incident photon is deflected by this interaction and is scattered in a new direction from the site of the collision. The energy of the scattered photon equals the energy of the incident photon minus the sum of the kinetic energy gained by the recoil electron and its binding energy. As with photoelectric absorption, Compton scattering results in the loss of an electron and ionization of the absorbing atom. Scattered photons continue on their new paths, causing further ionizations. The recoil electrons also give up their energy by ionizing other atoms.

The probability of a Compton interaction is directly proportional to the *electron density* of the absorber. The number of electrons in bone ($5.55 \times 10^{23}$/cc) is greater than in soft tissue ($3.34 \times 10^{23}$/cc); therefore the probability of Compton scattering is correspondingly greater in bone than in tissue. As a result, Compton interactions contribute to the formation of an image.

Scattered photons travel in all directions. The higher the energy of the incident photon, however, the greater the probability that the angle of scatter of the secondary photon will be small and its direction will be forward. These scattered photons darken and degrade the image while carrying no useful information.

## BEAM ATTENUATION

As an x-ray beam travels through matter, its intensity is reduced primarily through photoelectric absorption and Compton scattering. The absorption of the beam depends primarily on the thickness and density of the absorber and the energy of the beam. The reduction of beam intensity is predictable because it depends on physical characteristics of the beam and the absorber. A monochromatic beam of photons, a beam in which all the photons have the same energy, provides a useful example. When only the primary (not scattered) photons are considered, a constant fraction of the beam is attenuated as the beam moves through each unit thickness of an absorber. Therefore 1.5 cm of water may reduce a beam intensity by 50%, the next 1.5 cm by another 50% (to 25% of the original intensity), and so on. This is an exponential pattern of absorption (Fig. 1-26). The HVL described earlier in this chapter is a measure of beam energy describing the amount of an absorber that reduces the beam intensity by half; in the preceding example, the HVL is 1.5 cm of water.

Unlike the previous example, however, there is a wide range of photon energies in an x-ray beam. Low-energy photons are much more likely than high-energy photons to be absorbed. As a consequence, the superficial layers of an absorber tend to remove the low-energy photons and transmit the higher-energy photons. Therefore as an x-ray beam passes through matter, the intensity of the beam decreases, but the mean energy of the residual beam increases by preferential removal of low energy photons. In contrast to the absorption of a monochromatic beam, an x-ray beam is absorbed less and less by each succeeding unit

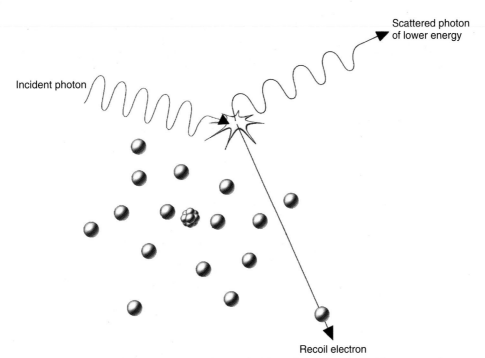

FIG. **1-25** Compton absorption occurs when an incident photon interacts with an outer electron, producing a scattered photon of lower energy than the incident photon and a recoil electron ejected from the target atom.

of absorber thickness. For example, the first 1.5 cm of water might absorb 50% of the photons in an incident x-ray beam having a mean energy of 50 kVp. The mean energy of the residual beam might increase 20% as a result of the loss of lower-energy photons. The next 1.5 cm of water removes only about 40% of the photons, and the average energy of the beam increases another 10%. If the water test object is thick enough, the mean energy of the residual beam eventually approaches the peak voltage applied across the tube.

As the energy of an x-ray beam increases, so does the transmission of the beam through an absorber. When the energy of the incident photon is raised to match the binding energy of the 1s orbital electrons of the absorber, however, then the probability of photoelectric absorption increases sharply and the number of transmitted photons is greatly decreased. This is called *K-edge absorption.* The probability that a photon will interact with an orbital electron is greatest when the energy of the photon equals the binding energy of the electron; it decreases as the photon energy increases. Photons with energy less than the binding energy of 1s orbital electrons interact photoelectrically only with electrons in the 2s or 2p orbitals and in orbitals even farther from the nucleus. Rare earth elements are sometimes used as filters because their 1s orbital binding energies (K edges) (50.24 keV for gadolinium) greatly increase the absorption of high-energy photons. This is desirable because these high-energy photons are not as likely as mid-energy photons to contribute to a radiographic image.

## Dosimetry

Determining the quantity of radiation exposure or dose is termed *dosimetry.* The term *dose* is used to describe the amount of energy absorbed per unit of mass at a site of interest. Exposure is a measure of radiation on the basis of its ability to produce ionization in air under standard conditions of temperature and pressure (STP).

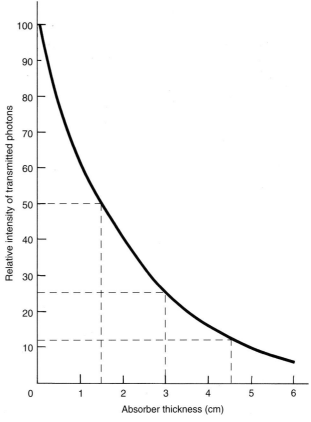

FIG. **1-26** Exponential decay of intensity in a homogeneous photon beam through the absorber, where the HVL is 1.5 cm of absorber. The curve for a heterogeneous x-ray beam does not drop quite as precipitously because of the preferential removal of low-energy photons and the increased mean energy of the resulting beam.

TABLE **1-3**
## Summary of Radiation Quantities and Units

| QUANTITY | SI UNIT | TRADITIONAL UNIT | CONVERSION |
|----------|---------|------------------|------------|
| Exposure | Coulomb/kilogram (C/kg) | Roentgen (R) | 1 C/kg = 3876 R |
| Absorbed dose | Gray (Gy) | rad | 1 Gy = 100 rad |
| Equivalent dose | Sievert (Sv) | rem | 1 Sv = 100 rem |
| Effective dose | Sievert (Sv) | — | — |
| Radioactivity | Becquerel (Bq) | Curie (Ci) | 1 Bq = $2.7 \times 10^{-11}$ Ci |

Data from The NIST Reference on Constants, Units, and Uncertainty: http://physics.nist.gov/cuu/Units/units.html.

## UNITS OF MEASUREMENT

Table 1-3 presents some of the more frequently used units for measuring quantities of radiation. In recent years a move has occurred to use a modernized version of the metric system called the *SI system* (Système International d'Unités).* This book uses SI units. The SI system uses *base units* including the kilogram (kg) (mass), the meter (length), the second (time), the ampere (electric current), and the mole (amount of substance). SI-derived units, including newton (force) and joule (energy), evolve from these base units. The following units are SI-derived units with special names.

### Exposure

Exposure is a measure of the capacity of x or gamma rays to ionize air. It is measured as the amount of charge per mass of air, namely, coulombs/kg. Historically this unit was called the Roentgen (where 1 R = $2.58 \times 10^{-4}$ C/kg. This unit measure the intensity of the radiation field as opposed to the amount of radiation absorbed, although there is a direct relationship. Largely exposure is being replaced by kerma.

### Kerma

When radiation interacts with matter it produces kinetic energy of electrons through phtotelectric absorption and Compton scattering. Ther kerma, an acronym for kinetic energy released in matter, measures the kinetic energy transferred from photons to electrons and is expressed in units of dose (gray [Gy]), where 1 Gy equals 1 joule/kg. Kerma is the sum of the initial kinetic energies of all the charged particles liberated by uncharged ionizing radiation (neurons and photons) in a sample of matter, divided by the mass of the sample. Kerma values made in air are called air kerma. The kerma is rapidly replacing exposure measured in coulombs/kg or R. An exposure of 1 R results in a tissue kerma of about 0.01 Gy (1 cGy).

### Absorbed Dose

Absorbed dose is a measure of the total energy absorbed by any type of ionizing radiation per unit of mass of any type of matter. It varies with the type and energy of radiation and the type of matter absorbing the energy. The SI unit is the Gy, where 1 Gy equals 1 joule/kg. The traditional unit of absorbed dose is the rad *(radiation absorbed dose)*, where 1 rad is equivalent to 100 ergs per gram (g) of absorber. One gray equals 100 rads.

### Equivalent Dose

The equivalent dose ($H_T$) is used to compare the biologic effects of different types of radiation on a tissue or organ. Particulate radiations have a high LET and are more damaging to tissue than is low-LET

radiation such as x rays. This relative biologic effectiveness of different types of radiation is called the radiation-weighting factor ($W_R$). For instance, deposition of 1 Gy of high-energy protons causes five times as much damage as 1 Gy of x-ray photons. The $W_R$ of photons, the reference, is 1. The $W_R$ of 5 keV neutrons and high-energy protons is 5 and the $W_R$ of α particles is 20. To account for this difference, the $H_T$ is computed as the product of the absorbed dose ($D_T$) averaged over a tissue or organ and the $W_R$:

$$H_T = W_R \times D_T$$

The unit of equivalent dose is the sievert (Sv). For diagnostic x-ray examinations 1 Sv equals 1 Gy. The traditional unit of equivalent dose is the rem *(roentgen equivalent man)*. One sievert equals 100 rem.

### Effective Dose

The effective dose (E) is used to estimate the risk in humans. For exposures to a part of the body, for instance, the jaws, the effective dose measures the equivalent whole-body dose. This allows the risk from exposure to one region of the body to be compared with the risk from exposure to another region. In addition to considering the relative biologic effectiveness of different types of radiation, it also considers the radiosensitivity of different tissues for cancer formation or heritable effect. The comparative radiosensitivities of different tissues are measured by the $W_T$. The tissue-weighting factors include red bone marrow, breast, colon, lung, and stomach, all 0.12; gonads 0.08; bladder, esophagus, liver, and thyroid, all 0.04; bone surface, brain, salivary glands, and skin, all 0.01; and other specified tissues totaling 0.12. Thus E is the sum of the products of the equivalent dose to each organ or tissue ($H_T$) and the tissue-weighting factor ($W_T$):

$$E = \Sigma W_T \times H_T$$

The unit of effective dose is the Sv.

### Radioactivity

The measurement of radioactivity (A) describes the decay rate of a sample of radioactive material. The SI unit is the becquerel (Bq); 1 Bq equals 1 disintegration/second. The traditional unit is the curie (Ci), which corresponds to the activity of 1 g of radium ($3.7 \times 10^{10}$ disintegrations/second). Accordingly, 1 mCi equals 37 megaBq and 1 Bq equals $2.7 \times 10^{-11}$ Ci.

## BIBLIOGRAPHY

Bushberg JT: *The essential physics of medical imaging,* ed 2, Baltimore, 2001, Lippincott Williams & Wilkins.
Bushong SC: *Radiologic science for technologists: physics, biology, and protection,* ed 7, St Louis, 2001, Mosby.
Wolbarst AB: *Physics of radiology,* ed 2, Madison, Wis, 2005, Medical Physics.

*The NIST Reference on Constants, Units, and Uncertainty: http://physics. nist.gov/cuu/Units/units.html.

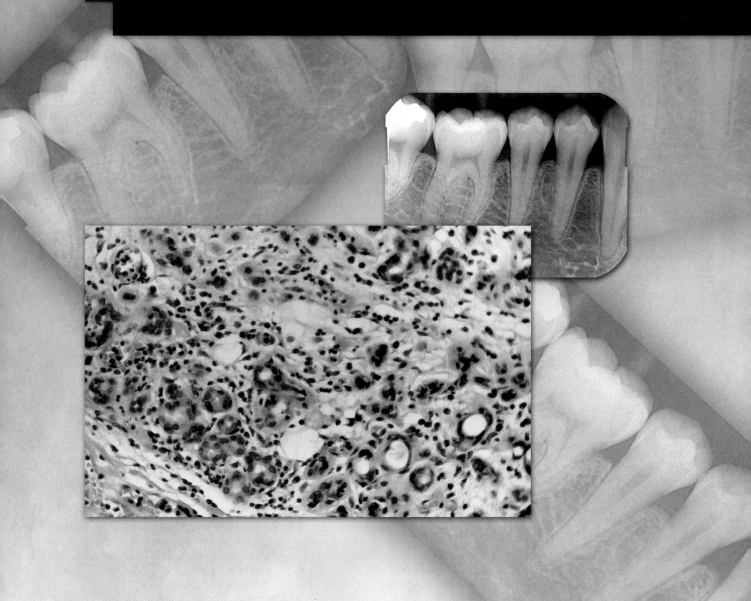

# PART TWO

# Biologic Effects
# of Radiation

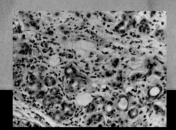

# CHAPTER 2

# Radiobiology

*R*adiobiology is the study of the effects of ionizing radiation on living systems. This discipline requires studying many levels of organization within biologic systems spanning broad ranges in size and temporal scale. The initial interaction between ionizing radiation and matter occurs at the level of the electron within the first $10^{-13}$ second after exposure. These changes result in modification of biologic molecules within the ensuing seconds to hours. In turn, the molecular changes may lead to alterations in cells and organisms that persist for hours, decades, and possibly even generations. These changes may result in injury or death.

## Radiation Chemistry

Radiation acts on living systems through direct and indirect effects. When the energy of a photon or secondary electron ionizes biologic macromolecules, the effect is termed *direct*. Alternatively, a photon may be absorbed by water in an organism, ionizing some of its water molecules. The resulting ions form free radicals (radiolysis of water) that in turn interact with and produce changes in biologic molecules. Because intermediate changes involving water molecules are required to alter the biologic molecules, this series of events is termed *indirect*.

### DIRECT EFFECT

In direct effects, biologic molecules (RH, where *R* is the molecule and *H* is a hydrogen atom) absorb energy from ionizing radiation and form unstable free radicals (atoms or molecules having an unpaired electron in the valence shell). Generation of free radicals occurs in less than $10^{-10}$ second after interaction with a photon. Free radicals are extremely reactive and have very short lives, quickly reforming into stable configurations by dissociation (breaking apart) or cross-linking (joining of two molecules). Free radicals play a dominant role in producing molecular changes in biologic molecules.

Free radical production:

$$RH + x\text{-radiation} \rightarrow R^{\cdot} + H^{+} + e^{-}$$

Free radical fates:
Dissociation:

$$R^{\cdot} \rightarrow X + Y^{\cdot}$$

Cross-linking:

$$R^{\cdot} + S^{\cdot} \rightarrow RS$$

Because the altered biologic molecules differ structurally and functionally from the original molecules, the consequence is a biologic change in the irradiated organism. *Approximately one third of the bio-logic effects of x-ray exposure result from direct effects.* However, direct effects are the most common outcome for particulate radiation such as neutrons and $\alpha$ particles.

### RADIOLYSIS OF WATER

Because water is the predominant molecule in biologic systems (about 70% by weight), it frequently participates in the interactions between x-ray photons and biologic molecules. A complex series of chemical changes occurs in water after exposure to ionizing radiation. Collectively these reactions result in the radiolysis of water.

$$photon + H_2O \rightarrow H^{\cdot} + OH^{\cdot}$$

Although the radiolysis of water is complex, on balance water is largely converted to hydrogen and hydroxyl free radicals. When dissolved oxygen is present in irradiated water, hydroperoxyl free radicals may also be formed:

$$H^{\cdot} + O_2 \rightarrow HO_2^{\cdot}$$

Hydroperoxyl free radicals contribute to the formation of hydrogen peroxide in tissues:

$$HO_2^{\cdot} + H^{\cdot} \rightarrow H_2O_2$$
$$HO_2^{\cdot} + HO_2^{\cdot} \rightarrow O_2 + H_2O_2$$

Both peroxyl radicals and hydrogen peroxide are oxidizing agents and are the primary toxins produced in the tissues by ionizing radiation.

### INDIRECT EFFECTS

*Indirect effects* are those in which hydrogen and hydroxyl free radicals, produced by the action of radiation on water, interact with organic molecules. The interaction of hydrogen and hydroxyl free radicals with organic molecules results in the formation of organic free radicals. About two thirds of radiation-induced biologic damage results from indirect effects. Such reactions may involve the removal of hydrogen:

$$RH + OH^{\cdot} \rightarrow R^{\cdot} + H_2O$$
$$RH + H^{\cdot} \rightarrow R^{\cdot} + H_2$$

The OH$^{\cdot}$ free radical is more important in causing such damage.

Organic free radicals are unstable and transform into stable, altered molecules as described in the earlier section in this chapter on direct effects (p. 18). These altered molecules have different chemical and biologic properties from the original molecules.

TABLE **2-1**
## *Comparison of Deterministic and Stochastic Effects of Radiation*

| | DETERMINISTIC EFFECTS | STOCHASTIC EFFECTS |
|---|---|---|
| Examples | Mucositis resulting from radiation therapy to oral cavity<br>Radiation-induced cataract formation | Radiation-induced cancer<br>Heritable effects |
| Caused by | Killing of many cells | Sublethal damage to DNA |
| Threshold dose? | Yes: sufficient cell killing required to cause a clinical response. | No: even one photon could cause a change in DNA that leads to a cancer or heritable effect. |
| Severity of clinical effects and dose | Severity of clinical effects is proportional to dose. The greater the dose the greater the effect. | Severity of clinical effects is independent of dose. All-or-none response; an individual either has effect or does not. |
| Probability of having effect and dose | Probability of effect independent of dose. All individuals show effect when dose is above threshold. | Frequency of effect proportional to dose. The greater the dose the greater the chance of having the effect. |

Both direct and indirect effects are completed within $10^{-5}$ second. The resulting damage may take hours to decades to become evident.

## CHANGES IN DEOXYRIBONUCLEIC ACID

Damage to a cell's deoxyribonucleic acid (DNA) is the primary cause of radiation-induced cell death, heritable (genetic) mutations, and cancer formation (carcinogenesis). Radiation-induced changes in protein, lipids, and carbohydrates after low or moderate doses (up to 10 Gy) of radiation are so slight that they do not contribute to radiation effects.

Radiation produces a number of different types of alterations in DNA, including the following:
- Breakage of one or both DNA strands
- Cross-linking of DNA strands within the helix to other DNA strands or to proteins
- Change or loss of a base
- Disruption of hydrogen bonds between DNA strands

The most important of these types of damage are single- and double-strand breakage. Most single-strand breakage is of little biologic consequence because the broken strand is readily repaired by using the intact second strand as a template. However, misrepair of a strand can result in a mutation and prevent cell division. If germ line cells are involved, this may lead to heritable effects. If somatic cells are involved, this may also lead to cancer. Double-strand breakage occurs when both strands of a DNA molecule are damaged. If the damaged sites on each strand are far apart, they are readily repaired. However, if the breaks are at the same location or within a few base pairs, then repair is complicated by the lack of an intact template strand and misrepair is common. Double-strand breakage is believed to be responsible for most cell killing, carcinogenesis, and heritable effects.

## Deterministic and Stochastic Effects

Radiation injury to organisms results from either the killing of large numbers of cells (deterministic effects) or sublethal damage to individual cells that results in cancer formation or heritable mutation (stochastic effects). The differences between deterministic and stochastic effects are shown in Table 2-1.

## Deterministic Effects on Cells
### EFFECTS ON INTRACELLULAR STRUCTURES

The effects of radiation on intracellular structures result from radiation-induced changes in their macromolecules. Although the initial molecular changes are produced within a fraction of a second after exposure, cellular changes resulting from moderate exposure require a minimum of hours to become apparent. These changes are manifest initially as structural and functional changes in cellular organelles. The changes may cause cell death.

### Nucleus
A wide variety of radiobiologic data indicate that the nucleus is more radiosensitive (in terms of lethality) than the cytoplasm, especially in dividing cells. *The sensitive site in the nucleus is the DNA within chromosomes.*

### Chromosome Aberrations
Chromosomes serve as useful markers for radiation injury. They may be easily visualized and quantified, and the extent of their damage is related to cell survival. Chromosome aberrations are observed in irradiated cells at the time of mitosis when the DNA condenses to form chromosomes. The type of damage that may be observed depends on the stage of the cell in the cell cycle at the time of irradiation.

Figure 2-1 shows the stages of the cell cycle. If radiation exposure occurs after DNA synthesis (i.e., in $G_2$ or mid and late S), only one arm of the affected chromosome is broken (*chromatid aberration*) (Fig. 2-2, *A*). However, if the radiation-induced break occurs before the DNA has replicated (i.e., in $G_1$ or early S), the damage manifests as a break in both arms (*chromosome aberration*) at the next mitosis (Fig. 2-2, *B*). Most simple breaks are repaired by biologic processes and go unrecognized. Figure 2-3 illustrates several common forms of chromosome aberrations resulting from incorrect repair. Formation of rings (Fig. 2-3, *A*) and dicentrics (Fig. 2-3, *B*) are lethal as the cell cannot complete mitosis. Translocations (Fig. 2-3, *C*) result in unequal

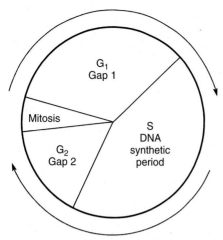

FIG. **2-1**   Cell cycle. A proliferating cell moves in the cycle from mitosis to gap 1 (G₁) to the period of DNA synthesis *(S)* to gap 2 (G₂) to the next mitosis.

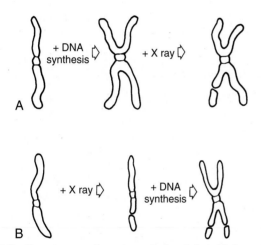

FIG. **2-2**   Chromosome aberrations. **A,** Irradiation of the cell after DNA synthesis results in a single-arm (chromatid) aberration. **B,** Irradiation before DNA synthesis results in a double-arm (chromosome) aberration.

distribution of chromatin material to daughter cells or they prevent completion of a subsequent mitosis. Chromosome aberrations have been detected in peripheral blood lymphocytes of patients exposed to medical diagnostic procedures. Moreover, the survivors of the atomic bombings of Hiroshima and Nagasaki have demonstrated chromosome aberrations in circulating lymphocytes more than two decades after the radiation exposure. The frequency of aberrations is generally proportional to the radiation dose received.

## EFFECTS ON CELL REPLICATION

Radiation is especially damaging to rapidly dividing cell systems, such as skin and intestinal mucosa and hematopoietic tissues. Irradiation of such cell populations will cause a reduction in size of the irradiated tissue as a result of mitotic delay (inhibition of progression of the cells through the cell cycle) and cell death (usually during mitosis). Reproductive death in a cell population is loss of the capacity for mitotic

division. The three mechanisms of reproductive death are DNA damage, bystander effect, and apoptosis.

### Deoxyribonucleic Acid Damage

Cell death is caused by damage to DNA, which in turn causes chromosome aberrations, which cause the cell to die during the first few mitoses after irradiation. It is the rate of cell replication in various tissues, and thus the rate of reproductive death, that accounts for the varying radiosensitivity of tissues. When a population of slowly dividing cells is irradiated, larger doses and longer time intervals are required for induction of deterministic effects than when a rapidly dividing cell system is involved.

### Bystander Effect

Cells that are damaged by radiation release into their immediate environment molecules that kill nearby cells. This bystander effect has been demonstrated for both α particles and x rays and causes chromosome aberrations, cell killing, gene mutations, and carcinogenesis.

### Apoptosis

Apoptosis, also known as programmed cell death, occurs during normal embryogenesis. Cells round up, draw away from their neighbors, and condense nuclear chromatin. This characteristic pattern, different from necrosis, can be induced by radiation in both normal tissue and in some tumors. Apoptosis is particularly common in hemopoietic and lymphoid tissues.

### Recovery

Cell recovery from DNA damage and the bystander effect involves enzymatic repair of single-strand breaks of DNA. Because of this repair, a higher total dose is required to achieve a given degree of cell killing when multiple fractions are used (e.g., in radiation therapy) than when the same total dose is given in a single brief exposure. Damage to both strands of DNA at the same site is usually lethal to the cell.

## RADIOSENSITIVITY AND CELL TYPE

Different cells from various organs of the same individual may respond to irradiation quite differently. This variation was recognized as early as 1906 by the French radiobiologists Bergonié and Tribondeau. They observed that the most radiosensitive cells have the following characteristics:

• A high mitotic rate
• Undergo many future mitoses
• Are most primitive in differentiation

Mammalian cells may be divided into three broad categories of radiosensitivity as shown in Table 2-2.

## Deterministic Effects on Tissues and Organs

The radiosensitivity of a tissue or organ is measured by its response to irradiation. Loss of moderate numbers of cells does not affect the function of most organs. However, with the loss of large numbers of cells, all affected organisms display an observable result. The severity of this change depends on the dose and thus the amount of cell loss. The following discussion pertains to the effect of irradiation of tissues and organs when the exposure is restricted to a small area. Moderate

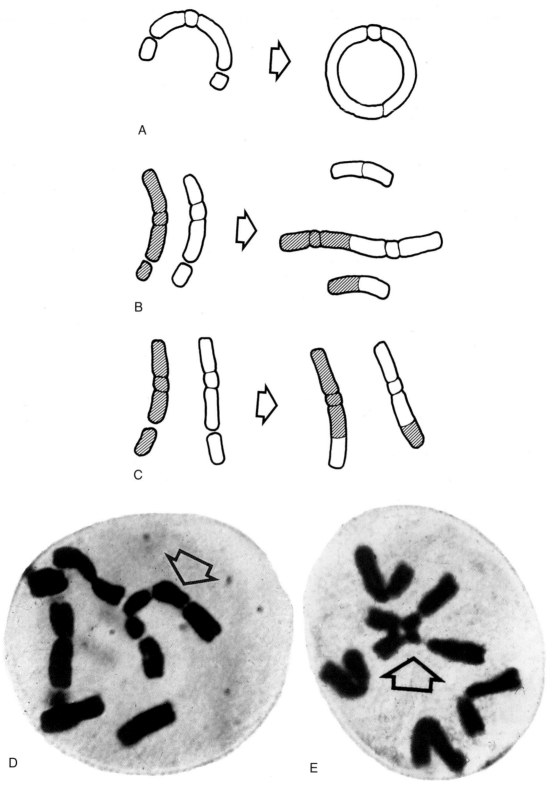

FIG. **2-3**  Chromosome aberrations. **A,** Ring formation plus acentric fragment. **B,** Dicentric formation. **C,** Translocation. In **D** and **E,** the *arrows* point to tetracentric exchange and chromatid exchange taking place in *Trandescantia,* an herb. (**D** and **E,** Courtesy Dr. M. Miller, Rochester, N.Y.)

TABLE **2-2**
*Relative Radiosensitivity of Various Cells*

|  | HIGH | INTERMEDIATE | LOW |
|---|---|---|---|
| Characteristics | Divide regularly<br>Long mitotic futures<br>Undergo no or little differentiation between mitoses | Divide occasionally in response to a demand for more cells | Highly differentiated<br>When mature are incapable of division |
| Examples | Spermatogenic and erythroblastic stem cells<br>Basal cells of oral mucous membrane | Vascular endothelial cells<br>Fibroblasts<br>Acinar and ductal salivary gland cells<br>Parenchymal cells of liver, kidney, and thyroid | Neurons<br>Striated muscle cells<br>Squamous epithelial cells<br>Erythrocytes |

BOX **2-1**
*Relative Radiosensitivity of Various Organs*

| High | Intermediate | Low |
|---|---|---|
| Lymphoid organs | Fine vasculature | Optic lens |
| Bone marrow | Growing cartilage | Muscle |
| Testes | Growing bone | |
| Intestines | Salivary glands | |
| Mucous membranes | Lungs | |
| | Kidney | |
| | Liver | |

doses to a localized area may lead to repairable damage. Comparable doses to the whole animal may result in death from damage to the most radiation-sensitive systems.

## SHORT-TERM EFFECTS

The short-term effects of radiation on a tissue (effects seen in the first days or weeks after exposure) are determined primarily by the sensitivity of its parenchymal cells. When continuously proliferating tissues (e.g., bone marrow, oral mucous membranes) are irradiated with a moderate dose, cells are lost primarily by reproductive death, bystander effect, and apoptosis. The extent of cell loss depends on damage to the stem cell pools and the proliferative rate of the cell population. The effects of irradiation on such tissues become apparent quickly as a reduction in the number of mature cells in the series. Tissues composed of cells that rarely or never divide (e.g., neurons or muscle) demonstrate little or no radiation-induced hypoplasia over the short term. The relative radiosensitivities of various tissues and organs are shown in Box 2-1.

## LONG-TERM EFFECTS

The long-term deterministic effects of radiation on tissues and organs (seen months and years after exposure) are a loss of parenchymal cells and replacement with fibrous connective tissue. These changes are caused by reproductive death of replicating cells and by damage to the fine vasculature. Damage to capillaries leads to narrowing and eventual obliteration of vascular lumens. This impairs the transport of oxygen, nutrients, and waste products and results in death of all cell types dependent on this vascular supply. Thus both dividing (radiosensitive) and nondividing (radioresistant) parenchymal cells are replaced by fibrous connective tissue, a progressive fibroatrophy of the irradiated tissue.

## MODIFYING FACTORS

The response of cells, tissues, and organs to irradiation depends on exposure conditions and the cell environment.

### Dose

The severity of deterministic damage seen in irradiated tissues or organs depends on the amount of radiation received. Very often a clinical threshold dose exists below which no adverse effects are seen. In all individuals receiving doses above the threshold level, the amount of damage is proportional to the dose.

### Dose Rate

The term *dose rate* indicates the rate of exposure. For example, a total dose of 5 Gy may be given at a high dose rate (5 Gy/min) or a low dose rate (5 mGy/min). Exposure of biologic systems to a given dose at a high dose rate causes more damage than exposure to the same total dose given at a lower dose rate. When organisms are exposed at lower dose rates, a greater opportunity exists for repair of damage, thereby resulting in less net damage. Although the total dose of diagnostic exposures is low, they are given at a high dose rate compared with background exposure.

### Oxygen

The radioresistance of many biologic systems increases by a factor of 2 or 3 when the exposure is made with reduced oxygen (hypoxia). The greater cell damage sustained in the presence of oxygen is related to the increased amounts of hydrogen peroxide and hydroperoxyl free radicals formed. This is important clinically because hyperbaric oxygen therapy may be used during radiation therapy of tumors having hypoxic cells.

### Linear Energy Transfer

In general, the dose required to produce a certain biologic effect is reduced as the linear energy transfer (LET) of the radiation is increased. Thus higher-LET radiations (e.g., α particles) are more efficient in damaging biologic systems because their high ionization density is more likely than x rays to induce double-strand breakage in DNA. Low-LET radiations such as x rays deposit their energy more sparsely, or uniformly, in the absorber and thus are more likely to cause single-strand breakage and less biologic damage.

## Radiotherapy in the Oral Cavity

### RATIONALE

The oral cavity is irradiated during radiation therapy of radiosensitive oral malignant tumors, usually squamous cell carcinomas. Radiation therapy for malignant lesions in the oral cavity is usually indicated when the lesion is radiosensitive, advanced, or deeply invasive and cannot be approached surgically. Combined surgical and radiotherapeutic treatment often provides optimal treatment. Increasingly, chemotherapy is being combined with radiation therapy and surgery.

Fractionation of the total x-ray dose into multiple small doses provides greater tumor destruction than is possible with a large single dose. Fractionation characteristically also allows increased cellular repair of normal tissues, which are believed to have an inherently greater capacity for recovery than tumor cells. Fractionation also increases the mean oxygen tension in an irradiated tumor, rendering the tumor cells more radiosensitive. This results from killing rapidly dividing tumor cells and shrinking the tumor mass after the first few fractions, reducing the distance that oxygen must diffuse from the fine vasculature through the tumor to reach the remaining viable tumor cells. The fractionation schedules currently in use have been established empirically.

### RADIATION EFFECT ON ORAL TISSUES

The following sections describe the complications (deterministic effects) of a course of radiotherapy on the normal tissue of the oral cavity (Fig. 2-4). Typically 2 Gy is delivered daily, bilaterally through 8- × 10-cm fields over the oropharynx, for a weekly exposure of 10 Gy. This continues typically for 6 to 7 weeks until a total of 64 to 70 Gy is administered.

Cobalt is often the source of γ radiation; however, on occasion small implants containing radon or iodine 125 are placed directly in a tumor mass. Such implants deliver a high dose of radiation to a relatively small volume of tissue in a short time. Recently a three-dimensional technique called intensity-modulated radiotherapy (IMRT) has been used to control the dose distribution with high accuracy.

#### Oral Mucous Membrane

The oral mucous membrane contains a basal layer composed of rapidly dividing, radiosensitive stem cells. Near the end of the second week of therapy, as some of these cells die, the mucous membranes begin to show areas of redness and inflammation (mucositis). As the therapy continues, the irradiated mucous membrane begins to separate from the underlying connective tissue, with the formation of a white to yellow pseudomembrane (the desquamated epithelial layer). At the end of therapy the mucositis is usually most severe, discomfort is at a maximum, and food intake is difficult. Good oral hygiene minimizes infection. Topical anesthetics may be required at mealtimes. Secondary yeast infection by *Candida albicans* is a common complication and may require treatment.

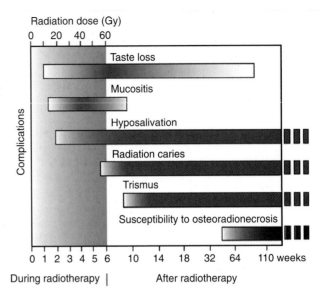

FIG. **2-4** Oral complications. Typical time course of complications seen during and after a course of radiation therapy to the head and neck. Shaded area in first 6 weeks represents accumulated dose. Shading within bars indicates severity of complication. Those changes persisting after 2 years pose lifelong risks. (Adapted from Kielbassa AM, Hinkelbein W, Hellwig E et al: Radiation-related damage to dentition, *Lancet Oncol* 7:326-335, 2006.)

After irradiation is completed, the mucosa begins to heal rapidly. Healing is usually complete by about 2 months. Later the mucous membrane tends to become atrophic, thin, and relatively avascular. This long-term atrophy results from progressive obliteration of the fine vasculature and fibrosis of the underlying connective tissue. These atrophic changes complicate denture wearing because they may cause oral ulcerations of the compromised tissue. Ulcers may also result from radiation necrosis or tumor recurrence. A biopsy may be required to make the differentiation.

#### Taste Buds

Taste buds are sensitive to radiation. Doses in the therapeutic range cause extensive degeneration of the normal histologic architecture of taste buds. Patients often notice a loss of taste acuity during the second or third week of radiotherapy. Bitter and acid flavors are more severely affected when the posterior two thirds of the tongue is irradiated and salt and sweet when the anterior third of the tongue is irradiated. Taste acuity usually decreases by a factor of 1000 to 10,000 during the course of radiotherapy. Alterations in the saliva may partly account for this reduction, which may proceed to a state of virtual insensitivity. Taste loss is reversible and recovery takes 60 to 120 days.

#### Salivary Glands

The major salivary glands are at times unavoidably exposed to 20 to 30 Gy during radiotherapy for cancer in the oral cavity or oropharynx. The parenchymal component of the salivary glands is rather radiosensitive (parotid glands more so than submandibular or sublingual glands). A marked and progressive loss of salivary secretion (hyposalivation) is usually seen in the first few weeks after initiation of radiotherapy. The extent of reduced flow is dose dependent and reaches

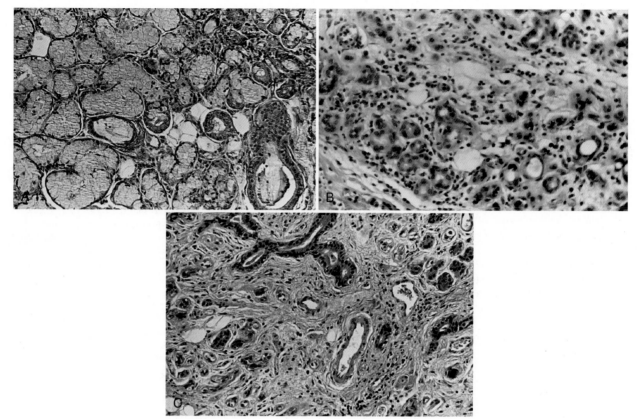

FIG. **2-5**    Radiation effects on human submandibular salivary glands. **A,** Normal gland. **B,** A gland 6 months after exposure to radiotherapy. Note the loss of acini and presence of chronic inflammatory cells. **C,** A gland 1 year after exposure to radiotherapy. Note the loss of acini and extensive fibrosis.

essentially zero at 60 Gy. The mouth becomes dry (xerostomia) and tender, and swallowing is difficult and painful. Patients with irradiation of both parotid glands are more likely to complain of dry mouth and difficulty with chewing and swallowing than are those with unilateral irradiation. Various saliva substitutes are available to help restore function. Use of IMRT has helped to spare the contralateral salivary glands and thus minimize the loss of salivary function.

The reduced volume of saliva in patients receiving radiation therapy that includes the major salivary glands is altered from normal. Because serous cells are more radiosensitive than mucous cells, the residual saliva is more viscous than usual. Further, the small volume of viscous saliva that is secreted usually has a pH value 1 unit below normal (i.e., an average of 5.5 in irradiated patients compared with 6.5 in unexposed individuals). This pH is low enough to initiate decalcification of normal enamel. In addition, the buffering capacity of saliva falls as much as 44% during radiation therapy. If some portions of the major salivary glands are spared, dryness of the mouth usually subsides in 6 to 12 months because of compensatory hypertrophy of residual salivary gland tissue. Reduced salivary flow that persists beyond a year is unlikely to show significant recovery.

Histologically, an acute inflammatory response may occur soon after the initiation of therapy, particularly involving the serous acini. In the months after irradiation the inflammatory response becomes more chronic, and the glands demonstrate progressive fibrosis, adiposis, loss of fine vasculature, and concomitant parenchymal degeneration (Fig. 2-5), thus accounting for the xerostomia.

## Teeth

Children receiving radiation therapy to the jaws may show defects in the permanent dentition such as retarded root development, dwarfed teeth, or failure to form one or more teeth (Fig. 2-6). If exposure precedes calcification, irradiation may destroy the tooth bud. Irradiation after calcification has begun may inhibit cellular differentiation, causing malformations and arresting general growth. Such exposure may retard or abort root formation, but the eruptive mechanism of teeth is relatively radiation resistant. Irradiated teeth with altered root formation still erupt. In general, the severity of the damage is dose dependent.

Adult teeth are resistant to the direct effects of radiation exposure. Pulpal tissue demonstrates long-term fibroatrophy after irradiation. Radiation has no discernible effect on the crystalline structure of enamel, dentin, or cementum, and radiation does not increase their solubility.

## Radiation Caries

Radiation caries is a rampant form of dental decay that may occur in individuals who receive a course of radiotherapy that includes exposure of the salivary glands. After radiotherapy that includes the major salivary glands, the microflora undergo a pronounced change, rendering them acidogenic in the saliva and plaque. Patients receiving radiation therapy to oral structures have increases in *Streptococcus mutans, Lactobacillus,* and *Candida.* Caries results from changes in the salivary glands and saliva, including reduced flow, decreased pH, reduced buffering capacity, increased viscosity, and altered flora. The residual saliva in individuals with xerostomia also has a low concentration of $Ca^{+2}$

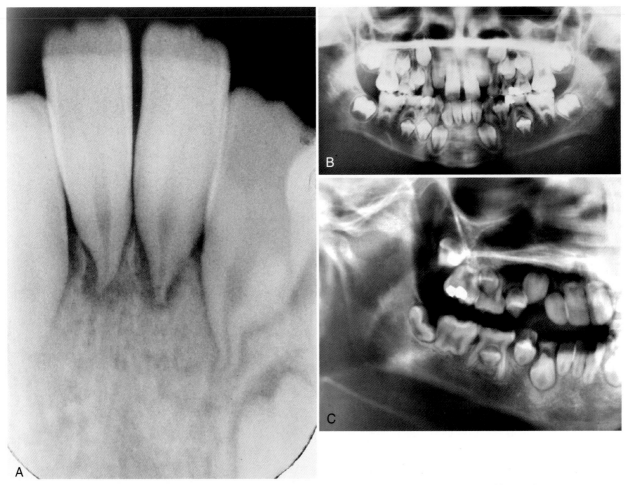

FIG. **2-6**  Dental abnormalities after radiotherapy in two patients. The first, a 9-year-old girl who received 35 Gy at the age of 4 years because of Hodgkin's disease, had severe stunting of the incisor roots with premature closure of the apices at 8 years **(A)** and retarded development of the mandibular second premolar crowns with stunting of the mandibular incisor, canine, and premolar roots at 9 years **(B).** The other patient **(C),** a 10-year-old boy who received 41 Gy to the jaws at age 4 years, had severely stunted root development of all permanent teeth with a normal primary molar. (**A** and **B,** Courtesy Mr. P.N. Hirschmann, Leeds, United Kingdom. **C,** Courtesy Dr. James Eischen, San Diego, Calif.)

ion. This results in greater solubility of tooth structure and reduced remineralization. Finally, because of the reduced or absent cleansing action of normal saliva, debris accumulates quickly. Irradiation of the teeth by itself does not influence the course of radiation caries.

Clinically, three types of radiation caries exist. The most common is widespread superficial lesions attacking buccal, occlusal, incisal, and palatal surfaces. Another type involves primarily the cementum and dentin in the cervical region. These lesions may progress around the teeth circumferentially and result in loss of the crown. A final type appears as a dark pigmentation of the entire crown. The incisal edges may be markedly worn. Combinations of all these lesions develop in some patients (Fig. 2-7). The histologic features of the lesions are similar to those of typical carious lesions. It is the rapid course and widespread attack that distinguish radiation caries.

The best method of reducing radiation caries is daily application for 5 minutes of a viscous topical 1% neutral sodium fluoride gel in custom-made applicator trays. Use of topical fluoride causes a 6-month delay in the irradiation-induced elevation of *S. mutans.* Avoidance of dietary sucrose, in addition to the use of a topical fluoride,

further reduces the concentrations of *S. mutans* and *Lactobacillus.* The best result is achieved from a combination of restorative dental procedures, excellent oral hygiene, a diet restricted in cariogenic foods, and topical applications of sodium fluoride. Patient cooperation in maintaining oral hygiene is extremely important because radiation caries is a lifelong threat. Teeth with gross caries or periodontal involvement are often extracted before irradiation.

### Bone

Treatment of cancers in the oral region often includes irradiation of the mandible or maxilla. The primary damage to mature bone results from radiation-induced damage to the vasculature of the periosteum and cortical bone, which are normally already sparse. Radiation also acts by destroying osteoblasts and, to a lesser extent, osteoclasts. Subsequent to irradiation, normal marrow may be replaced with fatty marrow and fibrous connective tissue. The marrow tissue becomes hypovascular, hypoxic, and hypocellular. In addition, the endosteum becomes atrophic, showing a lack of osteoblastic and osteoclastic activity, and some lacunae of the compact bone are empty, an indica-

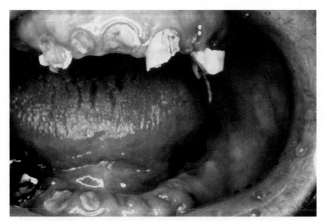

FIG. **2-7**  Radiation caries. Note the extensive loss of tooth structure in both jaws resulting from radiation-induced xerostomia.

tion of necrosis. The degree of mineralization may be reduced, leading to brittleness, or little altered from normal bone. When these changes are so severe that bone death results and the bone is exposed, the condition is termed *osteoradionecrosis*.

Osteoradionecrosis is the most serious clinical complication that occurs in bone after irradiation. The decreased vascularity of the mandible renders it easily infected by microorganisms from the oral cavity. This bone infection may result from radiation-induced breakdown of the oral mucous membrane, by mechanical damage to the weakened oral mucous membrane such as from a denture sore or tooth extraction, through a periodontal lesion, or from radiation caries. This infection may cause a nonhealing wound in irradiated bone that is difficult to treat (Fig. 2-8). It is more common in the mandible than in the maxilla, probably because of the richer vascular supply to the maxilla and the fact that the mandible is more frequently irradiated. The higher the radiation dose absorbed by the bone, the greater the risk for osteoradionecrosis.

Patients should be referred for dental care before undergoing a course of radiation therapy to minimize radiation caries and osteoradionecrosis. Radiation caries can be minimized by restoring all carious lesions before radiation therapy and initiating preventive techniques of good oral hygiene and daily topical fluoride. The risk for osteoradionecrosis and infection can be minimized by removing all teeth with extensive caries or with poor periodontal support (allowing sufficient time for the extraction wounds to heal before beginning radiation therapy) and adjusting dentures to minimize the risk of denture sores. Removal of teeth after irradiation should be avoided when possible. When teeth must be removed from irradiated jaws, the dentist should use atraumatic surgical technique to avoid elevating the periosteum and provide antibiotic coverage.

Often patients who have had radiation therapy require a radiographic examination to supplement clinical examinations. Radiographs are especially important to detect caries early. The amount of radiation from such diagnostic exposures is negligible compared with the amount received during therapy and should not serve as a reason to defer radiographs. Whenever possible, it is desirable to avoid taking radiographs during the first 6 months after completion of radiotherapy, however, to allow time for the mucous membrane to heal.

### Musculature
Radiation may causes inflammation and fibrosis resulting in contracture and trismus in the muscles of mastication. Usually the masseter

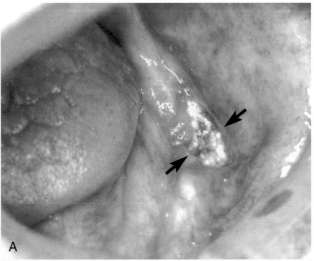

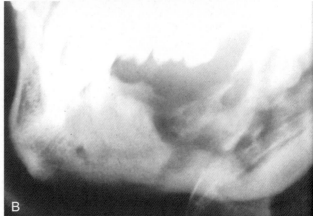

FIG. **2-8**  Osteoradionecrosis. **A,** Area of exposed mandible after radiotherapy. Note the loss of oral mucosa. **B,** Destruction of irradiated bone resulting from the spread of infection.

or pterygoid muscles are involved. Restriction in mouth opening usually starts about 2 months after radiotherapy is completed and progresses thereafter. An exercise program may be helpful in increasing opening distance.

## Deterministic Effects of Whole-Body Irradiation

### ACUTE RADIATION SYNDROME

The acute radiation syndrome is a collection of signs and symptoms experienced by persons after acute whole-body exposure to radiation. Information about this syndrome comes from animal experiments and human exposures in the course of medical radiotherapy, atom bomb blasts, and radiation accidents. Individually, the clinical symptoms are not unique to radiation exposure, but taken as a whole, the pattern constitutes a distinct entity (Table 2-3).

#### Prodromal Period
Within the first minutes to hours after exposure to whole-body irradiation of about 1.5 Gy, an individual may have anorexia, nausea, vomiting, diarrhea, weakness, and fatigue. These early symptoms constitute the prodromal period of the acute radiation syndrome. Their

cause is not clear but probably involves the autonomic nervous system. The severity and time of onset may be of significant prognostic value because they are dose related: the higher the dose, the more rapid the onset and the greater the severity of symptoms.

## Latent Period

After the prodromal reaction comes a latent period of apparent well-being during which no signs or symptoms of radiation sickness occur. The extent of the latent period is also dose related. It extends from hours or days after supralethal exposures (greater than approximately 5 Gy) to a few weeks after exposures of about 2 Gy.

## Hematopoietic Syndrome

Whole-body exposures of 2 to 7 Gy cause injury to the hematopoietic stem cells of the bone marrow and spleen. The high mitotic activity of these cells makes bone marrow a highly radiosensitive tissue. Doses in this range cause a rapid fall in the numbers of circulating granulocytes, platelets, and finally erythrocytes (Fig. 2-9). Although mature circulating granulocytes, platelets, and erythrocytes are radioresistant because they are nonreplicating cells, their paucity in the peripheral blood after irradiation reflects the radiosensitivity of their precursors. The rate of fall in the circulating levels of a cell depends on the life span of that cell in the peripheral blood. Granulocytes, with short lives

in circulation, fall off in a few days, whereas red blood cells, with long lives in circulation, fall off slowly.

The clinical signs of the hematopoietic syndrome include infection (from lymphopenia and granulocytopenia), hemorrhage (from loss of platelets), and anemia (from erythrocyte depletion). The probability of death is low after exposures at the low end of this range but much higher at the high end. When death results from the hematopoietic syndrome, it usually occurs 10 to 30 days after irradiation.

## Gastrointestinal Syndrome

The *gastrointestinal syndrome* is caused by whole-body exposures in the range of 7 to 15 Gy, which causes extensive damage to the gastrointestinal system in addition to the hematopoietic damage described previously. Exposure in this dose range causes considerable injury to the rapidly proliferating basal epithelial cells of the intestinal villi and leads to rapid loss of the epithelial layer of the intestinal mucosa. Because of the denuded mucosal surface, there is loss of plasma and electrolytes, loss of efficient intestinal absorption, and ulceration of the mucosal lining with hemorrhaging into the intestines. These changes are responsible for the diarrhea, dehydration, and loss of weight. Endogenous intestinal bacteria readily invade the denuded surface, producing septicemia.

At about the time that developing damage to the gastrointestinal system reaches a maximum, the effect of bone marrow depression is beginning to be manifested. The result is a marked lowering of the body's defense against bacterial infection and a decrease in effectiveness of the clotting mechanism. The combined effects of damage to these hematopoietic and gastrointestinal stem cell systems cause death within 2 weeks from fluid and electrolyte loss, infection, and possibly nutritional impairment. Thirty of the firefighters at the accident site at Chernobyl, Ukraine, died in the first few months of the hematopoietic or gastrointestinal syndrome.

## Cardiovascular and Central Nervous System Syndrome

Exposures in excess of 50 Gy usually cause death in 1 to 2 days. The few humans who have been exposed at this level showed collapse of the circulatory system with a precipitous fall in blood pressure in the hours preceding death. Autopsy revealed necrosis of cardiac muscle.

| TABLE **2-3** *Acute Radiation Syndrome* | |
|---|---|
| DOSE (Gy) | MANIFESTATION |
| 1 to 2 | Prodromal symptoms |
| 2 to 4 | Mild hematopoietic symptoms |
| 4 to 7 | Severe hematopoietic symptoms |
| 7 to 15 | Gastrointestinal symptoms |
| 50 | Cardiovascular and central nervous system symptoms |

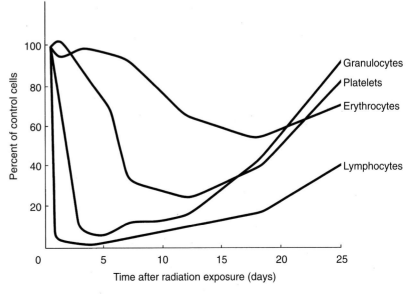

FIG. **2-9**  Radiation effects on blood cells. When whole-body exposure inhibits the replacement of circulating cells by stem cell proliferation, the duration of the circulating cells' survival is largely determined by their life span.

Victims also may show intermittent stupor, incoordination, disorientation, and convulsions suggestive of extensive damage to the nervous system. Although the precise mechanism is not fully understood, these latter symptoms most likely result from radiation-induced damage to the neurons and fine vasculature of the brain.

## Management of Acute Radiation Syndrome

The presenting clinical problems govern the management of different forms of acute radiation syndrome. Antibiotics are indicated when the granulocyte count falls. Fluid and electrolyte replacement is used as necessary. Whole blood transfusions are used to treat anemia, and platelets may be administered to arrest thrombocytopenia. Bone marrow grafts are indicated between identical twins because there is no risk for graft-versus-host disease.

## RADIATION EFFECTS ON EMBRYOS AND FETUSES

The effects of radiation on human embryos and fetuses have been studied in animals and in women exposed to diagnostic or therapeutic radiation during pregnancy and those exposed to radiation from the atomic bombs dropped at Hiroshima and Nagasaki. Embryos and fetuses are considerably more radiosensitive than adults because most embryonic cells are relatively undifferentiated and rapidly mitotic.

Exposures in the range of 2 to 3 Gy during the first few days after conception are thought to cause undetectable death of the embryo. The cells in the embryo are dividing rapidly and are highly sensitive to radiation. Lethality is common and many of these embryos fail to implant in the uterine wall. The first 15 weeks includes the period of organogenesis when the major organ systems form. The most common abnormalities among the Japanese children exposed early in gestation were reduced growth that persists through life and reduced head circumference (microcephaly), often associated with mental retardation. Other abnormalities included small birth size, cataracts, genital and skeletal malformations, and microphthalmia. The period of maximal sensitivity of the brain is 8 to 15 weeks after conception. The frequency of severe mental retardation after exposure to 1 Gy during this period is about 43%. These effects are deterministic in nature and are believed to have a threshold of about 0.1 to 0.2 Gy. This threshold dose is 400 to 800 times higher than the exposure from a dental examination (0.25 mGy from a full-mouth examination when a leaded apron is used).

## LATE EFFECTS

A number of late deterministic effects have been found in the survivors of the atomic bombing of Hiroshima and Nagasaki.

### Growth and Development

Children exposed in the bombings showed impairment of growth and development. They have reduced height, weight, and skeletal development. The younger the individual was at the time of exposure, the more pronounced the effects.

### Cataracts

The threshold for induction of cataracts (opacities in the lens of the eye) ranges from about 0.6 Gy when the dose is received in a single exposure to more than 5 Gy when the dose is received in multiple exposures over a period of weeks. These doses are much larger than those from dental radiography. Most affected individuals are unaware of their presence.

### Life Span Shortening

The survivors of the atomic bombings show a clear decrease in median life expectancy with increasing radiation dose. The reduction ranges from 2 months up to 2.6 years by dose group, with an overall mean of 4 months. Survivors demonstrate increased frequency of heart disease, stroke, and diseases of the digestive, respiratory, and hematopoietic systems.

## Stochastic Effects

Stochastic effects result from sublethal changes in the DNA of individual cells. The most important consequence of such damage is carcinogenesis. Heritable effects, although much less likely, can also occur.

## CARCINOGENESIS

Radiation causes cancer by modifying DNA. The most likely mechanism is radiation-induced gene mutation. Most investigators think that radiation acts as an initiator, that is, it induces a change in the cell so that it no longer undergoes terminal differentiation. Evidence also exists that radiation acts as a promoter, stimulating cells to multiply. Finally, it may also convert premalignant cells into malignant ones, for instance, conversion of proto-oncogenes to oncogenes. Gene mutations may also involve a loss of function in the case of tumor-suppressor genes. Data on radiation-induced cancers come primarily from populations of people who have been exposed to high levels of radiation; however, in principle, even low doses of radiation may initiate cancer formation in a single cell.

Estimation of the number of cancers induced by radiation is difficult. Radiation-induced cancers are not distinguishable from cancers produced by other causes. This means that the number of cancers can be estimated only as the number of excess cases found in exposed groups compared with the number in unexposed groups of people. The group of individuals most intensively studied for estimating the cancer risk from radiation is the Japanese atomic bomb survivors. The cases of more than 120,000 individuals have been followed since 1950, of whom 91,000 were exposed. The incidences of deaths from leukemias and solid cancers are shown in Tables 2-4 and 2-5. The risk for most solid cancers increases linearly with dose.

Most individuals in these studies received exposures far in excess of the diagnostic range. Thus the probability that a cancer will result from a small dose can be estimated only by extrapolation from the rates observed after exposure to larger doses (see Chapter 3). Box 2-2

### TABLE 2-4
### Cancer Mortality Rate in 86,611 Atomic Bomb Survivors Having 47,685 Deaths from All Causes (1950-2000)

| | LEUKEMIAS | SOLID CANCERS |
|---|---|---|
| Deaths | 296 | 10,127 |
| Radiation induced | 93 | 479 |

Data adapted from Preston DL, Pierce DA, Shimizu Y et al: Effect of recent changes in atomic bomb survivor dosimetry on cancer mortality risk estimates, *Radiat Res* 162:377-389, 2004.

### TABLE 2-5
## Comparison of Radiation-Induced Leukemias and Solid Tumors

| FEATURE | LEUKEMIAS | SOLID TUMORS |
|---|---|---|
| Onset | 2-3 years after exposure | 10 or more years after exposure |
| Peak incidence | 5-7 years after exposure, rarely occur more than 15 years after exposure | Elevated risk remains for the rest of the exposed individual's life |
| Demographics | The risk from exposure during childhood is about twice as great as the risk during adulthood. All forms except chronic lymphocytic leukemia. | The risk from exposure during childhood is about twice as great as the risk during adulthood. The number of cancers induced by radiation is most likely a multiple of their spontaneous frequency (see Box 2-2). |

### BOX 2-2
## Susceptibility of Different Organs to Radiation-Induced Cancer

| High | Intermediate | Low |
|---|---|---|
| Colon | Bladder | Bone surface |
| Stomach | Liver | Brain |
| Lung | Thyroid | Salivary glands |
| Bone marrow (leukemia) | | Skin |
| Female breast | | |

shows the radiosensitivity of various tissues in terms of susceptibility to radiation-induced cancer. The following discussion of radiation carcinogenesis pertains primarily to those organs exposed in the course of dental radiography.

### Leukemia

The incidence of leukemia (other than chronic lymphocytic leukemia) rises after exposure of the bone marrow to radiation. Atomic bomb survivors and patients irradiated for ankylosing spondylitis show a wave of leukemias beginning soon after exposure and peaking at around 7 years. For individuals exposed under age 30 years, the risk for development of leukemia ceases after about 30 years. For individuals exposed as adults, the risk persists throughout life. Leukemias appear sooner than solid cancers because of the higher rate of cell division and differentiation of hematopoietic stem cells compared with the other tissues. Persons younger than 20 years are more at risk than adults are.

Evidence also exists for a slightly increased risk for childhood cancer, both leukemia and solid tumors, after diagnostic irradiation in utero. The level of the risk is uncertain but thought to increase the absolute risk by about 0.06% per 0.1 Gy.

### Thyroid Cancer

The incidence of thyroid carcinomas (arising from the follicular epithelium) increases in humans after exposure. Only about 10% or less of individuals with such cancers die from their disease. The best-studied groups are Israeli children irradiated to the scalp for ring-worm; children in Rochester, New York, irradiated to the thymus gland; and survivors of the atomic bombs in Japan. Susceptibility to radiation-induced thyroid cancer is greater early in childhood than at any time later in life, and children are more susceptible than adults. Females are two to three times more susceptible than males to radiogenic and spontaneous thyroid cancers. The fallout from the accident at the Chernobyl nuclear power plant, primarily iodine 131, is thought to have caused about 4000 cases of thyroid cancer in children and 15 fatalities.

### Esophageal Cancer

Data pertaining to esophageal cancer are relatively sparse. Excess cancers are found in the Japanese atomic bomb survivors and in patients treated with x radiation for ankylosing spondylitis.

### Brain and Nervous System Cancers

Patients exposed to diagnostic x-ray examinations in utero and to therapeutic doses in childhood or as adults (average midbrain dose of about 1 Gy) show excess numbers of malignant and benign brain tumors. Additionally, a case-control study has shown an association between intracranial meningiomas and previous medical or dental radiography. The strongest association was with a history of exposure to full-mouth dental radiographs when younger than 20 years. Because of their age, it is likely that these patients received substantially more exposure than is the case today with contemporary imaging techniques.

### Salivary Gland Cancer

The incidence of salivary gland tumors is increased in patients treated with irradiation for diseases of the head and neck, in Japanese atomic bomb survivors, and in persons exposed to diagnostic x radiation. An association between tumors of the salivary glands and dental radiography has been shown, the risk being highest in persons receiving full-mouth examinations before the age of 20 years. Only individuals who received an estimated cumulative parotid dose of 0.5 Gy or more showed a significant correlation between dental radiography and salivary gland tumors.

### Cancer of Other Organs

Other organs such as the skin, paranasal sinuses, and bone marrow (with respect to multiple myeloma) also show excess neoplasia after exposure. However, the mortality and morbidity rates expected after head and neck exposure are much lower than for the organs described previously.

BOX **2-3**
*Basic Principles of Radiation Genetics*

- Radiation causes increased frequency of spontaneous mutations rather than inducing new mutations.
- The frequency of mutations increases in direct proportion to the dose, even at very low doses, with no evidence of a threshold.
- The majority of mutations are deleterious to the organism.
- Dose rate is important. At low dose rates the frequency of induced mutations is greatly reduced.
- Males are much more radiosensitive than females.
- The rate of mutations is reduced as the time between exposure and conception increases.

## HERITABLE EFFECTS

Heritable effects are changes seen in the offspring of irradiated individuals. They are the consequence of damage to the genetic material of reproductive cells. The basic findings of radiation-induced heritable effects are listed in Box 2-3. At low levels of exposure, such as encountered in dentistry, they are far less important than carcinogenesis.

### Effects on Humans

Our knowledge of heritable effects of radiation on humans comes largely from the atomic bomb survivors. To date, no such radiation-related genetic damage has been demonstrated. No increase has occurred in adverse pregnancy outcome, leukemia or other cancers, or impairment of growth and development in the children of atomic bomb survivors. Similarly, studies of the children of patients who received radiotherapy show no detectable increase in the frequency of genetic diseases. These findings do not exclude the possibility that such damage occurs but do show that it must be at a very low frequency.

### Doubling Dose

One way to measure the risk from genetic exposure is by determining the *doubling dose,* which is the amount of radiation a population requires to produce in the next generation as many additional muta-

tions as arise spontaneously. In humans, the genetic doubling dose is estimated to be approximately 1 sievert (Sv). Because the average person receives far less gonadal radiation, radiation contributes relatively little to genetic damage in populations. For comparison, the background dose is about 0.003 Sv per year and the gonadal dose to males from a full-mouth radiographic examination is about 0.001 Sv or less. This exposure is contributed largely by the maxillary views, which are angled caudally. The dose to the ovaries is about 50 times less, in the range of 0.00002 Sv.

## BIBLIOGRAPHY

Bushong SC: Radiologic science for technologists: physics, biology, and protection, ed 7, St. Louis, 2001, Mosby.

Gusev I, Guskova A, Mettler F: Medical management of radiation accidents, ed 2, Boca Raton, Fla, 2001, CRC.

Hall EJ, Giaccia AJ: Radiobiology for the radiologist, ed 6, Philadelphia, 2006, Lippincott Williams & Wilkins.

Steel GG: Basic clinical radiobiology, ed 3, London, 2002, Hodder Arnold.

## SUGGESTED READINGS

*GENETIC EFFECTS*

United Nations Scientific Committee on the Effects of Atomic Radiation: Hereditary effects of radiation (2001): http://www.unscear.org/unscear/en/publications/2001.html.

*ODONTOGENESIS*

Dahllof G: Craniofacial growth in children treated for malignant diseases, *Acta Odontol Scand* 56:378, 1998.

Kielbassa AM, Hinkelbein W, Hellwig E et al: Radiation-related damage to dentition, *Lancet Oncol* 7:326-335, 2006.

*ORAL SEQUELAE OF HEAD AND NECK RADIOTHERAPY*

Chung EM, Sung EC: Dental management of chemoradiation patients, *J Calif Dent Assoc* 34:735-742, 2006.

Sciubba JJ, Goldenberg D: Oral complications of radiotherapy, *Lancet Oncol* 7:175-183, 2006.

Teng MS, Futran ND: Osteoradionecrosis of the mandible, *Curr Opin Otolaryngol Head Neck Surg* 13:217-221, 2005.

*SOMATIC EFFECTS*

Committee to Assess Health Risks from Exposure to Low Levels of Ionizing Radiation: Health risks from exposure to low levels of ionizing radiation: BEIR VII—phase 2, Washington, DC, 2006, National Research Council, National Academies Press.

# PART
# THREE

## Radiation Safety and Protection

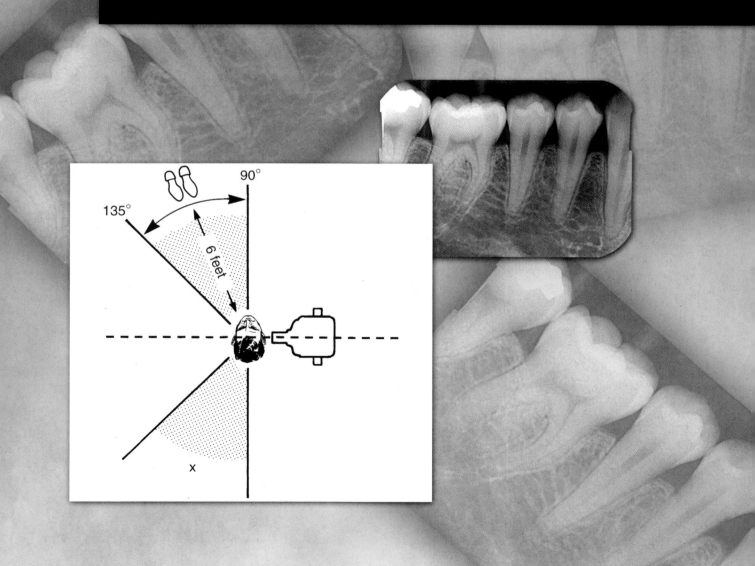

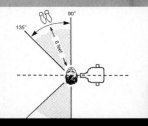

# CHAPTER 3

# Radiation Safety and Protection

Dentists must be prepared to intelligently discuss with patients the benefits and possible hazards involved with the use of x rays and to describe the steps taken to reduce the hazard. This chapter considers sources of exposure, estimates of risks from dental radiography, and means to minimize exposure from dental examinations.

## Sources of Radiation Exposure

The general population is exposed to radiation from natural and man-made sources (Table 3-1). Understanding these exposure sources provides a useful framework for considering dental exposure.

## NATURAL RADIATION

All life on earth has evolved in a continuous exposure to natural radiation (Fig. 3-1 and Table 3-1). Background radiation from cosmic and terrestrial sources yields an average annual effective dose of about 2.4 millisieverts (mSv) worldwide and 3.0 mSv in the United States because of higher radon levels.

### Cosmic Sources

Cosmic radiation includes energetic subatomic particles, photons from the sun and supernova, and to a lesser extent, the particles and photons (secondary cosmic radiation) generated by the interactions of primary cosmic radiation with atoms and molecules of the earth's atmosphere. Exposure from cosmic radiation is primarily a function of altitude, almost doubling with each 2000-meter (m) increase in elevation, because less atmosphere is present to attenuate the radiation. At sea level the exposure from cosmic radiation is about 0.24 mSv per year; at an elevation of 1600 m (approximately 1 mile, the elevation of Denver, Colorado), it is about 0.50 mSv per year. The global average is 0.4 mSv per year, about 16% of natural exposure.

Cosmic radiation also includes exposure resulting from airline travel. As more people travel frequently above the protection of the earth's atmosphere, cosmic radiation becomes a more significant contributor to exposure. An airline flight of 5 hours in the middle latitudes at an altitude of 12 km may result in a dose equivalent of about 25 μSv.

### Terrestrial Sources

Exposure from terrestrial sources comes from external sources such as soil and from internal sources, including radon and other radionuclides that are inhaled or ingested.

***External Radiation.*** Exposure from terrestrial sources comes from radioactive nuclides in the soil, primarily potassium 40 and the radioactive decay products of uranium 238 and thorium 232. Most of the γ radiation from these sources comes from the top 20 cm of soil. Indoor exposure from radionuclides is very close to that occurring outdoors because the shielding provided by structural materials balances the exposure from radioactive nuclides contained within these shielding materials. The average terrestrial exposure rate is about 0.5 mSv per year, or approximately 20% of the average annual background exposure.

***Radon.*** Radon, a decay product in the uranium series, is estimated to be responsible for approximately 52% of the radiation exposure of the world's population. As such, it is the largest single contributor to natural radiation (1.2 mSv). Radon is a gas (radon 222) that enters homes and buildings and by itself does little harm. However, radon decays to form solid products that emit α particles (porion 218, porion 214, lead 214, and bismuth 214). These decay products become attached to dust particles that can be inhaled and deposited on the bronchial epithelium in the respiratory tract. Exposure to this quantity of radiation may cause as many as 10,000 to 20,000 lung cancer deaths per year in the United States, mostly in smokers.

***Other Internal.*** Other sources of internal terrestrial exposure are radionuclides that are taken up from the external environment by ingestion. The greatest internal exposure comes from the ingestion of uranium and thorium and their decay products, primarily potassium 40 but also rubidium 87, carbon 14, tritium, and others. The total exposure from ingestion and inhalation other than radon is estimated at 0.3 mSv per year, about 12% of natural-origin exposure.

## MAN-MADE RADIATION

Humans have contributed many additional sources of radiation to the environment (Fig. 3-2). These may be categorized into three major groups: medical diagnosis and treatment, consumer and industrial products and sources, and other minor sources. Recent estimates suggest that medical exposure in the developed countries has grown rapidly in recent decades, particularly computed tomography (CT) of the chest and abdomen and increased use of cardiac nuclear medicine studies. It is estimated that the average doses from medical exposures are comparable to natural background exposure.

### Medical Diagnosis and Treatment

Well over one billion medical x-ray examinations are performed annually worldwide. This source of exposure contributes the large majority of exposures from man-made sources. Although sources in this group include radiation therapy and nuclear medicine, diagnostic medical exposure is the largest contributor, contributing most of this source. Dental x-ray examinations are responsible for less than 1% of the average annual exposures from man-made sources.

### Consumer and Industrial Products

Consumer and industrial products contain some of the most interesting and unsuspected sources. This group includes the domestic water

| TABLE 3-1 Average Annual Effective Dose of Ionizing Radiation | |
| --- | --- |
| SOURCE | DOSE (mSv) |
| *Natural* | |
| COSMIC | 0.4 |
| TERRESTRIAL | |
| External | 0.5 |
| Radon | 1.2 |
| Other | 0.3 |
| TOTAL | 2.4 |
| *Man-made* | |
| MEDICAL (ESTIMATED) | |
| X-ray diagnosis | 2 |
| Nuclear medicine | 0.5 |
| CONSUMER PRODUCTS OTHER | 0.08 |
| OTHER | |
| Occupational | 0.01 |
| Fallout | 0.01 |
| Nuclear fuel cycle | <0.01 |
| Dental radiology | ≤0.01 |
| TOTAL | 2.5 |

Natural exposures, consumer products and other from National Council on Radiation Protection and Measurements: NCRP Reports 93, 1987; 94, 1987. Medical exposures are estimated in recent unpublished data.

supply, tobacco products, combustible fuels, dental porcelain, television receivers, pocket watches, smoke alarms, and airport inspection systems but contributes only a small proportion of the total average annual man-made exposure.

### Other Man-made Sources

Individuals who work at medical and dental x-ray facilities, mining or milling, or with nuclear weapons are occupationally exposed to additional radiation exposure. Another source is the nuclear fallout from the nuclear weapons testing in the 1950s and early 1960s. Of these

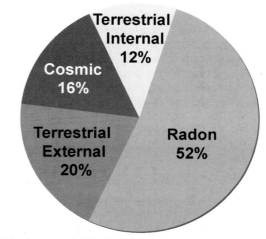

FIG. **3-1**  Sources of global background radiation contribute 2.4 mSv per year. Most exposure comes from radon, but there are significant contributions from cosmic and terrestrial sources including external from the soil and building materials and from ingested radionuclides. (Data modified from UNSCEAR 2000.)

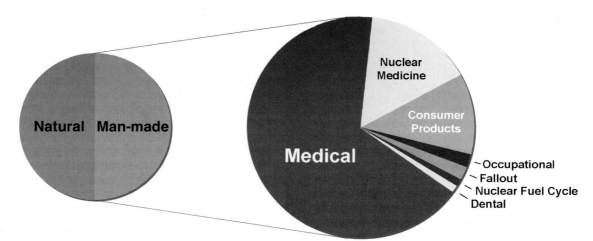

FIG. **3-2**  Sources of man-made radiation in the United States. The average person in the United States receives about as much radiation from man-made sources as from natural background exposure. Most man-made exposure comes from medical x-ray examinations, particularly CT, with significant contributions from nuclear medicine examinations, primarily cardiac imaging, and consumer products. Exposures from dental examinations and from occupational, fallout, and nuclear power sources are small.

sources, strontium 90 and iodine 131 are the most important. Because of its chemical similarity to calcium, strontium 90, a β emitter, is readily assimilated in the bones and teeth of children and young adults. Iodine 131, a γ emitter, accumulates in the thyroid gland. Fallout is no longer considered a significant source of exposure to the public because of the cessation of atmospheric testing of nuclear weapons.

Nuclear power (which contributes only about 0.01 mSv to the average annual exposure) is another man-made source of particular concern to the public. However, nuclear power and support facilities, in normal operation, add only about 10% of that contributed by the release of naturally occurring radionuclides from the combustion of coal, natural gas, and oil. In spite of this low contribution to the average annual exposure made by nuclear power, accidents have occurred. Between 1945 and 1987, 284 nuclear reactor accidents, excluding Chernobyl, were reported in several countries, resulting in the exposure of more than 1300 people, with 33 fatalities. The public was not directly affected in the majority of these accidents. The nuclear accident at Chernobyl in the Ukraine in 1986 made clear that the use of nuclear power facilities carries the real potential of causing considerable harm if not properly controlled. In that event, 29 persons in the immediate vicinity of the plant died of acute radiation injury in the first months after exposure. The long-term risk to the general population includes thyroid tumors that have resulted in 15 known fatalities.

## Dose and Risk in Radiography

This section considers governmental dose limits on individuals who are occupationally exposed and members of the general population, amounts of radiation received by patients in dental and medical radiography, and the estimated risks from these exposures.

## DOSE LIMITS

Recognition of the harmful effects of radiation and the risks involved with its use led the National Council on Radiation Protection and Measurements (NCRP) and the International Commission on Radiological Protection (ICRP) to establish guidelines for limitations on the amount of radiation received by both occupationally exposed individuals and the public. Since their establishment in the 1930s, these dose limits have been revised downward several times. These revisions reflect the increased knowledge concerning the harmful effects of radiation and the increased ability to use radiation more efficiently. The current occupational exposure limits have been established to ensure that no individuals will have deterministic effects and that the probability for stochastic effects is as low as reasonably and economically feasible (Table 3-2). Note that there are no limits on the exposure a patient can receive from diagnostic or therapeutic exposures.

Dose limits from man-made sources for members of the general public, not occupationally exposed, have been established at 10% of that of occupationally exposed individuals. The negligible individual dose, established by the NCRP, is considered to be the dose below which any effort to reduce the radiation exposure may not be cost-effective. In spite of the NCRP's endorsement of the nonthreshold hypothesis for purposes of radiation safety, it is thought that the impact on society of radiation exposure of this magnitude is negligible.

Dentists and their staff are occupationally exposed workers and are allowed to receive up to 50 mSv of whole-body radiation exposure per year (Table 3-2). Although this is considered to present only a minimal risk, every effort should be made to keep the dose to all individuals as low as practical. As a profession we do rather well. The average dose for individuals occupationally exposed in the operation

---

## TABLE **3-2**
### *Recommended Annual Limits for Human Exposure to Ionizing Radiation*

| RECOMMENDATION | NCRP | ICRP |
|---|---|---|
| ***Occupational Dose Limits*** | | |
| Relative to stochastic effects | 50 mSv annual effective dose limit and 10 mSv age (yr) cumulative effective dose limit | 50 mSv annual effective dose limit and 100 mSv in 5-yr cumulative effective dose limit |
| Relative to deterministic effects | 150 mSv annual equivalent dose limit to lens of eye and 500 mSv annual equivalent dose limit to skin and extremities | 150 mSv equivalent dose limit to lens of eye and 500 mSv annual equivalent dose limit to skin and extremities |
| ***Nonoccupational (Public) Dose Limits*** | | |
| Relative to stochastic effects | 5 mSv annual effective dose limit for infrequent exposure and 1 mSv annual effective dose limit for continuous exposure | 1 mSv annual effective dose limit and, if higher, not to exceed annual average of 1 mSv over 5 yr |
| Relative to deterministic effects | 50 mSv annual equivalent dose limit to lens of eye, skin, and extremities | 15 mSv annual equivalent dose limit to lens of eye and 50 mSv annual equivalent dose limit to lens of eye, skin, and extremities |
| Embryo-fetus | 0.5 mSv equivalent dose limit per month after pregnancy is known | 2 mSv equivalent dose limit after the pregnancy has been declared |
| Negligible individual dose* | 0.01 mSv annual effective dose | None established |

From National Council on Radiation Protection and Measurements: NCRP Report 116, 1993, and International Commission on Radiological Protection: Radiation protection, ICRP Publication 60, 1990.
*That dose below which any effort to reduce the radiation exposure cannot be justified.

| TABLE **3-3** | | |
| :--- | :--- | :--- |
| ***Effective Dose from Diagnostic X-Ray Examinations and Equivalent Background Exposure*** | | |
| EXAMINATION | EFFECTIVE DOSE (μSv) | EQUIVALENT BACKGROUND EXPOSURE (DAYS) |
| ***Intraoral**\* | | |
| Rectangular collimation | | |
|    Posterior bitewings – PSP or F-speed film | 5.0 | 0.6 |
|    FMX - PSP or F-speed film | 35 | 4 |
| Round collimation | | |
|    FMX - PSP or F-speed film | 171 | 21 |
|    FMX – D-speed film | 388 | 47 |
| ***Extraoral*** | | |
| Panoramic\*[†] | 9-26 | 1-3 |
| Cephalometric\*[‡] | 3-6 | 0.5-1 |
| Cone-beam imaging | | |
|    3D Accuitomo[§] | 20 | 3 |
|    NewTom 3G[‖] | 68 | 8 |
|    Gailieos[¶] | 70 | 9 |
|    Next Generation i-CAT Landscape mode\* | 74 | 9 |
|    PreXion[¶] | 185 | 23 |
|    i-CAT - Extended Scan\* | 235 | 29 |
|    CB Mercuray—Facial standard quality\* | 569 | 69 |
|    Iluma[¶] | 592 | 74 |
|    Promax 3D[¶] | 599 | 75 |
| Computed tomography[#] | | |
|    Somaton 64 MDCT\* | 860 | 105 |
|    Head | 2,000 | 243 |
|    Abdomen | 10,000 | 3 years |
|    Upper gastrointestinal tract[#] | 3,000 | 1 year |
|    Barium enema[#] | 7,000 | 2 years |
| Plain films | | |
|    Skull[#] | 70 | 9 |
|    Chest[#] | 20 | 2 |

\*Ludlow J: Personal communication, 2008.
[†]Lecomber AR, Yoneyama Y, Lovelock DJ et al: Comparison of patient dose from imaging protocols for dental implant planning using conventional radiography and computed tomography, *Dentomaxillofac Radiol* 30:255-259, 2001.
[‡]Gijbels F, Sanderink G, Wyatt J et al: Radiation doses of indirect and direct digital cephalometric radiography, *Br Dent J* 197:149-152, 2004.
[§]Hirsch E, Wolf U, Heinick F et al. Radiation doses from the cone beam CT-veraviewepocs 3D. 16th Int. Conf. Dentomaxillofacial Radiology, abstract OP-54, Beijing, 2007.
[‖]Ludlow JB, Davies-Ludlow LE, Brooks SL et al: Dosimetry of 3 CBCT devices for oral and maxillofacial radiology: CB Mercuray, NewTom 3G and i-CAT, *Dentomaxillofac Radiol* 35:219-226, 2006.
[¶]Ludlow J, Davies-Ludlow LE, Mol A: Dosimetry of recently introduced CBCT Units for Oral and Maxillofacial Radiology. 3D. 16th Int. Conf. Dentomaxillofacial Radiology, abstract OP-53, Beijing, 2007.
[#]Directorate-General for the Environment of the European Commission: Referral guidelines for imaging, Radiation Protection Report 118, European Commission, Luxembourg, 2000, and Shrimpton PC, Hillier MC, Lewis MA et al: National survey of doses from CT in the UK: 2003, *Br J Radiol* 79:968-980, 2006.

of dental x-ray equipment is far less than the limit: 0.2 mSv, or 0.4% of the allowable exposure.

## PATIENT EXPOSURE AND DOSE

Patient dose from dental radiography is usually reported as the amount of radiation received by a target organ. Although the actual exposures may vary considerably, Table 3-3 shows typical doses from various examinations. The equivalent exposure from natural and man-made background sources is shown. It may be seen that dental exposures are a small fraction of the annual average background exposure. The most radiosensitive target organs commonly studied include

bone marrow, thyroid gland, brain, and salivary glands. The mean active bone marrow dose is an important measurement because bone marrow is the target organ thought responsible for radiation-induced leukemia. Particular concern has been expressed over exposure of the thyroid because this gland has one of the highest radiation-induced cancer rates. There are also reports of brain and salivary gland tumors after therapeutic and diagnostic x-ray examinations.

## RISK ESTIMATES

The primary risk from dental radiography is radiation-induced cancer. The actual risk for cancer being induced in humans as a result of exposure to low doses of radiation is difficult to estimate for a number of reasons:

- The data for the cancer risk from radiation exposure involve exposures many times larger than those involved with dental radiology. Estimating cancer risk in dentistry thus requires extrapolating from high doses down to the low-dose range. A linear extrapolation is considered to be most appropriate, but the accuracy of this assumption is not known.
- Cancer is a common disease, accounting for about 20% of all deaths. It is estimated that in the United States in 2007 more than 1,400,000 new cases of cancer were diagnosed and that more than 560,000 people will die from this disease. The very low incidence that may result from dental exposure is impossible to detect by direct measurement.
- Radiation-induced cancers are clinically and histologically indistinguishable from cancers induced by other causes.
- The time between radiation exposure and the development of cancer may be years to decades, during which time individuals may be subjected to many other carcinogens.

In spite of these difficulties, the ICRP has developed an estimate that includes the probability for the induction of both fatal and nonfatal cancer and hereditary effects in an exposed population. On the basis of this estimate, 33 μSv for a full-mouth x ray delivered to 1,000,000 people would result in about two additional cancer deaths over the lifetime of the exposed individuals. This would be in addition to the 200,000 that would occur spontaneously. Such a calculation assumes a linear dose-response relationship and no threshold dose below which no risk exists. These assumptions may be in error and, if so, they most likely overestimate the actual risk.

This degree of risk from exposure to ionizing radiation may be expressed in multiple ways. It is helpful to compare the risk from dental exposures with that of equivalent natural exposures. Equivalent natural exposure is calculated as the product of the effective dose resulting from a specific radiographic examination and the average daily effective dose (8 μSv) delivered by natural sources. The dentist may point out to the patient that with optimal intraoral radiographic technique (E- or F-speed film or digital imaging, along with rectangular collimation) the days of equivalent exposure are only about 4 days for a full-mouth examination. For another example, the dependence of physical location within the United States on exposure to natural radiation may be used. The effective dose resulting from cosmic radiation in Denver is 0.24 mSv (240 μSv), higher than the average of the United States because of its high elevation and reduced atmospheric protection. This means that a person living in an average location in the United States who had one complete mouth survey and one panoramic image made by optimized techniques every year (total effective dose for these examinations = 42 μSv, see Table 3-3) would incur less than one fifth the risk for a person living in Denver who was not exposed to dental radiography. Put another way, if a person living in an average location in the United States had 14 complete mouth surveys (238 μSv) made by optimized techniques every year, he or she would incur only the same risk as a person living in Denver who was not exposed to dental radiography. There is no known risk from living in Denver pertaining to cosmic radiation.

Everyone is subject to risks in everyday life. Newspapers and news magazines occasionally publish articles dealing with the level of such risks. In consideration of the potential risk associated with dental radiography, it might be good to keep in mind that the average person's risk for death as a result of an accident while a patient in hospital is about 230 per million; choking to death, 13 per million; and dying in a boating accident, 4.6 per million. The risk from each of these events is greater than the risk from intraoral radiographic procedures.

In addition, people needlessly expose themselves to x radiation. There is a current trend for having full-body CT scans in hopes of detecting early signs of cancer, coronary artery disease, and other abnormalities. What most people do not realize is that a combined CT scan of the chest and abdomen delivers an *E* dose equal to almost 1000 chest radiographs. Furthermore, this increased exposure is often incurred for what is considered to be an unnecessary test: there is insufficient scientific evidence to justify CT screening for patients with no symptoms or family history suggesting disease.

Although the risk involved with dental radiography is certainly small in comparison with many other risks that are a common part of everyday life such as smoking or consumption of fatty foods, no basis exists to assume that it is zero. Although diagnostic radiation appears to be a weak carcinogen, the risk is increased because of the large number of people exposed. Practitioners must ensure that their patients avoid even the smallest unnecessary dose of radiation.

## Reducing Dental Exposure

There are three guiding principles in radiation protection; the first is the *principle of justification*. In making dental radiographs this principle obligates the dentist to do more good than harm. In radiology this means the dentist should identify those situations where the benefit to a patient from the diagnostic exposure exceeds the low risk of harm. In practice this principle influences what patients we select for radiographic examinations and what examinations we choose. These matters are considered in Chapter 15, Guidelines for Prescribing Dental Radiographs.

The second guiding rule is the *principle of optimization*. This principle holds that dentists should use every means to reduce unnecessary exposure to their patient and themselves. This philosophy of radiation protection is often referred to as the principle of ALARA (*As Low As Reasonably Achievable*). ALARA holds that exposures to ionizing radiation should be kept as low as reasonably achievable, economic and social factors being taken into account. The means to accomplish this end are considered later in this chapter.

The third principle is that of *dose limitation*. Dose limits are used for occupational and public exposures to ensure that no individuals are exposed to unacceptably high doses. There are no dose limits for individuals exposed for diagnostic or therapeutic purposes.

The dentist in each facility is responsible for the design and conduct of the radiation protection program. In this section, methods of exposure and dose reduction are described that can be used in dental radiography. Each subsection begins with a recommendation of the American Dental Association (ADA) Council on Scientific Affairs. This is followed by a discussion of ways in which these recommendations can be satisfied.

### PATIENT SELECTION CRITERIA

> Dentists should not prescribe routine dental radiographs at preset intervals for all patients. Instead, they should prescribe radiographs after an evaluation of the patient's needs that includes a health history review, a clinical dental history assessment, a clinical examination, and an evaluation of susceptibility to dental diseases. (ADA, 2006)

Radiographic selection criteria are clinical or historical findings that identify patients for whom a high probability exists that a radiographic examination will provide information affecting their treatment or prognosis. These criteria satisfy the principle of justification and are considered in Chapter 15.

## CONDUCTING THE EXAMINATION

When the decision has been made that a radiographic examination is justified (patient selection), the way in which the examination is conducted, the principle of optimization, greatly influences patient exposure to x radiation. The conduct of the examination may be divided into choice of equipment, choice of technique, operation of equipment, and processing and interpreting the radiographic image.

### Film and Digital Imaging

> Film of a speed slower than E-speed should not be used for dental radiographs. (ADA, 2006)

Currently, intraoral dental x-ray film is available in three speed groups: D, E, and F (Chapter 5). Clinically, film of speed group E is almost twice as fast (sensitive) as film of group D and about 50 times as fast as regular dental x-ray film (Fig. 3-3). The current F-speed films require about 75% the exposure of E-speed film and only about 40% that of D-speed. Faster films are desirable from the standpoint of exposure reduction. Multiple studies have found that F-speed film has the same useful density range, latitude, contrast, and image quality as D- and E-speed films and can be used in routine intraoral radiographic examinations without sacrifice of diagnostic information. Current digital sensors offer equal or greater dose savings than F-speed film and comparable diagnostic utility.

### Intensifying Screens and Film or Digital Imaging

> Rare-earth intensifying screens are recommended . . . combined with high-speed film of 400 or greater. (ADA, 2006)

Contemporary intensifying screens used in extraoral radiography use the rare earth elements gadolinium and lanthanum (see Chapter 5). These rare earth phosphors emit green light on interaction with x rays. Compared with the older calcium tungstate screens, rare earth screens decrease patient exposure by as much as 55% in panoramic and cephalometric radiography.

Unlike digital intraoral imaging, there is no significant dose reduction to be gained by replacing extraoral screen-film systems with digital imaging. Image resolution with digital systems is comparable to that obtained with rare earth screens matched with appropriate film.

### Source-to-Skin Distance

> Use of long source-to-skin distances of 40 cm, rather than short distances of 20 cm, decreases exposure by 10 to 25 percent. Distances between 20 cm and 40 cm are appropriate, but the longer distances are optimal. (ADA, 2006)

Two standard focal source-to-skin distances have evolved over the years for use in intraoral radiography, one 20 cm (8 inches) and the other 41 cm (16 inches). Use of the distance results in a 32% reduction in exposed tissue volume because the x-ray beam is less divergent (Fig. 3-4). One study reported a 30% decrease in the effective dose resulting from the use of a 30-cm distance instead of a 20-cm distance for a simulated 19-image complete mouth survey. Another study of patient exposures from intraoral radiographic examinations comparing a 40-cm distance with a 20-cm distance found a 38% to 45% decrease in thyroid exposure.

The use of a longer source-to-object distance also results in a smaller apparent focal spot size and thereby theoretically increases the

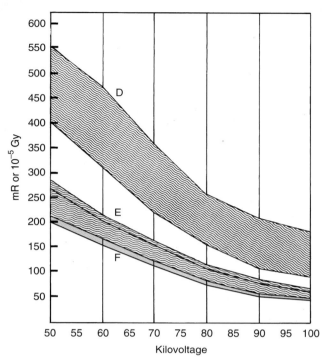

**Acceptable X-Ray Exposure Ranges**
**Speed Groups D, E, and F Film**

FIG. **3-3** Relationship between surface exposures delivered to a patient by exposure of groups D, E, and F (in light gray) intraoral films and diagnostic density at various kilovoltages. Note substantial overlap between E- and F-speed films. (Modified from HHS Publication [Food and Drug Administration] 85-8245, 1985.)

resolution of the radiograph (see Chapter 4). The clinical significance of the effect of focal spot size on image resolution, however, has been questioned.

### Rectangular Collimation

> Since a rectangular collimator decreases the radiation dose by up to fivefold as compared with a circular one, radiographic equipment should provide rectangular collimation for exposure of periapical and bitewing radiographs. (ADA, 2006)

The federal government requires that the x-ray beam used in intraoral radiography be collimated so that the field of radiation at the patient's skin surface is "contained in a circle having a diameter of no more than 7 cm (2¾ inches)" when the x-ray tube is operated above 50 kilovolts peak (kVp). In view of the dimensions of No. 2 intraoral film (3.2 × 4.1 cm) or digital sensor, a field size of this magnitude is almost three times that necessary to expose the image. Consequently, limiting the size of the x-ray beam even more than required by law may significantly reduce patient exposure. This results in not only decreased patient exposure but also increased image quality (Fig. 3-4). Additionally, the amount of radiation scatter generated is proportional to the area exposed. If scatter radiation is decreased, image fog is decreased and image quality is increased.

There are several means to limit of the size of the x-ray beam. First, a rectangular position-indicating device (PID) may be attached to the radiographic tube housing (Fig. 3-5). Use of a rectangular PID having

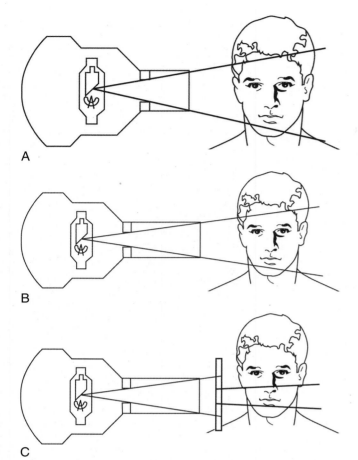

A

B

C

FIG. **3-4** Effect of source-to-skin distance and collimation on the volume of tissue irradiated. A larger volume of irradiated tissue results from **A** (with shorter source-to-skin distance) than from **B** (in which the longer source-to-skin distance produces a less divergent beam). In **C** the collimator between the round PID and the patient produces the effect of a rectangular PID on the tube housing or a rectangular collimating face shield on the film-holding instrument. This rectangular collimator (close to the patient in **C**) results in a smaller, less divergent beam and a smaller volume of tissue irradiated than in **A** or **B**.

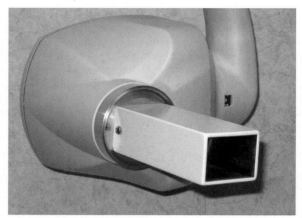

FIG. **3-5** A rectangular PID mounted on an x-ray machine provides a means to limit the shape of the x-ray beam to just larger than the film or digital sensor, thus minimizing the volume of tissue exposed. These devices are attached to an x-ray tube head to limit the size of the beam. They should be used with an external guide ring connected to the film or sensor to avoid cone cutting. (Courtesy Margraf Dental Manufacturing, Inc., www.margrafdental.com.)

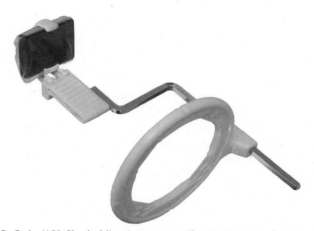

FIG. **3-6** XCP film-holding instrument. The aiming ring aligns a circular aiming cylinder from an x-ray machine with the sensor to assure that the image plane is perpendicular to the central ray and in the middle of the beam. Note notches to align rectangularly collimated aiming devices such as shown in Figures 3-5 or 3-7. Sensor is in plastic bag to prevent contamination from saliva. (Courtesy Dentsply Rinn, http://www.rinncorp.com/.)

an exit opening of 3.5 × 4.4 cm (1.38 × 1.34 inches) reduces the area of the patient's skin surface exposed by 60% over that of a round (7 cm) PID (see Fig. 3-4, *C*). This reduction in beam size, however, may make aiming the beam difficult. To avoid the possibility of unsatisfactory radiographs (cone cutting), a film-holding instrument that centers the beam over the film or sensor is recommended (Fig. 3-6).

Alternatively, film- and sensor-positioning devices with rectangular collimators may be used with round aiming cylinders (Figs. 3-7 and 3-8). These holders reduce patient exposure to the same degree as rectangular PIDs. In a study reviewing the effective dose delivered during complete mouth examinations made with film holders using round and rectangular collimation, rectangular collimation reduced the patient dose from intraoral examinations by about 60%.

## Filtration

The x-ray beam emitted from the radiographic tube consists of not only high-energy x-ray photons, but also many photons with relatively lower energy (see Chapter 1). Low-energy photons, which have little penetrating power, are absorbed mainly by the patient and contribute nothing to the information on the image. The purpose of filtration is to remove these low-energy x-ray photons selectively from the x-ray beam. This results in decreased patient exposure with no loss of radiographic information.

When an x-ray beam is filtered with 3 mm of aluminum, the surface exposure is reduced to about 20% of that with no filtration. In light of this and other information, the federal government has designated the specific amount of filtration, expressed as minimum half-value layer, required for dental x-ray machines operating at various kilovoltages. Practically, these requirements can be met by having 1.5 mm Al total filtration when operation from 50 to 70 kVp and with 2.5 mm Al total filtration when operating above 70 kVp.

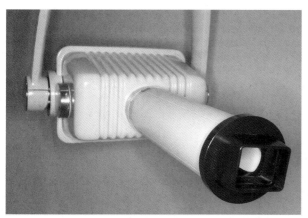

FIG. **3-7**   Rectangular collimation. An alternative means of limiting the size of an x-ray beam to a rectangle is to insert the device shown here into the end of a circular aiming cylinder that restricts the beam field to a rectangle.

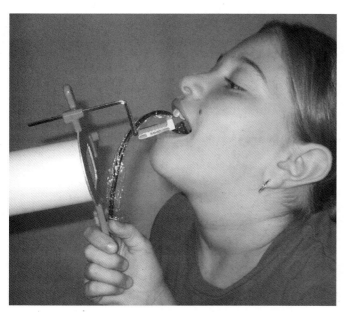

FIG. **3-8**   Rectangular collimation. Another means to collimate a round beam to a rectangle is to place a metallic shield in the path of the beam, thus limiting the size of the exposure field to an area just larger than the film or sensor. JADRAD Dental X-Ray Shield is illustrated. (Courtesy JADRAD Dental Diagnostics.)

## Leaded Aprons and Collars

> If all of the NCRP recommendations are followed rigorously, the use of a leaded apron on patients is not required. However, if any of the recommendations is not implemented, then a leaded apron should be used. Thyroid shielding with a leaded thyroid shield or collar is strongly recommended for children and pregnant women, as these patients may be especially susceptible to radiation effects. (ADA, 2006)

The function of leaded aprons and thyroid collars (Fig. 3-9) is to reduce radiation exposure of the gonads and thyroid gland. The NCRP 2003 recommendations referred to by the ADA are principally those already described, namely, use of patient selection criteria, fast

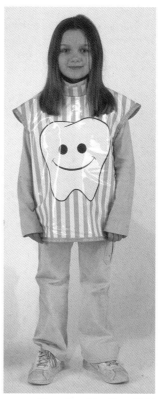

FIG. **3-9**   Leaded apron with a thyroid collar. Children are more sensitive to radiation than adults; thus the use of leaded aprons with thyroid collars is especially valuable. (Courtesy Dentsply Rinn.)

receptors, and rectangular collimators. The NCRP and ADA think that leaded aprons are not necessary because it is far more important in patient protection to place emphasis on reducing exposure of the primary beam to facial structures than to reduce the already very slight gonadal exposure. Recent research has shown that the risk of heritable effects from dental exposure is essentially insignificant (Chapter 2). Note, however, that most states currently require the use of leaded aprons.

There is, however, reason to be concerned about radiation exposure to the thyroid gland. Multiple studies, including those performed after the explosion of the Chernobyl reactor, have shown that the thyroid gland in children is especially sensitive to radiation. Accordingly, it is entirely appropriate to protect the thyroid glands of children during radiographic examinations. Again, the use of fast receptors and rectangular collimation is the best way to accomplish this aim, but thyroid collars further reduce dose to this organ.

## Film and Sensor Holders

> Film holders that align the film precisely with the collimated beam are recommended for periapical and bitewing radiographs. (ADA, 2006)

Film or digital sensor holders should be used when intraoral radiographs are made because they improve the alignment of the film, or digital sensor, with teeth and x-ray machine. Their use results in a significant reduction in unacceptable images. The use of film and sensor holders allows the operator to control the position and alignment of the film or sensor with respect to the teeth and jaws. This is especially important when the paralleling technique (Chapter 4) and digital imaging (Chapter 7) are used. In these cases it is often desirable to position the receptor away from the teeth so as to get the best image and reduce patient discomfort. This requires the use of a film or sensor holder. Most such devices have an external guide that shows the operator where to align the aiming cylinder (PID). As a result, the x-ray beam is properly directed toward the receptors. This greatly reduces the chance of the beam partially missing the image receptor (a "cone-cut") and also reduces image distortion (Chapter 4).

The decision as to which technique is used should be based on the diagnostic quality of the resultant radiographs, the efficiency of using radiation, and the convenience of the technique. The more efficient the technique, the fewer radiograph retakes will be required, along with less patient exposure. A study of comparative efficiencies of the bisection and parallel techniques found that the number of nondiagnostic radiographs was reduced by more than half when intraoral complete mouth examinations were made with the paralleling technique.

## Kilovoltage

> The operating potential of dental X-ray machines must range between 50 and 100 kilovolt peak but should range between 60 and 80 kVp. (ADA, 2006)

As the kVp is lowered, the mean energy of the beam decreases. This results in (1) an image with greater contrast (assuming that exposure time is increased), (2) a beam with more low-energy photons that carry the potential for risk but are not useful in making an image, and (3) reduced beam intensity requiring increased exposure time, thus increasing the risk of the patient moving and blurring the image. Although image diagnosis may be improved slightly with increased image contrast (low kVp) images, the patient dose is somewhat reduced with higher kVp exposures. The best balance is to use 60 to 80 kVp.

The availability of constant-potential (fully rectified), high-frequency or direct current (DC) dental x-ray units has made possible the production of radiographs with lower kilovoltage and at reduced levels of radiation. The surface exposure required to produce a comparable radiographic density using a constant-potential unit is approximately 25% less than that of a conventional self-rectified unit operating at the same kilovoltage. Currently several manufacturers produce DC units.

## Milliampere-Seconds

> The operator should set the amperage and time settings for exposure of dental radiographs of optimal quality. (ADA, 2006)

Of the three technical conditions (tube voltage, filtration, and exposure time), exposure time is the most crucial factor in influencing diagnostic quality. In terms of exposure, optimal image quality means that the radiograph is of diagnostic density, neither overexposed (too dark) nor underexposed (too light). Both overexposed and underexposed radiographs result in repeat exposures, thereby leading to needless additional patient exposure. Image density is controlled by the quantity of x rays produced, which in turn is best controlled by the combination of milliamperage and exposure time, termed *milliampere-seconds* (mAs) (Chapter 1). Typically, a radiograph of correct density will demonstrate very faint soft tissue outlines. Dentin will have an optical density of about 1.0. If your x-ray machine has a variable milliampere control, it should be set at the highest choice. Proper exposure times should be determined empirically by using optimal film processing conditions (Chapter 6) or manufacturer's recommendations for digital sensors. A chart showing optimal exposure times for each region of the arch in children and adults should be mounted by each x-ray machine. Because film-processing conditions are standardized, the only decision the dentist or the assistant needs to make is to select the proper exposure time.

## Film Processing

> Radiographs should not be overexposed and then underdeveloped, because this practice results in greater exposure to the patient and dental health care worker and can produce images of poor diagnostic quality. Dental radiographs should not be processed by sight, and manufacturers' instructions regarding time, temperature and chemistry should be followed. (ADA, 2006)

A major cause of unnecessary patient exposure is the deliberate overexposure of films compensated by underdevelopment of the film. This procedure results in both needless exposure of the patient and in films that are of inferior diagnostic quality (because of incomplete development). On the other hand, a properly exposed radiograph is of no value if all its diagnostic information is lost as a result of poor processing procedures. One dental insurance carrier reported that some 6% of the dental radiographs it received were not readable because of improper processing. Another study of 500 panoramic radiographs found that the average film contained at least one processing error. Time-temperature processing, in an adequately equipped and maintained darkroom, is the best way to ensure optimal film quality (see Chapter 6). To help ensure optimal image quality, the dental assistant should follow the film manufacturer's recommendation for processing solutions, not the solution manufacturer's directions.

The use of machines to process dental x-ray film has become widespread. More than 90% of dentists surveyed have reported using dental film processors. Automatic film processors should be used in a darkroom. Although some units have daylight loaders, allowing film to be placed in the machine in room light, such loaders are difficult to keep clean and free of contamination. Film processors, however, can actually increase patient exposure if not correctly maintained. Approximately 30% of all films retaken because of incorrect film density were directly related to processor variability. The introduction of a comprehensive maintenance program was found to reduce this retake rate significantly, resulting in a substantial savings in both patient exposure and operating costs.

## Interpreting the Images

> The dentist should view radiographs under appropriate conditions for analysis and diagnosis. (ADA, 2006)

Radiographs are best viewed in a semidarkened room with light transmitted through the films; all extraneous light should be eliminated. In addition, radiographs should be studied with the aid of a magnifying glass to detect even the smallest change in image density. A variable-intensity light source should also be available. Similarly, digital images are best interpreted on a computer screen in a darkened environment.

The diagnostic accuracy of radiographic caries diagnosis is only about 70% or less. This fact should stimulate individuals to place a greater emphasis on careful radiographic interpretation. Failure to diagnose problems is an increasing source of liability claims.

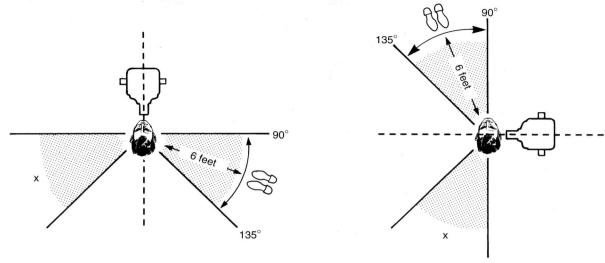

FIG. **3-10**   Position-and-distance rule. If no barrier is available, the operator should stand at least 6 feet from the patient, at an angle of 90 to 135 degrees to the central ray of the x-ray beam when the exposure is made.

## PROTECTING PERSONNEL

> Operators of radiographic equipment should use barrier protection when possible, and barriers should contain a leaded glass window to enable the operator to view the patient during exposure. When shielding is not possible, the operator should stand at least two meters from the tube head and out of the path of the primary beam. (ADA, 2006)

The methods of dose reduction discussed thus far have emphasized the effect on patient exposure. It should be apparent, however, that any procedure or technique that reduces radiation exposure to the patient also reduces the possibility of operator or office personnel exposure. In addition to those mentioned, several other steps can be taken to reduce the chance of occupational exposure.

Perhaps the single most effective way of limiting occupational exposure is the establishment of radiation safety procedures that are understood and followed by all personnel. Such written procedures are currently mandated by several states. First, every effort should be made so that the operator can leave the room or take a position behind a suitable barrier or wall during exposure of the image. Dental operatories should be designed and constructed to meet the minimal shielding requirement of the NCRP. This will require consultation with a qualified expert. This recommendation states that walls must be of sufficient density or thickness that the exposure to nonoccupationally exposed individuals (e.g., someone occupying an adjacent office) is no greater than 100 mGy per week. In most instances, it is not necessary to line the walls with lead to meet this requirement. Walls constructed of gypsum wallboard (drywall or sheet rock) are adequate for the average dental office.

If leaving the room or making use of some other barrier is impossible, strict adherence to what has been termed the *position-and-distance rule* is required: The operator should stand at least 6 feet (2 m) from the patient, at an angle of 90 to 135 degrees to the central ray of the x-ray beam (Fig. 3-10). When applied, this rule not only takes advantage of the inverse square law to reduce x-ray exposure to the operator but also take advantage of the fact that in this position the patient's head absorbs most scatter radiation. All practitioners should

check their state's regulations for use of ionizing radiation regarding operator position during x-ray exposures.

Second, the operator should never hold films or sensors in place. Film or sensor-holding instruments should be used (see Rectangular Collimation, p. 37). If correct film placement and retention are still not possible, a parent or other individual responsible for the patient should be asked to hold the sensor in place and, of course, be afforded adequate protection with a leaded apron. Under no circumstances should this person be one of the office staff.

Third, neither the operator nor patient should hold the radiographic tube housing during the exposure. Suspension arms should be adequately maintained to prevent housing movement and drift.

The best way to ensure that personnel are following office safety rules such as those described previously is with personnel-monitoring devices. Commonly referred to as *film badges,* these devices provide a useful record of occupational exposure. Their use is not only recommended but also required by law in certain states. Several companies in the United States offer dosimetry monitoring services. For a reasonable charge, these services provide badges that contain either a piece of sensitive film or a radiosensitive crystal (thermoluminescent dosimeter) and a printed report of accumulated exposure at regular intervals (Fig. 3-11). These reports indicate any undesirable change in work habits and help remove any apprehension office staff members may have about the possibility of exposure to x rays.

## QUALITY ASSURANCE

> Quality assurance protocols for the X-ray machine, imaging receptor, film processing, dark room, and leaded aprons and thyroid collars should be developed and implemented for each dental health care setting. (ADA, 2006)

*Quality assurance* may be defined as any planned activity to ensure that a dental office will consistently produce high-quality images with minimum exposure to patients and personnel (see Chapter 8). Studies have indicated that dentists may be needlessly exposing their patients to compensate for improper exposure techniques, film processing

# LANDAUER®

SAMPLE ORGANIZATION
RADIATION SAFETY OFFICER
2 SCIENCE ROAD
GLENWOOD, IL 60425

Landauer, Inc. 2 Science Road   Glenwood, Illinois 60425-1586
Telephone: (708) 755-7000   Facsimile: (708) 755-7016
www.landauerinc.com

**luxel**®

**RADIATION DOSIMETRY REPORT**

| ACCOUNT NO. | SERIES CODE | ANALYTICAL WORK ORDER | REPORT DATE | DOSIMETER RECEIVED | REPORT TIME IN WORK DAYS | PAGE NO. |
|---|---|---|---|---|---|---|
| 103702 | RAD | 992150087 | 06/13/03 | 06/09/03 | 4 | 1 |

| PARTICIPANT NUMBER | NAME | | | DOSIMETER | USE | RADIATION QUALITY | DOSE EQUIVALENT (MREM) FOR PERIODS SHOWN BELOW | | | YEAR TO DATE DOSE EQUIVALENT (MREM) | | | LIFETIME DOSE EQUIVALENT (MREM) | | | RECORDS FOR YEAR | INCEPTION DATE (MM/YY) |
|---|---|---|---|---|---|---|---|---|---|---|---|---|---|---|---|---|---|
| | ID NUMBER | BIRTH DATE | SEX | | | | DEEP DDE | EYE LDE | SHALLOW SDE | DEEP DDE | EYE LDE | SHALLOW SDE | DEEP DDE | EYE LDE | SHALLOW SDE | | |
| FOR MONITORING PERIOD: | | | | | | | 05/01/03 - 05/31/03 | | | 2003 | | | | | | | |
| 0000H | CONTROL | | | J | CNTRL | | M | M | M | | | | | | | 5 | 07/97 |
| | CONTROL | | | P | CNTRL | | M | M | M | | | | | | | | 07/97 |
| | CONTROL | | | U | CNTRL | | | | M | | | | | | | | 07/97 |
| 00189 | ADAMS, HEATHER | | | P | WHBODY | | M | M | M | 9 | 10 | 12 | 29 | 31 | 42 | 5 | 07/01 |
| | 336235619 | 08/31/1968 | F | | | | | | | | | | | | | | |
| 00191 | ADDISON, JOHN | | | J | WHBODY | PN | 90 | 90 | 90 | 100 | 100 | 100 | 200 | 200 | 200 | 5 | 07/01 |
| | 471563287 | 10/04/1968 | M | | | P | 60 | 60 | 60 | 70 | 70 | 70 | 170 | 170 | 170 | | |
| | | | | | | NF | 30 | 30 | 30 | 30 | 30 | 30 | 30 | 30 | 30 | | |
| 00202 | HARRIS, KATHY | | | P | WHBODY | | M | M | M | M | M | M | M | M | M | 5 | 02/02 |
| | 587582144 | 06/09/1960 | F | U | RFINGR | | | | M | | | 30 | | | 30 | | 02/02 |
| 00005 | MEYER, STEVE | | | P | COLLAR | PL | 119 | 119 | 113 | | | | | | | 5 | 08/97 |
| | 982778955 | 07/15/1964 | M | P | WAIST | P | 10 | 11 | 11 | | | | | | | | 08/97 |
| | | | | | ASSIGN | | 19 | 119 | 113 | 33 | 185 | 174 | 1387 | 2308 | 2320 | | |
| | | | | | NOTE | | ASSIGNED DOSE BASED ON EDE 1 CALCULATION | | | | | | | | | | |
| | | | | U | RFINGR | | | | 140 | | | 690 | | | 2180 | | 08/97 |
| 00203 | STEVENS, LEE | | | P | WHBODY | | ABSENT | | | M | M | M | M | M | M | 4 | 07/02 |
| | 335478977 | 08/25/1951 | M | U | RFINGR | | ABSENT | | | | | M | | | M | | 07/02 |
| 00204 | WALKER, JANE | | | P | WHBODY | | 3 | 3 | 3 | 12 | 11 | 11 | 22 | 21 | 21 | 5 | 11/02 |
| | 416995421 | 03/21/1947 | F | | | | | | | | | | | | | | |
| 00188 | WEBSTER, ROBERT | | | P | WHBODY | | 40 | 40 | 40 | 200 | 200 | 200 | 240 | 240 | 240 | 5 | 07/01 |
| | 355381469 | 05/15/1972 | M | | NOTE | | CALCULATED | | | | | | | | | | |

M: MINIMAL REPORTING SERVICE OF 1 MREM
ELECTRONIC MEDIA TO FOLLOW THIS REPORT

QUALITY CONTROL RELEASE: LMR                1 - PR   6774 - PT131 - N1                -21587

NVLAP®
NVLAP LAB CODE 100518-0 **

FIG. **3-11** Sample radiation dosimetry report showing that George Smith received an exposure of 0.60 μSv (60 mrem) during the month reported. The report also shows totals for the calendar quarter, year to date, and permanent or lifetime exposure. (Courtesy Landauer, Inc., Glenwood, Ill.)

practices, and darkroom procedures. One study reported that only 33% of panoramic radiographs that accompanied biopsy specimens were of acceptable diagnostic quality. However, when demands were placed on dentists to improve their techniques, the number of unsatisfactory radiographs was significantly reduced. Two studies by a dental insurance carrier demonstrated that after claims were rejected for unsatisfactory radiographs and the dentist was made aware of the errors and ways in which they could be corrected, the number of satisfactory radiographs submitted doubled. This suggests that when the dentist is presented with guidelines for quality assurance, along with proper motivation, patient exposure can be dramatically reduced.

Currently some states require dental offices to establish written guidelines for quality assurance and to maintain written records of quality assurance tests. Regardless of requirements, each dental office should establish maintenance and monitoring procedures as outlined in Chapter 8.

## CONTINUING EDUCATION

Practitioners should remain informed about safety updates and the availability of new equipment, supplies and techniques that could further improve the diagnostic quality of radiographs and decrease radiation exposure. (ADA, 2006)

Those who administer ionizing radiation must become familiar with the magnitude of exposure encountered in medicine, dentistry, and everyday life; the possible risks associated with such exposure; and the methods used to affect exposure and dose reduction. Although this chapter presents some of this information, acquiring knowledge and developing and maintaining skills is a life-long process.

## BIBLIOGRAPHY

American Dental Association Council on Scientific Affairs: The use of dental radiographs: update and recommendations, *J Am Dent Assoc* 137:1304-1312, 2006.

Code of Federal Regulations 21, Subchapter J: Radiological health, part 1000, Office of the Federal Register, General Services Administration, Washington, DC, 1994.

Committee to Assess Health Risks from Exposure to Low Levels of Ionizing Radiations: Health risks from exposure to low levels of ionizing radiation: BEIR VII, Washington, DC, 2006, National Academy Press.

Hall EJ, Giaccia AJ: Radiobiology for the radiologist, ed 6, Baltimore, 2006, Lippincott Williams & Wilkins.

Horner K, Rushton VE, Walker A et al: European guidelines on radiation protection in dental radiology: the safe use of radiographs in dental practice, *Radiat Protect* 136:1-115, 2004.

National Council on Radiation Protection and Measurements: Control of radon in houses, NCRP Report 103, Bethesda, Md, 1989, National Council on Radiation Protection and Measurements.

National Council on Radiation Protection and Measurements: *Quality assurance for diagnostic imaging*, NCRP Report 99, Bethesda, Md, 1990, National Council on Radiation Protection and Measurements.

National Council on Radiation Protection and Measurements: *Limitation of exposure to ionizing radiation*, NCRP Report 116, Bethesda, Md, 1993, National Council on Radiation Protection and Measurements.

National Council on Radiation Protection and Measurements: *Dental x-ray protection*, NCRP Report 145, Bethesda, Md, 2003, National Council on Radiation Protection and Measurements.

*Nationwide Evaluation of X-Ray Trends (NEXT), tabulation and graphical summary of the 1999 dental radiography survey*, CRCPD Publication E-03-6,Bethesda, Md, 2003, Center for Devices and Radiological Health, U.S. Food and Drug Administration.

Preston RJ: Radiation biology: concepts for radiation protection, *Health Phys* 88:545-556, 2005.

*Sources and effects of ionizing radiation*, volume 1: sources, New York, 2000, UNSCEAR, UN Publication.

Wall BF, Kendall GM, Edwards AA et al: What are the risks from medical X-rays and other low dose radiation? *Br J Radiol* 79:285-294, 2006.

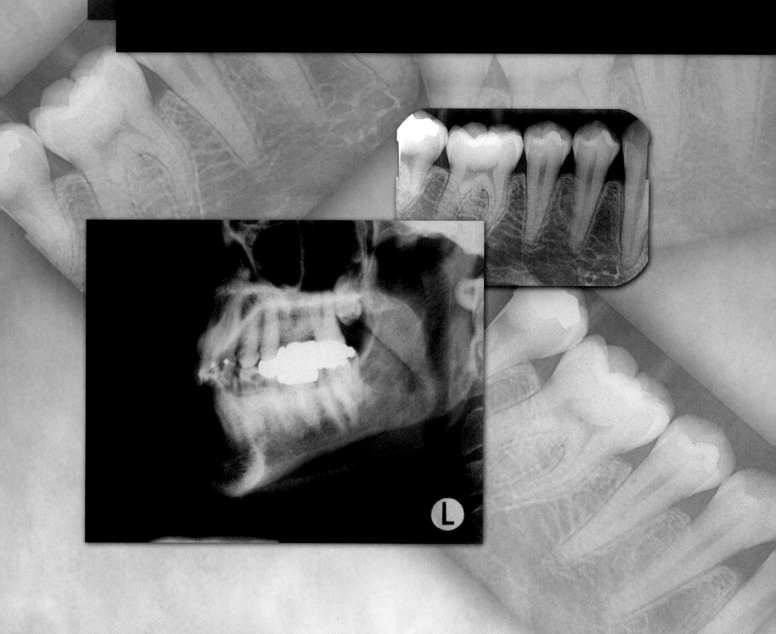

# PART
# FOUR

## Imaging Principles and Techniques

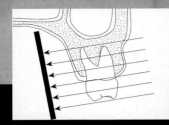

# CHAPTER 4

# Projection Geometry

A conventional radiograph is a two-dimensional projection image of a three-dimensional object. In such an image the entire volume of tissue between the x-ray source and the film or digital receptor is projected onto a two-dimensional image. To obtain the maximal value from a radiograph, a clinician must have a clear understanding of normal anatomy and then mentally reconstruct a three-dimensional image of the anatomic structures of interest from one or more of these two-dimensional views. Using high-quality radiographs greatly facilitates this task. The principles of projection geometry describe the effect of focal spot size and position (relative to the object and the film) on image clarity, magnification, and distortion. Clinicians use these principles to maximize image clarity, minimize distortion, and localize objects in the image field. Later chapters will consider different forms of tomographic imaging techniques that produce slices through tissue rather than projection images.

## Image Sharpness and Resolution

Several geometric considerations contribute to image clarity, particularly image sharpness and resolution. *Sharpness* measures how well a boundary between two areas of differing radiodensity is revealed. Image *spatial resolution* measures how well a radiograph is able to reveal small objects that are close together. Although sharpness and resolution are two distinct features, they are interdependent, being influenced by the same geometric variables. For clinical diagnosis it is desirable to optimize conditions that will result in images with high sharpness and resolution.

When x rays are produced at the target in an x-ray tube, they originate from all points within the area of the focal spot. Because these rays originate from different points and travel in straight lines, their projections of a feature of an object do not occur at exactly the same location on a film. As a result, the image of the edge of an object is slightly blurred rather than sharp and distinct. Figure 4-1 shows the path of photons that originate at the margins of the focal spot and provide an image of the edges of an object. The resulting blurred zone of unsharpness on an image causes a loss in image clarity by reducing sharpness and resolution. The larger the focal spot area, the greater the loss of clarity.

Three methods exist for minimizing this loss of image clarity and improving the quality of radiographs:

1. *Use as small an effective focal spot as practical.* Dental x-ray machines should have a nominal focal spot size of 1.0 mm or less. Some tubes used in extraoral radiography have effective focal spots measuring 0.3 mm, which greatly adds to image clarity. X-ray tube manufacturers use as small an effective focal spot size as is consistent with the requirements for heat dissipation. As described in Chapter 1,

the size of the effective focal spot is a function of the angle of the target with respect to the long axis of the electron beam. A large angle distributes the electron beam over a larger surface and decreases the heat generated per unit of target area, thus prolonging tube life. However, this results in a larger effective focal spot and loss of image clarity (Fig. 4-2). A small angle has a greater wearing effect on the target but results in a smaller effective focal spot, decreased unsharpness, and increased image sharpness and resolution. This angle of the face of the target to the central x-ray beam is usually between 10 and 20 degrees.

2. *Increase the distance between the focal spot and the object by using a long, open-ended cylinder.* Figure 4-3 shows how increasing the focal spot-to-object distance reduces image blurring by reducing the divergence of the x-ray beam. The longer focal spot-to-object distance minimizes blurring by using photons whose paths are almost parallel. The benefits of using a long focal spot-to-object distance support the use of long, open-ended cylinders as aiming devices on dental x-ray machines.

3. *Minimize the distance between the object and the film.* Figure 4-4 shows that, as the object-to-film distance is reduced, the unsharpness decreases, resulting in enhanced image clarity. This is the result of minimizing the divergence of the x-ray photons.

## Image Size Distortion

Image size distortion (magnification) is the increase in size of the image on the radiograph compared with the actual size of the object. The divergent paths of photons in an x-ray beam cause enlargement of the image on a radiograph. Image size distortion results from the relative distances of the focal spot-to-film and object-to-film (see Figs. 4-3 and 4-4). Accordingly, increasing the focal spot-to-film distance and decreasing the object-to-film distance minimizes image magnification. The use of a long, open-ended cylinder as an aiming device on an x-ray machine thus reduces the magnification of images on a periapical view. Furthermore, as previously mentioned, this technique also improves image clarity by increasing the distance between the focal spot and the object.

## Image Shape Distortion

Image shape distortion is the result of unequal magnification of different parts of the same object. This situation arises when not all the parts of an object are at the same focal spot-to-object distance. The physical shape of the object may often prevent its optimal orientation, resulting in some shape distortion. Such a phenomenon is seen by the differences in appearance of the image on a radiograph compared with the true shape. To minimize shape distortion, the practitioner

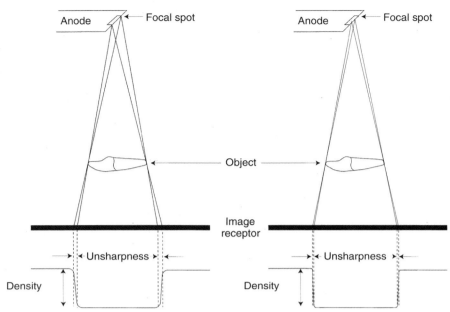

FIG. **4-1** Photons originating at different places on the focal spot result in a zone of unsharpness on the radiograph. The density of the image changes from a high background value to a low value in the area of an edge of enamel, dentin, or bone. On the left a large focal spot size results in a wide zone of unsharpness compared with a small focal spot size on the left that results in a narrow zone of unsharpness.

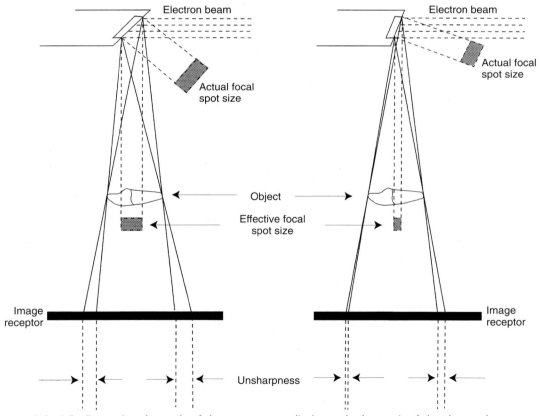

FIG. **4-2** Decreasing the angle of the target perpendicular to the long axis of the electron beam decreases the actual focal spot size and decreases heat dissipation and thereby tube life. It also decreases the effective focal spot size, thus increasing the sharpness of the image.

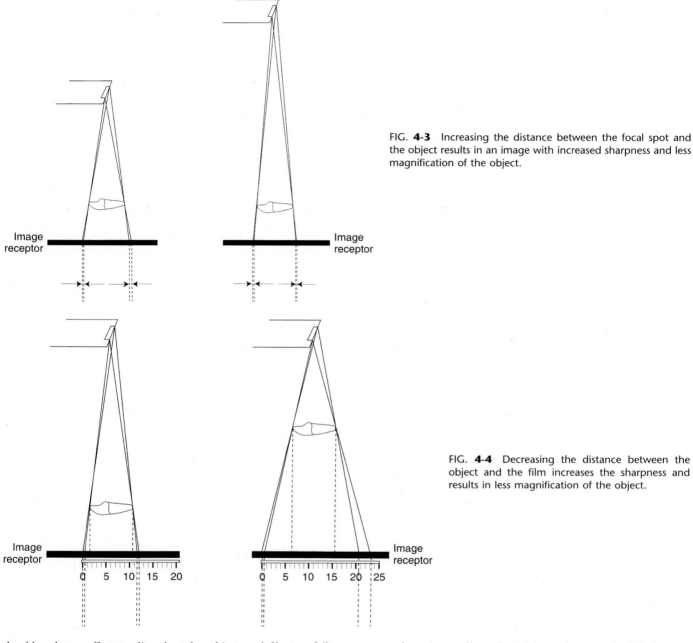

FIG. **4-3** Increasing the distance between the focal spot and the object results in an image with increased sharpness and less magnification of the object.

FIG. **4-4** Decreasing the distance between the object and the film increases the sharpness and results in less magnification of the object.

should make an effort to align the tube, object, and film carefully according to the following guidelines:

1. *Position the film parallel to the long axis of the object.* Image shape distortion is minimized when the long axes of the film and tooth are parallel. Figure 4-5 shows that the central ray of the x-ray beam is perpendicular to the film but the object is not parallel to the film. The resultant image is distorted because of the unequal distances of the various parts of the object from the film. This type of shape distortion is called *foreshortening* because it causes the radiographic image to be shorter than the object. Figure 4-6 shows the situation when the x-ray beam is oriented at right angles to the object but not to the film. This results in *elongation,* with the object appearing longer on the film than its actual length.

2. *Orient the central ray perpendicular to the object and film.* Image shape distortion occurs if the object and film are parallel but the

central ray is not directed at right angles to each. This is most evident on maxillary molar projections (Fig. 4-7). If the central ray is oriented with an excessive vertical angulation, the palatal roots appear disproportionately longer than the buccal roots.

The practitioner can prevent distortion errors by aligning the object and film parallel with each other and the central ray perpendicular to both.

## Paralleling and Bisecting-Angle Techniques

From the earliest days of dental radiography, a clinical objective has been to produce accurate images of dental structures that are normally visually obscured. An early method for aligning the x-ray

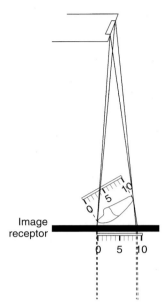

FIG. **4-5** Foreshortening of a radiographic image results when the central ray is perpendicular to the film but the object is not parallel with the film.

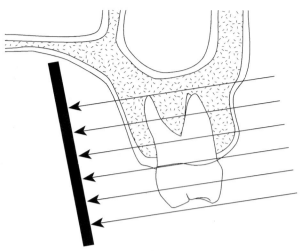

FIG. **4-7** The central ray should be perpendicular to the long axes of both the tooth and the film. If the direction of the x-ray beam is not at right angles to the long axis of the tooth, then the appearance of the tooth is distorted, as seen by apparent elongation of the length of the palatal roots. Additionally, distortion of the relationship of the height of the alveolar crest relative to the cementoenamel junction occurs. In this case the buccal alveolar crest appears to lie superior to the palatal cementoenamel junction.

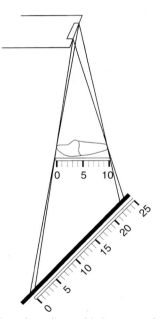

FIG. **4-6** Elongation of a radiographic image results when the central ray is perpendicular to the object but not to the film.

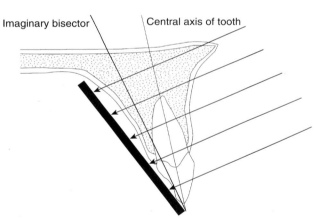

FIG. **4-8** In the bisecting-angle technique the central ray is directed at a right angle to the imaginary plane that bisects the angle formed by the film and the central axis of the object. This method results in an image that is the same length as the object.

beam and film with the teeth and jaws was the *bisecting-angle tech-nique* (Fig. 4-8). In this method the film is placed as close to the teeth as possible without deforming it. However, when the film is in this position, it is not parallel to the long axes of the teeth. This arrange-ment inherently causes distortion. Nevertheless, by directing the central ray perpendicular to an imaginary plane that bisects the angle between the teeth and the film, the practitioner can make the length of the tooth's image on the film correspond to the actual length of the tooth. This angle between a tooth and the film is especially apparent

when teeth are radiographed in the maxilla or anterior mandible. Although the projected length of a tooth is correct, the image is still distorted because the film and object are not parallel and the x-ray beam is not directed at right angles to them. This distortion tends to increase along the image toward the apex.

When the central ray is not perpendicular to the bisector plane, the length of the image of a projected tooth changes. If the central ray is directed at an angle that is more positive than perpendicular to the bisector, the image of the tooth is *foreshortened*. Likewise, if it is inclined with more negative angulation to the bisector, the image is *elongated*. In recent years, the bisecting-angle technique has been used less frequently for general periapical radiography as use of the paral-leling technique has increased.

Central axis of tooth

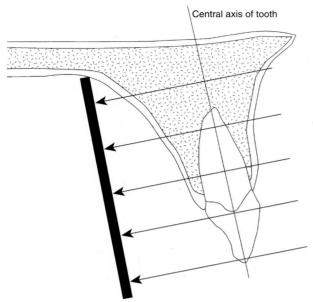

FIG. **4-9**  In the paralleling technique the central ray is directed at a right angle to the central axes of the object and the film.

The *paralleling technique* is the preferred method for making intraoral radiographs. It derives its name as the result of placing the film parallel to the long axis of the tooth (Fig. 4-9). This procedure minimizes image distortion and best incorporates the imaging principles described in the first three sections of this chapter.

To achieve this parallel orientation, the practitioner often must position the film toward the middle of the oral cavity, away from the teeth. Although this allows the teeth and film to be parallel, it results in some image magnification and loss of definition by increasing unsharpness. As a consequence, the paralleling technique also uses a relatively long open-ended aiming cylinder ("cone") to increase the focal spot-to-object distance. This directs only the most central and parallel rays of the beam to the film and teeth and reduces image magnification while increasing image sharpness and resolution. The paralleling technique has benefited from the development of fast-speed film emulsions, which allow relatively short exposure times in spite of an increased target-to-object distance.

Because it is desirable to position the film near the middle of the oral cavity with the paralleling technique, film holders should be used to support the film in the patient's mouth. Chapter 9 discusses film-holding instruments and techniques for intraoral radiography with the paralleling technique.

## Object Localization

In clinical practice, the dentist must often derive from a radiograph three-dimensional information concerning patients. The dentist may wish to use radiographs, for example, to determine the location of a foreign object or an impacted tooth within the jaw. Two methods are frequently used to obtain such three-dimensional information. The first is to examine two films projected at right angles to each other. The second method is to use the so-called tube shift technique.

Figure 4-10 shows the first method, in which *two projections taken at right angles to one another* localize an object in or about the maxilla

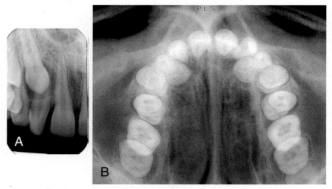

FIG. **4-10**  **A,** The periapical radiograph shows impacted canine lying apical to roots of lateral incisor and first premolar. **B,** The vertex occlusal view shows that the canine lies palatal to the roots of the lateral incisor and first premolar.

in three dimensions. In clinical practice the position of an object on each radiograph is noted relative to the anatomic landmarks. This allows the observer to determine the position of the object or area of interest. For example, if a radiopacity is found near the apex of the first molar on a periapical radiograph, the dentist may take an occlusal projection to identify its mediolateral position. The occlusal film may reveal a calcification in the soft tissues located laterally or medially to the body of the mandible. This information is important in determining the treatment required. The right-angle (or cross-section) technique is best for the mandible. On a maxillary occlusal projection the superimposition of features in the anterior part of the skull may frequently obscure the area of interest.

The second method used to identify the spatial position of an object is the *tube shift technique.* Other names for this procedure are the *buccal object rule* and *Clark's rule* (Clark described it in 1910). The rationale for this procedure derives from the manner in which the relative positions of radiographic images of two separate objects change when the projection angle at which the images were made is changed.

Figure 4-11 shows two radiographs of an object exposed at different angles. Compare the position of the object in question on each radiograph with the reference structures. If the tube is shifted and directed at the reference object (e.g., the apex of a tooth) from a more mesial angulation and the object in question also moves mesially with respect to the reference object, the object lies lingual to the reference object.

Alternatively, if the tube is shifted mesially and the object in question appears to move distally, it lies on the buccal aspect of the reference object (Fig. 4-12). These relationships can be easily remembered by the acronym *SLOB: Same Lingual, Opposite Buccal.* Thus, if the object in question appears to move in the same direction with respect to the reference structures as does the x-ray tube, it is on the lingual aspect of the reference object; if it appears to move in the opposite direction as the x-ray tube, it is on the buccal aspect. If it does not move with respect to the reference object, it lies at the same depth (in the same vertical plane) as the reference object.

Examination of a conventional set of full-mouth films with this rule in mind demonstrates that the incisive foramen is indeed located lingual (palatal) to the roots of the central incisors and that the mental foramen lies buccal to the roots of the premolars. This technique assists in determining the position of impacted teeth, the presence of

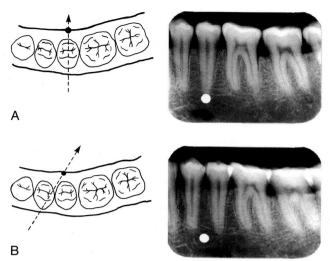

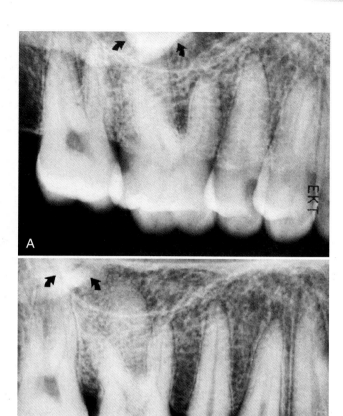

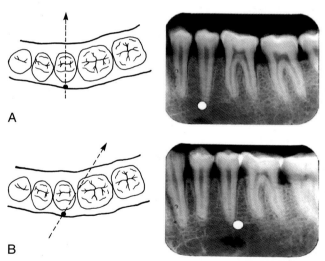

FIG. **4-11**  The position of an object may be determined with respect to reference structures with use of the tube shift technique. In **A,** an object on the lingual surface of the mandible may appear apical to the second premolar. When another radiograph is made of this region angulated from the mesial, **B,** the object appears to have moved mesially with respect to the second premolar apex ("same lingual" in the acronym *SLOB*).

FIG. **4-12**  The position of an object can be determined with respect to reference structures with use of the tube shift technique. In **A,** an object on the buccal surface of the mandible may appear apical to the second premolar. When another radiograph is made of this region angulated from the mesial, **B,** the object appears to have moved distally with respect to the second premolar apex ("opposite buccal" in the acronym *SLOB*).

FIG. **4-13**  The position of the maxillary zygomatic process in relation to the roots of the molars can help in identifying the orientation of projections. In **A,** the inferior border of the process lies over the palatal root of the first molar, whereas in **B** it lies posterior to the palatal root of the first molar. This indicates that when **A** was made the beam was oriented more from the posterior than when **B** was made. The same conclusion can be reached independently by examining the roots of the first molar. In **A,** the palatal root lies behind the distobuccal root, but in **B** it lies between the two buccal roots.

foreign objects, and other abnormal conditions. It works just as well when the x-ray machine is moved vertically as horizontally.

The dentist may have two radiographs of a region of the dentition that were made at different angles, but no record exists of the orientation of the x-ray machine. Comparison of the anatomy displayed on the images helps distinguish changes in horizontal or vertical angulation. The relative positions of osseous landmarks with respect to the teeth help identify changes in horizontal or vertical angulation. Figure 4-13 shows the inferior border of the zygomatic process of the maxilla over the molars. This structure lies buccal to the teeth and appears to move mesially as the x-ray beam is oriented more from the distal. Similarly, as the angulation of the beam is increased vertically, the zygomatic process is projected occlusally over the teeth.

## Peripheral Eggshell Effect

Projection images, those that project a three-dimensional volume onto a two-dimensional receptor, may produce a peripheral eggshell effect. Figure 4-14, *A,* shows a schematic view of an egg being exposed to an x-ray beam. The top photon has a tangential path through the apex of the egg and a much longer path through the shell of the egg than does the lower photon, which strikes the egg at right angles to the surface and travels through two thicknesses of the shell. As a result, photons traveling through the periphery of a curved surface are more attenuated than those traveling at right angles to the surface. Figure

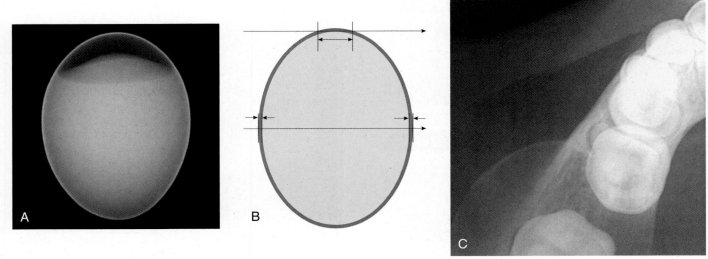

FIG. **4-14**   Peripheral eggshell effect. **A** is a radiograph of a hard-boiled egg. Note how the peripheral rim, the eggshell, is opaque even though the eggshell is uniform in thickness. **B** shows a schematic view of this egg being exposed to an x-ray beam. The top photon has a tangential path through the apex of the egg and a longer path through the shell of the egg than the lower photon. As a result, photons traveling through the periphery of a curved surface are more attenuated than those traveling at right angles to the surface. **C** shows an expansile lesion on the buccal surface of the mandible on an occlusal view. Note how the periphery of the expanded cortex is more opaque than the region inside the expanded border as a result of the peripheral eggshell effect.

4-14, *B,* shows an expansile lesion on the buccal surface of the mandible on an occlusal view. Note how the periphery of the expanded cortex is more opaque than the region inside the expanded border. The cortical bone in not thicker on the cortex than over the rest of the lesion, but rather the x-ray beam is more attenuated in this region because of the longer path length of photons through the bony cortex on the periphery. This peripheral eggshell effect accounts for why the lamina dura, the border of the maxillary sinuses and nasal fossa, and numerous other structures are well demonstrated on projection images. Note that soft tissue masses, such as the nose and tongue, do not show a peripheral eggshell effect because they are uniform rather then being composed of a dense layer surrounding a more lucent interior.

## BIBLIOGRAPHY

### *BUCCAL OBJECT RULE*

Chenail B, Aurelio JA, Gerstein H: A model for teaching the Buccal Object Moves Most Rule, *J Endod* 9:452-453, 1983.
Clark CA: A method of ascertaining the relative position of unerupted teeth by means of film radiographs, *Proc R Soc Med Odontol Sect* 3:87-90, 1910.

Goerig AC, Neaverth EJ: A simplified look at the buccal object rule in endodontics, *J Endod* 13:570-572, 1987.
Jacobs SG: Radiographic localization of unerupted maxillary anterior teeth using the vertical tube shift technique: the history and application of the method with some case reports, *Am J Orthod Dentofac Orthop* 116:415-423, 1999.
Jacobs SG: Radiographic localization of unerupted teeth: further findings about the vertical tube shift method and other localization techniques, *Am J Orthod Dentofac Orthop* 118:439-447, 2000.
Khabbaz MG, Serefoglou MH: The application of the buccal object rule for the determination of calcified root canals, *Int Endod J* 29:284-287, 1996.
Ludlow JB: The Buccal Object Rule, *Dentomaxillofac Radiol* 28:258, 1999.
Reader A: A teaching model for the buccal object rule, *J Dent Educ* 48:469-472, 1984.

### *PARALLELING TECHNIQUE*

Forsberg J: A comparison of the paralleling and bisecting-angle radiographic techniques in endodontics, *Int Endod J* 20:177-182, 1987.
Forsberg J, Halse A: Radiographic simulation of a periapical lesion comparing the paralleling and the bisecting-angle techniques, *Int Endod J* 27:133-138, 1994.
Schulze RK, d'Hoedt B: A method to calculate angular disparities between object and receptor in "paralleling technique," *Dentomaxillofac Radiol* 31:32-38, 2002.

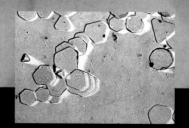

# CHAPTER 5

# X-Ray Film, Intensifying Screens, and Grids

A beam of x-ray photons that passes through the dental arches is reduced in intensity (attenuated) by absorption and scattering of photons out of the primary beam. The pattern of the photons that exits the subject, the remnant beam, conveys information about the structure and composition of the absorber. For this information to be useful diagnostically, the remnant beam must be recorded on an image receptor. The image receptor most often used in dental radiography is x-ray film. This chapter describes x-ray film and its properties and the use of intensifying screens and grids to modify radiographic images. Digital radiographic systems, which also may be used to make radiographs, are described in Chapter 7.

## X-Ray Film

### COMPOSITION

X-ray film has two principal components: emulsion and base. The emulsion, which is sensitive to x rays and visible light, records the radiographic image. The base is a plastic supporting material onto which the emulsion is coated (Fig. 5-1).

#### Emulsion

The two principal components of emulsion are silver halide grains, which are sensitive to x radiation and visible light, and a vehicle matrix in which the crystals are suspended. The *silver halide grains* are composed primarily of crystals of silver bromide. The composition of a dental film emulsion is shown in Table 5-1. Iodide is added to Ultra-Speed film because its large diameter (compared with bromine) disrupts the regularity of the silver bromide crystal structure, thereby increasing its sensitivity to x radiation. Iodide is not used in InSight film. The photosensitivity of the silver halide crystals also depends on the presence of trace amounts of a sulfur-containing compound. In addition, trace amounts of gold are sometimes added to silver halide crystals to improve their sensitivity.

The silver halide grains in InSight film are flat, tabular crystals with a mean diameter of about 1.8 μm (Fig. 5-2). Ultra-Speed film is composed of globular-shaped crystals about 1 μm in diameter. The tabular grains of the InSight film are oriented parallel with the film surface to offer a large cross-sectional area to the x-ray beam (Fig. 5-3). As a result, InSight film requires only about half the exposure of Ultra-Speed film.

In the manufacture of film, the silver halide grains are suspended in a surrounding *vehicle* that is applied to both sides of the supporting base. The vehicle, composed of gelatinous and nongelatinous materials, keeps the silver halide grains evenly dispersed. To ensure good adhesion of the emulsion to the film base, a thin layer of adhesive material is added to the base before the emulsion is applied. During film processing, the vehicle absorbs the processing solutions, allowing the chemicals to reach and react with the silver halide grains. An additional layer of vehicle is added to the film emulsion as an overcoat; this barrier helps protect the film from damage by scratching, contamination, or pressure from rollers when an automatic processor is used.

Film emulsions are sensitive to both x-ray photons and visible light. Film intended to be exposed by x rays is called *direct exposure film.* All intraoral dental film is direct exposure film. *Screen film,* which is sensitive to visible light, is used with intensifying screens that emit visible light. Screen film and intensifying screens are used for extraoral projections such as panoramic and skull radiographs. Intensifying screens are described later in this chapter.

#### Base

The function of the film base is to support the emulsion. The base must have the proper degree of flexibility to allow easy handling of the film. The base for dental x-ray film is 0.18 mm thick and is made of polyester polyethylene terephthalate. The film base is uniformly translucent and casts no pattern on the resultant radiograph. Some think that a base with a slight blue tint improves viewing of diagnostic detail. The film base must also withstand exposure to processing solutions without becoming distorted.

### INTRAORAL X-RAY FILM

A number of manufacturers around the world make intraoral dental x-ray film. In each case the film is made as a double-emulsion film, that is, coated with an emulsion on each side of the base. With a double layer of emulsion, less radiation can be used to produce an image. Direct exposure film is used for intraoral examinations because it provides higher-resolution images than screen-film combinations. Some diagnostic tasks, such as detection of incipient caries or early periapical disease, require this higher resolution.

One corner of each dental film has a small, raised dot that is used for film orientation (Fig. 5-4). The manufacturer orients the film in the packet so that the convex side of the dot is toward the front of the packet and faces the x-ray tube. The side of the film with the depression is thus oriented toward the patient's tongue. After the film has been exposed and processed, the dot is used to identify the image as showing the patient's right or left side. When the films are mounted with the images of the teeth in the anatomic position, each film is first oriented with the convex side of the dot toward the viewer. Then, on the basis of the features of the teeth and anatomic landmarks in the adjacent bone, the films are arranged in their normal sequential relationship in the mount.

Intraoral x-ray film packets contain either one or two sheets of film (Fig. 5-5). When double-film packs are used, the second film serves as a duplicate record that can be sent to insurance companies or to a colleague. The film is encased in a protective black paper wrapper and then in an outer white paper or plastic wrapping, which is resistant to moisture. The outer wrapping clearly indicates the location of the raised dot and identifies which side of the film should be directed toward the x-ray tube.

Between the wrappers in the film packet is a thin lead foil backing with an embossed pattern. The foil is positioned in the film packet behind the film, away from the tube. This lead foil serves several purposes. It shields the film from backscatter (secondary) radiation, which fogs the film and reduces subject contrast (image quality). It also reduces patient exposure by absorbing some of the residual x-ray beam. Perhaps most important, however, is the fact that if the film packet is placed backward in the patient's mouth so that the tube side of the film is facing away from the x-ray machine, the lead foil will be positioned between the subject and the film. In this circumstance most of the radiation is absorbed by the lead foil and the resulting radiograph is light and shows the embossed pattern in the lead foil. This combination of a light film with the characteristic pattern indicates that the film packet was put in the patient's mouth backward and that the patient's right side–left side designation indicated by the film dot was reversed.

Because intraoral direct exposure film packets have several uses and are used in large adults and small children, the film packets are made in a variety of sizes. The composition of the film is identical in each case.

### Periapical View

Periapical views are used to record the crowns, roots, and surrounding bone. Film packs come in three sizes: 0 for small children (22 × 35 mm); 1, which is relatively narrow and used for views of the anterior teeth (24 × 40 mm); and 2, the standard film size used for adults (31 × 41 mm) (Fig. 5-6).

### Bitewing View

Bitewing (interproximal) views are used to record the coronal portions of the maxillary and mandibular teeth in one image. They are

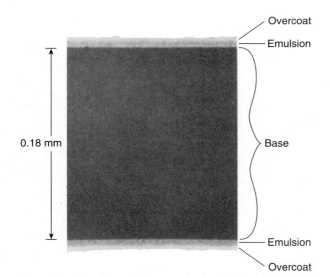

FIG. **5-1**   Scanning electron micrograph of Kodak InSight dental x-ray film (original magnification 300×). Note the overcoat, emulsion, and base on this double-emulsion film. (Courtesy Carestream Health, Inc., exclusive manufacturer of Kodak dental systems.)

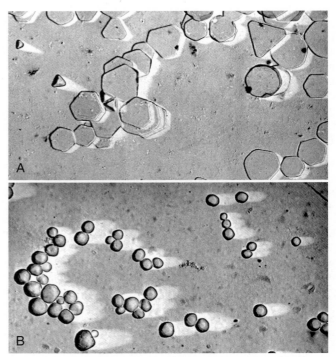

FIG. **5-2**   Scanning electron micrographs of emulsion comparing flat tabular silver bromide crystals of InSight film **(A)** with globular silver halide crystals of Ultra-Speed film **(B)**. (Courtesy Carestream Health, Inc., exclusive manufacturer of Kodak dental systems.)

### TABLE **5-1**
### *Typical Coating Weights per Film Side (mg/cm$^2$)* *

| FILM TYPE | SILVER | BROMIDE | IODIDE | EMULSION VEHICLE | OVERCOAT VEHICLE |
|---|---|---|---|---|---|
| InSight (F speed) | 0.8-1.1 | 0.6-0.75 | 0 | 0.6-0.8 | 0.1-0.2 |
| Ultra-Speed (D speed) | 0.6-0.9 | 0.6-0.75 | 0.0-0.02 | 0.4-0.7 | 0.1-0.2 |

*Courtesy Carestream Health, Inc., exclusive manufacturer of Kodak dental systems.

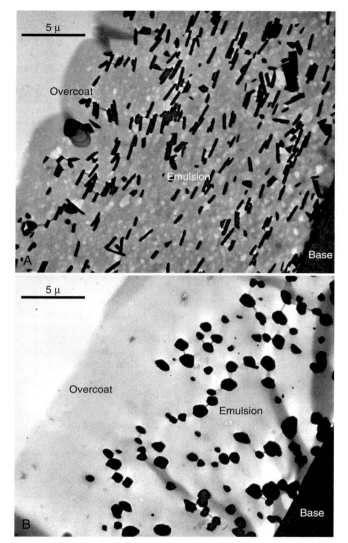

FIG. **5-3**  Cross-sectional electron microscopic image of emulsion of InSight film **(A)** and Ultra-Speed film **(B)**. Note that the orientation of the tabular crystals in the InSight film is essentially parallel to the film surface to increase the exposure surface area of the crystals to the x-ray beam. (Courtesy Carestream Health, Inc., exclusive manufacturer of Kodak dental systems.)

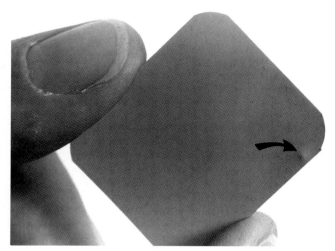

FIG. **5-4**  The raised film dot *(arrow)* indicates the tube side of the film and identifies the patient's right and left sides.

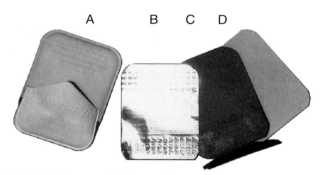

FIG. **5-5**  Moisture- and light-proof packet **(A)** contains an opening tab on the side opposite the tube. Inside is a sheet of lead foil **(B)** and a black, lightproof, interleaf paper wrapper **(C)** that is folded around the film **(D)**. Film is packaged with one or two sheets of film.

useful for detecting interproximal caries and evaluating the height of alveolar bone. Size 2 film is normally used in adults; the smaller size 1 is preferred in children. In small children, size 0 may be used. A relatively long size 3 also is available.

Bitewing films often have a paper tab projecting from the middle of the film on which the patient bites to support the film (Fig. 5-7). This tab is rarely visualized and does not interfere with the diagnostic quality of the image. Film-holding instruments for bitewing projections also are available.

## Occlusal View

Occlusal film is more than three times larger than size 2 film (57 × 76 mm) (see Fig. 5-6). It is used to show larger areas of the maxilla or mandible than may be seen on a periapical film. These films also are used to obtain right-angle views to the usual periapical view. The

FIG. **5-6**  Dental x-ray film is commonly supplied in various sizes. *Left,* Occlusal film; *top right,* adult posterior film; *middle right,* adult anterior film; *bottom right,* child-size film (in vinyl wrapping).

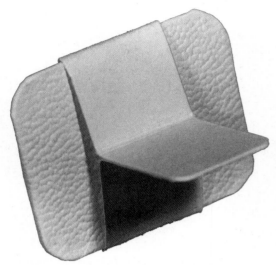

FIG. **5-7**   Paper loop placed around a size 2 adult film to support the film when the patient bites on the tab for a bitewing projection. This projection reveals the tooth crowns and alveolar crests.

name derives from the fact that the film usually is held in position by having the patient bite lightly on it to support it between the occlusal surfaces of the teeth (see Chapter 9).

## SCREEN FILM

The extraoral projections used most frequently in dentistry are the panoramic, cephalometric, and other skull views. For these projections and for virtually all other extraoral radiography, screen film is used with intensifying screens (described later in this chapter) to reduce patient exposure. Screen film is different from dental intraoral film. It is designed to be sensitive to visible light because it is placed between two intensifying screens when an exposure is made. The intensifying screens absorb x rays and emit visible light, which exposes the screen film. Silver halide crystals are inherently sensitive to ultraviolet (UV) and blue light (300 to 500 nm) and thus are sensitive to screens that emit UV and blue light. When film is used with screens that emit green light, the silver halide crystals are coated with sensitizing dyes to increase absorption. Because the properties of intensifying screens vary, the dentist should use the appropriate screen-film combination recommended by the screen and film manufacturer so that the emission characteristics of the screen match the absorption characteristics of the film.

Several general types of screen film are suitable for extraoral radiography. Several manufacturers supply high-contrast, medium-speed film suitable for skull radiography. Other films are available that are faster (i.e., they require less radiation exposure), but these provide less image detail. Such films should be considered for panoramic radiography when fine image detail is not available because of movement of the x-ray tube head during the exposure.

Another type of film provides less contrast and a wider latitude. This type reveals a wide range of densities and is most suitable for cephalometric radiography, when both bony and soft tissue details are desired.

Contemporary screen films use tabular-shaped (flat) grains of silver halide (Fig. 5-8) to capture the image. The tabular grains are oriented with their relatively large, flat surfaces facing the radiation

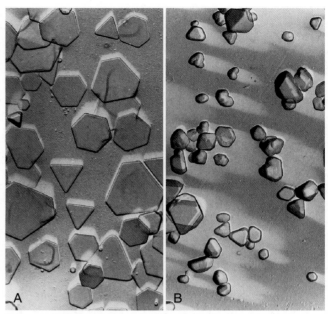

FIG. **5-8**   T grains of silver halide in an emulsion of T-Mat film **(A)** are larger and flatter than the smaller, thicker crystals in an emulsion of conventional film **(B)**. Note that the flat surfaces of the T grains are oriented parallel with the film surface, facing the radiation source. (Courtesy Carestream Health, Inc., exclusive manufacturer of Kodak dental systems.)

source, providing a larger cross-section (target) and resulting in increased speed without loss of sharpness. In addition, green-sensitizing dyes are added to the surface of the tabular grains, increasing their light-absorbing capability. Some manufacturers add an absorbing dye in the film emulsion to reduce crossover of light from one screen to the film emulsion on the opposite side. This increases the sharpness of the image.

## Intensifying Screens

Early in the history of radiography, scientists discovered that various inorganic salts or phosphors fluoresce (emit visible light) when exposed to an x-ray beam. The intensity of this fluorescence is proportional to the x-ray energy absorbed. These phosphors have been incorporated into intensifying screens for use with screen film. The sum of the effects of the x rays and the visible light emitted by the screen phosphors exposes the film in an intensifying cassette.

### FUNCTION

The presence of intensifying screens creates an image receptor system that is 10 to 60 times more sensitive to x rays than the film alone. Consequently, use of intensifying screens means a substantial reduction in the dose of x radiation to which the patient is exposed. Intensifying screens are used with films for virtually all extraoral radiography, including panoramic, cephalometric, and skull projections. In general, the resolving power of screens is related to their speed: the slower the speed of a screen, the greater its resolving power and vice versa. Intensifying screens are not used intraorally with periapical or occlusal films because their use would reduce the resolution of the resulting image below that necessary for diagnosis of much dental disease.

| TABLE **5-2** |  |
|---|---|
| **_Rare Earth Elements Used in Intensifying Screens_** | |
| EMISSION | PHOSPHOR |
| Green | Gadolinium oxysulfide, terbium activated |
| Blue and UV | Yttrium tantalite, niobium activated |

## COMPOSITION

Intensifying screens are made of a base supporting material, a phosphor layer, and a protective polymeric coat (Fig. 5-9). In all dental applications, intensifying screens are used in pairs, one on each side of the film, and they are positioned inside a cassette (Fig. 5-10). The purpose of a cassette is to hold each intensifying screen in contact with the x-ray film to maximize the sharpness of the image. Most cassettes are rigid, but they may be flexible.

### Base

The base material of most intensifying screens is some form of polyester plastic that is about 0.25 mm thick. The base provides mechanical support for the other layers. In some intensifying screens the base also is reflective; thus, it reflects light emitted from the phosphor layer back toward the x-ray film. This has the effect of increasing the light emission of the intensifying screen. However, it also results in some image "unsharpness" because of the divergence of light rays reflected back to the film. Some fine detail intensifying screens omit _the reflecting layer_ to improve image sharpness. In other intensifying screens the base is not reflective, and a separate coating of titanium dioxide is applied to the base material to serve as a reflecting layer.

### Phosphor Layer

The phosphor layer is composed of phosphorescent crystals suspended in a polymeric binder. When the crystals absorb x-ray photons, they fluoresce (see Fig. 5-9). The phosphor crystals often contain rare earth elements, most commonly lanthanum and gadolinium. Their fluorescence can be increased by the addition of small amounts of elements such as thulium, niobium, or terbium. Common phosphor combinations used in intensifying screens are shown in Table 5-2.

Some rare earth compounds are efficient phosphors. In the energy range typically used in dental radiography, a pair of rare earth intensifying screens absorbs about 60% of the photons that reach the cassette after passing through a patient. These phosphors are about 18% efficient in converting this x-ray energy to visible light. Rare earth screens convert each absorbed x-ray photon into about 4000 lower-energy, visible light (green or blue) photons. These visible photons then expose the film.

Different phosphors fluoresce in different portions of the spectrum. For example, light emission from Kodak Lanex (Fig. 5-11) rare earth intensifying screens ranges from 375 to 600 nm and peaks sharply at 545 nm (green). Figure 5-10 shows the spectral emission of a rare earth screen and the spectral sensitivity of an appropriate film. Other intensifying screens have a major peak at 350 nm (UV) and another at 450 nm (blue). It is important to match green-emitting screens with green-sensitive films and blue-emitting screens with blue-sensitive films.

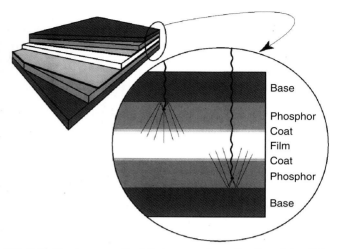

FIG. **5-9**    The image on the left shows a schematic of two intensifying screens (shades of gray) enclosing a film (white). The detailed view on the right shows x-ray photons entering at the top, traveling through the base, and striking phosphors in the base. The phosphors emit visible light, exposing the film. Some visible light photons may reflect off the reflecting layer of the base.

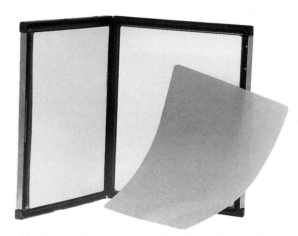

FIG. **5-10**    Cassette for 8- × 10-inch film. When the cassette is closed, the film is supported in close contact between two intensifying screens.

The speed and resolution of a screen depends on many factors, including the following:

- Phosphor type and phosphor conversion efficiency
- Thickness of phosphor layer and coating weight (amount of phosphor/unit volume)
- Presence of reflective layer
- Presence of light-absorbing dye in phosphor binder or protective coating
- Phosphor grain size

Fast screens have large phosphor crystals and efficiently convert x-ray photons to visible light but produce images with lower resolution. As the size of the crystals or the thickness of the screen decreases, the speed of the screen also declines, but image sharpness increases. Fast screens also have a thicker phosphor layer and a reflective layer, but these properties also decrease sharpness. In deciding on the combination to use, the practitioner must consider the resolution

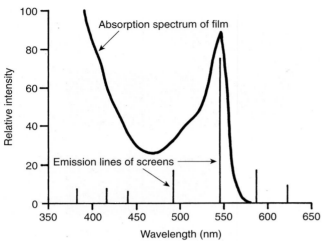

FIG. **5-11**   Relative sensitivity of Kodak T-Mat film *(continuous line)* and emission lines of a Kodak Lanex and Ektavision screens (gadolinium oxysulfide, terbium activated). Intensifying screens emit light as a series of relatively narrow line emissions. The maximal emission of the screen at 545 nm corresponds well to a high-sensitivity region of the film. (Data courtesy Carestream Health, Inc., exclusive manufacturer of Kodak dental systems.)

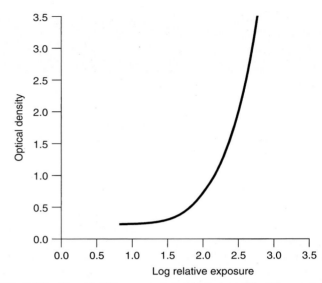

FIG. **5-12**   Characteristic curve of direct exposure film. The contrast (slope of the curve) is greater in the high-density region than in the low-density region.

requirements of the task for which the image will be used. Most dental extraoral diagnostic tasks can be accomplished with screen-film combinations that have a speed of 400 or faster.

### Protective Coat

A protective polymer coat (up to 15 μm thick) is placed over the phosphor layer to protect the phosphor and to provide a surface that can be cleaned. The intensifying screens should be kept clean because any debris, spots, or scratches may cause light spots on the resultant radiograph.

## Image Characteristics

Processing an exposed x-ray film causes it to become dark in the exposed area. The degree and pattern of film darkening depend on numerous factors, including the energy and intensity of the x-ray beam, composition of the subject imaged, film emulsion used, and characteristics of film processing. This section describes the major imaging characteristics of x-ray film.

### RADIOGRAPHIC DENSITY

When a film is exposed by an x-ray beam (or by light, in the case of screen-film combinations) and then processed, the silver halide crystals in the emulsion that were struck by the photons are converted to grains of metallic silver. These silver grains block the transmission of light from a viewbox and give the film its dark appearance. The overall degree of darkening of an exposed film is referred to as *radiographic density*. This density can be measured as the optical density of an area of an x-ray film where:

$$\text{Optical density} = \text{Log}_{10} \frac{I_o}{I_t}$$

where $I_o$ is the intensity of incident light (e.g., from a viewbox) and $I_t$ is the intensity of the light transmitted through the film. Thus the

measurement of film density also is a measure of the opacity of the film. With an optical density of 0, 100% of the light is transmitted; with a density of 1, 10% of the light is transmitted; with a density of 2, 1% of the light is transmitted, and so on.

A plot of the relationship between film optical density and exposure is called a *characteristic curve* (Fig. 5-12). It usually is shown as the relationship between the optical density of the film and the logarithm of the corresponding exposure. As exposure of the film increases, its optical density increases. A film is of greatest diagnostic value when the structures of interest are imaged on the relatively straight portion of the graph, between 0.6 and 3.0 optical density units. The characteristic curves of films reveal much information about film contrast, speed, and latitude.

An unexposed film, when processed, shows some density. This is caused by the inherent density of the base and added tint and the development of unexposed silver halide crystals. This minimal density is called *gross fog*, or *base plus fog*. The optical density of gross fog typically is 0.2 to 0.3.

Radiographic density is influenced by exposure and the thickness and density of the subject.

### Exposure

The overall film density depends on the number of photons absorbed by the film emulsion. Increasing the milliamperage (mA), peak kilovoltage (kVp), or exposure time increases the number of photons reaching the film and thus increases the density of the radiograph. Reducing the distance between the focal spot and film also increases film density.

### Subject Thickness

The thicker the subject, the more the beam is attenuated and the lighter the resultant image (Fig. 5-13). If exposure factors intended for adults are used on children or edentulous patients, the resultant films are dark because a smaller amount of absorbing tissue is in the path of the x-ray beam. The dentist should vary exposure (either kVp or time) according to the patient's size to produce radiographs of optimal density.

## Subject Density

Variations in the density of the subject exert a profound influence on the image. The greater the density of a structure within the subject, the greater the attenuation of the x-ray beam directed through that subject or area. In the oral cavity the relative densities of various natural structures, in order of decreasing density, are enamel, dentin and cementum, bone, muscle, fat, and air. Metallic objects (e.g., restorations) are far denser than enamel and hence better absorbers. Because an x-ray beam is differentially attenuated by these absorbers, the resultant beam carries information that is recorded on the radiographic film as light and dark areas. Dense objects (which are strong absorbers) cause the radiographic image to be light and are said to be *radiopaque*. Objects with low densities are weak absorbers. They allow most photons to pass through, and they cast a dark area on the film that corresponds to the *radiolucent* object.

## RADIOGRAPHIC CONTRAST

*Radiographic contrast* is a general term that describes the range of densities on a radiograph. It is defined as the difference in densities between light and dark regions on a radiograph. Thus an image that shows both light areas and dark areas has *high contrast*. This also is referred to as a *short gray scale of contrast* because few shades of gray are present between the black and white images on the film. A radiographic image composed only of light gray and dark gray zones has *low contrast*, also referred to as having a *long gray scale of contrast* (Fig. 5-14). The radiographic contrast of an image is the result of the interplay of subject contrast, film contrast, and scattered radiation.

## Subject Contrast

*Subject contrast* is the range of characteristics of the subject that influences radiographic contrast. It is influenced largely by the subject's thickness, density, and atomic number. The subject contrast of a patient's head and neck exposed in a lateral cephalometric view is high. The dense regions of the bone and teeth absorb most of the

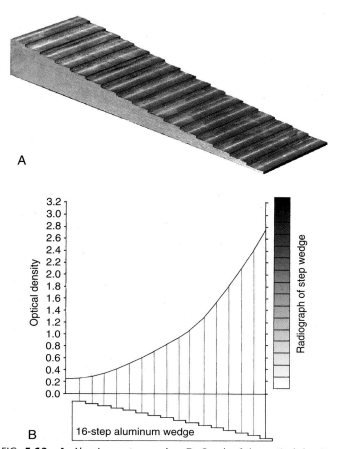

FIG. **5-13**  **A,** Aluminum step wedge. **B,** Graph of the optical density of a radiograph made by exposing the step wedge. Note that as the thickness of the aluminum decreases, more photons are available to expose the film and the image becomes progressively darker.

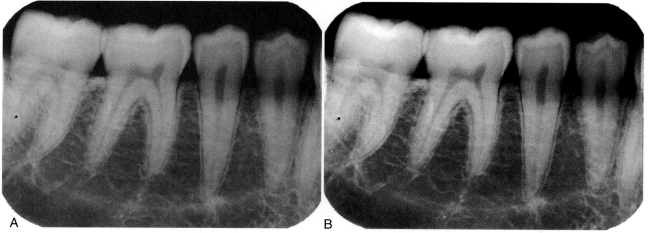

FIG. **5-14**  Radiograph of a dried mandible revealing low contrast **(A)** and high contrast **(B)**.

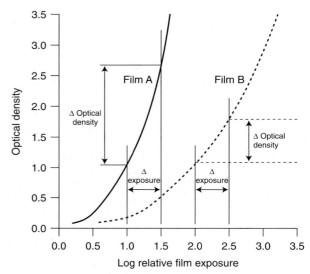

FIG. **5-16** Characteristic curves of two films demonstrating the greater inherent contrast of film *A* compared with film *B*. The slope of film *A* is greater than that of film *B*; thus film *A* shows a greater change in optical density than film *B* for a constant change in exposure. The fact that film *A* is faster than film *B* in this figure is unrelated to film contrast.

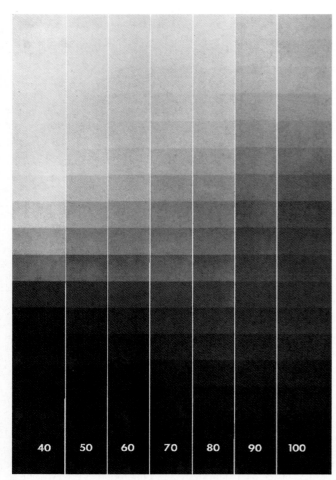

FIG. **5-15** Radiographs of a step wedge made at 40 to 100 kVp. As the kVp increases, the mA is reduced to maintain the uniform middle-step density. Note the long gray scale (low contrast) with high kVp. (Courtesy Carestream Health, Inc., exclusive manufacturer of Kodak dental systems.)

### Film Contrast

*Film contrast* describes the capacity of radiographic films to display differences in subject contrast, that is, variations in the intensity of the remnant beam. A high-contrast film reveals areas of small difference in subject contrast more clearly than does a low-contrast film. Film contrast usually is measured as the average slope of the diagnostically useful portion of the characteristic curve (Fig. 5-16): the greater the slope of the curve in this region, the greater the film contrast. In this illustration, film A has a higher contrast than film B. When the slope of the curve in the useful range is greater than 1, the film exaggerates subject contrast. This desirable feature, which is found in most diagnostic film, allows visualization of structures that differ only slightly in density. For example, the remnant beam in the region of a tooth pulp chamber will be more intense (greater exposure) than the beam from the surrounding enamel crown. A high-contrast film will show a greater contrast (difference in optical density) between these structures than will a low-contrast film. Films used with intensifying screens typically have a slope in the range of 2 to 3.

As can be seen in Figure 5-12, film contrast also depends on the density range being examined. With dental direct-exposure film, the slope of the curve continually increases with increasing exposure. As a result, properly exposed films have more contrast than do underexposed (light) films.

Film processing is another factor that influences film contrast. Film contrast is maximized by optimal film processing conditions. Mishandling of the film through incomplete or excessive development diminishes contrast of anatomic structures. Improper handling of film, such as storage at too high a temperature, exposure to excessively bright safelights, or light leaks in the darkroom, also degrades film contrast.

*Fog* on an x-ray film results in increased film density arising from causes other than exposure to the remnant beam. Film contrast is reduced by the addition of this undesirable density. Common causes

incident radiation, whereas the less dense soft tissue facial profile transmits most of the radiation.

Subject contrast also is influenced by beam energy and intensity. The energy of the x-ray beam, selected by the kVp, influences image contrast. Figure 5-15 shows an aluminum step wedge exposed to x-ray beams of differing energies. Because increasing the kVp increases the overall density of the image, the exposure time has been adjusted so that the density of the middle step in each case is comparable. As the kVp of the x-ray beam increases, subject contrast decreases. Similarly, when relatively low kVp energies are used, subject contrast increases. Most clinicians select a kVp in the range of 70 to 80. At higher values the exposure time is reduced, but the loss of contrast may be objectionable because subtle changes may be obscured.

Changing the time or mA of the exposure (and holding the kVp constant) also influences subject contrast. If the film is excessively light or dark, contrast of anatomic structures is diminished. Subtle changes in the mA may also slightly change subject contrast by changing the location of the radiographed structures on the characteristic curve, as described previously.

| TABLE 5-3 |  |
| :-- | :-- |
| **Intraoral Film Speed Classification** | |
| FILM SPEED GROUP | SPEED RANGE (RECIPROCAL ROENTGENS*) |
| C | 6-12 |
| D | 12-24 |
| E | 24-48 |
| F | 48-96 |

From National Council on Radiation Protection and Measurements, Report No. 145, Appendix E, 2004.
*Reciprocal Roentgens are the reciprocal of the exposure in Roentgens required to obtain a film with an optical density of 1.0 above base plus fog after processing.

of film fog are improper safelighting, storage of film at too high a temperature, and development of film at an excessive temperature or for a prolonged period. Film fog can be reduced by proper film processing and storage.

### Scattered Radiation

Scattered radiation results from photons that have interacted with the subject by Compton or coherent interactions. These interactions cause the emission of photons that travel in directions other than that of the primary beam. The consequent scattered radiation causes fogging of a radiograph, an overall darkening of the image that results in loss of radiographic contrast. In most dental applications the best means of reducing scattered radiation are to (1) use a relatively low kVp, (2) collimate the beam to the size of the film to prevent scatter from an area outside the region of the image, and (3) use grids in extraoral radiography.

## RADIOGRAPHIC SPEED

Radiographic speed refers to the amount of radiation required to produce an image of a standard density. Film speed frequently is expressed as the reciprocal of the exposure (in Roentgens) required to produce an optical density of 1 above gross fog. A fast film requires a relatively low exposure to produce a density of 1, whereas a slower film requires a longer exposure for the processed film to have the same density. Film speed is controlled largely by the size of the silver halide grains and their silver content.

The speed of dental intraoral x-ray film is indicated by a letter designating a particular group (Table 5-3). The fastest dental film currently available has a speed rating of F. Only films with a D or faster speed rating are appropriate for intraoral radiography. Currently the types of film used most often in the United States are Kodak Ultra-Speed (group D) and Kodak InSight (group E or F, depending on processing conditions). InSight film is preferred because it requires only about half the exposure of Ultra-Speed film and offers comparable contrast and resolution. F-speed film is faster than the D-speed film because tabular crystal grains are used in the emulsion of F-speed film. The characteristic curves in Figure 5-17 show that InSight film (curve on the left) is faster than Ultra-Speed film (curve on the right) because less exposure is required to produce the same level of density although the two films have similar contrast.

Although film speed can be increased slightly by processing the film at a higher temperature, this is achieved at the expense of increased

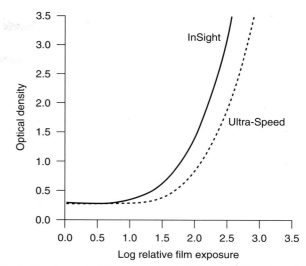

FIG. **5-17** Characteristic curves for InSight and Ultra-Speed film. InSight film is faster and has essentially the same contrast as Ultra-Speed film. (Courtesy Carestream Health, Inc., exclusive manufacturer of Kodak dental systems.)

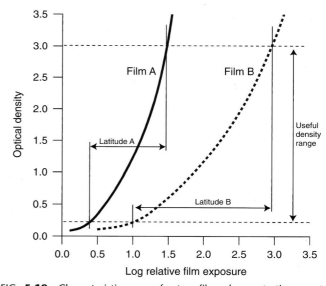

FIG. **5-18** Characteristic curves for two films demonstrating greater inherent latitude of film *B* compared with film *A*. The slope of film *B* is less steep than that of film *A*; therefore film *B* records a greater range of exposures within the useful density range than does film *A*.

film fog and graininess. Processing in depleted solutions can lower the effective speed. It is always preferable to use fresh processing solutions and follow the recommended processing time and temperature.

## FILM LATITUDE

Film latitude is a measure of the range of exposures that can be recorded as distinguishable densities on a film. A film optimized to display a wide latitude can record a subject with a wide range of subject contrast. A film with a characteristic curve that has a long straight-line portion and a shallow slope has a wide latitude (Fig. 5-18). As a consequence, wide variations in the amount of radiation exiting the subject can be recorded. Films with a wide latitude have lower contrast (i.e., a long gray scale) than do films with a narrow latitude. Wide-latitude films are useful when both the osseous structures of the skull and the soft tissues of the facial region must be recorded.

To some extent the operator can modify the latitude of an image. A high kVp produces images with a wide latitude and low contrast. Reduced exposure produces a somewhat lighter image and shows a slightly wider range of anatomic structures with lower contrast. Wide-latitude film is recommended for imaging structures with a wide range of subject densities.

## RADIOGRAPHIC NOISE

*Radiographic noise* is the appearance of uneven density of a uniformly exposed radiographic film. It is seen on a small area of film as localized variations in density. The primary causes of noise are radiographic mottle and radiographic artifact. Radiographic mottle is uneven density resulting from the physical structure of the film or intensifying screens. Radiographic artifacts are defects caused by errors in film handling, such as fingerprints or bends in the film, or errors in film processing, such as splashing developer or fixer on a film or marks or scratches from rough handling.

On intraoral dental film, mottle may be seen as *film graininess*, which is caused by the visibility of silver grains in the film emulsion, especially when magnification is used to examine an image. Film graininess is most evident when high-temperature processing is used.

Radiographic mottle is also evident when the film is used with fast intensifying screens. Two important causes of the phenomenon are *quantum mottle* and *screen structure mottle*. Quantum mottle is caused by a fluctuation in the number of photons per unit of the beam cross-sectional area absorbed by the intensifying screen. Quantum mottle is most evident when fast film-screen combinations are used. Under these conditions the relative nonuniformity of the beam is highest. The longer exposures required by slower film-screen combinations tend to average out the beam pattern and thereby reduce quantum mottle. Screen structure mottle is graininess caused by screen phosphors. It is most evident when fast screens with large crystals are used.

## RADIOGRAPHIC BLURRING

*Sharpness* is the ability of a radiograph to *define an edge precisely* (e.g., the dentin-enamel junction, a thin trabecular plate). *Resolution*, or resolving power, is the ability of a radiograph to record *separate structures* that are close together. It usually is measured by radiographing an object made up of a series of thin lead strips with alternating radiolucent spaces of the same thickness. The groups of lines and spaces are arranged in the test target in order of increasing numbers of lines and spaces per millimeter (Fig. 5-19). The resolving power is measured as the highest number of line pairs (a line pair being the image of an absorber and the adjacent lucent space) per millimeter that can be distinguished on the resultant radiograph when examined with low-power magnification. Typically, panoramic film-screen combinations can resolve about five line pairs per millimeter; periapical film, which has better resolving power, can delineate clearly more than 20 line pairs per millimeter.

Radiographic blur is caused by image receptor (film and screen) blurring, motion blurring, and geometric blurring.

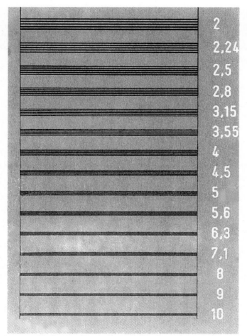

FIG. **5-19** Radiograph of a resolving power target consisting of groups of radiopaque lines and radiolucent spaces. Numbers at each group indicate the line pairs per millimeter represented by the group.

### Image Receptor Blurring

With intraoral dental x-ray film, the *size and number of the silver grains* in the film emulsion determines image sharpness: the finer the grain size, the finer the sharpness. In general, slow-speed films have fine grains and faster films have larger grains.

Use of *intensifying screens* in extraoral radiography has an adverse effect on image sharpness. Some degree of sharpness is lost because visible light and UV radiation emitted by the screen spread out beyond the point of origin and expose a film area larger than the phosphor crystal (see Fig. 5-9). The spreading light causes a blurring of fine detail on the radiograph. Intensifying screens with large crystals are relatively fast, but image sharpness is diminished. Furthermore, fast intensifying screens have a relatively thick phosphor layer, which contributes to dispersion of light and loss of image sharpness. Diffusion of light from a screen can be minimized and image sharpness maximized by ensuring as close a contact as possible between the intensifying screen and the film.

The presence of an image on each side of a double-emulsion film also causes a loss of image sharpness through *parallax* (Fig. 5-20). Parallax results from the apparent change in position or size of a subject when it is viewed from different perspectives. Because dental film has a double coating of emulsion and the x-ray beam is divergent, the images recorded on each emulsion vary slightly in size. In intraoral images, the effect of parallax on image sharpness is unimportant but is most apparent when wet films are viewed. Under these conditions the emulsion is swollen with water and the loss of image sharpness caused by parallax is more evident. When intensifying screens are used, parallax distortion contributes to image unsharpness because light from one screen may cross the film base and reach the emulsion on the opposite side. This problem can be solved by

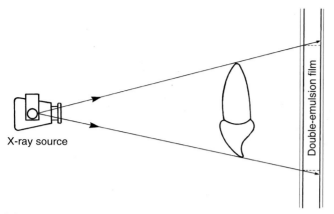

FIG. **5-20** Parallax unsharpness results when double-emulsion film is used because of the slightly greater magnification on the side of the film away from the x-ray source. Parallax unsharpness is a minor problem in clinical practice.

incorporating dyes into the base that absorb the light emitted by the screens.

### Motion Blurring

Image sharpness also can be lost through movement of the film, subject, or x-ray source during exposure. Movement of the x-ray source in effect enlarges the focal spot and diminishes image sharpness. Patient movement can be minimized by stabilizing the patient's head with the chair headrest during exposure. Use of a higher mA and kVp and correspondingly shorter exposure times also helps resolve this problem.

### Geometric Blurring

Several geometric factors influence image sharpness. Loss of image sharpness results in part because photons are not emitted from a point source (focal spot) on the target in the x-ray tube. The larger the focal spot, the greater the loss of image sharpness. Also, image sharpness is improved by increasing the distance between the focal spot and the object and reducing the distance between the object and the image receptor. Various means of optimizing projection geometry are discussed in Chapter 4.

## IMAGE QUALITY

*Image quality* describes the subjective judgment by the clinician of the overall appearance of a radiograph. It combines the features of density, contrast, latitude, sharpness, resolution, and perhaps other parameters. Various mathematic approaches have been used to evaluate these parameters further, but a thorough discussion of them is beyond the scope of this text. The *detective quantum efficiency (DQE)* is a basic measure of the efficiency of an imaging system. It encompasses image contrast, blur, speed, and noise. Often a system can be optimized for one of these parameters, but this usually is achieved at the expense of others. For instance, a fast system typically has a high level of noise. Even with these and other sophisticated approaches, however, more information is needed for complete understanding of all the factors responsible for the subjective impression of image quality.

## Grids

When an x-ray beam strikes a patient, many of the incident photons undergo Compton interactions and produce scattered photons. Typically the number of scattered photons in the remnant beam that reach the film is two to four times the number of primary photons that do not undergo absorption. The amount of scattered radiation increases with increasing subject thickness, field size, and kVp (energy of the x-ray beam). These scattered photons produce fog on the film and reduce the subject contrast.

### FUNCTION

The function of a grid is to reduce the amount of scattered radiation exiting a subject that reaches the film. The grid, which is placed between the subject and the film, preferentially removes the scattered radiation and spares primary photons; this reduces nonimaging exposure and increases subject contrast.

### COMPOSITION

A grid is composed of alternating strips of a radiopaque material (usually lead) and strips of radiolucent material (often plastic). The diagram in Figure 5-21 shows the interaction between a grid and an x-ray beam. When secondary photons generated in the subject are scattered toward the film, they usually are absorbed by the radiopaque material in the grid. This occurs because the direction of the scattered photons deviates from that of the primary beam, and consequently they cannot pass through the parallel plates of the grid. *Focused grids* are used most often. In a focused grid the strips of radiopaque material are all directed toward a common point, the focal spot of the x-ray tube, some distance away. Because the lead strips are angled toward the focal spot, their direction coincides with the paths of diverging photons in the primary x-ray beam. The lead strips absorb the scattered photons as their paths diverge from those of the primary photons. A focused grid can be used only within a range of distances from the focal spot where the alignment of lead strips closely coincides with the path of the diverging x-ray beam. The range of distances is specified on the grid.

Grids are manufactured with a varying number of line pairs of absorbers and radiolucent spaces per inch. Grids with 80 or more line pairs per inch do not show objectionable grid lines on the image. The ratio of grid thickness to the width of the radiolucent spacer is known as the *grid ratio*. The higher the grid ratio, the more effectively scattered radiation is removed from the x-ray beam. Grids with a ratio of 8 or 10 are preferred.

The image of the radiolucent grid lines on the film can be deleted by moving the grid perpendicular to the direction of the grid lines (but not moving the subject or the film) during exposure. This has the effect of blurring out the radiolucent lines and allowing a more uniform exposure. This movement does not interfere with the absorption of scattered photons. The apparatus for moving a grid is called a *Bucky*.

To compensate for the absorbing materials in the grid, the exposure required when a grid is used is approximately double that needed without a grid. Therefore grids should be used only when the improvement in diagnostic image quality is sufficient to justify the added exposure. For example, with lateral cephalometric examinations made for assessing the growth and development of the facial region (Chapter 12), use of a grid usually is not indicated because

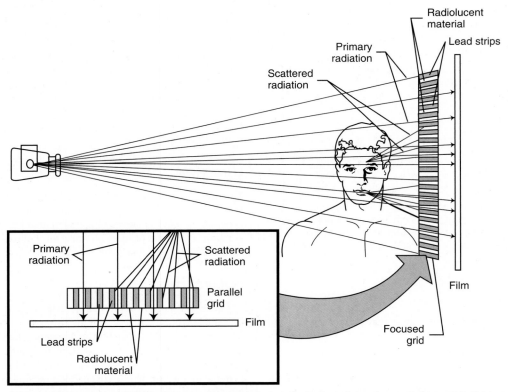

FIG. **5-21**  An x-ray grid absorbs scattered x-ray photons from the primary beam and prevents them from fogging the film. In a focused grid the absorber plates are angled toward the anode; in a parallel grid the absorber plates are parallel.

the improved contrast does not aid in identification of anatomic landmarks.

## BIBLIOGRAPHY

Bushberg JT: *The essential physics of medical imaging*, ed 2, Baltimore, 2001, Lippincott Williams & Wilkins.

Bushong SC: *Radiologic science for technologists: physics, biology, and protection*, ed 9, St. Louis, 2009, Mosby.

Ludlow JB, Platin E, Mol A: Characteristics of Kodak InSight, an F-speed intraoral film, *Oral Surg Oral Med Oral Pathol Oral Radiol Endod* 91: 120-129, 2001.

Nair MK, Nair UP: An in-vitro evaluation of Kodak InSight and Ektaspeed Plus film with a CMOS detector for natural proximal caries: ROC analysis, *Caries Res* 35:354-359, 2001.

Revised American Dental Association Specification No. 22 for intraoral dental radiographic film adapted. Council on Dental Materials and Devices, *J Am Dent Assoc* 80:1066-1068, 1970.

Thunthy KH, Ireland EJ: A comparison of the visibility of caries on Kodak F-speed (InSight) and D-speed (Ultra-speed) films, *LDA J* 60:31-32, 2001.

# CHAPTER 6

# Processing X-Ray Film

The recording medium (image receptor) most frequently used in dental radiography is radiographic film. Making excellent film radiographs will improve patient diagnoses and overall care. Making excellent radiographs requires using the proper film exposure times and optimizing film processing. This chapter describes these processes starting with the formation of the latent image, followed by conversion of the latent image into a visible image (film processing), and closing with how to establish the proper exposure time.

## Formation of the Latent Image

When a beam of photons exits an object and exposes an x-ray film, it chemically changes the photosensitive silver halide crystals in the film emulsion. These chemically altered silver bromide crystals constitute the latent (invisible) image on the film. Before exposure, film emulsion consists of photosensitive crystals containing primarily silver bromide suspended in a vehicle and layered on a thin sheet of transparent plastic base. Some crystals also contain small amounts of silver iodide. These silver halide crystals also contain a few free silver ions (interstitial silver ions) in the spaces between the crystalline lattice atoms (Fig. 6-1, *A*). The crystals are chemically sensitized by the addition of trace amounts of sulfur compounds, which bind to the surface of the crystals. The sulfur compounds play a crucial role in image formation. Along with physical irregularities in the crystal produced by iodide ions, sulfur compounds create *sensitivity sites*, the sites in the crystals that are sensitive to radiation. Each crystal has many sensitivity sites, which begin the process of image formation by trapping the electrons generated when the emulsion is irradiated. Exposure to radiation chemically alters the photosensitive silver halide crystals to produce the latent image. Processing the exposed film in developer and fixer converts the latent image into the visible radiographic image.

When the silver halide crystals are irradiated, x-ray photons interact primarily with the bromide ions by Compton and photoelectric interactions (Fig. 6-1, *B*). These interactions result in the removal of an electron from the bromide ions. By the loss of an electron, a bromide ion is converted into a neutral bromine atom. The free electrons move through the crystal until they reach a sensitivity site, where they become trapped and impart a negative charge to the site. The negatively charged sensitivity site then attracts positively charged free interstitial silver ions (Fig. 6-1, *C*). When a silver ion reaches the negatively charged sensitivity site, it is reduced and forms a neutral atom of metallic silver (Fig. 6-1, *D*). The sites containing these neutral silver atoms are now called *latent image sites*. This process occurs numerous times within a crystal. The overall distribution of latent image sites in a film after exposure constitutes the latent image.

Film processing converts the latent image into one that can be visualized (Fig. 6-2). The neutral silver atoms at each latent image site

(Fig. 6-2, *B*) render the crystals sensitive to development and image formation. The larger the aggregate of neutral silver atoms, the more sensitive the crystal is to the effects of the developer. Most latent image sites that are capable of being developed in an optimally exposed film have at least four or five silver atoms. Developer converts silver bromide crystals with neutral silver atoms deposited at the latent image sites into black, solid silver metallic grains (Fig. 6-2, *C*). These solid silver grains block light from a viewbox. Fixer removes unexposed, undeveloped silver bromide crystals (those without latent image sites), leaving the film clear in unexposed areas (Fig. 6-2, *D*). Thus the radiographic image is composed of the light (radiopaque) areas, where few photons reached the film, and dark (radiolucent) areas of the film that were struck by many photons.

## Processing Solutions

Film processing involves the following procedures:
1. Immerse exposed film in developer.
2. Rinse film in water bath.
3. Immerse film in fixer.
4. Wash film in water bath.
5. Dry film and mount for viewing.

This chapter first describes the function of developer and fixer. Procedures for each of these steps are described later.

### DEVELOPING SOLUTION

The developer reduces all silver ions in the exposed crystals of silver halide (those with a latent image) to metallic silver grains (see Fig. 6-2). To produce a diagnostic image, this reduction process must be restricted to crystals containing latent image sites. To accomplish this, the reducing agents used as developers are catalyzed by the neutral silver atoms at the latent image sites (see Fig. 6-2, *B*). The silver atoms act as a bridge by which electrons from the reducing agents reach silver ions in the crystal and convert them to solid grains of metallic silver. Individual crystals are developed completely or not at all during the recommended developing times (see Fig. 6-2, *C*). Variations in density on the processed radiographs are the result of different ratios of developed (exposed) and undeveloped (unexposed) crystals. Areas with many exposed crystals are denser because of their higher concentration of black metallic silver grains after development. If the developer remains too long in contact with silver bromide halide crystals that do not contain a latent image, it slowly reduces these crystals also, thereby overdeveloping the image.

When an exposed film is developed, the developer initially has no visible effect (Fig. 6-3). After this initial phase, the density increases, very rapidly at first and then more slowly. Eventually all the exposed crystals develop (become reduced to black metallic silver), and the

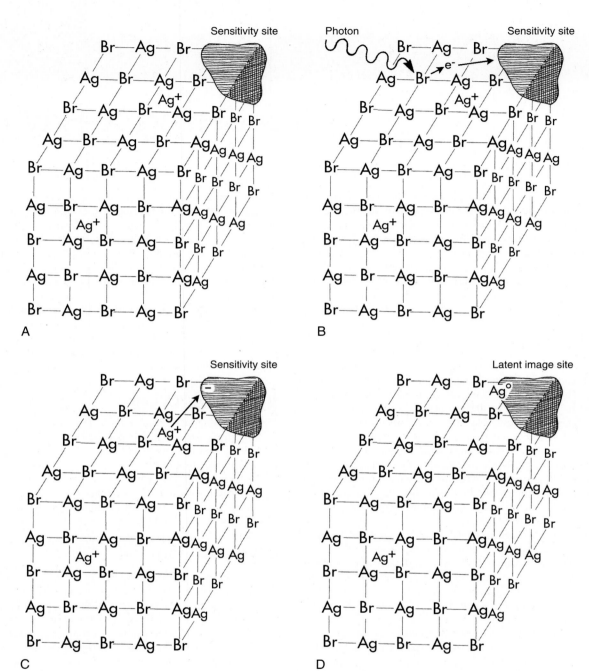

FIG. **6-1** **A,** A silver bromide crystal in the emulsion of an x-ray film contains mostly silver and bromide ions in a crystal lattice. There are also free interstitial silver ions and areas of trace chemicals that form sensitivity sites. **B,** Exposure of the crystal to photons in an x-ray beam results in the release of electrons, usually by interaction of the photon with a bromide ion. Bromide ions are converted to bromine atoms, and the recoil electrons have sufficient kinetic energy to move about in the crystal. When electrons reach a sensitivity site, they impart a negative charge to this region. **C,** Free interstitial silver ions (with a positive charge) are attracted to the negatively charged sensitivity site. **D,** When the silver ions reach the sensitivity site, they acquire an electron and become neutral silver atoms. These silver atoms now constitute a latent image site. The collection of latent image sites over the entire film constitutes the latent image. Developer causes the neutral silver atoms at the latent image sites to initiate the conversion of silver ions in the crystal into one large grain of metallic silver.

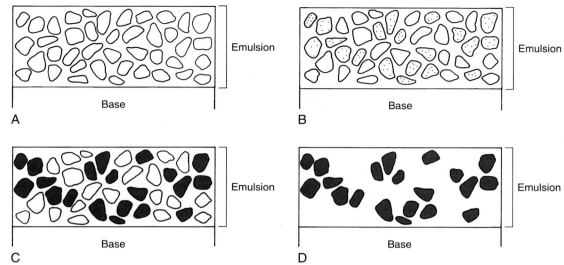

FIG. **6-2**  Emulsion changes during film processing. **A,** Before exposure, many silver bromide crystals are present in the emulsion. **B,** After exposure, the exposed crystals containing neutral silver atoms at latent image sites constitute the latent image (shaded areas in the crystals). **C,** The developer converts the exposed crystals containing neutral silver atoms at the latent image sites into solid grains of metallic silver. **D,** The fixer dissolves the unexposed, undeveloped silver bromide crystals, leaving only the solid silver grains. (Courtesy C.L. Crabtree, DDS, Bureau of Radiological Health, Rockville, Md.)

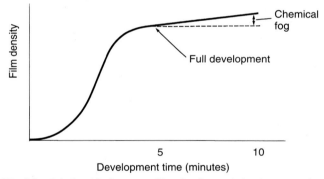

FIG. **6-3**  Relationship between film density and development time. The density of film rises quickly initially and then levels off, increasing more slowly because of chemical fogging.

developing agent starts to reduce the unexposed crystals. The development of unexposed crystals results in chemical fog on the film. The interval between maximal density and fogging explains why a properly exposed film does not become overdeveloped although it may be in contact with the developer longer than the recommended interval. Thus dark films usually are the result of overexposure rather than overdevelopment.

The developing solution contains four components, all dissolved in water: (1) developer, (2) activator, (3) preservative, and (4) restrainer.

## Developer

The primary function of the developing solution is to convert the exposed silver halide crystals into metallic silver grains. This process begins at the latent image sites, where electrons from the developing agents are conducted into the silver halide crystal and reduce the constituent silver ions (approximately 1 billion to 10 billion) to solid grains of metallic silver. Two developing agents are used in dental radiology: a pyrazolidone-type compound, usually Phenidone (1-phenyl-3-pyrazolidone), and hydroquinone (paradihydroxy benzene). Phenidone serves as the first electron donor that converts silver ions to metallic silver at the latent image site. This electron transfer generates the oxidized form of Phenidone. Hydroquinone provides an electron to reduce the oxidized Phenidone back to its original active state so that it can continue to reduce silver halide grains to metallic silver. Unexposed crystals, those without latent images, are unaffected during the time required for reduction of the exposed crystals.

## Activator

The developers are active only at alkaline pH values, usually around 10. This is achieved with the addition of alkali compounds (activators) such as sodium or potassium hydroxide. Buffers—usually sodium bicarbonate—are used to maintain this condition. The activators also cause the gelatin to swell so that the developing agents can diffuse more rapidly into the emulsion and reach the suspended silver bromide crystals.

## Preservative

The developing solution contains an antioxidant or preservative, usually sodium sulfite. The preservative protects the developers from oxidation by atmospheric oxygen and thus extends their useful life. The preservative also combines with the brown oxidized developer to produce a colorless soluble compound. If not removed, oxidation products interfere with the developing reaction and stain the film.

## Restrainer

Bromide, usually as potassium bromide, and benzotriazole are added to the developing solution to restrain development of unexposed silver halide crystals. Although bromide and benzotriazole depress the reduction of both exposed and unexposed crystals, they are much more effective in depressing the reduction of unexposed crystals. Consequently, the restrainers act as antifog agents and increase contrast.

## DEVELOPER REPLENISHER

In the normal course of film processing, Phenidone and hydroquinone are consumed, and bromide ions and other byproducts are released into solution. Developer also becomes inactivated by exposure to oxygen. These actions produce a "seasoned" solution, and the film speed and contrast stabilize. The developing solution of both manual and automatic developers should be replenished with fresh solution each morning to prolong the life of the seasoned developer. The recommended amount to be added daily is 8 ounces of fresh developer (replenisher) per gallon of developing solution. This assumes the development of an average of 30 periapical or 5 panoramic films per day. Some of the used solution may need to be removed to make room for the replenisher.

## RINSING

After development the film emulsion swells and becomes saturated with developer. At this point the films are rinsed in water for 30 seconds with continuous, gentle agitation before they are placed in the fixer. Rinsing dilutes the developer, slowing the development process. It also removes the alkali activator, preventing neutralization of the acid fixer. This rinsing process is typical for manual processing but is not used with automatic processing.

## FIXING SOLUTION

The primary function of fixing solution is to dissolve and remove the undeveloped silver halide crystals from the emulsion (see Fig. 6-2, D). The presence of unexposed crystals causes film to be opaque. If these crystals are not removed, the image on the resultant radiograph is dark and nondiagnostic. Figure 6-4 is a photomicrograph of film emulsion showing the solid silver grains after fixer has removed the

unexposed silver bromide crystals. (Compare it with Fig. 45-2, A, which shows the unprocessed emulsion.) A second function of fixing solution is to harden and shrink the film emulsion. As with developer, fixer should be replenished daily at the rate of 8 ounces per gallon.

Fixing solution also contains four components, all dissolved in water: (1) clearing agent, (2) acidifier, (3) preservative, and (4) hardener.

### Clearing Agent

After development the film emulsion must be cleared by dissolving and removing the unexposed silver halide. An aqueous solution of ammonium thiosulfate ("hypo") dissolves the silver halide grains. It forms stable, water-soluble complexes with silver ions, which then diffuse from the emulsion. The clearing agent does not have a rapid effect on the metallic silver grains in the film emulsion, but excessive fixation results in a gradual loss of film density because the grains of silver slowly dissolve in the acetic acid of the fixing solution.

### Acidifier

The fixing solution contains an acetic acid buffer system (pH 4 to 4.5) to keep the fixer pH constant. The acidic pH is required to promote good diffusion of thiosulfate into the emulsion and of silver thiosulfate complex out of the emulsion. The acid-fixing solution also inactivates any carryover developing agents in the film emulsion, blocking continued development of any unexposed crystals while the film is in the fixing tank.

### Preservative

Ammonium sulfite is the preservative in the fixing solution, as it is in the developer. It prevents oxidation of the thiosulfate clearing agent, which is unstable in the acid environment of the fixing solution. It also binds with any colored oxidized developer carried over into the fixing solution and effectively removes it from the solution, which prevents oxidized developer from staining the film.

### Hardener

The hardening agent most often used is aluminum sulfate. Aluminum complexes with the gelatin during fixing and prevents damage to the gelatin during subsequent handling. The hardeners also reduce swelling of the emulsion during the final wash. This lessens mechanical damage to the emulsion and limits water absorption, thus shortening drying time.

## WASHING

After fixing, the processed film is washed in a sufficient flow of water for an adequate time to ensure removal of all thiosulfate ions and silver thiosulfate complexes. Washing efficiency declines rapidly when the water temperature falls below 60° F. Any silver compound or thiosulfate that remains because of improper washing discolors and causes stains, which are most apparent in the radiopaque (light) areas. This discoloration results from the thiosulfate reacting with silver to form brown silver sulfide, which can obscure diagnostic information.

## Darkroom Equipment

The darkroom should be convenient to the x-ray machines and dental operatories and should be at least 4 × 5 feet (1.2 × 1.5 m) (Fig. 6-5). It must be well operated to ensure excellent radiographs.

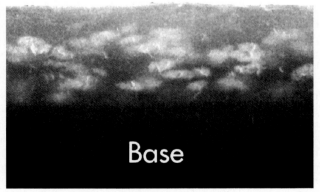

FIG. **6-4**   Scanning electron micrograph of a processed emulsion of Kodak Ultra-Speed dental x-ray film (5000×). Note the white-appearing solid silver grains above the base. (Courtesy Carestream Health, Inc., exclusive manufacturer of Kodak dental systems.)

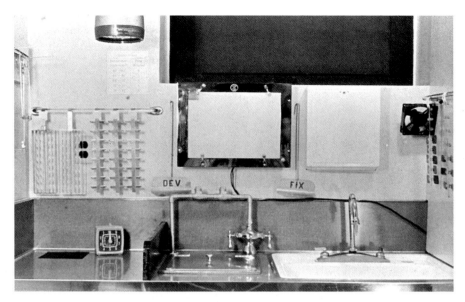

FIG. **6-5** Darkroom work area. *Left*, Film mounting area, timer, film racks, and safelight above. *Middle*, Developing and fixing tanks below the viewbox and stirring paddles. *Right*, Sink and drying racks with fan. (Courtesy C.L. Crabtree, DDS, Bureau of Radiological Health, Rockville, Md.)

## LIGHTPROOF

One of the most important requirements is that the darkroom be lightproof. If it is not, stray light will cause film fogging and loss of contrast. To make the darkroom lightproof, a light-tight door or doorless maze (if space permits) is used. The door should have a lock to prevent accidental opening, which might allow an unexpected flood of light that can ruin opened films.

The darkroom must also be well ventilated for the comfort of those working in the area and to exhaust the heat from the dryer and moisture from the drying films. Also, a comfortable room temperature helps maintain optimal conditions for developing, fixing, and washing solutions. If supplies (including unexposed x-ray film) are to be stored in the darkroom, ventilation is doubly important because temperatures of 90° F or higher can cause a generalized increase in density (film fog) on the film.

## SAFELIGHTING

The processing room should have both white illumination and safelighting. Safelighting is low-intensity illumination of relatively long wavelength (red) that does not rapidly affect open film but permits one to see well enough to work in the area (Fig. 6-6). To minimize the fogging effect of prolonged exposure, the safelight should have a 15-watt bulb and should be mounted at least 4 feet above the surface where opened films are handled. A new type of safelight uses a cluster of 20 red-emitting diodes, thus not needing a filter.

X-ray films are very sensitive to the blue-green region of the spectrum and are less sensitive to yellow and red wavelengths. Accordingly, the red GBX-2 filter is recommended as a safelight in darkrooms where either intraoral or extraoral films are handled because this filter transmits light only at the red end of the spectrum (Fig. 6-7). Film handling under a safelight should be limited to about 5 minutes because film emulsion shows some sensitivity to light from a safelight with prolonged exposure. The older ML-2 filters (yellow light) are not appropriate for fast intraoral dental film or extraoral panoramic or cephalometric film.

## MANUAL PROCESSING TANKS

All dental offices should have the capability to develop film by tank processing, if only as a backup for an automatic processor or digital imaging system. The tank must have hot and cold running water and a means of maintaining the temperature between 60° and 75° F. A practical size for a dental office is a master tank about 20 × 25 cm (8 × 10 inches) that can serve as a water jacket for two removable inserts that fit inside (Fig. 6-8). The insert tanks usually hold 3.8 L (1 gallon) of developer or fixer and are placed within the outer, larger master tank. The outer tank holds the running water for maintaining the temperature of the developer and fixer in the insert tanks and for washing films. The developer customarily is placed in the insert tank on the left side of the master tank and the fixer in the insert tank on the right. All three tanks should be made of stainless steel, which does not react with the processing solutions and is easy to clean. The master tank should have a cover to reduce oxidation of the processing solutions, protect the developing film from accidental exposure to light, and minimize evaporation of the processing solutions.

## THERMOMETER

The temperature of the developing, fixing, and washing solutions should be closely controlled. A thermometer can be left in the water circulating through the master tank to monitor the temperature and ensure that the water temperature regulator is working properly. The most desirable thermometers clip onto the side of the tank. Thermometers may contain alcohol or metal, but they should not contain mercury because they could break and contaminate the processor or solutions.

## TIMER

The x-ray film must be exposed to the processing chemicals for specific intervals. An interval timer is indispensable for controlling development and fixation times.

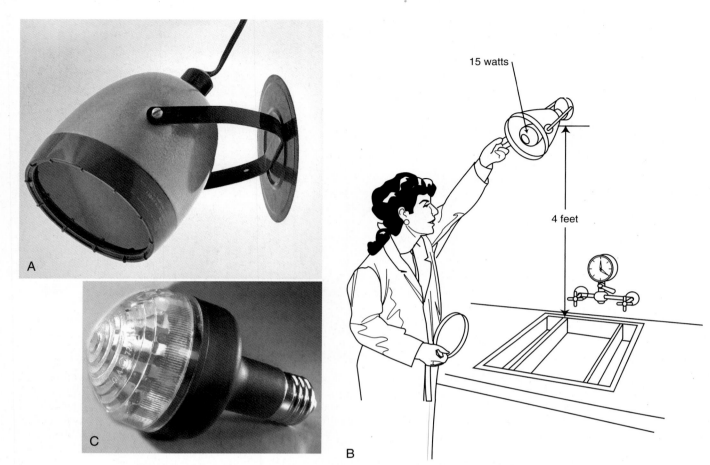

FIG. **6-6** **A,** A safelight may be mounted on the wall or ceiling in the darkroom and should be at least 4 feet from the work surface. **B,** The safelight uses a GBX-2 filter and 15-watt bulb. **C,** Bulb with cluster of 20 red-emitting diodes does not need a filter. (**C,** Courtesy Carestream Health, Inc., exclusive manufacturer of Kodak dental systems.)

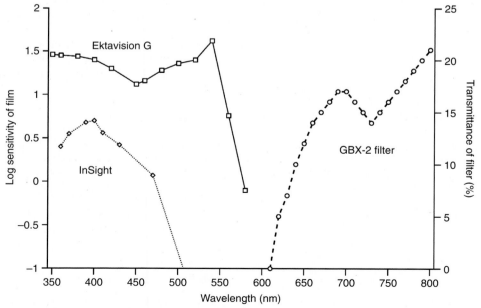

FIG. **6-7** Spectral sensitivities of Ektavision G film *(heavy line with squares)* and InSight film *(dotted line with diamonds)* shown with the transmission characteristics of a GBX-2 filter *(broken line with circles).* Note that the films are more sensitive in the blue-green portion of the spectrum (shorter than 600 nm); the GBX-2 filter transmits primarily red light (longer than 600 nm).

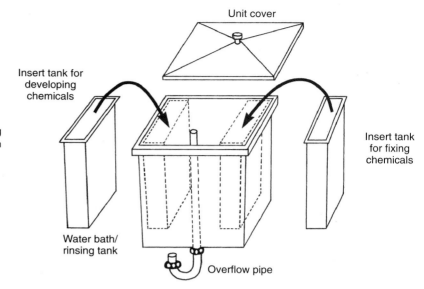

FIG. **6-8** Processing tank. The developing and fixing tanks are inserted into a bath of running water with an overflow drain.

## DRYING RACKS

Two or three drying racks can be mounted on a convenient wall for film hangers. Drip trays are placed underneath the racks to catch water that may run off the wet films. An electric fan can be used to circulate the air and speed the drying of films, but it should not be pointed directly at the films. Also, cabinet dryers are available that circulate warm air around the film and accelerate drying. Excessive heat must be avoided because it may damage the emulsion. If dryers are installed in the darkroom, they should be ventilated outside the darkroom to preclude high humidity and heat, which are detrimental to any unexposed film stored in the room.

## Manual Processing Procedures

Manual processing of film requires the following eight steps:
1. *Replenish solutions.* The first step in manual tank processing is to replenish the developer and fixer. Add fresh developer (replenisher) and fixer (8 ounces per gallon) to maintain the proper strength of each solution. Check the solution levels to ensure that the developer and fixer cover the films on the top clips of the film hangers.
2. *Stir solutions.* Next, stir the developer and fixing solution to mix the chemicals and equalize the temperature throughout the tanks. To prevent cross-contamination, use a separate paddle for each solution. It is best to label one paddle for the developer and the other for the fixer. Because proper developing time varies with the temperature of the solution, check the temperature of the developer after stirring.
3. *Mount films on hangers.* Using only safelight illumination in the darkroom, remove the exposed film from its lightproof packet or cassette. Hold the films only by their edges to avoid damage to the film surface. Clip the bare film onto a film hanger, one film to a clip (Fig. 6-9). To avoid any possible confusion later, label the film racks with the patient's name and the exposure date.
4. *Set timer.* Check the temperature of the developer and set the interval timer to the time indicated by the manufacturer for the solution temperature. For intraoral film processing in conventional solutions, use the following development times:

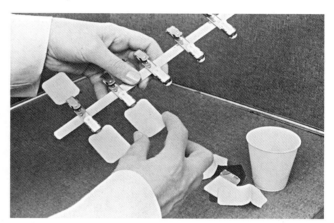

FIG. **6-9** Films are mounted securely on film clips. Film is always held by its edges to avoid fingerprints on the image. (Courtesy C.L. Crabtree, DDS, Bureau of Radiological Health, Rockville, Md.)

| TEMPERATURE | DEVELOPMENT TIME |
|---|---|
| 68° F | 5 minutes |
| 70° F | $4\frac{1}{2}$ minutes |
| 72° F | 4 minutes |
| 76° F | 3 minutes |
| 80° F | $2\frac{1}{2}$ minutes |

Processing films at either higher or lower temperatures and for longer or shorter times than recommended by the manufacturer reduces the contrast of the processed film. Also, processing too long or at temperatures higher than those recommended can result in film fog, which may diminish film contrast and diagnostic information.

5. *Develop.* Start the timer mechanism and immerse the hanger and films immediately in the developer. Agitate the hanger mildly for 5 seconds to sweep air bubbles off the film. Leave the films in the developer for the predetermined time without further

agitation. When removing the films, drain the excess developer into the wash bath.

6. *Rinse.* After development, remove the film hanger from the developer and place in the running water bath for 30 seconds. Agitate the films continuously in the rinse water to remove excess developer, thus slowing development and minimizing contamination of the fixer.

7. *Fix.* Place the hanger and film in the fixer solution for 2 to 4 minutes and agitate for 5 of every 30 seconds. This eliminates bubbles and brings fresh fixer into contact with the emulsion. Excess fixation (several hours) removes some of the metallic silver grains, diminishing the density of the film. When the films are removed, drain the excess fixer into the wash bath.

8. *Wash and dry.* After fixation of the films is complete, place the hanger in running water for at least 10 minutes to remove residual processing solutions. After the films have been washed, remove surface moisture by gently shaking excess water from the films and hanger. Dry the films in circulating, moderately warm air. If the films dry rapidly with small drops of water clinging to their surface, the areas under the drops dry more slowly than the surrounding areas. This uneven drying causes distortion of the gelatin, leaving a drying artifact in some cases. The result is spots that frequently are visible and detract from the usefulness of the finished radiograph. After drying, the films are ready to mount.

## Rapid-Processing Chemicals

In recent years a number of manufacturers have produced rapid-processing solutions. These solutions typically develop films in 15 seconds and fix them in 15 seconds at room temperature. They have the same general formulation as conventional processing solutions but often contain a higher concentration of hydroquinone. They also have a more alkaline pH than conventional solutions, which causes the emulsion to swell more, thus providing greater access to developer. These solutions are especially advantageous in endodontics and in emergency situations, when short processing time is essential. Although the resultant images may be satisfactory, they often do not achieve the same degree of contrast as films processed conventionally, and they may discolor over time if not fully washed. After viewing, rapidly processed films are placed in conventional fixing solution for 4 minutes and washed for 10 minutes. This improves the contrast and helps keep them stable in storage. Conventional solutions are preferred for most routine use.

## Changing Solutions

All processing solutions deteriorate as a result of continued use and exposure to air. Although regular replenishment of the developer and fixer prolongs their useful life, the buildup of reaction products eventually causes these solutions to cease functioning properly. Exhaustion of the developer results from oxidation of the developing agents, depletion of the hydroquinone, and buildup of bromide. Use of exhausted developer results in films that show reduced density and contrast. When the fixer becomes exhausted, silver thiosulfate complexes form and halide ions build up. The increased concentration of silver thiosulfate complexes slows the rate of diffusion of these complexes from the emulsion. The halide ions slow the rate of clearing of unexposed silver halide crystals. These changes result in films with incomplete clearing that turn brown with age. With regular replenishment, solutions may last 3 or 4 weeks before they must be changed. When the developer and fixer are replaced, the solutions must be prepared according to the directions on the containers.

A simple procedure can help determine when solutions should be changed. A double film packet instead of a single film packet is exposed on one projection for the first patient radiographed after new solutions have been prepared. One film is placed in the patient's chart, and the other is mounted on a corner of a viewbox in the darkroom. As successive films are processed, they are compared with this reference film. Loss of image contrast and density become evident as the solutions deteriorate, indicating when the time has come to change them. The fixer is changed when the developer is changed.

## Automatic Film Processing

Equipment that automates all processing steps is available (Fig. 6-10). Although automatic processing has a number of advantages, the most important is the time saved. Depending on the equipment and the temperature of operation, an automatic processor requires only 4 to 6 minutes to develop, fix, wash, and dry a film. Many dental automatic processors have a light-shielded (daylight loading) compartment in which the operator can unwrap films and feed them into the machine without working in a darkroom. This is desirable because the individual doing the developing does not have to work in the dark. However, special care must be taken to maintain infection control when using these daylight-loading compartments (see Chapter 8).

When extraoral films are processed, the light-shielded compartment is removed to provide room for feeding the larger film into the processor. Another attractive feature of the automatic system is that the density and contrast of the radiographs tend to be consistent. However, because of the higher temperature of the developer and the artifacts caused by rollers, the quality of films processed automatically often is not as high as that of those carefully developed manually. With automatically processed films, more grain usually is evident in the final image.

Whether automatic processing equipment is appropriate for a specific practice depends on the dentist and the nature and volume of the practice. The equipment is expensive and must be cleaned frequently. Also, the automated equipment may break down, and conventional darkroom equipment may still be needed as a backup system.

### MECHANISM

Automatic processors have an in-line arrangement. Typically, this consists of a transport mechanism that picks up the unwrapped film and passes it through the developing, fixing, washing, and drying sections (Fig. 6-11). The transport system most often used is a series of rollers driven by a constant-speed motor that operates through gears, belts, or chains. The rollers often consist of independent assemblies of multiple rollers in a rack, with one rack for each step in the operation. Although these assemblies are designed and positioned so that the film crosses over from one roller to the next, the operator may remove them independently for soaking, cleaning, and repairing.

The primary function of the rollers is to move the film through the developing solutions, but they also serve at least three other purposes. First, their motion helps keep the solutions agitated, which contributes to the uniformity of processing. Second, in the developer, fixer, and water tanks the rollers press on the film emulsion, forcing

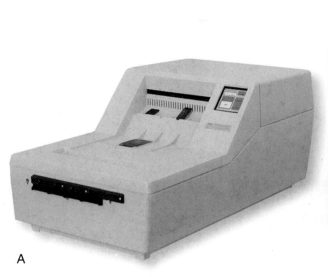
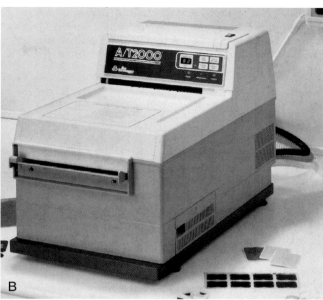

FIG. **6-10**    Automatic film processors. **A,** Dent-X 810 AR film processor. **B,** A/T 2000XR. (**A,** Courtesy AFP Imaging/Dent-X, Elmsford, N.Y.; **B,** courtesy Air Techniques, Inc., Hicksville, N.Y.)

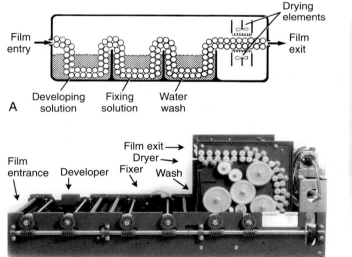
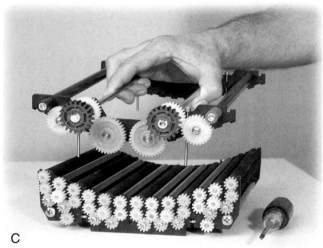

FIG. **6-11**    **A,** Automatic film processors typically consist of a roller assembly that transports the film through developing, fixing, washing, and drying stations. **B,** Assembly of film transport mechanism. **C,** Complete internal transport system. (**B** and **C,** Courtesy AFP Imaging/Dent-X, Elmsford, N.Y.)

some solution out of the emulsion. The emulsions rapidly fill again with solution, thus promoting solution exchange. Finally, the top rollers at the crossover point between the developer and fixer tanks remove developing solution, minimizing carryover of developer into the fixer tank. This feature helps maintain the uniformity of processing chemicals.

The chemical compositions of the developer and fixer are modified to operate at higher temperatures than those used for manual processing and to meet the more rapid development, fixing, washing, and drying requirements of automatic processing. The fixer has an addi-

tional hardener that helps the emulsion withstand the rigors of the transport system.

## OPERATION

Successful operation of an automatic processor requires standardized procedures and regular maintenance. The processor and surrounding area should always be kept clean so that no chemicals contaminate hands or films. Each morning the solution level and temperature should be checked before films are processed. Hands should be dry when handling film, and films should be touched only by their edges. The better processors have automatic replenishment systems. Once a week a maintenance routine should be followed, including cleaning the rollers and other working parts. It is also often useful to run a large film through the processor to clean the rollers.

## REPLENISHMENT

It is important to maintain the constituents of the developer and fixer carefully to preserve the optimal sensitometric and physical properties of the film emulsion within the narrow limits imposed by the speed and temperature of automatic processing. As the activity of the developing and fixing solutions lessens, its effect on the film diminishes. To compensate for this loss of activity, some automatic processors include an automatic replenishment system that adds fresh developer to the developer tank and fresh fixer to the fixer tank. As with manual processing, 8 ounces of fresh developer and fixer should be added per gallon of solution per day. This assumes an average workload of 30 intraoral or 5 extraoral films per day. Insufficient replenishment of the developer results in a loss of image contrast. Exhaustion of the fixing solution causes poor clearing of the film, insufficient hardening of the emulsion, and unreliable transport from the fixer assembly through the drying operation.

---

BOX 6-1
### Common Problems in Film Exposure and Development

**Light Radiographs** (Fig. 6-12)
**PROCESSING ERRORS**
Underdevelopment (temperature too low; time too short; thermometer inaccurate)
Depleted developer solution
Diluted or contaminated developer
Excessive fixation

**UNDEREXPOSURE**
Insufficient milliamperage
Insufficient peak kilovoltage
Insufficient time
Film-source distance too great
Film packet reversed in mouth (Fig. 6-13)

**Dark Radiographs** (Fig. 6-14)
**PROCESSING ERRORS**
Overdevelopment (temperature too high; time too long)
Developer concentration too high
Inadequate fixation
Accidental exposure to light
Improper safelighting

**OVEREXPOSURE**
Excessive milliamperage
Excessive peak kilovoltage
Excessive time
Film-source distance too short

**Insufficient Contrast** (Fig. 6-15)
Underdevelopment
Underexposure
Excessive peak kilovoltage
Excessive film fog

**Film Fog** (Fig. 6-16)
Improper safelighting (improper filter; excessive bulb wattage; inadequate distance between safelight and work surface; prolonged exposure to safelight)

Light leaks (cracked safelight filter; light from doors, vents, or other sources)
Overdevelopment
Contaminated solutions
Deteriorated film (stored at high temperature; stored at high humidity; exposed to radiation; outdated)

**Dark Spots or Lines** (Fig. 6-17)
Fingerprint contamination
Black wrapping paper sticking to film surface
Film in contact with tank or another film during fixation
Film contaminated with developer before processing
Excessive bending of film
Static discharge to film before processing
Excessive roller pressure during automatic processing
Dirty rollers in automatic processing

**Light Spots** (Fig. 6-18)
Film contaminated with fixer before processing
Film in contact with tank or another film during development
Excessive bending of film

**Yellow or Brown Stains**
Depleted developer
Depleted fixer
Insufficient washing
Contaminated solutions

**Blurring** (Fig. 6-19)
Movement of patient
Movement of x-ray tube head
Double exposure

**Partial Images** (Fig. 6-20)
Top of film not immersed in developing solution
Misalignment of x-ray tube head ("cone cut")

**Emulsion Peel**
Abrasion of image during processing
Excessive time in wash water

## Establishing Correct Exposure Times

When radiographs are first made with a new x-ray machine, it is important to examine the exposure guidelines that come with the machine. Typically such guidelines provide a table listing the various anatomic regions: incisors, premolars, or molars; patient size: adult or child; and the length of the aiming cylinder. For each of these combinations there will be a suggested exposure time. It is also important to start out using fresh processing chemicals and optimal processing conditions as previously described. After the first images are made on patients, it may be necessary to adjust exposure time. If optimal film processing techniques are being followed and the images are consistently dark, then exposure times should be decreased until optimal images are obtained. If images are consistently light, then exposure times should be increased. Once the optimal times have been determined, then these values should be posted by the control panel.

## Management of Radiographic Wastes

To prevent environmental damage, many communities and states have passed laws governing the disposal of wastes. Such laws often derive from the federal Resource Conservation and Recovery Act of 1976. Although dental radiographic waste constitutes only a small potential hazard, it should be discarded properly. The primary ingredient of concern in processing solutions is the dissolved silver found in used fixer. Another material of concern is the lead foil found in film packets.

Several means are available for properly disposing of the silver and lead. Silver may be recovered from the fixer by use of either the metallic replacement or electroplating methods. Metallic replacement uses cartridges through which waste solutions are poured. In this process, iron goes into the solution and the silver precipitates as sludge. In the electroplating method, the waste solutions come in contact with two electrodes through which a current passes. The cathode captures the silver. In either case, the scrap silver can be sold to silver refiners and buyers.

The lead foil is separated from the packet and collected until enough has been accumulated to sell to a scrap metal dealer. Dental offices also should consider using companies licensed to pick up waste materials. The names of such companies can be found in the telephone directory or obtained from the state hazardous waste management agency.

## Common Causes of Faulty Radiographs

Although film processing can produce radiographs of excellent quality, inattention to detail may lead to many problems and images that are diagnostically suboptimal. Poor radiographs contribute to a loss of diagnostic information and loss of professional and patient time. Box 6-1 presents a list of common causes of faulty radiographs. The steps necessary for correction are self-evident.

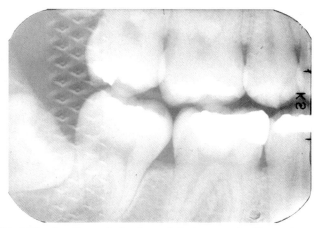

FIG. **6-13** A radiograph that is too light because the film packet was placed backward in the patient's mouth. Note the characteristic markings caused by exposure through the lead foil in the film packaging.

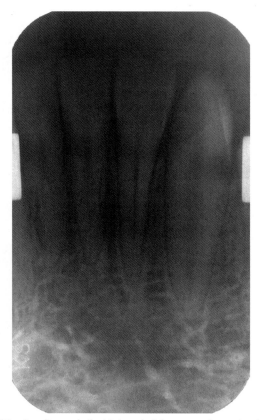

FIG. **6-14** A radiograph that is too dark because of overdevelopment or overexposure.

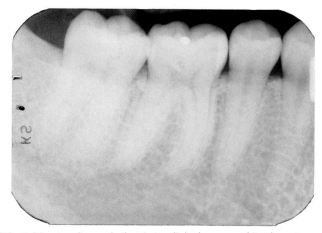

FIG. **6-12** A radiograph that is too light because of inadequate processing or insufficient exposure.

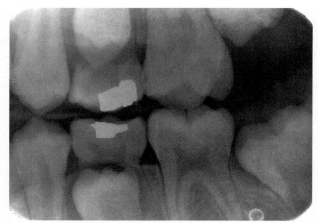

FIG. **6-15**   A radiograph with insufficient contrast, showing gray enamel and gray pulp chambers.

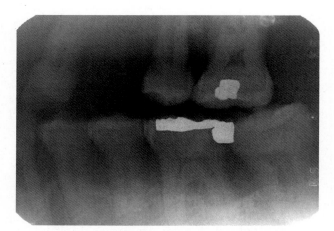

FIG. **6-16**   Fogged radiograph marked by lack of image detail.

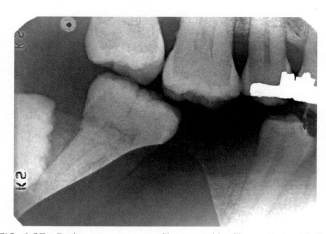

FIG. **6-17**   Dark spot on an x-ray film caused by film contact with the tank wall during fixation.

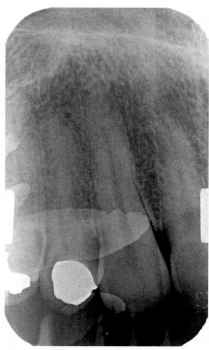

FIG. **6-18**   Light spots on an x-ray film caused by film contact with drops of fixer before processing.

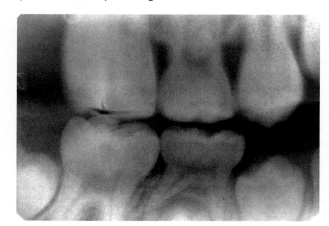

FIG. **6-19**   Blurred radiograph caused by movement of the patient during exposure.

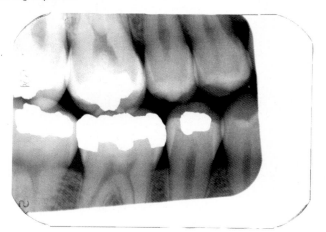

FIG. **6-20**   Partial image caused by poor alignment of the tube head with the film rectangular collimator.

## Mounting Radiographs

Radiographs must be preserved and maintained in the most satisfactory and useful condition. Periapical, interproximal, and occlusal films are best handled and stored in a film mount (Fig. 6-21). The operator can handle them with greater ease, and there is less chance of damaging the emulsion. Mounts are made of plastic or cardboard and may have a clear plastic window that covers and protects the film. However, the window may have scratches or imperfections that interfere with radiographic interpretation. The operator can arrange several films from the same individual in a film mount in the proper anatomic relationship. This facilitates correlation of the clinical and radiographic examinations. Opaque mounts are best because they prevent stray light from the viewbox from reaching the viewer's eyes.

The preferred method of positioning periapical and occlusal films in the film mount is to arrange them so that the images of the teeth are in the anatomic position and have the same relationship to the viewer as when the viewer faces the patient. The radiographs of the teeth in the right quadrants should be placed in the left side of the mount and those of the left quadrants in the right side. This system, advocated by the American Dental Association, allows the examiner's gaze to shift from radiograph to tooth without crossing the midline. The alternative arrangement, with the images of the right quadrants on the right side of the mount and those of the left quadrant on the left, is not recommended.

## Duplicating Radiographs

Occasionally radiographs must be duplicated; this is best accomplished with duplicating film. The film to be duplicated is placed against the emulsion side of the duplicating film, and the two films are held in position by a glass-topped cassette or photographic printing frame. The films are exposed to light, which passes through the clear areas of the original radiograph and exposes the duplicating film. The duplicating film is then processed in conventional x-ray processing solutions.

Unlike conventional x-ray film, duplicating film gives a positive image. Thus areas exposed to light come out clear, as on the original radiograph. Duplication typically results in images with less resolution and more contrast than the original radiograph. The best images are obtained when a circular, ultraviolet light source is used. In contrast to the usual negative film, images on duplicating film

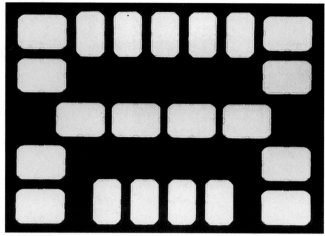

FIG. **6-21**  Film mount for holding nine narrow anterior periapical views, eight posterior periapical views, and four bitewing views.

that are too dark or too light are underexposed or overexposed, respectively.

## BIBLIOGRAPHY

Eikenberg S, Vandre R: Comparison of digital dental X-ray systems with self-developing film and manual processing for endodontic file length determination, *J Endod* 26:65-67, 2000.

Farman TT, Farman AG: Evaluation of a new F speed dental X-ray film: the effect of processing solutions and a comparison with D and E speed films, *Dentomaxillofac Radiol* 29:41-45, 2000.

Fitterman AS, Brayer FC, Cumbo PE: *Processing chemistry for medical imaging*, Technical and Scientific Monograph No. 5, N-327, Rochester, NY, 1995, Eastman Kodak.

Kodak: *Exposure and processing for dental film processing*: N-413: http://www.kodakdental.com/en/film/support. Accessed May 7, 2008.

Ludlow JB, Platin E, Delano EO et al: The efficacy of caries detection using three intraoral films under different processing conditions, *J Am Dent Assoc* 128:1401-1408, 1997.

Mees DEK, James TH: *The theory of the photographic process*, New York, 1977, Macmillan.

Syriopoulos K, Velders XL, Sanderink GC et al: Sensitometric evaluation of four dental x-ray films using five processing solutions, *Dentomaxillofac Radiol* 28:73-79, 1999.

# CHAPTER 7

# Digital Imaging

John B. Ludlow • André Mol

The advent of digital imaging has revolutionized radiology. This revolution is the result of both technologic innovation in image acquisition processes and the development of networked computing systems for image retrieval and transmission. Dentistry is seeing a steady increase in the use of these technologies, improvement of software interfaces, and introduction of new products. A number of forces are driving the shift from film to digital systems. The detrimental effects of inadequate film processing on diagnostic quality and the difficulty of maintaining high-quality chemical processing are well documented. Digital imaging eliminates chemical processing. Hazardous wastes in the form of processing chemicals and lead foil are eliminated with digital systems. Images can be electronically transferred to other health care providers without any alteration of the original image quality. In addition, digital intraoral receptors require less radiation than film, thus lowering patient exposure.

However, digital systems also have a number of disadvantages in comparison with film. The initial expense of setting up a digital imaging system is relatively high. Certain components such as the electronic x-ray receptor used in some intraoral systems are susceptible to rough handling and are costly to replace. Because digital systems use new or immature technologies, there is a risk—perhaps even a likelihood—of systems becoming obsolete or manufacturers going out of business. The excellent image quality and comparatively low cost of a properly exposed and processed film keeps film-based radiography competitive with digital alternatives.

The trends, however, are certain: computers play a role in the majority of dental practices, and that role is expanding as a variety of functions from appointment scheduling, procedure billing, and patient charting are integrated into seamless practice management software solutions. It is no longer a matter of *if* but rather *when* the majority of dental practices will use digital imaging. Already during this time of transition, film-based practices are confronted with digital images from practices that have implemented digital radiography. This chapter describes the characteristics of digital images, image receptors, display options, and storage devices, followed by a discussion of digital image processing.

## Analog Versus Digital

The term *digital* in digital imaging refers to the numeric format of the image content and its discreteness. Conventional film images can be considered an analog medium in which differences in the size and distribution of black metallic silver result in a continuous density spectrum. Digital images are numeric and discrete in two ways: (1) in terms of the spatial distribution of the picture elements (pixels) and

(2) in terms of the different shades of gray of each of the pixels. A digital image consists of a large collection of individual pixels organized in a matrix of rows and columns (Fig. 7-1). Each pixel has a row and column coordinate that uniquely identifies its location in the matrix. The formation of a digital image requires several steps, beginning with analog processes. At each pixel of an electronic detector, the absorption of x rays generates a small voltage. More x rays generate a higher voltage and vice versa. At each pixel, the voltage can fluctuate between a minimum and maximum value and is therefore an analog signal (Fig. 7-2, *A*).

Production of a digital image requires a process called *analog-to-digital conversion (ADC)*. ADC consists of two steps: sampling and quantization. *Sampling* means that a small range of voltage values are grouped together as a single value (Fig. 7-2, *B*). Narrow sampling better mimics the original signal but leads to larger memory requirements for the resulting digital image (Fig. 7-2, *C*). Once sampled, the signal is *quantized,* which means that every sampled signal is assigned a value. These values are stored in the computer and represent the image. For the clinician to see the image, the computer organizes the pixels in their proper locations and displays a shade of gray that corresponds to the number that was assigned during the quantization step.

To understand the strengths and weaknesses of digital radiography, the clinician establishes which elements of the radiographic imaging chain stay the same and which ones change. The imaging chain can be conceptualized as a series of interconnecting links beginning with the generation of x rays. Exposure factors, patient factors, and the projection geometry determine how the x-ray beam will be attenuated. A portion of the unattenuated x-ray beam is captured by the image receptor to form a latent image. This latent image is then processed and converted into a real image, which is viewed and interpreted by the clinician. The use of digital detectors changes the way we acquire, store, retrieve, and display images. However, besides an adjustment of the exposure time, digital detectors do not fundamentally change the way in which x rays are selectively attenuated by the tissues of the patient. The physics of the interaction of x rays with matter and the effects of the projection geometry on the appearance of the radiographic image are unaltered and remain critically important for understanding image content and for optimizing image quality.

## Digital Image Receptors

Digital image receptors encompass a number of different technologies and come in many different sizes and shapes. Unfortunately, a number of different and sometimes confusing names are in use to identify

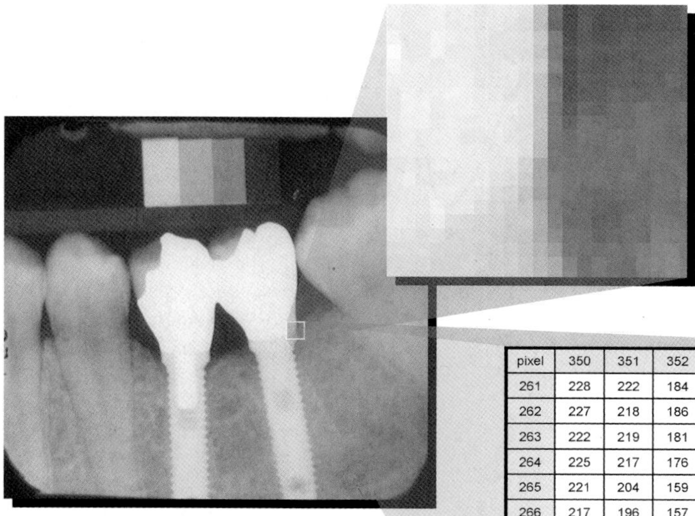

FIG. **7-1** The digital image is made up of a large number of discrete picture elements (pixels). Their size is so small that the image appears smooth at normal magnification. The location of each pixel is uniquely identified by a row and column coordinate within the image matrix. The value assigned to a pixel represents the intensity (gray level) of the image at that location.

| pixel | 350 | 351 | 352 | 353 | 354 | 355 | 356 | 357 |
|-------|-----|-----|-----|-----|-----|-----|-----|-----|
| 261 | 228 | 222 | 184 | 107 | 76 | 92 | 90 | 98 |
| 262 | 227 | 218 | 186 | 110 | 90 | 104 | 103 | 98 |
| 263 | 222 | 219 | 181 | 107 | 97 | 107 | 102 | 104 |
| 264 | 225 | 217 | 176 | 107 | 98 | 100 | 100 | 107 |
| 265 | 221 | 204 | 159 | 107 | 105 | 101 | 107 | 102 |
| 266 | 217 | 196 | 157 | 114 | 105 | 104 | 106 | 100 |
| 267 | 209 | 190 | 154 | 114 | 107 | 103 | 97 | 100 |
| 268 | 202 | 195 | 166 | 118 | 102 | 102 | 92 | 94 |
| 269 | 197 | 196 | 168 | 122 | 98 | 102 | 90 | 94 |
| 270 | 195 | 190 | 166 | 130 | 104 | 105 | 92 | 97 |
| 271 | 199 | 190 | 172 | 144 | 111 | 107 | 100 | 106 |
| 272 | 201 | 193 | 177 | 160 | 120 | 103 | 112 | 106 |
| 273 | 203 | 195 | 181 | 166 | 129 | 102 | 111 | 106 |
| 274 | 201 | 200 | 186 | 172 | 133 | 110 | 112 | 102 |

these receptors in medicine and dentistry. Currently, the most useful distinction is that between two main technologies: (1) solid-state technology and (2) photostimulable phosphor technology. Although solid-state detectors can be further subdivided, these detectors have in common certain physical properties and the ability to generate a digital image in the computer without any other external device. In medicine, the use of solid-state detectors is referred to as digital radiography. In dentistry, intraoral solid-state detectors are often called sensors. The other main technology, photostimulable phosphor (PSP), consists of a phosphor coated on top of a plate in which a latent image is formed after x-ray exposure. The latent image is converted to a digital image by a scanning device through stimulation by laser light. Some refer to this technology as storage phosphor on the basis of the notion that the image information is temporarily stored within the phosphor. Others use the term image plates to differentiate them from film and solid-state detectors. The use of PSP plates in medical radiology is referred to as computed radiography.

## SOLID-STATE DETECTORS

Solid-state detectors collect the charge generated by x rays in a solid semiconducting material. The key clinical feature of these detectors is the rapid availability of the image after exposure. The matrix and its associated readout and amplifying electronics of intraoral detectors are enclosed within a plastic housing to protect them from the oral environment. These elements of the detector consume part of the real estate of the sensor so that the active area of the sensor is smaller than its total surface area. Sensor bulk, although reduced by continued miniaturization of the electronic components, is a potential drawback of intraoral solid-state detectors. In addition, most detectors incorporate an electronic cable to transfer data to the computer. One manufacturer has produced a system that replaces the cable connection with

a radiofrequency transmitter. This frees the detector from a direct tether to the computer, but it necessitates some additional electronic components, thus increasing the overall bulk of the sensor.

A number of manufacturers produce detectors with varying active sensor areas roughly corresponding to the different sizes of intraoral film. Detectors without flaws are relatively expensive to produce, and the expense of the detector increases with increasing matrix size (total number of pixels). Pixel size varies from 20 to 70 micrometers (μm). Three types of solid-state sensors are in common use.

### Charge-Coupled Device

The charge-coupled device (CCD), introduced to dentistry in 1987, was the first digital image receptor to be adapted for intraoral imaging. The CCD uses a thin wafer of silicon as the basis for image recording. The silicon crystals are formed in a picture element (pixel) matrix (Fig. 7-3). When exposed to radiation, the covalent bonds between silicon atoms are broken, producing electron-hole pairs (Fig. 7-4). The number of electron-hole pairs that are formed is proportional to the amount of exposure that an area receives. The electrons are then attracted toward the most positive potential in the device, where they create "charge packets." Each packet corresponds to one pixel. The charge pattern formed from the individual pixels in the matrix represents the latent image (Fig. 7-5). The image is read by transferring each row of pixel charges from one pixel to the next in a "bucket brigade" fashion. As a charge reaches the end of its row, it is transferred to a readout amplifier and transmitted as a voltage to the analog-to-digital converter located within or connected to the computer. Voltages from each pixel are sampled and assigned a numeric value representing a gray level (ADC). Because CCD detectors are more sensitive to light than to x rays, most manufacturers use a layer of scintillating material coated directly on the CCD surface or coupled

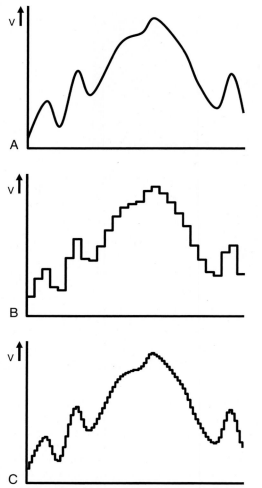

FIG. **7-2    A,** Illustration of an analog voltage signal generated by a detector. **B,** Sampling of the analog signal discards part of the signal. **C,** Sampling at a higher frequency preserves more of the original signal.

to the surface by fiberoptics. This increases the x-ray absorption efficiency of the detector. Gadolinium oxybromide compounds similar to those used in rare earth radiographic screens or cesium iodide are examples of scintillators that have been used for this purpose.

CCDs have also been made in linear arrays of a few pixels wide and many pixels long for panoramic and cephalometric imaging. In the case of panoramic units, the CCD is fixed in position opposite to the x-ray source with the long axis of the array oriented parallel to the fan-shaped x-ray beam. Some manufacturers provide CCD sensors that may be retrofitted to older panoramic units. Unlike film imaging, the mechanics for cephalometric imaging are different. Construction of a single CCD of a size that could simultaneously capture the area of a full skull would be prohibitively expensive. Combining a linear CCD array and a slit-shaped x-ray beam with a scanning motion permits scanning of the skull over several seconds. One disadvantage of this approach is the increased possibility of patient movement artifacts during the several seconds required to complete a scan.

### Complementary Metal Oxide Semiconductors

Complementary metal oxide semiconductor (CMOS) technology is the basis for typical consumer-grade video cameras. These detectors are also silicon-based semiconductors but are fundamentally different from CCDs in the way that pixel charges are read. Each pixel is isolated from its neighboring pixels and is directly connected to a transistor. Like the CCD, electron-hole pairs are generated within the pixel in proportion to the amount of x-ray energy that is absorbed. This charge is transferred to the transistor as a small voltage. The voltage in each transistor can be addressed separately, read by a frame grabber, and then stored and displayed as a digital gray value. CMOS technology is widely used in the construction of computer central processing unit chips and video camera detectors, and the technology is less expensive than that used in the manufacturing of CCDs. Several manufacturers are currently using this technology for intraoral imaging applications (Fig. 7-6).

### Flat Panel Detectors

Flat panel detectors are being used for medical imaging but have also been used in several extraoral imaging devices. The detectors can provide relatively large matrix areas with pixel sizes less than 100 μm. This allows direct digital imaging of larger areas of the body, including the head. Two approaches have been taken in selecting x-ray–sensitive materials for flat panel detectors. Indirect detectors are sensitive to

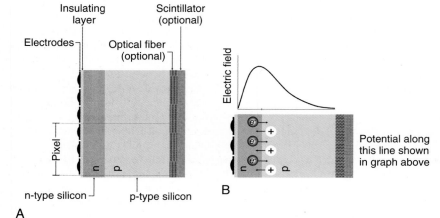

**A**

FIG. **7-3    A,** Basic structure of the CCD: electrodes insulated from an n-p silicon sandwich. The surface of the silicon may incorporate a scintillating material to improve x-ray capture efficiency and fiberoptics to improve resolution. One pixel utilizes three electrodes. **B,** Excess electrons from the n-type layer diffuse into the p-type layer while excess holes in the p-type layer diffuse into the n-type layer. The resulting charge imbalance creates an electric field in the silicon with a maximum just inside the n-type layer.

visible light, and an intensifying screen (gadolinium oxysulfide or cesium iodide) is used to convert x-ray energy into light. The performance of these devices is determined by the thickness of the intensifying screen. Thicker screens are more efficient but allow greater diffusion of light photons, leading to image unsharpness. Direct detectors use a photoconductor material (selenium) with properties similar to silicon and a higher atomic number, which permits more efficient absorption of x rays. Under the influence of an applied electrical field, the electrons that are freed during x-ray exposure of the selenium are conducted in a direct line to an underlying thin film transistor (TFT) detector element. Direct detectors using selenium (Z = 34) provide higher resolution but lower efficiency in comparison with indirect detectors using intensifying screens with gadolinium (Z = 64) or cesium (Z = 55). The electrical energy generated is proportional to the x-ray exposure and is stored at each pixel in a capacitor. The energy is released and read out by applying appropriate row and column voltages to a particular pixel's transistor. Currently, flat panel detectors are expensive and likely to be limited to specialized imaging tasks such as cone beam imaging.

## PHOTOSTIMULABLE PHOSPHOR

PSP plates absorb and store energy from x rays and then release this energy as light (phosphorescence) when stimulated by another light of an appropriate wavelength. To the extent that the stimulating light and phosphorescent light wavelengths differ, the two may be distinguished and the phosphorescence can be quantified as a measure of the amount of x-ray energy that the material has absorbed.

The PSP material used for radiographic imaging is "europium-doped" barium fluorohalide. Barium in combination with iodine, chlorine, or bromine forms a crystal lattice. The addition of europium ($Eu^{+2}$) creates imperfections in this lattice. When exposed to a sufficiently energetic source of radiation, valence electrons in europium can absorb energy and move into the conduction band. These electrons migrate to nearby halogen vacancies (F-centers) in the fluorohalide lattice and may become trapped there in a metastable state. While in this state, the number of trapped electrons is proportional to x-ray exposure and represents a latent image. When stimulated by red light of around 600 nm, the barium fluorohalide releases trapped electrons to the conduction band. When an electron returns to the $Eu^{+3}$ ion, energy is released in the green spectrum between 300 and 500 nm (Fig. 7-7). Fiberoptics conduct light from the PSP plate to a photomultiplier tube. The photomultiplier tube converts light into electrical energy. A red filter at the photomultiplier tube selectively removes the stimulating laser light, and the remaining green light is detected and converted to a varying voltage. The variations in voltage output from the photomultiplier tube correspond to variations in stimulated light intensity from the latent image. The voltage signal is quantified by an analog-to-digital converter and stored and displayed as a digital image. In practice, the barium fluorohalide material is

### Photoelectric Absorption in Silicon

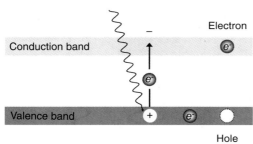

FIG. **7-4** X-ray or light photons impart energy to electrons in the valence band, releasing them into the conduction band. This generates an "electron-hole" charge pair.

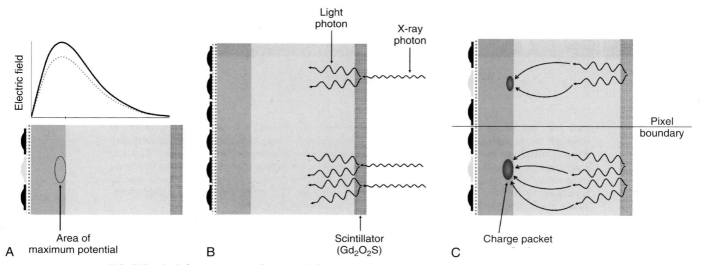

FIG. **7-5** **A,** Before exposure, the central electrode of each pixel is turned on, thus creating an area of maximum potential or potential well. **B,** X-ray photons are absorbed in the scintillating material and are converted to light photons. Light photons are absorbed in the silicon through photoelectric absorption. **C,** Electrons released from the valence band collect selectively near the n-p layer interface in the area of maximum potential to form a charge packet. During CCD readout, the electrical potential of the pixel electrodes are sequentially modulated to shift the charge packet from pixel to pixel.

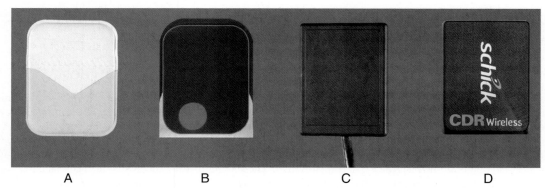

FIG. **7-6**  **A,** Kodak No. 2 film. **B,** Soredex Optime No. 2 PSP plate sitting on barrier envelope to demonstrate packaged size. **C,** Gendex No. 2 CCD sensor. **D,** Schick No. 2 CMOS wireless sensor.

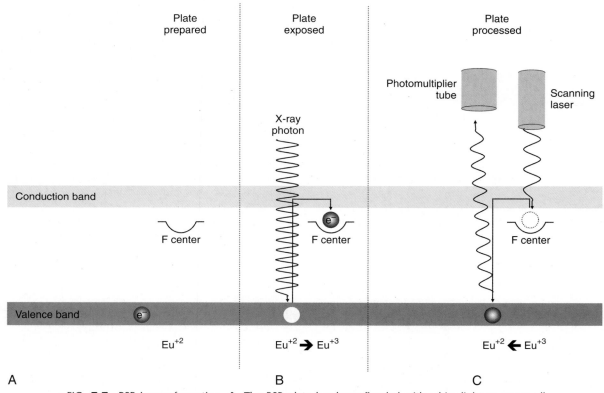

FIG. **7-7**  PSP image formation. **A,** The PSP plate has been flooded with white light to return all electrons to the valence band. **B,** Exposure to x rays imparts energy to europium valence electrons, moving them into the conduction band. Some electrons become trapped at "F centers." **C,** A red scanning laser imparts energy to electrons at the F centers, promoting them to the conduction band from which many return to the valence band. With the electron's return to the valence band, energy is released in the form of light photons in the green spectrum. This light is detected by a photomultiplier tube or diode with a red filter to screen out the scanning laser light.

combined with a polymer and spread in a thin layer on a base material to create a PSP. For intraoral radiography, a polyester base similar to radiographic film is used.

When they are manufactured in standard intraoral sizes, these plates provide handling characteristics similar to intraoral film. PSP plates are also made in sizes commonly used for panoramic and cephalometric imaging. Some PSP processors accommodate a full range of intraoral and extraoral plate sizes. Other processors are limited to intraoral or extraoral formats.

Before exposure, PSP plates must be erased to eliminate "ghost images" from prior exposures (note that this is a different type of ghost image than that associated with panoramic radiography). This is accomplished by flooding the plate with a bright light. Placing plates on a dental viewbox with the phosphor side of the plates facing the light for 1 or 2 minutes can accomplish this. More intense light sources can be used for shorter periods of time. Some PSP systems integrate automatic plate-erasing lights. Erased plates are placed in light-tight containers before exposure. In the case of intraoral plates, sealable polyvinyl envelopes that are impervious to oral fluids and light are used for packaging. For large-format plates, conventional cassettes (without intensifying screens) are used. After exposure, plates should be processed as soon as possible because trapped electrons spontaneously release over time. The rate of loss of electrons is greatest shortly after exposure. The rate varies depending on the composition of the storage phosphor and the environmental temperature. Some phosphors lose 23% of their trapped electrons after 30 minutes and 30% after an hour. Because loss of trapped electrons is fairly uniform across the plate surface, early loss of charge does not typically result in clinically meaningful image deterioration. However, underexposed images may suffer noticeable image degradation. Adequately exposed images may be stored for 12 to 24 hours and retain acceptable image quality. A more important source of latent image fading is exposure to ambient light during plate preparation for processing. A semidark environment is recommended for plate handling. The more intense the background light and the longer the exposure of the plate to this light, the greater is the loss of trapped electrons and the more degraded the resultant image. Red safelights found in most darkrooms are not safe for exposed PSP plates, which are most sensitive to the red light spectrum.

### Stationary Plate Scans

A number of approaches have been adopted for "reading" the latent images on PSP plates. An approach used by Soredex in its Digora system and Air Techniques in its ScanX system uses a rapidly rotating multifaceted mirror that reflects a beam of red laser light. As the mirror revolves, the laser light sweeps across the plate. The plate is advanced and the adjacent line of phosphor is scanned. The direction of the laser scanning the plate is termed the *fast scan direction*. The direction of plate advancement is termed the *slow scan direction*.

Both companies have also introduced image erasing into the scanner. This improves work flow and reduces potential plate damage from manual erasing. Furthermore, the mechanism used for plate intake in the Soredex Optime scanner requires a metal disk on the back of the plate. This disk also serves as a marker to indicate when a plate was exposed backward.

### Rotating Plate Scans

An alternate approach to plate reading used by Gendex in the DenOptix system and by Kodak in the CR 7400 system involves a rapidly rotating drum that holds the plate. The rotation of the drum past a fixed laser provides a rapid scan. Incremental movement of the laser in the slow scan direction allows image data to be acquired line by line.

## Digital Detector Characteristics

### CONTRAST RESOLUTION

Contrast resolution is the ability to distinguish different densities in the radiographic image. This is a function of the interaction of the following:

- Attenuation characteristics of the tissues imaged
- Capacity of the image receptor to distinguish differences in numbers of x-ray photons coming from different areas of the subject

FIG. **7-8**  Contrast resolution. Examples of gray-scale ramps representing distinct gray levels from black to white. Bit depth controls the number of possible gray levels in the image. The actual number of distinct gray levels that are displayed is dependent on the output device and image processing. The perceived number of gray levels is influenced by viewing conditions and the visual acuity of the observer. **A,** 6 bits/pixel—64 gray levels. **B,** 5 bits/pixel—32 gray levels. **C,** 4 bits/pixel—16 gray levels. **D,** 3 bits/pixel—8 gray levels.

- Ability of the computer display to portray differences in density
- Ability of the observer to recognize those differences

Current digital detectors capture data at 8, 10, 12, or 16 bits. The bit depth is a power of 2 (Fig. 7-8). This means that the detector can theoretically capture 256 ($2^8$) to 65,536 ($2^{16}$) different densities. In practice the actual number of meaningful densities that can be captured is limited by inaccuracies in image acquisition, that is, *noise*. Regardless of the number of density differences that a detector can capture, conventional computer monitors are capable of displaying a gray scale of only 8 bits. Because operating systems such as Windows reserve a number of gray levels for the display of system information, the actual number of gray levels that can be displayed on a monitor is 242. A more important limiting factor is the human visual system, which is capable of distinguishing only about 60 gray levels at any time under ideal viewing conditions. Considering the typical viewing environment in the dental operatory, the actual number of gray levels that can be distinguished falls to less than 30. Human visual limitations are also present for film viewing; however, the luminance (brightness) of a typical radiograph view box is much greater than that of a typical computer display. Therefore the ambient lighting of the room in which the image is viewed will theoretically have a lower impact on film than on digital displays.

### SPATIAL RESOLUTION

Spatial resolution is the capacity for distinguishing fine detail in an image. Resolution is often measured and reported in units of line-pairs per millimeter. Test objects consisting of sets of very fine radiopaque lines separated from each other by spaces equal to the width of a line are constructed with a variety of line widths (Fig. 7-9). A line and its associated space are called a *line pair (lp)*. At least two pixels are required to resolve a line pair, one for the dark line and one for the light space. Typical observers are able to distinguish about 6 lp/mm without benefit of magnification. Intraoral film is capable of providing more than 20 lp/mm of resolution. Unless a film image is magnified, the observer is unable to appreciate the extent of the detail in the image.

With solid-state digital imaging systems the theoretic resolution limit is determined by pixel size: the smaller the size of the pixel, the higher the resolution. With 20-μm pixels, a theoretical resolution of

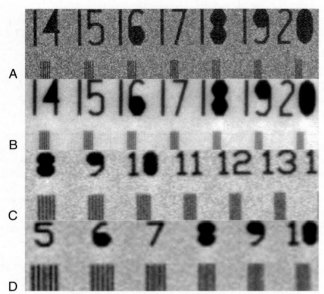

FIG. **7-9** Images of a line-pair resolution test phantom made with various receptors. **A,** Kodak InSight film. **B,** Trophy RVGui high-resolution CCD. **C,** Gendex DenOptix PSP scanned at 600 DPI. **D,** Gendex DenOptix PSP scanned at 300 DPI.

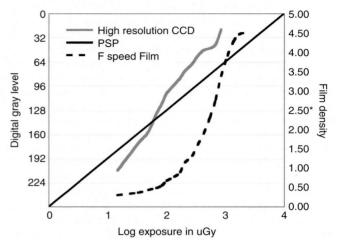

*An optical density of 2.5 is generally considered the upper limit of useful clinical density in the absence of special illumination or "hot lighting" of films.

FIG. **7-10** Representative exposure latitudes of CCD, PSP, and intra-oral film sensors. Note that the clinically useful optical density of film has an upper limit of 2.5. Use of a more intense viewbox or "hot light-ing" can extend the upper end of the usable density range and expand useful film latitude.

25 lp/mm can be obtained. In practice, however, actual resolution is usually lower because of a variety of sources of electronic noise, diffusion of photons in the scintillator coating, as well as potentially imperfect optical coupling in systems using fiber optics. Currently the highest resolution intraoral CCD for dentistry has a pixel size of approximately 20 μm. This compares with a silver grain size of 8 μm for intraoral film.

Resolution in PSP systems is influenced by the thickness of the phosphor material. Thicker phosphor layers cause more diffusion and yield a lower resolution. On the other hand, a thicker layer enhances x-ray absorption efficiency, resulting in a faster image receptor. Resolution is also inversely proportional to the diameter of the laser beam. Effective beam diameter is increased by vibration in the rotating mirror and drum scanner designs. Slow scan motion influences resolution by the increment of plate advancement. This increment may be adjusted to increase or reduce resolution in some systems. Current PSP systems are capable of providing more than 7 lp/mm of resolution.

Software displays of all digital images permit magnification of images. A periapical image filling the display of a computer monitor may be magnified by a factor of 10 times or more. At this level of magnification, the image takes on a building block pattern or pixelated appearance and the limits of resolution of the imaging system are evident.

## DETECTOR LATITUDE

The ability of an image receptor to capture a range of x-ray exposures is termed *latitude*. A desirable quality in intraoral image receptors is the ability to record a broad range of tissue densities, from gingiva to enamel. At the same time, subtle differences in density within these tissues should be visually apparent. The useful range of densities in film radiography is two orders of magnitude,

from 0.5 to 2.5. The dynamic range of film actually extends for more than four orders of magnitude, but densities of 3 and 4, which transmit only 1/1,000th to 1/10,000th of the incident light, require intensified illumination or hot lighting to be distinguished from a density of 2.5. Such devices are not commonly used in general practice. The latitude of CCD and CMOS detectors is similar to that of film and can be extended with digital enhancement of contrast and brightness. PSP receptors enjoy larger latitudes and have a linear response to five orders of magnitude of x-ray exposure (Fig. 7-10).

## DETECTOR SENSITIVITY

The sensitivity, or speed, of a detector is its ability to respond to small amounts of radiation. Intraoral film speed is classified according to speed group by criteria developed by the International Organization for Standardization. Extraoral screen-film combinations use a classification system developed by Eastman Kodak. Currently there are no classification standards for dental digital x-ray receptors. As a result, the reported sensitivity of systems by equipment manufacturers may exaggerate the performance that can actually be achieved in routine practice. The useful sensitivity of digital receptors is affected by a number of factors including detector efficiency, pixel size, and system noise. Current PSP systems for intraoral imaging allow dose reductions of about 50% in comparison with F-speed film with similar diagnostic performance. Subjectively, most observers prefer intraoral PSP images with a higher level of x-ray exposure. Paradoxically this can lead to increased patient doses if the level of x-ray exposure is determined by "most attractive" image criteria. In general, solid-state detectors require less exposure than PSP systems or film. CCD and PSP systems for extraoral imaging require exposures similar to those needed for 200-speed screen-film systems.

## Digital Image Viewing

### CATHODE RAY TUBE DISPLAY

Conventional computer monitors use cathode ray tube (CRT) designs. A beam of electrons emanating from an electron "gun" rapidly scans a phosphor-coated screen. The electron scan is horizontal and builds an image line by line. The image is repeated or refreshed at a rate of 60 times a second (hertz) or more to avoid the appearance of flicker. Color monitors use three electron guns, one each for red, blue, and green phosphors. The variable intensity of the electron beam is responsible for different shades of gray or color hue and intensity. High-quality monitors are able to display 256 different gray values or a combination of gray and color values. CRT displays involve conversion of digital information into analog voltages, which are supplied to the electron guns. Some loss of the original image information is inherent in the digital-to-analog conversion process. A number of factors affect the subjective quality of a monitor. The dot pitch is a measure of the distance between groups of subpixels (red, green, and blue phosphors) in the CRT. Smaller dot pitches, 0.28 mm or less, provide more pixels per area and sharper-looking images. The brightness of the monitor affects perceived contrast in the image. Bright monitors are essential in working environments with bright ambient lighting. Over time, the color phosphors in a CRT fade, reducing the brightness of the monitor and the contrast within the image.

### THIN FILM TRANSISTOR DISPLAY

TFT technology, which is used in flat panel detectors, is also used in laptop and flat panel computer displays. The process is somewhat reversed in that a signal is sent to the pixel's transistor, which in turn causes the associated liquid crystal display (LCD) to transmit light with an intensity proportional to the transistor voltage. Subpixels composed of red, green, and blue phosphors are subjected to varied voltages and in combination create a pixel output of a particular hue and intensity. The output of laptop displays is limited in intensity and does not have the dynamic range or contrast found in conventional desktop CRT or LCD displays. The viewing angle of laptop displays is also limited, and the observer needs to be positioned squarely in front of the display for optimum viewing quality. Current laptop displays are of sufficient quality to be used for typical dental diagnostic tasks. Desktop versions of TFT LCD displays have overcome brightness and viewing angle problems but consume more power and thus are not suited for laptop configurations. An increasing number of flat panel displays are actually brighter than conventional CRT displays and have viewing angles as wide as 160 degrees. Some flat panel displays incorporate a digital video interface, which allows direct display of digital information without digital-to-analog conversion. These displays virtually eliminate signal loss and distortion from digital-to-analog conversion.

### ELECTRONIC DISPLAY CONSIDERATIONS

The display of digital images on electronic devices is a fairly straightforward engineering issue. Positioning an image in the context of other diagnostic and demographic information and in useful relationships with other images is a more complex challenge that may vary according to diagnostic task, practice pattern, and practitioner preference. These challenges are answered with varying degrees of success by image display software. The quality, capabilities, and ease of use of display software vary from vendor to vendor. Even with the same software, the display of images can vary dramatically, depending on how the software handles resizing of windows or the size and resolutions of different displays. For instance, on some displays, it may be impossible to view a full-mouth series of images on a single screen at normal magnification (100%). Software may permit reduction in image size or scrolling around the window to compensate for smaller display areas. These approaches are not as fast or flexible as shifting a film mount around on a view box. The visibility of electronic displays is degraded by many of the same elements that degrade viewing of film images. Bright background illumination from windows or other sources of ambient light reduces visual contrast sensitivity. Light reflecting off a monitor surface may further reduce the visibility of image contrast. Images are best viewed in an environment in which lighting is subdued and indirect.

### HARD COPIES

Until all dental health care providers and third parties are able to send, receive, store, and display digital images from a variety of acquisition sources, there will be a need for a universal medium to exchange radiographic image information. With the development of digital photography as a mainstream technology, digital image printing has become an economical solution for making digital radiographs transferable. The question is whether the printed image provides adequate image quality to prevent loss of diagnostic information. Any time a digital image is modified, including the process of printing it in hard copy, there needs to be sufficient assurance that the image retains relevant diagnostic information. The requirements for quality vary with the diagnostic task at hand. For instance, assessment of the impaction status of a third molar puts a lower demand on the image quality than caries detection. Unfortunately, there is limited scientific evidence to support the diagnostic efficacy of printed images. The large number of variables that influence the quality of the printed image—for instance, the printing technology, printer quality, printer settings, and type of media—makes the printing process a much more complicated process than it initially appears to be. It is therefore imperative, when images must be printed, to use a printing system that is designed for its intended use and to follow the manufacturer's recommendations. Of course, it is always preferable to transfer images digitally when possible. The main types of printing technologies available for image printing include laser, inkjet, and dye sublimation with the use of either film or paper.

#### Film Printers

Radiologists have traditionally relied on film images for common interpretive tasks. Many radiologists still prefer film even for inherently digital technologies such as magnetic resonance and computed tomography imaging. Unfortunately, high-quality film printers that use laser or dye sublimation technologies are expensive, and low-cost alternatives suffer from reduced diagnostic quality. Current film transparencies produced with ink jet technology appear to be suboptimal for tasks such as caries diagnosis.

#### Paper Printers

Although printing on film allows radiographs to be evaluated in a traditional manner with the transmitted light of a viewbox, paper-printed digital radiographs require reflective light from a normally lit room. This offers a substantial advantage because most dental operatories are not well equipped to control the ambient light level for

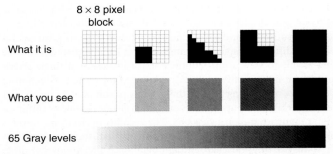

FIG. **7-11** Gray scale printing: Each image pixel is assigned to an 8 × 8 pixel array on the printed page. From 0 to 64 black ink dots can be used to fill each array, resulting in 65 potential gray levels. This means that an 8 bit (256 gray levels) is reduced to 6 bits with a concomitant loss of contrast resolution during the printing process.

viewing film images on a viewbox. Moreover, printing digital radiographs on paper allows the dentist to use technologies developed for the digital photography domain.

Photographic printers vary widely in price and quality. Although more costly models usually provide higher print resolution, printer resolution is only one of many factors determining the final quality of the printed image. Ink jet printers are by far the most dominant in the market and offer the most economical alternative. Dye sublimation printers provide excellent image quality but are generally more expensive.

For any printing technology, the printing resolution is usually defined as the number of dots per inch (DPI) the printer can print. A printer with a higher DPI number is capable of laying the ink down more tightly than a printer with a lower DPI number. As a result, printers with a higher DPI number can print smaller objects and thus are said to have "higher resolution." The resolution of the digital radiograph can never be increased by a printer that prints at a higher resolution than that of the image itself. On the other hand, printing digital radiographs at a lower resolution may reduce the final resolution of the image unless the printed size of the image is increased. Spatial resolution is preserved as long as the image prints pixel for pixel.

The same cannot be said of contrast resolution, which is always reduced by the printing process. The reason for this is that the printer is not actually printing with shades of gray but is instead printing varying numbers of black dots. Typically an 8 × 8 pixel page array is assigned to each image pixel (Fig. 7-11). The number of elements in the array that are filled with a black ink dot determines the relative gray level of the array. The 8 × 8 array provides for 0 to 64 ink dots or 65 gray values. With an 8 × 8 dot array, it may not be possible to print all pixels of an image on a single page. For instance, a PSP panoramic image with a physical size of 15 × 30 cm might be scanned at 150 DPI. For each pixel of this image to print within the same dimensions, a printer resolution of 1200 DPI (8 × 150) is required. If the maximum resolution of the printer is 1200 DPI, then images with higher resolutions must be printed at a larger size to obtain full spatial resolution. Likewise, a bitewing image scanned at 300 DPI must be printed at twice its physical size of 30 × 40 mm to preserve the original resolution. Resizing of an image to fit on a printed page leads to interpolation of pixels and can result in a significant loss of resolution.

## IMAGE PROCESSING

Any operation that acts to improve, restore, analyze, or in some way change a digital image is a form of image processing. The use of digital imaging in dental radiography involves a variety of image processing operations. Some of these operations are integrated in the image acquisition and image management software and are hidden from the user. Others are controlled by the user with the intention to improve the quality of the image or to analyze its contents.

## IMAGE RESTORATION

When the raw image data enter the computer, they are usually not yet ready for storage or display. A number of preprocessing steps need to be performed to correct the image for known defects and to adjust the image intensities so that they are suitable for viewing. For example, some of the pixels in a CCD sensor are always defective. The image is restored by substituting the gray values of the defective pixels with some weighted average of the gray values from the surrounding pixels. Depending on the quality of the sensor and the choices made by the manufacturer, a variety of other operations may be applied to the image before it becomes visible on the display. They are executed very rapidly and are unnoticed by the user. Most of the preprocessing operations are set by the manufacturer and cannot be changed.

## IMAGE ENHANCEMENT

The term *image enhancement* implies that the adjusted image is an improved version of the original one. Most image enhancement operations are applied to make the image visually more appealing (subjective enhancement). This can be accomplished by increasing contrast, optimizing brightness, and reducing unsharpness and noise. Subjective image enhancement does not necessarily improve the accuracy of image interpretation. Image enhancement operations are often task specific: what benefits one diagnostic task may reduce the image quality for another task. For example, increasing contrast between enamel and dentin for caries detection may make it more difficult to identify the contour of the alveolar crest. Image enhancement operations are also dependent on viewer preference.

### Brightness and Contrast

Digital radiographs do not always effectively use the full range of available gray values. They can be relatively dark or light, and they can show too much contrast in certain areas or not enough. Although this can be judged visually, the image histogram is a convenient tool to examine which of the available gray values the image is using (Fig. 7-12). The minimum and maximum values and the shape of the histogram indicate the potential benefit of brightness and contrast enhancement operations.

Digital imaging software commonly includes a histogram tool and tools for the adjustment of brightness and contrast. Some also allow adjustment of the γ value. Changing the gamma value of an image selectively enhances image contrast in either the brighter or darker areas of the image. Adjustment of brightness, contrast, and γ value changes the original intensity values of the image (input) to new values (output). The operator can choose to make these changes permanent or to restore the image to its original settings. Figure 7-13 is a graphic representation of the relationship between input values (horizontal axis) and output values (vertical axis) with the

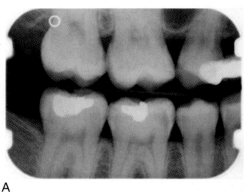
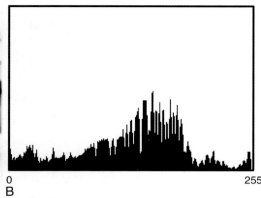

A                                              B

FIG. **7-12**   Digital image **(A)** with image histogram **(B).** Horizontal axis represents image gray levels (8 bits—256 levels); vertical axis represents number of pixels. Each bar indicates the number of pixels in the image with that particular gray level.

corresponding images and their histograms. Digital imaging software usually also includes tools for histogram equalization and contrast inversion. Histogram equalization is an enhancement operation that increases contrast between those image intensities abundantly present within the image while reducing contrast between image intensities that are used only sparsely. The actual effect of histogram equalization depends on the image content and may sometimes lead to unexpected degradation of image quality. Contrast inversion changes the radiographic positive image into a radiographic negative image. Although this may affect the subjective perception of the image content, the altered appearance is foreign to interpretive practice and is little used.

The effect of contrast enhancement on the diagnostic value of digital radiographs is controversial. Some studies show substantial benefits of contrast enhancement operations, whereas others have found only limited value or no improvement at all. The effect of contrast enhancement cannot easily be predicted. The key to successful image enhancement is to selectively enhance relevant radiographic signs without simultaneously enhancing distracting features.

### Sharpening and Smoothing

The purpose of sharpening and smoothing filters is to improve image quality by removing blur or noise. Noise is often categorized as high-frequency noise (speckling) or low-frequency noise (gradual intensity changes). Filters that smooth an image are sometimes called *despeckling filters* because they remove high-frequency noise. Filters that sharpen an image either remove low-frequency noise or enhance boundaries between regions with different intensities (edge enhancement). For the purposeful application of filters, it is important to know what type of noise the filters reduce and how that affects radiographic features of interest. Without this knowledge, important radiographic features may degrade or disappear as noise is removed. Similarly, edge enhancement of radiographic features of interest may enhance noise or enhance local contrast to the extent that it simulates disease. Sharpening and smoothing filters may make the dental radiographic images subjectively more appealing; however, there is no scientific evidence suggesting an increase in diagnostic value. The indiscriminate use of filters made available in most imaging software packages should be avoided if there is no scientific support for their clinical usefulness.

### Color

Most digital systems currently on the market provide opportunities for color conversion of gray-scale images, also called *pseudocolor.* Humans can distinguish many more colors than shades of gray. Transforming the gray values of a digital image into various colors could theoretically enhance the detection of objects within the image. However, this works only if all the gray values representing an object are unique for that object. Because this is rarely the case, boundaries between objects may change and new boundaries may be created. In most cases this will distract the observer from seeing the real content of the image and result in degraded image interpretation. Therefore color conversion of radiographs is neither diagnostically nor educationally useful. Some useful applications of color exist. When objects can be uniquely identified on the basis of a set of image features, color can be used to label or highlight these objects. The development of such criteria is a complex task, and only a limited number of successful studies have been reported in the literature.

### Digital Subtraction Radiography

When two images of the same object are registered and the image intensities of corresponding pixels are subtracted, a uniform difference image is produced. If there is a change in the radiographic attenuation between the baseline and follow-up examination, this change shows up as a brighter area when the change represents gain and as a darker area when the change represents loss (Fig. 7-14). The strength of digital subtraction radiography (DSR) is that it cancels out the complex anatomic background against which this change occurs. As a result, the conspicuousness of the change is greatly increased.

For DSR to be diagnostically useful, it is imperative that the baseline projection geometry and image intensities be reproduced. The projection geometry is defined by the position and orientation of the x-ray source, the patient, and the detector, relative to one another. If the projection geometry used for the follow-up image is different from the projection geometry used for the baseline image, the subtraction image will show these differences. They can be difficult to distinguish from actual changes within the patient, or they may hide actual change. Perfect reproduction of the projection geometry would be ideal but is impossible to achieve clinically. Although most changes can be reversed through image processing, horizontal and vertical beam angulation changes cannot be reversed and should be

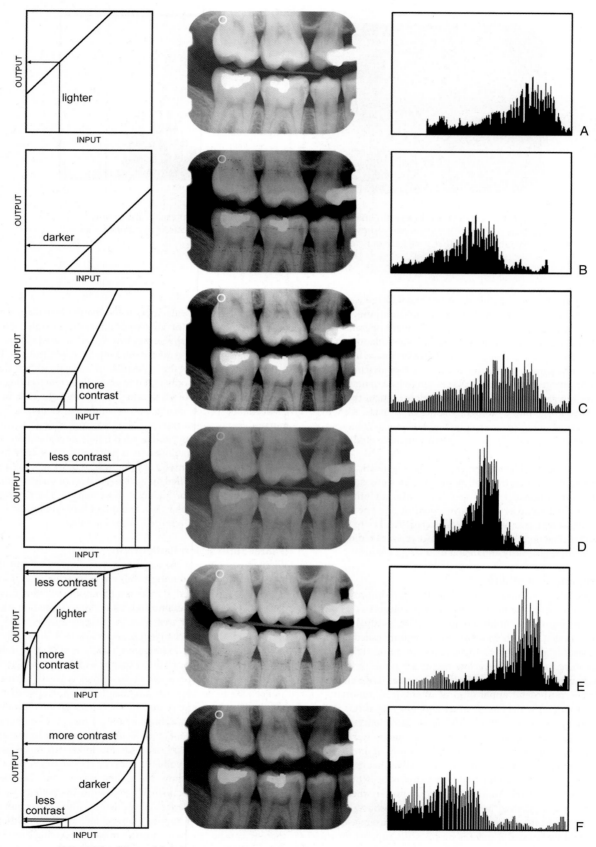

FIG. **7-13** Effect of brightness, contrast, and γ adjustment as illustrated by image transformation graphs *(left)*, digital images *(middle)*, and image histograms *(right)*. The image adjustments are relative to those of Figure 7-12. **A,** Increase in brightness. **B,** Decrease in brightness. **C,** Increase in contrast. **D,** Decrease in contrast. **E,** Increase in γ. **F,** Decrease in γ.

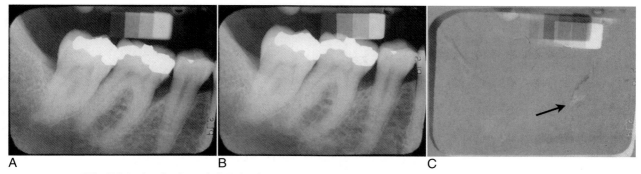

FIG. **7-14** Application of digital subtraction radiography for detection and quantification of periodontal bone healing. **A,** Baseline image. **B,** Standardized 1-year follow-up image. **C,** Subtraction image showing increase in bone *(arrow)*.

reproduced as accurately as possible. The actual tolerance of changes in the projection geometry depends on how much actual change needs to be detected. Although exact reproduction of the projection geometry is not strictly necessary, some form of mechanical standardization will reduce the reliance on image processing and will generally produce better results.

Subtraction images are well suited for acquiring quantitative information, such as linear, area, and density measurements. Methods used to make such measurements range from visual interpretation and manual measurement to computer-aided image analysis. Regardless of the analytic technique used, detecting and quantifying actual changes within a patient requires that factors affecting such measures be controlled.

## IMAGE ANALYSIS

Image analysis operations are designed to extract diagnostically relevant information from the image. This information can range from simple linear measurements to fully automated diagnosis. The use of image analysis tools brings with it the responsibility to understand their limitations. The accuracy and precision of a measurement are limited by the extent to which the image is a truthful and reproducible representation of the patient and by the operator's ability to make an exact measurement.

### Measurement

Digital imaging software provides a number of tools for image analysis. Digital rulers, densitometers, and a variety of other tools are readily available. These tools are usually digital equivalents of existing tools used in endodontics, orthodontics, periodontology, implantology, and other areas of dentistry (Fig. 7-15). Digital imaging has also added new tools that were not available with film-based radiography. The size and image intensity of any area within a digital radiograph can be measured. Tools are also being developed for measuring the complexity of the trabecular bone pattern. Such measurements can be useful as screening tools for osteoporosis assessment and for detecting other diseases.

### Diagnosis

One of the most challenging areas of research is the development of tools and procedures that automate the detection, classification, and quantification of radiographic signs of disease. The rationale for the use of such methods is to achieve early and accurate disease detection

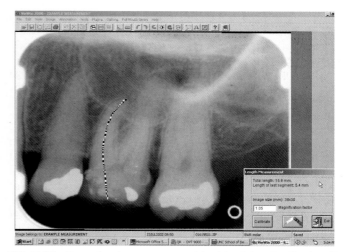

FIG. **7-15** Example of a measurement tool to determine the length of the crown and mesiobuccal root of the first molar. The measurement has been calibrated for a magnification factor of 1.05. The digital measurement tool is more versatile than the analog ruler; however, for both types of measurement tools, the apparent length remains dependent on the projection geometry.

by using reproducible and objective criteria. The development of automated image analysis operations is very complex and requires a thorough understanding of anatomy, pathology, and radiographic image formation. The three basic steps of image analysis are segmentation, feature extraction, and object classification. Of these, segmentation is the most critical step. The goal of segmentation is to simplify the image and reduce it to its basic components. This involves subdividing the image, thus separating objects from the background. Objects of interest are defined by the diagnostic task, for example, a tooth, a carious lesion, a bone level, or an implant. When image segmentation results in the detection of an object, a variety of features can be measured that assist in determining what the object represents. Such features may include measures of size and shape, relative location, average density, homogeneity, and texture. A unique set of values for a certain combination of features can lead to classification of the object. Automated cephalometric landmark identification is an example of this technology. Other dental examples include caries detection, classification of periodontal disease, and detection and quantification of periapical bone lesions. The success of many of these applications is highly dependent on specific imaging parameters. Very few provide reliable results when used clinically. This underscores the complexity of the radiographic image interpretation process.

## Image Storage

The use of digital imaging in dentistry requires an image archiving and management system that is very different from that used for conventional radiography. Storage of diagnostic images on magnetic or optical media raises a number of new issues that must be considered. The file size of dental digital radiographs varies considerably, ranging from approximately 200 kilobytes for intraoral images to as much as 6 megabytes for extraoral images. Storage and retrieval of these images in an average-sized dental practice is not a trivial issue. Fortunately, the development of new storage media and the continuing decrease in the price of a unit of storage has alleviated the capacity issue in dental radiography. The hard drive capacities of modern computers already exceed the storage needs of most dental practices.

The simplicity with which digital images can be modified through image processing poses a potential risk with respect to ensuring the integrity of the diagnostic information. Once in a digital format, critical image data can be deleted or modified. It is important that the software prevents the user from permanently deleting or modifying original image data, whether intentional or unintentional. Not all software programs provide such a safeguard. As the use of digital imaging in dentistry continues to expand, the implementation of standards for preserving original image data becomes urgent. It is also imperative that images and other important patient-related information are regularly stored on secondary external media. The use of computers for storing critical patient information mandates the design and use of a backup protocol. Box 7-1 shows some issues that need to be considered when a backup protocol is designed. Backup media suitable for external storage of digital radiographs include external hard drives, digital tapes, CDs, and DVDs. Downloading of data by telephone or dedicated data lines to off-site commercial storage sites is available through a number of vendors and provides essentially unlimited storage and backup. All these technologies are low in cost and have demonstrated reasonable reliability.

The purpose of image compression is to reduce the size of digital image files for archiving or transmission. In particular, storing extraoral images in a busy clinic may pose a challenge to storage capacity

and speed of image access. The purpose of file compression is to significantly reduce the file size while preserving critical image information.

Compression methods are generally classified as lossless or lossy. *Lossless* methods do not discard any image data, and an exact copy of the image is reproduced after decompression. Most compression techniques take advantage of redundancies in the image, which can be expressed in simpler terms. The maximum compression rate for lossless compression is usually less than 3:1. *Lossy* compression methods achieve higher levels of compression by discarding image data. Empiric evidence suggests that this does not necessarily affect the diagnostic quality of an image. Compression rates of 12:1 and 14:1 were shown to have no appreciable effect on caries diagnosis. For determining endodontic file length, a rate of 25:1 was diagnostically equivalent to the uncompressed image. A compression rate of 28:1 was acceptable for the subjective evaluation of image quality and the detection of artificial lesions in panoramic radiographs.

Version 3.0 of the DICOM (Digital Imaging and Communications in Medicine) standard adopted JPEG (Joint Photographic Experts Group) as the compression method, which provides a range of compression levels. Other types of image compression methods, such as wavelet compression, are being investigated for their use in medical imaging. Although the use of low and medium levels of lossy compression appear to have little effect on the diagnostic value of dental images, the application of lossy compression should be used with caution and only after its effect for specific diagnostic tasks has been evaluated. With the continuing increase in the capacity of storage media and the widespread use of high-speed data communication lines, lossy compression of dental radiographs is rapidly becoming obsolete. At the same time, new digital image receptors are generating images with more and more pixels and more bits per pixel, thus increasing storage needs. Image compression negates to some extent the gain from such high-end detectors. Whether we need high resolution detectors and whether we can use image compression should be dictated by diagnostic criteria. Current evidence suggests that detector quality and moderate image compression have a limited impact on diagnostic outcomes.

## Systems Compatibility

The development of digital imaging systems for dental radiography has largely been driven by industry. Manufacturers have adopted and developed technologies according to individual needs and philosophies. As a result, image formats among systems from different vendors are not standardized, and image archival, retrieval, and display systems are often incompatible. Despite the proprietary nature of imaging software, it is possible to transfer images from one vendor's system to the other. Most systems provide image export and import tools using a variety of generic image formats, such as JPEG and TIFF (tagged image file format). However, the process of transferring images through export-import procedures is cumbersome. It requires a number of steps, and the operator needs to ensure that the right images are imported into the proper patient folder. It can also not be assumed that the display and calibration of imported and native images will be the same.

Clearly, exporting and importing is not the method of choice when digital imaging is going to be used on a large scale. It has long been recognized that the adoption of a standard for transferring images and associated information between digital imaging devices in medicine

---

**BOX 7-1**
*Digital Image Backup Considerations*

- Type of backup media
- Time and method of backup
- Backup interval
- Storage location of backup media
- Recovery time
- Recovery reliability
- Future compatibility of backup technology

and dentistry is necessary. The American College of Radiology and the National Electrical Manufacturers Association formed a joint committee to develop a standard for digital imaging systems. A large number of professional organizations have contributed to this complex development process, which has resulted in the current standard, known as the *Digital Imaging and Communications in Medicine (DICOM) standard*. Various dental organizations, including the American Dental Association, are playing an active role in defining aspects of the standard related to dentistry. The DICOM standard is not a static set of rules dictating to manufacturers how to build imaging devices. Rather it is an evolving document addressing the interoperability of medical and dental imaging and information systems. Manufacturers of digital imaging systems for dental radiography are responding to the call to adopt the DICOM standard. Not all systems are currently conforming to the DICOM standard, and those that do may not conform to every aspect of the standard. The successful adoption of digital imaging in dentistry requires interoperability of all devices. It is likely that manufacturers do not want to be left behind and that the market will weed out those that are *noncompliant*. Dentists using different vendors with DICOM-compliant imaging devices will be able to exchange images seamlessly.

## Clinical Considerations

Some fundamental differences from film in the clinical handling of digital receptors should be noted (Table 7-1). Because digital receptors are intended to be reusable, they must be handled with greater care than their film counterparts. Indeed, in certain situations film may be intentionally damaged through bending to accommodate patient anatomy. This is never the case with digital receptors. Examples of common image artifacts found on images made with solid-state or PSP systems are shown in Box 7-2. PSP plates are susceptible to bending and scratching during handling that induce permanent artifacts in the receptor. These artifacts obscure information of potential diagnostic importance and may necessitate disposal of the receptor and repeat imaging of the patient. Because of the inability of digital detectors to be bent to accommodate patient anatomy, new imaging strategies must be used for some patients. It may not be possible to consistently capture the distal surface of the canine on premolar views. An additional projection may be required to adequately visualize this surface.

A significant potential problem with most PSP systems is the inability to distinguish images from plates that have been exposed backward. Unlike film packets, which incorporate a lead foil with

*Text continued on p. 98.*

---

### TABLE 7-1
### *Clinical Comparison of Intraoral Imaging Alternatives*

| IMAGING STEP | FILM | CCD/CMOS | PSP |
|---|---|---|---|
| Receptor preparation | None | (1) Place protective plastic sleeve over receptor<br>(2) Receptor must be connected to computer and patient identifying information entered for acquisition/archiving software | (1) "Erase" plates<br>(2) Package plates in protective plastic envelope |
| Receptor placement | (1) Numerous generic film holding devices are available<br>(2) Film may be bent to accommodate anatomy | (1) Specialized receptor holder specific for manufacturer's receptor may limit options<br>(2) Receptor inflexibility and bulk limit placement options<br>(3) Receptor cable must be carefully routed out of patient mouth<br>(4) Patient discomfort more likely than with film or PSP | (1) Many receptor holders used for film may be adapted for PSP plates<br>(2) Bending of receptor may irreversibly damage it |
| Exposure | Simple exposure | Computer must be activated before exposure | Simple exposure |
| Processing | (1) Dark, light-safe environment in form of darkroom or daylight loader required<br>(2) Processor chemistry must be prepared or replenished<br>(3) Chemical temperature must be warmed, or processing time must be adjusted to accommodate temperature<br>(4) Films must be removed from wrapper; lead foil must be separated for recycling | Image acquisition and display is almost immediate | (1) Dimly light environment desirable to prevent loss of image information<br>(2) Processor must be programmed with patient and detector information so that images are identified, preprocessed, and stored properly<br>(3) Protective wrapper must be removed from plates<br>(4) Plates must be loaded on drum systems |

*Continued*

TABLE **7-1**
*Clinical Comparison of Intraoral Imaging Alternatives—cont'd*

| IMAGING STEP | FILM | CCD/CMOS | PSP |
|---|---|---|---|
| Display preparation | (1) Films may be placed in a variety of film mounts<br>(2) Mounts must be labeled with patient-identifying information | (1) Software may be configured to place image in appropriate position in digital mount when exposures are made in a predetermined sequence; otherwise, images must be individually placed in mount | (1) Images must be individually placed in mount<br>(2) Images may need to be digitally rotated to achieve proper orientation |
| Display | (1) A room with subdued lighting and a masked viewbox are optimal<br>(2) Any light source (including the operatory window or ceiling light) will permit a quick evaluation of the image | Same considerations apply to all digital receptor types<br>(1) A room with subdued lighting is optimal for interpretation activities<br>(2) A computer and display with appropriate software are necessary; viewing is restricted to the location of the computer<br>(3) Laptop computers increase flexibility of computer placement but may reduce display quality<br>(4) Size of the display will restrict the numbers of images that may be viewed simultaneously; more time is required to open/close or expand contract images when interpreting a series of images | |
| Image duplication | Quality of duplication is always inferior to original and is sometimes nondiagnostic | (1) Electronic copies may be stored on a variety of media without loss of image quality<br>(2) Output on film or paper is inferior and is often nondiagnostic unless appropriate combinations of expensive printers and papers or film are used | |

BOX **7-2**
*Common Problems in Digital Image Receptor Exposure, Processing, and Handling*
Enrique Platin

### Noisy Images
Although the brightness of these images has been adjusted to display similar average gray values, notice the noisy appearance of the underexposed bitewing radiograph (Fig. 7-16, *A*, 0.032 second) compared with the properly exposed radiograph (Fig. 7-16, *B*, 0.32 second).

PSP image degradation as a result of excessive exposure to ambient light between image acquisition and plate scanning (Fig. 7-17). This type of noise resembles that of x-ray underexposure.

### Nonuniform Image Density
Partial exposure of PSP plates to excessive ambient light prior to scanning results in nonuniform image density (Fig. 7-18, *A*). This happens when plates are overlapped while exposed to ambient light (Fig. 7-18, *B*).

### Distorted Images
Bending of PSP plates during intraoral placement: moderate bending (Fig. 7-19, *A*), retake of *A* (Fig. 7-19, *B*), severe bending (Fig. 7-19, *C*), and retake of *C* (Fig. 7-19, *D*).

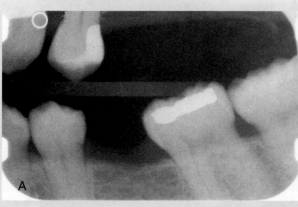
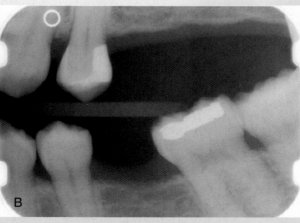

FIG. **7-16**

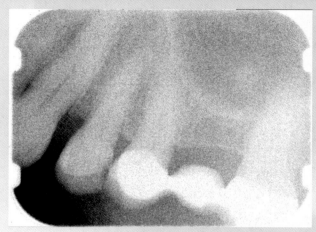

FIG. **7-17**

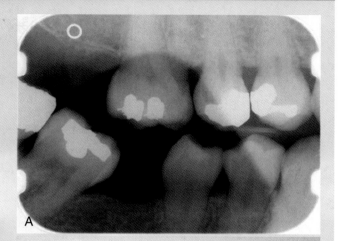

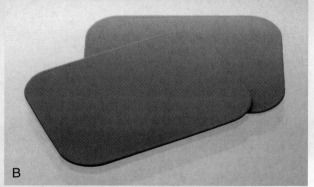

FIG. **7-18**

### Double Images

PSP double image on incisor periapical radiograph resulting from incomplete erasure of previous image of posterior periapical region (Fig. 7-20, *A*) and retake (Fig. 7-20, *B*).

More examples of double images resulting from incomplete erasure of PSP receptors: posterior periapical radiograph with double image (Fig. 7-21, *A*), retake of *A* (Fig. 7-21, *B*), anterior periapical radiograph with double image (Fig. 7-21, *C*), and retake of *C* (Fig. 7-21, *D*).

### Damaged Image Receptors

Scratched phosphor surface mimicking root canal filling (Fig. 7-22, *A*) and retake (Fig. 7-22, *B*).

Image artifacts resulting from excessive bending of the PSP plate (Fig. 7-23, *A*) and excessive bending has resulted in permanent damage to the phosphor plate (Fig. 7-23, *B*).

PSP circular artifact as a result of plate damage (Fig. 7-24, *A*) and localized swelling of the protective coating from disinfectant solution on work surface (Fig. 7-24, *B*).

PSP image artifact resulting from plate surface contamination (Fig. 7-25, *A*). This artifact was caused by a glove powder smudge that prevented proper scanning of the affected area of the PSP plate (Fig. 7-25, *B*). Contaminants combined with skin oils may permanently damage the phosphor plate surface.

Malfunctioning CCD sensor resulting from rough handling (dropped sensor). The sensor produces geometric image artifacts (Fig. 7-26, *A* and *B*).

### Improper Use of Image Processing

Improper use of image processing tools, such as filters, may result in false-positive findings. An edge enhancement filter was applied to the panoramic image, which produced radiolucencies at restoration edges simulating recurrent caries (Fig. 7-27, *A*). These radiolucencies are not present in a follow-up intraoral image (Fig. 7-27, *B*).

*Continued*

BOX **7-2**
*Common Problems in Digital Image Receptor Exposure, Processing, and Handling—cont'd*

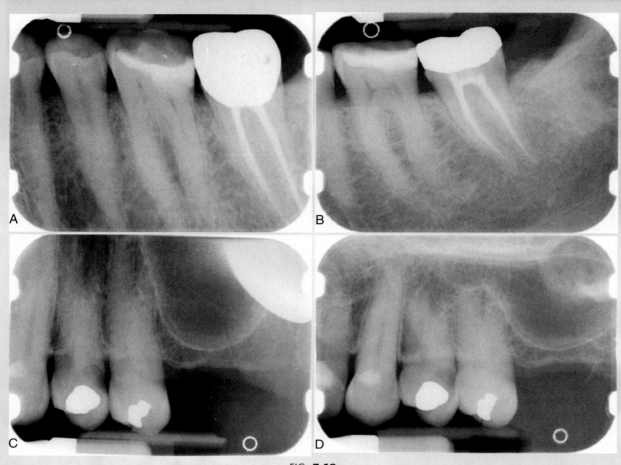

FIG. **7-19**

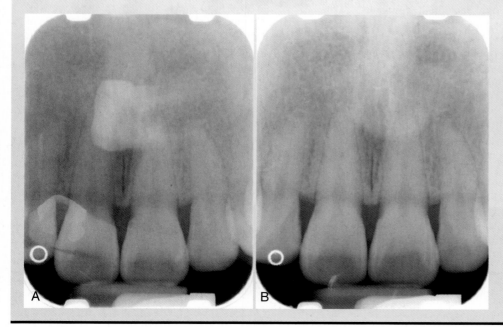

FIG. **7-20**

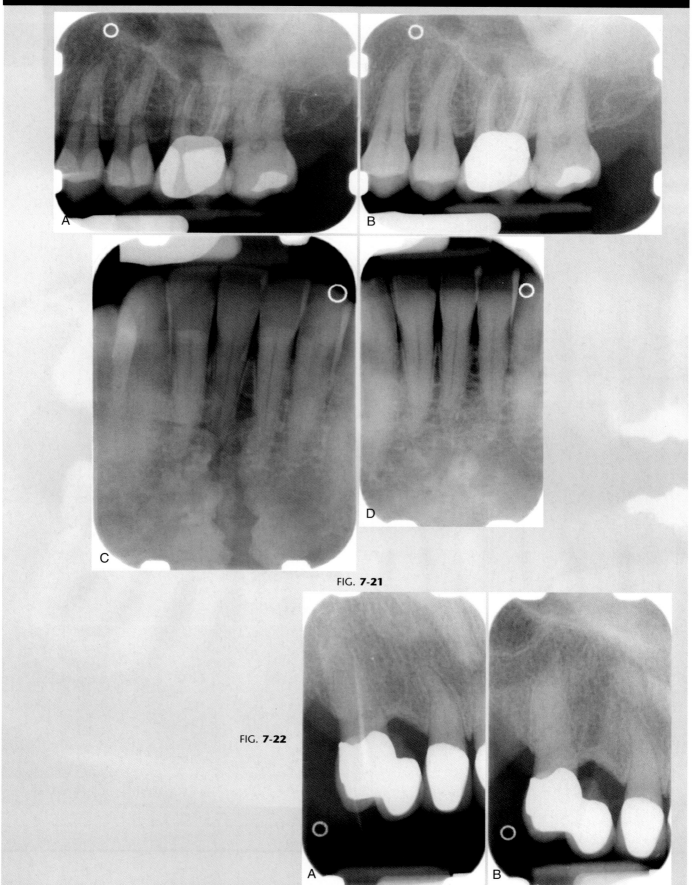

FIG. **7-21**

FIG. **7-22**

BOX **7-2**
*Common Problems in Digital Image Receptor Exposure, Processing, and Handling—cont'd*

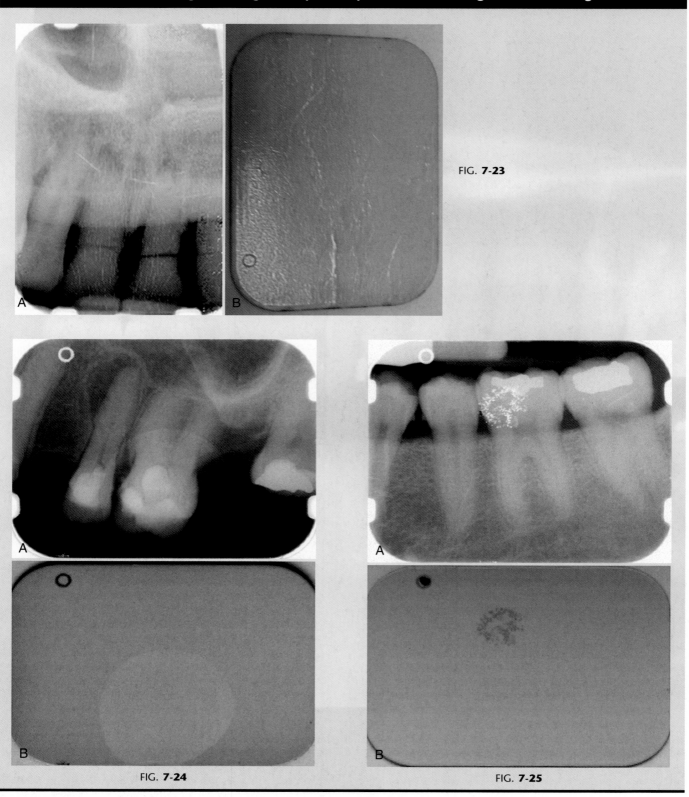

FIG. **7-23**

FIG. **7-24**

FIG. **7-25**

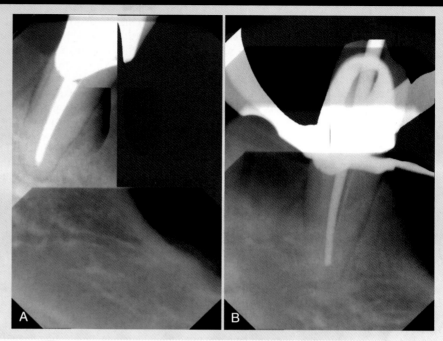

FIG. **7-26**

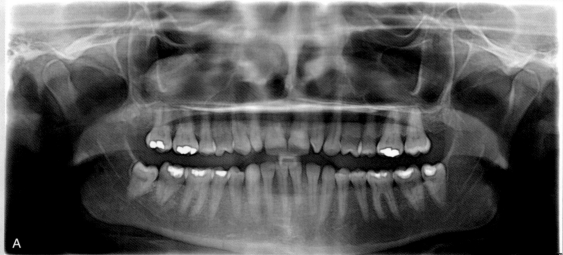

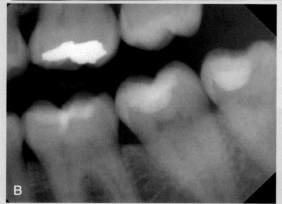

FIG. **7-27**

a characteristic embossed pattern that results in an underexposed image of the anatomy with the pattern artifact when exposed backward, PSP images have little x-ray attenuation from the polyester base. It is much too easy for inattentive radiographers to mount these digital images on the contralateral position from their true side. One can imagine the liability that could occur from diagnosing and treating disease on the opposite side of the actual lesion. To date, only the Soredex Optime system has addressed this issue by incorporating a round metal disk on the back of intraoral plates. (See Fig. 7-7.) This marker becomes visible on the image if the imaging plate is exposed backward. The appearance of the marker on the image does not fully obscure the anatomic information and these images can be "mirrored" with imaging software tools without the need for repeated exposure.

Infection control is also an issue with digital receptors. Digital receptors cannot be sterilized by conventional means. They may be disinfected by wiping with mild agents such as isopropyl alcohol but

should not be immersed in disinfecting solutions. The adage that "you can autoclave a digital receptor . . . once" stems from the fact that heat will ruin electronic components in CCD and CMOS sensors and will distort the polyester base of PSP plates. Another potential drawback to drum-based PSP systems is the 2- to 5-minute cycle time required by some devices for plate scanning. During this time, no additional plates may be processed. With film and non–drum-based PSP scanners, there is less delay between the times when additional films or plates may be "fed" into the processor. Although each of the preceding concerns are of potential importance, the advantage of eliminating chemical processing in digital systems should not be overlooked. The time required to properly monitor and maintain a film processor is significant. Too often, insufficient attention is paid to this critical aspect of film radiography. Digital systems may not save the time gained by eliminating film processing, but they will eliminate the loss in diagnostic quality that occurs when insufficient time and effort is spent on film processing quality assurance.

TABLE **7-2**

## Comparison of Physical Properties of Film, Charge-Coupled Device, Complementary Metallic Oxide Semiconductor, and Photostimulable Phosphor Receptors

| FEATURE | TECHNICAL COMMENT | CLINICAL COMMENT |
|---|---|---|
| Spatial resolution | Intraoral systems:<br>Film > CCD = CMOS > PSP<br>Panoramic systems:<br>Film = CCD = PSP<br>Cephalometric systems:<br>Film > CCD = PSP | The limits of resolution for digital systems are readily appreciated when magnifying these images. With magnification a "blocky" or "pixelated" appearance is evident. Resolution of panoramic systems is limited by mechanical motion to about 5 lp/mm. |
| Exposure latitude | PSP >> CCD = CMOS ≥ film | Because of the wide latitude of PSP and the automatic brightness and contrast "optimization" by image acquisition software, use of more x-ray exposure than is necessary is possible. |
| Receptor dimensions | For equivalent imaged area, Film = PSP < CCD = CMOS | The "active area" of CCD and CMOS receptors is smaller than the surface area because of other electronic components within the plastic housing. |
| Time for image acquisition | CCD = CMOS << PSP = film | Rapid image acquisition may be important for endodontic procedures or during implant placement. |
| Image quality | Subjective quality is best with film when carefully exposed and well processed. | Digital and film imaging are not significantly different when used for common diagnostic tasks. |
| Image adjustment/processing | Improves appearance of digital images. | Takes time; may not improve diagnostic performance. |
| Cost | Initial costs of digital systems are greater than film. Subsequent costs vary greatly depending on receptor wear and tear or abuse. | Manufacturers' estimates of life expectancy of reusable receptors are perhaps overly optimistic. |
| Reliability | Mechanical problems affect digital PSP and film systems. Software reliability varies greatly among manufacturers. Changes in unrelated computer components and software can cause digital systems to malfunction. | Digital systems fail when problems occur with receptors during image acquisition, or with computers during image processing, archiving, and display. |
| Image storage and retrieval | Data backup is critical for digital systems. | Films can be misfiled and lost or be damaged by poor storage conditions. Digital data can be lost as a result of failures in power supplies or storage media and operator error. |
| Transmitting images to others | Rapidly done with digital images. | Facilitates communication between colleagues or with insurance companies. |

## Conclusion

Dental practitioners commonly ask, "Which is better, film or digital imaging?" There is no simple answer to this question (Tables 7-1 and 7-2). Reported technical properties of resolution, contrast, and latitude are confounded by a lack of standardization in the assessment of these characteristics. From a diagnostic standpoint most studies suggest that digital performance is not clinically different from film for typical diagnostic tasks such as caries diagnosis. The "look and feel" of digital displays is distinctly different from film viewing, and some practitioners may find this difference disconcerting. A basic understanding of computers and a mastery of common computing skills is essential for viewing digital images. Beyond this, learning the peculiarities and vagaries of a particular acquisition and display software will take time and may not be intuitive. Multiple mouse clicks through multiple menus may be required to view a full-mouth series of images. This may modestly increase the time required to complete the interpretative process.

In selecting an imaging system, other issues should be considered. Digital images avoid environmental pollutants encountered with film processing, but what about the environmental impact associated with the disposal of broken or obsolete electronic equipment? The initial financial outlay for digital imaging hardware makes these systems more expensive than film. Manufacturers are quick to point out that the costs of film or digital systems should be amortized over the life of the equipment and consumables; however, the life expectancy of newer digital systems is highly speculative. Mishandling of digital system components can catastrophically shorten any projected life expectancy. And what price should we place on the ability to instantly transmit images and to integrate them into a fully electronic record? There are no universal answers to these questions. They must be asked and answered according to the needs and objectives of individual dental practices. As practice patterns and technology change with time, the answers will also change. Although the details of the image in our crystal ball have yet to resolve, the trends of increasing adoption of digital imaging and continuing technologic innovation makes the future of digital imaging in dentistry certain.

## BIBLIOGRAPHY
### DIGITAL DETECTORS AND DISPLAYS

Abreu M Jr, Mol A, Ludlow JB: Performance of RVGui sensor and Kodak Ektaspeed Plus film for proximal caries detection, *Oral Surg Oral Med Oral Pathol Oral Radiol Endod* 91:381-385, 2001.

Couture RA, Hildebolt C: Quantitative dental radiography with a new photostimulable phosphor system, *Oral Surg Oral Med Oral Pathol Oral Radiol Endod* 89:498-508, 2000.

Hildebolt CF, Couture RA, Whiting BR: Dental photostimulable phosphor radiography, *Dent Clin North Am* 44:273-297, 2000.

Sanderink GC, Miles DA: Intraoral detectors: CCD, CMOS, TFT, and other devices, *Dent Clin North Am* 44:249-255, v, 2000.

Van der Stelt PF: Principles of digital imaging, *Dent Clin North Am* 44:237-248, v, 2000.

### IMAGE PROCESSING

Analoui M: Radiographic image enhancement, I: spatial domain techniques, *Dentomaxillofac Radiol* 30:1-9, 2001.

Analoui M: Radiographic digital image enhancement, II: transform domain techniques, *Dentomaxillofac Radiol* 30:65-77, 2001.

Baxes GA: *Digital image processing: principles and applications*, New York, 1994, John Wiley.

Gonzalez R, Wood R: *Digital image processing*, ed 3, 2007, Upper Saddle River, NJ, Prentice Hall.

Gröndahl H-G, Gröndahl K, Webber R: A digital subtraction technique for dental radiography, *Oral Surg Oral Med Oral Pathol* 55:96-102, 1983.

Lehmann T, Gröndahl H-G, Benn D: Computer-based registration for digital subtraction in dental radiology, *Dentomaxillofac Radiol* 29:323-346, 2000.

Mol A: Image processing tools for dental applications, *Dent Clin North Am* 44:299-318, 2000.

Russ JC: *The image process handbook*, ed 4, Boca Raton, Fla, 2002, CRC Press.

Ruttimann U, Webber R, Schmidt E: A robust digital method for film contrast correction in subtraction radiography, *J Periodont Res* 21:486-495, 1986.

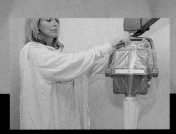

# CHAPTER 8

# Radiographic Quality Assurance and Infection Control

A quality assurance program in radiology is a series of procedures designed to ensure optimal and consistent operation of each component in the imaging chain. When all components are functioning properly, the result is consistently high-quality radiographs made with low exposure to patients and office personnel.

The goal of an *infection control program in radiology* is a series of procedures designed to avoid cross-contamination among patients and between patients and operators.

## Radiographic Quality Assurance

Because radiographs are indispensable for patient diagnosis, the dentist must ensure that optimal exposure and film processing conditions are maintained. To reach this goal, a quality assurance program includes evaluation of the performance of x-ray machines, manual and automatic processing procedures, image receptors, and viewing conditions. Optimization of these components results in the most diagnostic images and the lowest exposure for patients. It is best if one individual is given the responsibility for implementing the quality assurance program and to take corrective action when indicated. Most of these steps are quickly accomplished yet can have a significant influence on radiographic quality (Box 8-1).

### DAILY TASKS

Several tasks should be performed daily to ensure excellent radiographs.

### Compare Radiographs with Reference Film

One of the most common causes of poor radiographs is poor film processing in the darkroom, in particular the use of depleted solutions. A simple and effective means for constant monitoring of the quality of images produced in an office is to check daily films against a reference film. Soon after film-processing solutions are replaced, mount a patient film that has been properly exposed and processed with exact time-temperature technique on a corner of the viewbox. This image, with optimal density and contrast, serves as a reference for the radiographs made in the following days and weeks (Fig. 8-1). All subsequent images should be compared with this reference film.

Comparison of daily images with the reference film may reveal problems before they interfere with the diagnostic quality of the images. When a problem is identified, it is important to determine the probable source and to take corrective action. For instance, if the processing solutions have become depleted, the resultant radiographs are light and have reduced contrast. Both developer and fixer should be changed when degradation of the image quality is evident. Light images may also result from cold solutions or insufficient developing time. Dark images may be caused by excessive developing time, developer that is too warm, or light leaks.

There are two methods that are more accurate than a reference film but require additional equipment and more time to perform. These are sensitometry/densitometry and the use of a step wedge.

### Make Step-Wedge Test of Processing System

The most accurate and rigorous method of testing film-processing solutions is to use a sensitometer and densitometer. A sensitometer exposes film to a calibrated light pattern. After processing, a densitometer is used to measure the optical density of each step in the test pattern of the film exposed by the sensitometer. A change in the density readings from day to day indicates a problem in the darkroom.

For most dental offices a variation of this method using a step-wedge test provides accurate monitoring of day-to-day processing conditions. This information is used to measure the speed of the imaging system and image contrast. Both are sensitive measures of the processing environment. A step wedge is readily made with the lead foil from film packets. Stack five sheets together and staple at one end (Fig. 8-2). Cut off four fifths of the top layer, three fifths of the second layer, two fifths of the third layer, and one fifth of the fourth layer to create a five-step wedge. Lay the wedge on top of a film packet and expose with the usual setting for an adult bitewing view. The resultant image should show five steps from dark to light. Save the first film after changing to fresh processing solution for comparison with images made on subsequent days. Monitor the processing solutions at the beginning of each day with a step-wedge image to ensure that the processing system is operational for patient care.

### Enter Findings in Retake Log

Another simple and effective means of reducing the number of faulty radiographs is to keep a retake log. Record all errors for images that must be re-exposed.

### Replenish Processing Solutions

At the beginning of each work day, check the levels of the processing solutions and replenish if necessary. Replenish the developer with fresh developing solution and the fixer with fresh fixing solution.

### Check Temperature of Processing Solutions

At the beginning of each work day, check the temperature of the processing solutions. The solutions must reach the optimal temperature before use—68° F (20° C) for manual processing and 82° F (28° C) for heated automatic processors. The instructions accompanying the film and processor verify the optimal temperature. Unheated automatic processors should be located away from windows or heaters that may cause their temperature to vary during the day. Proper temperature regulation is required for accurate time-temperature processing.

## BOX 8-1
### Schedule of Radiographic Quality Assurance Procedures

#### Daily
- Check processing by comparing radiographs with reference film or with step wedge
- Enter causes of retakes in a log
- Replenish processing solutions
- Check temperature of processing solutions

#### Weekly
- Replace processing solutions
- Clean processing equipment
- Clean viewboxes
- Review retake log

#### Monthly
- Check darkroom safelighting
- Clean intensifying screens
- Rotate film stock
- Check exposure charts
- Inspect leaded aprons and thyroid collars

#### Yearly
- Calibrate x-ray machine

## WEEKLY TASKS

### Replace Processing Solutions
The replacement frequency of processing solutions depends primarily on the rate of use of the solutions but also on the size of tanks, whether a cover is used, and the temperature of the solutions. In most offices the solutions should be changed weekly or every other week. The results of the step-wedge test will help determine the proper frequency.

### Clean Processing Equipment
Regular cleaning of the processing equipment is necessary for optimal operation. Clean the solution tanks of manual and automatic processing equipment when the solutions are changed. Clean the rollers of automatic film processors weekly according to the manufacturer's instructions. After cleaning, rinse the tanks and rollers twice as long as the manufacturer recommends to prevent the cleaner from interfering with the action of the film-processing solutions.

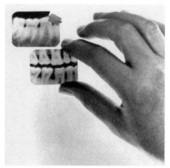

FIG. **8-1** Radiographs should be checked daily against a reference film made with fresh solutions. As processing solutions become exhausted, the daily images become increasingly light and lose contrast. When these changes are clear, both the developer and the fixer should be changed. (Courtesy C.L. Crabtree, DDS, Bureau of Radiological Health, Rockville, Md.)

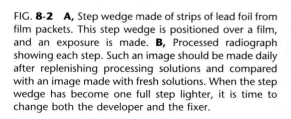
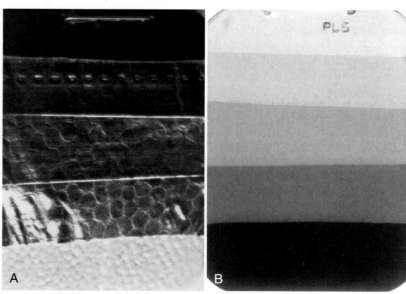

FIG. **8-2   A,** Step wedge made of strips of lead foil from film packets. This step wedge is positioned over a film, and an exposure is made. **B,** Processed radiograph showing each step. Such an image should be made daily after replenishing processing solutions and compared with an image made with fresh solutions. When the step wedge has become one full step lighter, it is time to change both the developer and the fixer.

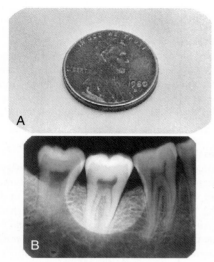

FIG. **8-3** Penny test for unsafe illumination. **A,** A penny is left on the exposed duplicate film from the double-film pack on the working surface during the time that any film would be opened (usually about 5 minutes). **B,** If the processed radiograph shows an outline of the penny, the film is being fogged by inappropriate safelighting conditions.

### Clean Viewboxes

Clean viewboxes weekly to remove any particles or defects that may interfere with film interpretation.

### Review Retake Log

Review the retake record weekly and identify any recurring problems with film processing conditions or operator technique. Use this information to educate staff or to initiate corrective actions.

## MONTHLY TASKS

### Check Darkroom Safelighting

Film becomes fogged in the darkroom because of inappropriate safelight filters, excessive exposure to safelights, and stray light from other sources. Such films are dark, show low contrast, and have a muddy gray appearance. Inspect the darkroom monthly to assess the integrity of the safelights (preferably GBX-2 filters with 15-watt bulbs). The glass filter should be intact, with no cracks. To check for light leaks in a darkroom, turn off all lights, allow vision to accommodate to the dark, and check for light leaks, especially around doors and vents. Mark light leaks with chalk or masking tape. Weather stripping is useful for sealing light leaks under doors.

The following simple penny test can be used monthly to evaluate for fogging caused by inappropriate safelighting conditions (Fig. 8-3):

1. Open the packet of an exposed film and place the test film in the area where the films are usually unwrapped and clipped on the film hanger.
2. Place a penny on the film and leave it in this position for the approximate time required to unwrap and mount a full-mouth set of films, usually about 5 minutes.
3. Develop the test film as usual. If the image of the penny is visible on the resultant film, the room is not light-safe for the particular film tested. Each type of film used in the office should be tested to measure the integrity of the darkroom.

| Projection | Exposure time | |
| | Seconds | Impulses |
| --- | --- | --- |
| Adult periapicals | | |
| Incisors | 0.25 | 15 |
| Premolars | 0.30 | 18 |
| Molars | 0.35 | 21 |
| Occlusal | 0.40 | 24 |
| Adult bitewings | | |
| Premolar | 0.30 | 18 |
| Molar | 0.35 | 21 |
| Edentulous periapicals | | |
| Incisors | 0.20 | 12 |
| Premolars | 0.25 | 15 |
| Molars | 0.30 | 18 |
| Occlusal | 0.35 | 21 |
| Children | | |
| Anterior periapicals | 0.25 | 15 |
| Posterior periapicals | 0.25 | 15 |
| Bitewing | 0.25 | 15 |
| Occlusal | 0.30 | 18 |

X-ray machine: brand name
Location: room
mA: 15
kVp: 70
E-speed film: brand name

FIG. **8-4** Sample wall chart showing identification information for x-ray machine, film type, mA and kVp settings, and appropriate exposure times for various anatomic locations and patient sizes. The optimal exposure times must be determined empirically in each office because they vary with the machine settings used, source-to-skin distance, and other factors.

### Clean Intensifying Screens

Clean all intensifying screens in panoramic and cephalometric film cassettes monthly. The presence of scratches or debris results in recurring light areas on the resultant images. The foam supporting the screens must be intact and capable of holding both screens closely against the film. If close contact between the film and screens is not maintained, the image loses sharpness.

### Rotate Film Stock

Dental x-ray film is quite stable when it is properly handled. Store it in a cool, dry facility away from a radiation source. Rotate stock when new film is received so that old film does not accumulate in storage. Always use the oldest film first, but never after its expiration date.

### Check Exposure Charts

Each month inspect exposure tables listing the proper peak kilovoltage (kVp), milliamperes (mA), and exposure times for making radiographs of each region of the oral cavity that are posted by each x-ray machine (Fig. 8-4). Verify that the information is legible and accurate. These tables help ensure that all operators use the appropriate exposure factors. Typically the mA is fixed at its highest setting; the kVp is fixed, usually at 70 kVp; and the exposure time is varied to account for patient size and location of the area of interest in the mouth. Exposure times are initially determined empirically. Careful time-temperature processing (described in Chapter 6) must be used with fresh solutions during this initial determination of exposure times.

## Check Leaded Aprons and Collars

Visually inspect leaded aprons and collars for evidence of cracking. A fluoroscopic examination performed by a qualified individual can confirm any cracks in the lead shielding. Replace as necessary. Such cracking is usually caused by folding the shields when not in use. It can be minimized by hanging the aprons from a hook or draping them over a handrail.

## YEARLY TASKS: CALIBRATE X-RAY MACHINE

X-ray machines are generally quite stable, and only rarely is a malfunction of the machine the cause of poor radiographs. Accordingly, machines need to be calibrated only annually unless a specific problem is identified or substantive repair is necessary that may affect operation. Usually dental service companies or health physicists should make these machine measurements because of the specialized equipment and knowledge required. The following parameters should be measured:

1. X-ray output. Use a radiation dosimeter to measure the intensity and reproducibility of radiation output (Fig. 8-5). Acceptable values are shown in Figure 3-3.
2. Collimation and beam alignment. The field diameter for dental intraoral x-ray machines should be no greater than 2¾ inches. The tip of the position-indicating device (PID), or aiming cylinder, should be closely aligned with the x-ray beam.

   For panoramic machines, the beam exiting the patient should not be larger than the film slit holding the film cassette. This may be tested by taping dental films in front of and behind the slit. A pin stick should be made through both films to allow subsequent realignment. Expose, process, and realign both films. The exposure to the film in front of the slit should be comparable in size to the film exposure behind the slit. Service is required if the front film exposure is larger than or not well oriented with the film exposure behind the slit.

3. Beam energy. The kVp or half-value layer (HVL) of the beam should be measured to ensure that the beam has sufficient energy for film exposure without excessive soft tissue dosage. Measurement of kVp requires specialized equipment. It should be accurate within 5 kVp. Measurement of HVL requires a dosimeter. The HVL should be at least 1.5 mm aluminum (Al) at 70 kVp and 2.5 mm Al at 90 kVp.
4. Timer. Electric pulse counters count the number of pulses generated by an x-ray machine during a preset time interval. The timer should be accurate and reproducible.
5. mA. Verify the linearity of the mA control if two or more mA settings are available on the machine. Make an exposure using the usual adult bitewing setting. Then reduce the mA to the lower value and select another exposure time, ensuring that the product of the mA and time in seconds (impulses) is the same as for the adult bitewing. For example, if the machine has 10- and 15-mA settings, and 15 mA and 24 impulses are used for adult bitewings, select 15 mA and 24 impulses for the first exposure and measure the dose. Make a second exposure at 10 mA and 36 impulses and measure the dose. The dose at each exposure combination should be the same (15 × 24 = 10 × 36). A discrepancy implies nonlinearity in the mA control or a fault in the timer. The step wedge described previously may also be used in place of the dosimeter. In this case the density of each step of each image should be the same.

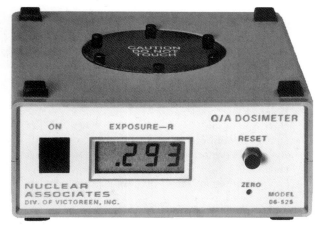

FIG. **8-5**  Device for measuring exposure output of an x-ray machine. The aiming cylinder of the x-ray machine is positioned on the center of the top and an exposure made. The display on the front gives the output in roentgens.

6. Tube head stability. The tube head should be stable when placed around the patient's head, and it should not drift during the exposure. When the tube head is not stable, service is necessary to adjust the suspension mechanism.
7. Focal spot size. Measure the size of the focal spot because it may become enlarged with excessive heat buildup within an x-ray machine. An enlarged focal spot contributes to geometric fuzziness in the resultant image. A specialized piece of equipment is required for this test.

## Infection Control

Dental personnel and patients are at increased risk for acquiring tuberculosis, herpes viruses, upper respiratory infections, and hepatitis strains A through E. After the recognition of acquired immunodeficiency syndrome (AIDS) in the 1980s, rigorous hygienic procedures were introduced in dental offices. The primary goal of infection control procedures is to prevent cross-contamination between patients and between patients and health care providers. The potential for cross-contamination in dental radiography is great. An operator's hands may become contaminated by contact with a patient's mouth and saliva-contaminated films and film holders. The operator then must adjust the x-ray tube head and x-ray machine control panel settings to make the exposure. Cross-contamination also may occur when operators open film packets to process the films in the darkroom. The procedures described in the following sections minimize or eliminate cross-contamination (Box 8-2). Each dental office or practice should have a written policy describing its infection control practices. It is best if one individual in a practice, usually the dentist, assumes responsibility for implementing these procedures. This person also educates other members of the practice.

### APPLY UNIVERSAL PRECAUTIONS

Universal precautions are infection control guidelines designed to protect workers from exposure to diseases spread by blood and certain body fluids. Under universal precautions, all human blood and saliva are treated as if known to be infectious for human immunodeficiency

Apply universal precautions
- Wear gloves during all radiographic procedures
- Disinfect and cover x-ray machine, working surfaces, chair, and apron
- Sterilize nondisposable instruments
- Use barrier-protected film (sensor) or disposable container
- Prevent contamination of processing equipment

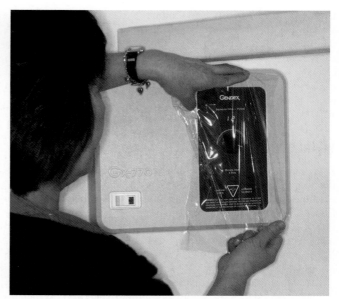

FIG. **8-7**  Plastic wrap covers parts of console that are touched during the radiographic examination.

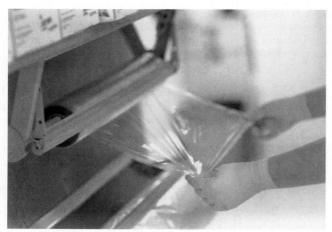

FIG. **8-6**  Plastic wrap from a dispenser is used to cover countertops and the x-ray machine console.

virus (HIV) and hepatitis B virus. Accordingly, the means used to protect against cross-contamination are used universally, that is, for all individuals. The American Dental Association and the Centers for Disease Control and Prevention stress the use of universal precautions because many patients are unaware that they are carriers of infectious disease or choose not to reveal this information.

### Wear Gloves During All Radiographic Procedures

The practitioner should always wear gloves when making radiographs or handling contaminated film packets or associated materials such as cotton rolls and film-holding instruments or when removing barrier protections from surfaces and radiographic equipment. After the patient is seated, the practitioner should wash his or her hands and put on disposable gloves in sight of the patient if the operatory arrangement permits. Dental assistants should wear eyewear or a mask or faceshield if exposure to bodily fluids is anticipated.

Charts should be kept away from sources of contamination and not handled during the radiographic examination. Chair adjustments should be made in advance, or adjustments should be made on control surfaces that are covered, such as the headrest control.

### Disinfect and Cover X-Ray Machine, Working Surfaces, Chair, and Apron

The goal of preventing cross-contamination is addressed in part by disinfecting all surfaces and by using barriers to isolate equipment

from direct contact. Although barriers greatly aid infection control, they do not replace the need for effective surface cleaning and disinfection. Experience has demonstrated that, during the daily activity of treatment, failure of mechanical barriers is common. It is advantageous and reassuring to the operator to know that whenever this happens, the surfaces that may become accidentally exposed are clean and disinfected. Any surface that may be contaminated should be surface disinfected. This includes the x-ray machine control panel, tube head, and beam alignment device, dental chair and headrest, surfaces on which film is placed, leaded apron and thyroid collar, and the doorknob of the operatory. Operators should avoid touching walls and other surfaces with contaminated gloves. Good surface disinfectants include iodophors, chlorines, and synthetic phenolic compounds. Although the American Dental Association does not recommend specific chemical disinfectants and sterilants, it does suggest that when dentists use a chemical agent for disinfection or sterilization, the agent should be an Environmental Protection Agency (EPA) registered hospital disinfectant of low to intermediate activity. The agent should also be tuberculocidal—an effective killer of tuberculosis—and capable of preventing other infectious diseases, including hepatitis B and HIV.

Barriers should cover working surfaces that were previously cleaned and disinfected. Barriers protect the underlying surface from becoming contaminated. An effective barrier for the countertops and x-ray control console is plastic wrap, which may be conveniently stored in a butcher's paper dispenser mounted on a wall (Fig. 8-6). When covering the x-ray control console, the operator should be sure to include the exposure switch and the exposure time control if they are integral parts of the unit (Fig. 8-7). An x-ray exposure switch that is independent of the console should be covered with a sandwich bag or food storage bag or wrapped with plastic wrap.

The dental chair headrest, headrest adjustments, and chair back may be easily covered with a plastic bag (Fig. 8-8). The x-ray tube head, PID, and yoke should be covered while they are still wet with disinfectant with a barrier to stop any dripping (Fig. 8-9). The bag

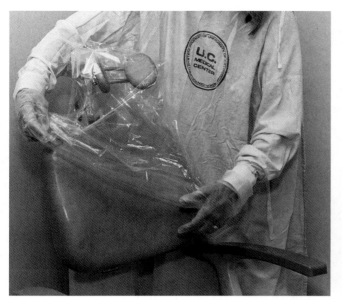

FIG. **8-8**   A new plastic bag is placed over the chair and headrest for each patient.

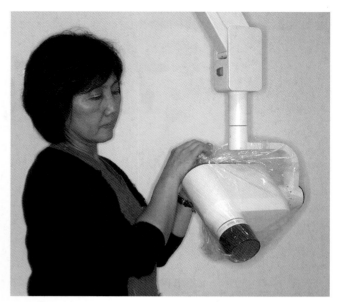

FIG. **8-9**   A plastic bag is slipped over the x-ray tube head with a large rubber band just proximal to the swivel or tie ends, as shown here. The plastic is pulled tight over the PID and secured with a light rubber band slipped over the PID and placed next to the head.

should be secured by tying a knot in the open end or by placing a heavy rubber band over the x-ray tube head just proximal to the swivel. Also, the leaded apron should be cleaned, disinfected, and covered between patients because it is frequently contaminated with saliva as the result of handling (readjusting its position) during a radiographic procedure. The apron should be suspended on a heavy coat hanger to permit turning front to back. It should be sprayed with a detergent-containing disinfectant and then wiped and covered with the same type of plastic garment bag used for the x-ray head and chair back (Fig. 8-10). The operatory is now prepared for radiography.

Panoramic and cephalometric equipment should receive the same maintenance for decontamination and disinfection as other equipment. Panoramic bite blocks, chin rest, and patient handgrips should be cleaned with detergent-iodine disinfectant and covered with a plastic bag. Disposable bite blocks may be used. The head-positioning guides, control panel, and exposure switch should be carefully wiped with a paper towel that is well moistened with disinfectant. The radiographer should wear disposable gloves while positioning and exposing the patient. The gloves should be removed before the cassette is removed from the machine for processing because the cassette and film remain extraoral and should not be handled with contaminated disposable gloves. Cephalostat ear posts, ear post brackets, and forehead support or nasion pointer should be cleaned and disinfected with iodine-detergent disinfectant. These may then also be covered in plastic.

After patient exposures are completed, the barriers should be removed, contaminated working surfaces (including those in the darkroom) and the apron sprayed with disinfectant and wiped as described previously. Then the barriers should be replaced in preparation for the next patient.

### Sterilize Nondisposable Instruments
It is best to use film-holding instruments that are heat sterilizable. After sterilization, the instruments should be kept in bags for storage and subsequent transport to the radiography area. When the instruments are taken to the radiography area, it is good technique to remove them from the bag immediately before use. After use, instru-

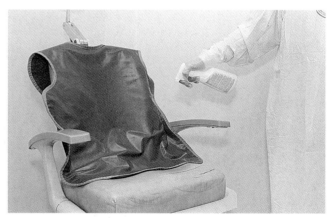

FIG. **8-10**   Hanging apron is sprayed with disinfectant and then dried and covered with a garment bag.

ments should be replaced in the bag to reinforce cleanliness in the area. The same sterilization bag should be used to transport the contaminated instruments back to the cleaning and sterilizing room.

### Use Barrier-Protected Film (Sensor) or Disposable Container
Film should be obtained in advance from a central source. To prevent contamination of bulk supplies of film, they should be dispensed in procedure quantities. The required number of films for a full-mouth or interproximal series should be prepackaged in coin envelopes or paper cups in the central preparation room. These envelopes of films should be dispensed with the film-holding instruments. For unanticipated occasions in which an unusual number of films are required, a small container of films can be on hand in the central preparation and sterilizing room. No one wearing contaminated gloves should retrieve

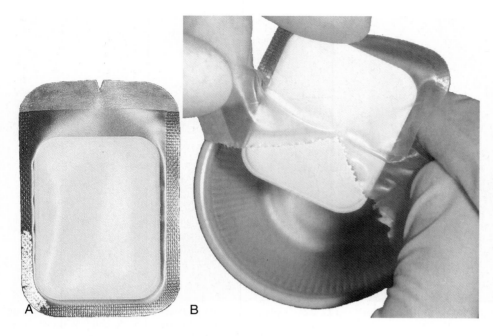

FIG. **8-11** Dental film with a plastic barrier to protect film from contact with saliva. **A,** Note notch on side of plastic envelope for opening. **B,** During opening, the plastic is removed and the clean film allowed to drop into a container.

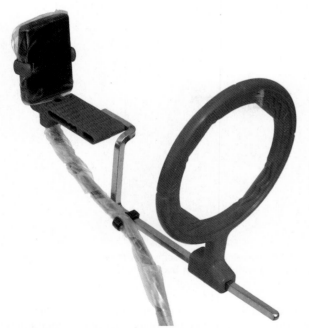

FIG. **8-12** Film-holding instrument with barrier wrapping protecting sensor and cord from saliva.

a film from this supply. Films should be dispensed only by staff members with clean hands or wearing clean gloves.

Film packets may be packaged in a plastic envelope (Fig. 8-11), which protects the film from contact with saliva and blood during exposure. Barrier-protected film fits in most film-holding instruments. An attractive feature of the protective envelopes is the ease with which they may be opened and the film extracted. For best results, the packet should be immersed in a disinfectant after the films have been exposed in the patient's mouth. Then the packet should be dried and

opened, allowing the film to drop out. The barrier envelopes can be conveniently opened in a lighted area, the film dropped onto a clean work area or into a clean paper or plastic cup, and the film transferred to the daylight loader or darkroom for processing.

If barrier-protected film is not used, the exposed film should be placed in a disposable container for later transport to the darkroom for processing. Paper film packets are exposed to saliva and possibly blood during exposure in the patient's mouth. To prevent saliva from seeping into a paper film packet, a paper towel should be placed beside the container for exposed films. The practitioner should use this towel to wipe each film as it is removed from the patient's mouth and before it is placed with the other exposed films. This problem may also be avoided by using film packaged in vinyl.

Sensors for digital imaging are not able to be sterilized; thus it is important to use a barrier to protect them from contamination when placed in the patient's mouth (Fig. 8-12). Typically the manufacturers of these sensors recommend the use of plastic barrier sheaths. The supplemental use of latex finger cots provides significant added protection and is recommended for routine use when using digital sensors. Because such barriers may fail, the sensors should be cleaned and disinfected with an EPA-registered intermediate-level hospital disinfectant after every patient. The manufacturer of such equipment should be consulted for proper disinfectant.

### Prevent Contamination of Processing Equipment

After all exposures are made, the operator should remove his or her gloves and take the container of contaminated films to the darkroom. The goal in the darkroom is to break the infection chain so that only clean films are placed into processing solutions. Two towels should be placed on the darkroom working surface. The container of contaminated films should be placed on one of these towels. After the exposed film is removed from its packet, it should be placed on the second towel. The film packaging is discarded on the first towel with the container.

Removing film from a packet without touching (contaminating) it is a relatively simple procedure. Figure 8-13 illustrates the method

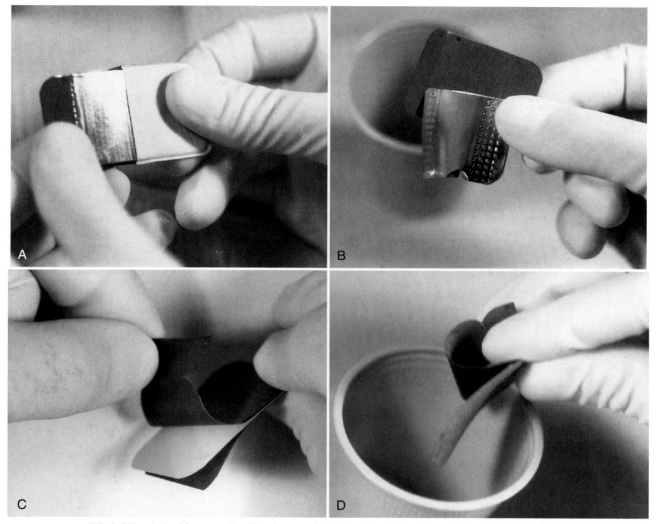

FIG. **8-13**  Method for removing films from packet without touching them with contaminated gloves. **A,** Packet tab is opened and lead foil and black interleaf paper are slid from wrapping. **B,** Foil is rotated away from black paper and discarded. **C,** Paper wrapping is opened. **D,** Film falls into a clean cup.

for opening a contaminated film packet while wearing contaminated gloves without touching the film. The practitioner dons a clean pair of gloves, picks up the film packet by the color-coded end, and pulls the tab upward and away from the packet to reveal the black paper tab wrapped over the end of the film. Now, holding the film over the second towel, he or she carefully grasps the black paper tab that wraps the film and pulls the film from the packet. When the film is pulled from the packet, it will fall from the paper wrapping onto the clean towel. The paper wrapper may need to be shaken lightly to cause the film to fall free. The packaging materials should be placed on the first paper towel. After all films are opened, the practitioner gathers the contaminated packaging and container and discards them along with the contaminated gloves. The clean films are processed in the usual manner. It is not necessary to wear gloves when handling processed films, film mounts, or patient charts.

An alternate procedure when exposing films in vinyl packaging is to place the exposed film, still in the protective plastic envelope, in an approved disinfecting solution when it is removed from the mouth and after wiping it with a paper towel. It should remain in the disinfectant after the exposure of the last film for the recommended time. Immersion for 30 seconds in a 5.25% solution of sodium hypochlorite is effective.

Automatic film processors with daylight loaders offer a special problem because of the risk for contaminating the sleeves with contaminated gloves or film packets. One approach is to clean the films by immersion in a disinfectant, with or without a plastic envelope, as previously described. With this method the operator cleans the films, puts on clean gloves, and then takes only cleaned film packets into the daylight loader. An alternate approach is to open the top of the loader, place a clean barrier on the bottom, and insert the cup of exposed film packets and a clean cup. The operator then closes the top, puts on clean gloves, pushes his or her hands through the sleeve, and opens the film packets, allowing the film to drop into the clean cup. After all film packets have been opened, the contaminated gloves are removed, the films are loaded into the developer, and hands are removed. Then the top of the loader may be removed and the contaminated materials removed.

# BIBLIOGRAPHY

## *QUALITY ASSURANCE*

American Dental Association Council on Scientific Affairs: The use of dental radiographs: update and recommendations, *J Am Dent Assoc* 137:1304-1312, 2006.

Goren AD, Lundeen RC, Deahl ST II et al: Updated quality assurance self-assessment exercise in intraoral and panoramic radiography, American Academy of Oral and Maxillofacial Radiology, Radiology Practice Committee, *Oral Surg Oral Med Oral Pathol Oral Radiol Endod* 89: 369-374, 2000.

Kodak Dental Radiography Series: *Quality assurance in dental radiography,* N-416, Rochester, NY, 1995, Eastman Kodak.

Michel R, Zimmerman TL: Basic radiation protection considerations in dental practice, *Health Phys* 77:S81-S83, 1999.

National Radiological Protection Board: *Guidance notes for dental practitioners on the safe use of x-ray equipment* (2001): www.nrpb.org.uk.

## *INFECTION CONTROL*

American Academy of Oral and Maxillofacial Radiology infection control guidelines for dental radiographic procedures, *Oral Surg Oral Med Oral Pathol* 73:248-249, 1992.

American Dental Association Council on Scientific Affairs and American Dental Association Council on Dental Practice: Infection control recommendations for the dental office and the dental laboratory, *J Am Dent Assoc* 127:672-680, 1996.

Hubar JS, Gardiner DM: Infection control procedures used in conjunction with computed dental radiography, *Int J Comput Dent* 3:259-267, 2000.

Kohn WG, Collins AS, Cleveland JL et al; Centers for Disease Control and Prevention: Guidelines for infection control in dental health-care settings—2003, *MMWR Morb Mortal Wkly Rep* 52(RR-17):1-61, 2003.

Miller CH, Palenik CJ: *Infection control and management of hazardous materials for the dental team,* ed 4, St. Louis, Mosby (in press).

U.S. Department of Labor, Occupational Safety and Health Administration: Occupational exposure to bloodborne pathogens, needlestick and other sharp injuries, final rule, *Fed Reg* 66:5317-5325, 2001.

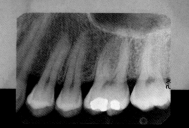

# CHAPTER 9

# Intraoral Radiographic Examinations

Intraoral radiographic examinations are the backbone of imaging for the general dentist. Intraoral radiographs can be divided into three categories: periapical projections, bitewing projections, and occlusal projections. Periapical radiographs should show all of a tooth, including the surrounding bone. Bitewing radiographs show only the crowns of teeth and the adjacent alveolar crests. Occlusal radiographs show an area of teeth and bone larger than periapical radiographs.

A full-mouth set of radiographs consists of periapical and bitewing projections (Fig. 9-1). These projections, when well exposed and properly processed, can provide considerable diagnostic information to complement the clinical examination. As with any clinical procedure, the operator must clearly understand the goals of dental radiography and the criteria for evaluating the quality of performance.

Radiographs should be made only when a clear diagnostic need exists for the information the radiograph may provide. Accordingly, the frequency of such examinations varies with the individual circumstances of each patient (see Chapter 15).

## Criteria of Quality

Every radiographic examination should produce radiographs of optimal diagnostic quality, incorporating the following features:
- Radiographs should record the complete areas of interest on the image. In the case of intraoral periapical radiographs, the full length of the roots and at least 2 mm of periapical bone must be visible. If evidence of a pathologic condition is present, the area of the entire lesion plus some surrounding normal bone should show on one radiograph. If this is not possible to achieve on a periapical radiograph, an occlusal projection may be required as well as an extraoral projection. Bitewing examinations should demonstrate each posterior proximal surface at least once.
- Radiographs should have the least possible amount of distortion. Most distortion is caused by improper angulation of the x-ray beam rather than by the curvature of the structures being examined or inappropriate positioning of the receptor. Close attention to proper positioning of the receptor and x-ray tube results in diagnostically useful images.
- Radiographs should have optimal density and contrast to facilitate interpretation. Although milliamperage (mA), peak kilovoltage (kVp), and exposure time are crucial parameters influencing density and contrast, faulty processing can adversely affect the quality of a properly exposed radiograph.

When evaluating radiographs and considering whether to retake a view, the practitioner should consider the initial reason for making the image. When a full-mouth set is indicated, it is not necessary to retake a view that fails to open a contact or show a periapical region if the missing information is available on another view. If a single view or only a few views are needed, they should be repeated only if they fail to reveal the desired information.

## Periapical Radiography

Two intraoral projection techniques are commonly used for periapical radiography: the paralleling technique and the bisecting-angle technique. Most clinicians prefer the paralleling technique because it provides a less distorted view of the dentition. The paralleling technique is the most appropriate technique for digital imaging. The following discussion describes the principles and uses of the paralleling technique to obtain a full-mouth set of radiographs. When anatomic configuration (e.g., palate and floor of the mouth) precludes strict adherence to the paralleling concept, slight modifications may have to be made. If the anatomic constraints are extreme, some of the principles of the bisecting-angle technique may be used to accomplish the required receptor placement and determine the vertical angulation of the tube. The bisecting-angle technique is described later in the chapter.

The term *image receptor* refers to any medium that can capture an image including film, charge-coupled device (CCD) or complementary metal oxide semiconductors (CMOS) sensors, or storage phosphor plates. The principles for making radiographs are the same for each of these receptor types; thus this chapter uses the general term *receptor* to refer any of the image receptors.

### GENERAL STEPS FOR MAKING AN EXPOSURE

- *Prepare unit for exposure.* Place barriers for universal infection control and have receptors and receptor-holding instruments ready at chairside (see Chapter 9).
- *Greet and seat the patient.* Position the patient upright in the chair with the back and head well supported and briefly describe the procedures that are to be performed. Position the dental chair low for maxillary projections and elevated for mandibular projections. Ask the patient to remove eyeglasses and all removable appliances. Drape the patient with a lead apron regardless of whether a single image or a full series is to be made. Do not comment on any discomfort the patient may feel during the procedure. If it seems necessary to apologize for any discomfort, do it after the examination.
- *Adjust the x-ray unit setting.* Set the x-ray machine for the proper kVp, mA, and exposure time. Generally only the exposure time is adjusted for the various anatomic locations.
- *Wash hands thoroughly.* Wash your hands with soap and water, preferably in front of the patient or at least in an area where the patient can observe or be aware of the washing. Put on disposable gloves.

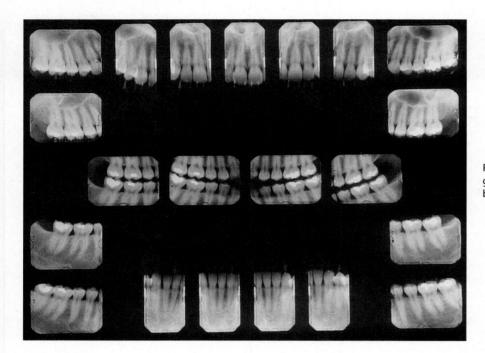

FIG. **9-1** Mounted full-mouth set of radiographs consisting of 17 periapical views and four bitewing views.

- *Examine the oral cavity.* Before placing any receptors in the mouth, examine the teeth to estimate their axial inclination, which influences the placement of the receptor. Also note tori or other obstructions that modify receptor placement.
- *Position the tube head.* Bring the tube head to the side to be examined so that it is readily available for final positioning after the receptor has been placed in the mouth.
- *Position the receptor.* Insert receptor into the holding device and position the receptor and holding device in the region of the patient's mouth to be examined. Leading with the apical end of the receptor, rotate it into the oral cavity. Place the receptor as far from the teeth as possible. This provides the maximal space available in the midline of the palate and the greatest depth toward the center of the floor of the mouth. The added space allows the receptor to be oriented parallel to the long axis of the teeth. With the receptor now in the mouth, place it gently on the palate or floor of the mouth. Next, rotate the receptor-holding instrument either up or down until the bite-block rests on the teeth to be radiographed. Place a cotton roll between the bite-block and the teeth opposite those being radiographed. This helps stabilize the receptor-holding instrument and in many cases contributes to the patient's comfort. Then ask the patient to close his or her mouth gently, holding the instrument and receptor in place. If the bite-block is not on the teeth when the patient closes, the receptor may move into the palate or floor of the mouth and may cause discomfort from faulty positioning.
- *Position the x-ray tube.* Adjust the vertical and horizontal angulation of the tube head to correspond to the receptor-holding instrument. The end of the aiming cylinder of the x-ray machine must be flush or parallel to the guide ring instrument. Alignment is satisfactory when the aiming cylinder covers the port and is within the limits of the face shield. Caution the patient not to move.
- *Make the exposure.* Make the exposure with the preset exposure time. If the receptor is a film or storage phosphor plate, then after exposure remove the receptor from the patient's mouth, dry it with

---

**BOX 9-1**
*Projections*

***Anterior Periapical (Use No. 1 Receptor)***
- Maxillary central incisors: one projection
- Maxillary lateral incisors: two projections
- Maxillary canines: two projections
- Mandibular centrolateral incisors: two projections
- Mandibular canines: two projections

***Posterior Periapical (Use No. 2 Receptor)***
- Maxillary premolars: two projections
- Maxillary molars: two projections
- Maxillary distomolar (as needed): two projections
- Mandibular premolars: two projections
- Mandibular molars: two projections
- Mandibular distomolar (as needed): two projections

***Bitewing (Use No. 2 Receptor)***
- Premolars: two projections
- Molars: two projections

---

a paper towel, and place it in an appropriate receptacle outside the exposure area. If the receptor is a CCD or CMOS sensor, then you may be able to keep it in the patient's mouth and reposition it for the next view. Encourage the patient along the way.

A typical full-mouth set of radiographs consists of 21 images (Box 9-1, see also Fig. 9-1). Establish a regular sequence when making exposures to avoid overlooking individual projections. Make the anterior views before the posterior views because the former causes less discomfort for the patient. The following description of procedures pertains to the paralleling technique.

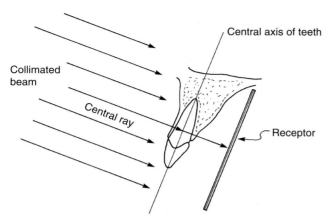

FIG. **9-2** Paralleling technique illustrates the parallelism between the long axis of the tooth and the receptor. The central ray is directed perpendicular to each.

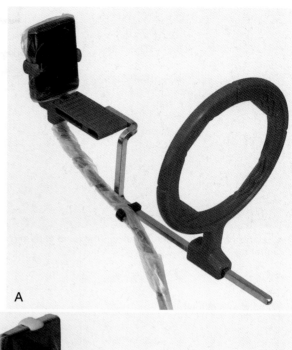

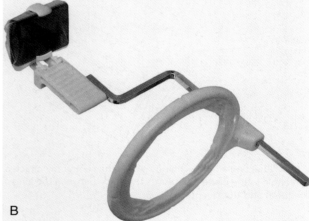

FIG. **9-3** Receptor-holding instruments. **A,** XCP instrument for anterior views with wired sensor. **B,** XCP instrument for posterior views with wireless sensor. (**A** and **B,** Courtesy Dentsply Rinn, Elgin, Ill.)

## PARALLELING TECHNIQUE

The central concept of the paralleling technique (also called the *right-angle* or *long-cone technique*) is that the x-ray receptor is supported parallel to the long axis of the teeth and the central ray of the x-ray beam is directed at right angles to the teeth and receptor (Fig. 9-2). This orientation of the receptor, teeth, and central ray minimizes geometric distortion and presents the teeth and supporting bone in their true anatomic relationships. To reduce geometric distortion, the x-ray source should be located relatively distant from the teeth. The use of a long source-to-object distance reduces the apparent size of the focal spot, thus increasing image sharpness, and provides images with minimal magnification. The paralleling method works equally well for film, CCD or CMOS sensors, or storage phosphor plates.

### Receptor-Holding Instruments

Use instruments to allow precise positions of the receptor in the patient's mouth. Many of these receptor holders are specific for various brands of digital sensors, storage phosphor plates, or film. It is also important to use a receptor-holding instrument that has an external guiding ring. This guiding ring is used to align the x-ray aiming cylinder and ensures that the receptor is centered in the beam behind the teeth of interest and that the receptor and teeth are perpendicular to the x-ray beam (Fig. 9-3). These should be used with rectangular collimators to reduce patient exposure (Chapter 3).

### Receptor Placement

For the best images, the receptor should be positioned parallel to the teeth and deep in the patient's mouth. This is particularly important when rigid sensors are used because they may be larger than film. For maxillary projections, the superior border of the receptor generally rests at the height of the palatal vault in the midline. Similarly, for mandibular projections, the receptor should be used to displace the tongue posteriorly or toward the midline to allow the inferior border of the receptor to rest on the floor of the mouth away from the mucosa on the lingual surface of the mandible. Especially for digital sensors, patient acceptance and comfort are best when the receptor is placed in the center of the mouth.

### Angulation of the Tube Head

The orientation of the x-ray machine's aiming cylinder in the vertical and horizontal planes should be adjusted to align with the aiming ring. The horizontal direction of the beam primarily influences the degree of overlapping of the images of the crowns at the interproximal spaces (Fig. 9-4).

## BISECTING-ANGLE TECHNIQUE

The bisecting-angle technique was used often in the first half of the 1900s but has been largely replaced by the paralleling technique. This method may be useful when the operator is unable to apply the paralleling technique because of large rigid sensors or the anatomy of the patient. The bisecting-angle technique is based on a simple geometric theorem, Cieszynski's rule of isometry, which states that two triangles are equal when they share one complete side and have two equal angles. Dental radiography applies the theorem as follows. The

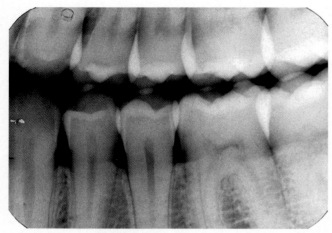

FIG. **9-4** Horizontal overlapping of crowns is the result of misdirection of the central ray.

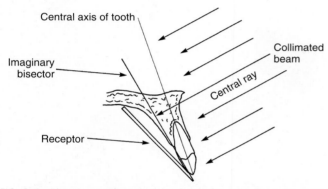

FIG. **9-5** Bisecting-angle technique shows the central ray directed at a right angle to the plane that bisects the angle between the long axis of the tooth and the receptor.

receptor is positioned as close as possible to the lingual surface of the teeth, resting in the palate or in the floor of the mouth (Fig. 9-5). The plane of the receptor and the long axis of the teeth form an angle with its apex at the point where the receptor is in contact with the teeth along an imaginary line that bisects this angle and directs the central ray of the beam at right angles to this bisector. This forms two triangles with two equal angles and a common side (the imaginary bisector). Consequently, when these conditions are satisfied, the images cast on the receptor theoretically are the same length as the projected object. To reproduce the length of each root of a multirooted tooth accurately, the central beam must be angled differently for each root. Another limitation of this technique is that the alveolar ridge often projects more coronally than its true position, thus distorting the apparent height of the alveolar bone around the teeth.

## Receptor-Holding Instruments

Several methods can be used to support receptors intraorally for bisecting-angle projections. The preferred method is to use a receptor-holding bisecting-angle instrument that provides an external device for localizing the x-ray beam. The bisecting-angle instrument uses a fixed average bisecting angle. It is not desirable to have the patient support the receptor from the lingual surface with his or her forefinger. Patients often use excessive force and bend the receptor, causing distortion of the image. Also, the receptor might slip without the operator's expertise, resulting in an improper image field. Finally, without an external guide to the position of the receptor, the x-ray beam may miss part of the receptor, resulting in a partial image *(cone cut)*.

## Positioning of the Patient

For radiographs of the maxillary arch, the patient's head should be positioned upright with the sagittal plane vertical and the occlusal plane horizontal. When the mandibular teeth are to be radiographed, the head is tilted back slightly to compensate for the changed occlusal plane when the mouth is opened.

## Receptor Placement

The projections described for the paralleling technique may also be used for the bisecting-angle technique. The receptor is positioned behind the area of interest, with the apical end against the mucosa on the lingual or palatal surface. The occlusal or incisal edge is oriented against the teeth with an edge of the receptor extending just beyond the teeth. If necessary for the patient's comfort, the anterior corner of a film can be softened by bending it before it is placed against the mucosa. Care must be taken not to bend the film excessively because this may result in considerable image distortion and pressure defects in the emulsion that are apparent on the processed receptor. Such bending is not possible with CCD or CMOS sensors or storage phosphor plates.

*Text continued on p. 135.*

## PARALLELING TECHNIQUE • **MAXILLARY CENTRAL INCISOR PROJECTION***

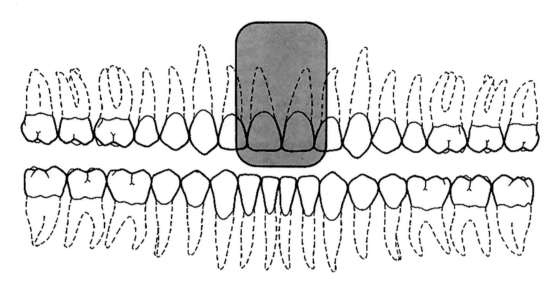

**Image Field.** The field of view on these radiographs *(shaded area)* should include both central incisors and their periapical areas.

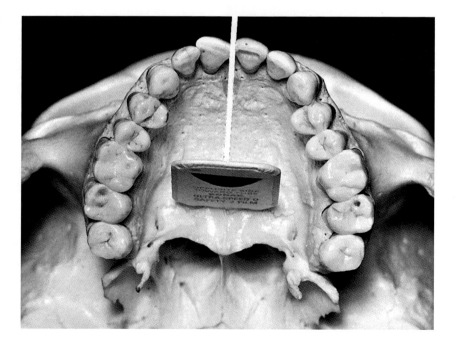

**Receptor Placement.** Place a No. 1 receptor at about the level of the second premolars or first molars to take advantage of the maximal palatal height so that the entire length of the teeth can be projected on it. Have the receptor resting on the palate with its midline centered with the midline of the arch. Position the packet's long axis parallel to the long axis of the maxillary central incisors.

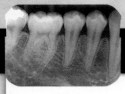

## PARALLELING TECHNIQUE • **MAXILLARY CENTRAL INCISOR PROJECTION*—cont'd**

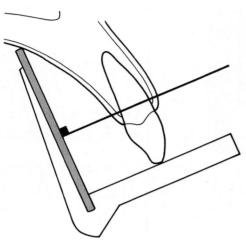

**Projection of Central Ray.**[†] Direct the central ray through the contact point of the central incisors and perpendicular to the plane of the receptors and roots of the teeth. Because the axial inclination of the maxillary incisors is about 15 to 20 degrees, the vertical angulation of the tube should be at the same positive angle. The tube should have 0 horizontal angulation.

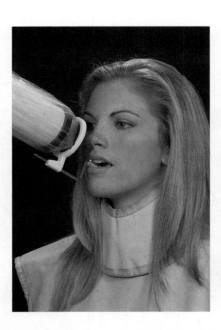

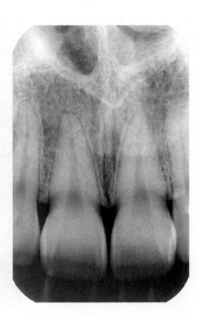

**Point of Entry.**  Direct the point of entry of the central ray high on the lip, in the midline, just below the septum of the nostril. If the palatal vault is unusually low or a palatal torus is present, it may be necessary to tilt the receptor holder positively and compromise a completely parallel relationship between the receptor and the teeth to ensure that the periapical region is included on the image.

---

*Patient photos for the paralleling technique on pages 114, 116, 118, 120, 122, 124, 126, 128, 130, 132, and 134 are from Iannucci J, Jansen Howerton L: *Dental radiography: principles and techniques,* ed 3, St. Louis, 2006, Saunders.
[†]Projection of the central ray and point of entry are described in the discussion of the paralleling technique for instances when a receptor-holding device without a tube alignment ring or face shield is used. When using a receptor-holding device with a tube-alignment ring or face shield, position the device in the mouth to give the appropriate horizontal and vertical angulation.

## PARALLELING TECHNIQUE • **MAXILLARY LATERAL PROJECTION**

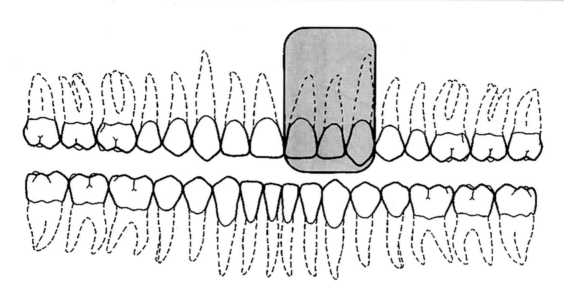

**Image Field.** This projection should show the lateral incisor and its periapical field centered on the radiograph. Include the mesial interproximal area with the distal aspect of the central incisor on the radiograph so that no overlap is evident.

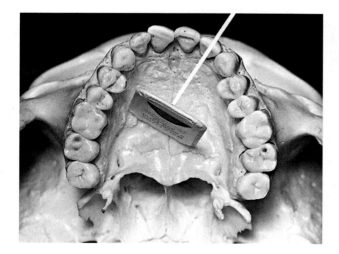

**Receptor Placement.** Place a No. 1 receptor deep in the oral cavity parallel with the long axis and the mesiodistal plane of the maxillary lateral incisor.

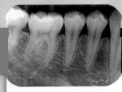

## PARALLELING TECHNIQUE • **MAXILLARY LATERAL PROJECTION—cont'd**

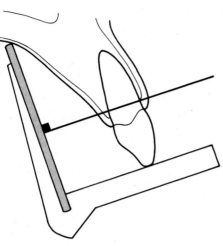

**Projection of Central Ray.** Direct the central ray through the middle of the lateral incisor, with no overlapping of the margins of the crowns at the interproximal space on its mesial aspect. Do not attempt to visualize the distal contact with the canine.

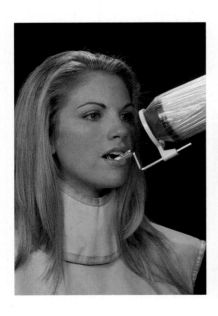

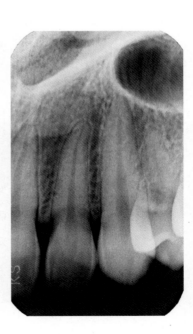

**Point of Entry.** Orient the central ray to enter high on the lip about 1 cm from the midline.

## PARALLELING TECHNIQUE • **MAXILLARY CANINE PROJECTION**

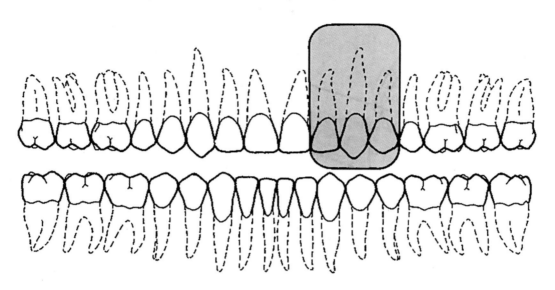

**Image Field.** This projection should demonstrate the entire canine, with its periapical area, in the midline of the radiograph. Open the mesial contact area. Ignore the distal contact because it will be visualized on other projections.

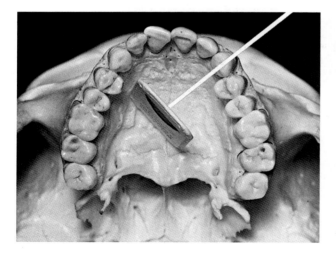

**Receptor Placement.** Place a No. 1 receptor against the palate, well away from the palatal surface of the teeth. Orient the receptor packet with its anterior edge at about the middle of the lateral incisor and its long axis parallel with the long axis of the canine.

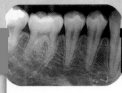

## PARALLELING TECHNIQUE • **MAXILLARY CANINE PROJECTION—cont'd**

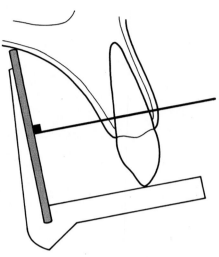

**Projection of Central Ray.** Position the holding instrument so that it directs the beam through the mesial contact of the canine. Do not attempt to open the distal contact.

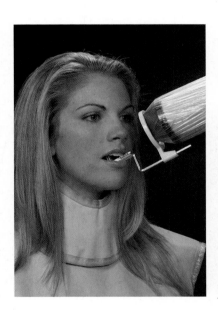

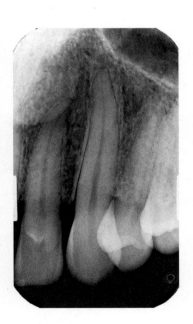

**Point of Entry.** Direct the central ray through the canine eminence. The point of entry will be at about the intersection of the distal and inferior borders of the ala of the nose.

PARALLELING TECHNIQUE • **MAXILLARY PREMOLAR PROJECTION**

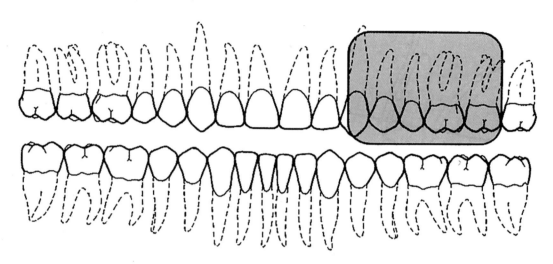

**Image Field.** The radiograph of this region should include the images of the distal half of the canine and the premolars, with room for at least the first molar.

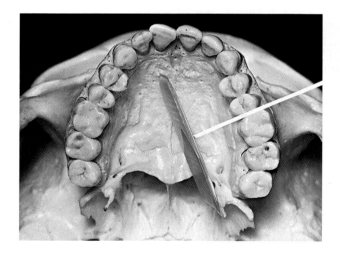

**Receptor Placement.** Place a No. 2 receptor in the mouth with the long dimension parallel with the occlusal plane and in the midline and near the palatal midline. The packet should extend far enough forward to cover the distal half of the canine. It will also include the premolars and the first molar and maybe the mesial portion of the second molar. The plane of the receptor should be nearly vertical to correspond with the long axis of the premolar teeth. Position the receptor-holding device so that the long axis of the receptor is parallel with the mean buccal plane of the premolars. This establishes the proper horizontal angulation.

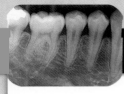

## PARALLELING TECHNIQUE • **MAXILLARY PREMOLAR PROJECTION—cont'd**

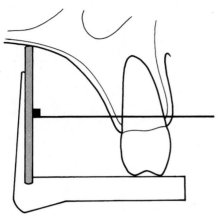

**Projection of Central Ray.** Direct the central ray perpendicular to the receptor. The horizontal angulation of the holding instrument should be adjusted to permit the beam to pass through the interproximal area between the first and second premolars.

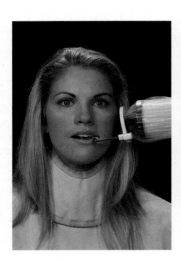

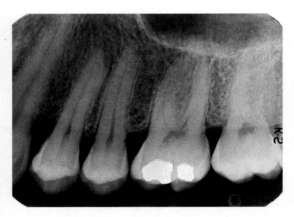

**Point of Entry.** Place the holding instrument so that the central ray passes through the center of the second premolar root. This point usually is below the pupil of the eye.

## PARALLELING TECHNIQUE • **MAXILLARY MOLAR PROJECTION**

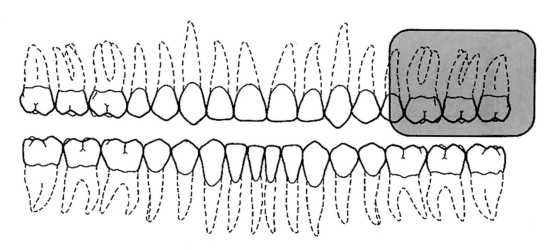

**Image Field.** The radiograph of this region should show the images of the distal half of the second premolar, the three maxillary permanent molars, and some of the tuberosity. Include the same area on the receptor even if some or all molars are missing. If the third molar is impacted in an area other than the region of the tuberosity, a distal oblique or extraoral projection (e.g., panoramic or oblique lateral jaw view) may be required.

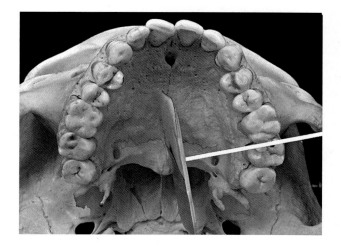

**Receptor Placement.** When placing the No. 2 receptor for this projection, position the wide dimension of the receptor nearly horizontal to minimize brushing the palate and dorsum of the tongue. When the receptor is in the region to be examined, rotate it into position with a firm and definite motion. This maneuver is important in avoiding the gag reflex, and resolute action by the operator enhances the patient's confidence. Place the receptor far enough posterior to cover the first, second, and third molar areas and some of the tuberosity. The anterior border should just cover the distal aspect of the second premolar. To cover the molars from crown to apices, place the receptor at the midline of the palate. In this position room should be available to orient the receptor parallel with the molar teeth. The mesial or distal rotation of the receptor-holding device should ensure that the long axis of the receptor is parallel with the mean buccal plane of the molars (to establish the proper horizontal angulation). A shallow palate may require slight tipping of the holding instrument to avoid bending the receptor.

NOTE: In some cases the size of the mouth (length of the arch) does not allow positioning of the receptor (holding device) as far posterior as recommended for the molar projection. However, by placing the receptor-holding device so that half the tube alignment ring or face shield is behind the outer canthus of the eye, the molars and part of the tuberosity usually can be included in the image of the molar projection.

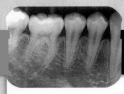
PARALLELING TECHNIQUE • **MAXILLARY MOLAR PROJECTION—cont'd**

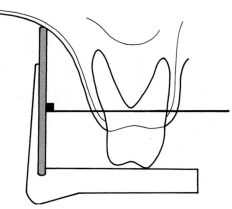

**Projection of Central Ray.** Direct the central ray perpendicular to the receptor. Adjust the horizontal angulation of the receptor-holding instrument to direct the beam at right angles to the buccal surfaces of the molar teeth.

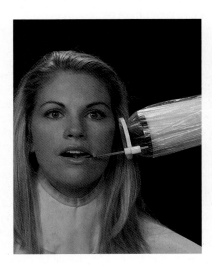

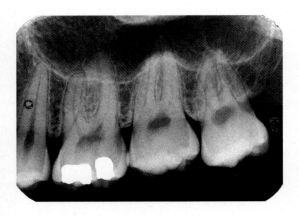

**Point of Entry.** The point of entry of the central ray should be on the cheek below the outer canthus of the eye and the zygoma at the position of the maxillary second molar.

## PARALLELING TECHNIQUE • **MAXILLARY DISTAL OBLIQUE MOLAR PROJECTION**

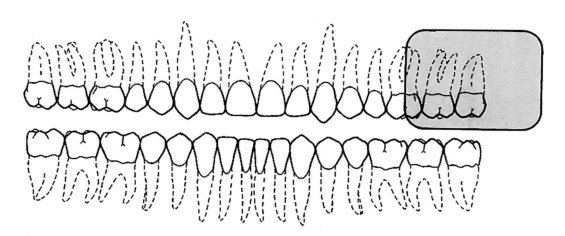

**Image Field.** This projection provides a view of the maxillary tuberosity region more posterior than usually is seen in the molar projection. It allows detection or evaluation of impacted teeth or pathologic conditions in the bone of this area.

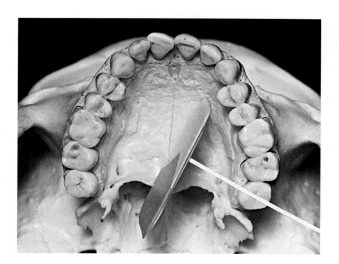

**Receptor Placement.** Position the holding device with a No. 2 receptor in the molar region of the maxilla and rotate distally, angling the receptor across the midline so that the posterior border is away from the teeth of interest and the anterior border is near the molars on the side being radiographed. Position this receptor with a definite movement to minimize patient discomfort.

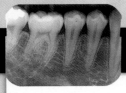

## PARALLELING TECHNIQUE • MAXILLARY DISTAL OBLIQUE MOLAR PROJECTION—cont'd

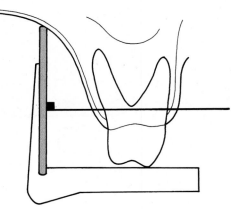

**Projection of Central Ray.** Direct the central ray from the posterior aspect through the third molar region and perpendicular to the angled receptor, projecting the more posterior objects anteriorly onto the receptor.

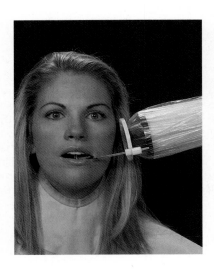

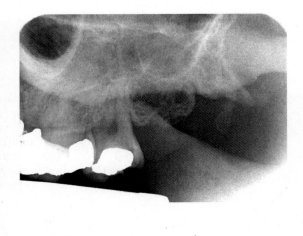

**Point of Entry.** The central ray enters the maxillary third molar region just below the middle of the zygomatic arch, distal to the lateral canthus of the eye.

NOTE: Occasionally a hypersensitive patient gags when a receptor is placed for the usual maxillary molar projection. However, if a modified distal oblique projection is used, moving the posterior border of the receptor more medially frequently is less irritating to the patient, and the image is obtained with comfort. The patient's reaction of relief indicates when a sufficient rotation has been achieved. Although this maneuver may result in some overlapping of the molar contact areas, these surfaces will be apparent on the bitewing projection. Slight overlapping of contact areas is preferable to no radiograph of the region.

## PARALLELING TECHNIQUE • **MANDIBULAR CENTROLATERAL PROJECTION**

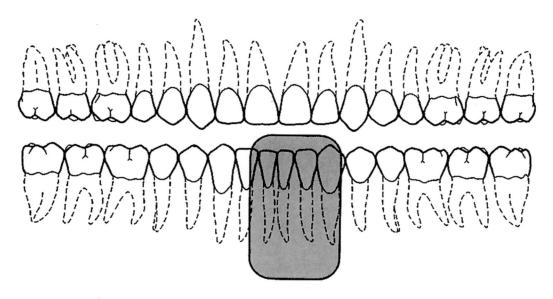

**Image Field.** Center the image of the mandibular central and lateral incisors and their periapical areas on the receptor. Because the space in this area frequently is restricted, use two of the narrower anterior periapical receptors for the incisors to provide good coverage with minimal discomfort. In addition, the incisor contact areas are better visualized on two narrower anterior receptors because the angulation of the central ray can be adjusted for the contact area on each side.

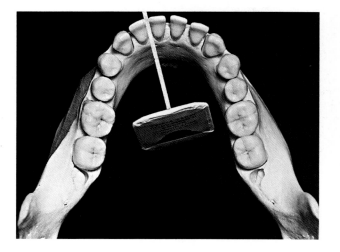

**Receptor Placement.** Place the long dimension of the No. 1 receptor vertically behind the central and lateral incisors with the contact area centered and the lower border below the tongue. Position the receptor posteriorly as far as possible, usually between the premolars. With the receptor resting gently on the floor of the mouth as the fulcrum, tip the instrument downward until the receptor-holder bite-block is resting on the incisors. Instruct the patient to close the mouth slowly. As the patient is closing slowly and the floor of the mouth is relaxing, rotate the instrument with the teeth as the fulcrum to align the receptor to be more parallel with the teeth.

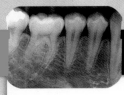

## PARALLELING TECHNIQUE • **MANDIBULAR CENTROLATERAL PROJECTION—cont'd**

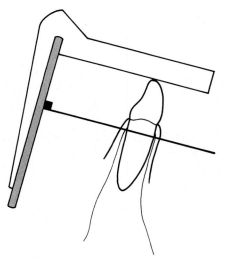

**Projection of Central Ray.** Orient the central ray through the interproximal space between the central and lateral incisors.

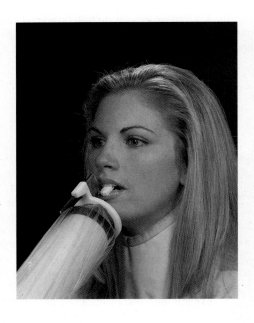

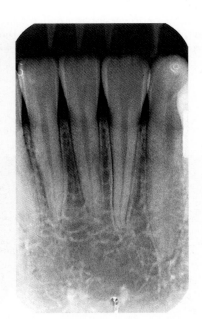

**Point of Entry.** The central ray enters below the lower lip and about 1 cm lateral to the midline.

## PARALLELING TECHNIQUE • **MANDIBULAR CANINE PROJECTION**

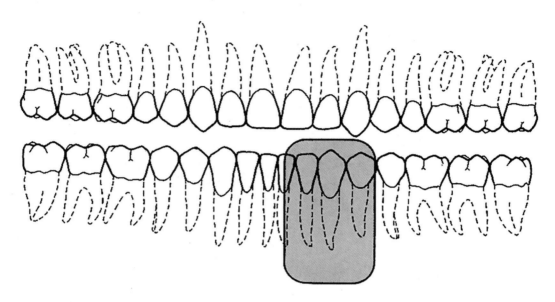

**Image Field.** This image should show the entire mandibular canine and its periapical area. Open its mesial contact area. The distal contact is included on other projections.

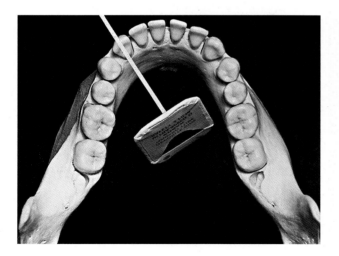

**Receptor Placement.** Place a No. 1 receptor packet in the mouth with its long dimension vertical and the canine in the midline of the receptor. Position it as far lingual as the tongue and contralateral alveolar process permit, with its long axis parallel and in line with the canine. The instrument must be tipped with the bite-block on the canine before the patient is asked to close.

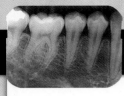

## PARALLELING TECHNIQUE • MANDIBULAR CANINE PROJECTION—cont'd

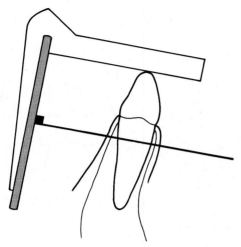

**Projection of Central Ray.** Direct the central ray through the mesial contact of the canine without regard to the distal contact.

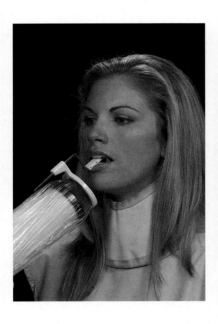 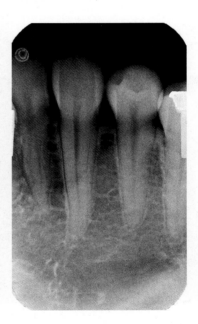

**Point of Entry.** The point of entry is nearly perpendicular to the ala of the nose, over the position of the canine, and about 3 cm above the inferior border of the mandible.

PARALLELING TECHNIQUE • **MANDIBULAR PREMOLAR PROJECTION**

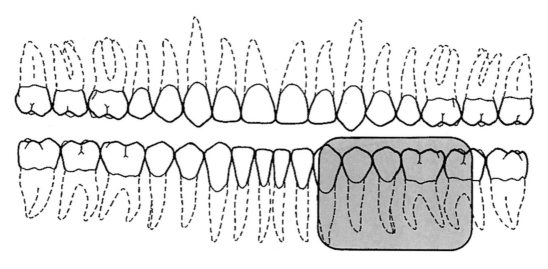

**Image Field.** The radiograph of this area should show the distal half of the canine, the two premolars, and the first molar.

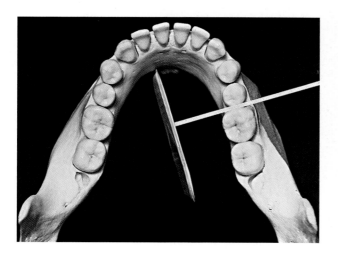

**Receptor Placement.** Bring the No. 2 receptor into the mouth with its plane nearly horizontal. Rotate the lead edge to the floor of the mouth between the tongue and the teeth with the anterior border near the midline of the canine. Place the receptor away from the teeth to position it in the deeper portion of the mouth. Placing the receptor toward the midline also provides more room for the anterior border of the receptor in the curvature of the jaw as it sweeps anteriorly. Prevent the anterior border from contacting the very sensitive attached gingiva on the lingual surface of the mandible.

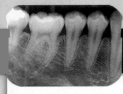

## PARALLELING TECHNIQUE • **MANDIBULAR PREMOLAR PROJECTION—cont'd**

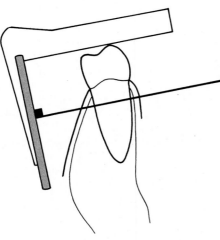

**Projection of Central Ray.** Position the receptor-holding instrument to project the central ray through the second premolar-molar area. The vertical angulation should be small, nearly parallel with the occlusal plane, to keep the receptor as nearly parallel with the long axis of the teeth as possible. Adjust the horizontal angulation and the placement of the receptor-holding device to direct the beam through the premolar contact points.

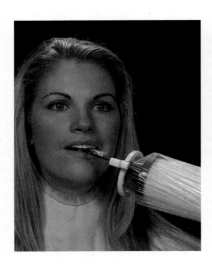
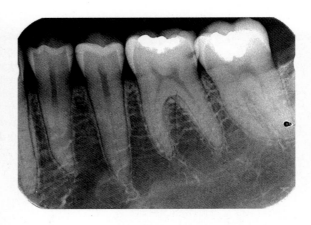

**Point of Entry.** The point of entry of the central ray is below the pupil of the eye and about 3 cm above the inferior border of the mandible.

## PARALLELING TECHNIQUE • **MANDIBULAR MOLAR PROJECTION**

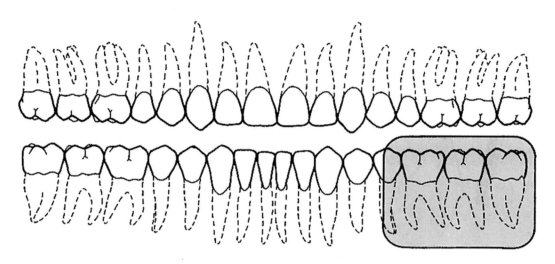

**Image Field.** The radiograph of this region should include the distal half of the second premolar and the three mandibular permanent molars. In the case of an impacted third molar or a pathologic condition distal to the third molar, a distal oblique molar projection or even additional extraoral projections (panoramic or lateral ramus) may be required to demonstrate the area adequately. If the molar area is edentulous, place the receptor far enough posterior to include the retromolar area in the examination.

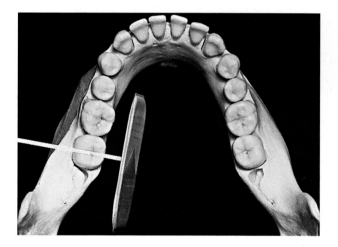

**Receptor Placement.** Place the No. 2 receptor in the mouth with its plane nearly horizontal. Rotate the inferior edge downward beneath the lateral border of the tongue, displacing it medially. The anterior edge of the receptor should be at about the middle of the second premolar. In most cases the tongue forces the receptor near the alveolar process and molars, aligning it parallel with the long axis of the teeth and the line of occlusion.

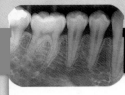

## PARALLELING TECHNIQUE • **MANDIBULAR MOLAR PROJECTION—cont'd**

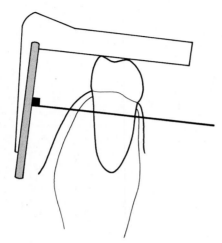

**Projection of Central Ray.** Proper placement of the holding instrument directs the central ray through the second molar. Adjust the horizontal angulation to project the beam through the contact areas. Because of the slight lingual inclination of the molars, the central ray may have some slight positive angulation (approximately 8 degrees).

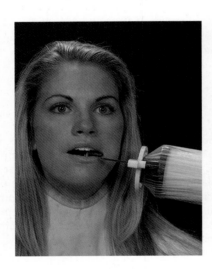 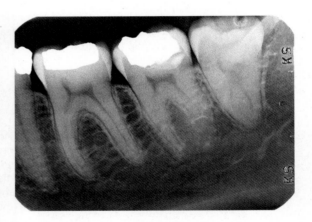

**Point of Entry.** Direct the point of entry of the central ray below the outer canthus of the eye about 3 cm above the inferior border of the mandible.

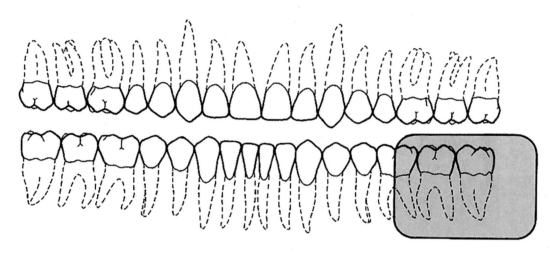

**Image Field.** The distal oblique projection provides a view of the third molar and the retromolar area of the mandible that usually is not included in the molar radiograph. It is intended primarily for detection or examination of impacted teeth and pathologic conditions in the bone in this area rather than for the teeth themselves; the images of the teeth are distorted and overlap because of the oblique path of the x-ray beam. This projection may eliminate the requirement for an extraoral radiograph of the area.

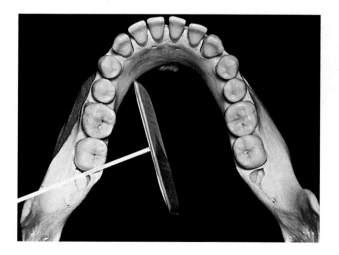

**Receptor Placement.** Place the receptor holder in the floor of the mouth between the tongue and alveolar process and parallel with the long axis of the molars. Position the instrument as far posteriorly as possible and then rotate the receptor-holding device distally, moving the posterior margin of the receptor toward the midline. The beam is directed posteroanteriorly, and more distal objects are projected anteriorly onto the receptor.

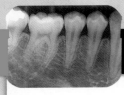

## PARALLELING TECHNIQUE • MANDIBULAR DISTAL OBLIQUE MOLAR PROJECTION—cont'd

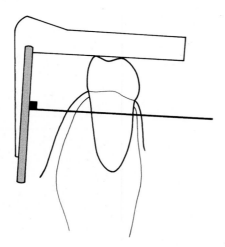

**Projection of Central Ray.** The position of the holding instrument projects the central ray from a more posterior aspect through the third molar area to the receptor.

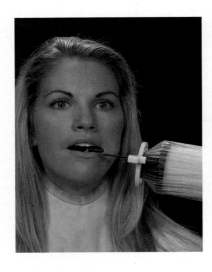

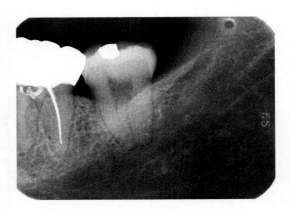

**Point of Entry.** Orient the point of entry about 3 cm above the antegonial notch on the inferior border of the mandible, in line with the anterior border of the ramus.

TABLE **9-1**
*Angulation Guidelines for Bisecting-Angle Projections**

| PROJECTION | MAXILLA | MANDIBLE |
| --- | --- | --- |
| Incisors | +40 degrees | −15 degrees |
| Canines | +45 degrees | −20 degrees |
| Premolars | +30 degrees | −10 degrees |
| Molars | +20 degrees | −5 degrees |

NOTE: With a positive (+) angulation the aiming tube is pointed downward, and with a negative (−) angulation it is pointed upward.
*When the occlusal plane is oriented parallel with the floor.

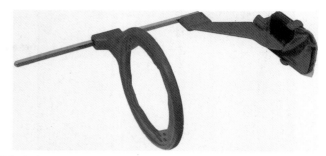

FIG. **9-6**   Receptor-holding device for bitewing radiographs. Note the external localizing ring, which is used to position the aiming tube of the x-ray machine to ensure that the entire receptor is in the x-ray beam. (Courtesy Dentsply Rinn, Elgin, Ill.)

## Angulation of the Tube Head

*Horizontal Angulation.*  When a receptor-holding device with a beam-localizing ring is used, the instrument is positioned horizontally so that when the tube is aligned with the ring, the central ray is directed through the contacts in the region being examined. If the receptor-holding device does not have a beam-localizing feature, the tube is pointed so as to direct the central ray through the contacts. In this situation the radiation beam is also centered on the receptor. This angulation usually is at right angles (in the horizontal projection) to the buccal or facial surfaces of the teeth in each region.

*Vertical Angulation.*  In practice, the clinician's goal is to aim the central ray of the x-ray beam at right angles to a plane bisecting the angle between the receptor and the long axis of the tooth. This principle works well with flat, two-dimensional structures, but teeth that have depth or are multirooted show evidence of distortion. Excessive vertical angulation results in foreshortening of the image, whereas insufficient vertical angulation results in image elongation. The angle that directs the central ray perpendicular to the bisecting plane varies with the individual's anatomy. Several measurements can be used as a general guide when the occlusal plane is oriented parallel with the floor (Table 9-1).

## BITEWING EXAMINATIONS

Bitewing (also called *interproximal*) radiographs include the crowns of the maxillary and mandibular teeth and the alveolar crest on the same receptor. Bitewing receptors are particularly valuable for detecting interproximal caries in the early stages of development before it becomes clinically apparent. Because of the horizontal angle of the x-ray beam, these radiographs also may reveal secondary caries below restorations that may escape recognition in the periapical views. Bitewing projections are also useful for evaluating the periodontal condition. They provide a good perspective of the alveolar bone crest, and changes in bone height can be assessed accurately through comparison with the adjacent teeth. In addition, because of the angle of projection directly through the interproximal spaces, the bitewing receptor is especially effective and useful for detecting calculus deposits in interproximal areas. (Because of its relatively low radiodensity, calculus is better visualized on radiographs made with reduced exposure.) The long axis of bitewing receptors usually is oriented horizontally but may be oriented vertically.

## Horizontal Bitewing Receptors

To obtain the desirable characteristics of the bitewing examination described, the beam is carefully aligned between the teeth and parallel with the occlusal plane. As the receptor or receptor-holding instrument is placed in the mouth, the portion of the mandibular quadrant that is being radiographed is in view. The position of the teeth in this segment of the mandibular quadrant is evaluated, and the beam is directed through the contacts. Some difference may exist in the curvature of the mandibular and maxillary arches. However, when the x-ray beam is accurately directed through the mandibular premolar contacts, overlapping is minimal or absent in the maxillary premolar segment. A few degrees of tolerance are available in the horizontal angulation before overlapping becomes critical. The contact between the maxillary first and second molars often is angled a few degrees more anteriorly than between the mandibular first and second molars. The aiming cylinder is positioned about +10 degrees to project the beam parallel with the occlusal plane (occlusal dentinoenamel junction [DEJ]). This minimizes overlapping of the opposing cusps onto the occlusal surface and thus improves the probability of detecting early occlusal lesions at the DEJ.

The XCP bitewing instrument has an external guide ring for positioning the tube head. This reduces the possibility of cone cutting the receptor (Fig. 9-6). To position the XCP instrument properly, the guide bar is placed parallel with the direction of the beam that opens the contacts of the dentition being examined.

A receptor fitted with a bitewing tab or loop may be used instead of a holding device (Fig. 9-7). The receptor is placed in a comfortable position lingual to the teeth to be examined. The aiming cylinder is oriented in the predetermined direction that passes the x-ray beam through the interproximal spaces. To help prevent cone cutting, the central ray is directed toward the center of the bitewing tab, which protrudes to the buccal side. The beam is angulated +7 to +10 degrees vertically to preclude overlap of the cusps onto the occlusal surface.

Two posterior bitewing views, a premolar and a molar, are recommended for each quadrant. However, for children aged 12 years or younger, one bitewing receptor (No. 2 receptor) usually suffices. The premolar projection should include the distal half of the canines and the crowns of the premolars. Because the mandibular canines usually are more mesial than the maxillary canines, the mandibular canine is used as the guide for placement of the premolar bitewing receptor. The molar bitewing receptor is placed 1 or 2 mm beyond the most distally erupted molar (maxillary or mandibular).

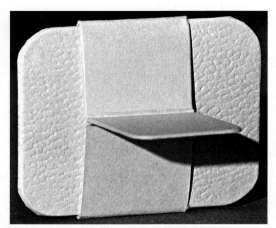

FIG. **9-7**   Bitewing loop, showing the tab that the patient bites on to support the receptor (film) during exposure.

## Vertical Bitewing Receptors

Vertical bitewing receptors usually are used when the patient has moderate to extensive alveolar bone loss. Orienting the length of the receptor vertically increases the likelihood that the residual alveolar crests in the maxilla and the mandible will be recorded on the radiograph (Fig. 9-8). The principles for positioning the receptor and orienting the x-ray beam are otherwise the same as for horizontal bitewing projections.

*Text continued on p. 147.*

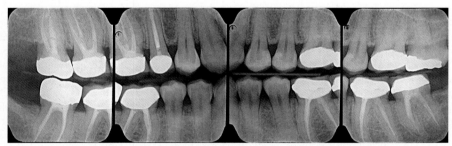

FIG. **9-8**   A set of vertical bitewings. Orienting the length of the receptor vertically increases the likelihood that, even in patients with extensive alveolar bone loss, the residual alveolar crests in the maxilla and the mandible will be recorded on the radiograph.

# PREMOLAR BITEWING PROJECTION*

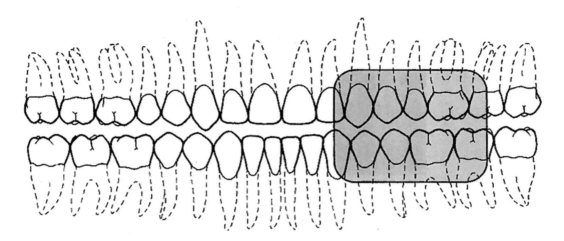

**Image Field.** This projection should cover the distal portion of the mandibular canine anteriorly and show equally the crowns of the maxillary and mandibular premolar teeth.

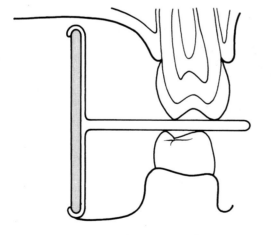

**Receptor Placement.** Place the receptor between the tongue and the teeth, far enough from the lingual surface of the teeth to prevent interference by the palate on closing and parallel to the long axes of the teeth. The anterior border of the receptor should extend beyond the contact area between the mandibular canine and the first premolar. Hold the receptor in place until the patient's mouth is completely closed. Holding the receptor while closing prevents it from being displaced distally.

*Patient photos for the bitewing projections on pages 138 and 140 are from Iannucci J, Jansen Howerton L: *Dental radiography: principles and techniques,* ed 3, St. Louis, 2006, Saunders.

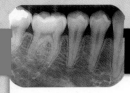

## PREMOLAR BITEWING PROJECTION—cont'd

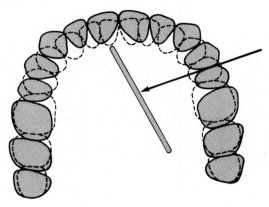

**Projection of Central Ray.** Adjust the horizontal angulation of the cone to project the central ray to the center of the receptor through the premolar contact areas. To compensate for the slight inclination of the receptor against the palatal mucosa, the vertical angulation should be about +5 degrees. (In the drawing, the mandibular teeth are in dashed lines.)

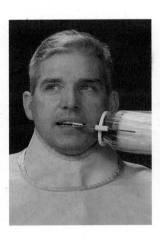

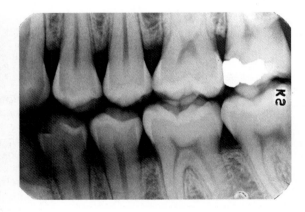

**Point of Entry.** Identify the point of entry by retracting the cheek and determining that the central ray will enter the line of occlusion at the point of contact between the second premolar and the first molar.

## MOLAR BITEWING PROJECTION

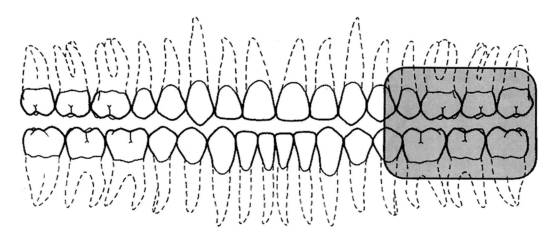

**Image Field.** This projection should show the distal surface of the most posterior erupted molar and equally the crowns of the maxillary and mandibular molars. Because the maxillary and mandibular molar contact areas may not be open from the same horizontal angulation, they may not be visible on one receptor. In this case it may be desirable to open the maxillary molar contacts because the mandibular molar contacts usually are open on the periapical receptors.

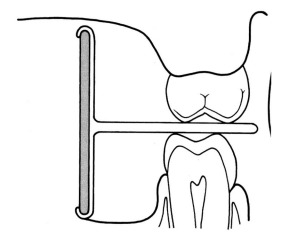

**Receptor Placement.** Place the receptor between the tongue and teeth, as far lingual as practical to avoid contacting the sensitive attached gingiva. The distal margin of the receptor should extend 1 to 2 mm beyond the most posterior erupted molar. When using the XCP, adjust the horizontal angulation by placing the guide bar parallel with the direction of the central ray to open the contact area between the first and second molars.

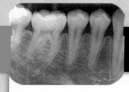

## MOLAR BITEWING PROJECTION—cont'd

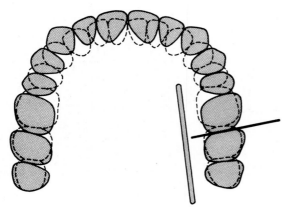

**Projection of Central Ray.** Project the central ray to the center of the receptor and through the contact of the first and second maxillary molars. Angle the central ray slightly from the anterior because the molar contacts usually are not oriented at right angles to the buccal surfaces of these teeth. A vertical angulation of +10 degrees is recommended. (In the drawing, the mandibular teeth are in *dashed lines*.)

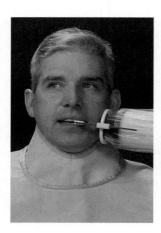

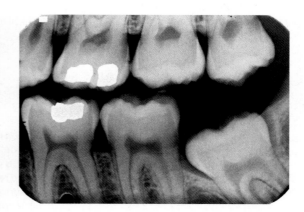

**Point of Entry.** The central ray should enter the cheek below the lateral canthus of the eye at the level of the occlusal plane.

## ANTERIOR MAXILLARY OCCLUSAL PROJECTION

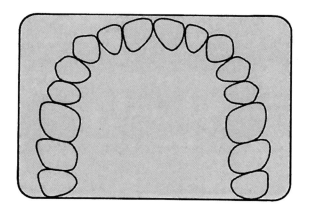

**Image Field.** The primary field of this projection includes the anterior maxilla and its dentition and the anterior floor of the nasal fossa and teeth from canine to canine.

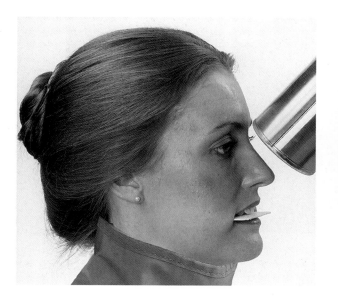

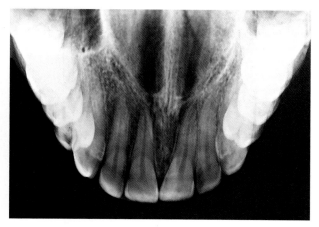

**Receptor Placement.** Adjust the patient's head so that the sagittal plane is perpendicular and the occlusal plane is horizontal to the floor. Place the receptor in the mouth with the exposure side toward the maxilla, the posterior border touching the rami, and the long dimension of the receptor perpendicular to the sagittal plane. The patient stabilizes the receptor by gently closing the mouth or using gentle bilateral thumb pressure.

**Projection of Central Ray.** Orient the central ray through the tip of the nose toward the middle of the receptor with approximately +45 degrees vertical angulation and 0 degrees horizontal angulation.

**Point of Entry.** The central ray enters the patient's face approximately through the tip of the nose.

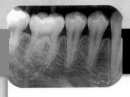

# CROSS-SECTIONAL MAXILLARY OCCLUSAL PROJECTION*

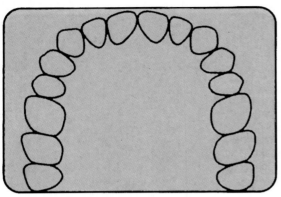

**Image Field.** This projection shows the palate, zygomatic processes of the maxilla, anteroinferior aspects of each antrum, nasolacrimal canals, teeth from second molar to second molar, and nasal septum.

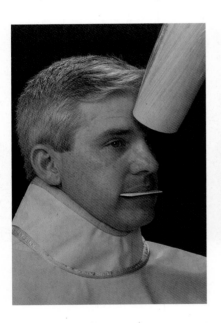

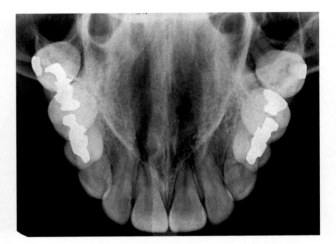

**Receptor Placement.** Seat the patient upright with the sagittal plane perpendicular to the floor and the occlusal plane horizontal. Place the receptor, with its long dimension perpendicular to the sagittal plane, crosswise in the mouth. Gently push the receptor in backward until it contacts the anterior border of the mandibular rami. The patient stabilizes the receptor by gently closing the mouth.

**Projection of Central Ray.** Direct the central ray at a vertical angulation of +65 degrees and a horizontal angulation of 0 degrees, to the bridge of the nose just below the nasion, toward the middle of the receptor.

**Point of Entry.** Generally, the central ray enters the patient's face through the bridge of the nose.

*Patient photo for this occlusal projection is from Iannucci J, Jansen Howerton L: *Dental radiography: principles and techniques,* ed 3, St. Louis, 2006, Saunders.

# LATERAL MAXILLARY OCCLUSAL PROJECTION*

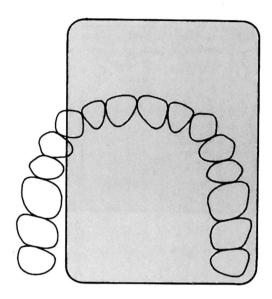

**Image Field.** This projection shows a quadrant of the alveolar ridge of the maxilla, inferolateral aspect of the antrum, tuberosity, and teeth from the lateral incisor to the contralateral third molar. In addition, the zygomatic process of the maxilla superimposes over the roots of the molar teeth.

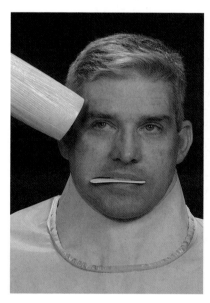

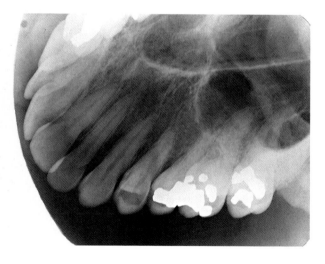

**Receptor Placement.** Place the receptor with its long axis parallel to the sagittal plane and on the side of interest, with the tube side toward the side of the maxilla in question. Push the receptor posteriorly until it touches the ramus. Position the lateral border parallel with the buccal surfaces of the posterior teeth, extending laterally approximately 1 cm past the buccal cusps. Ask the patient to close gently to hold the receptor in position.

**Projection of Central Ray.** Orient the central ray with a vertical angulation of +60 degrees, to a point 2 cm below the lateral canthus of the eye, directed toward the center of the receptor.

**Point of Entry.** The central ray enters at a point approximately 2 cm below the lateral canthus of the eye.

*Patient photo for this occlusal projection is from Iannucci J, Jansen Howerton L: *Dental radiography: principles and techniques,* ed 3, St. Louis, 2006, Saunders.

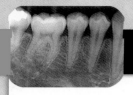

# ANTERIOR MANDIBULAR OCCLUSAL PROJECTION*

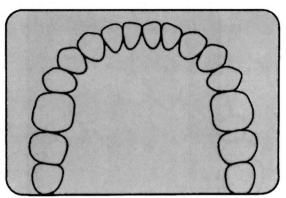

**Image Field.** This projection includes the anterior portion of the mandible, the dentition from canine to canine, and the inferior cortical border of the mandible.

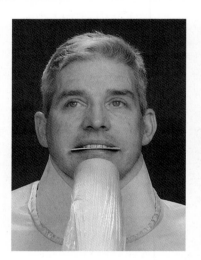

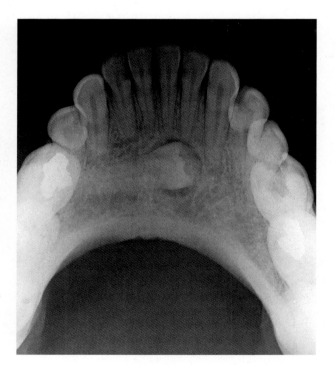

**Receptor Placement.** Seat the patient tilted back so that the occlusal plane is 45 degrees above horizontal. Place the receptor in the mouth with the long axis perpendicular to the sagittal plane and push it posteriorly until it touches the rami. Center the receptor with the pebbled side (tube side) down and ask the patient to bite lightly to hold the receptor in position.

**Projection of Central Ray.** Orient the central ray with −10 degrees angulation through the point of the chin toward the middle of the receptor; this gives the ray −55 degrees of angulation to the plane of the receptor.

**Point of Entry.** The point of entry of the central ray is in the midline and through the tip of the chin.

*Patient photo for this occlusal projection is from Iannucci J, Jansen Howerton L: *Dental radiography: principles and techniques,* ed 3, St. Louis, 2006, Saunders.

# CROSS-SECTIONAL MANDIBULAR OCCLUSAL PROJECTION*

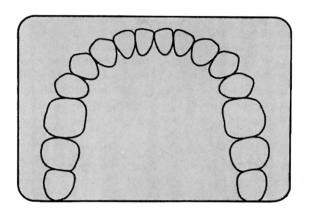

**Image Field.** This projection includes the soft tissue of the floor of the mouth and reveals the lingual and buccal plates of the mandible from second molar to second molar. When this view is made to examine the floor of the mouth (e.g., for sialoliths), the exposure time should be reduced to half the time used to create an image of the mandible.

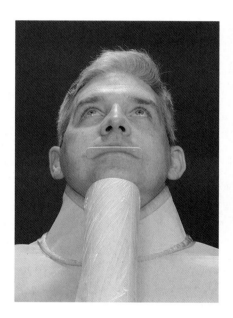

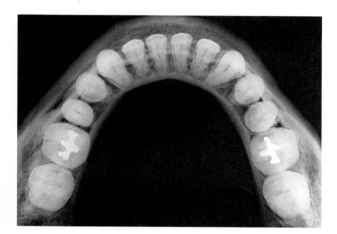

**Receptor Placement.** Seat the patient in a semireclining position with the head tilted back so that the ala-tragus line is almost perpendicular to the floor. Place the receptor in the mouth with its long axis perpendicular to the sagittal plane and with the tube side toward the mandible. The anterior border of the receptor should be approximately 1 cm beyond the mandibular central incisors. Ask the patient to bite gently on the receptor to hold it in position.

**Projection of Central Ray.** Direct the central ray at the midline through the floor of the mouth approximately 3 cm below the chin, at right angles to the center of the receptor.

**Point of Entry.** The point of entry of the central ray is in the midline through the floor of the mouth approximately 3 cm below the chin.

*Patient photo for this occlusal projection is from Iannucci J, Jansen Howerton L: *Dental radiography: principles and techniques,* ed 3, St. Louis, 2006, Saunders.

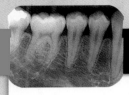

## LATERAL MANDIBULAR OCCLUSAL PROJECTION

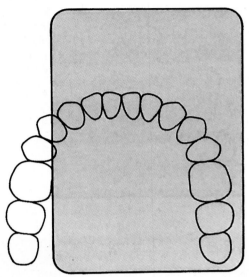

**Image Field.** This projection covers the soft tissue of half the floor of the mouth, the buccal and lingual cortical plates of half of the mandible, and the teeth from the lateral incisor to the contralateral third molar. When this view is used to provide an image of the floor of the mouth, the exposure time should be reduced to half that used to provide an image of the mandible.

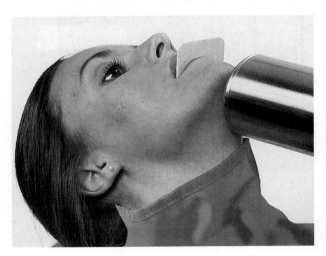

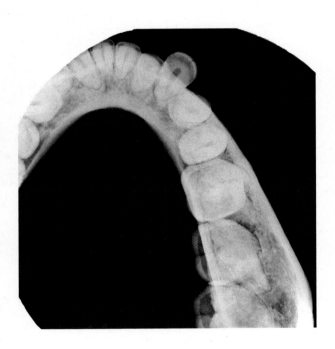

**Receptor Placement.** Seat the patient in a semireclining position with the head tilted back so that the ala-tragus line is almost perpendicular to the floor. Place the receptor in the mouth with its long axis initially parallel with the sagittal plane and with the pebbled side down toward the mandible. Place the receptor as far posterior as possible, then shift the long axis buccally (right or left) so that the lateral border of the receptor is parallel with the buccal surfaces of the posterior teeth and extends laterally approximately 1 cm.

**Projection of Central Ray.** Direct the central ray perpendicular to the center of the receptor through a point beneath the chin, approximately 3 cm posterior to the point of the chin and 3 cm lateral to the midline.

**Point of Entry.** The point of entry of the central ray is beneath the chin, approximately 3 cm posterior to the chin and approximately 3 cm lateral to the midline.

## Occlusal Radiography

An occlusal radiograph displays a relatively large segment of a dental arch. It may include the palate or floor of the mouth and a reasonable extent of the contiguous lateral structures. Occlusal radiographs also are useful when patients are unable to open wide enough for periapical radiographs or for other reasons cannot accept periapical receptors. Because occlusal radiographs are exposed at a steep angulation, they may be used with conventional periapical radiographs to determine the location of objects in all three dimensions. Typically, the occlusal radiograph is especially useful in the following cases:

- To precisely locate roots and supernumerary, unerupted, and impacted teeth (this technique is especially useful for impacted canines and third molars)
- To localize foreign bodies in the jaws and stones in the ducts of sublingual and submandibular glands
- To demonstrate and evaluate the integrity of the anterior, medial, and lateral outlines of the maxillary sinus
- To aid in the examination of patients with trismus, who can open their mouths only a few millimeters; this condition precludes intraoral radiography, which may be impossible or at least extremely painful for the patient
- To obtain information about the location, nature, extent, and displacement of fractures of the mandible and maxilla
- To determine the medial and lateral extent of disease (e.g., cysts, osteomyelitis, malignancies) and to detect disease in the palate or floor of the mouth

To make an occlusal radiograph, a relatively large receptor (7.7 × 5.8 cm [3 × 2.3 inches]) is inserted between the occlusal surfaces of the teeth. Occlusal receptors are made only of film or storage phosphor plates. Neither CCD nor CMOS sensors exist this large. As its name implies, the receptor lies in the plane of occlusion. The "tube" side of this receptor is positioned toward the jaw to be examined, and the x-ray beam is directed through the jaw to the receptor. Because of its size, the receptor allows examination of relatively large portions of the jaw. Standardized projections are used, which stipulate a desired relationship between the central ray, receptor, and region being examined. However, the clinician should feel free to modify these relationships to meet a specific clinical requirement.

## Radiographic Examination of Children

Concern about radiation protection is most important for children because of their greater sensitivity to irradiation. The best way to reduce unnecessary exposure is for the dentist to make the minimal number of receptors required for the individual patient. These judgments are based on a careful clinical examination and consideration of the patient's age, medical history, growth considerations, and general oral health, as well as whether caries is present and the time elapsed since previous examinations. Prudence suggests making bitewing examinations for caries assessment at periodic intervals after the patient's contacts have closed. The frequency should be determined partly by the patient's caries rate. A periapical survey is often recommended for children early in the mixed dentition stage. Special attention should be paid to procedures that reduce exposure (see Chapter 3), including use of fast receptor, proper processing, beam-limiting devices, and leaded aprons and thyroid shields.

Radiography in a child can be an interesting and challenging experience. Although the principles of periapical radiography for children

are the same as for adults, in practice children present special considerations because of their small anatomic structures and possible behavioral problems. The smaller size of the arches and dentition requires the use of smaller periapical receptors. The relatively shallow palate and floor of the mouth may require further modification of receptor placement. Special radiographic examinations using occlusal receptor for extraoral projections have been suggested.

## PATIENT MANAGEMENT

Children are often apprehensive about the radiographic examination, much as they are about many other types of dental procedures. The radiographic examination usually is the first manipulative procedure performed on a young patient. If this examination is nonthreatening and comfortable, subsequent dental experiences usually are accepted with little or no apprehension. This apprehension is best allayed by familiarizing children with the procedure, which is done by explaining it in a manner they can comprehend. It often is wise to describe the x-ray machine as a camera used to take pictures of teeth. The child can become more comfortable with the receptor and x-ray machine by touching them before the examination. The operator should carry on a conversation with children to distract them and gain their confidence. It may be advantageous for the child to watch an older brother or sister being radiographed or to have the parent or dental assistant serve as a model. For children who feel a gagging sensation, the clinician can have them breathe through the nose, curl their toes, make a fist, or follow other such devices to distract their attention from the radiographic procedure. However, if the procedure is postponed until the next appointment, the gag reflex may not be encountered or often is much easier for the patient to control. It is especially important to explain to the patient that the procedure will be much easier the next time—plant the positive thought.

## EXAMINATION COVERAGE

When a complete radiographic survey is necessary, it should show the periapical region of all teeth, the proximal surfaces of all posterior teeth, and the crypts of the developing permanent teeth. The number of projections required depends on the child's size. Also, an exposure appropriate to the child's size should be used. For example, a 50% reduction in the mA used for the usual young adult gives the proper density for patients younger than 10 years. Exposure is reduced about 25% for those aged between 10 and 15 years.

### Primary Dentition (3 to 6 Years)

A combination of projections can be used to provide adequate coverage for the pedodontic patient. This examination may consist of two anterior occlusal receptors, two posterior bitewing receptors, and up to four posterior periapical receptors as indicated (Fig. 9-9). For the maxillary and interproximal projections, the child is seated upright with the sagittal plane perpendicular to and the occlusal plane parallel with the floor (horizontal plane). For mandibular projections, except the occlusal, the child is seated upright with the sagittal plane perpendicular. The tragus corner of the mouth line is oriented parallel to the floor. Some find that a panoramic view, rather than the four periapicals, is more informative and results in less exposure to the child (see Chapter 3).

*Maxillary Anterior Occlusal Projection.* A No. 2 receptor should be placed in the mouth with its long axis perpendicular to the sagittal plane and the pebbled surface toward the maxillary teeth. The

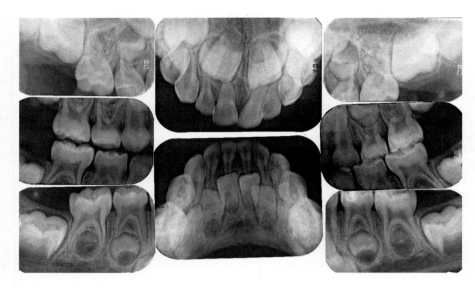

FIG. **9-9**  Radiographic examination of primary dentition consists of two anterior occlusal views, four posterior periapical views, and two bitewing views.

receptor is centered on the midline with the anterior border extending just beyond the incisal edges of the anterior teeth. The central ray is directed at a vertical angulation of +60 degrees through the tip of the nose toward the center of the receptor.

*Mandibular Anterior Occlusal Projection.* The child should be seated with the head tipped back so that the occlusal plane is about 25 degrees above the plane of the floor. A No. 2 receptor is placed with the long axis perpendicular to the sagittal plane and the pebbled surface toward the mandibular teeth. The central ray is oriented at −30 degrees vertical angulation and through the tip of the chin toward the receptor.

*Bitewing Projection.* A No. 0 receptor is used with a paper loop receptor holder. The receptor is placed in the child's mouth as in the adult premolar bitewing projection. The image field should include the distal half of the canine and the deciduous molars. A positive vertical angulation of +5 to +10 degrees should be used. The horizontal angle is oriented to direct the beam through the interproximal spaces.

*Deciduous Maxillary Molar Periapical Projection.* A No. 0 receptor in a modified XCP or BAI bite-block, either with or without the aiming ring and indicator bar, is used. The receptor is positioned in the midline of the palate with the anterior border extending to the maxillary primary canine. The image field of this projection should include the distal half of the primary canine and both primary molars.

*Deciduous Mandibular Molar Projection.* A No. 0 receptor is positioned in a modified XCP or BAI bite-block, with or without the aiming ring and indicator bar, between the posterior teeth and tongue. The exposed radiograph should show the distal half of the mandibular primary canine and the primary molar teeth.

### Mixed Dentition (7 to 12 Years)

A complete examination of the mixed dentition, if indicated, consists of two incisor periapical views, four canine periapical views, four posterior periapical views, and two or four posterior bitewings (Fig. 9-10). For the maxillary and interproximal projections, the child should be seated upright with the sagittal plane perpendicular and the occlusal plane parallel to the floor. For the mandibular projections, the child should be seated upright with the sagittal plane perpendicu-

lar and the ala-tragus line parallel to the floor. XCP instruments are used for larger children. The bisecting-angle bite-blocks may be more comfortable for smaller individuals.

*Maxillary Anterior Periapical Projection.* A No. 1 receptor should be centered on the embrasure between the central incisors in the mouth behind the maxillary central and lateral incisors. The receptor should be centered on the midline.

*Mandibular Anterior Periapical Projection.* A No. 1 receptor should be positioned behind the mandibular central and lateral incisors.

*Canine Periapical Projection.* A No. 1 receptor should be positioned behind each of the canines.

*Deciduous and Permanent Molar Periapical Projection.* A No. 1 or No. 2 receptor (if the child is large enough) should be positioned with the anterior edge behind the canine.

*Posterior Bitewing Projection.* Bitewing projections should be exposed in the premolar region with a No. 1 or No. 2 receptor as previously described, using either bitewing tabs or the Rinn bitewing instrument. Four bitewing projections should be exposed when the second permanent molars have erupted.

### Mobile Radiography

There are occasions when it is difficult to have a patient come to a conventional wall-mounted dental x-ray machine. For instance, in remote sites such as nursing homes, hospitals, or at disaster scenes, it could be highly advantageous to have a portable machine that could be taken directly to the patient. Combining such a portable x-ray generator with digital imaging provides rapid, self-contained imaging capability. In recent years such a portable battery-powered x-ray generator has been approved by the Food and Drug Administration (Fig. 9-11). Clinical trials have shown that this unit can be held stable and produces clinically acceptable images. This machine uses a high-frequency, constant potential x-ray generator (60 kilowatt constant potential) and has a short focal spot to skin distance (20 cm). Both these factors allow for short exposure times compared with conventional units. It has a small focus spot (0.4 mm). The operator dose is mitigated by the use of internal shielding materials in the unit to reduce leakage exposure and a shield on the aiming cylinder to

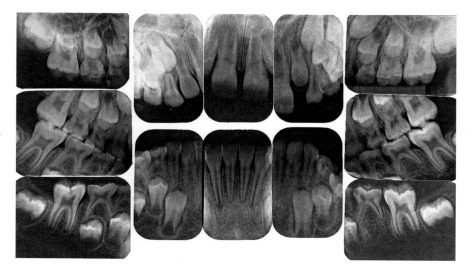

FIG. **9-10** Radiographic examination of mixed dentition consists of two incisor views, four canine views, four posterior views, and two bitewing views.

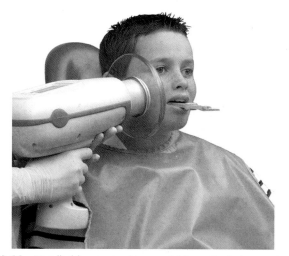

FIG. **9-11** Handheld x-ray machine useful for patients in remote situations. Operator dose is reduced by internal shielding and shield on aiming cylinder to reduce backscatter. (Courtesy Aribex, Inc.)

minimize backscatter from the patient. These units are approved for use in many but not all states in the United States.

## Special Considerations

The radiographic procedures that have been described in this chapter are for the "well" patient. These procedures may need to be modified for patients who have unusual difficulties. Specific modifications depend on the patient's physical and emotional characteristics. As with any dental procedure, however, the dental assistant begins the examination by showing appreciation of the patient's condition and sympathy for any problems that might occur for either of them. If the assistant is kind but firm, the patient's confidence increases, which helps the patient relax and cooperate. Following are a few conditions and circumstances that may be encountered, with some recommenda-

tions and suggestions that may help the clinician achieve an adequate radiographic examination.

## INFECTION

Infection in the orofacial structures may result in edema and lead to trismus of some of the muscles of mastication. As a result, intraoral radiography may be painful to the patient and difficult for both the patient and radiologist. Under such circumstances extraoral or occlusal techniques may offer the only possibility of an examination. The choice of a specific extraoral projection depends on the condition and the areas to be examined. Although the resulting radiograph may not be ideal in many respects, it usually provides more useful information than the diagnostician would have without it. In the case of edema in an area to be examined, exposure time should be increased to compensate for the tissue swelling.

## TRAUMA

A patient who has undergone trauma may have a dental or facial fracture. Dental fractures are best appreciated by using periapical or occlusal radiographs. Special care must be taken when making these views because of the condition of the patient. Skeletal fractures are usually best seen with panoramic or other extraoral views or a computed tomography examination. In some cases patients with fractures of the facial skeleton may be bedridden because of involvement of other injuries. Consequently, an extraoral radiographic examination with the patient in the supine position is necessary. However, the circumstances need not compromise the techniques, and satisfactory intraoral radiographs can be produced if the proper relative positions of the tube, patient, and receptor are observed.

## PATIENTS WITH MENTAL DISABILITIES

Patients with mental disabilities may cause some difficulty for the radiologist who is attempting an examination. The difficulty usually is the result of the patient's lack of coordination or inability to comprehend what is expected. However, when the radiographic examination is performed speedily, unpredictable moves by the patient can be minimized. In some cases sedation may be required.

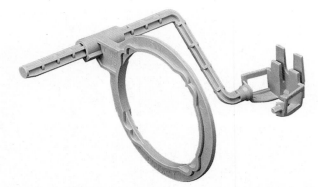

FIG. **9-12**    EndoRay receptor holder used for endodontic radiographs. (Courtesy Dentsply Rinn, Elgin, Ill.)

## PATIENTS WITH PHYSICAL DISABILITIES

Patients with physical disabilities (e.g., loss of vision, loss of hearing, loss of the use of any or all extremities, congenital defects such as cleft palate) may require special handling during a radiographic examination. These patients usually are cooperative and eager to assist. They may be accustomed to so much discomfort and inconvenience that their tolerance level is high, and they are not challenged by the relatively slight irritation represented by the x-ray procedures. Generally, intraoral and extraoral radiographic examinations may be performed for these patients if a good rapport between the patient and radiology technician is established and maintained. Members of the patient's family often are very helpful in assisting the patient into and out of the examination chair and in receptor positioning and holding, inasmuch as they usually are familiar with the patient's condition and accustomed to coping with it.

## GAG REFLEX

Occasionally, patients who need a radiographic examination manifest a gag reflex at the slightest provocation. These patients usually are very apprehensive and frightened by unknown procedures; others simply seem to have very sensitive tissue that precipitates a gag reflex when stimulated. This sensitivity is manifested when the receptor is placed in the oral cavity. To overcome this disability, the radiologist should make an effort to relax and reassure the patient. The radiologist can describe and explain the procedures. Often gagging can be controlled if the operator bolsters the patient's confidence by demonstrating technical competence and showing authority tempered with compassion. The gag reflex often is worse when a patient is tired; therefore it is advisable to perform the examination in the morning, when the individual is well rested, especially in the case of children.

Stimulating the posterior dorsum of the tongue or the soft palate usually initiates the gag reflex. Consequently, during the placement of the receptor, the tongue should be very relaxed and positioned well to the floor of the mouth. This can be accomplished by asking the patient to swallow deeply just before opening the mouth for placement of the receptor. (The dentist should never mention the tongue, nor ask patients to relax the tongue; this usually makes them more conscious of it and precipitates involuntary movements.) The

receptor is carried into the mouth parallel to the occlusal plane. When the desired area is reached, the receptor is rotated with a decisive motion, bringing it into contact with the palate or the floor of the mouth. Sliding it along the palate or tongue is likely to stimulate the gag reflex. Also, the dentist must keep in mind that the longer the receptor stays in the mouth, the greater the possibility that the patient will start to gag. The patient should be advised to breathe rapidly through the nose because mouth breathing usually aggravates this condition.

Any little exercise that can be devised that does not interfere with the x-ray examination but shifts the patient's attention from the receptor and the mouth is likely to relieve the gag reaction. Asking patients to hold their breath often can create such a distraction or to keep a foot or arm suspended during receptor placement and exposure. In extreme cases, topical anesthetic agents in mouthwashes or spray can be administered to produce temporary numbness of the tongue and palate to reduce gagging. However, in our experience this procedure gives limited results. The most effective approach is to reduce apprehension, minimize tissue irritation, and encourage rapid breathing through the nose. If all measures fail, an extraoral examination may be the only means, short of administering general anesthesia, to examine the patient radiographically.

## RADIOGRAPHIC TECHNIQUES FOR ENDODONTICS

Radiographs are essential to the practice of endodontics. Not only are they indispensable for determining the diagnosis and prognosis of pulp treatment, they also are the most reliable method of managing endodontic treatment. The presence of a rubber dam, rubber dam clamp, and root canal instruments may complicate an intraoral periapical examination by impairing proper receptor positioning and aiming cylinder angulation. Despite these obstacles, certain requirements must be observed:

1. The tooth being treated must be centered in the image.
2. The receptor must be positioned as far from the tooth and apex as the region permits to ensure that the apex of the tooth and some periapical bone are apparent on the radiograph.

For maxillary projections, the patient is seated so that the sagittal plane is perpendicular and the occlusal plane is parallel to the floor. For mandibular projections, the patient is seated upright with the sagittal plane perpendicular and the tragus-to-corner of the mouth line parallel to the floor. Specially designed receptor holders for endodontic radiographs are available (Fig. 9-12). These instruments fit over files, clamps, and the rubber dam without touching the subject tooth. The aiming cylinder is aligned so as to direct the central ray perpendicular to the center of the receptor.

Often a single radiograph of a multirooted tooth made at the normal vertical and horizontal projection does not display all the roots. In these cases, when it is necessary to separate the roots on multirooted teeth, a second projection may be made. The horizontal angulation is altered 20 degrees mesially for maxillary premolars, 20 degrees mesially or distally for maxillary molars, or 20 degrees distally for an oblique projection of mandibular molar roots.

If a sinus tract is encountered, its course is tracked by threading a No. 40 gutta-percha cone through the tract before the radiograph is made. It also is possible to localize and determine the depth of periodontal defects with this gutta-percha tracking technique.

A final radiograph of the treated tooth is made to demonstrate the quality of the root canal filling and the condition of the periapical tissues after removal of the clamp and rubber dam.

## PREGNANCY

Although a fetus is sensitive to ionizing radiation, the amount of exposure received by an embryo or fetus during dental radiography is extremely low. No incidences have been reported of damage to a fetus from dental radiography. Regardless, prudence suggests that such radiographic examinations be kept to a minimum consistent with the mother's dental needs. As with any patient, radiographic examination is limited during pregnancy to cases with a specific diagnostic indication. With the low patient dose afforded by use of optimal radiation safety techniques (see Chapter 3), an intraoral or extraoral examination can be performed whenever a reasonable diagnostic requirement exists.

## EDENTULOUS PATIENTS

Radiographic examination of edentulous patients is important, whether the area of interest is one tooth or an entire arch. These areas may contain roots, residual infection, impacted teeth, cysts, or other pathologic entities that may adversely affect the usefulness of prosthetic appliances or the patient's health. After a determination has been made that these entities are not present, repeated examinations to detect them are not warranted in the absence of signs or symptoms.

If available, a panoramic examination of the edentulous jaws is most convenient. If abnormalities of the alveolar ridges are identified, the higher resolution of periapical receptor is used to make intraoral projections to supplement the panoramic examination.

In a completely or partly edentulous patient, a receptor-holding device is used for intraoral radiography of the alveolar ridges. Placement of the receptor-holding instrument may be complicated by its tipping into the voids normally occupied by the crowns of the missing teeth. To manage this difficulty, cotton rolls are placed between the ridge and the receptor holder, supporting the holder in a horizontal position. An orthodontic elastic band to hold cotton rolls to the bite-block on the receptor holder often is useful when several such projections must be exposed. With elastics, it is simple to maneuver the cotton rolls into the areas that require support. The patient may steady the receptor-holding instrument with a hand or an opposing denture.

If panoramic equipment is not available, an examination consisting of 14 intraoral views provides an excellent survey. The exposure required for an edentulous ridge is approximately 25% less than that for a dentulous ridge. This examination consists of seven projections in each jaw (adult No. 2 receptor) as follows:

Central incisors (midline): one projection
Lateral canine: two projections
Premolar: two projections
Molar: two projections

## BIBLIOGRAPHY

Adriaens PA, De Boever J, Vande Velde F: Comparison of intra-oral long-cone paralleling radiographic surveys and orthopantomographs with special reference to the bone height, *J Oral Rehabil* 9:355-365, 1982.

Biggerstaff RH, Phillips JR: A quantitative comparison of paralleling long-cone and bisection-of-angle periapical radiography, *Oral Surg Oral Med Oral Pathol* 62:673-677, 1976.

Dubrez B, Jacot-Descombes S, Cimasoni G: Reliability of a paralleling instrument for dental radiographs, *Oral Surg Oral Med Oral Pathol Oral Radiol Endod* 80:358-364, 1995.

Forsberg J, Halse A: Radiographic simulation of a periapical lesion comparing the paralleling and the bisecting-angle techniques, *Int Endod J* 27:133-138, 1994.

Iannucci J, Jansen Howerton L: *Dental radiography: principles and techniques,* ed 3, St. Louis, Saunders, 2006.

Scandrett FR, Tebo HG, Miller JT et al: Radiographic examination of the edentulous patient, 1: review of the literature and preliminary report comparing three methods, *Oral Surg Oral Med Oral Pathol* 35:266-274, 1973.

Schulze RK, d'Hoedt B: A method to calculate angular disparities between object and receptor in "paralleling technique," *Dentomaxillofac Radiol* 31:32-38, 2002.

Weclew TV: Comparing the paralleling extension cone technique and the bisecting angle technique, *J Acad Gen Dent* 22:18-20, 1974.

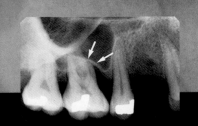

# CHAPTER 10

# Normal Radiographic Anatomy

The radiographic recognition of disease requires a sound knowledge of the radiographic appearance of normal structures. Intelligent diagnosis mandates an appreciation of the wide range of variation in the appearance of normal anatomic structures. Similarly, most patients demonstrate many of the normal radiographic landmarks, but it is a rare patient who shows them all. Accordingly, the absence of one or even several such landmarks in any individual should not necessarily be considered abnormal.

## Teeth

Teeth are composed primarily of dentin, with an enamel cap over the coronal portion and a thin layer of cementum over the root surface (Fig. 10-1). The enamel cap characteristically appears more radiopaque than the other tissues because it is the most dense, naturally occurring substance in the body. Because it is 90% mineral, it causes the greatest attenuation of x-ray photons. Its radiographic appearance is uniformly opaque and without evidence of the fine structure. Only the occlusal surface reflects the complex gross anatomy. The dentin is about 75% mineralized, and because of its lower mineral content, its radiographic appearance is roughly comparable to that of bone. Dentin is smooth and homogeneous on radiographs because of its uniform morphologic features. The junction between enamel and dentin appears as a distinct interface that separates these two structures. The thin layer of cementum on the root surface has a mineral content (50%) comparable to that of dentin. Cementum is not usually apparent radiographically because the contrast between it and dentin is so low and the cementum layer is so thin.

Diffuse radiolucent areas with ill-defined borders may be apparent radiographically on the mesial or distal aspects of teeth in the cervical regions between the edge of the enamel cap and the crest of the alveolar ridge (Fig. 10-2). This phenomenon, called *cervical burnout*, is caused by the normal configuration of the affected teeth, which results in decreased x-ray absorption in the areas in question. Close inspection will reveal intact edges of the proximal surfaces. Furthermore, the perception of these radiolucent areas results from the contrast with the adjacent, relatively opaque enamel and alveolar bone. Such radiolucencies should be anticipated in almost all teeth and should not be confused with root surface caries, which frequently have a similar appearance.

The pulp of normal teeth is composed of soft tissue and consequently appears radiolucent. The chambers and root canals containing the pulp extend from the interior of the crown to the apices of the roots. Although the shape of most pulp chambers is fairly uniform within tooth groups, great variations exist among individuals in the size of the pulp chambers and the extent of pulp horns. The practitioner must anticipate such variations in the proportions and distribution of the pulp and verify them radiographically when planning restorative procedures.

In normal, fully formed teeth the root canal may be apparent, extending from the pulp chamber to the apex of the root. An apical foramen is usually recognizable (Fig. 10-3). In other normal teeth the canal may appear constricted in the region of the apex and not discernible in the last millimeter or so of its length (Fig. 10-4). In this case the canal may occasionally exit on the side of the tooth, just short of the radiographic apex. Lateral canals may occur as branches of an otherwise normal root canal. They may extend to the apex and end in a normal, discernible foramen or may exit the side of the root. In either case, two or more terminal foramina might cause endodontic treatment to fail if they are not identified.

At the end of a developing tooth root the pulp canal diverges and the walls of the root rapidly taper to a knife edge (Fig. 10-5). In the recess formed by the root walls and extending a short distance beyond is a small, rounded, radiolucent area in the trabecular bone, surrounded by a thin layer of hyperostotic bone. This is the dental papilla bounded by its bony crypt. The papilla forms the dentin and the primordium of the pulp. When the tooth reaches maturity, the pulpal walls in the apical region begin to constrict and finally come into close apposition. Awareness of this sequence and its radiographic pattern is often useful in evaluating the stage of maturation of the developing tooth; it also helps avoid misidentifying the apical radiolucency as a periapical lesion.

In a mature tooth, the shape of the pulp chamber and canal may change. With aging occurs a gradual deposition of secondary dentin. This process begins apically, proceeds coronally, and may lead to pulp obliteration. Trauma to the tooth (e.g., from caries, a blow, restorations, attrition, or erosion) also may stimulate dentin production, leading to a reduction in size of the pulp chamber and canals. Such cases usually include evidence of the source of the pathologic stimulus. In the case of a blow to the teeth, however, only the patient's recollection may suggest the true reason for the reduced pulp chamber size.

## Supporting Structures

### LAMINA DURA

A radiograph of sound teeth in a normal dental arch demonstrates that the tooth sockets are bounded by a thin radiopaque layer of dense bone (Fig. 10-6). Its name, *lamina dura* ("hard layer"), is derived from its radiographic appearance. This layer is continuous with the shadow of

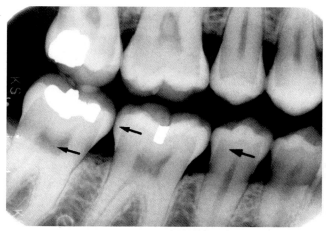

FIG. **10-1**   Teeth are composed of pulp (*arrow* on the second molar), enamel (*arrow* on the first molar), dentin (*arrow* on the second premolar), and cementum (usually not visible radiographically).

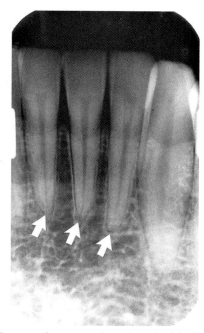

FIG. **10-3**   Root canals open at the apices of adult incisors *(arrows).*

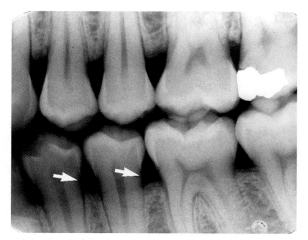

FIG. **10-2**   Cervical burnout caused by overexposure of the lateral portion of teeth between the enamel and alveolar crest *(arrows).*

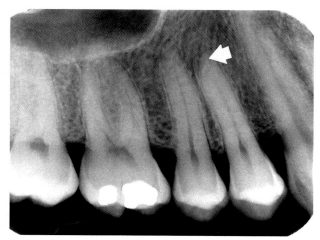

FIG. **10-4**   Although the root canal is not radiographically visible in the apical 2 mm of a tooth, anatomically it is present *(arrow).*

the cortical bone at the alveolar crest. It is only slightly thicker and no more highly mineralized than the trabeculae of cancellous bone in the area. Its radiographic appearance is caused by the fact that the x-ray beam passes tangentially through many times the thickness of the thin bony wall, which results in its observed attenuation (the egg-shell effect). Developmentally the lamina dura is an extension of the lining of the bony crypt that surrounds each tooth during development.

The appearance of the lamina dura on radiographs may vary. When the x-ray beam is directed through a relatively long expanse of the structure, the lamina dura appears radiopaque and well defined. When the beam is directed more obliquely, however, the lamina dura appears more diffuse and may not be discernible. In fact, even if the supporting bone in a healthy arch is intact, identification of a lamina dura completely surrounding every root on each film is frequently difficult, although it usually is evident to some extent about the roots on each film (Fig. 10-7). In addition, small variations and disruptions in the continuity of the lamina dura may result from superimpositions of cancellous bone and small nutrient canals passing from the marrow spaces to the periodontal ligament.

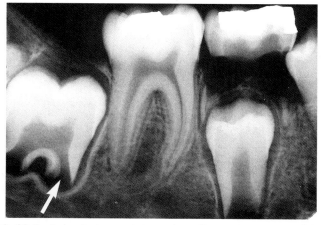

FIG. **10-5**   A developing root shown by a divergent apex around the dental papilla *(arrow),* which is enclosed by an opaque bony crypt.

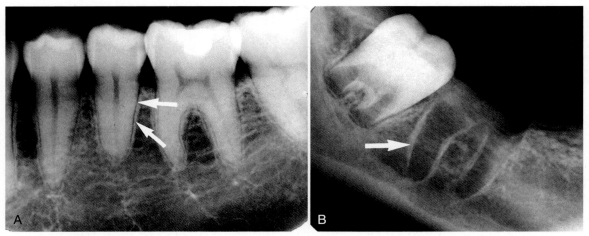

FIG. **10-6** The lamina dura *(arrows)* appears as a thin opaque layer of bone around teeth, **A,** and around a recent extraction socket, **B.**

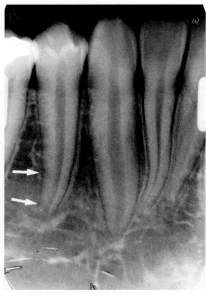

FIG. **10-7** The lamina dura is poorly visualized on the distal surface of this premolar *(arrows)* but is clearly seen on the mesial surface.

The thickness and density of the lamina dura on the radiograph vary with the amount of occlusal stress to which the tooth is subjected. The lamina dura is wider and more dense around the roots of teeth in heavy occlusion and thinner and less dense around teeth not subjected to occlusal function.

The image of a double lamina dura is not uncommon if the mesial or distal surfaces of roots present two elevations in the path of the x-ray beam. A common example of this is seen on the buccal and lingual eminences on the mesial surface of mandibular first molar roots (Fig. 10-8).

The appearance of the lamina dura is a valuable diagnostic feature. The presence of an intact lamina dura around the apex of a tooth strongly suggests a vital pulp. Because of the variable appearance of the lamina dura, however, the absence of its image around an apex on a radiograph may be normal. Rarely, in the absence of disease the

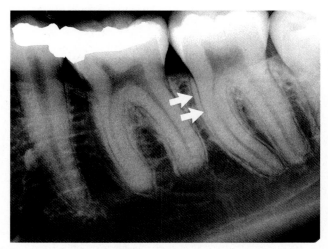

FIG. **10-8** A double periodontal ligament space and lamina dura *(arrows)* may be seen when there is a convexity of the proximal surface of the root.

lamina dura may be absent from a molar root extending into the maxillary sinus. The clinician is therefore advised to consider other signs and symptoms, as well as the integrity of the lamina dura, when establishing a diagnosis and treatment.

## ALVEOLAR CREST

The gingival margin of the alveolar process that extends between the teeth is apparent on radiographs as a radiopaque line, the alveolar crest (Fig. 10-9). The level of this bony crest is considered normal when it is not more than 1.5 mm from the cementoenamel junction of the adjacent teeth. The alveolar crest may recede apically with age and show marked resorption with periodontal disease. Radiographs can demonstrate only the position of the crest; determining the significance of its level is primarily a clinical problem (see Chapter 18).

The length of the normal alveolar crest in a particular region depends on the distance between the teeth in question. In the anterior region the crest is reduced to only a point of bone between the

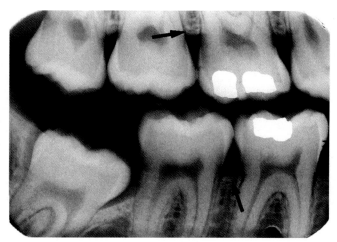

FIG. **10-9**  The alveolar crests *(arrows)* are seen as cortical borders of the alveolar bone.

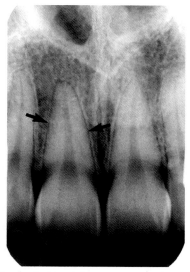

FIG. **10-10**  The periodontal ligament space *(arrows)* is seen as a narrow radiolucency between the tooth root and lamina dura.

close-set incisors. Posteriorly it is flat, aligned parallel with and slightly below a line connecting the cementoenamel junctions of the adjacent teeth. The crest of the bone is continuous with the lamina dura and forms a sharp angle with it. Rounding of these sharp junctions is indicative of periodontal disease.

The image of the crest varies from a dense layer of cortical bone to a smooth surface without cortical bone. In the latter case the trabeculae at the surface are of normal size and density. In the posterior regions this range of radiodensity of the crest is presumed to be normal if the bone is at a proper level in relation to the teeth. The absence of an image of cortex between the incisors, however, is considered by many to be an indication of incipient disease, even if the level of the bone is not abnormal.

## PERIODONTAL LIGAMENT SPACE

Because the periodontal ligament (PDL) is composed primarily of collagen, it appears as a radiolucent space between the tooth root and the lamina dura. This space begins at the alveolar crest, extends around the portions of the tooth roots within the alveolus, and returns to the alveolar crest on the opposite side of the tooth (Fig. 10-10).

The PDL varies in width from patient to patient, from tooth to tooth in the individual, and even from location to location around one tooth (Fig. 10-11). Usually it is thinner in the middle of the root and slightly wider near the alveolar crest and root apex, suggesting that the fulcrum of physiologic movement is in the region where the PDL is thinnest. The thickness of the ligament relates to the degree of function because the PDL is thinnest around the roots of embedded teeth and those that have lost their antagonists. The reverse is not necessarily true, however, because an appreciably wider space is not regularly observed in persons with especially heavy occlusion or bruxism.

The shape of the tooth creates the appearance of a double PDL space. When the x-ray beam is directed so that two convexities of a root surface appear on a film, the double PDL space is seen (see Fig. 10-8).

## CANCELLOUS BONE

The cancellous bone (also called *trabecular bone* or *spongiosa*) lies between the cortical plates in both jaws. It is composed of thin radi-

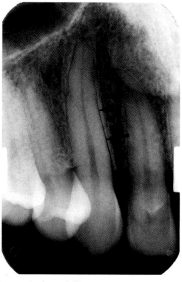

FIG. **10-11**  The periodontal ligament space appears wide on the mesial surface of this canine *(arrows)* and thin on the distal surface.

opaque plates and rods (trabeculae) surrounding many small radiolucent pockets of marrow. The radiographic pattern of the trabeculae comes from two anatomic sources. First is the cancellous bone itself. The second is the endosteal surface of the outer cortical bone where the cancellous bone fuses with the cortical bone. At this surface trabecular plates are relatively thick and make a significant contribution to the radiographic image. The trabecular pattern shows considerable intrapatient and interpatient variability, which is normal and not a manifestation of disease. To evaluate the trabecular pattern in a specific area, the practitioner should examine the trabecular distribution, size, and density and compare them throughout both jaws, and especially to the corresponding region on the opposite side. This frequently demonstrates that a particularly suspect region is characteristic for the individual.

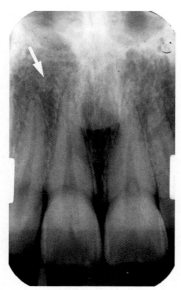

FIG. **10-12**   The trabecular pattern in the anterior maxilla is characterized by fine trabecular plates and multiple small trabecular spaces *(arrow)*.

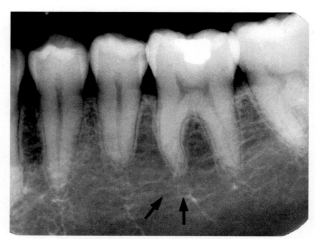

FIG. **10-14**   The trabecular pattern in the posterior mandible is quite variable, generally showing large marrow spaces and sparse trabeculation, especially inferiorly *(arrows)*.

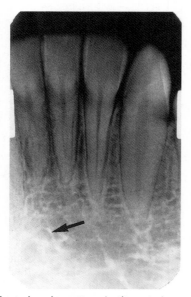

FIG. **10-13**   The trabecular pattern in the anterior mandible is characterized by coarser trabecular plates and larger marrow spaces *(arrow)* than in the anterior maxilla.

The trabeculae in the anterior maxilla are typically thin and numerous, forming a fine, granular, dense pattern (Fig. 10-12), and the marrow spaces are consequently small and relatively numerous. In the posterior maxilla the trabecular pattern is usually quite similar to that in the anterior maxilla, although the marrow spaces may be slightly larger.

In the anterior mandible the trabeculae are somewhat thicker than in the maxilla, resulting in a coarser pattern (Fig. 10-13) with trabecular plates that are oriented more horizontally. The trabecular plates are also fewer than in the maxilla, and the marrow spaces are correspondingly larger. In the posterior mandible the periradicular trabeculae and marrow spaces may be comparable to those in the anterior mandible but are usually somewhat larger (Fig. 10-14). The trabecular plates are oriented mainly horizontally in this region also. Below the apices of the mandibular molars the number of trabeculae dwindles still more. In some cases the area from just below the molar roots to the inferior border of the mandible may appear to be almost devoid of trabeculae. The distribution and size of the trabeculae throughout both jaws show a relationship to the thickness (and strength) of the adjacent cortical plates. It may be speculated that where the cortical plates are thick (e.g., in the posterior region of the mandibular body) internal bracing by the trabeculae is not required, so there are relatively few except where required to support the alveoli. By contrast, in the maxilla and anterior region of the mandible, where the cortical plates are relatively thin and less rigid, trabeculae are more numerous and lend internal bolstering to the jaw. Occasionally the trabecular spaces in this region are very irregular, with some so large that they mimic pathologic lesions.

If trabeculae are apparently absent, suggesting the presence of disease, it is often revealing to examine previous radiographs of the region in question. This helps determine whether the current appearance represents a change from a prior condition. An abnormality is more likely when the comparison indicates a change in the trabecular pattern. If prior films are not available, it is frequently useful to repeat the radiographic examination at a reduced exposure because this often demonstrates the presence of an expected but sparse trabecular pattern that was overexposed and burned out in the initial projection. Finally, if prior films are not available and reduced exposure does not allay the examiner's apprehension, it may be appropriate to expose another radiograph at a later time to monitor for ominous changes. Again, considerable variation may exist in trabecular pattern among patients, so examining all regions of the jaws is important in evaluating a trabecular pattern for any individual. This enables the dentist to determine the general nature of the particular pattern and whether any areas deviate appreciably from that norm.

The buccal and lingual cortical plates of the mandible and maxilla do not cast a discernible image on periapical radiographs.

## MAXILLA

### Intermaxillary Suture

The intermaxillary suture (also called the *median suture*) appears on intraoral periapical radiographs as a thin radiolucent line in the midline between the two portions of the premaxilla (Fig. 10-15). It extends from the alveolar crest between the central incisors superiorly through the anterior nasal spine and continues posteriorly between the maxillary palatine processes to the posterior aspect of the hard palate. It is not unusual for this narrow radiolucent suture to terminate at the alveolar crest in a small rounded or V-shaped enlargement (Fig. 10-16). The suture is limited by two parallel radiopaque borders of thin cortical bone on each side of the maxilla. The radiolucent region is usually of uniform width. The adjacent cortical margins may be either smooth or slightly irregular. The appearance of the intermaxillary suture depends on both anatomic variability and the angulation of the x-ray beam through the suture.

### Anterior Nasal Spine

The anterior nasal spine is most frequently demonstrated on periapical radiographs of the maxillary central incisors (Fig. 10-17). Located in the midline, it lies some 1.5 to 2 cm above the alveolar crest, usually at or just below the junction of the inferior end of the nasal septum and the inferior outline of the nasal aperture. It is radiopaque because of its bony composition and it is usually V shaped.

### Nasal Aperture

Because the air-filled nasal aperture (and cavity) lies just above the oral cavity, its radiolucent image may be apparent on intraoral radiographs of the maxillary teeth, especially in central incisor projections. On periapical radiographs of the incisors the inferior border of the fossa aperture as a radiopaque line extending bilaterally away from the base of the anterior nasal spine (Fig. 10-18). Above this line is the radiolucent space of the inferior portion of the cavity. If the radiograph was made with the x-ray beam directed in the sagittal plane, the relatively radiopaque nasal septum is seen arising in the midline from the anterior nasal spine (Fig. 10-19). The shadow of the septum may appear wider than anticipated and not sharply defined because the image is a superimposition of septal cartilage and vomer bone. Also, the septum frequently deviates slightly from the midline, and its plate of bone (the vomer) is somewhat curved.

The nasal cavity contains the opaque shadows of the inferior conchae extending from the right and left lateral walls for varying distances toward the septum. These conchae fill varying amounts of the lateral portions of the cavity (Fig. 10-20). The floor of the nasal aperture and a small segment of the nasal cavity are occasionally projected high onto a maxillary canine radiograph (Fig. 10-21). Also, in the posterior maxillary region, the floor of the nasal cavity may be seen in the region of the maxillary sinus. (It is not possible from a single radiograph to determine which of two superimposed structures is in front of or behind the other unless the conclusion is based on an

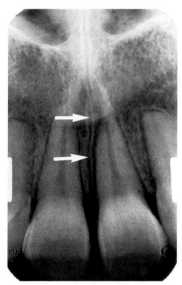

FIG. **10-15**  The intermaxillary suture *(arrows)* appears as a curving radiolucency in the midline of the maxilla.

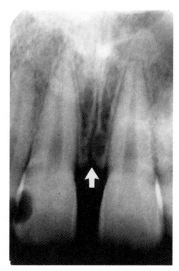

FIG. **10-16**  The intermaxillary suture may terminate in a V-shaped widening *(arrow)* at the alveolar crest.

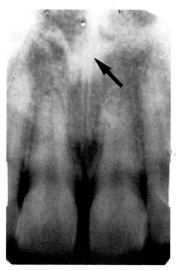

FIG. **10-17**  The anterior nasal spine is seen as an opaque V-shaped projection from the floor of the nasal aperture in the midline *(arrow)*.

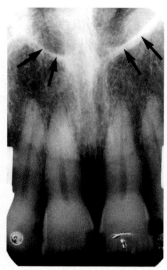

FIG. **10-18**   The anterior floor of the nasal aperture *(arrows)* appears as opaque lines extending laterally from the anterior nasal spine.

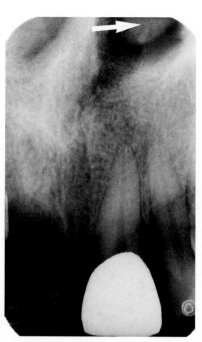

FIG. **10-20**   The mucosal covering of the inferior concha *(arrow)* is occasionally visualized in the nasal cavity.

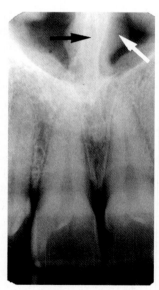

FIG. **10-19**   The nasal septum *(black arrow)* arises directly above the anterior nasal spine and is covered on each side by nasal mucosa *(white arrow).*

awareness of the anatomic features and relationships.) It may falsely convey the impression of a septum in the sinus or a limiting superior sinus wall (Fig. 10-22).

## Incisive Foramen

The incisive foramen (also called the *nasopalatine* or *anterior palatine foramen*) in the maxilla is the oral terminus of the nasopalatine canal. This canal originates in the anterior floor of the nasal fossa. The incisive foramen transmits the nasopalatine vessels and nerves (which may participate in the innervation of the maxillary central incisors) and lies in the midline of the palate behind the central incisors at approximately the junction of the median palatine and incisive sutures. Its radiographic image is usually projected between the roots

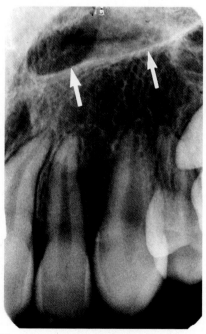

FIG. **10-21**   The floor of the nasal aperture *(arrows)* may often be seen extending above the maxillary lateral incisor and canine.

and in the region of the middle and apical thirds of the central incisors (Fig. 10-23). The foramen varies markedly in its radiographic shape, size, and sharpness. It may appear smoothly symmetric, with numerous forms, or very irregular, with a well-demarcated or ill-defined border. The position of the foramen is also variable and may be recognized at the apices of the central incisor roots, near the alveolar crest, anywhere in between, or extending over the entire distance. The great variability of its radiographic image is primarily the result of (1) the differing angles at which the x-ray beam is directed for the maxillary central incisors and (2) some variability in its anatomic size.

Familiarity with the incisive foramen is important because it is a potential site of cyst formation. An incisive canal cyst is radiographically discernible because it frequently causes a readily perceived enlargement of the foramen and canal. The presence of a cyst is presumed if the width of the foramen exceeds 1 cm or if enlargement can be demonstrated on successive radiographs. Also, if the radiolucency of the normal foramen is projected over the apex of one central incisor, it may suggest a pathologic periapical condition. The absence of disease is indicated by a lack of clinical symptoms and an intact lamina dura around the central incisor in question.

The lateral walls of the nasopalatine canal are not usually seen on periapical views but on occasion can be visualized on a projection of the central incisors as a pair of radiopaque lines running vertically from the superior foramina of the nasopalatine canal to the incisive foramen (Fig. 10-24, *A*). Cone-beam images of this region, however, regularly demonstrate the borders of the nasopalatine canal (Figs. 10-24, *B* and *C*). Visualization of these structures is important when placing an implant in this region is considered.

### Superior Foramina of the Nasopalatine Canal

The nasopalatine canal originates at two foramina in the floor of the nasal cavity. The openings are on each side of the nasal septum, close to the anteroinferior border of the nasal cavity, and each canal passes downward somewhat anteriorly and medially to unite with the canal from the other side in a common opening, the incisive (nasopalatine) foramen. The superior foramina of the canal occasionally appear in projections of the maxillary incisors, especially when an exaggerated vertical angle is used (Fig. 10-25). They are usually round or oval, although they make take a variety of outlines, depending on the angle of projection.

### Lateral Fossa

The lateral fossa (also called *incisive fossa*) is a gentle depression in the maxilla near the apex of the lateral incisor (Fig. 10-26). On periapical projections of this region it may appear diffusely radiolucent. The image will not be misinterpreted as a pathologic condition, however, if the radiograph is examined for an intact lamina dura around the root of the lateral incisor. This finding, coupled with absence of clinical symptoms, suggests normalcy of the bone.

### Nose

The soft tissue of the tip of the nose is frequently seen in projections of the maxillary central and lateral incisors, superimposed over the roots of these teeth. The image of the nose has a uniform, slightly opaque appearance with a sharp border (Fig. 10-27). Occasionally the radiolucent nares can be identified, especially when a steep vertical angle is used.

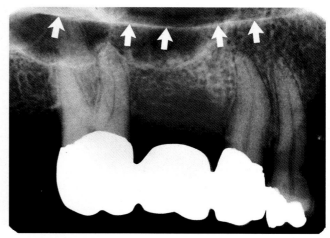

FIG. **10-22** The floor of the nasal aperture *(arrows)* extends posteriorly, superimposed with the maxillary sinus.

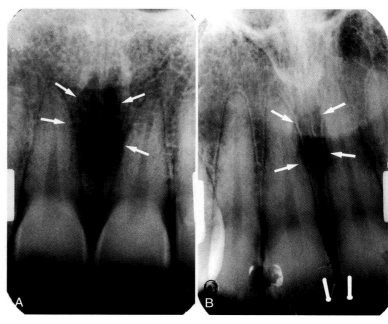

FIG. **10-23** **A,** The incisive foramen appears as an ovoid radiolucency *(arrows)* between the roots of the central incisors. **B,** Note its borders, which are diffuse but within normal limits.

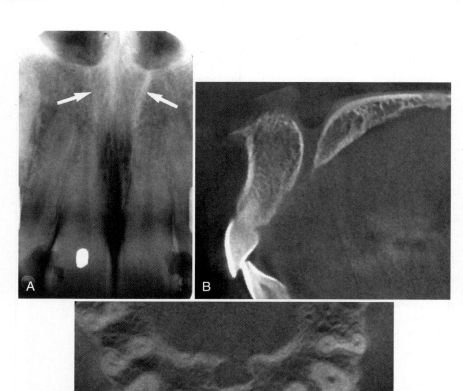

FIG. **10-24  Nasopalatine Canal. A,** The lateral walls of the nasopalatine canal *(arrows)* extend from the incisive foramen to the floor of the nasal fossa. **B,** Cone-beam image in the sagittal plane demonstrates superior foramina in the floor of the nasal fossa, the anterior and posterior borders of the canal, and the incisive foramen opening onto the hard palate. **C,** Cone-beam image in the axial plane at the level of the incisive foramen demonstrates anterior and lateral borders of the incisive canal lying palatal to the incisor roots seen in cross section. (**B** and **C** made with 3DX Accuitomo, J. Morita.)

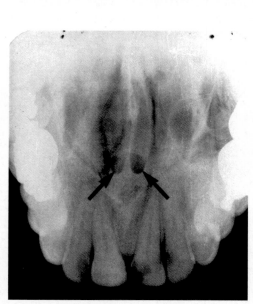

FIG. **10-25**   The superior foramina of the nasopalatine canal *(arrows)* appear just lateral to the nasal septum and posterior to the anterior nasal spine.

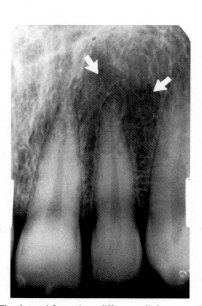

FIG. **10-26**   The lateral fossa is a diffuse radiolucency *(arrows)* in the region of the apex of the lateral incisor. It is formed by a depression in the maxilla at this location.

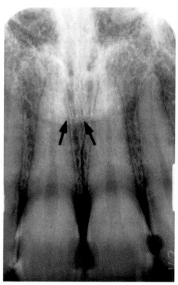

FIG. **10-27**   The soft tissue outline of the nose *(arrows)* is superimposed on the anterior maxilla.

## Nasolacrimal Canal

The nasal and maxillary bones form the nasolacrimal canal. It runs from the medial aspect of the anteroinferior border of the orbit inferiorly to drain under the inferior concha into the nasal cavity. Occasionally it can be visualized on periapical radiographs in the region above the apex of the canine, especially when steep vertical angulation is used (Fig. 10-28). The nasolacrimal canals are routinely seen on maxillary occlusal projections (see Chapter 9) in the region of the molars (Fig. 10-29).

## Maxillary Sinus

The maxillary sinus, like the other paranasal sinuses, is an air-containing cavity lined with mucous membrane. It develops by the invagination of mucous membrane from the nasal cavity. The largest of the paranasal sinuses, it normally occupies virtually the entire body of the maxilla. Its function is unknown.

The sinus may be considered as a three-sided pyramid, with its base the medial wall adjacent to the nasal cavity and its apex extending laterally into the zygomatic process of the maxilla. Its three sides are (1) the superior wall forming the floor of the orbit, (2) the anterior wall extending above the premolars, and (3) the posterior wall bulging above the molar teeth and maxillary tuberosity. The sinus communicates with the nasal cavity by the ostium, some 3 to 6 mm in diameter positioned and under the posterior aspect of the middle concha of the ethmoid bone.

The borders of the maxillary sinus appear on periapical radiographs as a thin, delicate, tenuous radiopaque line (actually a thin layer of cortical bone) (Fig. 10-30). In the absence of disease it appears continuous, but on close examination it can be seen to have small interruptions in its smoothness or density. These discontinuities are probably illusions caused by superimposition of small marrow spaces. In adults the sinuses are usually seen to extend from the distal aspect of the canine to the posterior wall of the maxilla above the tuberosity.

The maxillary sinuses show considerable variation in size. They enlarge during childhood, achieving mature size by the age of 15 to 18 years. They may change during adult life in response to environ-

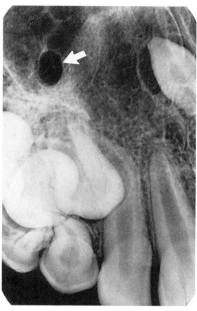

FIG. **10-28**   The nasolacrimal canal *(arrow)* is occasionally seen near the apex of the canine when steep vertical angulation is used. Note the mesiodens (supernumerary tooth) superior to the central incisor.

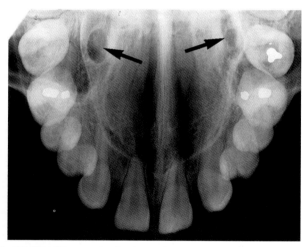

FIG. **10-29**   The nasolacrimal canals are commonly seen as ovoid radiolucencies *(arrows)* on maxillary occlusal projections.

mental factors. The right and left sinuses usually appear similar in shape and size, although marked asymmetry is occasionally present. The floors of the maxillary sinus and nasal cavity are seen on dental radiographs at approximately the same level around the age of puberty. In older individuals the sinus may extend farther into the alveolar process, and in the posterior region of the maxilla its floor may appear considerably below the level of the floor of the nasal cavity. Anteriorly each sinus is restricted by the canine fossa and is usually seen to sweep superiorly, crossing the level of the floor of the nasal cavity in the premolar or canine region. Consequently, on periapical radiographs of the canine, the floors of the sinus and nasal cavity are often superimposed and may be seen crossing one another, forming an inverted Y in the area (Fig. 10-31).

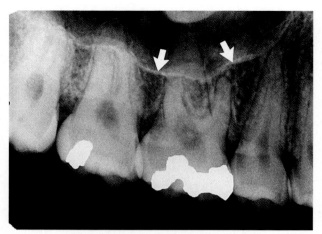

FIG. **10-30**   The inferior border of the maxillary sinus *(arrows)* appears as a thin radiopaque line near the apices of the maxillary premolars and molars.

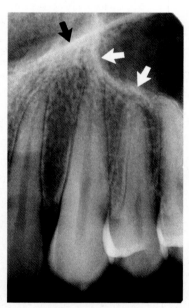

FIG. **10-31**   The anterior border of the maxillary sinus *(white arrows)* crosses the floor of the nasal fossa *(black arrow).*

The outline of the nasal fossa is usually heavier and more diffuse than that of the thin, delicate cortical bone denoting the sinus. The degree of extension of the maxillary sinus into the alveolar process is extremely variable. In some projections the floor of the sinus will be well above the apices of the posterior teeth; in others it may extend well beyond the apices toward the alveolar ridge. In response to a loss of function (associated with the loss of posterior teeth) the sinus may expand farther into the alveolar bone, occasionally extending to the alveolar ridge (Fig. 10-32).

The roots of the molars usually lie in close apposition to the maxillary sinus. Root apices may project anatomically into the floor of the sinus, causing small elevations or prominences. The thin layer of bone covering the root is seen as a fusion of the lamina dura and the floor of the sinus. Rarely, defects may be present in the bony covering of the root apices in the sinus floor, and a periapical radiograph will fail to show lamina dura covering the apex.

When the rounded sinus floor dips between the buccal and palatal molar roots and is medial to the premolar roots, the projection of the apices is superior to the floor. This appearance conveys the impression that the roots project into the sinus cavity, which is an illusion. As the positive vertical angle of the projection is increased, the roots medial to the sinus appear to project farther into the sinus cavity. In contrast, the roots that are lateral to the sinus appear to move either out of the sinus or farther away from it as the angle is increased.

The intimate relationship between sinus and teeth leads to the possibility that clinical symptoms originating in the sinus may be perceived in the teeth and vice versa. This proximity of sinus and teeth is in part a consequence of the gradual developmental expansion of the maxillary sinus, which thins the sinus walls and opens the canals that traverse the anterolateral and posterolateral walls and carry the superior alveolar nerves. The nerves are then in intimate contact with the membrane lining the sinus. As a result, an acute inflammation of the sinus is frequently accompanied by pain in the maxillary teeth innervated by that portion of the nerve proximal to the insult. Subjective symptoms in the area of the maxillary posterior teeth may require careful analysis to differentiate tooth pain from sinus pain.

Frequently, thin radiolucent lines of uniform width are found within the image of the maxillary sinus (Fig. 10-33). These are the shadows of neurovascular canals or grooves in the lateral sinus walls that accommodate the posterior superior alveolar vessels, their branches, and the accompanying superior alveolar nerves. Although

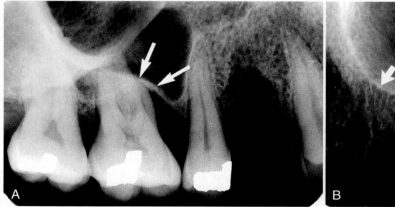

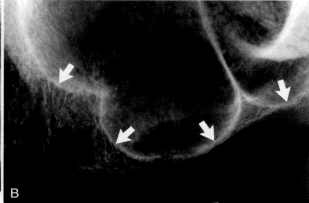

FIG. **10-32**   The floor of the maxillary sinus *(arrows)* extends toward the crest of the alveolar ridge in response to missing teeth.

they may be found coursing in any direction (including vertically), they are usually seen running a curved posteroanterior course that is convex toward the alveolar process. On occasion they may be found to branch and rarely also to extend outside the image of the sinus and continue as an interradicular channel. Because such vascular markings are not seen in the walls of cysts, they may serve to distinguish a healthy sinus from a cyst.

Often one or several radiopaque lines traverse the image of the maxillary sinus (Fig. 10-34). These opaque lines are called *septa*. They are thin folds of cortical bone that projecting a few millimeters away from the floor and wall of the antrum or they may extend across the sinus. They are usually oriented vertically vary in number, thickness, and length. They appear on many periapical intraoral radiographs and frequently on cone-beam images. Although septa appear to separate the sinuses into distinct compartments, this is seldom the case. Rather, the septa typically extend only a few millimeters into the central volume of the sinus. Septa deserve attention because they sometimes mimic periapical disease, and the chambers they create in

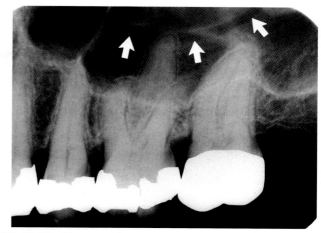

FIG. **10-33** Neurovascular canals *(arrows)* in the lateral wall of the maxillary sinus.

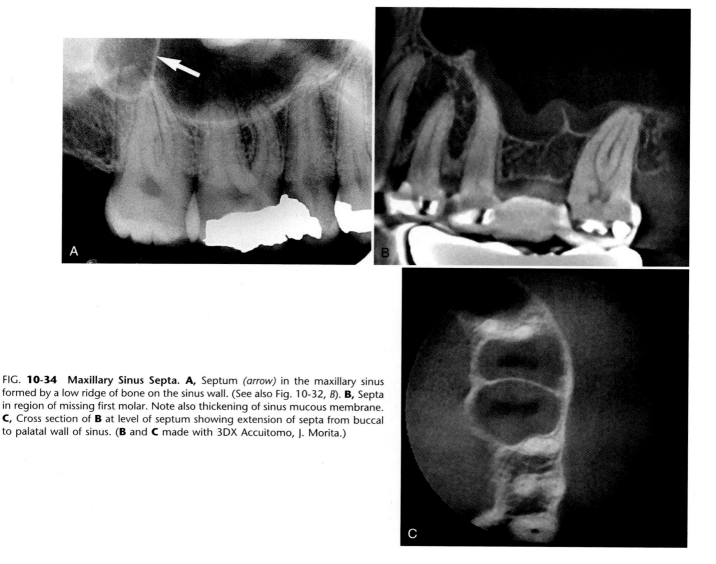

FIG. **10-34 Maxillary Sinus Septa. A,** Septum *(arrow)* in the maxillary sinus formed by a low ridge of bone on the sinus wall. (See also Fig. 10-32, *B*). **B,** Septa in region of missing first molar. Note also thickening of sinus mucous membrane. **C,** Cross section of **B** at level of septum showing extension of septa from buccal to palatal wall of sinus. (**B** and **C** made with 3DX Accuitomo, J. Morita.)

the alveolar recess may complicate the search for a root fragment displaced into the sinus.

The floor of the maxillary sinus occasionally shows small radiopaque projections, which are nodules of bone (Fig. 10-35). These must be differentiated from root tips, which they resemble in shape. In contrast to a root fragment, which is quite homogeneous in appearance, the bony nodules often show trabeculation; and although they may be quite well defined, at certain points on their surface they blend with the trabecular pattern of adjacent bone. A root fragment may also be recognized by the presence of a root canal. It is not uncommon to see the floor of the nasal fossa in periapical views of the posterior teeth superimposed on the maxillary sinus (see Fig. 10-22). The floor of the nasal fossa is usually oriented more or less horizontally, depending on film placement, and is superimposed high on maxillary views. The image, a solid opaque line, frequently appears somewhat thicker than the adjacent sinus walls and septa.

### Zygomatic Process and Zygomatic Bone

The zygomatic process of the maxilla is an extension of the lateral maxillary surface that arises in the region of the apices of the first and second molars and serves as the articulation for the zygomatic bone.

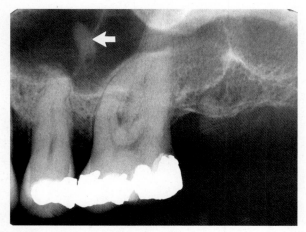

FIG. **10-35**   This bony nodule *(arrow)* is a normal variant of the floor of the maxillary sinus.

On periapical radiographs the zygomatic process appears as a U-shaped radiopaque line with its open end directed superiorly. The enclosed rounded end is projected in the apical region of the first and second molars (Fig. 10-36). The size, width, and definition of the zygomatic process are quite variable, and its image may be large, depending on the angle at which the beam was projected. The maxillary antrum may expand laterally into the zygomatic process of the maxilla (and even into the zygomatic bone after the maxillozygomatic suture has fused), thereby resulting in a relatively increased radiolucent region within the U-shaped image of the process.

When the sinus is recessed deep within the process (and perhaps into the zygomatic bone), the image of the air space within the process is dark, and typically, the walls of the process are rather thin and well defined (in contrast to the very dark radiolucent air space). When the sinus exhibits relatively little penetration of the maxillary process (usually in younger individuals or those who have maintained their posterior teeth and vigorous masticatory function), the image of the walls of the zygomatic process tends to be somewhat thicker, and the appearance of the sinus in this region is somewhat smaller and more opaque.

The inferior portion of the zygomatic bone may be seen extending posteriorly from the inferior border of the zygomatic process of the maxilla (thereby completing the zygomatic arch between the zygomatic processes of the maxillary and temporal bones). It can be identified as a uniform gray or white radiopacity over the apices of the molars (Fig. 10-37). The prominence of the molar apices superimposed on the shadow of the zygomatic bone, and the amount of detail supplied by the radiograph, depends in part on the degree of aeration (pneumatization) of the zygomatic bone that has occurred, on the bony structure, and on the orientation of the x-ray beam.

### Nasolabial Fold

An oblique line demarcating a region that appears to be covered by a veil of slight radiopacity frequently traverses periapical radiographs of the premolar region (Fig. 10-38). The line of contrast is sharp, and the area of increased radiopacity is posterior to the line. The line is the nasolabial fold, and the opaque veil is the thick cheek tissue superimposed on the teeth and the alveolar process. The image of the fold becomes more evident with age as the repeated creasing of the skin along the line (where the elevator of the lip, zygomatic head, and orbicularis all insert into the skin) and the degeneration of the elastic

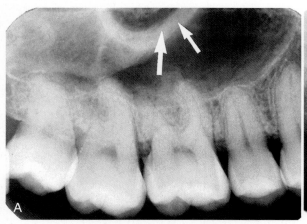
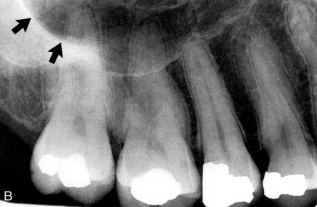

FIG. **10-36**   The zygomatic process of the maxilla *(arrows)* protrudes laterally from the maxillary wall.
Its size may be quite variable: small with thick borders **(A)** or large with thin borders **(B)**.

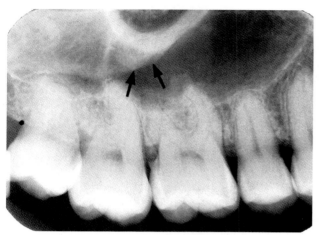

FIG. **10-37**   The inferior border of the zygomatic arch *(arrows)* extends posteriorly from the inferior portion of the zygomatic process of the maxilla.

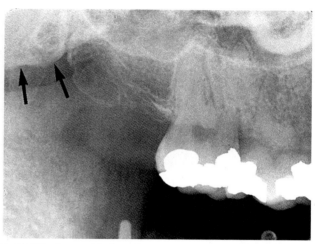

FIG. **10-39**   Pterygoid plates *(arrows)* located posterior to the maxillary tuberosity.

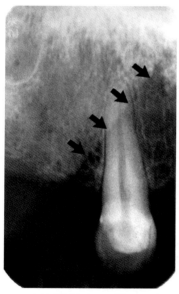

FIG. **10-38**   The nasolabial fold *(arrows)* extends across the canine-premolar region.

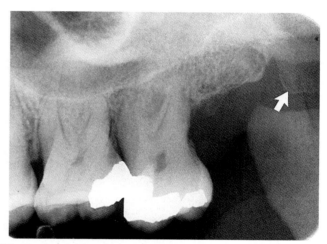

FIG. **10-40**   The hamular process *(arrow)* extends downward from the medial pterygoid plate.

fibers finally lead to the formation and deepening of permanent folds. This radiographic feature frequently proves useful in identifying the side of the maxilla represented by a film of the area if it is edentulous and few other anatomic features are demonstrated.

## Pterygoid Plates

The medial and lateral pterygoid plates lie immediately posterior to the tuberosity of the maxilla. The image of these two plates is extremely variable, and on many intraoral radiographs of the third molar area they do not appear at all. When they are apparent, they almost always cast a single radiopaque homogeneous shadow without any evidence of trabeculation (Fig. 10-39). Extending inferiorly from the medial pterygoid plate is the hamular process (Fig. 10-40), which on close inspection can show trabeculae.

## MANDIBLE

### Symphysis

Radiographs of the region of the mandibular symphysis in infants demonstrate a radiolucent line through the midline of the jaw between the images of the forming deciduous central incisors (Fig. 10-41). This suture usually fuses by the end of the first year of life, after which it is no longer radiographically apparent. It is not frequently encountered on dental radiographs because few young patients have cause to be examined radiographically. If this radiolucency is found in older individuals, it is abnormal and may suggest a fracture or a cleft.

### Genial Tubercles

The genial tubercles (also called the *mental spine*) are located on the lingual surface of the mandible slightly above the inferior border and in the midline. They are bony protuberances, more or less spine shaped, that often are divided into a right and left prominence and a superior and inferior prominence. They serve to attach the genioglossus muscles (at the superior tubercles) and the geniohyoid muscles (at

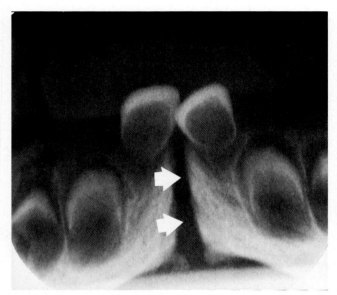

FIG. **10-41**   Mandibular symphysis *(arrows)* in a newborn infant. Note the bilateral supernumerary primary incisors adjacent to it.

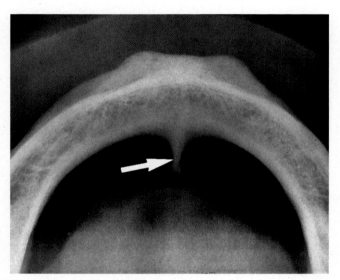

FIG. **10-42**   Genial tubercles *(arrow)* on the lingual surface of the mandible in this cross-sectional mandibular occlusal view.

the inferior tubercles) to the mandible. They are well visualized on mandibular occlusal radiographs as one or more small projections (Fig. 10-42). Their appearance on periapical radiographs of the mandibular incisor region is variable: often they appear as a radiopaque mass (up to 3 to 4 mm in diameter) in the midline below the incisor roots (Fig. 10-43). They also may not be apparent at all.

### Lingual Foramen

There is usually a foramen on the lingual surface of the midline of the mandible in the region of the genial tubercles, the lingual foramen. Often there are two or even more such foramina. The superior foramen contains a neurovascular bundle from the lingual arteries and nerve, whereas the inferior foramen is supplied from the sublin-

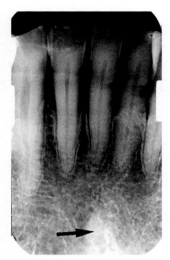

FIG. **10-43**   The genial tubercles *(arrow)* appear as a radiopaque mass, in this case without evidence of the lingual foramen.

gual or submental arteries and from the mylohyoid nerve. The lingual foramen (Fig. 10-44) is typically visualized as a single round radiolucent canal with a well-defined opaque border lying in the midline below the level of the apices of the incisors.

### Mental Ridge

On periapical radiographs of the mandibular central incisors, the mental ridge (protuberance) may occasionally be seen as two radiopaque lines sweeping bilaterally forward and upward toward the midline (Fig. 10-45). They are of variable width and density and may be found to extend from low in the premolar area on each side up to the midline, where they lie just inferior to or are superimposed on the mandibular incisor tooth roots. The image of the mental ridge is most prominent when the beam is directed parallel with the surface of the mental tubercle (as when using the bisecting-angle technique).

### Mental Fossa

The mental fossa is a depression on the labial aspect of the mandible extending laterally from the midline and above the mental ridge. Because of the resulting thinness of jawbone in this area, the image of this depression may be similar to that of the submandibular fossa (see later) and may, likewise, be mistaken for periapical disease involving the incisors (Fig. 10-46).

### Mental Foramen

The mental foramen is usually the anterior limit of the inferior dental canal that is apparent on periapical radiographs (Fig. 10-47). Its image is quite variable, and it may be identified only about half the time because the opening of the mental canal is directed superiorly and posteriorly (Fig. 10-48). As a result, the usual view of the premolars is not projected through the long axis of the canal opening. This circumstance is responsible for the variable appearance of the mental foramen. Although the wall of the foramen is of cortical bone, the density of the foramen's image varies, as does the shape and definition of its border. It may be round, oblong, slitlike, or very irregular and partially or completely corticated. The foramen is seen about halfway between the lower border of the mandible and the crest of the alveolar process, usually in the region of the apex of the second premolar. Also, because it lies on the surface of the mandible, the position of its image

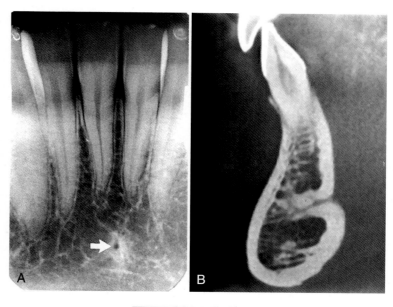

FIG. **10-44** **Lingual Foramen. A,** Lingual foramen on a periapical view *(arrow),* with a sclerotic border, in the symphyseal region of the mandible. **B,** Cone-beam image showing sagittal section of anterior mandible and superior lingual foramen extending deep into mandible from lingual surface. (**B** made with 3DX Accuitomo, J. Morita.)

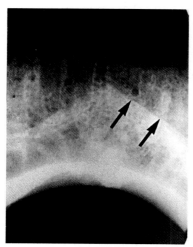

FIG. **10-45** Mental ridge *(arrows)* on the anterior surface of the mandible, seen as a radiopaque ridge.

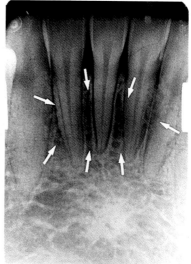

FIG. **10-46** The mental fossa is a radiolucent depression on the anterior surface of the mandible *(arrows)* between the alveolar ridge and mental ridge.

in relation to the tooth roots is influenced by projection angulation. It may be projected anywhere from just mesial of the permanent first molar roots to as far anterior as mesial of the first premolar root. The image of two mental foramina, one above the other, has also been observed.

When the mental foramen is projected over one of the premolar apices, it may mimic periapical disease (Fig. 10-49). In such cases, evidence of the inferior dental canal extending to the suspect radiolucency or a detectable lamina dura in the area would suggest the true nature of the dark shadow. It is well to point out, however, that the relative thinness of the lamina dura superimposed with the radiolucent foramen may result in considerable "burnout" of the lamina dura image, which will complicate its recognition. Nevertheless, a second radiograph from another angle is likely to show the lamina dura clearly, as well as some shift in position of the radiolucent foramen relative to the apex.

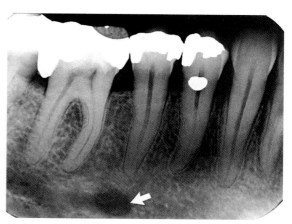

FIG. **10-47** The mental foramen *(arrow)* appears as an oval radiolucency near the apex of the second premolar.

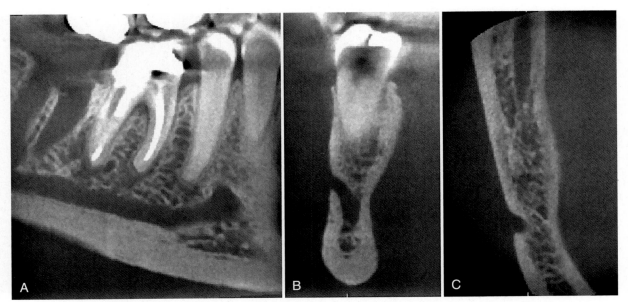

FIG. **10-48** **Cone-Beam Images Through Mental Foramen. A,** Oblique through body of mandible showing mandibular canal rising toward the mental foramen lying just anterior to apex of second premolar. **B,** Coronal section through mental foramen shows how the mandibular canal ascends to the mental foramen. This is important if implants are to be placed in this region. **C,** Axial section through mental foramen demonstrating posterior inclination of opening on mandibular surface. Note also section through mandibular canal posteriorly *(top of image).* (Images made with 3DX Accuitomo, J. Morita.)

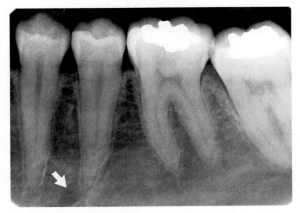

FIG. **10-49** The mental foramen *(arrow)* (over the apex of the second premolar) may simulate periapical disease. Continuity of the lamina dura around the apex, however, indicates the absence of periapical abnormality.

## Mandibular Canal

The radiographic image of the mandibular canal is a dark linear shadow with thin radiopaque superior and inferior borders cast by the lamella of bone that bounds the canal (Fig. 10-50). Sometimes the borders are seen only partially or not at all. The width of the canal shows some interpatient variability but is usually rather constant anterior to the third molar region. The canal's course may be apparent between the mandibular foramen and the mental foramen. Only rarely is the image of its anterior continuation toward the midline discernible on the radiograph.

The relationship of the mandibular dental canal to the roots of the lower teeth may vary, from one in which there is close contact with all molars and the second premolar to one in which the canal has no intimate relationship to any of the posterior teeth. In the usual picture, however, the canal is in contact with the apex of the third molar, and the distance between it and the other roots increases as it progresses anteriorly. When the apices of the molars are projected over the canal, the lamina dura may be overexposed, conveying the impression of a missing lamina or a thickened PDL space that is more radiolucent than apparently normal for the patient (Fig. 10-51). To ensure the soundness of such a tooth, other clinical testing procedures must be used (e.g., vitality testing). Because the canal is usually located just inferior to the apices of the posterior teeth, altering the vertical angle for a second film of the area is not likely to separate the images of the apices and canal.

Histologic studies have shown that the inferior alveolar nerve typically courses through the mandible as one major trunk with branches extending to the apices of the teeth. There are, however, multiple smaller branches of the inferior alveolar nerve running roughly parallel to the major trunk. Occasionally these branches are large enough that they have a secondary mandibular canal. Such bifid canals are seen most commonly on panoramic and cone-beam images (Fig. 10-52). Patients with bifid canals are at greater risk of inadequate anesthesia or difficulties with jaw surgery, including implants, or trauma.

## Nutrient Canals

Nutrient canals carry a neurovascular bundle and appear as radiolucent lines of fairly uniform width. They are most often seen on mandibular periapical radiographs running vertically from the inferior dental canal directly to the apex of a tooth (Fig. 10-53) or into the interdental space between the mandibular incisors (Fig. 10-54). They

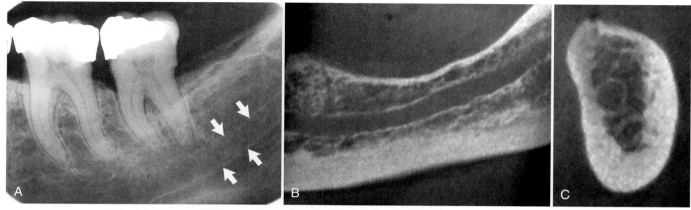

FIG. **10-50  Mandibular Canal. A,** Arrows denote its radiopaque superior and inferior cortical borders on periapical view. **B,** Cone-beam section through body of mandible demonstrating corticated borders of mandibular canal. **C,** Cone-beam cross-sectional view demonstrating circular mandibular canal with corticated borders lying adjacent to lingual plate. (**B** and **C** made with 3DX Accuitomo, J. Morita.)

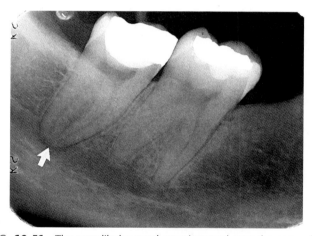

FIG. **10-51**   The mandibular canal superimposed over the apex of a molar causes the image of the periodontal ligament space to appear wider *(arrow)*. The presence of an intact lamina dura, however, indicates that there is no periapical disease.

are visible in about 5% of all patients and are more frequent in blacks, males, older persons, and individuals with high blood pressure or advanced periodontal disease. They also indicate a thin ridge, useful in implant assessment. Because they are anatomic spaces with walls of cortical bone, their images occasionally have hyperostotic borders. At times a nutrient canal will be oriented perpendicular to the cortex and appear as a small round radiolucency simulating a pathologic radiolucency.

## Mylohyoid Ridge

The mylohyoid ridge is a slightly irregular crest of bone on the lingual surface of the mandibular body. Extending from the area of the third molars to the lower border of the mandible in the region of the chin, it serves as an attachment for the mylohyoid muscle. Its radiographic image runs diagonally downward and forward from the area of the third molars to the premolar region, at approximately the level of the apices of the posterior teeth (Fig. 10-55). Sometimes this image is

superimposed on the images of the molar roots. The margins of the image are not usually well defined but appear quite diffuse and of variable width. The contrary is also observed, however, where the ridge is relatively dense with sharply demarcated borders (Fig. 10-56). It will be more evident on periapical radiographs when the beam is positioned with excessive negative angulation. In general, as the ridge becomes less defined, its anterior and posterior limits blend gradually with the surrounding bone.

## Submandibular Gland Fossa

On the lingual surface of the mandibular body, immediately below the mylohyoid ridge in the molar area, there is frequently a depression in the bone. This concavity accommodates the submandibular gland and often appears as a radiolucent area with the sparse trabecular pattern characteristic of the region (Fig. 10-57). This trabecular pattern is even less defined on radiographs of the area because it is superimposed on the relatively reduced mass of the concavity. The radiographic image of the fossa is sharply limited superiorly by the mylohyoid ridge and inferiorly by the lower border of the mandible but is poorly defined anteriorly (in the premolar region) and posteriorly (at about the ascending ramus). Although the image may appear strikingly radiolucent, accentuated as it is by the dense mylohyoid ridge and inferior border of the mandible, awareness of its possible presence should preclude its being confused with a bony lesion by the inexperienced clinician.

## External Oblique Ridge

The external oblique ridge is a continuation of the anterior border of the mandibular ramus. It follows an anteroinferior course lateral to the alveolar process; it is relatively prominent in its upper part and juts considerably on the outer surface of the mandible in the region of the third molar (Fig. 10-58). This bony elevation gradually flattens, and usually disappears, at about where the alveolar process and mandible join below the first molar. The ridge is a line of attachment of the buccinator muscle. Characteristically, it is projected onto posterior periapical radiographs superior to the mylohyoid ridge, with which it runs an almost parallel course. It appears as a radiopaque line of varying width, density, and length, blending at its anterior end with the shadow of the alveolar bone.

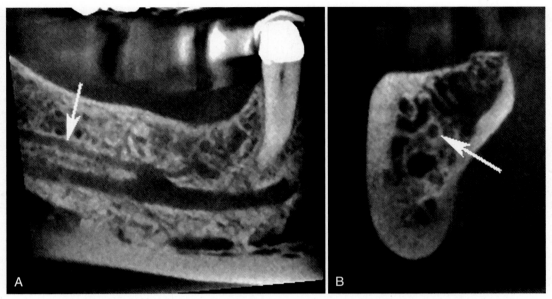

FIG. **10-52**  **Bifid Mandibular Canals. A,** Cone-beam section through body of mandible showing bifid mandibular canal. Superior branch has smaller diameter than the primary canal *(arrow)*. **B,** Cross-sectional image showing primary canal and superior secondary canal *(arrow)*. (Images made with 3DX Accuitomo, J. Morita.)

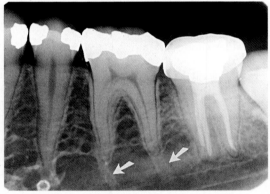

FIG. **10-53**  Nutrient canals *(arrows)*, demonstrated by radiopaque cortical borders, descend from the mandibular first molar.

### Inferior Border of the Mandible

Occasionally the inferior mandibular border will be seen on periapical projections (Fig. 10-59) as a characteristically dense, broad radiopaque band of bone.

### Coronoid Process

The image of the coronoid process of the mandible is frequently apparent on periapical radiographs of the maxillary molar region as a triangular radiopacity, with its apex directed superiorly and somewhat anteriorly, superimposed on the region of the third molar (Fig. 10-60). In some cases it may appear as far forward as the second molar and be projected above, over, or below these molars, depending on the position of the jaw and the projection of the x-ray beam. Usually the shadow of the coronoid process is homogeneous, although internal trabeculation can be seen in some cases. Its appearance on maxil-

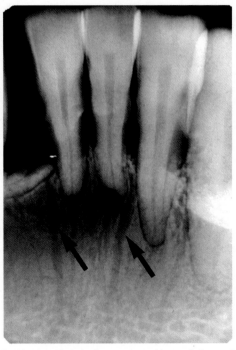

FIG. **10-54**  Nutrient canals demonstrated by radiolucencies *(arrows)* in the anterior mandible of a patient with severe periodontal disease.

lary molar radiographs results from the downward and forward movement of the mandible when the mouth is open. Consequently, if the opacity reduces the diagnostic value of a film and the film must be remade, the second view should be acquired with the mouth minimally open. (This contingency must be considered whenever this area

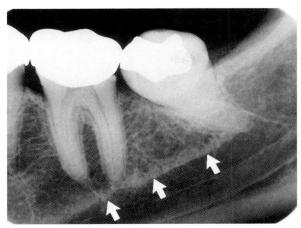

FIG. **10-55** Mylohyoid ridge *(arrows)* running at the level of the molar apices and above the mandibular canal.

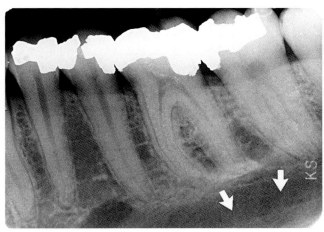

FIG. **10-57** Submandibular gland fossa *(arrows)*, indicated by a poorly defined radiolucency and sparse trabecular bone below the mandibular molars.

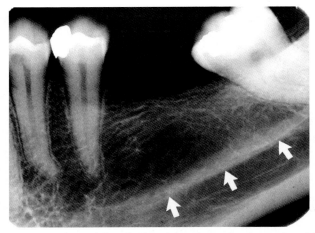

FIG. **10-56** The mylohyoid ridge *(arrows)* may be dense, especially when a radiograph is exposed with excessive negative angulation.

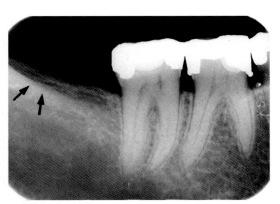

FIG. **10-58** External oblique ridge *(arrows)*, seen as a radiopaque line near the alveolar crest in the mandibular third molar region.

is radiographically examined.) On occasion, and especially when its shadow is dense and homogeneous, the coronoid process is mistaken for a root fragment by the neophyte clinician. The true nature of the shadow can be easily demonstrated by obtaining two radiographs with the mouth in different positions and noting the change in position of the suspect shadow.

## Restorative Materials

Restorative materials vary in their radiographic appearance, depending primarily on their thickness, density, and atomic number. Of these, the atomic number is most influential.

A variety of restorative materials may be recognized on intraoral radiographs. The most common, silver amalgam, is completely radiopaque (Fig. 10-61). Gold is equally opaque to x rays, whether cast as a crown or an inlay (Fig. 10-62) or condensed as gold foil. Stainless steel pins also appear radiopaque (Fig. 10-63). Often a calcium hydroxide base is placed in a deep cavity to protect the pulp. Although such base material may be radiolucent, most is radiopaque (Fig. 10-64). Another material of comparable radiopacity is gutta-percha,

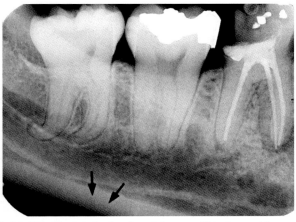

FIG. **10-59** The inferior border of the mandible *(arrows)* is seen as a dense, broad radiopaque band.

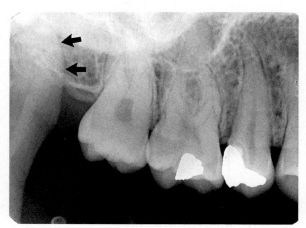

FIG. **10-60**   Coronoid process of the mandible *(arrows)* superimposed on the maxillary tuberosity.

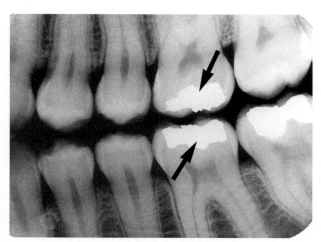

FIG. **10-61**   Amalgam restorations appear completely radiopaque *(arrows)*.

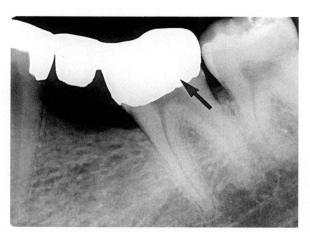

FIG. **10-62**   A cast gold crown, appearing completely radiopaque *(arrow)*, serves as the terminal abutment of a bridge.

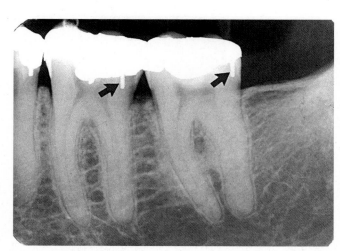

FIG. **10-63**   Stainless steel pins *(arrows)* provide retention for amalgam restorations.

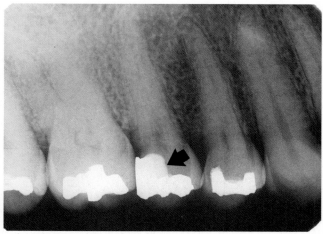

FIG. **10-64**   Base material *(arrow)* is usually radiopaque but less opaque than the amalgam restoration.

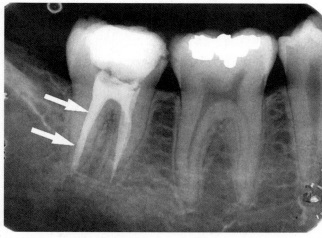

FIG. **10-65**   Gutta-percha *(arrows)* is a radiopaque rubberlike material used in endodontic therapy.

a rubberlike substance used to fill tooth canals during endodontic therapy (Fig. 10-65). Silver points were previously used to obliterate canals during endodontic therapy (Fig. 10-66). Other restorative materials that appear rather radiolucent on intraoral films include silicates, usually in combination with a base but now seldom used (Fig. 10-67), composite, usually in anterior teeth (Fig. 10-68), and porcelain, now usually fused to a metallic coping (Fig. 10-69). Composite restorative materials may also be opaque (Fig. 10-70). In addition, stainless steel crowns (Fig. 10-71) and orthodontic appliances around teeth (Fig. 10-72) are relatively radiopaque.

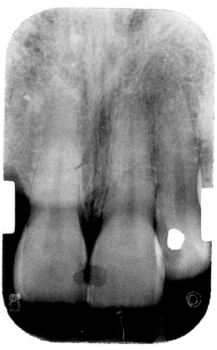

FIG. **10-68**   Composite restorations may be radiolucent and may suggest caries but can be recognized by their well-demarcated border with dentin.

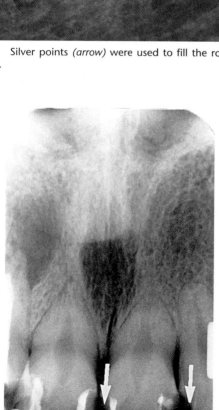

FIG. **10-66**   Silver points *(arrow)* were used to fill the root canals in this patient.

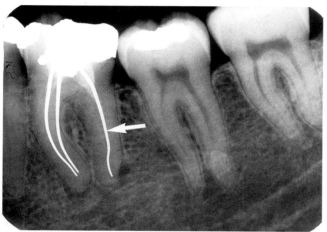

FIG. **10-67**   Radiolucent silicate restorations *(arrows)* were placed over a base to protect the pulp in this patient.

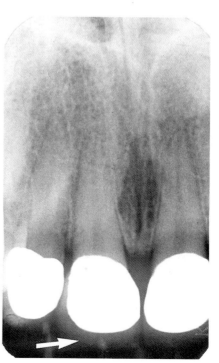

FIG. **10-69**   Porcelain appears radiolucent *(arrow)* over a metal coping.

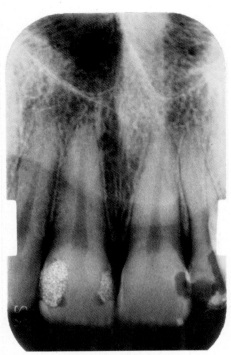

FIG. **10-70**    Composite restorations containing particles of barium glass are radiopaque and not likely to be confused with caries.

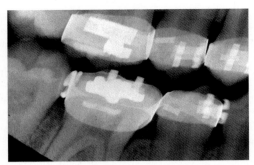

FIG. **10-72**    Orthodontic appliances have a characteristic radiopaque appearance.

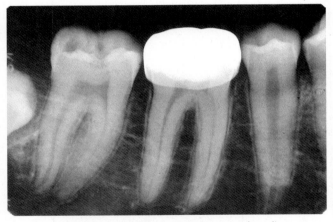

FIG. **10-71**    Stainless steel crowns appear mostly radiopaque.

## BIBLIOGRAPHY

Berkovitz BKB, Holland GR, Moxham BL: *Oral anatomy, histology and embryology,* ed 3, London, 2002, Mosby.

Claeys V, Waskens G: Bifid mandibular canal: literature review and case report, *Dentomaxilofac Radiol* 34:55-58, 2005.

Kasle MJ: *An atlas of dental radiographic anatomy,* ed 4, Philadelphia, 1994, WB Saunders.

Liang X, Jacobs R, Lambrichts I et al: Lingual foramina on the mandibular midline revisited: a macroanatomical study, *Clin Anat* 20:246-251, 2007.

Lusting JP, London D, Dor BL et al: Ultrasound identification and quantitative measurement of blood supply to the anterior part of the mandible, *Oral Surg Oral Med Oral Pathol Oral Radiol Endod* 96:625-629, 2003.

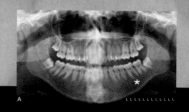

# Panoramic Imaging

Alan G. Lurie

Panoramic imaging (also called *pantomography*) is a technique for producing a single tomographic image of the facial structures that includes both the maxillary and mandibular dental arches and their supporting structures (Fig. 11-1). This is a curvilinear variant of conventional tomography and is also based on the principle of the reciprocal movement of an x-ray source and an image receptor around a central point or plane, called the image layer, in which the object of interest is located. Objects in front of or behind this image layer are not clearly captured because of their movement relative to the centers of rotation of the receptor and x-ray source.

The principal advantages of panoramic images include the following:

- Broad coverage of the facial bones and teeth
- Low patient radiation dose
- Convenience of the examination for the patient
- Use in patients unable to open their mouths
- Short time required to make a panoramic image, usually in the range of 3 to 4 minutes (This includes the time necessary for positioning the patient and the actual exposure cycle.)
- Patients readily understand panoramic films; thus they are also a useful visual aid in patient education and case presentation.

Panoramic images are most useful clinically for diagnostic problems requiring broad coverage of the jaws. Common examples include evaluation of trauma, location of third molars, extensive dental or osseous disease, known or suspected large lesions, tooth development (especially in the mixed dentition), retained teeth or root tips (in edentulous patients), temporomandibular joint (TMJ) pain, and developmental anomalies. These tasks do not require the high resolution and sharp detail available on intraoral images. Panoramic imaging is often used as the initial evaluation image that can provide the required insight or assist in determining the need for other projections. Panoramic images are also useful for patients who do not tolerate intraoral procedures well. However, when a full-mouth series of radiographs is available for a patient receiving general dental care, typically little or no additional useful information is gained from a simultaneous panoramic examination.

The main disadvantage of panoramic radiology is that the image does not display the fine anatomic detail available on intraoral periapical radiographs. Thus it is not as useful as periapical radiography for detecting small carious lesions, fine structure of the marginal periodontium, or periapical disease. The proximal surfaces of premolars also typically overlap. Accordingly, the availability of a panoramic radiograph for an adult patient often does not preclude the need for intraoral films for the diagnoses of most commonly encountered dental diseases. Other problems associated with panoramic radiography include unequal magnification and geometric distortion across the image. Occasionally the presence of overlapping structures, such as the cervical spine, can hide odontogenic lesions, particularly in the incisor regions. Further, clinically important objects may be situated outside the plane of focus (image layer) and may appear distorted or not present at all.

## Principles of Panoramic Image Formation

Paatero and, working independently, Numata were the first to describe the principles of panoramic radiography. The following illustrations explain the operation of a panoramic machine. Two adjacent disks are rotating at the same speed in opposite directions as an x-ray beam passes through their centers of rotation (Fig. 11-2). Lead collimators in the shape of a slit, located at the x-ray source and at the image receptor, limit the central ray to a narrow vertical beam. Radiopaque objects A, B, C, and D stand upright on disk 1 and rotate past the slit. Their images are recorded on the receptor, which also moves past the slit at the same time. The objects are displayed sharply on the receptor because they are moving past the slit at the same rate and in the same direction as the receptor. This causes their moving shadows to appear stationary in relation to the moving receptor. Other objects between the letters and the center of rotation of disk 1 rotate with a slower velocity and are blurred on the receptor. Any objects between the x-ray source and the center of rotation of disk 1 move in the opposite direction of the receptor, and their shadows are also blurred on the receptor.

Figure 11-3 shows that the same relationship of moving film to image is achieved if disk 1 is held stationary and the x-ray source is rotated so that the central ray constantly passes through the center of rotation of disk 1 and, simultaneously, both disk 2 and the lead collimator *(Pb)* rotate around the center of disk 1. Note that, although disk 2 moves, the receptor on this disk also rotates past the slit. In this situation, as before, the objects A through D move through the x-ray beam in the same direction and at the same rate as the receptor. To obtain optimal image definition, it is crucial that the speed of the receptor passing the collimator slit *(Pb)* be maintained equal to the speed at which the x-ray beam sweeps through the objects of interest.

In the case where the receptor is a charge-coupled device (CCD) array, the image is electronically transmitted to the controlling

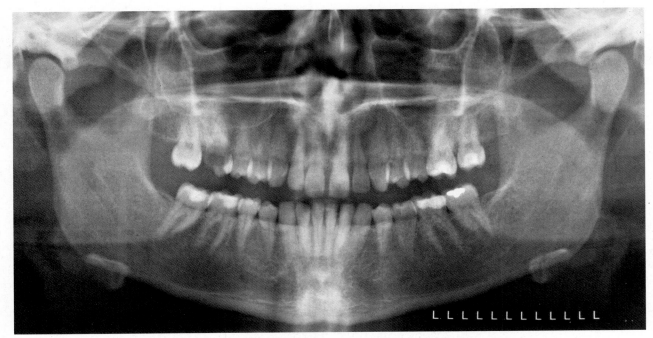

FIG. **11-1** Maxilla, mandible, and dentition in an adult patient (panoramic view).

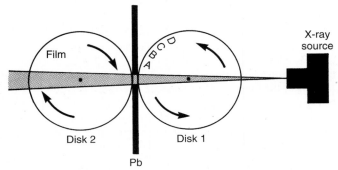

FIG. **11-2** Movement of the film and objects (*A, B, C,* and *D*) about two fixed centers of rotation. *Pb,* Lead collimator.

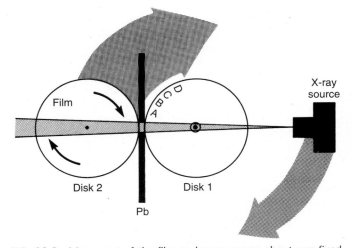

FIG. **11-3** Movement of the film and x-ray source about one fixed center of rotation. *Pb,* Lead collimator.

computer as the x-ray beam hits it, and this transmission is continuous as the x-ray source and receptor are traveling around the patient. The resulting geometric projection characteristics are the same as if film or a photostimulable phosphor plate (PSP) had been used. This holds true for geometric distortions such as magnification and elongation, the presence of ghost images, superimposition of the cervical spine over midline structures, overlap of teeth, and left-right size variations from lack of proper positioning of the patient's sagittal plane in the instrument.

Figure 11-4 shows that a patient may replace disk 1 and that objects A through D represent teeth and surrounding bone. In practice, the center of rotation is located off to the side, away from the objects being imaged. During the exposure cycle, the machine automatically shifts to one or more additional rotation centers. The rate of movement of the receptor behind the slit is regulated to be the same as that of the central ray sweeping through the dental structures on the side of the patient nearest the receptor. Structures on the opposite side of the patient (near the x-ray tube) are distorted and appear out of focus because the x-ray beam sweeps through them in the direction opposite that in which the image receptor is moving. In addition, structures near the x-ray source are so magnified (and their borders so blurred) that they are not seen as discrete images on the resultant image. These structures appear only as diffuse phantom or ghost images. Because of both these circumstances, only structures near the receptor are usefully captured on the resultant image. Structures located more centrally in the body relative to the jaws, such as the hyoid bone and epiglottis, appear on the right, left, and sometimes central areas of the final image.

Most panoramic machines now use a continuously moving center of rotation rather than multiple fixed locations. Figure 11-5 shows a continually moving center of rotation. This feature optimizes the shape of the image layer to reveal the teeth and supporting bone. This center of rotation is initially near the lingual surface of the right body of the mandible when the left TMJ is imaged. The rotation center moves forward along an arc that ends just lingual to the symphysis of the mandible when the midline is imaged. The arc is reversed as the opposite side of the face is imaged. In some contemporary panoramic machines, the shape of the image layer can be adjusted to better conform to the shape of the patients' mandibulofacial anatomy or to better show specific anatomic areas such as the TMJ or the maxillary sinuses. This is accomplished through varying the shape of the moving center of rotation, and allows better representation of children, unusually configured patients, and specific anatomic sites of interest.

## IMAGE LAYER

The image layer is a three-dimensional curved zone, or "focal trough," where the structures lying within this layer are reasonably well defined on final panoramic image. The structures seen on a panoramic image are primarily those located within the image layer. Objects outside the image layer are blurred, magnified, or reduced in size and are sometimes distorted to the extent of not being recognizable. The shape of the image layer varies with the brand of equipment used. Figure 11-6 shows the general shape of the image layer used in panoramic machines. The factors that affect its size are variables that influence image definition: arc path, velocity of the receptor and x-ray tube head, alignment of the x-ray beam, and collimator width. The location of the image layer can change with extensive machine use, so recalibration may be necessary if consistently suboptimal images are produced.

As the position of an object is moved within the image layer, the size and shape of the resultant image change. Figure 11-7, *A* through *F*, illustrates the influence of patient positioning on image size and shape. Figure 11-7, *A* and *B*, shows a mandible supporting a brass ring properly aligned in the middle of the image layer. Note the even

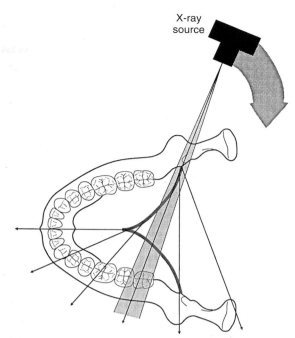

FIG. **11-5** Movement of the x-ray source and beam. The dark line shows a continuously moving center of rotation. As the source moves behind the patient's neck and the anterior teeth are imaged, the center of rotation moves forward along the arc *(dark line)* toward the sagittal plane. The x-ray source continues to move around the patient to image the opposite side.

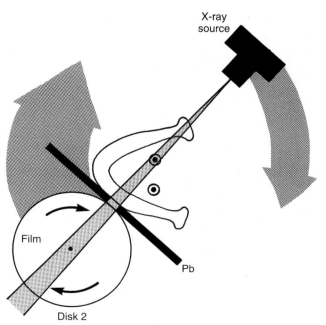

FIG. **11-4** Movement of the film and x-ray source about a shifting center of rotation. *Pb,* Lead collimator.

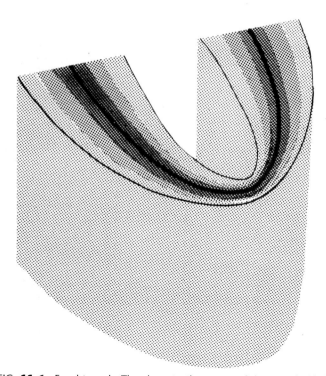

FIG. **11-6** Focal trough. The closer to the center of the trough *(dark zone)* an anatomic structure is positioned, the more clearly it is imaged on the resulting radiograph.

magnification of the ring and the images of the anterior teeth in proper proportion. Figure 11-7, *C* and *D*, shows the same mandible positioned 5 mm anterior to the middle of the center of the image layer. This position causes distortion of the ring in the horizontal dimension, with the ring appearing thinner and a commensurate decreased width of the images of the teeth. Figure 11-7, *E* and *F*, shows the same mandible positioned 5 mm posterior to the middle of the focal trough. Now the horizontal distortion results in the ring appear-

ing wider and a commensurate increased width of the projected teeth. On these images the vertical dimension, in contrast to the horizontal dimension, is little altered, although it appears to be. These distortions result from the reciprocal horizontal movements of the receptor and x-ray source. Thus, as a general rule, when the structure of interest, in this case the mandible, is displaced to the lingual side of its optimal position in the image layer, toward the x-ray source, the beam passes more slowly through it than the speed at which the receptor moves.

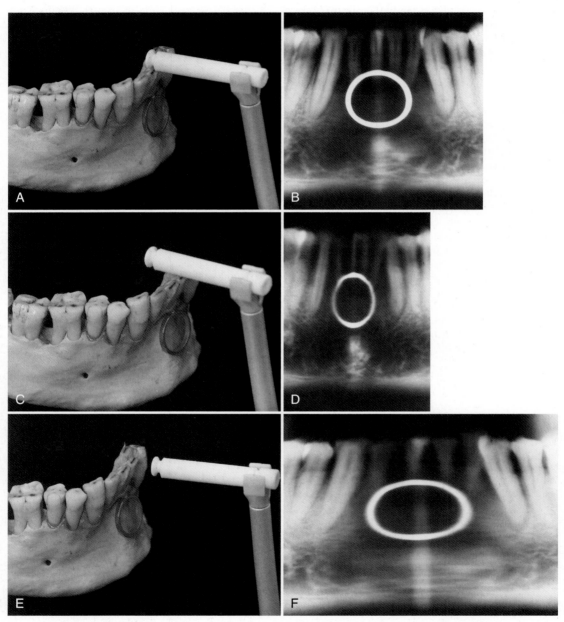

FIG. **11-7** **A,** Mandible supporting a metal ring positioned at the center of the focal trough. The incisal edges of the mandibular teeth are indexed by a bite rod–positioning device. The mandible is positioned at the center of the trough. **B,** Resultant panoramic radiograph. **C,** Mandible and ring positioned 5 mm anterior to the focal trough. The incisal edges of the teeth are anterior to the trough. **D,** Resultant panoramic radiograph demonstrating the horizontal minification of both ring and mandibular teeth. **E,** Mandible and ring positioned 5 mm posterior to the focal trough. The incisal edges of the teeth are also posterior to the trough. **F,** Resultant panoramic radiograph demonstrating the horizontal magnification of both ring and mandibular teeth.

Consequently, the images of the structures in this region are elongated horizontally on the image and they appear wider. Alternatively, when the mandible is displaced toward the buccal aspect of the image layer, the beam passes at a rate faster than normal through the structures. In the example shown, because the receptor is moving at the proper rate, the representations of the anterior teeth are compressed horizontally on the image, and they appear thinner. Special attention must be paid to these considerations in following the progress of a bony lesion, especially in the anterior region. As a result of improper patient positioning the lesion may appear greater (enlarging) (see Figure 11-7, *F*) or reduced (healing) (see Figure 11-7, *D*) on successive images. Thus the importance of careful alignment and positioning of the patient's dental arches within the area of the image layer is apparent.

The same principle applies to the patient's sagittal plane being rotated in the image layer. The posterior structures on the side to which the patient's head is rotated will be magnified in the horizontal dimension because the posterior structures will be moved away from the image receptor, whereas posterior structures on the opposite side will be moved closer to the image receptor and will be reduced in horizontal dimension. The resulting image will have horizontally large molar teeth and mandibular ramus, and severe premolar overlap, on one side and horizontally smaller molar teeth and mandibular ramus on the other side. This must not be confused with a congenital or developmental facial asymmetry (This positioning artifact is demonstrated in Figure 11-8).

## PANORAMIC MACHINES

A number of companies manufacture high-quality film-based and digital panoramic machines. The Othoralix 8500 (KaVo Dental Corp.,

Gendex Dental Systems, Lake Zurich, Ill. [Fig. 11-9]), the Proline XC (Planmeca Oy, Helsinki, Finland [Fig. 11-10]), and the Orthophos XG-Plus (Sirona Dental Systems GmbH, Bensheim, Germany [Fig. 11-11]) are all highly versatile. In addition to producing standard panoramic images of the jaws, they have the capability of adjusting to patients of various sizes and making frontal and lateral images of TMJs. These machines also are capable of producing tomographic views through the sinuses and cross-sectional views of the maxilla and mandible. These views are acquired by having special tube head and film movements programmed into the machine. Each machine also has the capability for adding on a cephalometric attachment to allow exposure of standardized skull views. Some machines further have the capability of automated exposure control. This is accomplished by measuring the amount of radiation passing through the patient's mandible during the initial part of the exposure and adjusting the imaging factors (peak kilovoltage [kVp], milliamperage [mA], and speed of imaging movements) to obtain a correctly exposed image. Finally, all of these machines are available in CCD-digital configurations.

There are now computer-controlled multimodality machines in which the direction and speed of movement of the tube head and film are highly variable, in some cases including multidirectional tomography. This allows the machines to be programmed to make tomographic views through many areas of the head. For instance, they can be programmed to image frontal or lateral views of the TMJs, coronal or sagittal sections through the maxillary sinuses, and cross-sectional cuts through a predetermined portion of the maxilla or mandible. These machines have much greater versatility than the conventional panoramic machines, and they are more expensive. Most of the special examinations made on these machines use circular or hypocycloidal

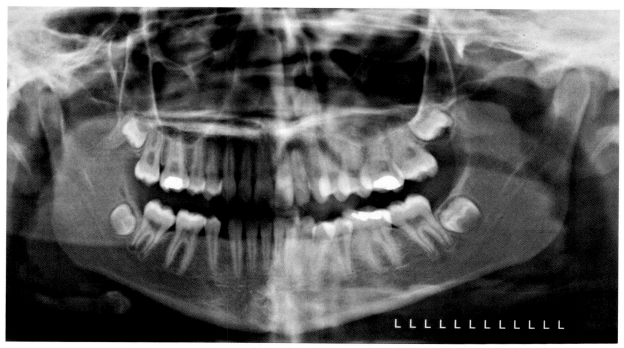

FIG. **11-8** Panoramic image showing positioning error-rotation of the sagittal plane. The patient's head was rotated to the left, moving the right side closer to the receptor and the left side further from the receptor. Note the relative magnification of the left-sided molar teeth, mandibular ramus, and condyle and the severe overlap of the posterior teeth. It is important to recognize this fairly common distortion and not to mistake it for a skeletal asymmetry.

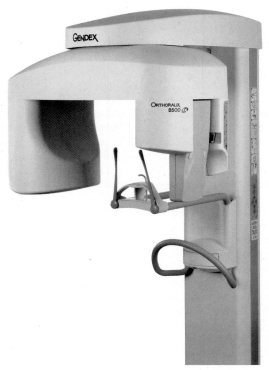

FIG. **11-9** Orthoralix 8500 panoramic machine. (Courtesy Orthoralix 8500, KaVo Dental Corp., Gendex Dental Systems, Lake Zurich, Ill.)

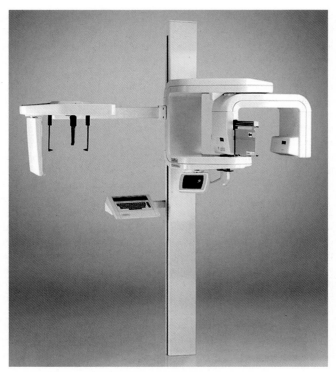

FIG. **11-10** Proline XC panoramic machine. (Courtesy Planmeca Inc., Wood Dale, Ill.)

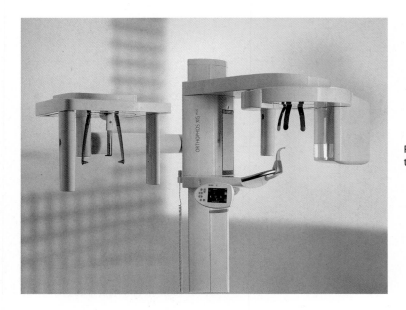

FIG. **11-11** Orthophos XG-PLUS panoramic machine. (Courtesy Sirona Dental Systems GmbH, Bensheim, Germany.)

tomography (see Chapter 13). The use of such instruments has substantially diminished in recent years with the steadily increasing use of cone-beam computed tomography (CBCT, see Chapter 14). Several new panoramic machines are also capable of accomplishing some degree of CBCT imaging.

## Patient Positioning and Head Alignment

To obtain diagnostically useful panoramic radiographs, it is necessary to properly prepare patients and to position their heads carefully in the image layer. Dental appliances, earrings, necklaces, hairpins, and any other metallic objects in the head and neck region should be removed. It may also be wise to demonstrate the machine to the patient by cycling it while explaining the need to remain still during the procedure. This is particularly true for children, who may be anxious. Children should be instructed to look forward and to not follow the tube head with their eyes.

The anteroposterior position radiograph of the patient is achieved typically by having patients place the incisal edges of their maxillary and mandibular incisors into a notched positioning device (the bite-block). Patients should not shift the mandible to either side when making this protrusive movement. The midsagittal plane must be centered within the image layer of the particular x-ray unit.

Placement of the patient either too far anterior or posterior results in significant dimensional aberrations in the images. Too far posterior results in magnified mesiodistal dimensions through the anterior sextants and resulting "fat" teeth (see Figure 11-7, F). Too far anterior results in reduced mesiodistal dimensions through the anterior sextants and resulting "thin" teeth (see Figure 11-7, D). Failure to position the midsagittal plane in the rotational midline of the machine results in a radiograph showing right and left sides that are unequally magnified in the horizontal dimension (see Fig. 11-8). Poor midline posi-

tioning is a common error, causing horizontal distortion in the posterior regions, excessive tooth overlap in the premolar regions and, on occasion, nondiagnostic, clinically unacceptable images. A simple method for evaluating the degree of horizontal distortion of the image is to compare the apparent width of the mandibular first molars bilaterally. The smaller side is too close to the receptor and the larger side is too close to the x-ray source.

The patient's chin and occlusal plane must be properly positioned to avoid distortion. The occlusal plane is aligned so that it is lower anteriorly, angled 20 to 30 degrees below the horizontal. A general guide for chin positioning is to place the patient so that a line from the tragus of the ear to the outer canthus of the eye is parallel with the floor. If the chin is tipped too high, the occlusal plane on the radiograph appears flat or inverted, and the image of the mandible is distorted (Fig. 11-12, A). In addition, a radiopaque shadow of the hard palate is superimposed on the roots of the maxillary teeth. If the chin is tipped too low, the teeth become severely overlapped, the symphyseal region of the mandible may be cut off the film, and both mandibular condyles may be projected off the superior edge of the film (Fig. 11-12, B). Patients are positioned with their backs and spines as erect as possible and their necks extended. Having patients place their

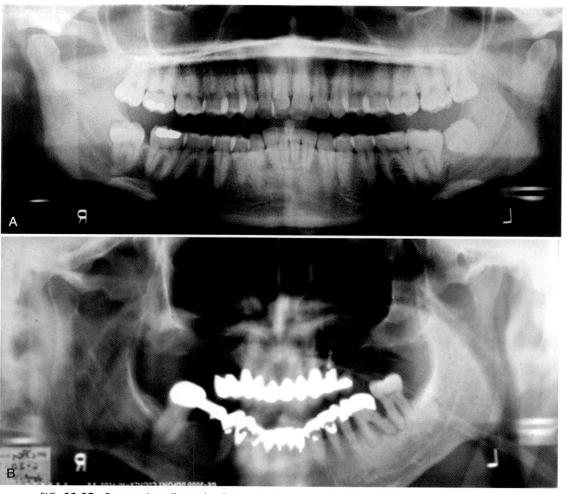

FIG. **11-12** Panoramic radiographs demonstrating poor patient head alignment. **A,** The chin and occlusal plane are rotated upward, resulting in overlapping images of the teeth and an opaque shadow (the hard palate) obscuring the roots of the maxillary teeth. **B,** The chin and occlusal plane are rotated downward, cutting off the symphyseal region on the radiograph and distorting the anterior teeth.

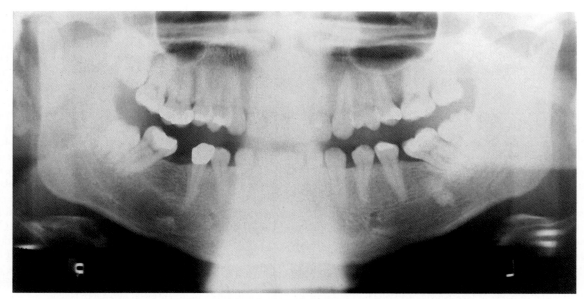

FIG. **11-13**  Panoramic radiograph of an improperly positioned patient. Note the large radiopaque region in the middle. This artifact ("spine-shadow ghost") could have been eliminated by having the patient sit straight and align or stretch the neck.

feet on a foot support and using a cushion for back support may facilitate proper back positioning in seated units. These devices help straighten the spine, minimizing the artifact produced by a shadow of the spine.

Proper neck extension is best accomplished by using a gentle upward force on the mastoid eminences when positioning the head in a manner similar to applying cervical traction. Allowing patients to slump their heads and necks forward causes a large opaque artifact in the midline created by the superimposition of an increased mass of cervical spine. This shadow obscures the entire symphyseal region of the mandible and may require that the radiograph be retaken (Fig. 11-13). Finally, after patients are positioned in the machine, they should be instructed to swallow and hold the tongue on the roof of the mouth. This raises the dorsum of the tongue to the hard palate, eliminating the air space and providing optimal visualization of the apices of the maxillary teeth.

## Image Receptors

Intensifying screens (see Chapter 5) are routinely used in panoramic radiography because they significantly reduce the amount of radiation required for properly exposing a radiograph. Fast films combined with high-speed (rare earth) screens are indicated for most examinations. In most cases, the manufacturer provides panoramic machines with intensifying screens. The type of screen (manufacturer and model) is printed in black letters on each screen and clearly projected onto the radiograph. With rare earth screens and fast films, the patient's skin exposure from panoramic radiography is approximately equivalent to four bitewing views made with F-speed film.

Most manufacturers have developed direct digital acquisition panoramic machines. The receptor on such a machine is either an array of CCDs or a film-sized PSP plate rather than film. The CCD array transmits an electronic signal to the controlling computer, which displays the image on the viewscreen as it is being acquired. The software of the unit makes internal adjustments to the acquired data to

render an interpretable image on the screen. The PSP plate is processed in the same manner as an intraoral PSP, and a similar image characteristic adjustment is automatically performed by the software package. Both these digital modalities allow the user to perform postprocessing modifications on the image, including linear contrast and density adjustments, black/white reversal, area of interest magnification, edge enhancement, and color rendering. Most units acquire and store their electronic data in DICOM format (*D*igital *I*maging and *CO*mmunication in *M*edicine); this allows for rapid telecommunication of images worldwide to all DICOM compliant workstations. DICOM is the international standard language for the electronic communication of digital images, be they radiographs, photographs, histopathologic slides, or any other type of "picture image." The American Dental Association recommended that all digital x-ray units manufactured after 2004 be DICOM compliant. These units are becoming more widely used as dentistry increases its use of direct digital imaging and electronic patient records.

All panoramic images should have some mechanism for automatically marking the patient's left or right sides on the image. Also, the patient's name, age, and the date the image was acquired should be indicated, with markers, photographic imprinting, or glued labels. The dentist's name must be on the image. No significant anatomic structures should be obscured by any of these labels or markings. Also, no parts of the image are trimmed to make the film fit the patient's chart.

## Panoramic Film Darkroom Techniques

Special darkroom procedures are needed when panoramic film is being processed. These films are far more light sensitive than intraoral films, especially after they have been exposed. A reduction in darkroom lighting from that used for conventional intraoral film is necessary. A Kodak GBX-2 filter can be installed with a 15-watt bulb at least 4 feet from the working surface. An ML-2 filter should not be used because it fogs panoramic film. Panoramic film should be developed either manually or in automatic film processors according to the manufacturer's recommendations. Obtaining optimal results relies on the same care to develop, rinse, fix, and wash panoramic films as is taken with intraoral films.

## Interpreting the Panoramic Image

As with all image interpretation, the starting points are the systematic analysis of the image and a thorough understanding of the appearances of the normal anatomic structures and their variants on the image. Panoramic images are quite different from intraoral images and demand a disciplined and focused approach to their interpretation. Recognizing normal anatomic structures on panoramic radiographs is challenging because of the complex anatomy of the midface, the superimposition of various anatomic structures, and the changing projection orientation. The many potential artifacts associated with machine and patient movement, patient positioning, and unusual patient anatomy must be identified and understood. *The absence of a normal anatomic structure may be the most important finding on the image.* Thus it is essential to identify the presence and integrity of all the major anatomic structures.

Most images in dentistry are two-dimensional representations of three-dimensional structures. Thus, on a posteroanterior (PA) skull film, orbital rims, nasal conchae, teeth, cervical vertebrae, and petrous ridges are all in sharp focus on the image, although they may be as much as a foot apart from each other. Although this presents less of an interpretation problem with panoramic images, which are curved image "slices" of the mandibulofacial tissues, there is still a thickness to the tomogram which must be considered, and the clinician must relate the structures on the image to their relative positions in the midfacial skeleton. An example of this three-dimensionality is the relative positioning of the external oblique and mylohyoid ridges in the mandible: on the panoramic image, they generally both appear sharp, whereas physically the external oblique ridge is on the mandibular buccal surface and the mylohyoid ridge is on the mandibular lingual surface, separated by several millimeters. When panoramic images are viewed, it is important for the clinician to remember this principle and to attempt to visualize the structures three-dimensionally in his or her mind.

It is helpful to view the image as if looking at the patient, with the structures on the patient's right side positioned on the viewer's left (Fig. 11-14). Thus the image is presented in the same orientation as that of periapical and bitewing images, making the interpretation more comfortable. It is extremely important to recognize the planes of the patient that are represented in different parts of the panoramic image. The panoramic image is actually three images in one: left and right lateral images posterior to the canines and a PA image anterior to the canines. The anterior sextants are also subject to the most dimensional distortion and to superimposition artifacts from the cervical vertebrae. Thus a useful mental approach to the panoramic image is to consider it as two lateral views surrounding a PA view in the middle, a sort of Mercator projection of the mid and lower face. This mental approach to viewing the panoramic image is illustrated by the panoramic and lateral and PA cephalometric images in Figure 11-15 and by the opened skull in Figure 11-16.

As with all image viewing, you should mask out extraneous light from around the image, dim the room lights, and when possible, work seated in a quiet room. This applies equally to viewing digital images on a computer display and traditional film radiographs on a viewbox.

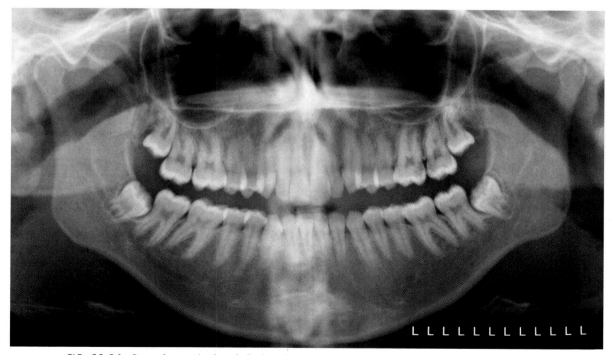

FIG. **11-14** Properly acquired and displayed panoramic image of an adult patient. Note that the patient's left side is indicated on the image and that the image is oriented as if the clinician were facing the patient. This is the same orientation used with a full mouth series, making it easier for the clinician to orient himself or herself and to interpret the image.

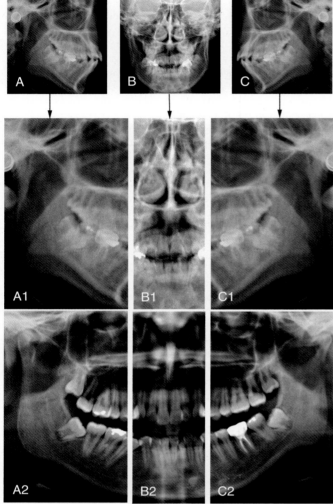

FIG. **11-15 Intellectual Segmentation of the Panoramic Image.** The panoramic image is composed of right and left lateral images connected in the middle by a PA image; it looks similar to a Mercator projection of the globe. This is appreciated by comparing the segmented panoramic image and the labeled structures to the matching cephalometric films acquired on the same patient. **A-C,** Left lateral, PA, and right lateral cephalometric images. These images are cropped and aligned to produce **A1-C1. A2-C2** show a segmented panoramic image on the same patient. Note the similarities between the lateral cephalometric images and the panoramic image posterior to the canines, and between the PA cephalometric image and the panoramic image between the canines. Thus, when interpreting a panoramic image, the clinician should think of viewing left and right lateral projections of the midface, connected in the middle by a PA projection.

## THE MANDIBLE

Studying the mandible (Figs. 11-17 and 11-18) can be compartmentalized into the major anatomic areas of this curved bone:

- Condylar process and temporomandibular joint
- Coronoid process
- Ramus
- Body and angle

- Anterior sextant
- Mandibular dentition and supporting alveolus

The clinician should be able to follow a cortical border around the entire bone, with the exception of the dentate areas. This border should be smooth, without interruptions ("step deformities") and should have symmetric thicknesses in comparable anatomic areas (e.g., angles, inferior borders of bodies, posterior borders of rami). The trabeculation of the mandible tends to be more plentiful in the anterior regions, whereas the marrow compartment increases toward the angle and into the ramus; however, these trabecular patterns and densities should be relatively symmetric. This is especially true in children, who have very sparse trabeculation throughout the deciduous and mixed dentition stages.

The mandibular condyle is generally positioned slightly anteroinferior to its normal closed position because the patient has to slightly open and protrude the mandible to engage the positioning device in most panoramic machines. The TMJ can be assessed for gross anatomic changes of the condylar head and glenoid fossa; the soft tissues, such as the articular disc and posterior ligamentous attachment, cannot be evaluated. The glenoid fossa is part of the temporal bone, and as such it can be pneumatized by the mastoid air cells. This can result in the appearance of a multilocular radiolucency in the articular eminence and the roof of the glenoid fossa, a variant of normal. More definitive osseous assessment of the TMJ is accomplished by using complex motion tomography, CBCT, or computed tomography (CT), and magnetic resonance imaging (MRI) is the examination of choice for evaluation of the disc and pericondylar soft tissues (Brooks, 1997).

Shadows of other structures that can be superimposed over the mandibular ramal area include the following:

- Pharyngeal airway shadow, especially when the patient is unable to expel the air and place the tongue in the palate during the exposure
- Posterior wall of the nasopharynx
- Cervical vertebrae, especially in patients with pronounced anterior lordosis, typically seen in severely osteoporotic individuals
- Ear lobe and ear decorations
- Nasal cartilage and nasal decorations
- Soft palate and uvula
- Dorsum of the tongue and tongue decorations
- Ghost shadows of the opposite side of the mandible and metallic decorations

From the angle of the mandible, viewing should be continued anteriorly toward the symphyseal region. A fracture often manifests as a discontinuity (step deformity) in the inferior border; a sharp change in the level of the occlusal plane indicates that the fracture passes through the tooth-bearing area, whereas a cant in the entire occlusal table without a step deformity in the occlusal plane indicates that the fracture is posterior to the tooth-bearing area. The width of the cortical bone at the inferior border of the mandible should be at least 3 mm in adults and of uniform density. The bone may be thinned locally by an expansile lesion such as a cyst or thinned generally by systemic diseases such as hyperparathyroidism and osteoporosis. The outlines of both sides of the mandible should be compared for symmetry, noting any changes. Asymmetry of size may result from improper patient positioning or conditions such as hemifacial hyperplasia or hypoplasia. The hyoid bone may be projected below or onto the inferior border of the mandible.

Trabeculation is most evident within the alveolar process. The mandibular canals and mental foramina are usually clearly visualized in the ramus and body regions of the body of the mandible. Typically

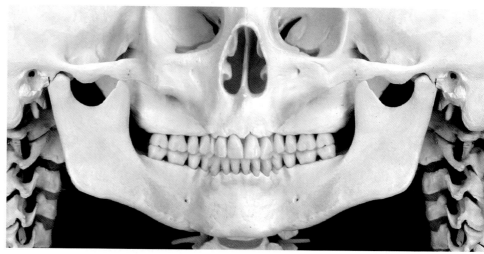

FIG. **11-16** This figure shows the bones of the mandible, midface, cervical spine and skull base as they appear on a panoramic image. Most important, this appearance is composed of left and right lateral views of the skeleton posterior to the canines, and an anterior view anterior to the premolars.

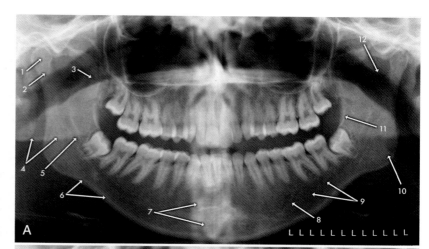

FIG. **11-17 Mandibular Bony Anatomic Structures on the Panoramic Image.** The labeled **(A)** and unlabeled **(B)** images are duplicate images of the same patient. *1,* Mandibular condyle. *2,* Neck of mandibular condyle. *3,* Coronoid process of mandible. *4,* Ghost image, posterior aspect of inferior border of left side of mandible. *5,* Inferior alveolar (mandibular) canal. *6,* Inferior border of mandible. *7,* Superimposed shadow of cervical vertebrae. *8,* Mental foramen. *9,* Submandibular fossa (lingual salivary gland depression) (also see Fig. 11-19). *10,* Mandibular angle. *11,* External oblique ridge. *12,* Sigmoid notch.

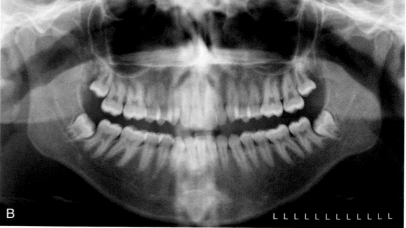

the canals exhibit uniform width or gentle tapering from the mandibular foramina to the mental foramina. They may be less well seen in the first molar and premolar regions. When only one border of the canal is seen, it is typically the inferior border. The canals usually rise to meet the mental foramina, often looping several millimeters anterior of the mental foramina; this is termed the "anterior loop" of the mandibular canal, and its position and extent are considerations when planning dental implants in the mandibular canine regions. A bulging of the canal suggests a neural tumor; however, it should be noted that slight widening at the point that the canal bends to enter the body of the mandible from the ramus is a variation of normal. The mandible should be examined for radiolucencies or

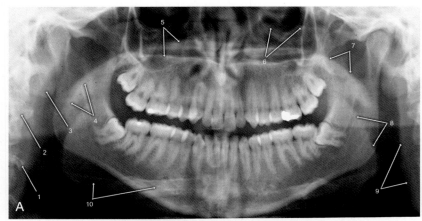

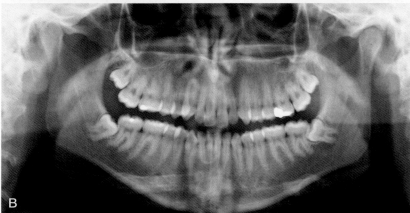

FIG. **11-18** **Spinal, Neck, and Soft Tissue Anatomic Structures on the Panoramic Image.** The labeled **(A)** and unlabeled **(B)** images are duplicate images of the same patient. *1,* Schmörl's Node (variant of normal anatomy of the vertebral body). *2,* Cervical vertebra. *3,* Ear lobe. *4,* Soft palate and uvula. *5,* Hard palate (the lower line is the junction of the hard palate and the lateral wall of the nasal cavity on the tube side, and the upper line is the junction of the hard palate and lateral wall of the nasal cavity on the receptor side). *6,* Orbital rim. *7,* Floor of nasopharynx (upper surface of soft palate). *8,* Posterior surface of tongue. *9,* Posterior pharyngeal wall. *10,* Hyoid bone.

opacities. The midline is more opaque because of the mental protuberance, increased trabecular numbers, and attenuation of the beam as it passes through the cervical spine. Many modern panoramic machines automatically increase the exposure factors as they pass across the cervical spine region in an attempt to minimize this opacity; nevertheless, some opacity is generally seen in the anterior regions of the image. There are often depressions on the lingual surfaces of the mandible, which are occupied by the submandibular and sublingual glands: these depressions are termed the lingual salivary gland depressions, or fossae, and are often more radiolucent. This anatomic feature is shown on a panoramic image, a periapical image, a coronal CT image, and a dry skull in Figure 11-19.

## MIDFACIAL REGION

The midface is a complex mixture of bones, air cavities and soft tissues, all of which appear on panoramic images (Figs. 11-20 and 11-21). Individual bones that may appear the panoramic image of the midface include temporal, zygoma, mandible, frontal, maxilla, sphenoid, ethmoid, vomer, nasal, turbinate, and palate; thus, it is somewhat of a misnomer to refer to the midfacial region on the panoramic image as "the maxilla." Maintaining the discipline and focus of a systemic examination of all aspects of the midfacial images is difficult and critical in the overall examination of the panoramic image.

As with the mandible, the maxilla can be compartmentalized into major sites for examination:

- Cortical boundary of the maxilla, including the posterior border and the alveolar ridge
- Pterygomaxillary fissure
- Maxillary sinuses
- Zygomatic complex, including inferior and lateral orbital rims, zygomatic process of maxilla, and anterior portion of zygomatic arch
- Nasal cavity and conchae
- Temporomandibular joint (already viewed in the mandible, but revisiting important structures is always a good idea in image interpretation)
- Maxillary dentition and supporting alveolus

Examining the cortical outline of the maxilla is a good way to center the examination of the midface. The posterior border of the maxilla extends from the superior portion of the pterygomaxillary fissure down to the tuberosity region and around to the other side. The posterior border of the pterygomaxillary fissure is the pterygoid spine of the sphenoid bone (the anterior border of the pterygoid plates). Occasionally, the sphenoid sinus may extend into this structure. The pterygomaxillary fissure itself has an inverted teardrop appearance; it is very important to identify this area on both sides of the image because maxillary sinus mucoceles and carcinomas will characteristically destroy the posterior maxillary border, which is then manifested as loss of the anterior border of the pterygomaxillary fissure. Also, LeFort fractures of the maxilla by definition involve the pterygoid plate(s), and this will often be initially diagnosed by disturbances of the integrity of the pterygomaxillary fissure on the panoramic image. In fact, this may be the only evidence for such a fracture on the panoramic image. To clarify the three-dimensional anatomy of the pterygomaxillary fissure, Figure 11-22 shows this

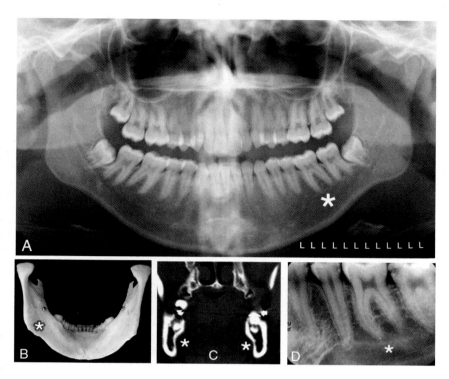

FIG. **11-19** The submandibular fossa (lingual salivary gland depression), a concavity often found on the posterior lingual surface of the mandible. This triangularly shaped area is bounded anatomically by the mylohyoid ridge, the inferior border of the mandibular body, and the posterior border of the mandibular ramus. *Asterisk* indicates the area of the submandibular fossa on the various images. **A,** Panoramic image. **B,** Photograph of the lingual side of a dried mandible. **C,** Coronal CT scan through the molar region of the mandible. **D,** Mandibular molar periapical image.

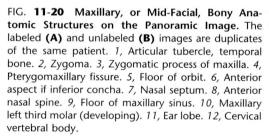

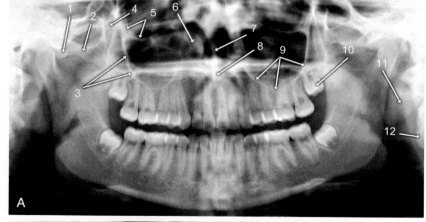

FIG. **11-20** Maxillary, or Mid-Facial, Bony Anatomic Structures on the Panoramic Image. The labeled **(A)** and unlabeled **(B)** images are duplicates of the same patient. *1,* Articular tubercle, temporal bone. *2,* Zygoma. *3,* Zygomatic process of maxilla. *4,* Pterygomaxillary fissure. *5,* Floor of orbit. *6,* Anterior aspect if inferior concha. *7,* Nasal septum. *8,* Anterior nasal spine. *9,* Floor of maxillary sinus. *10,* Maxillary left third molar (developing). *11,* Ear lobe. *12,* Cervical vertebral body.

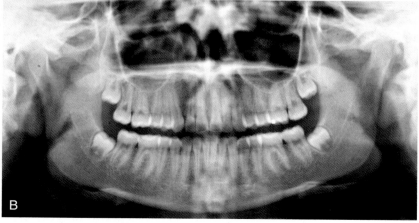

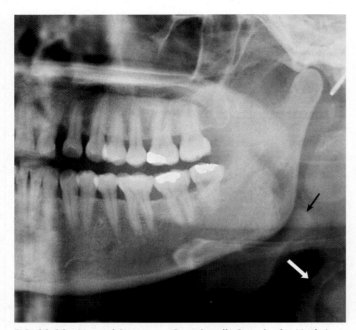

FIG. **11-21    Normal Structures Occasionally Seen in the Neck Area on Panoramic Images.** The *white arrow* indicates the superior aspect of the thyroid cartilage, which can be mistaken for a vascular calcification. The *black arrow* indicates the epiglottis. Also note the ear decoration posterior to the mandibular condylar head.

structure in a dried skull, in an axial CT image, and in the panoramic image.

The maxillary sinuses are usually well visualized on panoramic images. The clinician should identify each of the borders (posterior, anterior, floor, roof) and then note whether they are entirely outlined with cortical bone, roughly symmetric, and comparable in radiographic density. The borders should be present and intact. The medial border of the maxillary sinus is the lateral border of the nasal cavity; however, this interface is not demonstrated on the panoramic image. The superior border, or roof, of the maxillary sinus is the floor of the orbit; this interface is demonstrated on the panoramic image in its most anterior aspect. Although it is useful to compare right and left maxillary sinuses when looking for abnormalities, it is important to remember that the sinuses are frequently nonpathologically asymmetric relative to size, shape, and presence and numbers of septae. The posterior aspect of the sinus is more opaque because of superimposition of the zygoma. Each sinus should be examined for evidence of a mucous retention cyst, mucoperiosteal thickening, and other sinus abnormalities.

The zygomatic complex, or "buttress" of the midface, is a very complex anatomic area, with contributions from the frontal, zygomatic, and maxillary bones. It includes the lateral and inferior orbital rims, the zygomatic process of the maxilla, and the zygomatic arch. The zygomatic process of the maxilla arises over the maxillary first and second molars. The maxillary sinus can pneumatize the zygomatic process of the maxilla up to the zytomaticomaxillary suture. This can result in the appearance of an elliptical, corticated radiolucency in the maxillary sinus, possibly superimposed over the roots of a molar tooth, on a panoramic image. The inferior border of the zygomatic arch extends posteriorly from the inferior portion of the zygomatic process of the maxilla and continues posteriorly to the articular tubercle and glenoid fossa of the temporal bone. The superior border of the zygomatic arch, which curves anterosuperiorly to

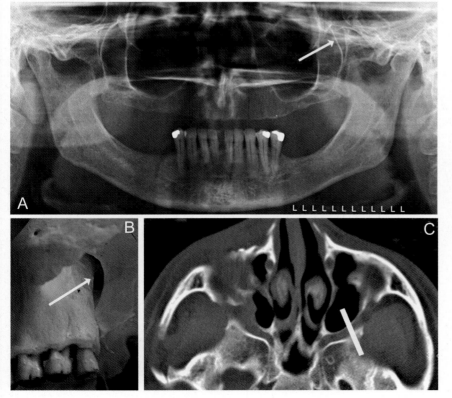

FIG. **11-22** The pterygomaxillary fissure, a space between the posterior surface of the maxilla and the anterior border of the pterygoid plates. **A,** The inverted teardrop shape of the fissure on a panoramic image *(arrow).* **B,** The fissure on a dried skull *(arrow).* **C,** The approximate image section of the panoramic image layer through the pterygomaxillary fissure on an axial CT section *(white bar).*

form the lateral aspect of the lateral orbital rim, should also be noted. The zygomaticotemporal suture lies in the middle of the zygomatic arch and may simulate a fracture if visualized on the image. Additionally, the mastoid air cells will occasionally pneumatize the temporal bone all the way to the zygomaticotemporal suture, giving the glenoid fossa of the TMJ the appearance of having a multilocular, or "soap-bubbly," radiolucency that is, in fact, a variant of normal.

The nasal fossa may show the nasal septum and inferior concha, including both the bone and its mucosal covering. The conchae, composed of an internal bone, the turbinate, and covering cartilage and mucosa, are seen in a coronal manner in the anterior portion of the image and in a sagittal manner in the posterior portions of the panoramic image. They can appear as very large, homogeneous, soft-tissue densities superimposed over the maxillary sinuses and occasionally the anterior nasopharynx.

## SOFT TISSUES

A number of opaque soft tissue structures may be identified on panoramic radiographs (see Figs. 11-20 and 11-21), including the tongue arching across the film under the hard palate, roughly from the region of the right angle of the mandible to the left angle), lip markings (in the middle of the film), the soft palate extending posteriorly from the hard palate (see Fig. 11-18, No. 7) over each ramus, the posterior wall of the oral and nasal pharynx, the nasal septum, ear lobes, nose, and nasolabial folds. Radiolucent airway shadows superimpose on normal anatomic structures and may be demonstrated by the borders of adjacent soft tissues. They include the nasal fossa, nasopharynx, oral cavity, and oropharynx. The epiglottis and thyroid cartilage are often seen in panoramic images. Occasionally the air space between the dorsum of the tongue and the soft palate simulates a fracture through the angle of the mandible.

## SUPERIMPOSITIONS AND GHOST IMAGES

Many radiopaque objects out of the image layer superimpose on the images of normal anatomic structures. This results when the x-ray beam projects through a dense object (e.g., an earring, the spinal column, the mandibular ramus, or the hard palate) that is in the path of the x-ray beam but out of the portion of the focal trough being imaged. The object typically appears blurred and projects either over the midline structures, as with the cervical vertebrae, or onto the opposite side of the radiograph with reversed configuration and more cranially positioned than the real structure (see Fig. 11-18). These contralateral images are termed "ghost images," and they may obscure normal anatomy or be mistaken for pathologic conditions.

## DENTITION

Finally, the teeth and supporting alveolar bone should be evaluated. Excessively wide or narrow anterior teeth suggest malposition of the patient in the image layer. Similarly, teeth that are wider on one side than the other suggest that the patient's sagittal plane was rotated. Although gross caries and periapical and periodontal disease may be evident, subtle disease requires intraoral images for diagnosis. The proximal surfaces of the premolar teeth often overlap, which further interferes with caries interpretation.

One of the strengths of the panoramic image is the demonstration of the complete dentition. Although there is a rare situation where positioning of the patient and of an ectopic tooth place the tooth out of the image layer, all the teeth are generally seen on the image. Thus the interpretation must always include identification of all erupted and developing teeth (Fig. 11-23). The teeth should be examined for gross abnormalities of number, position, and anatomy. Existing

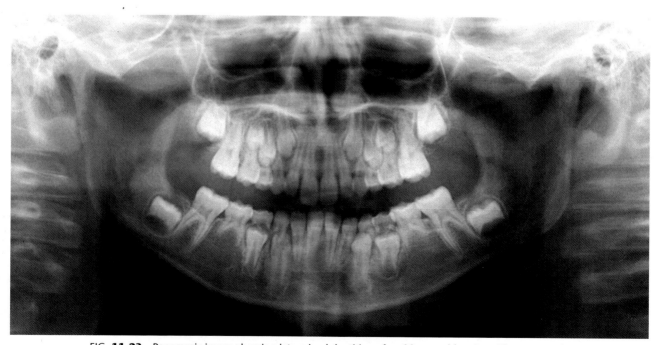

FIG. **11-23**  Panoramic image showing late mixed dentition of an 11-year-old patient. The panoramic image can be useful in identifying the presence or absence, as well as developmental status, of the permanent dentition. In this patient, the mandibular second premolars are congenitally absent, and the mandibular deciduous second molars are not undergoing root resorption, indicating that they will be retained. The permanent canines, second molars, and first and second premolars are in various stages of mineralization, with most of them beginning to erupt.

dentistry, including endodontic obturations, crowns, and other fixed restorations, should be noted.

It is particularly important to closely examine impacted third molars. Their orientation, the numbers and configurations of the roots, the relationships of the tooth components to critical anatomic structures such as the mandibular canal, the floor and posterior wall of the maxillary sinus, the maxillary tuberosity, and adjacent teeth, and the presence of abnormalities in the pericoronal or periradicular bone must be carefully studied. Suspected abnormalities of the dentition seen on panoramic images will generally require intraoral imaging for a more definitive demonstration of the area.

## BIBLIOGRAPHY

Brooks SL, Brand JW, Gibbs SJ et al: Imaging of the temporomandibular joint: a position paper of the American Academy of Oral and Maxillofacial Radiology, *Oral Surg Oral Med Oral Pathol Oral Radiol Endod* 83:609-618, 1997.

Chomenko AG: *Atlas for maxillofacial pantomographic interpretation,* Chicago, 1985, Quintessence.

Farman AG, editor: *Panoramic radiology: seminars on maxillofacial imaging and interpretation,* 2007, Berlin, Springer.

Langland OE, Langlais RP, McDavid WD et al: *Panoramic radiology,* ed 2, Philadelphia, 1989, Lea & Febiger.

Moore WE, editor: *Successful panoramic radiography:* KODAK Dental Radiography Series (2001): www.kodakdental.com/documentation/film/N-406SuccPanRad.pdf. Accessed February 20, 2008.

Numata H: Consideration of the parabolic radiography of the dental arch, *J Shimazu Stud* 10:13, 1933.

Paatero YV: The use of a mobile source of light in radiography, *Acta Radiol* 29:221, 1948.

Paatero YV: A new tomographic method for radiographing curved outer surfaces, *Acta Radiol* 32:177, 1949.

# CHAPTER 12

# Extraoral Radiographic Examinations

Sotirios Tetradis • Mel L. Kantor

In extraoral radiographic examinations both the x-ray source and image receptor (film or electronic sensor) are placed outside the patient's mouth. This chapter describes the most common extraoral radiographic examinations in which the source and sensor remain static. These include the *lateral cephalometric* projection of the sagittal or median plane; the *submentovertex* projection of the transverse or horizontal plane; the *Waters, posteroanterior cephalometric,* and *reverse-Towne* projections of the coronal or frontal plane; and the *oblique lateral* projections of the mandibular body and ramus. Panoramic radiography is described in Chapter 11, and other more complex imaging modalities are described in Chapters 13 and 14.

## Technique

The first step in obtaining a radiograph is the selection of the appropriate projection for the pertinent diagnostic task. However, for pedagogic reasons, this chapter begins with the technical facets of obtaining the extraoral views to make the reader familiar with the various projections.

Extraoral radiographs are produced with conventional dental x-ray machines, certain models of panoramic machines, or higher-capacity medical x-ray units. Cephalometric and skull views require at least a 20 × 25 cm (8 × 10 inch) image receptor, whereas oblique lateral projections of the mandible can be obtained with a 13 × 18 cm (5 × 7 inch) image receptor. It is critical to correctly and clearly label the right and left sides of the image. This usually is done by placing a metal marker (an *R* or an *L*) on the outside of the cassette in a corner in which the marker does not obstruct diagnostic information.

The proper exposure parameters depend on the patient's size, anatomy, and head orientation; image receptor speed; x-ray source-to-receptor distance; and whether grids are used. In cases of known or suspected disease, medium- or high-speed rare-earth screen-film combinations provide optimal balance between diagnostic information and patient exposure. For orthodontic purposes, high-speed combinations reduce patient exposure without compromising the identification of anatomic landmarks necessary for cephalometric analysis. Although radiographic grids reduce scattered radiation and improve contrast and resolution, they result in higher patient exposure. Cephalometry does not require the use of grids. However, grids could improve the radiographic appearance of fine structures, such as trabecular architecture, and aid in the diagnosis of disease.

Proper positioning of the x-ray source, patient, and image receptor requires patience, attention to detail, and experience. The main anatomic landmark used in patient positioning during extraoral radiography is the canthomeatal line, which joins the central point of the external auditory canal to the outer canthus of the eye. The canthomeatal line forms approximately a 10-degree angle with the Frankfort plane, the line that connects the superior border of the external auditory canal with the infraorbital rim. The image receptor and patient placement, central beam direction, and resultant image for the lateral, submentovertex, Waters, posteroanterior, reverse-Towne, and mandibular oblique lateral projections are summarized in Table 12-1 and are described in detail in the following sections.

## LATERAL SKULL PROJECTION (LATERAL CEPHALOMETRIC PROJECTION)

Of the extraoral radiographs described in this chapter, the lateral cephalometric projection is by far the most commonly used in dentistry. All cephalometric radiographs, including the lateral view, are made with a cephalostat that helps maintain a constant relationship among the skull, the film, and the x-ray beam. Skeletal, dental, and soft tissue anatomic landmarks delineate lines, planes, angles, and distances that are used to generate measurements and to classify patient craniofacial morphologic features. At the beginning of treatment, these measurements are often compared with an established standard; during treatment, the measurements are usually compared with those from previous cephalometric radiographs of the same patient to monitor growth and development as well as treatment.

### Image Receptor and Patient Placement
The image receptor is positioned parallel to the patient's midsagittal plane. The site of interest is placed toward the image receptor to minimize distortion. In cephalometric radiography, the patient is placed with the left side toward the image receptor (U.S. standards), and a wedge filter at the tube head is positioned over the anterior aspect of the beam to absorb some of the radiation and to allow visualization of soft tissues of the face.

### Position of the Central X-Ray Beam
The central beam is perpendicular to the midsagittal plane of the patient and the plane of the image receptor and is centered over the external auditory meatus.

### Resultant Image (Fig. 12-1)
Exact superimposition of right and left sides is impossible because structures on the side near the image receptor are magnified less than the same structures on the side far from the image receptor. Bilateral

**TABLE 12-1**
*Technical Aspects of Extraoral Radiographic Projections and Resultant Images*

| | Lateral Ceph | SMV | Waters | PA Ceph | Reverse Towne | Oblique Lateral Body | Oblique Lateral Ramus |
|---|---|---|---|---|---|---|---|
| Patient placement | Film parallel to midsagittal plane | Canthomeatal line parallel to film | Canthomeatal line at 37° with film | Canthomeatal line at 10° with film | Canthomeatal line at −30° with film | Film in contact with cheek at molar area | Film in contact with cheek at ramus area |
| Central beam | Beam perpendicular to film | Beam perpendicular to film | Beam perpendicular to film | Beam perpendicular to film | Beam perpendicular to film | Beam aims at the molar-premolar area | Beam aims at the ramus area |
| Diagram of patient placement | | | | | | | |
| Illustration of patient placement | | | | | | | |
| Skull view | | | | | | | |
| Resultant image | | | | | | | |

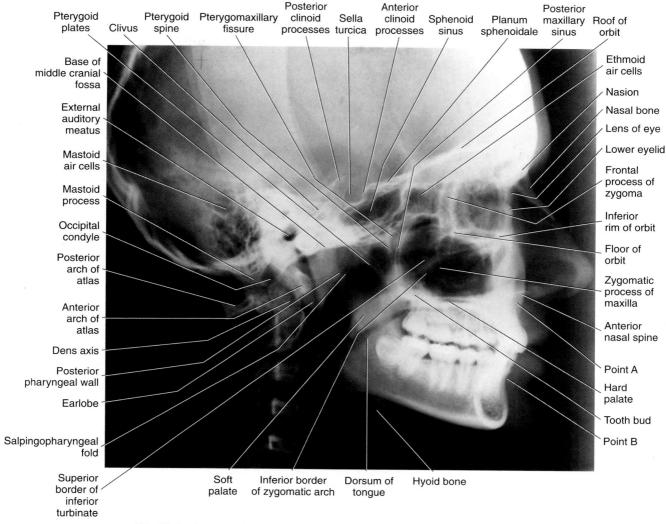

FIG. **12-1** Anatomic landmarks identified in the lateral cephalometric projection.

structures close to the midsagittal plane demonstrate less discrepancy in size compared with bilateral structures farther away from the midsagittal plane. Structures close to the midsagittal plane (e.g., the clinoid processes and inferior turbinates) should be nearly superimposed.

There are many cephalometric analyses that are based on a variety of anatomic landmarks. Steiner and Ricketts analyses are two commonly used analyses that use the skeletal, dental, and soft tissue landmarks included in Box 12-1. Precise identification of the various landmarks on the lateral cephalometric radiograph is necessary to generate accurate cephalometric measurements. The landmarks in Box 12-1 are shown in Figure 12-2, *A*, on a side view of a skull and in Figure 12-2, *B*, on a 5-mm wide midline section of an orthodontic patient imaged by cone-beam computed tomography. Finally, Figure 12-2, *C*, depicts the projected landmark position on the lateral cephalogram of an orthodontic patient. Although taken for a specific purpose, a lateral cephalometric radiograph is still a lateral *skull* film and should be interpreted as such. It is not sufficient to limit the interpretation to the cephalometric analysis.

## SUBMENTOVERTEX (BASE) PROJECTION

### Image Receptor and Patient Placement
The image receptor is positioned parallel to patient's transverse plane and perpendicular to the midsagittal and coronal planes. To achieve this, the patient's neck is extended as far backward as possible, with the canthomeatal line forming a 10-degree angle with the image receptor.

### Position of the Central X-Ray Beam
The central beam is perpendicular to the image receptor, directed from below the mandible toward the vertex of the skull (hence the name *submentovertex,* or *SMV*), and centered about 2 cm anterior to a line connecting the right and left condyles.

### Resultant Image (Fig. 12-3)
The midsagittal plane (represented by an imaginary line extending from the interproximal space of the maxillary central incisors through the nasal septum, to the middle of the anterior arch of the atlas, and to the dens) should divide the skull image in two symmetric halves.

## BOX 12-1
### Definition of Cephalometric Landmarks

#### Skeletal Landmarks

1. Porion (P): The most superior point of the external auditory canal
2. Sella (S): Center of the hypophyseal fossa
3. Nasion (N): Frontonasal suture
4. Orbitale (O): The most inferior point of the infraorbital rim
5. PT point: The most posterior point of the pterygomaxillary fissure
6. Basion (Ba): The most anterior point of the foramen magnum
7. PNS: The tip of the posterior nasal spine
8. ANS: The tip of the anterior nasal spine
9. A point: The deepest point of the anterior border of the maxillary alveolar ridge concavity
10. B point (B): The deepest point in the concavity of the anterior border of the mandible
11. Pogonion (Po): The most anterior point of the symphysis
12. Gnathion: The midpoint of the symphysis outline between pogonion and menton
13. Menton (M): The most inferior point of the symphysis
14. Gonion: The most convex point along the inferior border of the mandibular ramus
15. Ramus point: The most posterior point of the posteroinferior border of the mandibular ramus
16. R1: Most inferior point of the sigmoid notch
17. R2: An arbitrary point on the lower border of the mandible below R1
18. R3: The most concave point of the anterior border of the mandibular ramus
19. R4: The most convex point of the posterior border of the mandibular ramus
20. Articulare (Ar): The point of intersection between the basisphenoid and the posterior border of the condylar head
21. Condyle top: The most superior point of the condyle
22. DC point: The center of the condylar head

#### Dental Landmarks

23. U6 mesial cusp: Tip of the maxillary first molar mesial buccal cusp
24. U6 mesial: Contact point on the mesial surface of the maxillary first molar
25. U6 distal: Contact point on the distal surface of the maxillary first molar
26. L6 mesial cusp: Tip of the mandibular first molar mesial buccal cusp
27. L6 mesial: Contact point on the mesial surface of the mandibular first molar
28. L6 distal: Contact point on the distal surface of the mandibular first molar
29. UI incisal: Incisal edge of maxillary central incisor
30. UI facial: The most convex point of the buccal surface of the maxillary central incisor
31. UI root: Root tip of the maxillary central incisor
32. LI incisal: Incisal edge of mandibular central incisor
33. LI facial: The most convex point of the buccal surface of the mandibular central incisor
34. LI root: Root tip of the mandibular central incisor

#### Soft Tissue Landmarks

35. SofttTissue glabella: Most anterior point of the soft tissue covering the frontal bone
36. Soft tissue nasion: Most concave point of soft tissue outline at the bridge of the nose
37. Tip of nose: The most anterior point of the nose
38. Subnasale: The soft tissue point where the curvature of the upper lip connects to the floor of the nose
39. Soft tissue A point: The most concave point of the upper lip between subnasale and the upper lip point
40. Upper lip: The most anterior point of the upper lip
41. Stomion superius: Most inferior point of the upper lip
42. Stomion inferius: Most superior point of the upper lip
43. Lower lip: The most anterior point of the lower lip
44. Soft tissue B point: The most concave point of the lower lip between chin and lower lip point
45. Soft tissue pogonion: The most anterior point of the soft tissue of the chin
46. Soft tissue gnathion: The midpoint of the chin soft tissue outline between soft tissue pogonion and soft tissue menton
47. Soft tissue menton: The most inferior point of the soft tissue of the chin

---

The buccal and lingual cortical plates of the mandible should be projected as uniform opaque lines. An underexposed view is required for the evaluation of the zygomatic arches because they will be overexposed or "burned out" on radiographs obtained with normal exposure factors.

## WATERS PROJECTION

### Image Receptor and Patient Placement
The image receptor is placed in front of the patient and perpendicular to the midsagittal plane. The patient's head is tilted upward so that the canthomeatal line forms a 37-degree angle with the image receptor. If the patient's mouth is open, the sphenoid sinus will be seen superimposed over the palate.

### Position of the Central X-Ray Beam
The central beam is perpendicular to the image receptor and centered in the area of the maxillary sinuses.

### Resultant Image (Fig. 12-4)
The midsagittal plane (represented by an imaginary line extending from the interproximal space of the maxillary central incisors through

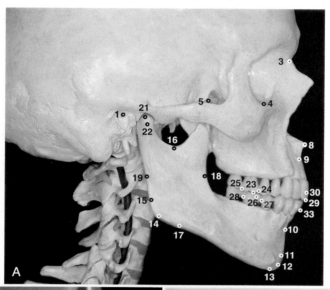

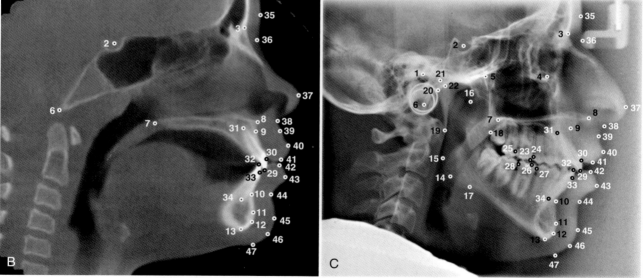

FIG. **12-2  A,** Anatomic cephalometric landmarks shown on a side view of the skull. **B,** Midline anatomic cephalometric landmarks depicted on a 5-mm-wide CBCT (cone-beam computed tomography) scan section of an orthodontic patient. **C,** Cephalometric landmarks used in Steiner and Ricketts cephalometric analyses.

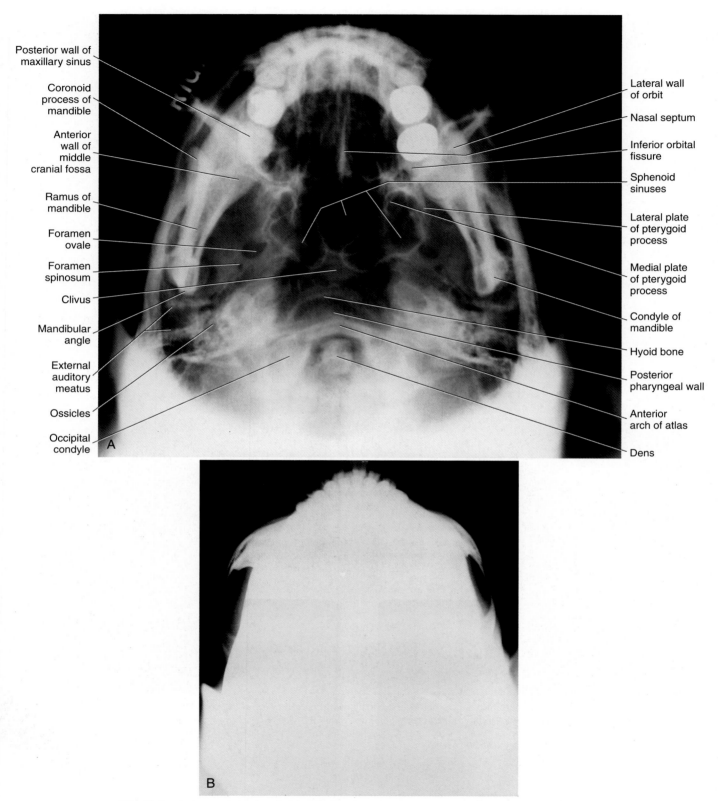

Posterior wall of maxillary sinus

Coronoid process of mandible

Anterior wall of middle cranial fossa

Ramus of mandible

Foramen ovale

Foramen spinosum

Clivus

Mandibular angle

External auditory meatus

Ossicles

Occipital condyle

Lateral wall of orbit

Nasal septum

Inferior orbital fissure

Sphenoid sinuses

Lateral plate of pterygoid process

Medial plate of pterygoid process

Condyle of mandible

Hyoid bone

Posterior pharyngeal wall

Anterior arch of atlas

Dens

A

B

FIG. **12-3   A,** Anatomic landmarks identified in the submentovertex projection. **B,** An underexposed submentovertex view reveals the zygomatic arches.

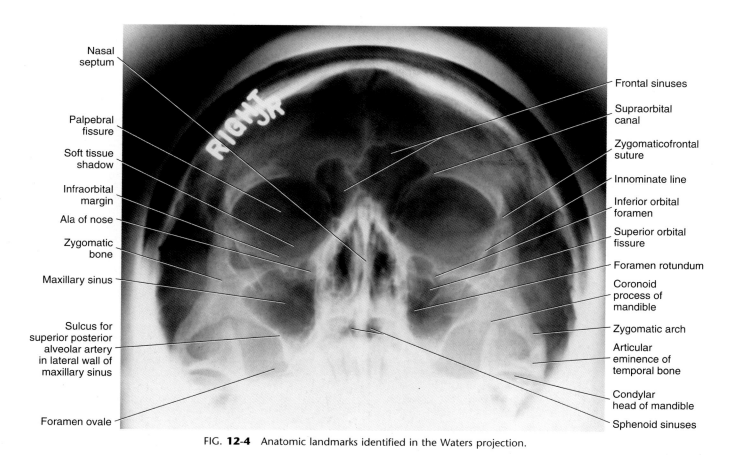

Nasal septum
Palpebral fissure
Soft tissue shadow
Infraorbital margin
Ala of nose
Zygomatic bone
Maxillary sinus
Sulcus for superior posterior alveolar artery in lateral wall of maxillary sinus
Foramen ovale

Frontal sinuses
Supraorbital canal
Zygomaticofrontal suture
Innominate line
Inferior orbital foramen
Superior orbital fissure
Foramen rotundum
Coronoid process of mandible
Zygomatic arch
Articular eminence of temporal bone
Condylar head of mandible
Sphenoid sinuses

FIG. **12-4** Anatomic landmarks identified in the Waters projection.

the nasal septum and the middle of the bridge of the nose) should divide the skull image in two symmetric halves. The petrous ridge of the temporal bone should be projected below the floor of the maxillary sinus.

## POSTEROANTERIOR SKULL PROJECTION (POSTEROANTERIOR CEPHALOMETRIC PROJECTION)

### Image Receptor and Patient Placement
The image receptor is placed in front of the patient, perpendicular to the midsagittal plane and parallel to the coronal plane. The patient is placed so that the canthomeatal line forms a 10-degree angle with the horizontal plane and the Frankfort plane is perpendicular to the image receptor. In the posteroanterior (PA) skull projection, the canthomeatal line is perpendicular to the image receptor.

### Position of the Central X-Ray Beam
The central beam is perpendicular to the image receptor, directed from the posterior to the anterior (hence the name *posteroanterior,* or *PA*), parallel to patient's midsagittal plane, and is centered at the level of the bridge of the nose.

### Resultant Image (Fig. 12-5)
The midsagittal plane (represented by an imaginary line extending from the interproximal space of the central incisors through the nasal septum and the middle of the bridge of the nose) should divide the

skull image into two symmetric halves. The superior border of the petrous ridge should lie in the lower third of the orbit.

## REVERSE-TOWNE PROJECTION (OPEN-MOUTH)

### Image Receptor and Patient Placement
The image receptor is placed in front of the patient, perpendicular to the midsagittal and parallel to the coronal plane. The patient's head is tilted downward so that the canthomeatal line forms a 25- to 30-degree angle with the image receptor. To improve the visualization of the condyles, the patient's mouth is opened so that the condylar heads are located inferior to the articular eminence. When the clinician requests this image to evaluate the condyles, it is necessary to specify "open-mouth, reverse-Towne" otherwise a standard Towne view of the occiput may result.

### Position of the Central X-Ray Beam
The central beam is perpendicular to the image receptor and parallel to patient's midsagittal plane and it is centered at the level of the condyles.

### Resultant Image (Fig. 12-6)
The midsagittal plane (represented by an imaginary line extending from the middle of the foramen magnum and the posterior arch of the atlas through the middle of the bridge of the nose and the nasal septum) should divide the skull image into two symmetric halves. The

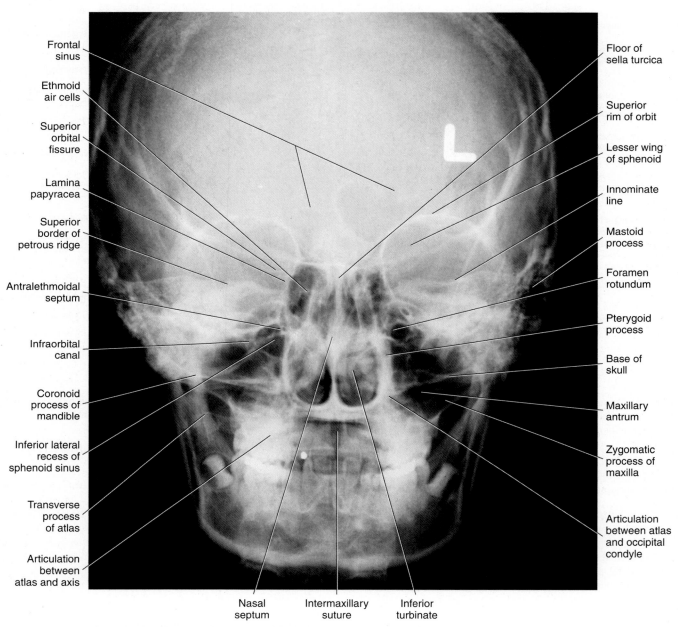

Frontal sinus

Ethmoid air cells

Superior orbital fissure

Lamina papyracea

Superior border of petrous ridge

Antralethmoidal septum

Infraorbital canal

Coronoid process of mandible

Inferior lateral recess of sphenoid sinus

Transverse process of atlas

Articulation between atlas and axis

Floor of sella turcica

Superior rim of orbit

Lesser wing of sphenoid

Innominate line

Mastoid process

Foramen rotundum

Pterygoid process

Base of skull

Maxillary antrum

Zygomatic process of maxilla

Articulation between atlas and occipital condyle

Nasal septum

Intermaxillary suture

Inferior turbinate

FIG. **12-5**   Anatomic landmarks identified in the PA cephalometric projection.

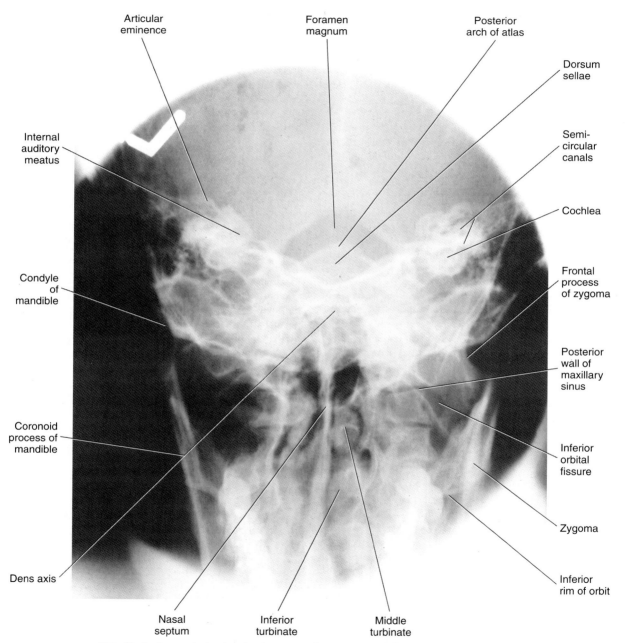

FIG. **12-6**  Anatomic landmarks identified in the open-mouth reverse-Towne projection.

petrous ridge of the temporal bone should be superimposed at the inferior part of the occipital bone, and the condylar heads should be projected inferior to the articular eminence.

## MANDIBULAR OBLIQUE LATERAL PROJECTIONS

### Mandibular Body Protection

#### Image Receptor and Patient Placement

The image receptor is placed against the patient's cheek on the side of interest and centered in the molar-premolar area. The lower border of the cassette is parallel and at least 2 cm below the inferior border of the mandible. The head is tilted toward the side being examined, and the mandible is protruded.

#### Position of the Central X-Ray Beam

The central beam is directed toward the molar-premolar region from a point 2 cm below the angle of the opposite side of the mandible.

#### Resultant Image (Fig. 12-7)

A clear image of the teeth, the alveolar ridge, and the body of the mandible should be obtained. If significant distortion is present, the head was tilted excessively. If the contralateral side of the mandible is superimposed over the area of interest, the head was not tilted sufficiently.

### Mandibular Ramus Projection

#### Image Receptor and Patient Placement

The image receptor is placed over the ramus and far enough posteriorly to include the condyle. The lower border of the cassette is parallel and at least 2 cm below the inferior border of the mandible. The head is tilted toward the side being examined so that the condyle of the area of interest and the contralateral angle of the mandible form a horizontal line. The mandible is protruded.

#### Position of the Central X-Ray Beam

The central beam is directed toward the center of the imaged ramus, from 2 cm below the inferior border of the opposite side of the mandible at the area of the first molar.

#### Resultant Image (Fig. 12-8)

A clear image of the third molar–retromolar area, angle of the mandible, ramus, and condyle head should be obtained. If significant distortion is present, the head was tilted excessively. If the contralateral side of the mandible is superimposed over the area of interest, the head was not tilted sufficiently.

### Evaluating the Image

Extraoral images should first be evaluated for overall quality. Proper exposure and processing will result in an image with good contrast and density. Proper patient positioning prevents unwanted superimpositions and distortions and facilitates identification of anatomic landmarks. Interpreting poor-quality images can lead to diagnostic errors and subsequent treatment errors.

The first step in the interpretation of radiographic images is the identification of anatomy. A thorough knowledge of normal radiographic anatomy and the appearance of normal variants is critical for the identification of pathology. Abnormalities cause disruptions of normal anatomy. Detecting the altered anatomy precedes classifying the type of change and developing a differential diagnosis. What is not detected cannot be interpreted. Figures 12-1 through 12-8 present

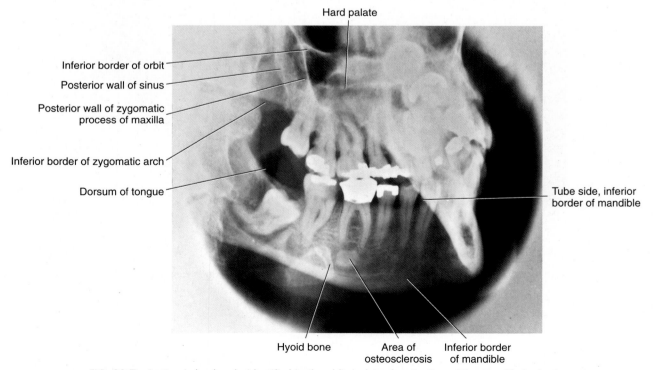

FIG. **12-7**  Anatomic landmarks identified in the oblique lateral projection of the mandibular body.

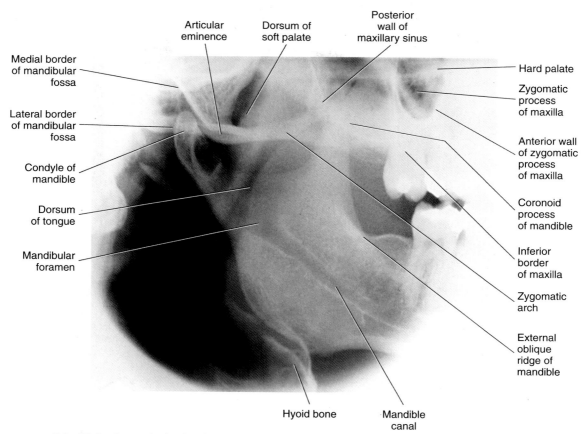

FIG. **12-8** Anatomic landmarks identified in the oblique lateral projection of the mandibular ramus.

the major anatomic landmarks that can be identified in the various extraoral projections.

Interpretation of extraoral radiographs should be thorough, careful, and meticulous. Images should be interpreted in a room with reduced ambient light, and peripheral light from the viewbox or monitor should be masked. A systematic, methodical approach should be used for the visual exploration or interrogation of the diagnostic image. A method for the visual interrogation of extraoral projections is presented below. This method is not the only approach to examining radiographic images. Any technique that reliably ensures that the entire image will be examined is equally appropriate.

## LATERAL PROJECTION (FIG. 12-9)

*Step 1* Evaluate the base of the skull and calvarium. Identify the mastoid air cells, clivus, clinoid processes, sella turcica, sphenoid sinuses, and roof of the orbit. In the calvarium, assess vessel grooves, sutures, and diploic space. Look for intracranial calcifications.

*Step 2* Evaluate the upper and middle face. Identify the orbits, sinuses (frontal, ethmoid, and maxillary), pterygomaxillary fissures, pterygoid plates, zygomatic processes of the maxilla, anterior nasal spine, and hard palate (floor of the nose). Evaluate the soft tissues of the upper and middle face, nasal cavity (turbinates), soft palate, and dorsum of tongue.

*Step 3* Evaluate the lower face. Follow the outline of the mandible, starting from the condylar and coronoid processes, to the rami, angles, and bodies, and finally to the anterior mandible. Evaluate the soft tissue of the lower face.

*Step 4* Evaluate the cervical spine, airway, and area of the neck. Identify each individual vertebra, confirm that the skull-C1 and C1-C2 articulations are normal, and assess the general alignment of the vertebrae. Assess soft tissues of the neck, hyoid bone, and airway.

*Step 5* Evaluate the alveolar bone and teeth.

## SMV PROJECTION (FIG. 12-10)

*Step 1* Evaluate the calvarium and posterior cranial fossa. Assess the foramen magnum, atlas, dens, and occipital condyles. Identify the petrous ridge of the right and left temporal bones, the external auditory canals, and the mastoid air cells. In this and all subsequent steps, compare the right and left sides and look for symmetry.

*Step 2* Evaluate the middle cranial fossa. Identify the foramina ovale and spinosum. Assess the clivus and sphenoid sinuses.

*Step 3* Evaluate the upper and middle face. Assess the nasal cavity, nasal septum, maxillary and ethmoid sinuses, and orbits. Assess both the bony borders and antra or contents of these structures.

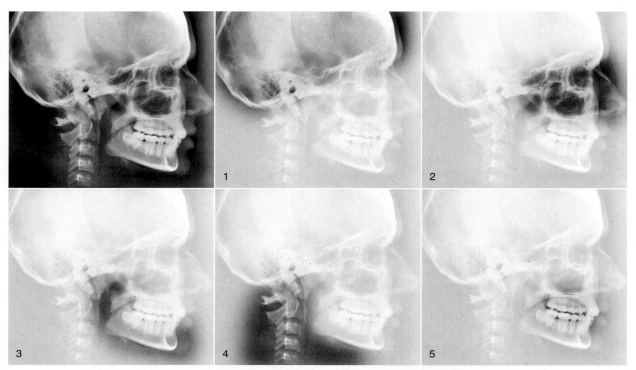

FIG. **12-9** Interrogating the lateral cephalometric projection. The radiograph in the upper left demonstrates the whole image. Subsequent radiographs correspond to the steps of interrogation.

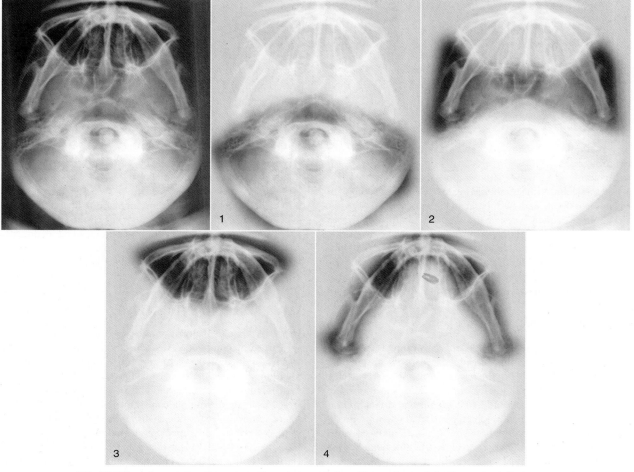

FIG. **12-10** Interrogating the submentovertex projection. The radiograph in the upper left demonstrates the whole image. Subsequent radiographs correspond to the steps of interrogation.

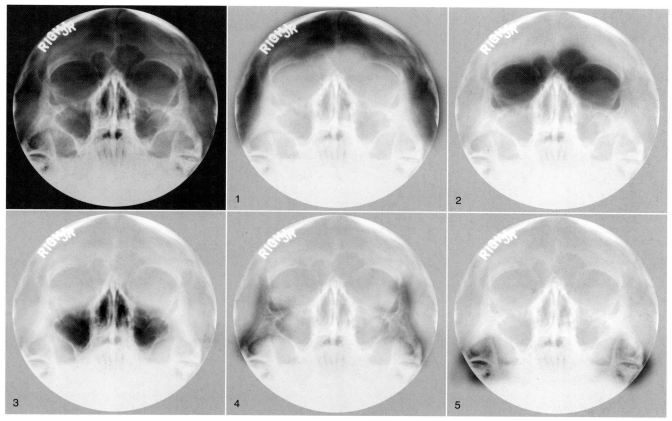

FIG. **12-11**   Interrogating the Waters projection. The radiograph in the upper left demonstrates the whole image. Subsequent radiographs correspond to the steps of interrogation.

**Step 4** Evaluate the mandible. Follow the outline from the right condylar head, coronoid process, ramus, angle, and body through the anterior mandible to the left body, angle, ramus, coronoid process, and condyle.

## WATERS PROJECTION (FIG. 12-11)

**Step 1** Evaluate the calvarium and sutures, starting in the left temporal area over the supraorbital ridges to the right temporal area. Look for intracranial calcifications. In this and all subsequent steps, compare the right and left sides and look for symmetry.

**Step 2** Evaluate the orbits and the frontal sinuses. Identify the supraorbital and infraorbital rim, the inferior orbital foramen, the floor of the orbit, the zygomaticofrontal sutures, and the innominate line of the infratemporal fossa crossing on the lateral aspect of each orbit.

**Step 3** Evaluate the maxillary sinuses and nasal cavity. Identify the superior, medial, and lateral walls and the floor of the maxillary sinuses; the nasal septum; and the floor and lateral walls of the nasal cavity. Try to identify the foramen rotundum projected toward the mesial wall of the sinus.

**Step 4** Evaluate the zygomatic arches. Identify the frontal, maxillary, and temporal processes of the zygoma and the zygomaticofrontal

suture. Confirm continuity of outlines and symmetry with the contralateral side.

**Step 5** Evaluate the condylar and coronoid processes of the mandible. This is one of the best PA views of the coronoid process.

## POSTEROANTERIOR PROJECTION (FIG. 12-12)

**Step 1** Evaluate the calvarium, sutures, and diploic space starting in the area of the left external auditory meatus (EAM), over the top of the calvarium, to the right EAM. Look for intracranial calcifications. Identify the mastoid air cells and petrous ridge of the right and left temporal bones. In this and all subsequent steps, compare the right and left sides and look for symmetry.

**Step 2** Evaluate the upper and middle face. Identify the orbits, sinuses (frontal, ethmoid, and maxillary), and zygomatic processes of the maxilla. Assess the nasal cavity, middle and inferior turbinates, nasal septum, and hard palate.

**Step 3** Evaluate the lower face. Follow the outline of the mandible starting from the right condylar and coronoid processes, ramus, angle, and body through the anterior mandible to the left body, angle, ramus, coronoid process, and condyle.

**Step 4** Evaluate the cervical spine. Identify the dens, the superior border of C2, and the inferior border of C1.

**Step 5** Evaluate the alveolar bone and teeth.

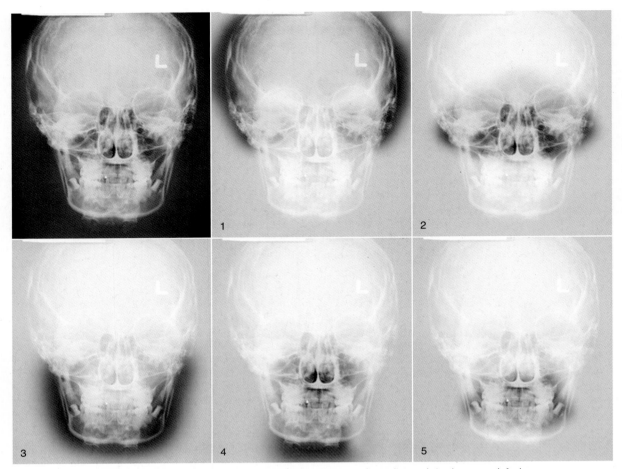

FIG. **12-12**  Interrogating the PA cephalometric projection. The radiograph in the upper left demonstrates the whole image. Subsequent radiographs correspond to the steps of interrogation.

## REVERSE-TOWNE PROJECTION (FIG. 12-13)

*Step 1* Evaluate the calvarium and look for intracranial calcifications. Identify the foramen magnum and the posterior arch of the atlas. In this and all subsequent steps, compare the right and left sides and look for symmetry.

*Step 2* Evaluate the middle cranial fossa, petrous ridges, and mastoid air cells. The anatomy in this area is difficult to discern. Look for displacement, interruption of outlines, radiolucencies, and loss of symmetry. Identify the odontoid process (dens) of the axis (C2) in the midline.

*Step 3* Evaluate the nasal cavity. Identify the outline of the nasal cavity, the nasal septum, and the inferior and middle turbinates.

*Step 4* Evaluate the condylar and coronoid process. In the open-mouth projection, the condylar head, including its superior surface and condylar neck, should be identified.

## Selection Criteria

Although this section appears toward the end of this chapter, in practice, selecting the appropriate extraoral radiographic examination is the *first* step in obtaining and interpreting a radiograph.

Extraoral radiographs are used to examine areas not fully covered by intraoral films or to evaluate the cranium, face (including the maxilla and mandible), or cervical spine for diseases, trauma, or abnormalities. Before an extraoral radiograph is obtained, it is essential to evaluate the patient's complaints and clinical signs in detail. The clinician must first decide which anatomic structures need to be evaluated and then select the appropriate projection(s). Usually, at least two radiographs taken at right angles to each another are obtained for spatial localization of pathologic conditions. Figure 12-14 summarizes the use of extraoral radiographs for the evaluation of various anatomic structures. Although panoramic radiography is the subject of another chapter, it is included in Figure 12-14 for comparison.

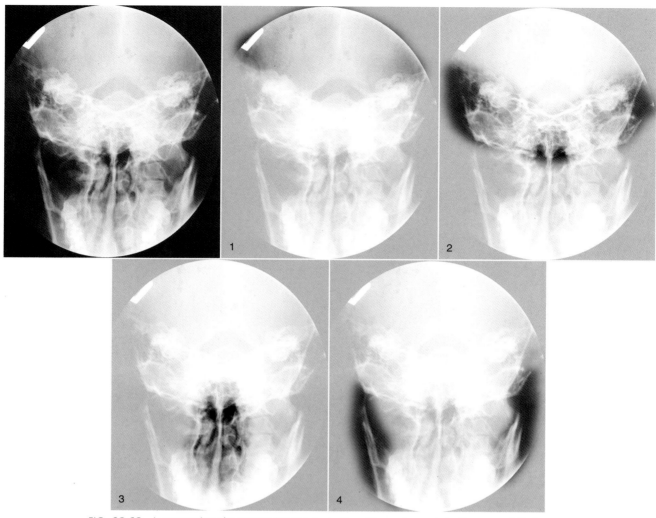

FIG. **12-13** Interrogating the reverse-Towne projection. The radiograph in the upper left demonstrates the whole image. Subsequent radiographs correspond to the steps of interrogation.

| AREA OF INTEREST | Lateral Ceph | SMV | Waters | PA Ceph | Reverse Towne | Oblique Body | Lateral Ramus | Panoramic |
|---|---|---|---|---|---|---|---|---|
| Anterior mandible | ▨ | ▨ | | ▨ | | | | ☐ |
| Mandibular body | ☐ | ☐ | | ▨ | | ■ | | ■ |
| Ramus | | | | ▨ | | ☐ | ■ | ■ |
| Coronoid process | | | ■ | ▨ | ☐ | | ■ | ▨ |
| Condylar neck | | | | ▨ | ■ | | ■ | |
| Condylar head | | ▨ | ☐ | ☐ | ■ | | ▨ | ☐ |
| Anterior maxilla | ▨ | | ☐ | ▨ | | | | ▨ |
| Posterior maxilla | ☐ | ▨ | ☐ | ☐ | | ☐ | | ■ |
| Orbit | ▨ | ☐ | ■ | ■ | | | | |
| Zygoma | ☐ | ☐ | ■ | ☐ | | | | ▨ |
| Zygomatic arch | | ■ | ▨ | | | | | ☐ |
| Nasal bones | ■ | | ▨ | ☐ | | | | |
| Nasal cavity | ☐ | ☐ | ▨ | ■ | ☐ | | | ☐ |
| Maxillary sinus | ▨ | ☐ | ■ | ☐ | | | | ▨ |
| Frontal sinus | ■ | ☐ | ▨ | ■ | | | | |
| Ethmoid sinus | ☐ | ▨ | ▨ | ▨ | | | | |
| Sphenoid sinus | ■ | ■ | ☐ | | | | | |

☐ Low usefulness
▨ Medium usefulness
■ High usefulness
No symbol: Not recommended

FIG. **12-14** Relative usefulness of extraoral radiographic projections to display various anatomic structures.

## BIBLIOGRAPHY

Ballinger PW, Frank ED: *Merrill's atlas of radiographic positions and radiologic procedures,* vol 2, ed 10, pp 353-399, St. Louis, 2003, Mosby.

Kantor ML, Norton LA: Normal radiographic anatomy and common anomalies seen in cephalometric films, *Am J Orthod Dentofac Orthop* 91:414-426, 1987.

Keats TE, Anderson MW: *Atlas of normal roentgen variants that may simulate disease,* ed 7, pp 3-275, St. Louis, 2001, Mosby.

Miyashita K: *Contemporary cephalometric radiography,* pp 245-266, Tokyo, 1996, Quintessence.

Shapiro R: *Radiology of the normal skull,* Chicago, 1981, Year Book Medical.

Swischuk LE: *Imaging of the cervical spine in children,* New York, 2002, Springer-Verlag.

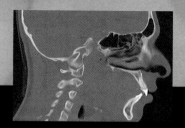

# CHAPTER 13

# Advanced Imaging

In collaboration with Neil L. Frederiksen

The imaging modalities described in this chapter use equipment and techniques that are beyond the routine needs of most general dental practitioners. Each of these techniques makes a tomographic image, that is, a slice through tissue, rather than a simple projection image. The most versatile of these modalities are computed tomography (CT) and magnetic resonance imaging (MRI). Nuclear medicine and ultrasonography are used for more specialized applications. Film tomography, a mainstay imaging technique during the twentieth century, is being rapidly replaced by CT, MRI, and cone-beam imaging (Chapter 14). Each of these imaging modalities is used to aid in the diagnosis of conditions in the oral cavity; thus everyone involved in providing oral health care must have a basic understanding of their operating principles and clinical applications.

## Computed Tomography

In 1972 Godfrey Hounsfield, an engineer, announced the invention of a revolutionary imaging technique that used image reconstruction mathematics developed by Alan Cormack in the 1950s and 1960s to produce cross-sectional images of the head. Currently this form of imaging is called *computed tomography,* abbreviated as *CT.* Hounsfield and Cormack shared the Nobel Prize in Physiology or Medicine in 1979 for their pioneering work.

### COMPUTED TOMOGRAPHY SCANNERS

In its simplest form a CT scanner consists of an x-ray tube that emits a finely collimated, fan-shaped x-ray beam directed through a patient to a series of scintillation detectors or ionization chambers (Fig. 13-1, *A*). These detectors measure the number of photons that exit the patient. This information can be used to produce a cross-sectional image of the patient. In early versions of CT scanners, both the x-ray tube and detectors rotated synchronously about the patient. In more recent design the detectors form a continuous ring about the patient and the x-ray tube moves in a circle within the fixed detector ring (Fig. 13-1, *B*). Originally patients would lie on a stationary table while the x-ray source rotated one cycle around them. Then the table would move 1 to 5 mm for the next scan. CT scanners that used this type of "step and shoot" movement for image acquisition are called *incremental scanners.* The final image set consists of a series of contiguous or overlapping axial images, made at right angles to the long axis of the patient's body. These two-dimensional slices are cross sections, typically 1 mm thick.

In 1989 CT scanners were introduced that acquire image data in a *helical* (sometimes inaccurately called *spiral*) fashion (Fig. 13-2). With helical scanners the gantry containing the x-ray tube and detectors continuously revolves around the patient, whereas the table on which the patient is lying continuously advances through the gantry. This results in the acquisition of a continuous helix of data as the x-ray beam moves down the patient. Helical CT is now the standard. In helical CT scanners, *pitch* refers to the amount of patient movement compared with the width of the image acquired. More precisely,

$$\text{Pitch} = \frac{\text{Table travel per x-ray tube rotation}}{\text{Image thickness}}$$

A pitch of 1 means that the image width is equal to the amount of patient movement per slice. A pitch of 2 means that the patient moves twice as far as the detector is wide and only half the tissue is exposed. A pitch of 0.5 means that half the image is overlapped each slice. Overlapping reconstructions results in the highest spatial resolution but also the highest patient dose. Compared with incremental CT scanners, helical scanners provide improved multiplanar image reconstructions, reduced examination time, and a reduced radiation dose.

Multidetector helical CT (MDCT, multislice CT, or multirow CT) scanners were introduced in 1998. MDCT imaging has become widely used and has had a pronounced clinical impact. With this method, anywhere from four to 64 adjacent detector arrays are used in conjunction with helical CT (see Fig. 13-1, *C*). Additionally, the time for the x-ray tube to make a full cycle around the patient has been reduced to as little as 0.35 second. These developments allow images from multiple slices to be captured quickly and simultaneously, thus greatly reducing both exposure time and motion artifact from breathing, peristalsis, or heart contractions. This is important for patients who cannot hold their breath for long periods of time and for pediatric and trauma patients. The quality of axial, reformatted, and three-dimensional images is also greatly improved with MDCT compared with single-slice scanners. The meaning of pitch with MDCT varies with the individual manufacturer but often means that table travel per x-ray tube rotation divided by total active detector width. In general, the patient dose is higher with MDCT than with single-slice machines.

The most recent CT development is an electron beam CT. In this machine an electron gun generates an electron beam that is focused electrostatically on a fixed tungsten target circling halfway around the patient. The x rays that are generated expose the detector array circling

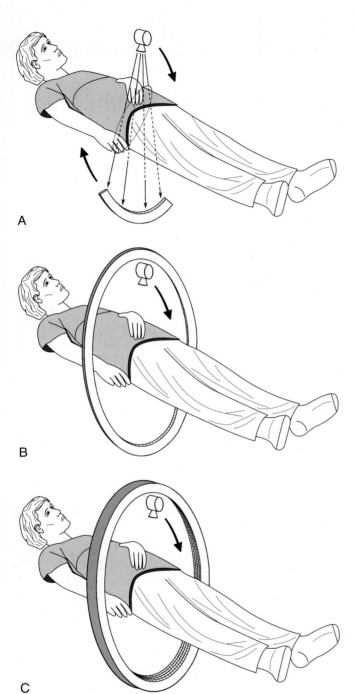

FIG. **13-1** **Mechanical Geometry of CT Scanners. A,** In CT scanners the x-ray source emits a fan beam. In early CT scanners both the x-ray source and the detector array revolved around the patient. **B,** In current scanners the x-ray tube revolves around the patient and the remnant beam is detected by a fixed circular array. **C,** In contemporary CT multidetector scanners the detector array has 4 to 64 rows of detectors.

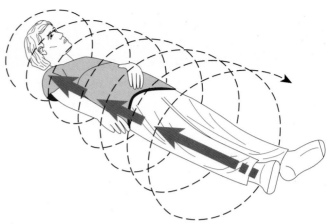

FIG. **13-2** **Helical CT.** In helical scanners the patient is moves continuously through the gantry and the x-ray source moves continuously around the patient in a circle. The net effect is to describe a helical beam, and image, path through the patient.

the other half of the patient. Because there are no moving parts, an image may be acquired in less that 100 microseconds. This technique is primarily used for cardiac imaging to "stop" heart motion.

## X-RAY TUBES

CT scanners use x-ray tubes with rotating anodes (see Fig. 1-10). These tubes have a high heat capacity, up to 8 million heat units]; (compare with dental tubes of 20 kilo heat units). They operate at 120 to 140 kilovolts peak (kVp) and 200 to 800 milliamperes. Focal spot sizes range from 0.5 to 2.0 mm. The high x-ray output minimizes exposure time and improves image quality by increasing the signal-to-noise ratio. The high kVp also provides a wide dynamic range by reducing bone absorption compared with soft tissue and extends tube life by reducing tube loading. The tubes operate continuously by using three-phase or high-frequency generators. The x-ray beam is collimated both before and after the patient. Prepatient collimation adjusts patient exposure. Postpatient collimation controls slice thickness. Slice thickness is typically between 1 and 3 mm. Thinner slices result in higher spatial resolution and contrast, less partial volume effect (see later), and higher patient dose.

## DETECTORS

The x-ray beam exiting the patient is captured by an array of detectors. These detectors are usually gas filled or solid state. Gas-filled ion chamber detectors are usually made of high-pressure xenon. The ion chamber sends a signal proportional to the number of photons captured. Gas-filled ion chambers respond quickly but only capture about 50% of the photons in the beam. Solid-state detectors are used more commonly. These are usually made of cadmium tungstate, are optically coupled to a photodiode, and are as small as 0.625 mm across. These detectors are about 80% efficient. The signal from either type of detector is amplified, digitized, and sent to a computer for analysis.

## IMAGE RECONSTRUCTION

The photons recorded by the detectors represent a composite of the absorption characteristics of all elements of the patient in the path of the x-ray beam. Computer algorithms use these photon counts to construct one, or more often, many digital cross-sectional images. The CT image is recorded and displayed as a matrix of individual blocks called *voxels* (volume elements) (Fig. 13-3). Each square of the image matrix is a *pixel*. Images are typically 512 × 512 or 1024 × 1024 pixels. Although the size of the pixel (about 0.6 mm or less) is determined partly by the computer program used to construct the image, the length of the voxel (about 1 to 20 mm) is determined by the width of the x-ray beam, which in turn is controlled by the prepatient and postpatient collimators. Next an interpolator algorithm is used to correct for the helical motion of the scanner and to construct planar cross sections from the helical information.

The methods used to reconstruct images are complex. Initially an object with four compartments, as shown in Figure 13-4, should be pictured. The linear attenuation coefficients (densities) of each of the four cells can be computed by using four simultaneous equations to solve for four unknowns. This method becomes computationally impracticable when there are $512^2$ or $1024^2$ cells. Instead, methods called *filtered back-projection* algorithms involving Fourier transformations are used for rapid image reconstruction. A modification of these methods, called the Feldkamp reconstruction, is used for MDCT

and cone-beam reconstructions to account for the diverging x-ray beam. After reconstruction various image-processing filters are applied. Typically these are smoothing filters to minimize noise in low-contrast objects such as soft tissue and edge-sharpening filters to improve visualization of fine bony detail.

## COMPUTED TOMOGRAPHIC IMAGE

For image display, each pixel is assigned a CT number representing tissue density. This number is proportional to the degree to which the material within the voxel has attenuated the x-ray beam. CT numbers, also known as *Hounsfield units* (HU, named in honor of the inventor Sir Godfrey Hounsfield), range from −1000 to +1000, each corresponding to a different level of beam attenuation (Table 13-1). Some newer CT machines have a range of up to 4000 HU. Because the human eye can only detect about 40 shades of gray, it is useful to adjust the range and mean of CT numbers displayed on a monitor (Fig. 13-5). An image optimized for viewing bone, a "bone window," may have a range (window width, or WW) of 700 units and mean of 500 (window level, or WL). Alternatively, an image optimized to view soft tissues may have a WW of 400 units and a WL of 40. In these

FIG. **13-3 CT Image Formation. A,** Data for a single-plane image are acquired from multiple projections made during the course of a 360-degree rotation around the patient. Slice thickness c is controlled by the width of the postpatient collimator. **B,** A single-plane image is constructed from absorption characteristics of the subject and displayed as differences in optical density, ranging from −1000 to +1000 HU. Several planes may be imaged from multiple contiguous scans. **C,** The image consists of a matrix of individual pixels representing the face of a volume called a *voxel.* Although dimensions a and b are determined partly by the computer program used to construct the image, dimension c is controlled by the collimator as in **A. D,** Cuboid voxels can be created from the original rectangular voxel by computer interpolation. This allows the formation of multiplanar and three-dimensional images **(E).**

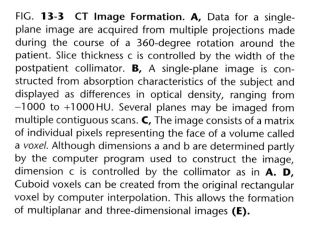
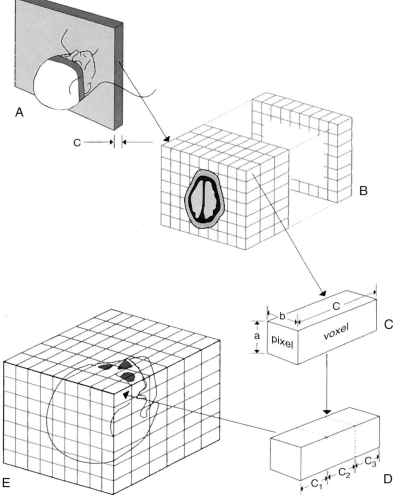

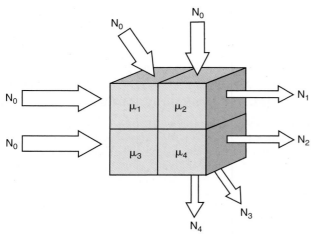

FIG. **13-4**    **Image Reconstruction.** Assume four volumes with differing linear attenuation coefficients ($\mu$). A beam entering the object with $N_0$ photons is reduced in intensity by object. The intensity of the remnant beam is measured by the detector array. The value of each cell in the object can be determined by solving four (or more) independent simultaneous equations. Such a brute-force approach is computationally intensive and in practice much faster algorithms are used to reconstruct images.

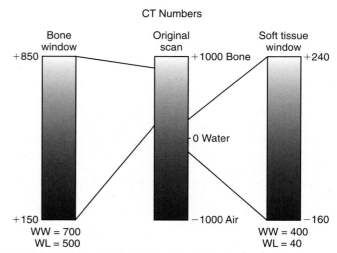

FIG. **13-5**    **Window Width and Level.** CT numbers, also called Hounsfield units (HU), are scaled on cortical bone (+1000), water (0), and air (−1000). Viewing bone or soft tissue is optimized by improving the contrast of the appropriate region of the original image. Window width (*WW*) is the range of CT numbers used, and window level (*WL*) is the mid portion of the range. Bone and soft tissue window views are used to enhance visualization of those tissues. In this example, a bone window may have a range of 700 and a mean of 500, whereas a soft tissue window may have a range of 400 and a mean of 40.

TABLE **13-1**
*Typical Hounsfield Units for Air and Tissues*

| TISSUE | HOUNSFIELD UNITS (CT NUMBERS) |
|---|---|
| Bone | +400 to +1000 |
| Soft tissue | +40 to +80 |
| Water | 0 |
| Fat | −60 to −100 |
| Lung | −400 to −600 |
| Air | −1000 |

images bone is light, soft tissue is gray, and air is black. By convention, these images are displayed as if the clinician is standing at the feet of the patient who is lying on his or her back. Thus the patient's right side will appear on the left and anterior will appear at the top (Fig. 13-6, *A*).

CT has several advantages over conventional film radiography and tomography. First, CT eliminates the superimposition of images of structures outside the area of interest. Second, because of the inherent high-contrast resolution of CT, differences between tissues that differ in physical density by less than 1% can be distinguished; conventional radiography requires a 10% difference in physical density to distinguish between tissues. Third, data from a single CT imaging procedure, consisting of either multiple contiguous or one helical scan, can be viewed as images in the axial, coronal, or sagittal planes, or in any arbitrary plane, depending on the diagnostic task. This is referred to as *multiplanar reformatted imaging*. Having the capability of viewing normal anatomy or pathologic processes simultaneously in three orthogonal planes greatly facilitates radiographic interpretation (Fig. 13-6).

Multiplanar images are two dimensional and require a certain degree of mental integration by the viewer for interpretation. This

limitation has led to the development of computer programs that reformat data acquired from axial CT scans into three-dimensional images. The use of three-dimensional images has been boosted by the use of MDCT as a means of reviewing large amounts of information collected at each examination.

Three-dimensional reformatting requires that each original voxel, shaped as a rectangular solid, be dimensionally altered into multiple cuboidal voxels. This process, called *interpolation*, creates sets of evenly spaced cuboidal voxels (cuberilles) that occupy the same volume as the original voxel (see Fig. 13-4, *D*). The CT numbers of the cuberilles represent the average of the original voxel CT numbers surrounding each of the new voxels. Isotropic voxels as small as 0.24 mm can be achieved. Creation of these new cuboidal voxels allows the image to be reconstructed in any plane without loss of resolution by locating the position of each voxel in space relative to one another. In constructing the three-dimensional CT image, only cuberilles representing the surface of the object scanned are displayed on the monitor. The surface formed by these cuberilles is made to appear as if illuminated by a light source located behind the viewer (Fig. 13-7). In this manner the visible surface of each pixel is assigned a gray-level value, depending on its distance from and orientation to the light source. Thus pixels that face the light source or are closer to it appear brighter than those that are turned away from the source or are farther away. Once constructed, three-dimensional CT images may be further manipulated by rotation about any axis to display the structure imaged from any angle. Also, external surfaces of the image can be removed electronically to reveal concealed deeper anatomy.

## ARTIFACTS

Different types of artifacts may degrade CT images. *Partial volume artifact* occurs because a voxel has finite dimensions. When a voxel

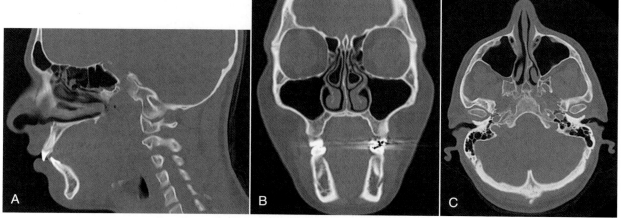

FIG. **13-6 Multiplanar Reconstruction Views Facilitate Interpretation of Complex Anatomy.**
**A,** CT images demonstrating sagittal plane through lateral incisors and foramen lacerum. Note frontal, ethmoid, and sphenoid sinuses. **B,** Coronal view through ethmoid and maxillary sinuses and mental foramen in left mandible. **C,** Axial view through level of maxillary sinuses and mandibular condyles. Patient's right side appear on the left side of the coronal and sagittal images as if the patient is lying on the back with the toes pointed toward the observer.

contains tissues of differing densities, for example, bone and soft tissue, the resulting CT number for that voxel is an intermediate value that does not represent either tissue. This may result in the resulting image as a blurring of the junction of the tissues or as a loss of part of a thin cortical layer of bone. *Beam-hardening artifact* results by the preferential absorption of lower energy photons in the heterogeneous x-ray beam. Because the distance through the center of the head is longer than along a path closer to the surface, there will be beam hardening seen as darkening in the middle of an axial slice. Software algorithms may minimize this artifact. *Metal artifacts* occur because of the near complete absorption of x-ray photons by metallic restorations. They appear as opaque streaks in the occlusal plane (see Fig. 13-6, *B* and *C*).

## CONTRAST AGENTS

Contrast agents are substances used to improve visualization of structure. CT imaging frequently uses iodine, administered intravenously, to enhance soft tissue and vascular image detail. The iodine in the contrast medium has a large atomic number and thus effectively absorbs x rays (Fig. 13-8). Often malignant facial tumors are more vascularized than surrounding normal tissues; thus the presence of the iodine perfusing these tissues increases their radiographic density and makes their margins more detectable. Contrast medium also helps to visualize enlarged lymph nodes containing metastatic carcinoma. It should be remembered that contrast dye can be toxic to the kidneys in elderly individuals with kidney disease.

## APPLICATIONS

CT is useful for the diagnosis of and for determining the extent of a wide variety of infections, osteomyelitis, cysts, benign and malignant tumors, and trauma in the maxillofacial region. The ability of CT imaging to display fine bone detail makes it an ideal modality for lesions involving bone. Three-dimensional CT has been applied to trauma and craniofacial reconstructive surgery and has been

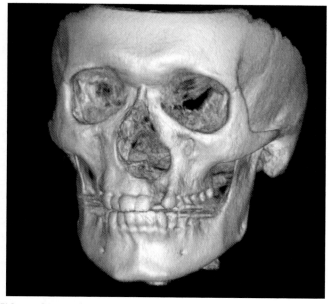

FIG. **13-7 Three-dimensional Surface Rendering.** Three-dimensional images can be reconstructed from the cuberilles, oriented in any arbitrary direction, and made to appear to have depth by highlighting structures near the front and shadowing structures near the back. Note cleft in left alveolar ridge of the left maxilla. Artifact from metallic restorations is also evident extending laterally from the occlusal plane. This image reconstructed from cone-beam data; see Chapter 14.

used both for treatment of congenital and acquired deformities. The availability of data in a three-dimensional format also has allowed the construction of life-sized models that can be used for trial surgeries and the construction of surgical stents for guiding dental implant placement and for the creation of accurate implanted prostheses.

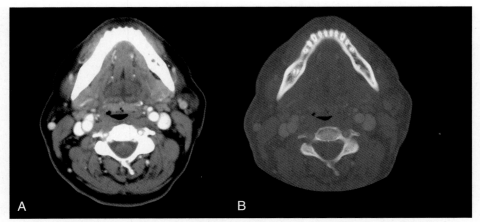

FIG. **13-8**  **Contrast Agents.** Iodine may be administered intravenously to enhance blood vessels and structures with a rich vascular supply, including the periphery of some tumors. **A,** CT through mandible in soft tissue window and after administration of iodine. Note prominent great vessels lying just anterior and lateral to cervical vertebrae and muscles of floor of mouth and neck. **B,** Same axial slice displayed in bone window. Note presence of fine detail in mandible and cervical spine including cortical and cancellous bone and teeth, including their pulp chambers, but loss of soft tissue contrast.

## Magnetic Resonance Imaging

Paul Lauterbur described the first magnetic resonance image in 1973 and Peter Mansfield further developed use of the magnetic field and the mathematical analysis of the signals for image reconstruction. MRI was developed for clinical use around 1980. In 2003 Lauterbur and Mansfield were awarded the Nobel Prize in Physiology or Medicine.

To make a magnetic resonance image, the patient is first placed inside a large magnet. This magnetic field causes the nuclei of many atoms in the body, particularly hydrogen, to align with the magnetic field. The scanner then directs a radiofrequency (RF) pulse into the patient, causing some hydrogen nuclei to absorb energy (resonate). When the RF pulse is turned off, the stored energy is released from the body and detected as a signal in a coil in the scanner. This signal is used to construct the magnetic resonance image, in essence a map of the distribution of hydrogen.

MRI has the particular advantages of being noninvasive, using nonionizing radiation, and making high-quality images of soft tissue resolution in any imaging plane. Disadvantages of MRI include its high cost, long scan times, and the fact that various metals in the imaging field either will distort the image or may move in the strong magnetic field, injuring the patient.

### PROTONS

Individual protons and neutrons (nucleons) in the nuclei of all atoms possess a spin, or angular momentum. In nuclei having equal numbers of protons and neutrons the spin of each nucleon cancels that of another, producing a net spin of zero. However, nuclei containing an unpaired proton or neutron have a net spin. Because spin is associated with an electrical charge, a magnetic field is generated in nuclei with unpaired nucleons, causing these nuclei to act as magnets with north and south poles (magnetic dipoles) and having a magnetic moment. The most common of these atoms, the magnetic resonance active nuclei, are hydrogen, carbon 13, nitrogen 15, oxygen 17, fluorine 19,

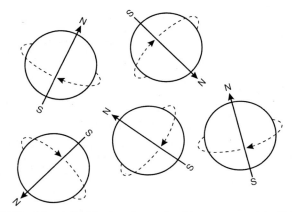

FIG. **13-9**  **Magnetic Dipoles.** A sample of hydrogen nuclei within a patient showing randomly oriented dipoles, thus no net magnetic vector.

sodium 23, and phosphorus 31. Hydrogen is by far the most abundant of these atoms in the body.

A hydrogen nucleus consists of a single unpaired proton and therefore acts as a magnetic dipole. Normally these magnetic dipoles are randomly oriented in space (Fig. 13-9). When an external magnetic field is applied, the hydrogen nuclear axes align in the direction of the magnetic field (Fig. 13-10). Two states are possible: *spin-up,* which parallels the external magnetic field, and *spin-down,* which is antiparallel with the field. Because more energy is required to align antiparallel with the magnetic field, those hydrogen nuclei are considered to be at a higher energy state than those aligned parallel with the field. Nuclei prefer to be in a lower energy state, and usually more are aligned parallel with the magnetic field. This results in a net magnetization vector in the direction of the magnetic field. Increasing the magnetic field strength increases the magnitude of the net magnetization vector.

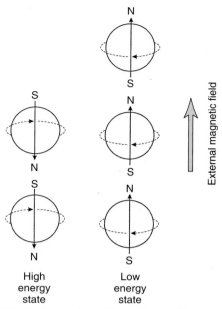

FIG. **13-10** **Hydrogen Nuclei in an External Magnetic Field.** In the presence of an applied strong external magnetic field, most nuclei are in the lower energy state and are aligned parallel with the magnetic field, whereas others align in the higher energy state antiparallel to the magnetic field.

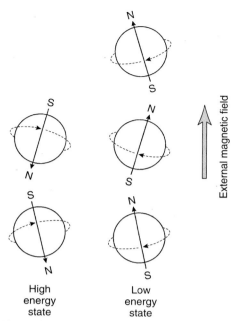

FIG. **13-11** **Hydrogen Nuclei in an External Magnetic Field.** The magnetic dipoles are not aligned exactly with the external magnetic field. Instead, the axes of spinning protons actually oscillate or wobble with a slight tilt from being absolutely parallel with the flux of the external magnet.

## PRECESSION

The magnetic moments of hydrogen nuclei in a magnetic field do not align exactly with the direction of the magnetic field. Instead, the orientations of the axes of spinning protons actually oscillate with a slight tilt from a position absolutely parallel with the flux of the external magnet (Fig. 13-11). This tilting of the spin axis, called *precession*, is similar to that of a spinning toy top, which rotates around an upright position as it slows down. Similarly, the presence of the magnetic field causes the axis of the spinning proton to wobble (or precess) around the lines of the applied magnetic field (Fig. 13-12). The rate or frequency of precession is called the *precessional, resonance,* or *Larmor frequency.* The precessional frequency depends on the species of nucleus (hydrogen nucleus or other) and is proportional to the strength of the external magnetic field. The magnetic field in a magnetic resonance scanner is provided by an external permanent magnet. Magnetic resonance field strengths range from 0.1 to 4 Tesla (T) with 1.5 T being the most common. (1.5 T is about 30,000 times the strength earth's magnetic field.) The Larmor precession frequency of hydrogen is 63.86 megahertz in a magnetic field of 1.5 T. Other magnetic resonance active nuclei precess at different frequencies in the same magnetic field.

## RESONANCE

Nuclei can be made to undergo transition from one energy state to another by absorbing or releasing energy. Energy required for transition from the lower to the higher energy level can be supplied by electromagnetic energy in the RF portion of the electromagnetic spectrum. In an MRI scanner the RF broadcast from an antenna coil is directed to tissue with protons (hydrogen nuclei) aligned in the Z axis (long axis of a patient) by the external static magnetic field

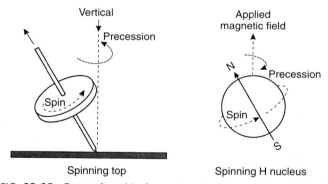

FIG. **13-12** **Precession.** Much as a top rotates around a vertical axis when spinning, a spinning hydrogen nucleus rotates around the direction of the external magnetic field. This movement is called precession and the rate or frequency of precession is called the precessional, resonance, or Larmor frequency. The Larmor frequency depends on the strength of the external magnetic field and is specific for the nuclear species.

(Fig. 13-13). When the frequency of the RF pulse matches the Larmor frequency of the protons in the tissue, the protons resonate and absorb the RF energy. This causes some of the low-energy nuclei (parallel) to gain energy to convert to the high-energy (antiparallel) state. As a consequence, the longitudinal magnetic vector is reduced. The longer the RF pulse is applied, the less the longitudinal magnetic vector. The RF pulse also causes the protons to precess in phase with each other, resulting in a net tissue magnetization vector in the transverse plane (XY plane) perpendicular to longitudinal alignment (Z axis) (Fig. 13-14). If the RF pulse is of sufficient intensity and duration, the longitudinal magnetic vector is reduced to zero. An RF pulse that

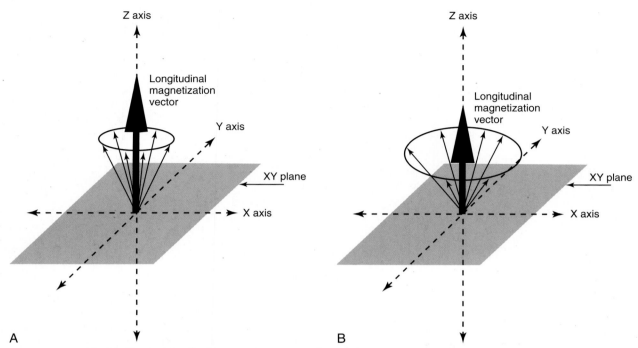

FIG. **13-13   Longitudinal Magnetic Vector.** When hydrogen nuclei are in an external magnetic field, two energy states result: spin-up, which is parallel to the direction of the field, and spin-down, which is antiparallel to the direction of the field. **A,** The combined effect of these two energy states is a weak net magnetic moment, or magnetization vector parallel with the applied magnetic field. **B,** When the frequency of the RF pulse matches the Larmor frequency of the protons absorb the RF energy causing some low-energy nuclei to convert to the high-energy state, thereby reducing the net longitudinal magnetic vector, vertical black arrow in Z axis.

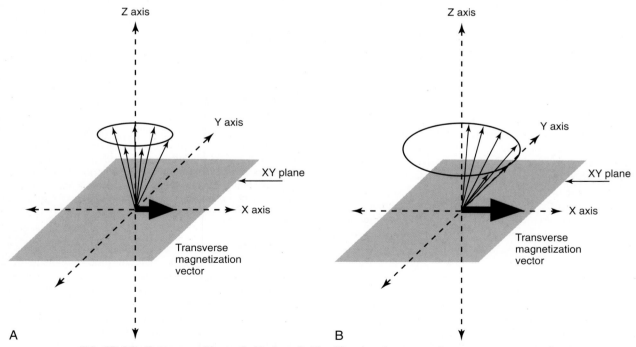

FIG. **13-14   Transverse Magnetic Vector. A,** The RF pulse also causes the protons to precess in phase with each other, resulting in a net tissue magnetization vector in the transverse plane (XY plane). **B,** Increasing the intensity and duration RF of the pulse increases the transverse magnetization vector because the nuclei are more nearly in phase, horizontal black arrow in X axis.

accomplished this is called a *90-degree RF pulse* or having a *flip angle of 90 degrees.* At this time the net magnetic vector in the transverse plane is maximized because the magnetic moments of all nuclei are in phase.

## MAGNETIC RESONANCE SIGNAL

The precession of the net magnetic vector, that is, the precession of the magnetic moments of the hydrogen nuclei in phase in the transverse plane, induces a current flow in a receiver coil (Fig. 13-15), the MR signal. The frequency of this alternating current signal matches the frequency of the RF pulse and the Larmor precessional frequency of hydrogen nuclei. The magnitude of this signal is proportional to the overall concentration of hydrogen nuclei (proton density) in the tissue. This strength of the signal also depends on the degree to which hydrogen is bound within a molecule. Tightly bound hydrogen atoms, such as those present in bone, do not align themselves with the external magnetic field and produce only a weak signal. Loosely bound or mobile hydrogen atoms such as those in soft tissues and liquids react to the RF pulse and thus produce a detectable signal at the end of the RF pulse. The concentration of loosely bound hydrogen nuclei available to create the signal is referred to as the *proton density* or *spin density* of the tissue in question. The higher the concentration of these nuclei of loosely bound hydrogen atoms, the stronger the net transverse magnetization, the more intense the recovered signal, and the brighter the corresponding part of the magnetic resonance image.

When the RF pulse is turned off, the nuclei begin to return to their original lower-energy spin state, a condition called *relaxation.* As they give up the energy absorbed by the RF pulse, some of the high-energy nuclei return to the low-energy state and the net longitudinal magnetic vector returns to its original state. Additionally, and independently, the individual magnetic moments of the protons begin to interact with each other and dephase. This results in reduction of the magnetization in the transverse plane, a condition called *decay.* As a result of the loss of transverse magnetization and the dephasing of the hydrogen nuclei, there is a loss of intensity of the magnetic resonance signal. The reduced voltage induced in the receiving coil is called the *free induction decay (FID)* signal. In sum, the FID of the MR signal results from the loss of the transverse net magnetization vector. This results from return of the net magnetization vector to the longitudinal plane and dephasing of the hydrogen nuclei.

## T1 AND T2 RELAXATION

Relaxation at the end of the RF pulse results in recovery of the longitudinal magnetization. This is accomplished by a transfer of energy from individual hydrogen nuclei (spin) to the surrounding molecules (lattice). This is an exponential process and the time required for 63% of the net magnetization to return to equilibrium (the time constant) by this transfer of energy is called the *T1 relaxation time* or *spin-lattice relaxation time.* The T1 relaxation time varies with different tissues and reflects the ability of their nuclei to transfer their excess energy to surrounding molecules (Table 13-2).

Additionally, and the end of the RF pulse, the magnetic moments of adjacent hydrogen nuclei begin to interfere with one another, causing the nuclei to dephase with a resultant loss of transverse magnetization. The time constant that describes the exponential rate of loss of transverse magnetization is called the *T2 relaxation time* or the *spin-spin relaxation time.* As the transverse magnetization rapidly decays to zero, so does the amplitude and duration of the detected radio signal. T2 relaxation occurs more rapidly than T1 relaxation. Note that both T1 and T2 times are features of the tissues being examined.

## RADIOFREQUENCY PULSES SEQUENCES (AND IMAGE CONTRAST)

The components of the RF pulse sequence are set by the operator and determine the appearance of the resultant image. The most basic features of a pulse sequence are the repetition time (TR) and echo time (TE). The TR time is the duration between repeat RF pulses (Fig. 13-16). The time between pulse repetitions determines the amount of T1 relaxation that has occurred at the time the signal is

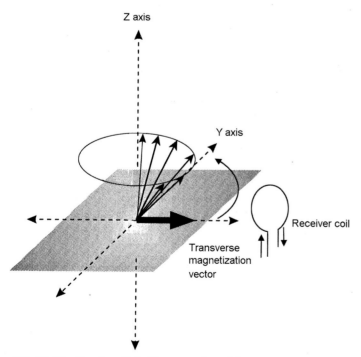

FIG. **13-15**  **Receiver Coil.** The precession of the net transverse magnetic vector in the XY plane induces a current flow in a receiver coil, the magnetic resonance signal. The frequency of this induced alternating current signal matches the frequency of the RF pulse and the Larmor precessional frequency of hydrogen nuclei.

| TABLE **13-2** *T1 and T2 Relaxation Times in a Main Field of 1.5 Tesla* | | |
|---|---|---|
| **TISSUE TYPE** | **T1 TIME (MS)** | **T2 TIME (MS)** |
| Fat | 240-250 | 60-80 |
| Bone marrow | 550 | 50 |
| White matter of cerebrum | 780 | 90 |
| Gray matter of cerebrum | 920 | 100 |
| Muscle | 860-900 | 50 |
| CSF (similar to water) | 2200-2400 | 500-1400 |

*CSF*, Cerebrospinal fluid.

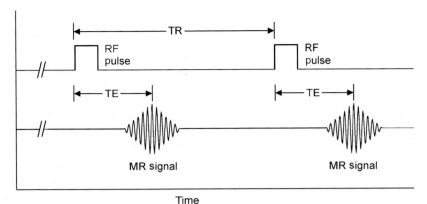

FIG. **13-16** **RF Pulses Sequences.** The most basic features of a pulse sequence are the TR, the duration between repeat RF pulses, and the TE, the time after application of the RF pulse when the magnetic resonance signal is read. TR determines amount of T1 relaxation that has occurred at the time the signal is collected, whereas TE controls the amount of T2 relaxation that has occurred when the signal is collected.

collected. The TE time is the time after application of the RF pulse when the magnetic resonance signal is read. It controls the amount of T2 relaxation that has occurred when the signal is collected. There are many sequences that can be used to emphasize various features of the tissues being examined.

## TISSUE CONTRAST

Image contrast between tissues is governed by intrinsic features of the tissues, including proton density, T1 and T2 times of the issues being imaged, and how the TR and TE times are adjusted to emphasize these features. For instance, a tissue that has a high proton density and strong transverse magnetization vector (protons precessing in phase) at TE will produce a strong magnetic resonance signal that will appear bright on a magnetic resonance image. Conversely, a tissue with a low proton density or low transverse magnetization vector at TE produces a weak signal and appears dark on a magnetic resonance image.

### T1-Weighted Image

A T1-weighted image emphasizes differences in T1 values of tissues (Fig. 13-17, *A*). This is accomplished by use of short TR times, typically 300 to 700 ms, and short TE times (20 ms). In such images tissues with fast T1 times, such as fat, will appear bright, whereas those with long T1 times, such as cerebrospinal fluid (CSF) (water), will appear dark. T1-weighted images are more commonly used to demonstrate anatomy.

### T2-Weighted Image

A T2-weighted image emphasizes differences in T2 values of tissues (Fig. 13-17, *B*). This is accomplished by use of long TR times (2000 ms) and long TE times, typically 60 ms or more. In such images tissues with long T2 times, such as CSF for temporomandibular (TMJ) joint fluid, will appear bright, whereas tissues with short T2 times, such as fat, will appear dark. Images with T2 weighting are most commonly used for identifying inflammatory or other pathologic changes.

There are many pulse sequences involving varying the strength and timing of the RF pulses that emphasize or suppress various tissues in the resultant images. Techniques such as spin echo and gradient echo allow images to be captured rapidly. Other techniques allow the signal from fat, or water, to be enhanced or suppressed. A technique called "fat saturation" nulls the signal from fat.

## Contrast Agents

Contrast agents, most commonly gadolinium, may be administered intravenously to improve tissue contrast (Fig. 13-17, *C*). Gadolinium is not imaged itself, but rather it shortens the T1 relaxation times of enhancing tissues, making them appear brighter. It is useful for enhancing some tumors by allowing them to be better differentiated from surrounding normal tissue. For imaging the head and neck, it is common practice to obtain T1, T1 postgadolinium administration and with fat saturation, and T2 with fat saturation images. It should be noted that just recently there is evidence that gadolinium-based contrast media could be a cause of a debilitating disease called nephrogenic systemic fibrosis in some patients with renal dysfunction. The implications of this finding are under active study.

## SCANNER GRADIENTS

To generate an image, a magnetic resonance signal must be collected from a discrete slice of tissue in the patient. This is accomplished by using three gradient coils within the bore of the imaging magnet oriented in the X (left to right), Y (anterior to posterior), and Z (head to toe) planes. The intensity of the magnetic field surrounding a patient may be modified with these gradient coils. When one of coils is turned on, it creates a gradient in the intensity of the magnetic field. Thus in a 1.5 T scanner, when the Z-axis gradient is turned on, the strength of the magnetic field at the head might be 1.4 T and that at the toe 1.6 T. When this gradient field is applied, the precessional frequency of hydrogen nuclei will vary linearly along the magnetic gradient. Accordingly, when an RF pulse is applied, only those nuclei precessing at the same frequency as the applied signal will resonate. This allows selecting the desired slice of tissue along the patient's long axis (Z gradient). The slope of the gradient applied and the bandwidth of the RF pulse determine the thickness of this slice. The location of the signal within the X and Y (transverse) planes of the selected longitudinal plane is derived by switching off the Z-gradient coil followed by rapidly turning on the X- and then the Y-gradient coils (phase encoding and frequency encoding, respectively). This sequence alters the phase and precessional frequencies of the nuclei in the selected slice. The resulting magnetic resonance signal from the patient is read out while the frequency-encoding gradient is applied. The signal from the patient contains many frequencies that is decomposed by the fast Fourier transform into amplitude and frequency. This information, which reflects the number of hydrogen nuclei and their T1 and T2

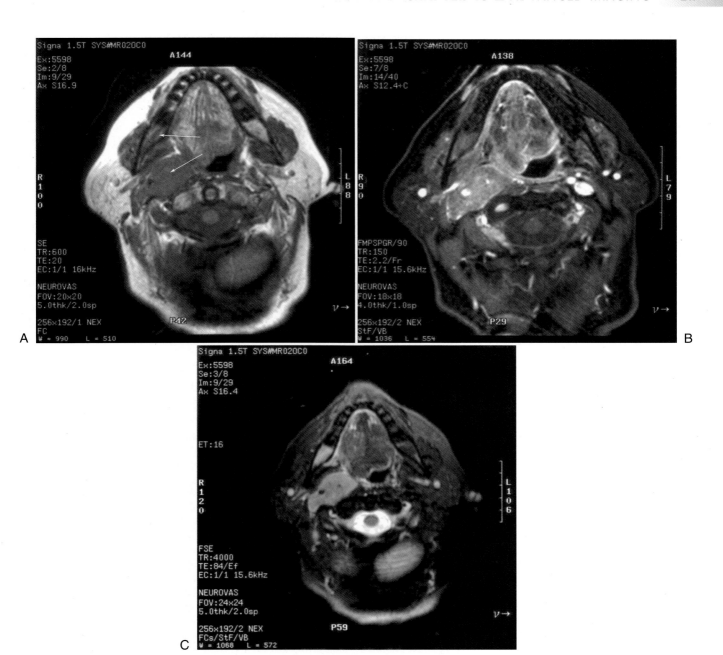

FIG. **13-17** **MRI Images.** MRI examination performed to evaluate neck mass in a patient with known diagnosis of multiple myeloma. **A,** Axial T1 precontrast (no fat saturation) image through mandible. Note abnormally dark marrow in posterior right mandible (*arrow,* compare with left side) and mass in right carotid space (*other arrow*). **B,** Axial T1 postcontrast image with fat saturation. Note abnormal enhancement of both marrow in right mandible and of the mass in the right carotid space. **C,** Axial T2 with fat saturation demonstrating abnormally bright signal in both marrow in right mandible and of the mass in the right carotid space. (Courtesy Dr. Thomas Underhill, Radiology Associates, Richmond, Va.)

properties at each X and Y location in the selected longitudinal plane, is reconstructed into magnetic resonance images.

## MAGNETIC RESONANCE IMAGES

MRI has several advantages over other diagnostic imaging procedures. First, it offers the best contrast resolution of soft tissues. Although x-ray attenuation coefficients of soft tissues may vary by no more than

1%, T1 and T2 relaxation times may vary by up to 40%. Second, no ionizing radiation is involved with MRI. Third, because the region of the body imaged in MRI is controlled with the gradient coils, direct multiplanar imaging is possible without reorienting the patient. Disadvantages of MRI include relatively long imaging times and the potential hazard imposed by the presence of ferromagnetic metals in the vicinity of the imaging magnet. This latter disadvantage excludes from MRI any patient with implanted metallic foreign objects or medical devices that consist of or contain ferromagnetic metals (e.g., cardiac pacemakers, some cerebral aneurysm clips or ferrous foreign bodies in the eye). The strong magnetic fields may move these objects and harm patients. Metals used in dentistry for restorations or orthodontics will not move but may distort the image in their vicinity. Titanium implants cause only minor image degradation. Finally, some patients have claustrophobia when positioned in an MRI machine.

## APPLICATIONS

Because of its excellent soft tissue contrast resolution, MRI is useful in evaluating soft tissue conditions, for instance, the position and integrity of the disk in the TMJ (Fig. 13-18); for soft tissue disease especially neoplasia involving the soft tissues, such as tongue, cheek, salivary glands, and neck; determining malignant involvement of lymph nodes; and determining perineural invasion by malignant neoplasia. Similar to CT imaging, a contrast agent such as gadolinium can be added to enhance the image resolution of neoplasia (Fig 13-19). Also, it is customary to remove the high signal of surrounding fat tissue (fat suppression) to enhance the appearance of the neoplasm. A typical protocol would include T1, T1 postgadolinium (with fat suppression), and T2 (with fat suppression) images.

## Nuclear Medicine

Film radiography, CT, MRI, and diagnostic ultrasonography are morphologic imaging techniques in that each requires a macroscopic anatomic change for information to be recorded by an image receptor. However, in some human diseases abnormal biochemical processes occur without anatomic change. Radionuclide imaging (a form of functional imaging) provides a means of assessing such physiologic change. Nuclear medicine examinations are commonly used for assign function of the brain, thyroids, heart, lungs, and gastrointestinal system as well as for diagnosis and follow-up of metastatic disease, bone tumors, and infection (Fig. 13-20).

Radionuclide imaging uses radioactive atoms or molecules that emit gamma rays. These atoms behave in an organism in a manner comparable to their stable counterparts because they are chemically indistinguishable. Radionuclides allow measurement of tissue function in vivo and provide an early marker of disease through measurement of biochemical change. After the radionuclides are administered, they distribute in the body according to their chemical properties. The γ-scintillation camera detects gamma rays and forms planar images showing the locations of the radionuclides in the body. Single photon emission computed tomography (SPECT) and positron emission tomography (PET) imaging are advanced nuclear medicine techniques that form tomographic views. Recently molecular imaging of individual gene expression is being accomplished in the laboratory.

## RADIONUCLIDES

The ideal radionuclide has a short half-life, emits γ rays but no charged particles, and is capable of binding to a variety of pharmaceuticals. Although many γ-emitting isotopes are used in radionuclide imaging, including iodine ($^{131}$I), gallium ($^{67}$Ga), and selenium ($^{74}$Se), the most commonly used is technetium 99m ($^{99m}$Tc). Technetium 99m has a half-life of 6 hours and emits primarily 140 kiloelectron volt (keV) photons. As technetium pertechnetate, $^{99m}$Tc mimics iodine distribution when injected intravenously and is concentrated by the salivary and thyroid glands and gastric mucosa. When it is attached to various carrier molecules, it can be used to examine virtually every organ of the body.

To image bone, $^{99m}$Tc is typically bound to methylene diphosphonate (MDP) and a dose of 20 to 30 mCi (740 to 1110 mega-Becquerels [MBq]) is injected intravenously. Immediately after injection the tracer distributes intravascularly. Images made during this flow phase, the first 60 to 90 seconds, are called radionuclide angiography. In the second, or blood pool phase, the tracer quickly moves into the extracellular space. The third, or bone scintigraphy phase, is made 2 to 3 hours after injection. The MDP deposition in the skeleton depends both on osteoclastic activity and blood flow (Fig. 13-20). Images made 2 to 3 hours after injection show most of the tracer activity in the skeleton, kidneys, and bladder. Most metastatic tumors in bone induce formation of new bone and thus may be detected on such an examination.

Radionuclide-labeled tracers are used in quantities well below amounts that are lethal to cells. However, although radionuclide imaging is considered noninvasive, the radiation dose the patient receives as a result of intravenous injection of radionuclide-labeled tracers should be considered. Injection of 740 MBq of $^{99m}$Tc pertechnetate delivers a whole-body radiation dose of 2 milliGrays (mGy). This quantity is less than the average annual effective dose resulting from natural radiation (see Chapter 3).

## γ-SCINTILLATION CAMERA

γ-Scintillation cameras (also called *Anger cameras*) are the most common means of forming an image (Fig. 13-21). These cameras capture photons and convert them to light and then to a voltage signal. This signal is reconstructed to a planar image that shows the distribution of the radionuclide in the patient. The first part of the gamma camera is a collimator. It absorbs γ rays that do not travel parallel to the plates, thus improving image resolution. The γ rays that pass through the collimator then strike a scintillation crystal. This crystal, often made of sodium iodide with trace amounts of thallium, fluoresces when it absorbs γ rays. These flashes of light are detected by an array of photomultiplier tubes coupled to the crystal with light pipes. The photomultiplier tubes capture the flash and amplify the signal. The size of the signal is proportional to the energy of the absorbed photon. The signals from the photomultiplier tubes go through an analog to digital converter and then to a pulse height analyzer. This device detects the intensity of the signal, and thus the energy of the incident absorbed photons, and only uses those from the radionuclide when forming the final image. Many of the γ rays released from the radionuclide in the patient undergo Compton absorption at some distant site and result in a new scattered photon. If these scattered, lower-energy photons pass through the collimator of the gamma camera, they may degrade image resolution. However, these scattered photons are detected by the pulse height analyzer and are rejected so that they do not contribute to the image. Gamma cameras have a spatial resolution of up 3 to 5 mm. Use of a scintillation crystal for acquisition of data for image formation has led to the labeling of this technique as *scintigraphy*.

## SINGLE PHOTON EMISSION COMPUTED TOMOGRAPHY

SPECT is a method of acquiring tomographic slices through a patient. Most gamma cameras have SPECT capability. In this technique either a single or multiple gamma camera is rotated 360 degrees about the patient. Image acquisition takes about 30 to 45 minutes. The acquired

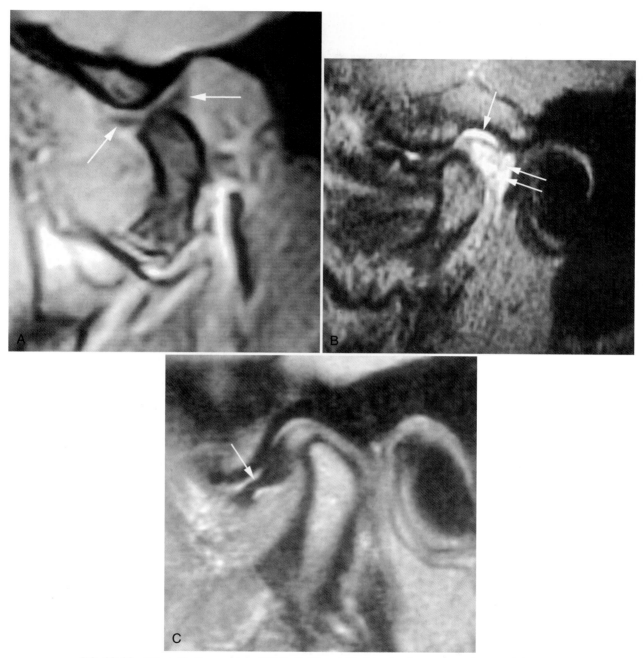

FIG. **13-18**   **Magnetic Resonance of TMJ. A,** T1-weighted magnetic resonance image of the TMJ. In this image the jaw is partly open, as indicated by the location of the condyle relative to the articular eminence. The articular disk, which has a "bow tie" appearance *(arrows)*, is in a normal position relative to the translating condyle. **B,** T2-weighted magnetic resonance image of the TMJ. This image illustrates both inflammatory effusion into the superior joint space *(arrow)* and hyperemia caused by increased vasculature in the retrodiskal tissues *(double arrows)*. **C,** Proton or spin density magnetic resonance image of the TMJ. In this image the disk is anteriorly displaced *(arrow)*, with the posterior band in the 9 o'clock position relative to the condylar head. (**B** and **C,** Courtesy Richard Harper, DDS, Dallas, Tex.)

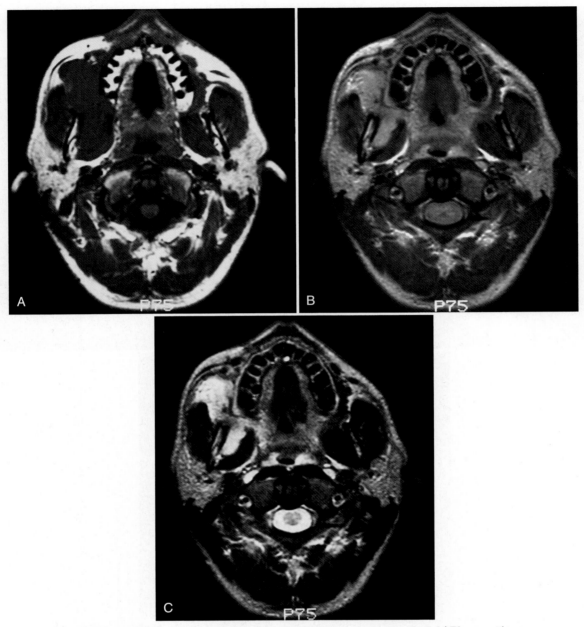

FIG. **13-19**    Gadolinium Enhancement of Magnetic Resonance Image.  **A,** Axial T1 magnetic resonance image of a rabdomyosarcoma involving the soft tissues of the right face. The tumor cannot be
distinguished from the adjacent masseter and pterygoid muscles because both have the same tissue
signal. **B,** Axial T1 postgadolinium magnetic resonance image of same case. Note that the tumor now
has a brighter signal (lighter) than the adjacent muscles because of its greater vascularity, enhanced
by the gadolinium. **C,** Axial T2 magnetic resonance image of same case. Note that the tumor has a
brighter signal than adjacent muscles because of greater fluid content of the tumor.

data are processed by filtered back projection and, more recently,
iterative reconstruction algorithms, to form a number of contiguous
axial slices, similar to CT by x ray. These data can then be used to
construct multiplanar images of the study area (see Fig. 13-20).
Tomography enhances contrast and removes superimposed activity.
Recently SPECT images have been fused with CT images to improve
identifying of the location of the radionuclide.

## APPLICATIONS

The maxillofacial region most common use of nuclear medicine is to
investigate abnormal metabolic bone activity, for instance, in assessing
growth activity in cases of condylar hyperplasia and presence of metastatic lesions. Traditionally a combination of $^{99m}$Tc MDP and gallium
citrate was used to diagnose osteomyelitis, but CT imaging is now
used more frequently.

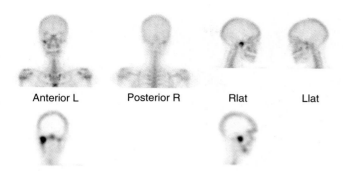

Anterior L      Posterior R      Rlat      Llat

FIG. **13-20  Radionuclide Image.** The increased uptake of $^{99m}$Tc-MDP in the region of the right TMJ. The top row images were captured with a γ-scintillation camera. The lower two tomographic images were captured with SPECT.

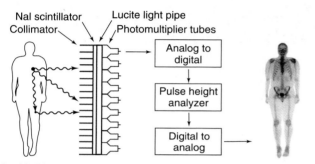

FIG. **13-21  Gamma Scintillation Camera.** The principal components of a gamma scintillation camera are a collimator to limit γ rays to those perpendicular to the surface of the camera, a scintillator to absorb the γ rays and emit a flash of visible light, photomultiplier tubes to count the flashes of light and measure their energy, a pulse height analyzer to select only those flashes from the administered radionuclide, and a monitor to display the resultant image. The most superior γ ray will pass through the collimator and contribute to the image and the collimator will block the second γ ray. The photon resulting from Compton scattering in the leg will be rejected by the pulse height analyzer and not contribute to the image. Image of patient is anterior view of patient after intravenous injection of $^{99m}$Tc-MDP.

## POSITRON EMISSION TOMOGRAPHY

PET is a more advanced imaging modality in nuclear medicine. PET, which is reported to have a sensitivity nearly 100 times that of a gamma camera, relies on positron-emitting radionuclides generated in a cyclotron. The utility of PET is based not only on its sensitivity but also on the fact that the most commonly used radionuclides ($^{11}$C, $^{13}$N, $^{15}$O, $^{18}$F) are isotopes of elements that occur naturally in organic molecules. Although fluorine does not technically fit into this category, it is a chemical substitute for hydrogen. These radionuclides are used as is, or more commonly, incorporated into a radiopharmaceutical such as glucose or amino acids by use of a medical cyclotron. After the radiopharmaceutical is injected into the patient, the isotope distributes within the body's tissue according to the carrier molecule and emits a positron. This positron then interacts with a free electron and mutual annihilation occurs, resulting in the production of two 551-keV photons emitted at 180 degrees to each other. The PET scanner consists of a ring of many detectors in a circle around the patient (Fig. 13-22). The detector crystals are often made of bismuth germinate.

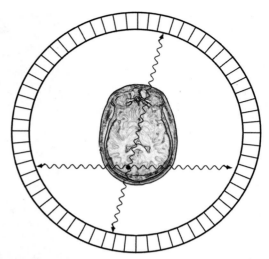

FIG. **13-22  PET Scanner.** A PET scanner consists of a ring of detectors that measure pairs of 511 keV γ rays traveling in opposite directions from positron annihilation. Each pair is recorded simultaneously; thus the location of the radionuclide can be determined as the intersection of the pairs of detectors recording simultaneous events. The location of the common source of the radionuclide is thus readily determined as the intersection of the flight paths of the γ rays.

Electronically coupled opposing detectors simultaneously identify the pair of γ photons using coincidence detection circuits that measure events within 10 to 20 nanoseconds. The annihilation event is thus known to have occurred along the line joining the two detectors. Raw PET scan data consist of a number of these coincidence lines, which are reorganized into projections that identify where isotope is concentrated within the patient. The spatial resolution of a PET scanner is about 5 mm. PET is useful in skeletal imaging for assessing primary bone tumors, locating metastases in bone, and detecting osteomyelitis. For instance, $^{18}$F-fluoro-2-deoxyglucose ($^{18}$F-FDG) is a radiopharmaceutical commonly used for studying glucose use in the brain and heart and to look for cancer metastases (Fig. 13-23). PET images are often fused with CT scans to facilitate anatomic localization of radionuclide. The PET/CT combination has been shown to be quite helpful in staging and treatment planning of squamous cell carcinoma in the head and neck.

## Ultrasonography

Sonography is a technique based on sound waves that acquires images in real time and without the use of ionizing radiation. The phenomenon perceived as sound is the result of periodic changes in the pressure of air against the eardrum. The periodicity of these changes lies anywhere between 1500 and 20,000 Hz. By definition, ultrasound has a periodicity greater than 20 kHz, greater than the audible range. Diagnostic ultrasonography (sonography), the clinical application of ultrasound, uses vibratory frequencies in the range of 1 to 20 MHz.

Scanners used for sonography generate electrical impulses that are converted into ultra-high-frequency sound waves by a transducer, a device that can convert one form of energy into another—in this case, electrical energy into sonic energy. The most important component of the transducer is a thin piezoelectric crystal or material made up of a great number of dipoles arranged in a geometric pattern. A dipole may be thought of as a distorted molecule that appears to have a

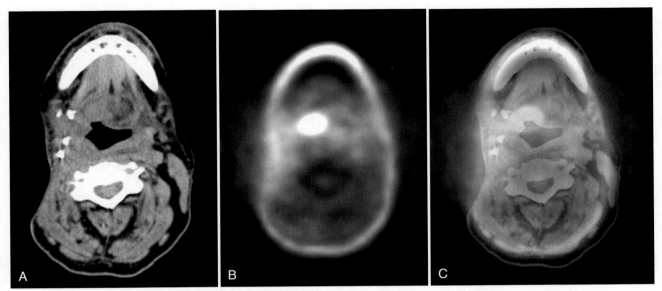

FIG. **13-23**    **PET Scan and Fused PET-CT.** This patient has a known recurrent carcinoma at the base of the tongue. **A,** Soft-tissue algorithm CT at level of inferior border of mandible. The four metallic objects on the patient's right side posterior to the mandible represent vascular clips from prior surgery. **B,** FDG PET scan showing oval-shaped region of high metabolic activity of tumor at the right tongue base. The FDG activity in the anterior mandible is related to low level metabolic activity in the vicinity of a reconstruction plate. **C,** Fused images **A** and **B** demonstrating the region of high metabolic activity superimposed on the CT anatomy. Images acquired on combined PET-CT scanner. (Courtesy Dr. Todd W. Stultz, Cleveland Clinic, Ohio.)

positive charge on one end and a negative charge on the other. Currently, the most widely used piezoelectric material is lead zirconate titanate. The electrical impulse generated by the scanner causes the dipoles in the crystal to realign themselves with the electrical field and thus suddenly change the crystal's thickness. This abrupt change begins a series of vibrations that produce the sound waves that are transmitted into the tissues being examined.

The transducer emitting ultrasound is held against the body part being examined. The ultrasonic beam passes through or interacts with tissues of different acoustic impedance. Sonic waves that reflect (echo) toward the transducer cause a change in the thickness of the piezoelectric crystal, which in turn produces an electrical signal that is amplified, processed, and ultimately displayed as an image on a monitor. Typically the transducer serves as both a transmitter and a receiver. Current techniques permit echoes to be processed at a sufficiently rapid rate to allow perception of motion; this is referred to as *real-time imaging.*

The ultrasound signal transmitted into a patient is attenuated by a combination of absorption, reflection, refraction, and diffusion. The higher the frequency of the sound waves, the higher the image resolution but the less the penetration of the sound through soft tissue. The fraction of the beam that is reflected to the transducer depends on the acoustic impedance of the tissue, which is a product of its density (and thus the velocity of sound through it) and the beam's angle of incidence. Because of its acoustic impedance, a tissue has a characteristic internal echo pattern. Consequently, not only can changes in echo patterns distinguish between different tissues and boundaries, but they also can be correlated with pathologic changes within a tissue. Tissues that do not produce signals, such as fluid-filled cysts, are said to be *anechoic* and appear black. Tissues that produce a weak signal are *hypoechoic,* whereas tissues that produce intense signals such as ligaments, skin, or needles or catheters are *hyperechoic* and appear bright. Interpretation of sonograms thus relies on knowledge of both the physical properties of ultrasound and the anatomy of the tissues being scanned.

Ultrasonography is used in the head and neck region for evaluating for neoplasms in the thyroid, parathyroid or salivary glands or lymph nodes, for stones in salivary glands or ducts, Sjögren's syndrome, and the vessels of the neck, including the carotid for atherosclerotic plaques (Figs. 13-24 and 13-25). Ultrasonography is also used to guide fine-needle aspiration in the neck. Recent advances include three-dimensional imaging to allow multiplanar reformatting, surface renderings (for example of a fetal face), and color Doppler sonography for evaluation blood flow.

## Conventional Tomography

Conventional tomography is a radiographic technique, usually using film, designed to image a slice or plane of tissue. This is accomplished by blurring the images of structures lying outside the plane of interest through the process of motion "unsharpness." Since the introduction of CT, MRI, and cone-beam imaging, which have superior contrast resolution, film-based tomography has been used less frequently. When conventional tomography is used in dentistry it is applied primarily to high-contrast anatomy, such as that encountered in TMJ and dental implant imaging.

Conventional tomography uses an x-ray tube and radiographic film rigidly connected and capable of moving about a fixed axis or fulcrum (Fig. 13-26). The examination begins with the x-ray tube and film positioned on opposite sides of the fulcrum, which is located

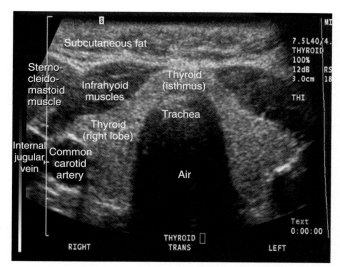

FIG. **13-24** Ultrasound examination (transverse section) of a healthy thyroid gland. This image shows glandular, muscular, adipose, and vascular tissues because of the different acoustic impedance of these tissues. (Courtesy Dr. Christos Angelopoulos, Columbia University, College of Dental Medicine, N.Y.)

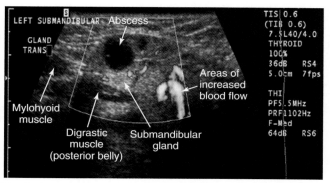

FIG. **13-25** Doppler Ultrasound. Transverse view of submandibular gland showing abscess formation and increased blood flow. (Courtesy Dr. Christos Angelopoulos, Columbia University, College of Dental Medicine, N.Y.)

within the body's plane of interest (focal plane). As the exposure begins, the tube and film move in opposite directions simultaneously through a mechanical linkage. With this synchronous movement of tube and film, the images of objects located within the focal plane (at the fulcrum) remain in fixed positions on the radiographic film throughout the length of tube and film travel and are clearly imaged. On the other hand, the images of objects located outside the focal plane have continuously changing positions on the film; as a result, the images of these objects are blurred beyond recognition by motion unsharpness. The resulting zone of sharp image is called the *tomographic layer*. Blurring of overlying structures is greatest (and the tomographic layer the thinnest) under the following circumstances:
- Overlying structures lie far from the focal plane
- The focal plane lies far from the film
- The long axis of the structure to be blurred is oriented perpendicular to the direction of tube travel
- The distance of tube travel is large

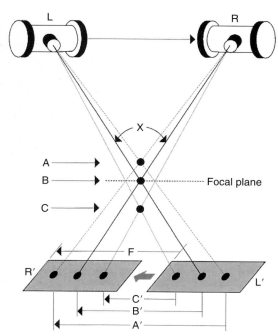

FIG. **13-26** **Tomographic Techniques.** As the x-ray tube moves from left to right, the film moves in the opposite direction. In the figure, points *A* and *C* lie outside the focal plane (the plane that contains the fulcrum), whereas object *B* lies at the center of tube/film movement. Only objects that lie in the focal plane (i.e., *B*) remain in sharp focus because the image of *B* moves exactly the same distance (*B'*) as the film travels (*F*), and thus its image remains stationary on the film. The image of point *A* moves more than the film (distance *A'*) and the image of point *C* less than the film (distance *C'*); therefore the images of both are blurred. *X* is the tomographic angle. The greater the tomographic angle, the thinner the tomographic layer.

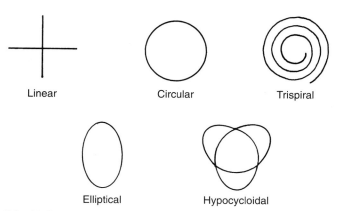

FIG. **13-27** **Tomographic Movements.** Linear movements, either vertical or horizontal, are mechanically simple but result in streaking artifacts. The more complex motions result in fewer streaking artifacts and sharper images.

There are at least five types of tomographic movement: linear, circular, elliptic, hypocycloidal, and spiral (Fig. 13-27). Mechanically, the simplest tomographic motion is linear. More complex movements such as circular, elliptic, hypocycloidal, and spiral produce images without streaking artifacts common to the linear movements. Many of the more expensive panoramic units are capable of making tomographic sections of the jaws (Fig. 13-28).

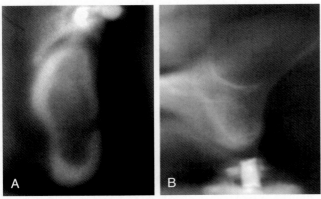

FIG. **13-28** **Linear Tomographic Images Made by Panoramic Units. A,** Mandibular tomogram in the region of the mental foramen. **B,** Maxillary tomograms in the premolar region acquired with an Instrumentarium Orthopantomograph 100 panoramic unit. Note the dome-shaped opacity in the floor of the maxillary sinus consistent with a mucous retention phenomenon. (**B,** Courtesy Brad Potter, DDS, Augusta, Ga.)

# BIBLIOGRAPHY

## COMPUTED TOMOGRAPHY

Bononmo L, Foley D, Imhof H et al: *Multidetector computed tomography technology: advances in imaging techniques,* ed 1, London, 2003, Royal Society of Medicine Press.

Bushberg JT, Seibert JA, Leidholdt EM Jr et al: *The essential physics of medical imaging,* ed 2, Baltimore, 2002, Williams & Wilkins.

Bushong, SC: *Computed tomography,* ed 1, New York, 2000, McGraw-Hill.

Fishman EK, Jeffrey RB Jr: *Multidetector CT: principles, techniques, and clinical applications,* ed 1, Philadelphia, 2004, Lippincott Williams & Wilkins.

Kalender W: *Computed tomography: fundamentals, systems technology, image quality, applications,* ed 2, Erlangen, 2005, Publicis Corporate Publishing.

Knollmann F, Coakley FV: *Multislice CT: principles and protocols,* ed 1, Philadelphia, 2006, Elsevier.

Marchal G, Vogl TJ, Heiken JP et al: *Multidetector-row computed tomography,* ed 1, Milan, 2005, Springer.

Silverman PM: *Multislice computed tomography: a practical approach to clinical protocols,* ed 1, Philadelphia, 2002, Lippincott Williams & Wilkins.

## MAGNETIC RESONANCE IMAGING

Bushberg JT, Seibert JA, Leidholdt EM Jr et al: *The essential physics of medical imaging,* ed 2, Baltimore, 2002, Williams & Wilkins.

Westbrook C, Roth CK, Talbot J: *MRI in practice,* ed 3, Oxford, 2005, Blackwell Publishing.

## NUCLEAR MEDICINE

Mettler FA, Guiberteau MJ: *Essentials of nuclear medicine,* ed 5, Philadelphia, 2006, WB Saunders.

Schiepers C: *Diagnostic nuclear medicine,* ed 2, Berlin, 2006, Springer.

Sharp PF, Gemmell HG, Murray AD: *Practical nuclear medicine,* ed 3, London, 2005, Springer-Verlag.

Wilson MA: *Nuclear medicine,* ed 1, Philadelphia, 1998, Lippincott-Raven.

## ULTRASOUND

Brant WE: *Ultrasound,* ed 1, Philadelphia, 2001, Lippincott Williams & Wilkins.

Emshoff R, Bertram S, Strobl H: *Ultrasonographic cross-sectional characteristics of muscles of the head and neck, Oral Surg Oral Med Oral Pathol Oral Radiol Endod* 87:93-106, 1999.

Goldman LW, Fowlkes JB, editors: *Categorical course in diagnostic radiology physics: CT and US cross-sectional imaging,* Oak Brook, Ill, 2000, RSNA Publications.

Middleton WD, Kurtz AB, Hertzberg BA: *Ultrasound: the requisites,* ed 2, St. Louis, 2004, Mosby.

Shimizu M, Okamura K, Yoshiura K et al: Sonographic diagnostic criteria for screening Sjögren's syndrome, *Oral Surg Oral Med Oral Path Oral Radiol Endod* 102:85-93, 2006.

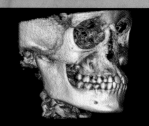

# CHAPTER **14**

# Cone-Beam Computed Tomography

William C. Scarfe • Allan G. Farman

Cone-beam computed tomography (CBCT) is a recent technology initially developed for angiography in 1982 and subsequently applied to maxillofacial imaging. It uses a divergent or "cone"-shaped source of ionizing radiation and a two-dimensional area detector fixed on a rotating gantry to acquire multiple sequential projection images in one complete scan around the area of interest (Fig. 14-1). It is only since the late 1990s that it has become possible to produce clinical systems that are both inexpensive and small enough to be used in the dental office. Four technologic factors have converged to make this possible: (1) the development of compact high-quality flat-panel detector arrays, (2) reductions in the cost of computers capable of image reconstruction, (3) development of inexpensive x-ray tubes capable of continuous exposure and, (4) limited-volume scanning (e.g., head and neck), eliminating the need for subsecond gantry rotation speeds.

This technology has been given several names including dental volumetric tomography, cone-beam volumetric tomography, dental computed tomography, and cone-beam imaging. The most frequently applied and preferred term is *cone-beam computed tomography* because it is a digital analog of film tomography in a more exact way than is traditional computed tomography (CT), the x-ray is either conical or pyramidal, and the technology is not limited to dentistry. The principal feature of CBCT is that multiple planar projections are acquired by rotational scan to produce a volumetric dataset from which interrelational images can be generated.

## Principles of Cone-Beam Computed Tomography

All CT scanners consist of an x-ray source and detector mounted on a rotating gantry. During rotation of the gantry, the receptor detects x rays attenuated by the patient. These recordings constitute "raw data" that is reconstructed by a computer algorithm to generate cross-sectional images whose component picture element *(pixel)* values correspond to linear attenuation coefficients. CT can be divided into two categories on the basis of acquisition x-ray beam geometry, namely, fan beam (Fig. 14-1) and cone beam (Fig. 14-2).

Cone-beam scanners use a two-dimensional digital array providing an area detector rather than a linear detector as CT does. This is combined with a three-dimensional (3D) x-ray beam with circular collimation so that the resultant beam is in the shape of a cone, hence the name "cone beam." Because the exposure incorporates the entire region of interest (ROI), only one rotational scan of the gantry is necessary to acquire enough data for image reconstruction. Cone-beam geometry has inherent quickness in volumetric data acquisition and therefore the potential for significant cost savings compared with CT. CBCT produces an entire volumetric dataset from which the voxels are extracted. Voxel dimensions are dependent on the pixel size on the area detector. Therefore CBCT units in general provide voxel resolutions that are *isotropic*—equal in all three dimensions.

## Image Acquisition

The cone-beam technique involves a rotational scan exceeding 180 degrees of an x-ray source and a reciprocating area detector moving synchronously around the patient's head. During the rotation, many exposures are made at fixed intervals, providing single projection images known as *basis images*. These are similar to lateral cephalometric radiographic images, each slightly offset from one another. The complete series of basis images is referred to as the *projection data*. Software programs incorporating sophisticated algorithms including back-filtered projection are applied to these projection data to generate a 3D volumetric data set that can be used to provide primary reconstruction images in three orthogonal planes (axial, sagittal, and coronal).

There are four components to CBCT image acquisition:
• X-ray generation
• Image detection system
• Image reconstruction
• Image display

The image generation and image detection specifications of currently available systems (Tables 14-1 and 14-2) reflect proprietary variations in these parameters.

### X-RAY GENERATION

Although CBCT is technically simple in that only a single scan of the patient is made to acquire a data set, a number of clinically important parameters should be considered in x-ray generation.

#### Patient Positioning

CBCT can be performed with the patient in three possible positions: sitting, standing, and supine. Equipment that requires the patient to lie supine physically occupies a larger surface area or physical *footprint* and may not be accessible for patients with some physical disabilities. Standing units may not be able to be adjusted to a height to accommodate wheelchair-bound patients. Seated units are the most comfortable; however, fixed seats may also not allow scanning of physically disabled or wheelchair-bound patients. Because scan times are often

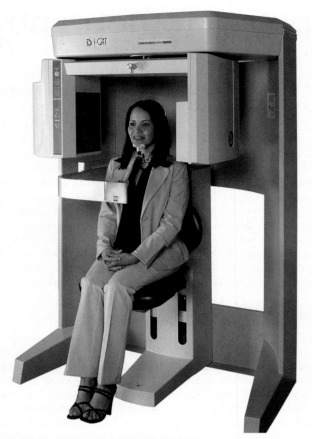

FIG. **14-1  Example of CBCT Unit.** Imaging may be performed with the patient seated, supine, or standing. The patient's head is positioned and stabilized between the x-ray generator and detector by a head-holding apparatus. The detector may be a flat panel (this example) or image intensifier. During exposure the generator and detector rotate fully or partially around the patient's head. Scan time is as fast as 5 seconds. Most CBCT units have a small "footprint" enabling in-office placement. (Courtesy Imaging Sciences International, Hatfield, Pa.)

greater than that used with panoramic imaging, perhaps more important than patient orientation is the head restraint mechanism used. With all systems it is important to immobilize the patient's head because any movement degrades the final image.

### X-ray Generator

During the scan rotation, each projection image is made by sequential single-image capture of the remnant x-ray beam by the detector. Technically, the easiest method of exposing the patient is to use a constant beam of radiation during the rotation and allow the x-ray detector to sample the attenuated beam in its trajectory. However, this results in a continuous radiation exposure to the patient, much of which does not contribute to the formation of the image. It is preferable to pulse the x-ray beam to coincide with the detector sampling. This means that actual exposure time is markedly less than scanning time. This technique reduces patient radiation dose considerably.

The ALARA (*As Low As Reasonably Achievable*) principle of dose optimization necessitates that CBCT exposure factors should be adjusted on the basis of patient size. This can be achieved by appropriate selection of either tube current (milliamperes [mA]), tube voltage (kilovolts peak [kVp]), or both. On some CBCT units both kVp and mA are automatically modulated in near real time by a feedback mechanism detecting the intensity of the transmitted beam, a process known generically as *automatic exposure control*. On others, exposure settings are automatically determined by the initial scout exposure. This feature is highly desirable because it is operator independent. The variation in exposure parameters together with the presence of pulsed x-ray beam and size of the image field are the primary determinants of patient exposure.

### Scan Volume

The dimensions of the *field of view* or *scan volume* able to be covered are primarily dependent on the detector size and shape, beam projection geometry, and the ability to collimate the beam. The shape of the scan volume can be either a cylinder or spherical. Collimating the primary x-ray beam limits x-radiation exposure to the ROI. Limiting field size therefore ensures that an optimal field of view can be selected for each patient on the basis of individual needs. Scanning of the entire craniofacial region is difficult to incorporate into cone-beam design because of the high cost of large area detectors. One manufacturer has expanded the scan volume height by software addition of two rotational scans to produce a single volume with a 22-cm height.

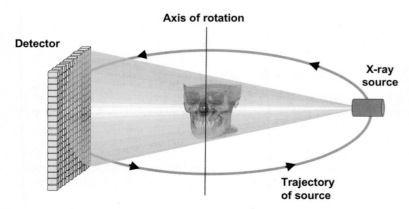

FIG. **14-2  Cone-Beam Imaging Geometry.** A 3D cone (this example) or pyramidal (if collimation is rectangular) divergent x-ray beam is directed through a central object onto a detector (either solid-state flat panel or image intensifier/charge-coupled device). After a single two-dimensional projection is acquired by the detector, the x-ray source and detector rotate a small distance around a trajectory arc. At this second angular position another basis projection image or frame is captured. This sequence continues around the object for the entire 360 degrees (full trajectory) or a reduced or partial trajectory.

## IMAGE DETECTION

Current CBCT units can be divided into two groups on the basis of detector type: image intensifier tube/charge-coupled device combination or flat-panel imager. The former configuration comprises an x-ray image intensifier tube coupled to a charge-coupled device with a fiber optic coupling. Flat-panel imaging consists of detection of x rays with an "indirect" detector that is based on a large area solid-state sensor panel coupled to an x-ray scintillator layer (see Chapter 7). The most common flat-panel configuration consists of a cesium iodide scintillator applied to a thin film transistor made of amorphous silicon.

### Voxel Size

The principal determinants of nominal voxel size in CBCT are the x-ray tube focal spot size, x-ray geometric configuration, and the matrix and pixel size of the solid state detector. Both the focal spot size and the geometric configuration of the x-ray source determine the degree of geometric unsharpness, a limiting factor in spatial resolution. However, the cost of x-ray tubes, and therefore of the CBCT unit, increases substantially with smaller focal spot size. Reducing the object-to-detector distance and increasing source-to-object distance also minimizes geometric unsharpness. In maxillofacial CBCT the detector position is limited because it must be located far enough from the patient's head so that it freely rotates and clears the patient's shoulders. Limitations also exist in extending the source-to-object distance because this increases the size of the CBCT unit. However, reducing source-to-object distance produces a magnified projected image on the detector, increasing potential spatial resolution.

### Grayscale

The ability of CBCT to display differences in attenuation is related to the ability of the detector to detect subtle contrast differences. This parameter is called the *bit depth* of the system and determines the number of shades of gray available to display the attenuation. At the time of writing, all available CBCT units used detectors capable of recording grayscale differences of 12 bits or higher. If a 12-bit detector ($2^{12}$) is used to define the scale, 4096 shades are available to display contrast. Although higher bit-depth images in CBCT are possible, this added information comes at the expense of increased computational time and substantially larger file sizes.

## RECONSTRUCTION

Once the basis projection frames have been acquired, it is necessary to process these data to create the volumetric data set. This process is called *primary reconstruction*. Although a single cone-beam rotation may take less than 30 seconds, it produces 100 to more than 600 individual projection frames, each with more than a million pixels with 12 to 16 bits of data assigned to each pixel. The reconstruction of these data is computationally complex. To facilitate data handling, data are usually acquired by one computer (acquisition computer) and transferred by an Ethernet connection to a processing computer (workstation). In contrast to conventional CT, cone-beam data reconstruction is performed by personal computer–based rather than workstation platforms.

Reconstruction times vary depending on the acquisition parameters (voxel size, size of the image field, and number of projections), hardware (processing speed, data throughput from acquisition to

### Scan Factors

The speed with which individual images are acquired is called the *frame rate* and is measured in frames, projected images, per second. The maximum frame rate of the detector and rotational speed determines the number of projections that may be acquired. The number of projection images comprising a single scan may be fixed or variable. With a higher frame rate, more information is available to reconstruct the image; therefore, primary reconstruction time is increased. However, higher frame rates increase the signal-to-noise ratio, producing images with less noise. In the maxillofacial region, another advantage of a higher frame rate is that it reduces metallic artifact. Note that higher frame rates are usually accomplished with a longer scan time and hence higher patient dose.

Most CBCT imaging systems use a complete circular trajectory or a scan arc of 360 degrees to acquire projection data. This physical requirement is usually necessary to produce adequate projection data for 3D reconstruction. However, it is theoretically possible to reduce the completeness of the scanning trajectory to less than a full circle and still reconstruct a volumetric data set. This approach potentially reduces the scan time and is mechanically easier to perform.

It is desirable to reduce CBCT scan times to as short as possible to reduce motion artifact resulting from subject movement. This can be substantial and may be a limiting factor in voxel resolution. Decreased scanning times may be achieved by increasing the detector frame rate, reducing the number of projections, or reducing the scan arc. The latter two possibilities produce data with higher noise, whereas the first is optimal.

## TABLE 14-2
### Comparative Specifications of Food and Drug Administration–Approved Cone-Beam Computed Tomography Systems

| VENDOR, HEADQUARTERS | AFP IMAGING CORP. ELMSFORD, N.Y. | J. MORITA MANUFACTURING CORP., KYOTO, JAPAN | IMAGING SCIENCES INT., HATFIELD, PA. | HITACHI MEDICAL SYSTEMS, TOKYO, JAPAN | IMTEC IMAGING (DISTRIBUTED BY KODAK DENTAL SYSTEMS), ARDMORE, OKLA. | SIRONA DENTAL SYSTEMS, CHARLOTTE, N.C. | PLANMECA OY, HELSINKI, FINLAND | TERARECON INC., SAN MATEO, CALIF. | EWOO TECHNOLOGY CO., LTD., GYEONGGI-DO, KOREA |
|---|---|---|---|---|---|---|---|---|---|
| CBCT name | NewTom 3G | 3D Accuitomo | i-CAT | CB MercuRay | ILUMA Ultra Cone Beam CT Scanner | Galileos | ProMax 3D | PreXion 3D | Picasso Trio |
| Grayscale (bit depth) | 12 | 12 | 14 | 12 | 14 | 12 reduced from 16 | 12 | 16 | 12 |
| Image detector | II/CCD | CsI/a-Si | CsI/a-Si | II/CCD | CsII/a-Si | PST | CsII/CMOS | CsI/a-Si | CsI/a-Si |
| Voxel size | 0.07-0.2 | 0.125-2.0 | 0.12-0.4 | 0.1-0.5 | 0.1/0.2/0.3/0.4 | 0.15/0.3 | 0.15 | 0.07 | 0.1 |
| Scan factors (No./degrees/frames) | 1/360°/x | 1/180°,360°/x | 1 or 2/360°/ 156,306,612 | 1/360°/x | 1/360°/x | 1/210°/200 | 1/194°/x | 1/360°/ 512,1024 | 1/360°/ 256,320 |
| Patient positioning | Supine | Seated | Seated | Seated | Seated | Standing/ sitting | Standing | Seated | Standing |
| Preinstalled software | NewTom 3G | i-Dixel | Xoran Cat / iVision | CBWorks | ILUMA VISION3D | GALAXIS 3D | Romexis 3D Explorer | — | EasyDent |
| Scan time (s) | 5.6-36 | 8.5, 17 | 10-40 | 9.6 | 20-40 | 14 | 18 | 19/37 | 15/24 |
| X-ray source (all DC) | Pulsed | Constant | Pulsed | Constant | Constant | Pulsed | Pulsed | Constant | Constant |
| mA/kVp | 15 max/110 max | 1-10/60-80 | 3-5/120 | 2-15/60-120 | 4-7/120 | 5-7/85 | 8-16/84 | 4/90 | 4-10/60-90 |
| AEC | Yes | No | Yes | Yes | Yes | — | — | — | — |
| Scan volume (height × diameter) (cm) | 15 × 25 | 6 × 6, 4 × 4 | (6, 8, 13, 27.4) × 17 | (5.12, 11.7, 15) × 25 | (10-19) × (17-19) | 15 × 15 | 8 × 8, 5 × 8, 5 × 4 | 8 × 8 | 8 × 5, 12 × 7 |
| Primary reconstruction (min) | 7-20 | 0.5 | 1-10 | 6 | 2.5 | 4.5 | 3 | 1.5-3 | 3-6 |

II/CCD, Area image intensifier/charge coupled device; CsI/a-Si, cesium iodide/amorphous silicon flat panel; CMOS, complementary metal oxide semiconductor; PST, proprietary Siemens Technology; AEC, automatic exposure control; min, minutes; cm, centimeter; s, seconds; No., number; DC, direct current; PD, photo diode; —, data unavailable at time of printing. Data current as of June 21, 2007.

workstation computer), and software (reconstruction algorithms) used. Reconstruction should be accomplished in an acceptable time (less than 5 minutes) to complement patient flow.

The reconstruction process consists of two stages (Fig. 14-3):
1. Acquisition stage. This stage is performed at the acquisition computer. Once the multiple planar projection images are acquired, these images must be corrected by for inherent pixel imperfections and uneven exposure. Image calibration should be performed routinely to remove these defects.
2. Reconstruction stage. The remaining data-processing steps are performed on the reconstruction computer. The corrected images are converted into a special representation called a *sinogram,* a composite image developed from extracting a row of pixels from each projection image. Therefore the first sinogram will comprise a series of the first rows from each projection. If there are 300 projections, then the sinogram will have 300 rows. This process is referred to as the *radon transformation.* The resulting image comprises multiple sine waves of different amplitude. The sinogram is then reconstructed with a filtered back-projection algorithm for CBCT-acquired volumetric data called the Feldkamp algorithm. Once all slices have been reconstructed, they are combined into a single volume for visualization.

## DISPLAY

The volumetric data set is a compilation of all available voxels and, for most CBCT devices, is presented to the clinician on screen as secondary reconstructed images in three orthogonal planes (axial, sagittal, and coronal), usually at a thickness defaulted to the native resolution (Fig. 14-4). Optimum visualization of orthogonal reconstructed images is dependent on the adjustment of window level and window width to favor bone and the application of specific filters.

### Multiplanar Reformation

Because of the isotropic nature of the volumetric dataset, data sets can be sectioned nonorthogonally. Most software provides for various nonaxial two-dimensional images, referred to as *multiplanar reformation* (MPR). Such MPR modes include oblique, curved planar reformation and, serial transplanar reformation (Fig. 14-5). Because of the large number of component orthogonal images in each plane and the difficulty in relating adjacent structures, two methods have been developed to visualize adjacent voxels.

Most simply, any multiplanar image can be "thickened" by increasing the number of adjacent voxels included in the display. This creates an image slab that represents a specific volume of the patient, referred to as a *ray sum.* Full-thickness perpendicular ray sum images can be used to generate simulated projections such as lateral cephalometric images (Fig. 14-6). Unlike conventional radiographs, these ray sum images are without magnification and parallax distortion. However, this technique uses the entire volumetric data set and interpretation suffers from the problems of "anatomic noise"—the superimposition of multiple structures.

### Three-Dimensional Volume Rendering

Volume rendering refers to techniques that allow the visualization of 3D data by integration of large volumes of adjacent voxels and selective display. Two specific techniques are available.

*Indirect volume rendering* is a complex process requiring selection of the intensity or density of the grayscale level of the voxels to be displayed within an entire data set (called "segmentation"). This is technically demanding and computationally difficult, requiring specific software; however, it provides a volumetric surface reconstruction with depth (Fig. 14-7).

*Direct volume rendering* is a much simpler process. The most common technique is *maximum intensity projection* (MIP). MIP visualizations are achieved by evaluating each voxel value along an imaginary projection ray from the observer's eyes within a particular volume of interest and then representing only the highest value as the display value. Voxel intensities that are below an arbitrary threshold are eliminated (Fig. 14-8).

## Clinical Considerations

For each image acquisition there are procedural steps and numerous operator-controlled exposure parameters that must be specified. Consistent and methodic imaging technique minimizes patient radiation exposure and optimizes the resultant image quality.

### PATIENT SELECTION CRITERIA

Cone beam exposure provides a radiation dose to the patient higher than those of other dental radiographic procedures. Accordingly, the principal tenet of the ALARA principle must be applied: there should be justification of the exposure to the patient so that the total potential

FIG. **14-3 Image Acquisition and Reconstruction.** The acquisition stage involves acquisition of individual basis projections and subsequent modification of these images to correct for inconsistencies. Image correction is sequential and consists of the removal of signal voids from individual or linear pixel defects, image normalization by histogram equalization so that a full range of voxel intensity values are used, and removal of inherent electronic detector artifacts. After correction, images undergo reconstruction that includes converting the corrected basis projection images into sinograms and application of the Feldkamp reconstruction to the corrected sinograms, which includes weighting the information according to location, applying specific filters to the image, and finally use of back-projection techniques to reconstitute the image.

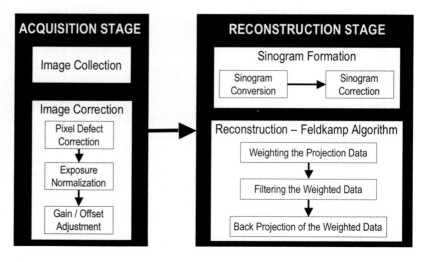

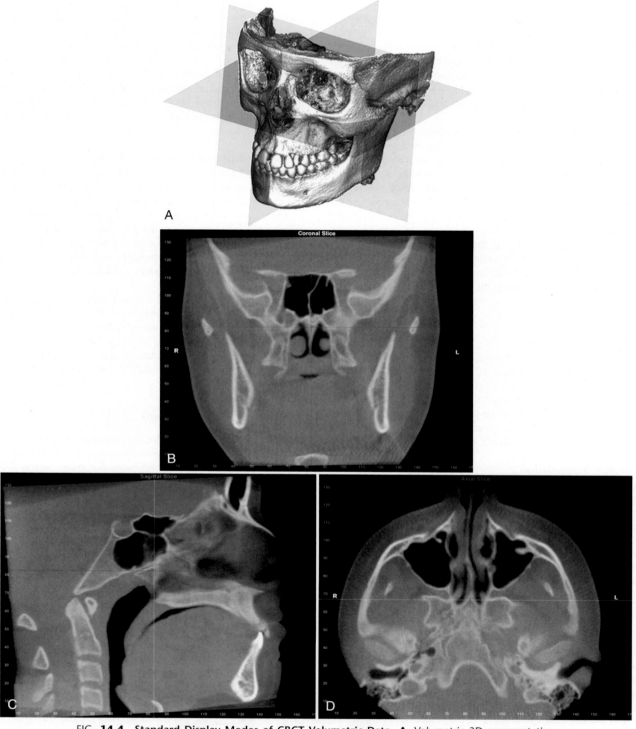

FIG. **14-4**  **Standard Display Modes of CBCT Volumetric Data. A,** Volumetric 3D representation of hard tissue showing the three orthogonal planes in relation to the reconstructed volumetric data set: coronal, sagittal, and axial. Each orthogonal plane has multiple thin slice sections in each plane. **B,** Representative coronal image. **C,** Representative sagittal image. **D,** Representative axial image. (Images produced using Dolphin 3D, Chatsworth, Calif.)

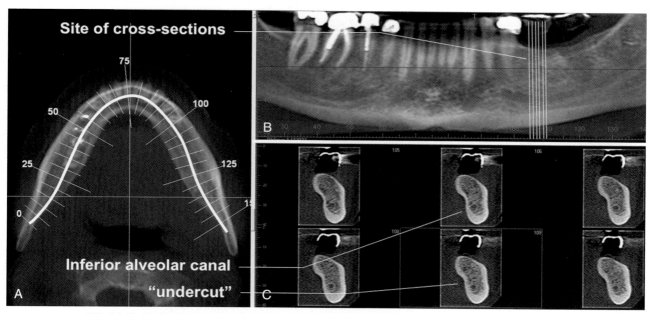

FIG. **14-5** **Multiplanar Reformation.** A thick axial image simulating an occlusal image **(A)** with an MPR oblique curved line *(white solid)* and resultant "panoramic" **(B)** and serial cross-sectional 1-mm-thick images **(C)** of a potential implant site in the lower left mandible. The axial and panoramic images are used as reference images to show the location of the cross-sectional images. The cross-sectional images demonstrate the amount of undercut and location of the inferior alveolar canal.

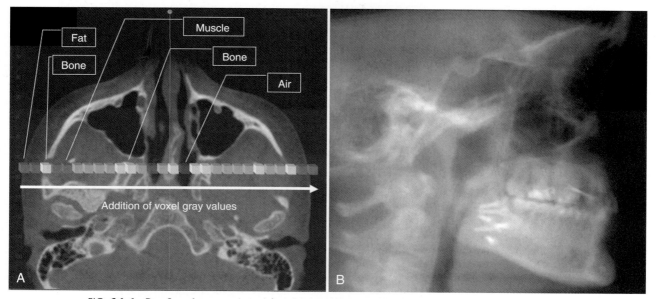

FIG. **14-6** **Ray Sum Images.** An axial projection **(A)** is used as the reference image. A section slice is identified that, in this case, corresponds to the mid sagittal plane and the thickness of this increased to include both left and right sides of the volumetric data set. As the thickness of the "slab" increases, adjacent voxels representing elements such as air, bone, and soft tissues are added. The resultant image generated **(B)** from a full-thickness ray sum provides a simulated lateral cephalometric image.

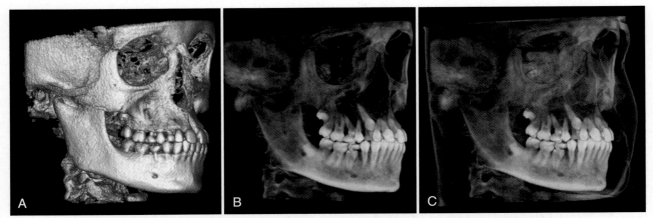

FIG. **14-7   3D Volumetric Surface Rendering.** Manual segmentation is often accomplished by an adjustable scale determining the upper and lower limit and range of intensity values to include in the segmentation. The visual result of changes in this scale is displayed in "real time" so that the effects of incremental changes can be visualized. The segmentation may be optimized to reveal the objects of interest including **(A)** bone as a solid surface or shaded surface display, **(B)** bone and the dentition under the bone as a transparency using volumetric imaging, or **(C)** bone, the dentition, and the soft tissue surface using volumetric imaging. (Segmentation performed with Dolphin 3D, Chatsworth, Calif.)

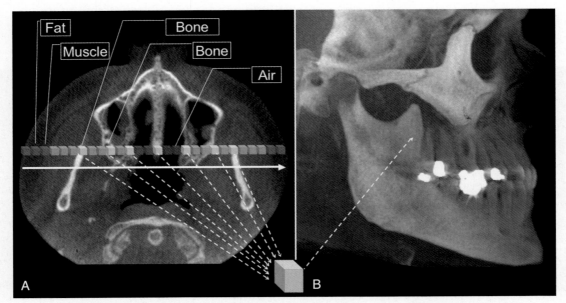

FIG. **14-8   Maximum Intensity Projection.** This method produces a "pseudo" 3D image by evaluating each voxel value along an imaginary projection ray from the observer's eyes within the data set and then representing only the highest value as the display value. In this example, an axial projection **(A)** is used as the reference image. A projection ray is identified throughout the entire volumetric data set along which individual voxels are identified, each with varying grayscale intensity corresponding to various tissue densities such as fat, muscle, air, and bone. The MIP algorithm selects only those values along the projection ray that have the highest values (usually corresponding to bone) and represents this as only one pixel on the resultant image **(B).**

diagnostic benefits are greater than the individual detriment radiation exposure might cause. Currently CBCT is most commonly used in the assessment of pathologic conditions and structural maxillofacial deformity, the preoperative assessment of orthodontics, and in the assessment of available bone for implant placement. It is advisable that the indication for the CBCT examination be documented by entry in the patient's chart or on the written request or prescriptive order for the CBCT examination.

## PATIENT PREPARATION

Patients should be escorted into the scanner unit and before head stabilization provided with appropriate personal radiation barrier protection. Although the mandatory use of these devices is regulated by regional (state) or federal legislation, it is recommended that at least a leaded torso apron be applied correctly (above the collar) to the patient. This is particularly advisable for pregnant patients and for children. It is highly recommended that a lead thyroid collar also be used, provided that this will not interfere with the scan, to reduce thyroid exposure.

Each CBCT unit has a unique method of head stabilization, varying from chin cups to posterior or lateral head supports to head restraints. Patient motion can be minimized by application of one or more methods simultaneously. Image quality is severely degraded by head movement, so it is important to obtain patient compliance.

Alignment of the area of interest with the x-ray beam is critical in imaging the appropriate field, thereby reducing patient radiation exposure and optimizing image quality by reducing scattered radiation. Often facial topographic reference planes (e.g., the mid sagittal plane, Frankfort horizontal) or internal references (e.g., occlusal plane, palatal plane) are adjusted to coincide or be aligned with external laser lights to position the patient correctly.

Immediately before the scan, the patient should be asked to remove all metallic objects form the head and neck areas. This includes eyeglasses, jewelry (including earrings and piercings), and metallic partial dentures. It is not necessary to remove plastic completely removable prostheses. Unless specifically indicated otherwise (e.g., closed temporomandibular [TMJ] views or orthodontic views), it is desirable that the dentition be separated but held together firmly during the scan. This can be performed with a tongue depressor or cotton rolls. Separation of the teeth is particularly useful in single arch scans where scatter from metallic restorations in the opposing arch can be reduced. The patient should be directed to remain as still as possible before exposure, to breathe slowly through the nose, and to close the eyes. This latter suggestion reduces the possibility of the patient moving as a result of following the detector as it passes in front of the face.

## IMAGING PROTOCOL

An imaging protocol is a set of technical exposure parameters for CBCT dependent on the specified purpose of the examination. An imaging protocol is developed to produce images of optimal quality with the least amount of radiation exposure to the patient. For specific cone beam units, manufacturer-provided imaging protocols are usually available. Most commonly they involve modifications in imaging field, number of basis projections, and voxel resolution. Operators should be aware of the effects of all parameters on image quality and patient dose when choosing imaging protocols.

### Voxel Size
The voxel size with which projection images are acquired varies from manufacturer to manufacturer principally on the basis of the matrix size of the detector and projection geometry. In addition, CBCT units may offer a selection of voxel sizes. For these choices the image detector collects information over a series of pixels in the horizontal and vertical directions and averages the data. This collation or pixel binning results in a substantial reduction in data processing, reducing secondary reconstruction times. Therefore voxel size should be specified as either acquisition or reconstruction. Generally, decreasing voxel size increases spatial resolution, but because of the pixel fill factor of a particular flat panel, a higher radiation dose may be required.

### Scan Time and Number of Projections
Adjusting the frame rate to increase the number of basis image projections provides reconstructed images with fewer artifacts and better image quality (Fig. 14-9). However, increasing the number of projections increases patient radiation exposure proportionately.

### Scanning Trajectory
Reconstructed images from incomplete, limited, or truncated scanning trajectories may suffer from strong limited-angle artifacts because of missing information. Images created with incomplete scanning arcs suffer from greater peripheral unidirectional streaking artifacts and more pronounced mid plane cupping and photon starvation artifacts. Missing data can be somewhat compensated for with a number of approaches, including use of statistical knowledge of the patient's anatomy and use of a number of algorithm projection completion techniques.

### Field of View
Collimation of the CBCT primary x-ray beam enables limitation of the x radiation to the area of interest. This functionality provides dose savings by limiting the irradiation field to fit the field of view (FOV), with a reduced exposure dose to the patient and improved image quality because of reduced scattered radiation (see Fig. 14-9).

## IMAGE OPTIMIZATION

Most programs offer the user means to adjust brightness, contrast, and edge sharpening. To optimize image presentation and facilitate diagnosis, it is necessary to adjust contrast (window) and brightness (level) parameters to favor bony structures. Great variability exists in cone beam imaging between CBCT units and within the same unit depending on the number of scans performed. Although CBCT proprietary software may provide for window/level presets, it is advisable that this be adjusted for each scan. After these parameters are set, further enhancements can be performed by the application of sharpening, filtering, and edge algorithms. The use of these functions must be weighed against the visual effects of increased noise in the image (Fig. 14-10).

## REPORTS

Cone-beam imaging comprises not only the technical component of patient exposure but a responsibility for interpreting the resultant volumetric data set. Documentation of an imaging examination is an important part of a patient's medical record. The mechanics of image reporting include the development of a series of images formatted to display the condition/region appropriately (image report) and a

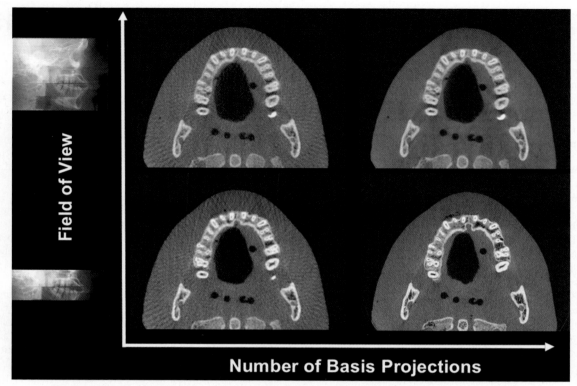

FIG. **14-9    Pictorial Plot of the Effect of Number of Basis Projection Images and Size of FOV on Image Quality.** Increasing number of projections in one 360-degree scan (x-axis) provides more data and reduces image noise; however, it increases patient dose proportionately. Reducing the number of projections creates undersampling and produces streaks. Minimizing the FOV reduces patient exposure and resultant scatter radiation and decreases image noise.

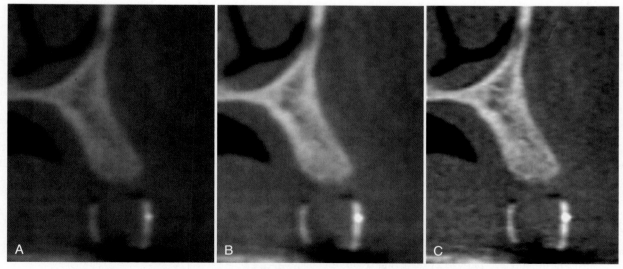

FIG. **14-10    Effect of Image Enhancement on CBCT Images.** The visual effect of three sequential adjustments on corrected MPR cross-sectional images. **A,** Default image after interpolation algorithm—smoothens edges of cortical bone but adds blur to high-contrast structures. **B,** Adjustment of window level and width to bone preset (W/L: 3000/500). **C,** Addition of mild sharpen algorithm. (Images captured with i-CAT, ISI, Hatfield, Pa, created with XoranCat software, Xoran Technologies, Inc., Ann Arbor, Mich.)

cognitive interpretation of the significance of the imaging findings (interpretive report).

## ARCHIVING, EXPORT, AND DISTRIBUTION

The process of CBCT imaging produces two data products, the volumetric image data from the scan and the image report generated by the operator. Both sets of data must be archived and distributed. Scan data backup is usually performed in its native or proprietary image format. However, export of image data is usually in the DICOM (*D*igital *I*maging and *C*ommunications in *M*edicine) file format standard for use in specialized software.

## Image Artifacts

The fundamental factor that impairs CBCT image quality is image artifact. An artifact is any distortion or error in the image that is unrelated to the subject being studied. Artifacts can be classified according to their etiology.

### ACQUISITION ARTIFACTS

Artifacts can arise from limitations in the physical processes involved in the acquisition of CBCT data. As an x-ray beam passes through an object, lower energy photons are absorbed in preference to higher energy photons. This phenomenon, called *beam hardening,* results in two types of artifact: (1) distortion of metallic structures as a result of differential absorption, known as a *cupping* artifact, and (2) streaks and dark bands that can appear between two dense objects (Fig. 14-11). In clinical practice it is advised to reduce the field size, modify patient position, or separate the dental arches to avoid scanning regions susceptible to beam hardening (e.g., metallic restorations, dental implants).

### PATIENT-RELATED ARTIFACTS

Patient motion can cause misregistration of data, which appear as unsharpness in the reconstructed image. This can be minimized by restraining the head and using as short a scan time as possible. It is also important to remove metallic objects such as jewelry before scanning because of the beam-hardening artifacts described previously.

### SCANNER-RELATED ARTIFACTS

Typically scanner-related artifacts present as circular or ring streaks resulting from imperfections in scanner detection or poor calibration (Fig. 14-12). Either of these problems will result in a consistently and repetitive reading at each angular position of the detector, resulting in a circular artifact.

### CONE BEAM–RELATED ARTIFACTS

The beam projection geometry of CBCT and image reconstruction method produce three types of cone-beam–related artifacts:
- Partial volume averaging
- Undersampling
- Cone-beam effect

*Partial volume averaging* is a feature of both conventional fan and CBCT imaging. It occurs when the selected voxel size of the scan is larger than the size of the object being imaged. For instance, a voxel 1 mm on a side may contain both bone and adjacent soft tissue. In this case, the displayed pixel is not representative of either bone or soft tissue but rather becomes a weighted average of the different brightness values. Boundaries in the resultant image may present with a "step" appearance or homogeneity of pixel intensity levels. Partial volume averaging artifacts occur in regions where surfaces are rapidly changing in the z direction, for example, in the temporal bone. Selection of the smallest acquisition voxel can reduce the presence of these effects.

*Undersampling* of the object can occur when too few basis projections are provided for image reconstruction. A reduced data sample leads to misregistration, sharp edges, and noisier images as a result of *aliasing,* which appear as fine striations in the image (see Fig. 14-9). Because increasing the number of basis projections is proportional to patient exposure, the importance of this artifact should be considered in relation to the diagnostic information.

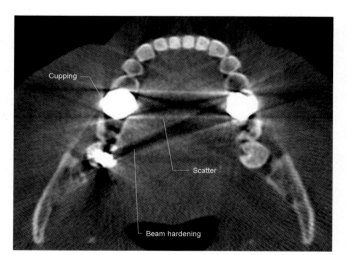

FIG. **14-11**   **CBCT Artifacts.** Axial view demonstrating beam hardening *(dark bands),* scatter *(white streaks),* and cupping (image distortion) artifacts. (Images captured with i-CAT, ISI, Hatfield, Pa.)

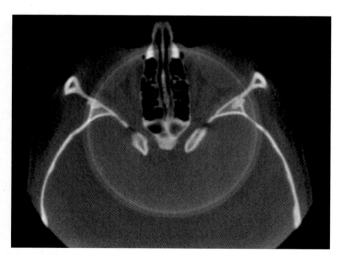

FIG. **14-12**   **CBCT Artifacts.** Visual appearance of scanner-related artifacts as circular rings on axial image indicating imperfections in scanner detection as a result of poor calibration. (Images captured with i-CAT, ISI, Hatfield, Pa.)

The *cone beam effect* is a potential source of artifacts, especially in the peripheral portions of the scan volume. Because of the divergence of the x-ray beam as it rotates around the patient in a horizontal plane, structures at the top or bottom of the image field will only be exposed when the x-ray source is on the opposite side of the patient. This results in image distortion, streaking artifacts, and greater peripheral noise. This effect is minimized by manufacturers incorporating various forms of cone-beam reconstruction. Clinically it can be reduced by positioning the region of interest in the horizontal plane of the x-ray beam.

## Strengths and Limitations

Cone-beam imaging has a number of features that make it suitable for many dental applications, but it also has a number of limitations.

## STRENGTHS

### Size and Cost
CBCT equipment has a greatly reduced size and physical footprint compared with conventional CT and it is approximately one fourth to one fifth the cost. Both these features make it available for the dental office.

### High-Speed Scanning
Compared with conventional CT, the time for the CBCT scanning is substantially reduced and, for most equipment, is less than 30 seconds. This is because the CBCT requires only a single scan to capture the necessary data compared with conventional CT scanners, where several fan beam rotations are required to complete the imaging of an object.

### Submillimeter Resolution
Currently all CBCT units use megapixel solid-state devices for x-ray detection. These devices provide submillimeter pixel resolution of component basis projection images. The size of these voxels determines the resolution of the image. CBCT produces images with submillimeter voxel resolution ranging from 0.4 mm to as low as 0.125 mm. Because of this characteristic, coronal and subsequent MPR of CBCT data has the same resolution as axial data. This level of spatial resolution is applicable for maxillofacial applications.

### Low Patient Radiation Dose
Published reports indicate that the effective dose (2005 International Committee on Radiation Protection) for various CBCT devices ranges from 52 to 1025 microsieverts ($\mu$Sv) depending on the type and model of CBCT equipment and imaging protocol used. These values are approximately equivalent to 4 to 77 digital panoramic radiographs (approximately 13.3 $\mu$Sv) or 5 to 103 days equivalent per capita background dose (approximately 3600 $\mu$Sv in the United States). Patient radiation dose can be lowered by collimating the beam, elevating the chin, and using thyroid and cervical spine shielding. CBCT provides a range of dose reductions of between 96% and 51% compared with conventional head CT (range 1400 to 2100 $\mu$Sv).

### Interactive Analysis
CBCT data reconstruction and viewing is performed natively by use of a personal computer. In addition, some manufacturers provide software with extended functionality for specific applications such as implant placement or orthodontic analysis. Finally, the availability of cursor-driven measurement algorithms provides the practitioner with an interactive capability for real-time dimensional assessment, annotation, and measurements.

## LIMITATIONS

Although there has been enormous interest in CBCT, this technology has limitations related to the cone beam projection geometry, detector sensitivity, and contrast resolution that produce images that lack the clarity and utility of conventional CT images.

### Image Noise
The cone beam projection acquisition geometry results in a large volume being irradiated with every basis image projection. A large portion of the photons undergo Compton scattering interactions and produce scattered radiation. Most scattered radiation is produced omnidirectionally and recorded by pixels on the cone beam area detector; it does not reflect the actual attenuation of an object along a specific path of the x-ray beam. This additional recorded x-ray attenuation, reflecting nonlinear attenuation, is called *noise* and contributes to image degradation. The amount of scattered radiation is generally proportional to the total mass of tissue contained within the primary x-ray beam; this increases with increasing object thickness and field size. The contribution of this scattered radiation to production of the CBCT image may be greater than the primary beam. In clinical applications, the scatter-to-primary ratios are about 0.01 for single-ray CT and 0.05 to 0.15 for fan-beam and spiral CT and may be as large as 0.4 to 2 in CBCT.

Additional sources of image noise in CBCT are variations in the homogeneity of the incident x-ray beam (quantum mottle) and added noise of the detector system (electronic). The inhomogeneity of x-ray photons depends on the number of the primary and scattered x-ray absorbed, the primary and scattered x-ray spectra incident on the detector and the number of views (projections). Electronic noise is due to the inherent degradations of the detector system related to the x-ray absorption efficiency of energy at the detector.

In addition, because of the increased divergence of the x-ray beam over the area detector, there is a pronounced *heel effect*. This produces a large variation or *nonuniformity* of the incident x-ray beam on the patient and resultant nonuniformity in absorption with greater signal-to-noise ratio (noise) on the cathode side of the image relative to the anode side.

### Poor Soft Tissue Contrast
Contrast is the spatial variation of the x-ray photon intensities that are transmitted through the patient; contrast thus gives a measure of difference between regions in an image. The variation in transmitted intensities is a result of differential attenuation of x rays by tissues that differ in density, atomic number, and thickness. Two principal factors limit the contrast resolution of CBCT. Although scattered radiation contributes to increased noise of the image, it is also a significant factor in reducing the contrast of the cone beam system. X-ray scatter reduces subject contrast by adding background signals that are not representative of the anatomy, thereby reducing image quality.

Second, there are numerous inherent flat panel detector-based artifacts that affect its linearity or response to x radiation. Saturation (nonlinear pixel effects above a certain exposure), dark current (charge that accumulates over time with or without exposure), and bad pixels (pixels that do not react to exposure) contribute to nonlinearity. In addition, the sensitivity of different regions of the panel to radiation (pixel-to-pixel gain variation) may not be uniform over the entire region.

## Specific Applications in Dentistry

CBCT technology has had a substantial impact on maxillofacial imaging. It has been applied to diagnosis in all areas of dentistry and is now expanding into treatment applications. CBCT should not be considered a replacement for panoramic or conventional projection radiographic applications but rather as a complementary modality for specific applications.

### IMPLANT SITE ASSESSMENT

Perhaps the greatest impact of CBCT has been on the planning of dental implant placements. CBCT provides cross-sectional images of the alveolar bone height, width, and angulation and accurately depicts vital structures such as the inferior alveolar dental nerve canal in the mandible or the sinus in the maxilla. The most useful series of images for implant site assessment include the axial, reformatted panoramic, and serial transplanar images at the specific location (Fig. 14-13). In many instances a diagnostic stent is made with radiographic markers and inserted at the time of the scan (Fig. 14-14). This provides a precise reference of the location of the proposed implants or teeth.

DICOM data can be imported into third-party software applications that provide many useful tools that can be used to assess and plan both the surgical and prosthetic components of implant therapy. In addition, the data set may then be used to construct a surgical implant guidance stent to facilitate the precise placement of implants.

### ORTHODONTICS AND THREE-DIMENSIONAL CEPHALOMETRY

CBCT imaging is being used in the diagnosis, assessment, and analysis of maxillofacial orthodontic and orthopedic anomalies. CBCT provides display of the position of impacted and supernumerary teeth and their relationships to adjacent roots or other anatomic structures. This facilitates surgical exposure and planning of subsequent movement. Also, information regarding palatal morphologic features and dimensions, tooth inclination and torque, root resorption, and available alveolar bone width for buccolingual movement of teeth can be obtained. CBCT also provides adequate visualization of the TMJ, the pharyngeal airway space, and soft tissue relationships.

Perhaps the greatest potential use of CBCT in orthodontics is that it is capable of providing both conventional two- and three-dimensional cephalometric images in one acquisition. CBCT data sets can be manipulated by the ray sum technique to generate simulated panoramic, lateral, submentovertex, and posteroanterior

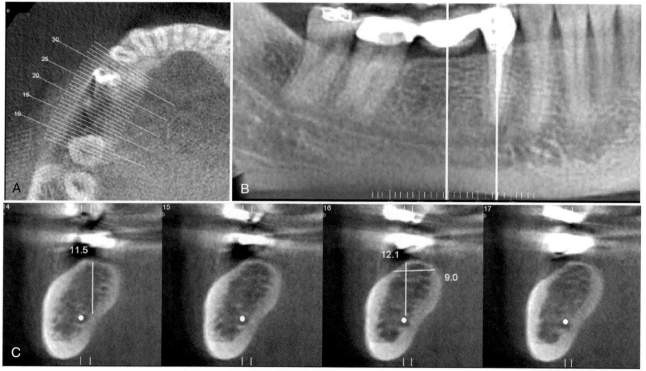

FIG. **14-13** **CBCT for Implant Site Assessment.** A curved planar MPR is accomplished by aligning the long axis of the imaging plane with the dental arch **(A)**, providing a region panorama-like thin-slice image **(B)**. In addition, serial thin-slice transplanar images are often generated **(C)**, useful in the assessment of specific morphologic features such as the location of the inferior alveolar canal (shown with a *white dot*) for implant site assessment and for allowing measurement of the available alveolar bone height and width. (Images captured and created with Newtom 3G, AFP Imaging Corp., Elmsford, N.Y.)

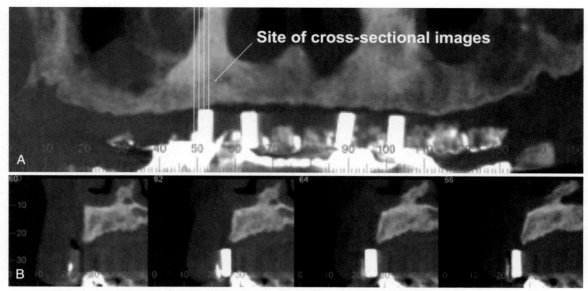

FIG. **14-14**    **Use of a Diagnostic Stent.** Stents provide fiducial radiographic landmarks that can be used to correlate proposed clinical location and angulation of implants with the available alveolar bone. The panoramic projection **(A)** provides an overview of location, whereas serial cross-sectional images **(B)** indicate alveolar bone height. In this example, the four transplanar images of the maxillary right canine region indicate that the proposed placement is too far buccal and too perpendicular to engage the available bone. (Images captured with i-CAT, ISI, Hatfield, Pa, created with XoranCat software, Xoran Technologies, Inc., Ann Arbor, Mich.)

cephalometric images (Fig. 14-15). Alternatively, it is possible to extract the topographic features of the skull and air/soft tissue interfaces in high detail by using a variety of orthodontic-centered products. There are numerous potential benefits to 3D cephalometry including accuracy of linear measurements, visual demonstration of dentoskeletal relationships and facial esthetics, and the potential for assessment of growth and development (Fig. 14-16).

## LOCALIZATION OF THE INFERIOR ALVEOLAR CANAL

The relationship of the inferior alveolar canal to the roots of mandibular third molar teeth is of importance when attempting to minimize the likelihood of nerve damage that may lead to permanent loss of sensation to one side to the lower lip. Thus accurate assessment of the position of the canal in relation to the impacted third molar may reduce injuries to this nerve. Traditional panoramic imaging may be adequate when the third molar is clear of the canal, but in the case of radiographic superimposition it is advisable to use a 3D imaging approach. This can be achieved at comparatively low radiation dose with CBCT combined either with the proprietary software accompanying the imaging device or with a third-party diagnostic software (Fig. 14-17).

## TEMPOROMANDIBULAR JOINT

CBCT provides multiplanar and potentially 3D images of the condyle and surrounding structures to facilitate analysis and diagnosis of bone morphologic features, joint space and dynamic function, critical keys to providing appropriate treatment outcomes in patients with TMJ signs and symptoms. Imaging can depict the features of degenerative joint disease (Fig. 14-18), developmental anomalies of the condyle, ankylosis,

and rheumatoid arthritic disease. Appropriate imaging protocols should include reformatted panoramic and axial reference images, corrected parasagittal and paracoronal transerial slices, and for those cases in which asymmetry or surgery is contemplated, 3D reconstructions.

## CONDITIONS OF THE MAXILLOFACIAL COMPLEX

CBCT can assist in the assessment of many conditions of the jaws, most notably dental conditions such as impacted canines and supernumerary teeth, fractured or split teeth, periapical lesions, and periodontal disease (Fig. 14-19). Benign calcifications (e.g., tonsilloliths, lymph nodes, salivary gland stones) can also be identified by location and differentiated from potentially significant calcifications of the arteries such as carotid artery calcifications or veins (e.g., phleboliths). Although CBCT does not provide suitable soft tissue contrast to distinguish the contents of paranasal opacifications, the morphologic characteristics and extent of these lesions are particularly well seen (e.g., mucous extravasation cyst).

Most important, the location, size, shape, extent, and full involvement of jaw conditions can be visualized with a combination of two- and three-dimensional images. CBCT has been found to be particularly useful for trauma (Fig. 14-20) and for visualizing the extent and degree of involvement of osteomyelitis.

## RAPID PROTOTYPING

Rapid prototyping (RP) is broad term used to describe a group of related processes and techniques that are used to fabricate physical scale models directly from 3D computer-assisted design data. The purpose of RP in maxillofacial imaging is to create a life-size, dimensionally accurate model of an anatomic structure. These models are

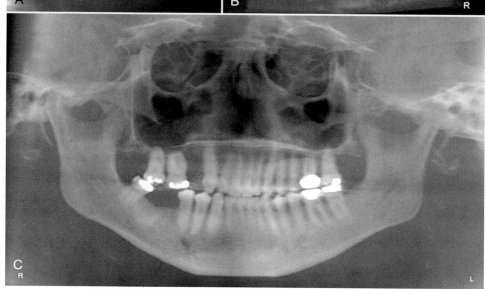

FIG. **14-15** Two-dimensional Projections Generated with Cone Beam Data Set. This patient had an asymmetry of one side of the face. Ray sum reformation of the CBCT data was performed to provide multiple conventional images such as the lateral cephalometric **(A)**, frontal cephalometric or posteroanterior **(B)**, and panoramic **(C)** projections. (Images generated with Dolphin 3D, Chatsworth, Calif.)

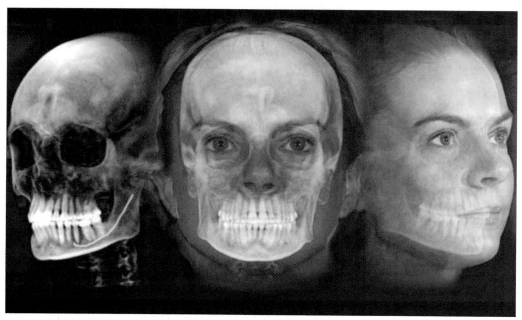

FIG. **14-16** Fusion. 3D anatomic views demonstrating imaging possibilities with fusion of CBCT data and photographic image sets. (Images created with 3DMD, Atlanta, Ga. courtesy Dr. Chester Wang).

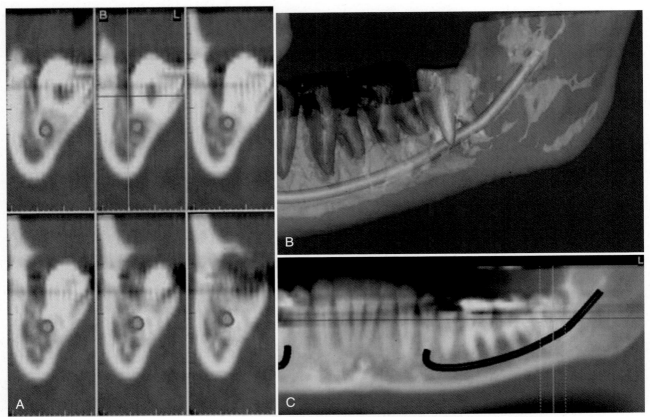

FIG. **14-17   Region Reconstructed. A,** Cross-sectional views. **B,** Third-party software used to demonstrate location of inferior alveolar canal to an impacted third molar in 3D images. **C,** MPR reformatted images using proprietary software demonstrating proximity of the root of an unerupted and impacted third molar associated with the inferior alveolar canal. (Images created with Simplant, Materialise, Leuven, Belgium, courtesy 3DDX, Brighton, Mass.)

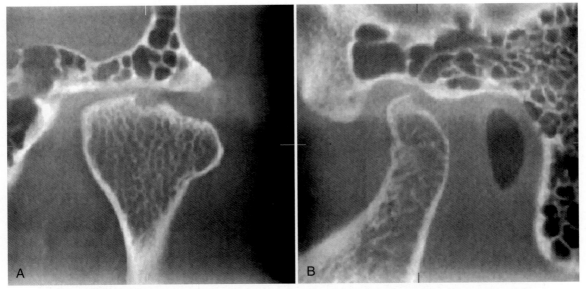

FIG. **14-18   Regional Cone-Beam Imaging. A,** Corrected coronal and, **B,** sagittal images of a right TMJ with erosive defects on the superior surface of the condyle associated with active mild degenerative joint disease. (Images captured and created with 3DX Accuitomo, J. Morita Mfg. Corp., Kyoto, Japan.)

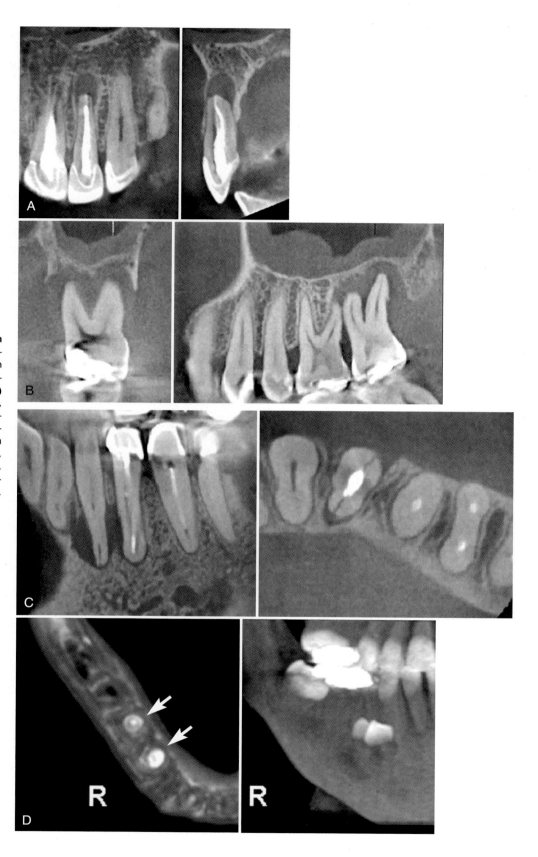

FIG. **14-19 Regional Cone-Beam Imaging.** Numerous dental conditions can be demonstrated in high resolution with regional CBCT, including **(A)** periapical condition, **(B)** periodontal and periapical disease, **(C)** root fracture and associated alveolar bone loss, and **(D)** supernumerary teeth. (Images **A-C** captured with 3DX Accuitomo, J. Morita Mfg. Corp., Kyoto, Japan. **D** captured with i-CAT, ISI, Hatfield, Pa., created using XoranCat software, Xoran Technologies, Inc., Ann Arbor, Mich.)

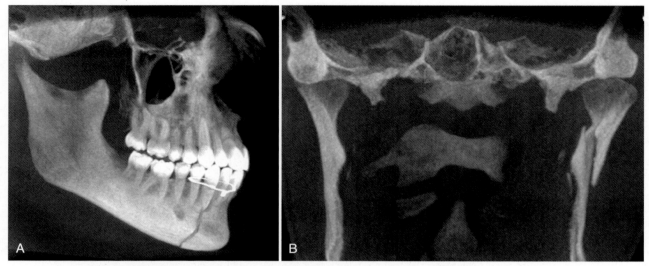

FIG. **14-20** **Fracture Demonstration.** Use of MIP projections in the assessment of complex mandibular fractures. **A,** an oblique thin slab MPR image with a MIP application demonstrates a simple, slightly displaced fracture of the right parasymphyseal region, whereas, **B,** a coronal thin slab MIP image demonstrates a comminuted displaced left subcondylar neck fracture. (Images captured with i-CAT, ISI, Hatfield, Pa., created using XoranCat software, Xoran Technologies, Inc., Ann Arbor, Mich.)

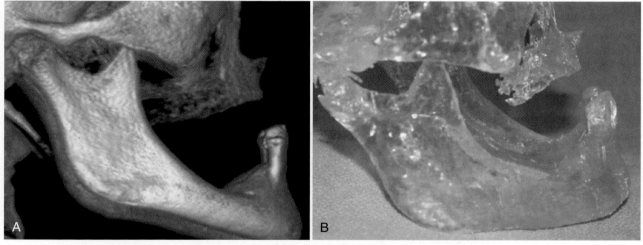

FIG. **14-21** **Rapid Prototype.** **A,** 3D volumetric reconstruction from CBCT data. **B,** Rapid prototype constructed model of patient with right-sided chemically induced osteonecrosis. Modeling was performed before surgical resection and reconstruction to provide addition of bone in the right mandibular premolar area. (Volumetric rendering performed with 3DVR, AlloVision LLC, Greenville, S.C.)

also referred to as *biomodels*. DICOM data imported to proprietary software can be used to compute 3D images generated by thresholding the intensity of the voxel values to be displayed and segmenting these from the background. The models produced are used for presurgical planning of a number of complex maxillofacial surgical cases, including craniofacial reconstruction for correction of deformity caused by trauma, tumor resection, distraction osteogenesis, and, more widely, dental implants (Fig. 14-21). The models provide the practitioner with a higher level of confidence before he or she performs a surgical procedure and may reduce surgical and anesthetic time.

## Conclusion

CBCT imaging systems have been recently been introduced for imaging hard tissues of the maxillofacial region. CBCT is capable of providing accurate, submillimeter resolution images at shorter scan times, lower dose, and lower costs compared with medical fan-beam CT. Increasing availability of this technology provides the practitioner with an imaging modality capable of providing a 3D representation that is extending maxillofacial imaging from diagnosis to image guidance of operative and surgical procedures.

# BIBLIOGRAPHY

## RADIATION DOSE

Dula K, Mini R, van der Stelt PF et al: Hypothetical mortality risk associated with spiral computed tomography of the maxilla and mandible, *Eur J Oral Sci* 104:503-510, 1996.

Ludlow JB, Davies-Ludlow LE, Brooks SL: Dosimetry of two extraoral direct digital imaging devices: NewTom cone beam CT and Orthophos Plus DS panoramic unit, *Dentomaxillofac Radiol* 32:229-234, 2003.

Ludlow JB, Davies-Ludlow LE, Brooks SL et al: Dosimetry of 3 CBCT devices for oral and maxillofacial radiology: CB Mercuray, NewTom 3G and i-CAT, *Dentomaxillofac Radiol* 35:219-226, 2006 [erratum in *Dentomaxillofac Radiol* 35:392, 2006].

Mah JK, Danforth RA, Bumann A et al: Radiation absorbed in maxillofacial imaging with a new dental computed tomography device, *Oral Surg Oral Med Oral Pathol Oral Radiol Endod* 96:508-513, 2003.

Nakajima A, Sameshima GT, Arai Y et al: Two- and three-dimensional orthodontic imaging using limited cone beam-computed tomography, *Angle Orthod* 75:895-903, 2005.

Schulze D, Heiland M, Thurmann H et al: Radiation exposure during midfacial imaging using 4- and 16-slice computed tomography, cone beam computed tomography systems and conventional radiography, *Dentomaxillofac Radiol* 33:83-86, 2004.

## IMAGE RECONSTRUCTION

Endo M, Tsunoo T, Nakamori N et al: Effect of scattered radiation on image noise in cone beam CT, *Med Phys* 28:469-474, 2001.

Feldkamp LA, Davis LC, Kress JW: Practical cone-beam algorithm, *J Opt Soc Am* 1:612-619, 1984.

Siewerdsen JH, Jaffray DA: Cone-beam computed tomography with a flat-panel imager: magnitude and effects of x-ray scatter, *Med Phys* 28:220-231, 2001.

## CLINICAL APPLICATIONS

Cotton TP, Geisler TM, Holden DT et al: Endodontic applications of cone-beam volumetric tomography, *J Endod* 33:1121-1132, 2007.

D'Urso PS, Barker TM, Earwaker WJ et al: Stereolithography biomodelling in cranio-maxillofacial surgery: a prospective trial, *J Craniomaxillofac Surg* 27:30-37, 1999.

Holberg C, Steinhauser S, Geis P et al: Cone-beam computed tomography in orthodontics: benefits and limitations, *J Orofacac Orthop* 66:434-444, 2005.

Scarfe WC, Farman AG, Sukovic P: Clinical applications of cone-beam computed tomography in dental practice, *J Can Dent Assoc* 72:75-80, 2006.

Swennen GR, Schutyser F: Three-dimensional cephalometry: spiral multi-slice vs cone-beam computed tomography, *Am J Orthod Dentofacial Orthop* 130:410-416, 2006.

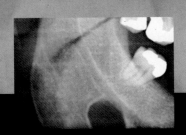

# Guidelines for Prescribing Dental Radiographs

Sharon L. Brooks

The decision to conduct a radiographic examination should be based on the individual needs of the patient. These needs are determined by findings from the dental history and clinical examination and modified by patient age and general health. A radiographic examination is necessary when the history and clinical examination have not provided enough information for complete evaluation of a patient's condition and formulation of an appropriate treatment plan. Radiographic exposures are necessary only when, in the dentist's judgment, it is reasonably likely that the patient will benefit by the discovery of clinically useful information on the radiograph.

## Role of Radiographs in Disease Detection and Monitoring

The goal of dental care is to preserve and improve patients' oral health while minimizing other health-related risks. Although the diagnostic information provided by radiographs may be of definite benefit to the patient, the radiographic examination does carry the potential for harm from exposure to ionizing radiation. One of the most effective means of reducing possible harm is to avoid making radiographs that will not contribute information pertinent to patient care. The judgment that underlies the decision to make a radiographic examination centers on several factors, including the following:

- Prevalence of the diseases that may be detected radiographically in the oral cavity
- Ability of the clinician to detect these diseases clinically and radiographically
- Consequences of undetected and untreated disease
- Impact of asymptomatic anatomic and pathologic variations detected radiographically on patient treatment

As a general principle, radiographs are indicated when a reasonable probability exists that they will provide valuable information about a disease that is not evident clinically. Conversely, radiographs are not indicated when they are unlikely to yield information contributing to patient care. Radiographic information considered clinically useful includes data that are valuable in detecting disease and in monitoring the progression of known diseases.

For many clinical situations it is not readily apparent to the practitioner whether radiographs have a reasonable probability of providing valuable information. In these situations it is up to the practitioner's clinical judgment after weighing the patient factors to decide whether radiographs are indicated.

The philosophy of taking radiographs only when there is a high probability of obtaining clinically useful information has been advocated by all the organizations responsible for developing or endorsing guidelines for ordering radiographs. However, many dentists use radiographs as a screening tool, simply to see "what's there," without having a specific suspicion of disease arising from the dental history or clinical examination. There are probably a number of reasons for doing this. Some dentists think that they have not provided an adequate service to their patients if they cannot assure them that they have searched diligently for disease with all reasonable diagnostic methods, including radiographs. They may state that having complete information, regardless of whether it affects the treatment plan, is of such benefit that it outweighs the risk of the radiation exposure. Other dentists raise medicolegal issues, stating fear of lawsuits if they fail to detect disease. Others express concern about the effect on the efficiency of the dental office of the extended examinations required for prescribing radiographs on the basis of signs and symptoms. The next few paragraphs will address these concerns.

Unlike their use in dentistry, screening radiographs are rarely used in medicine, with the exception of mammography for women above a certain age or with increased risk factors for breast cancer, and there is controversy over whether even this type of examination should be used as frequently as it is today. Breast cancer is a relatively common yet serious disease that should be detected early, before the cancer becomes large enough to be found clinically. On the other hand, diseases of the jaws (with the exceptions of caries, periapical and periodontal disease) are rare and concentrated in certain ages, sexes, and ethnicities. These diseases are unlikely to be discovered on routine screening radiographs before they have produced signs or symptoms that could be found on a thorough clinical examination and history. Periodontal disease can be diagnosed clinically, although radiographs are used to determine the extent of bone loss and the presence of other factors that may affect prognosis. Periapical disease is usually associated with extensive restorations or caries that can be detected clinically. Dental caries on proximal surfaces, however, may not be detectable on clinical examination until it has reached an advanced stage; thus this is one occult disease for which screening radiographs are considered appropriate. Regarding the threat of lawsuits for failure to diagnose, dentists who follow guidelines on radiographs developed or endorsed by authoritative bodies that help establish the standard of care should have no concerns. Although lawsuits can be filed for many reasons, it is unlikely that they will be successful if it can be shown that the practitioner did a *thorough* clinical examination and history and carefully considered the guidelines when determining whether to order radiographs.

Some dentists set up their practices so that new patients are automatically seen first by the dental hygienist, who takes a predetermined set of radiographs at the first appointment, before the dentist sees the patient. Although this may make efficient use of the dentist's time, it is contrary to the recommendations of the American Dental Association (ADA) that the selection of radiographs should be based on the findings of the clinical examination. Performing a thorough examination before radiographs are ordered should not be an insurmountable obstacle for an efficient dental practice.

Regarding the issue of cost versus benefit of radiographs, for any individual patient there is little risk of harm from a set of radiographs, even if no important diagnostic information is revealed. However, there is a large societal cost, both in terms of health care dollars and radiation risk, if millions of dental patients receive unproductive radiographic examinations, as would happen if routine screening were widespread.

Our philosophy is that radiographs should be based on the need for diagnostic information for patients on a case-by-case basis. For that reason, the next section will discuss some of the clinical situations that may call for a radiographic examination.

## CARIES

Dental caries is the most common dental disease, affecting people of all ages. Although the caries prevalence rates of developed countries have been decreasing since the 1970s, probably partially as a result of the widespread use of fluoride, increasing numbers of older adults are maintaining their teeth throughout their lifetimes, leaving them at risk for developing both coronal and root caries. Although occlusal, buccal, and lingual carious lesions are reasonably easy to detect clinically, interproximal caries and caries associated with existing restorations are much more difficult to detect with only a clinical examination (see Chapter 17). Studies have repeatedly demonstrated that clinicians using radiographs detect caries not evident clinically, both in enamel and in dentin. Although a radiographic examination is very important for diagnosis of dental caries, the optimal frequency for such an examination should be based on mitigating features such as the patient's age, medical condition, diet, oral hygiene practices, oral health status, and the nature of the caries process itself.

Carious lesions demonstrate one of three behaviors: progression, arrest, or regression. Only about 50% of lesions progress beyond the initial, just-detectable defect, and in most instances the lesions demonstrate a slow rate of progression through enamel (months to years). Mechanisms are also in use to enhance remineralization of early enamel lesions. However, the rate of caries progression is significantly faster in deciduous than in permanent enamel, and patients vary widely in their rates of formation of caries and in their rates of caries progression.

Because the presence of caries cannot be determined with confidence by clinical examination alone, it is necessary to expose patients periodically through bitewing radiography to monitor dental caries. The length of the exposure intervals varies considerably because of different patient circumstances. For most patients in good physical health with adequate oral hygiene, an infrequent radiographic examination is needed to monitor dental caries. However, if the patient history and clinical examination suggest that the individual has a relatively high caries experience, shorter intervals allow careful monitoring of disease.

## PERIODONTAL DISEASES

Some form of periodontal disease affects most people at some point during their lives, gingivitis more often in younger individuals and periodontitis more commonly in older adults. Periodontal diseases are responsible for a substantial portion of all teeth lost. A consensus exists among practitioners that radiographic examinations play an important role in the evaluation of patients with periodontal disease after the disease is initially detected on clinical examination (see Chapter 18). In addition to providing a picture of the extent of alveolar bone support for the dentition, radiographic examinations help demonstrate local factors that complicate the disease, including the presence of gingival irritants such as calculus and faulty restorations. Occasionally the length and morphologic features of roots, visible on periapical radiographs, are crucial factors in the prognosis of the disease. These observations suggest that, when clinical evidence exists of periodontal disease other than nonspecific gingivitis, it is appropriate to make radiographs, generally a combination of periapicals and bitewings, to help establish the severity of the disease. Follow-up radiographs after therapy is complete will help the clinician monitor the progression of disease and determine whether the destruction of alveolar bone has been halted.

## DENTAL ANOMALIES

Abnormal formation of teeth may be manifested as deviations in number, size, and composition. These abnormalities in dental development occur more frequently, and are more likely to have a serious impact, in the permanent dentition than in the primary dentition. The most frequently encountered anomalies are the presence of supernumerary teeth, usually mesiodens, or developmentally absent teeth, usually second premolars (see Chapter 19).

Few anomalies exist for which orthodontic treatment or surgical correction or modification must start at an early age. When the dentist suspects an abnormality requiring treatment, radiographs to confirm and localize it are not required until the time when the treatment is most appropriate. For example, a panoramic examination of a 5-year-old child to determine the presence or absence of permanent teeth may be ill timed. Although the examination provides evidence that one or more second premolars or lateral incisors are developmentally missing, this information usually does not influence the current treatment plan. When examination for dental anomalies is appropriate, both the radiation dose and the anticipated diagnostic benefit should be considered. Projections that best demonstrate the required diagnostic information should be selected. A panoramic radiograph of the lower face is usually best for observing the presence or absence of teeth in all quadrants, although a periapical film or an occlusal film is sufficient for an examination limited to one area.

## GROWTH AND DEVELOPMENT AND DENTAL MALOCCLUSION

Children and adolescents are often examined to assess the growth and development of the teeth and jaws. This assessment considers the relationship of one jaw to the other and to the soft tissues. An examination of occlusion, growth, and development requires an individualized radiographic examination that may include periapicals or a panoramic examination to supplement any radiographs ordered to assess dental disease. In addition, a patient of any age group who is being considered for orthodontic treatment may need other radiographs, such as a lateral or frontal cephalograph, occlusal view, carpal index, or temporomandibular joint (TMJ) radiograph, depending on the clinical findings (Fig. 15-1).

Cone-beam computed tomography (CBCT) is being used increasingly frequently for orthodontic evaluation, to provide three-dimensional information about jaw relationships, and to substitute for multiple other imaging examinations (see Chapter 14). At this time it is not yet clear which patients will benefit from CBCT in terms of treatment considerations.

The dentist who is the primary provider of orthodontic treatment should select the number and type of radiographs needed. The needs of each patient should be considered individually. Selected radiographs should allow a maximal diagnostic yield with a minimal radiographic exposure after consideration of the clinical examination, the study of plaster models and photographs, and the optimal time to initiate treatment.

## OCCULT DISEASE

*Occult disease* refers to disease that presents no clinical signs or symptoms. Occult diseases in the jaws include a combination of dental and intraosseous findings. Dental findings may include incipient carious lesions, resorbed or dilacerated roots, and hypercementosis. Intraosseous findings include osteosclerosis, unerupted teeth, periapical disease, and a wide variety of cysts and benign and malignant tumors

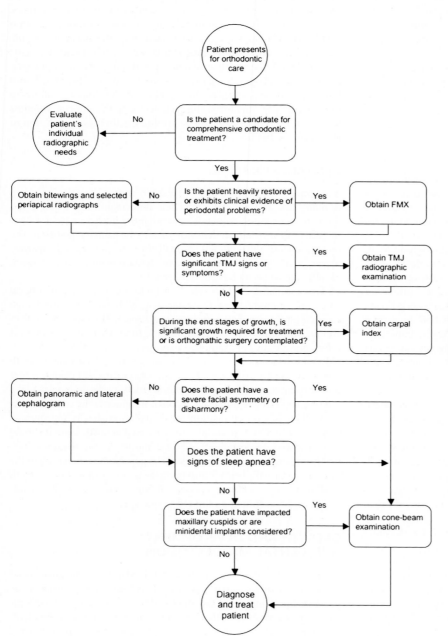

FIG. **15-1** An example of a clinical algorithm to order radiographs for orthodontic patients. Selected radiographs are ordered after the dentist's consideration of the patient's history and clinical characteristics.

(see Chapters 20 through 25). Small carious lesions, resorption of root structure, and bony lesions may go unnoticed until signs and symptoms develop.

Although the consequences of some occult diseases may be quite serious, most serious diseases are rare. Often a historical or clinical sign or symptom of intraosseous disease suggests its presence. For instance, an unusual contour of bone or an absent third molar, not explained by a history of extraction, suggests the possibility of an impaction with the potential for an associated dentigerous cyst. Although patient history and clinical signs and symptoms do not always accurately predict the finding of dental and intraosseous findings, the majority of these true occult diseases are not clinically relevant or they are so rare that, except for caries as described previously, the dentist need not obtain a radiographic examination of the jaws solely to screen for them in dentate individuals in the absence of unusual clinical signs or symptoms. Caries is an exception because of its much higher prevalence than other occult diseases.

There is a considerable difference of opinion on whether asymptomatic edentulous patients seen for routine denture construction should have screening radiographs taken to look for occult disease. Several studies have demonstrated a relatively large number of lesions on radiographs of edentulous patients, including retained root tips and areas of sclerotic bone, but almost all these findings required no treatment and did not affect the outcome of care. For that reason, some recommend no radiographs of edentulous patients if the clinical examination is negative for signs and symptoms of disease. Others still think that screening radiographs of these patients are of value. As the standard of care for completely or partially edentulous patients moves toward dental implants rather than removable prosthetics, imaging to assess the quantity and quality of bone available for implants is gaining in importance.

There has been increasing interest in the last few years in using panoramic radiographs to screen patients for the presence of calcified atheromas in the bifurcation of the carotid artery, a finding that may indicate an increased risk for the development of a cerebrovascular accident (stroke). However, the value of this finding has been questioned recently because a noncalcified vulnerable plaque, which is not visible on panoramic radiographs, may put the patient at more risk for stroke than a more stable calcified plaque. Nevertheless, the general consensus at this time is that panoramic radiographs made for dental purposes should be evaluated for this calcification, particularly in patients older than 55 years, but that these radiographs should not be made simply to screen for atheromas without other dental indications. (See Chapter 28 for more details.)

## JAW DISEASE

Imaging of known jaw lesions, such as fibro-osseous diseases or neoplastic diseases, before biopsy and definitive treatment is also important for appropriate management of the patient. For small lesions of the jaws, periapical or panoramic radiographs may be enough as long as the lesion can be seen in its entirety. If clinical evidence of swelling exists, some type of radiograph at 90 degrees to the original plane should be made to determine whether there is expansion of the jaw or perforation of the buccal or lingual cortical bone. If lesions are too large to fit on standard dental films, extend into the maxillary sinus or other portions of the head outside the jaws, or are suspected of malignancy, additional imaging such as computed tomography (CT) or CBCT is appropriate before biopsy (see Chapters 13 and 14). This type of imaging can define the extent of the lesion, suggest an operative approach, and provide information about the nature of the lesion. The person performing the biopsy or managing the patient should order the advanced images to decrease confusion and increase coordination of care.

## TEMPOROMANDIBULAR JOINT

Many types of diseases affect the TMJ, including congenital and developmental malformations of the mandible and cranial bones; acquired disorders such as disk displacement, neoplasms, fractures, and dislocations; inflammatory diseases that produce capsulitis or synovitis; and arthritides of various types, including rheumatoid arthritis and osteoarthritis. The goal of TMJ imaging, similar to that for imaging other body parts, should be to obtain new information that will influence patient care. Radiologic examination may not be needed for all patients with signs and symptoms referable to the TMJ region, particularly if no treatment is contemplated (see Chapter 26). The decision of whether and how to image the joints should depend on the results of the history and clinical findings, the clinical diagnosis, and results of prior examinations, as well as the tentative treatment plan and expected outcome.

The cost of the examination and the radiation dose should also influence the decision if more than one type of examination can provide the desired information. For example, information about the status of the osseous tissues can be obtained from panoramic radiographs, plain films, conventional tomography, CT, CBCT, and magnetic resonance imaging (MRI). The subtlety of the expected findings and the amount of detail required should be considered when selecting the examination to perform. If soft tissue information such as disk position is necessary for patient care, MRI or arthrography is appropriate.

## IMPLANTS

An increasingly common method of replacing missing teeth is with osseointegrated implants, metal screws that are inserted into the mandible or maxilla. Prosthetic appliances are then affixed to the screws after a period of healing. Preoperative planning is crucial to ensure success of the implants. The dentist must evaluate the adequacy of the height and thickness of bone for the desired implant; the quality of the bone, including the relative proportion of medullary and cortical bone; the location of anatomic structures such as the mandibular canal or maxillary sinus; and the presence of structural abnormalities such as undercuts that may affect placement or angulation of the implant (see Chapter 32).

Standard periapical and panoramic radiographs can supply information regarding the vertical dimensions of the bone in the proposed implant site. However, some type of cross-sectional imaging (conventional tomography, CT, or CBCT) is recommended before implant placement for visualization of important anatomic landmarks, determination of size and path of insertion of implant, and evaluation of the adequacy of the bone for anchorage of the implant. There is also increasing use of implant planning software and preparation of surgical drilling guides, which require the three-dimensional data from CT or CBCT. Postoperative evaluation of implants may be needed at later times to judge healing, assess complete seating of fixtures, and ensure continued health of the surrounding bone.

## PARANASAL SINUSES

Because dentists are not usually the primary providers of treatment for acute or chronic sinus disease, the necessity to perform sinus imaging may be limited in general dental practice. However, because sinus disease can present as pain in the maxillary teeth and because periapical inflammation of maxillary molars and premolars can also lead to changes in the mucosa of the maxillary sinus, circumstances occur in which the dentist needs to obtain an image of the maxillary sinus. Another reason to image this area is to assess the need for bone augmentation/sinus lift before implant placement in the posterior maxilla. Periapical and panoramic radiographs demonstrate the floor of the maxillary sinus well, but visualization of other walls requires additional imaging techniques such as occipitomental (Waters) view, CBCT, or CT. These radiographs are best ordered by the person treating the patient so that diagnostic and therapeutic measures may be coordinated (see Chapter 27).

## TRAUMA

Patients who have sustained trauma to the oral region may visit a dentist for evaluation and management of the injuries. For proper management it is important to determine the full extent of the injuries. Periapical or panoramic radiographs are helpful for evaluation of fractures of the teeth. If a suspected root fracture is not visible on a periapical radiograph, a second radiograph made with a different angulation may be helpful. A fracture that is not perpendicular to the beam may not be detectable unless root resorption is present. Thus a tooth with a history of trauma should be monitored and evaluated radiographically on a periodic basis, even if the original radiograph is negative.

Fractures of the mandible can frequently be detected with panoramic radiographs, supplemented by images at 90 degrees such as a posteroanterior or reverse-Towne view (see Chapter 29). Trauma to the maxilla and midface may require CT or CBCT for a thorough evaluation. Affected patients are more likely to report to a hospital emergency department than to a general dental office. The hospital may have a standard protocol for trauma cases. Ideally the clinician responsible for managing care determines the appropriate radiographs for the specific case.

## Radiographic Examinations

After concluding that a patient requires a radiograph, the dentist should consider which radiographic examination is most appropriate to meet all the patient's diagnostic and treatment planning needs. A variety of radiographic projections is available. In choosing one, the dentist should consider the anatomic relationships, the size of the field, and the radiation dose from each view. Table 15-1 summarizes the more common types of radiographic examinations for general

### TABLE 15-1
### Dental Radiographic Examinations and Their Properties

| TYPE OF EXAMINATION | COVERAGE | RESOLUTION | RELATIVE EXPOSURE* | DETECTABLE DISEASE |
|---|---|---|---|---|
| **Intraoral Radiographs** | | | | |
| Periapical | Limited | High | 1 | Caries, periodontal disease, occult disease |
| Bitewings | Limited | High | 10 | Caries, periodontal bone level |
| Full-mouth periapical | Limited | High | 14-17 | Caries, periodontal disease, dental anomalies, occult disease |
| Occlusal | Moderate | High | 2.5 | Dental anomalies, occult disease, salivary stones, expansion of jaw |
| **Extraoral Radiographs** | | | | |
| Panoramic | Broad | Moderate | 1-2 | Dental anomalies, occult disease, extensive caries, periodontal disease, periapical disease, TMJ |
| Conventional tomography/slice | Moderate | Moderate | 0.2-0.6 | TMJ, implant site assessment |
| CBCT | Broad | Moderate to high | 4-42 | Implant, TMJ, craniofacial relationships, dental anomalies, extent of disease, fracture |
| CT/head | Broad | High | 25-800 | Extent of craniofacial disease, fracture, implants |
| MRI | Broad | Moderate | — | Soft tissue disease, TMJ |
| Skull | Broad | Moderate | 30 | Fracture, anatomic relation, jaw disease |

From Frederiksen N, Benson B, Sokolowski T: Effective dose and risk assessment from computed tomography of the maxillofacial complex, *Dentomaxillofac Radiol* 24:55-58, 1995; Scaf G, Lurie AG, Mosier KM et al: Dosimetry and cost of imaging osseointegrated implants with film-based and computed tomography, *Oral Surg Oral Med Oral Pathol Oral Radiol Endod* 83:41-48, 1997; White SC: 1992 assessment of radiation risks from dental radiology, *Dentomaxillofac Radiol* 21:118-126, 1992; Ludlow JB, Davies-Ludlow LE, Brooks SL et al: Dosimetry of 3 CBCT devices for oral and maxillofacial radiology: CB Mercuray, NewTom 3G and i-CAT, *Dentomaxillofac Radiol* 35:219-226, 2006.
*The parameters assume use of F-speed film and rectangular collimation for periapical films, round collimation for bitewings and occlusal views, and rare-earth screens for panoramic examinations. With D-speed film the intraoral values are more than doubled compared with F-speed film, and with round collimation the periapical values increase by 2.5 times compared with rectangular collimation.

dental patients and factors to consider in choosing the most appropriate one. For example, a panoramic radiograph provides broad area coverage with moderate resolution. Intraoral films give more detailed information but a significantly higher radiation dose per unit area exposed. The clinician must use clinical judgment to weigh these factors. Examples of all these radiographs can be found in previous chapters.

## INTRAORAL RADIOGRAPHS

Intraoral radiographs are examinations made by placing the x-ray film within the patient's mouth during the exposure. These exposures offer the dentist a high-detail view of the teeth and bone in the area exposed. Such views are most appropriate for revealing caries and periodontal and periapical disease in a localized region. A complete-mouth or full-mouth examination (FMX) consists of periapical views of all the tooth-bearing regions as well as interproximal views (see Chapter 9).

### Periapical Radiographs

Periapical views show all of a tooth and the surrounding bone and are very useful for revealing caries and periodontal and periapical disease. These views may be made of a specific tooth or region or as part of an FMX.

### Interproximal Radiographs

Interproximal views (bitewings) show the coronal aspects of both the maxillary and mandibular dentition in a region, as well as the surrounding crestal bone. These views are most useful for revealing proximal caries and evaluating the height of the alveolar bony crest. They can be made in either the anterior or posterior region of the mouth.

### Occlusal Radiographs

Occlusal views are intraoral radiographs in which the film is positioned in the occlusal plane. They are often used in lieu of periapical views in children because the small size of the patient's mouth limits film placement. In adults, occlusal radiographs may supplement periapical views, providing visualization of a greater area of teeth and bone. They are useful for demonstrating impacted or abnormally placed maxillary anterior teeth or visualizing the region of a palatal cleft. Occlusal views may also demonstrate buccal or lingual expansion of bone or presence of a sialolith in the submandibular duct.

## EXTRAORAL RADIOGRAPHS

Extraoral radiographs are examinations made of the orofacial region by use of films located outside the mouth. The relationships among patient position, film location, and beam direction vary depending on the specific radiographic information desired. The standard technique for making several extraoral radiographs is discussed in Chapter 12. Only the panoramic radiograph is described here because it has common use as a radiographic examination for general dental patients.

### Panoramic Radiographs

Panoramic radiographs provide a broad view of the jaws, teeth, maxillary sinuses, nasal fossa, and TMJs (see Chapter 11). They show which teeth are present, their relative state of development, the presence or absence of dental abnormalities, and many traumatic and pathologic lesions in bone. Panoramic radiographs are the technique of choice for initial examinations of edentulous patients. Because this system is an extraoral technique and uses intensifying screens, the resolution of the images is less than with the intraoral nonscreen films (see Chapter 5). Panoramic radiographs are also susceptible to artifacts from improper patient positioning that negatively affect the image. Consequently this system is generally considered inadequate for independent diagnosis of caries, root abnormalities, and periapical changes.

In the majority of dental patients, oral disease involving the teeth or jaw bones lies within the area imaged by periapical radiographs. Therefore when a full-mouth set of radiographs is available, a panoramic examination is usually redundant because it does not add information that alters the treatment plan. However, situations may exist in which a panoramic radiograph may be preferred over a periapical examination, such as for assessing growth and development in a child or adolescent. Panoramic views are most useful when the required field of view is large but the need for high resolution is of less importance. Although the selection of a radiographic examination should be based on the extent of the expected information it is likely to provide, the relatively low dose of radiation from the panoramic examination should also be a qualifying factor.

### Advanced Imaging Procedures

A variety of advanced imaging procedures such as CT, CBCT, MRI, ultrasonography, and nuclear medicine scans may be required in specific diagnostic situations. These techniques are discussed in Chapter 13, although in general the dentist refers the patient to a hospital or other imaging center for these procedures rather than performing them in the dental office.

## Guidelines for Ordering Radiographs

The ADA has issued guidelines recommending which radiographs to make and how often to repeat them:
- Make radiographs only after a clinical examination.
- Order only those radiographs that directly benefit the patient in terms of diagnosis or treatment plan.
- Use the least amount of radiation exposure necessary to generate an acceptable view of the imaged area.

## PREVIOUS RADIOGRAPHS

Most patients have been seen previously by a dentist and have already had radiographs made. These radiographs are helpful regardless of when they were exposed. If they are relatively recent, they may be adequate to the diagnostic problem at hand. Even if they were made so long ago that they are not likely to reflect the current status of the patient, they may still prove useful. These previous radiographs may demonstrate whether a condition has worsened, has remained unchanged, or has shown healing, such as in the progression of caries or periodontal disease.

## ADMINISTRATIVE RADIOGRAPHS

Administrative radiographs are those made for reasons other than diagnosis, including those made for an insurance company or for an examining board. We think that it is appropriate to expose patients only when it benefits their health care. Most administrative radiographs do not serve such an objective. Unfortunately, this recommendation is often not adhered to in practice, and dentists are left to sort out the most appropriate criteria to use in their practices.

## Use of Guidelines to Order Dental Radiographs

At any time, patients generally have a combination of diseases that the clinician must consider. Therefore guidelines specify not only which examinations to order but also which specific patient factors influence the number and type of x-ray films to order.

A panel of individuals was convened in the mid 1980s at the request of a branch of the Food and Drug Administration (FDA) to develop a set of guidelines for the making of dental radiographs. The panel addressed the topic of appropriate radiographs for an adequate evaluation of a new or recall asymptomatic patient seeking general dental care. The guidelines were updated in 2004 to reflect changes in technology and to address situations not considered in the first document (Table 15-2). However, there was no change in philosophy between the original and current guidelines.

The guidelines describe circumstances (patient age, medical and dental history, and physical signs) that suggest the need for radiographs. These circumstances are called *selection criteria*. The guidelines also suggest the types of radiographic examinations most likely to benefit the patient in terms of yielding diagnostic information. They recommend that radiographs not be made unless some expectation exists that they will provide evidence of diseases that will affect the treatment plan. The ADA was an equal partner with the FDA in the revision of the guidelines and recommends their use.

These guidelines also form the basis of the recommendations in this chapter. However, the practitioner, who is the only one who knows the patient's dental history and susceptibility to oral disease, must make the ultimate decision on whether to order radiographs, using the guidelines as a resource, not as a standard of care or a regulation.

Central to the guidelines is the idea that dentists should expose patients to radiation only when they reasonably expect that the resulting radiograph will benefit patient care. Accordingly, two situations mandate a radiograph: some clinical evidence of an abnormality that requires further evaluation for a complete assessment or a high probability of disease that warrants a screening examination.

Selection criteria for radiographs are those signs or symptoms found in the patient history or clinical examination that suggest that a radiographic examination will yield clinically useful information. A key concept in the use of selection criteria is recognition of the need to consider each patient individually. Prescription of radiographs should be decided on an individual basis according to the patient's demonstrated need.

The guidelines include a description of clinical situations in which radiographs are likely to contribute to the diagnosis, treatment, or prognosis. Two examples highlight the differences between ordering radiographs for dental diseases with clinical signs and symptoms and dental diseases with no clinical indicators but high prevalences. In the first case, a patient has a hard swelling in the premolar region of the mandible with expansion of the buccal and lingual cortical plates. The clinical sign of swelling alerts the dentist to the need for a radiograph to determine the nature of the abnormality causing the swelling.

An example of the second situation is the patient who comes seeking general dental care after having not seen a dentist for many years. Even without clinical evidence of caries, bitewings are indicated because of the prevalence of dental caries in the population. Because this patient has not had interproximal radiographs for many years, it is reasonable to assume that the patient may benefit from the radiograph by the detection of interproximal caries. Although no clinical signs exist that predict the presence of early caries, the dentist relies on clinical knowledge of the prevalence of caries to decide that this radiograph has a reasonable probability of finding disease.

Without some specific indication, it is inappropriate to expose the patient "just to see if there is something there." The major exception to this rule is the use of interproximal films for caries when no clinical signs exist of early lesions. The probability of finding occult disease in a patient with all permanent teeth erupted and no clinical or historical evidence of abnormality or risk factors is so low that making a periapical or panoramic radiographic survey just to look for such disease is not indicated.

## PATIENT EXAMINATION

The ordering of radiographs requires a reasonable expectation that they will provide information that will contribute to solving the diagnostic problem at hand. Accordingly, the first step is a careful examination of the patient, including transillumination of the anterior teeth to evaluate for interproximal decay. The clinical examination provides indications as to the nature and extent of the radiographic examination appropriate to the situation.

A team of dentists tested the ability of the ADA guidelines to reduce the number of intraoral radiographs while still offering adequate diagnostic information. This testing of the use of selection criteria demonstrated that a small but significant number of radiographic findings was not 100% covered in the anterior region if only posterior interproximal and selected periapical radiographs were used. The testing suggested that anterior interproximal radiographs or anterior periapicals are also indicated to detect interproximal caries and periodontal disease in the anterior region, specifically for patients with high levels of dental disease. A panoramic radiograph could be made in place of the periapical radiographs to supplement the posterior bitewings if the totality of the disease expected indicates a broad area of coverage and fine detail is not required.

In the ADA/FDA guidelines patients are classified by stage of dental development, by whether they are being evaluated for the first time (without previous documentation) or being reevaluated during a recall visit, and by an estimate of their risk for having dental caries or periodontal disease. A footnote to Table 15-2 also outlines some other clinical findings that indicate when radiographs are likely to contribute to a complete description of the asymptomatic patient.

Applying these guidelines to the specific circumstances with each patient requires clinical judgment and an amalgamation of knowledge, experience, and concern. Clinical judgment is also required to recognize situations that are *not* described by the guidelines but in which patients will need radiographs nonetheless.

### Initial Visit

The guidelines recommend that a child with primary dentition who is cooperative and has closed posterior contacts have only interproximal radiographs to examine for caries. Additional periapical/occlusal views are recommended only in the case of clinically evident diseases or specific historic or clinical indications such as those listed at the footnote of Table 15-2. If the molar contacts are not closed, interproximal radiographs are not necessary because the proximal surfaces may be examined directly.

For radiographic examination of a new patient in the transitional dentition, after eruption of the first permanent tooth the guidelines recommend interproximal radiographs to assess for dental caries and a panoramic radiograph or selected periapical/occlusal views to evaluate growth and development, this being a time when management of dental anomalies might begin.

The guidelines group adolescents and dentate adults together to identify the kind and extent of appropriate radiographic examination. The guidelines recommend that these patients receive an individualized examination consisting of interproximal views and panoramic or periapical views selected on the basis of specific historical or clinical indications. The presence of generalized dental disease often indicates the need for a full-mouth examination. Alternatively, the presence of only a few localized abnormalities or diseases suggests that a more limited examination consisting of interproximal and selected periapical views may suffice. In circumstances with no evidence of current or past dental disease, only interproximal views may be necessary for caries examination.

For the edentulous patient presenting for prosthetic treatment, an individualized examination that is based on clinical signs and symptoms should be performed. This may include a panoramic radiograph or selected periapical/occlusal views, with some type of cross-sectional examination if dental implants are being considered.

### Recall Visit

Patients who are returning after initial care require careful examination before determining the need for radiographs. As at the initial examination, selected periapical views should be obtained if any of the historical or clinical signs or symptoms listed in the footnote to Table 15-2 are present and need further evaluation.

The guidelines recommend interproximal radiographs for recall patients to detect interproximal caries. The optimal frequency for these views depends on the age of the patient and the probability of finding this disease. If the patient has clinically demonstrable caries or the presence of high-risk factors for caries (poor diet, poor oral hygiene, and those listed in the footnote to Table 15-2), then bitewings are exposed at fairly frequent intervals (6 to 12 months for children and adolescents and 6 to 18 months for adults) until no carious lesions are clinically evident. The recommended intervals are longer for individuals not at high risk for caries: 12 to 24 months for the child, 18 to 36 months for the adolescent, and 24 to 36 months for the adult. Note that individuals can change risk category, going from high to low risk or the reverse.

Clinical judgment about need for and type of radiographic examination should be used for other circumstances, such as evaluating the status of periodontal disease, monitoring growth and development, and endodontic or restorative considerations. The interproximal examination may be supplemented by a panoramic, selected periapical/occlusal, or an advanced imaging examination, depending on the patient's specific needs.

A radiographic examination may be required in a number of other situations, such as for patients contemplating orthodontic or implant treatment or patients with intraosseous lesions. The goal should be to obtain the necessary diagnostic information with the minimal radiation dose and financial cost, which can be substantial for advanced imaging procedures such as MRI. The dentist should determine specifically what type of information is needed and the most appropriate technique for obtaining it. An example of a clinical algorithm for ordering radiographs before orthodontic treatment is shown in Figure 15-1, using guidelines endorsed by the American Academy of Orthodontics. Because guidelines for ordering radiographs for other situations are not as well developed, the dentist must rely on clinical judgment.

## SPECIAL CONSIDERATIONS

### Pregnancy

Occasionally it is desirable to obtain radiographs of a woman who is pregnant. The x-ray beam is largely confined to the head and neck region in dental x-ray examinations; thus, fetal exposure is only about 1 microgray ($\mu$Gy) for a full-mouth examination. This exposure is quite small compared with that received normally from natural background sources. However, concerns have been raised about a possible relationship between maternal radiation dose to the thyroid gland from dental radiographs and low birth-weight babies, prompting the ADA to recommend the use of protective thyroid collars and aprons during dental radiography, especially of children, women of childbearing age, and pregnant women. Because the use of radiographs in all patients is predicated on there being a diagnostic need for them, the guidelines apply to patients who are pregnant as well as those who are not.

### Radiation Therapy

Patients with a malignancy in the oral cavity or perioral region often receive radiation therapy for their disease. Some oral tissues receive 50 Gy or more. Although such patients are often apprehensive about receiving additional exposure, dental exposure is insignificant compared with what they have already received. The average skin dose from a dental radiograph is approximately 3 milligrays (mGy), less if faster film or digital imaging is used. Furthermore, patients who have received radiation therapy may have radiation-induced xerostomia and thus are at a high risk for development of radiation caries, which may produce serious consequences if extractions are needed in the future. Accordingly, patients who have had radiation therapy to the oral cavity should be carefully followed up because they are at special risk for dental disease.

## EXAMPLES OF USE OF THE GUIDELINES

Consider the ways in which the guidelines can be applied to different clinical situations:

- The first visit of a 5-year-old boy to a dental office. A careful clinical examination reveals that the patient is cooperative and that the posterior teeth are in contact. Posterior bitewings are recommended to detect caries. If all of this patient's teeth are present, no evidence exists of decay, a reasonably good diet is being observed, and the parent(s) seem(s) well motivated to promote good oral hygiene, no further radiographic examination is required at this time. Radiographs for the detection of development abnormalities are not in order at this age because a complete appraisal cannot be made at age 5 years. Even if it could be made, it is too early to initiate treatment for such abnormalities.

- A 25-year-old woman receiving a 6-month checkup after her last treatment for a fractured incisor. No caries is evident on interproximal radiographs made 6 months ago; currently no clinical signs suggest caries, nor does the patient have high-risk factors for caries. No evidence exists of periodontal disease or other remarkable signs or symptoms in general or associated with the recently fractured tooth. As long as the fractured incisor

**TABLE 15-2**
## U.S. Food and Drug Administration Guidelines for Prescribing Dental Radiographs*

*The recommendations in this table are subject to clinical judgment and may not apply to every patient. They are to be used by dentists only after reviewing the patient's health history and completing a clinical examination. Because every precaution should be taken to minimize radiation exposure, protective thyroid collars and aprons should be used whenever possible. This practice is strongly recommended for children, women of childbearing age and pregnant women.*

| TYPE OF ENCOUNTER | PATIENT AGE AND DENTAL DEVELOPMENTAL STAGE | |
| --- | --- | --- |
| | CHILD WITH PRIMARY DENTITION (PRIOR TO ERUPTION OF FIRST PERMANENT TOOTH) | CHILD WITH TRANSITIONAL DENTITION (AFTER ERUPTION OF FIRST PERMANENT TOOTH) |
| New patient[†] being evaluated for dental diseases and dental development | Individualized radiographic examination consisting of selected periapical/occlusal views and/or posterior bitewings if proximal surfaces cannot be visualized or probed; patients without evidence of disease and with open proximal contacts may not require a radiographic examination at this time | Individualized radiographic examination consisting of posterior bitewings with panoramic examination or posterior bitewings and selected periapical images |
| Recall patient[†] with clinical caries or at increased risk for caries[‡] | Posterior bitewing examination at six- to 12-month intervals if proximal surfaces cannot be examined visually or with a probe | |
| Recall patient* with no clinical caries and not at increased risk of developing caries[‡] | Posterior bitewing examination at 12- to 24-month intervals if proximal surfaces cannot be examined visually or with a probe | |
| Recall patient[†] with periodontal disease | Clinical judgment as to the need for and type of radiographic images for the evaluation of periodontal disease; imaging may consist of, but is not limited to, selected bitewing and/or periapical images of areas in which periodontal disease (other than nonspecific gingivitis) can be demonstrated clinically | |
| Patient for monitoring of growth and development | Clinical judgment as to need for and type of radiographic images for evaluation and/or monitoring of dentofacial growth and development | |
| Patient with other circumstances including, but not limited to, proposed or existing implants, pathology, restorative/endodontic needs, treated periodontal disease and caries remineralization | Clinical judgment as to need for and type of radiographic images for evaluation and/or monitoring of these conditions | |

*Reprinted from U.S. Department of Health and Human Services, Public Health Service, Food and Drug Administration; and American Dental Association, Council on Dental Benefit Programs, Council on Scientific Affairs.
[†]Clinical situations for which radiographs may be indicated, but are not limited to, include the following: **Positive historical findings:** Previous periodontal or endodontic treatment, history of pain or trauma, familial history of dental anomalies, postoperative evaluation of healing, remineralization monitoring, presence of implants or evaluation for implant placement. **Positive clinical signs/symptoms:** clinical evidence of periodontal disease, large or deep restorations, deep carious lesions, malposed or clinically impacted teeth, swelling, evidence of dental/facial trauma, mobility of teeth, sinus tract ("fistula"), clinically suspected sinus pathology, growth abnormalities, oral involvement in known or suspected systemic disease, positive neurologic findings in the head and neck, evidence of foreign objects, pain and/or dysfunction of the temporomandibular joint, facial asymmetry, abutment teeth for fixed or removable partial prosthesis, unexplained bleeding, unexplained sensitivity of teeth, unusual eruption, spacing or migration of teeth, unusual tooth morphology, calcification or color, missing teeth with unknown reason, clinical erosion.

## PATIENT AGE AND DENTAL DEVELOPMENTAL STAGE

| ADOLESCENT WITH PERMANENT DENTITION (PRIOR TO ERUPTION OF THIRD MOLARS) | ADULT, DENTATE OR PARTIALLY EDENTULOUS | ADULT, EDENTULOUS |
|---|---|---|
| Individualized radiographic examination consisting of posterior bitewings with panoramic examination or posterior bitewings and selected periapical images; a full-mouth intraoral radiographic examination is preferred when the patient has clinical evidence of generalized dental disease or a history of extensive dental treatment | | Individualized radiographic examination based on clinical signs and symptoms |
| Posterior bitewing examination at six- to 12-month intervals if proximal surfaces cannot be examined visually or with a probe | Posterior bitewing examination at six- to 18-month intervals | Not applicable |
| Posterior bitewing examination at 18- to 36-month intervals | Posterior bitewing examination at 24- to 36-month intervals | Not applicable |
| Clinical judgment as to the need for and type of radiographic images for the evaluation of periodontal disease; imaging may consist of, but is not limited to, selected bitewing and/or periapical images of areas in which periodontal disease (other than nonspecific gingivitis) can be demonstrated clinically | | Not applicable |
| Clinical judgment as to need for and type of radiographic images for evaluation and/or monitoring of dentofacial growth and development; panoramic or periapical examination to assess developing third molars | Usually not indicated | |
| Clinical judgment as to need for and type of radiographic images for evaluation and/or monitoring of these conditions | | |

‡Factors increasing risk for caries may include, but are not limited to, the following: high level of caries experience or demineralization, history of recurrent caries, high titers of cariogenic bacteria, existing restoration of poor quality, poor oral hygiene, inadequate fluoride exposure, prolonged nursing (bottle or breast), diet with high sucrose frequency, poor family dental health, developmental or acquired enamel defects, developmental or acquired disability, xerostomia, genetic abnormality of teeth, many multisurface restorations, chemotherapy/radiation therapy, eating disorders, drug/alcohol abuse, irregular dental care.

shows normal vitality testing, no radiographs are recommended for this patient. If the incisor is nonvital, a periapical view of this tooth should be exposed.

- A 45-year-old man returning to the dentist's office after 1 year. At his last visit you placed two mesial, occlusal, distal amalgam restorations on premolars and performed root canal therapy on number 30. The patient has a 5-mm pocket in the buccal furcation of number 3 but no other evidence of periodontal disease. The guidelines recommend that this patient receive interproximal radiographs to see whether he still has active caries and periapical views of numbers 3 and 30 to evaluate the extent of the periodontal disease and periapical disease, respectively.

- A 65-year-old woman coming to the office for the first time. No previous radiographs are available. A history exists of root canal therapy in two teeth, although the patient is not aware which teeth were treated. Clinical examination reveals multiple carious teeth, multiple missing teeth, and pockets of more than 3 mm involving most of the remaining teeth. The guidelines recommend a full-mouth examination, including interproximal radiographs, for this patient because of the high probability of finding caries, periodontal disease, and periapical disease.

# BIBLIOGRAPHY

## GUIDELINES FOR ORDERING RADIOGRAPHS

Åkerblom A, Rohlin M, Hasselgren G: Individualised restricted intraoral radiography versus full-mouth radiography in the detection of periradicular lesions, *Swed Dent J* 12:151-159, 1988.

American Dental Association Council on Scientific Affairs: The use of dental radiographs: update and recommendations, *J Am Dent Assoc* 137:1304-1312, 2006.

Atchison KA, Luke LS, White SC: An algorithm for ordering pretreatment orthodontic radiographs, *Am J Orthod Dentofac Orthop* 102:29-44, 1992.

Atchison KA, White SC, Flack VF et al: Assessing the FDA guidelines for ordering dental radiographs, *J Am Dent Assoc* 126:1372-1383, 1995.

Bohay RN, Stephens RG, Kogon SL: A study of the impact of screening or selective radiography on the treatment and post delivery outcome for edentulous patients, *Oral Surg Oral Med Oral Pathol Oral Radiol Endod* 86:353-359, 1998.

Brooks SL: A study of selection criteria for intraoral dental radiography, *Oral Surg Oral Med Oral Pathol* 62:234-239, 1986.

Brooks SL, Brand JW, Gibbs SJ et al: Imaging of the temporomandibular joint: a position paper of the American Academy of Oral and Maxillofacial Radiology, *Oral Surg Oral Med Oral Pathol Oral Radiol Endod* 83:609-618, 1997.

Bruks A, Enberg K, Nordqvist I et al: Radiographic examinations as an aid to orthodontic diagnosis and treatment planning, *Swed Dent J* 23:77-85, 1999.

European Commission: Radiation protection 136, European guidelines on radiation protection in dental radiology: the safe use of radiographs in dental practice, 2004: http://ec.europa.eu/energy/nuclear/radioprotection/publication/doc/136_en.pdf. Accessed May 11, 2008.

Hollender L: Decision making in radiographic imaging, *J Dent Educ* 56:834-843, 1992.

Keur JJ: Radiographic screening of edentulous patients: sense or nonsense? A risk-benefit analysis, *Oral Surg Oral Med Oral Pathol* 62:463-467, 1986.

Luke LS, Lee P, Atchison KA et al: Orthodontic residents' indications for use of the lateral TMJ tomogram and the posteroanterior cephalogram, *J Dent Educ* 61:29-36, 1997.

Molander B: Panoramic radiography in dental diagnostics, *Swed Dent J* 119(Suppl):1-26, 1996.

Pitts NB, Kidd EA: Some of the factors to be considered in the prescription and timing of bitewing radiography in the diagnosis and management of dental caries, *J Dent* 20:74-84, 1992.

Rushton VE, Horner K, Worthington HV: Routine panoramic radiography of new adult patients in general dental practice: relevance of diagnostic yield to treatment and identification of radiographic selection criteria, *Oral Surg Oral Med Oral Pathol Oral Radiol Endod* 93:488-495, 2002.

Stephens RG, Kogon SL: New U.S. guidelines for prescribing dental radiographs: a critical review, *J Can Dent Assoc* 56:1019-1024, 1990.

Tyndall DA, Brooks SL: Selection criteria for dental implant site imaging: a position paper of the American Academy of Oral and Maxillofacial Radiology, *Oral Surg Oral Med Oral Pathol Oral Radiol* 89:630-637, 2000.

U.S. Department of Health and Human Services, Public Health Service, Food and Drug Administration, and American Dental Association, Council on Dental Benefit Programs, Council on Scientific Affairs: The selection of patients for dental radiographic examinations, revised ed (2004): www.ada.org/prof/resources/topics/radiography.asp. Accessed August 22, 2007.

White SC, Heslop EW, Hollender LG et al: Parameters of radiologic care: an official report of the American Academy of Oral and Maxillofacial Radiology, *Oral Surg Oral Med Oral Pathol Oral Radiol Endod* 91:498-511, 2001.

## DISEASE DETECTION

Atchison KA, White SC, Flack VF et al: Efficacy of the FDA selection criteria for radiographic assessment of the periodontium, *J Dent Res* 74:1424-1432, 1995.

Backer Dirks O: Posteruptive changes in dental enamel, *J Dent Res* 45(Suppl):503-511, 1966.

Friedlander AH, Freymiller EG: Detection of radiation-accelerated atherosclerosis of the carotid artery by panoramic radiography: a new opportunity for dentists, *J Am Dent Assoc* 134:1361-1365, 2003.

Hall WB: *Decision making in periodontology,* ed 3, St. Louis, 1998, Mosby.

Madden RP, Hodges JS, Salmen CW et al: Utility of panoramic radiographs in detecting cervical calcified carotid atheroma, *Oral Surg Oral Med Oral Pathol Oral Radiol Endod* 103:543-548, 2007.

Moles DR, Downer MC: Optimum bitewing examination recall intervals assessed by computer simulation, *Commun Dent Health* 17:14-19, 2000.

Reddy MS, Geurs NC, Jeffcoat RL et al: Periodontal disease progression, *J Periodontol* 71:1583-1590, 2000.

Shwartz M, Gröndahl H-G, Pliskin JS et al: A longitudinal analysis from bitewing radiographs of the rate of progression of approximal carious lesions through human dental enamel, *Arch Oral Biol* 29:529-536, 1984.

White SC, Atchison KA, Hewlett ER et al: Clinical and historical predictors of dental caries on radiographs, *Dentomaxillofac Radiol* 24:121-127, 1995.

White SC, Atchison KA, Hewlett ER et al: Efficacy of FDA guidelines for ordering radiographs for caries detection, *Oral Surg Oral Med Oral Pathol* 77:531-540, 1994.

## RADIATION DOSAGE AND EFFECTS

Frederiksen N, Benson B, Sokolowski T: Effective dose and risk assessment from computed tomography of the maxillofacial complex, *Dentomaxillofac Radiol* 24:55-58, 1995.

Hujoel PP, Bollen AM, Noonan CJ et al: Antepartum dental radiography and infant low birth weight, *JAMA* 291:1987-1993, 2004.

Ludlow JB, Davies-Ludlow LE, Brooks SL et al: Dosimetry of 3 CBCT devices for oral and maxillofacial radiology: CB Mercuray, NewTom 3G and i-CAT, *Dentomaxillofac Radiol* 35:219-226, 2006

Scaf G, Lurie AG, Mosier KM et al: Dosimetry and cost of imaging osseointegrated implants with film-based and computed tomography, *Oral Surg Oral Med Oral Pathol Oral Radiol Endod* 83:41-48, 1997.

White SC: 1992 assessment of radiation risks from dental radiology, *Dentomaxillofac Radiol* 21:118-126, 1992.

# PART FIVE

# Radiographic Interpretation

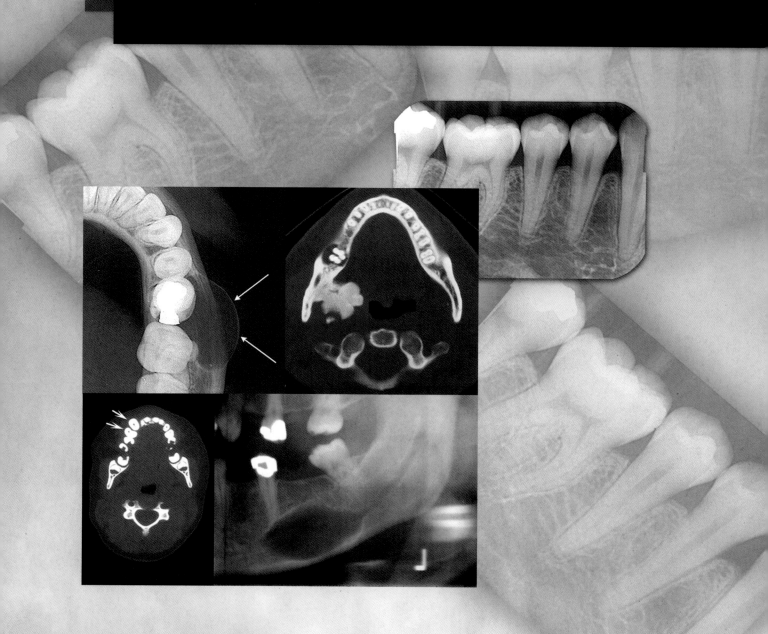

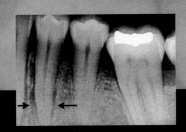

# CHAPTER 16

# Principles of Radiographic Interpretation

The objective of this chapter is to provide a step-by-step analytic process that can be applied to the interpretation of diagnostic images. However, reading this chapter, by itself, will not instantly bestow the ability to interpret radiographic films correctly; rather, it will equip the reader with a systematic method of image analysis. Proficiency comes only with practice.

## Clinical Examination

Radiographs are prescribed when the dentist thinks that they are likely to offer useful diagnostic information that will influence the treatment plan. Often some clinical sign or symptom or finding from the patient's history indicates the need for a radiologic examination. This clinical information should be used first to select the type of radiographs and later to aid in their interpretation.

### ACQUIRING APPROPRIATE DIAGNOSTIC IMAGES

An insufficient number or inadequate quality of radiographs limits the information available from diagnostic imaging. Because the general practitioner often is responsible both for prescribing and interpreting radiographs, inadequate films should be recognized and supplemental images obtained before proceeding with the analysis.

#### Quality of the Diagnostic Image
Before the analysis is started, the quality of the images is examined. Is the image distorted? For instance, if the image is elongated, greater error occurs in measuring the length of a root canal. Because of the inherent frequency of image distortion in panoramic films, this factor must always be taken into consideration. For example, a region of image magnification involving the mandibular condyle may be diagnosed erroneously as condylar hyperplasia. For this reason, a thorough knowledge of all possible image distortions is a prerequisite for analysis of panoramic images.

The practitioner also should check to see whether the density or contrast of the image has been degraded by exposure or developing errors. It may be impossible, for example, to diagnose osteoporosis in an overexposed image, or detail may be obscured in an underexposed film. If the images are of poor quality, it might be prudent to obtain better quality images before proceeding to the analysis.

#### Number and Type of Available Images
Initially the clinical examination indicates the number and types of films required (see Chapter 14). The interpretation of these films in turn may suggest the need for additional imaging. Caution should be exercised in attempting to make an interpretation on the basis of a single film, especially if the only film is a panoramic view. Also, a bitewing or periapical projection often can be supplemented by another view produced by altering the horizontal or vertical angulation of the x-ray beam. For example, detection of recurrent caries around a heavily restored dentition may benefit from an additional view taken by altering the angle of the x-ray beam. One of the benefits of a full-mouth series of intraoral films is that it provides a second view of most areas at a slightly different angle.

Conventional dental radiography produces images in only two dimensions, usually in the mesiodistal direction. In some cases a view at right angles to the plane of the original film is beneficial. For instance, if a condylar neck fracture is suspected, a lateral view of the condylar region (e.g., a panoramic view) should be supplemented with an anteroposterior view. In a similar fashion, occlusal projections of the jaws can provide a supplementary right-angle view for the periapical film. Use of a vertex occlusal view follows this principle in establishing the location of impacted maxillary cuspids. In some cases an investigation requires other images in addition to intraoral radiography or panoramic images. Techniques such as tomography, sialography, nuclear imaging, cone-beam computed tomography, conventional computed tomography, and magnetic resonance imaging may be required (see Chapter 15). These techniques are available through consultation with an oral and maxillofacial radiologist.

Diagnostic imaging should be completed before a biopsy procedure or treatment is provided. Diagnostic imaging can aid in the selection of the most appropriate site for a biopsy procedure to obtain the most representative tissue sample. Also, the biopsy procedure may alter the tissue by inducing inflammatory changes, which in turn alter the imaging characteristics of the tissue. This compromises the diagnostic information that can be obtained, such as determining the extent of a disease.

#### Viewing Conditions
Ideally, viewing conditions should include the following characteristics:
- Ambient light in the viewing room should be reduced.
- Intraoral radiographs should be mounted in a film holder.
- Light from the viewbox should be of equal intensity across the viewing surface.
- The size of the viewbox should accommodate the size of the film. If the viewing area is larger than the film, an opaque mask should be used to eliminate all light from around the periphery of the film. This mask can be fabricated from a sheet of opaque material cut to fit the entire viewbox, leaving an opening for one film.

- An intense light source is essential for evaluating dark regions of the film.
- A magnifying glass allows detailed examination of small regions of the film.

When images in a digital format are viewed, both room lighting and quality of the monitor are important.

## Image Analysis

When the quality and number of films are satisfactory, analysis of the image begins.

### SYSTEMATIC RADIOGRAPHIC EXAMINATION

The first step in image analysis is to use a systematic approach to identify all the normal anatomy present in an image or set of images. A profound knowledge of the variation of normal appearance is required to be able to recognize an abnormal appearance. Because no textbook can display all possible variations, the best learning method is to identify normal anatomy in every film analyzed. In this way the observer can build up a large mental database of the spectrum of normal anatomic appearances. An additional benefit of this procedure is that it forces the observer to examine the entire film. Practitioners should avoid limiting their attention to one particular region of the film; rather, all aspects of each image should be examined systematically. More than one abnormality may be present. For instance, a bitewing radiograph made to detect caries and alveolar bone loss also may reveal just the edge of an unsuspected intraosseous lesion that will be seen only if the dentist examines the radiograph thoroughly.

### INTRAORAL IMAGES

For almost all dental patients, treatment planning includes some combination of periapical and bitewing images. This chapter presents a systematic method for analyzing these images. This method may be used to analyze a single image or a full-mouth set. It is most important for the practitioner to develop a particular method and to use it regularly. A thorough examination is best accomplished when a specific sequence of analysis is used to enhance the scrutiny of all parts of images.

To follow the method presented here, the practitioner should examine the periapical images before the bitewing images, starting in the right maxilla and working across to the left and then dropping down and continuing in the left mandible to the right, concentrating on one anatomic structure at a time. First, the bone is examined. All anatomic landmarks appropriate for the region are identified. In the posterior maxilla, for example, the maxillary sinus, tuberosity, and zygomatic process of the maxilla should be examined. In what way does their appearance change as the angle of each projection is altered? Also, the character of the trabecular bone should be examined. Are the density and size of the trabeculae normal for the region? The same areas should be compared on adjacent images and with the corresponding area on images of the other side.

Next, a second visual circuit should be made through all the images, examining the bone of the alveolar process. In particular, the height of the alveolar crest relative to the teeth and the cortication should be examined. Loss of height of the alveolar bone (more than 1.5 mm from the adjacent cementoenamel junctions) may indicate active or past periodontal disease. All regions of the alveolar process should be examined to gain an overall appreciation for the extent and severity of alveolar bone loss. Any areas of erosion of the alveolar crest and the thickness of the overlying mucosa should be noted. Carcinomas arising from the epithelial covering may cause erosive lesions with ill-defined borders in the alveolar bone. The trabecular pattern of the alveolar process should be examined. The lamina dura may be examined later together with the periodontal membrane space and tooth roots.

Finally, a third visual circuit should be made, examining the dentition and associated structures. Each tooth should be studied in sequence, using all images available. The way the tooth's appearance and root structure change with different orientations of the x-ray beam should be noted. The teeth should be counted, looking for missing or supernumerary teeth. The crowns should be examined for normal development of the enamel and for caries. Particular attention should be paid to the interproximal regions at or below the contact points. Restorations should be checked carefully for signs of recurrent caries. Often lesions found on one view cannot be detected on another because of superimposition of the restoration. The pulp chamber should be examined for size and contents. The roots should be examined for shape and form to detect developmental or acquired abnormalities such as external resorption. The width of the periodontal ligament space around the roots of the tooth should be inspected. The width should be fairly uniform, with very subtle widening toward the cervical region of the tooth. In particular, the lamina dura around each tooth should be examined. Is it intact? The most common abnormalities found in the bone are radiolucent or radiopaque lesions at the apices of teeth.

### EXTRAORAL RADIOGRAPHY

The extraoral radiographs most commonly used in dentistry are panoramic images, cephalometric views, and examinations of the temporomandibular joint. Specific methods for examining these images are covered in the chapters pertaining to these types of images. The same general principles of thorough, systematic coverage described earlier should be used. For viewing each of these types of images, it is important to develop a definite sequence that considers all the hard and soft tissues in the field. The practitioner should always focus on one component at a time and examine it thoroughly. Only with such a pattern can the likelihood of detecting all abnormalities be maximized.

When an intraosseous lesion is identified, the following five steps should be used to analyze the lesion as fully as possible.

## Analysis of the Intraosseous Lesions

Two basic approaches can be used to analyze images of a lesion. One is the picture matching, or "Aunt Minnie," method. This involves trying to match the radiographic image with a mental picture or with an image in a favorite textbook. Although all radiologists probably use this technique to a certain extent, it has significant limitations. For instance, the observer's experience and memory limit the mental image of a particular disorder. Similarly, the appearance of different abnormalities in a textbook is limited by the author's knowledge and experience and, of course, by the number of images printed. Also, figures in a textbook usually represent the most ideal examples of the abnormality. For example, the term *periapical cemental dysplasia* often evokes a mental image of a radiolucent or mixed radiolucent-radiopaque lesion at the apex of a mandibular incisor because this

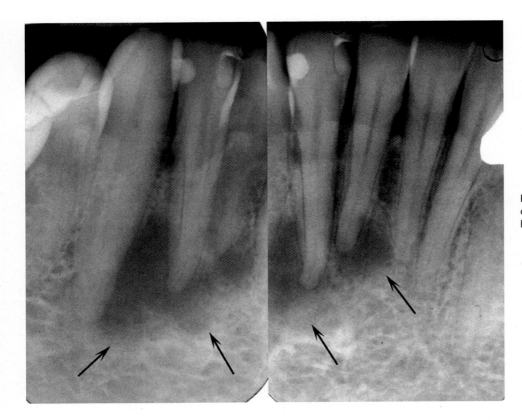

FIG. **16-1** The typical location of lesions of periapical cemental dysplasia. Early lesions are radiolucent *(arrows)*.

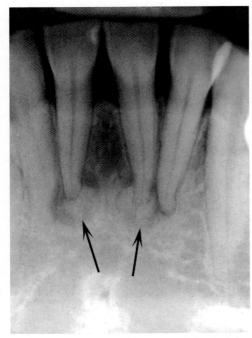

FIG. **16-2** Late lesions of periapical cemental dysplasia have a more radiopaque interior surrounded by a more radiolucent margin.

appearance is the one used most often in textbooks (Figs. 16-1 and 16-2). Although this is a common location, this concept limits recognition and acceptance of this lesion in other areas of the jaws or where teeth have been extracted (Fig. 16-3). Therefore using this technique limits the scope of possible entities to be considered in the interpretation.

The preferred method of radiographic interpretation is presented here. It is a step-by-step analysis of all the radiographic characteristics of the abnormality and production of a radiographic interpretation on the basis of these findings. This procedure helps ensure recognition and collection of all the information contained in the image and in turn improves the accuracy of interpretation.

## STEP 1: LOCALIZE THE ABNORMALITY

### Localized or Generalized

The anatomic location and limits of the abnormality should be described. This information aids in starting to select various disease categories. Many abnormalities are localized to a specific region. If an abnormal appearance affects all the osseous structures of the maxillofacial region, generalized conditions such as metabolic or endocrine abnormalities of bone are considered. If the abnormality is localized, it may be unilateral or bilateral (Fig. 16-4). Often variations of normal anatomy are more commonly bilateral, whereas abnormal conditions are more commonly unilateral. For instance, a bilateral mandibular radiolucency may indicate normal anatomy, such as extensive submandibular gland fossa, whereas fibrous dysplasia commonly is unilateral. However, a few abnormalities such as Paget's disease are always seen bilaterally in the mandible.

## Position in the Jaws

Is the abnormality in soft tissue or is it contained within the jaws? When the lesion is in bone, the point of origin, or epicenter, can be estimated on the basis of the assumption that the abnormality grew equally in every direction (this becomes less accurate with very large lesions). The point of origin may indicate the tissue types that compose the abnormality. However, determining the exact location may be difficult in some circumstances if the nature of the abnormality is not well defined. The following are a few examples:

- If the epicenter is coronal to a tooth, the lesion probably is composed of odontogenic epithelium (Fig. 16-5).
- If it is above the inferior alveolar nerve canal (IAC), the likelihood is greater that it is composed of odontogenic tissue (Fig. 16-6).
- If the epicenter is below the IAC, it is unlikely to be odontogenic in origin (Fig. 16-7).
- If it originates within the IAC, the tissue of origin probably is neural or vascular in nature (Fig. 16-8).

- The probability of cartilaginous lesions and osteochondromas occurring is greater in the condylar region.
- If the epicenter is within the maxillary antrum, the lesion is not of odontogenic tissue, as opposed to a lesion that has grown into the antrum from the alveolar process of the maxilla (Fig. 16-9).

Particular lesions tend to be found in specific locations:

- The epicenters of central giant cell granulomas commonly are located anterior to the first molars in the mandible and anterior to the cuspid in the maxilla in young patients.
- Osteomyelitis occurs in the mandible and rarely in the maxilla.
- Periapical cemental dysplasia occurs in the periapical region of teeth (see Figs. 16-1 and 16-2).

### Single or Multifocal

Establishing whether an abnormality is multifocal aids in interpretation because the list of possible multifocal abnormalities is short. Some examples are periapical cemental dysplasia, odontogenic keratocysts, metastatic lesions, multiple myeloma (Fig. 16-10), and leukemic infiltrates.

Occasionally exceptions to all these points occur. However, in the majority of cases these criteria will serve as a guide to an accurate interpretation.

### Size

Finally, consider the size of the lesion. There are very few size restrictions for a particular lesion, but the size may aid in the differential diagnosis. For instance, a dentigerous cyst is often larger than a hyperplastic follicle.

## STEP 2: ASSESS THE PERIPHERY AND SHAPE

Study the periphery of the lesion. Is the periphery well defined or ill defined? If an imaginary pencil can be used to draw confidently the limits of the lesion, the margin is well defined (Fig. 16-11). Do not become concerned if some small regions are ill defined; these may be due to the shape or direction of the x-ray beam at that particular location. A well-defined lesion is one in which most of the periphery is well defined. In contrast, it is difficult to draw an exact delineation

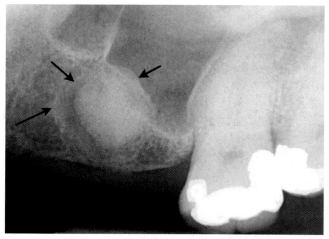

FIG. **16-3** A periapical film revealing a lesion of cemental dysplasia left behind after extraction of the associated tooth.

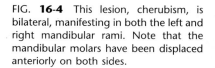

FIG. **16-4** This lesion, cherubism, is bilateral, manifesting in both the left and right mandibular rami. Note that the mandibular molars have been displaced anteriorly on both sides.

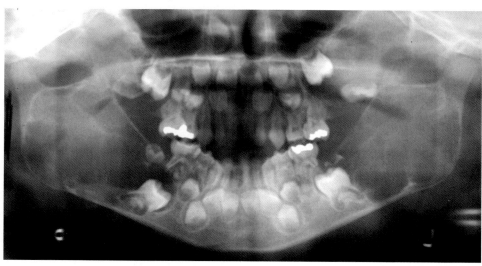

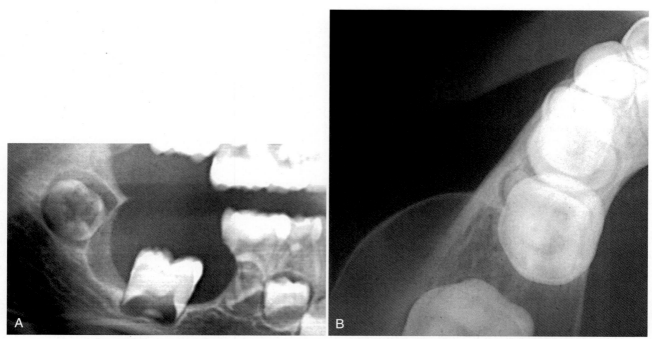

FIG. **16-5**   **A,** A cropped panoramic image of a lesion where the epicenter is coronal to the unerupted mandibular first molar. **B,** An occlusal projection providing a right-angled view of the same lesion.

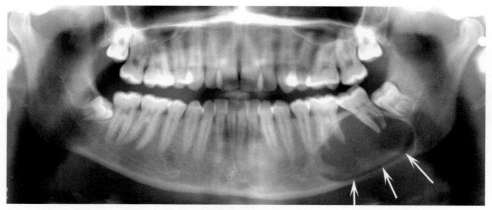

FIG. **16-6**   A panoramic image revealing a cystic ameloblastoma within the body of the left mandible. Note that the inferior alveolar nerve canal has been displaced inferiorly to the inferior cortex *(arrows)*, indicating that the lesion started superior to the canal.

around most of an ill-defined periphery (Fig. 16-12). These two types of peripheries or borders can be further broken down under two subcategories: well-defined borders and ill-defined borders.

### Well-Defined Borders

A punched-out border is one that has a sharp boundary in which no bone reaction is apparent immediately adjacent to the abnormality. This is analogous to punching a hole in a radiograph with a paper punch. The border of the resulting hole is well defined, and the surrounding bone has a normal appearance up to the edge of the hole. This type of border sometimes is seen in multiple myeloma (see Fig. 16-10).

A corticated margin is a thin, fairly uniform radiopaque line of reactive bone at the periphery of a lesion. This is commonly seen with cysts (see Fig. 16-5).

A sclerotic margin is a wide, radiopaque border of reactive bone that usually is not uniform in width. This may be seen with periapical cemental dysplasia and may indicate a very slow rate of growth or the potential for the lesion to stimulate the production of surrounding bone (see Figs. 16-2 and 16-3).

A radiopaque lesion may have a soft tissue capsule, which is indicated by the presence of a radiolucent line at the periphery. This may be seen in conjunction with a corticated periphery, as is observed with odontomas and cementoblastomas (Figs. 16-13 and 16-14).

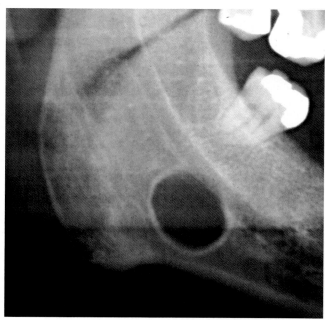

FIG. **16-7**   A cropped panoramic image displaying a lesion (developmental salivary gland defect) below the inferior alveolar canal and thus unlikely to be of odontogenic origin.

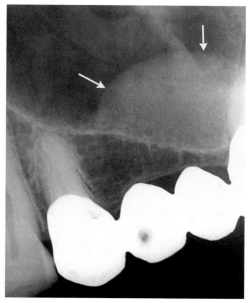

FIG. **16-9**   The lack of a peripheral cortex on this retention pseudocyst indicates that it originated in the sinus and not in the alveolar process. It therefore is unlikely to be of odontogenic origin.

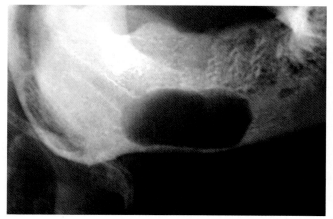

FIG. **16-8**   A lateral oblique view of the mandible revealing a lesion within the inferior alveolar canal. The smooth fusiform expansion of the canal indicates a neural lesion.

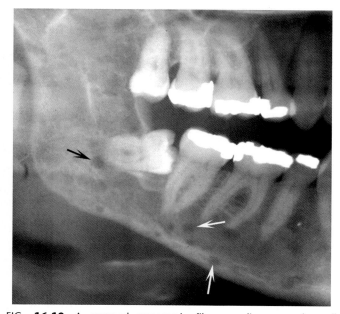

FIG. **16-10**   A cropped panoramic film revealing several small punched-out lesions of multiple myeloma (a few indicated by *arrows*) involving the body and ramus of the mandible.

## Ill-Defined Borders

A blending border is ill defined because of the gradual transition between normal-appearing bone trabeculae and the abnormal-appearing trabeculae of the lesion. The focus of this observation is on the trabeculae and not on the radiolucent marrow spaces. Some conditions with this type of margin are sclerosing osteitis (Fig. 16-15) and fibrous dysplasia.

An invasive border usually is associated with rapid growth and can be seen with malignant lesions. Usually an area of radiolucency with fewer or no trabeculae representing bone destruction can be seen just behind the margin (Fig. 16-16). In contrast to the blending border,

the focus of this observation is on the enlarging radiolucency at the expense of bone trabeculae. These borders have also been described as permeative because the lesion grows around existing trabeculae, producing radiolucent, fingerlike, or bay-type extensions at the periphery. This may result in enlargement of the marrow spaces at the periphery (Fig. 16-17).

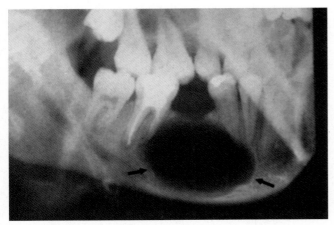

FIG. **16-11** A lateral oblique projection of the mandible showing the well-defined border of a residual cyst.

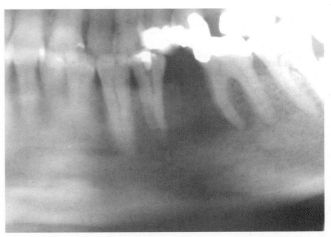

FIG. **16-12** A cropped panoramic radiograph showing the poorly defined border of a malignant neoplasm that has destroyed bone between the first molar and the first bicuspid.

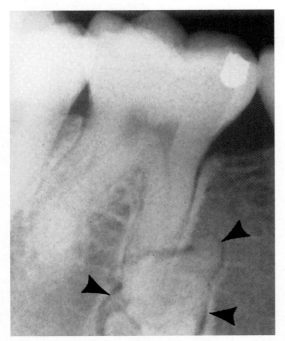

FIG. **16-13** Note the thin, radiolucent periphery positioned between the internal radiopaque structure of this odontoma and the radiopaque outer cortical boundary *(arrows)*.

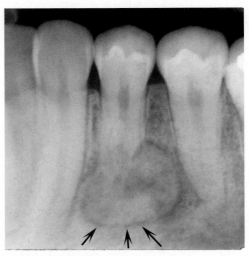

FIG. **16-14** A periapical film revealing a radiopaque mass associated with the root of the first bicuspid. Note the prominent radiolucent periphery *(arrows)* of this benign cementoblastoma.

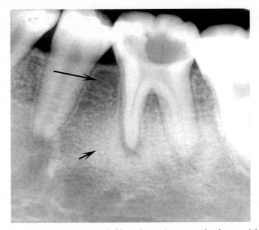

FIG. **16-15** In this periapical film there is a gradual transition from the dense trabeculae of sclerosing osteitis *(short arrow)* to the normal trabecular pattern near the crest of the alveolar process *(long arrow)*. This is an example of an ill-defined, blending border.

## Shape

The lesion may have a particular shape, or it may be irregular. The following are some examples:

- A circular or fluid-filled shape, much like an inflated balloon, which sometimes is referred to as hydraulic, is characteristic of a cyst (see Fig. 16-5).
- A scalloped shape is a series of contiguous arcs or semicircles that may reflect the mechanism of growth (Fig. 16-18). This shape may be seen in cysts (e.g., odontogenic keratocysts), cystlike lesions (e.g., simple bone cysts), and some tumors. Occasionally a lesion with a scalloped periphery is referred to as multilocular; however, in this text the term *multilocular* is reserved for the description of the internal structure.

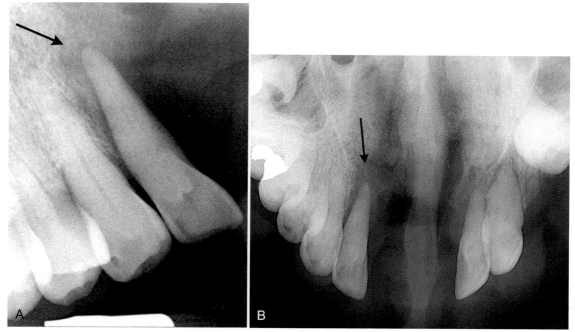

FIG. **16-16**   Periapical **(A)** and occlusal **(B)** films revealing a squamous cell carcinoma in the anterior maxilla. Note the invasive margin that extends beyond the lateral incisor *(arrow)* and the radiolucent region with no apparent trabeculae representing bone destruction behind this margin.

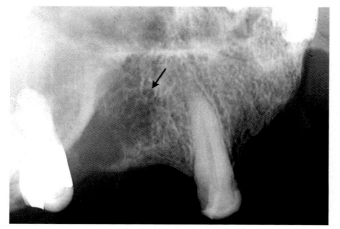

FIG. **16-17**   Lateral occlusal view of a lesion revealing an ill-defined periphery with enlargement of the small marrow spaces at the margin *(arrow)*. This is characteristic of a malignant neoplasm, in this case a lymphoma.

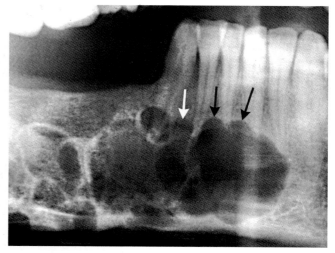

FIG. **16-18**   A cropped panoramic film of an odontogenic keratocyst displaying a scalloped border, especially around the apex of the associated teeth *(arrows)*.

## STEP 3: ANALYZE THE INTERNAL STRUCTURE

The internal appearance of a lesion can be classified into one of three basic categories: totally radiolucent, totally radiopaque, or mixed radiolucent and radiopaque (mixed density).

A radiolucent interior is common in cysts (see Fig. 16-5, *A*), and a totally radiopaque interior is observed in osteomas. The mixed density internal structure is seen as the presence of calcified structures against a radiolucent (black) backdrop. A challenging aspect of this analysis may be the decision concerning whether a calcified structure is in the internal aspect of the lesion or resides on either side. This is difficult to determine by using images that are two-dimensional representations of three-dimensional structures. The calcified structures should be examined and an attempt made to identify the structure by its shape, size, and pattern. For example, bone can be identified by the presence of trabeculae. Also, the degree of radiopacity may help; for instance, enamel is more radiopaque than bone. The following is a list of most radiolucent to most radiopaque material seen in plain radiographs:

- Air, fat, and gas
- Fluid
- Soft tissue
- Bone marrow
- Trabecular bone
- Cortical bone and dentine
- Enamel
- Metal

This list is useful but may be compromised by the amount of material, for instance, a large amount of cortical bone may be as radiopaque as enamel.

The following list presents a few possible internal structures that may be seen in mixed density lesions:

- Abnormal bone may have a variety of trabecular patterns different from normal bone. These variations result from a difference in the number, length, width, and orientation of the trabeculae. For instance, in fibrous dysplasia the trabeculae usually are greater in number, shorter, and not aligned in response to applied stress to the bone but are randomly oriented, resulting in patterns described as have an orange-peel or a ground-glass appearance (Fig. 16-19). Another example is the stimulation of new bone formation on existing trabeculae in response to inflammation. The result is thick trabeculae, giving the area a more radiopaque appearance (see Fig. 16-15).
- Septa represent residual trapped bone that has been organized into long strands or walls within the lesion. If these septa divide the internal structure into at least two compartments, the term *multilocular* is used. The length, width, and orientation of the septa can be assessed. For instance, curved, coarse septa may be seen in ameloblastoma and sometimes in odontogenic kerato-

cysts (Fig. 16-20), giving the internal pattern a multilocular, "soap bubble" appearance. The septa seen in giant cell granulomas are described as wispy or granular; odontogenic myxomas may display a small number of straight, thin septa.

- Dystrophic calcification is a calcification that occurs in damaged soft tissue. This is most commonly seen in calcified lymph nodes that appear as dense, cauliflower-like masses in the soft tissue. In chronically inflamed cysts the calcification may have a very delicate, particulate appearance without a recognizable pattern.
- Cementum usually has a homogeneous, dense, amorphous structure and sometimes is organized into round or oval shapes (see Figs. 16-2 and 16-3).
- Tooth structure usually can be identified by the organization into enamel, dentin, and pulp chambers. Also, the internal density is equivalent to tooth structure and greater than the surrounding bone (see Fig. 16-13).

## STEP 4: ANALYZE THE EFFECTS OF THE LESION ON SURROUND STRUCTURES

Evaluating the effects of the lesion on surrounding structures allows the observer to infer its behavior. The behavior may aid in identification of the disease, but this requires knowledge of the mechanisms of various diseases. For instance, inflammatory disease, as is seen in periapical osteitis, can stimulate bone resorption or formation. Bone formation may occur on the surface of existing trabeculae, resulting in thick trabeculae, which is reflected in the trabecular pattern and in an overall increase in the radiopacity of the bone (see Fig. 16-15). The term *space occupying* is used to describe a lesion that slowly creates its own space by displacing teeth and other surrounding structures. The following sections give examples of effects on surrounding structures and the conclusions that may be inferred from the behavior of the lesions.

### Teeth, Lamina Dura, and Periodontal Membrane Space

Displacement of teeth is seen more commonly with slower-growing, space-occupying lesions. The direction of tooth displacement is significant. Lesions with an epicenter above the crown of a tooth (i.e., follicular cysts and occasionally odontomas) displace the tooth apically (see Fig. 16-5, *A*). Lesions that start in the ramus, such as cherubism (see Fig. 16-4), may push teeth in an anterior direction. Some lesions (e.g., lymphoma, leukemia, Langerhans' cell histiocytosis) grow in the papilla of developing teeth and may push the developing tooth in a coronal direction (Fig. 16-21).

Widening of the periodontal membrane space may be seen with many different kinds of abnormalities. It is important to observe whether the widening is uniform or irregular and whether the lamina dura is still present. For instance, orthodontic movement of teeth results in widening of the periodontal membrane space, but the lamina dura remains intact. Malignant lesions can quickly grow down the ligament space, resulting in an irregular widening and destruction of the lamina dura (Fig. 16-22).

Resorption of teeth usually occurs with a more chronic or slowly growing process (see Fig. 16-5) and may result from chronic inflammation. Although tooth resorption is more commonly related to benign processes, malignant tumors occasionally resorb teeth.

### Surrounding Bone Density and Trabecular Pattern

The presence of reactive bone at the periphery of a lesion, whether corticated or sclerotic, usually signifies slow, benign growth and pos-

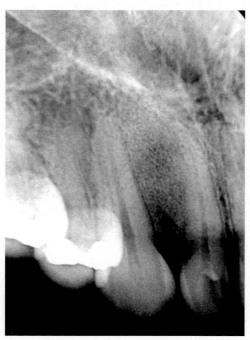

FIG. **16-19** A periapical film of a small lesion of fibrous dysplasia between the lateral incisor and cuspid demonstrating a change in bone pattern. Note the presence of a greater number of trabeculae per unit area and that the trabeculae are small and thin and randomly oriented in an orange-peel pattern.

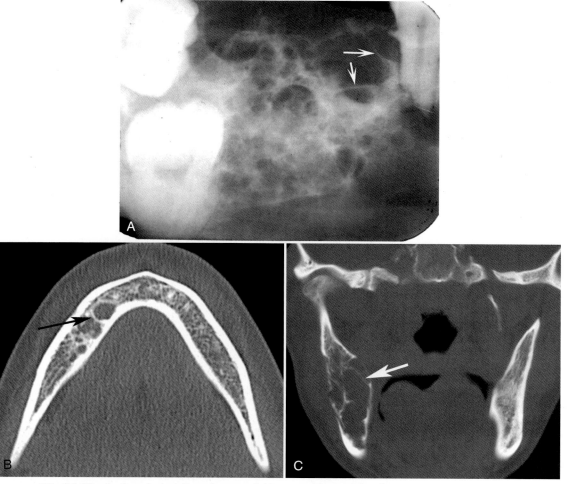

FIG. **16-20** **A,** A periapical film of an ameloblastoma. The multilocular pattern created by septa *(arrows)* divides the internal structure into small soap-bubble-like compartments. **B,** An axial CT image of an ameloblastoma has typically curved septa *(arrow),* whereas in **C,** a coronal CT image of a myxoma has typically straight septa *(arrow).*

sibly the ability to stimulate osteoblastic activity in the surrounding bone (see Fig. 16-3).

### Inferior Alveolar Nerve Canal and Mental Foramen

Some changes tend to be characteristic. For example, superior displacement of the inferior alveolar canal is strongly associated with fibrous dysplasia. Widening of the inferior alveolar canal with the maintenance of a cortical boundary may indicate the presence of a benign lesion of vascular or neural origin (see Fig. 16-8). Irregular widening with cortical destruction may indicate the presence of a malignant neoplasm growing down the length of the canal.

### Outer Cortical Bone and Periosteal Reactions

The cortex of bone may remodel in response to a lesion. A slowly growing lesion may allow time for the outer periosteum to manufacture new bone so that the resulting expanded bone appears to have maintained an outer cortical plate (see Fig. 16-5). On the other hand,

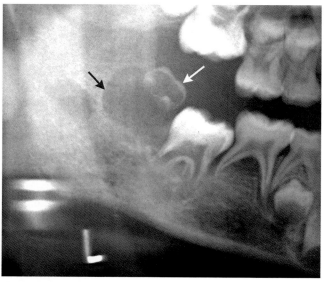

FIG. **16-21** Leukemic infiltration of the mandible showing coronal displacement of the developing second molar *(white arrow)* from the remnants of its crypt *(black arrow).* There is a lack of a lamina dura around the apex of the first molar and widening of the periodontal ligament space around the second deciduous molar.

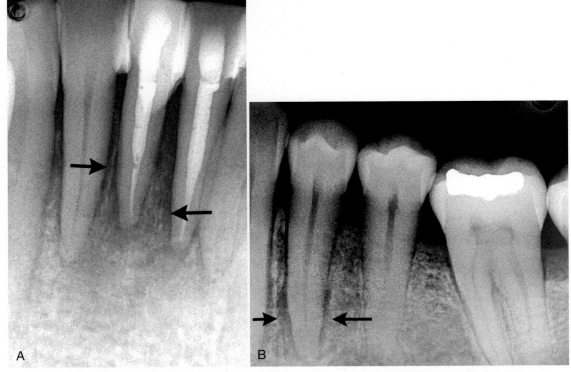

FIG. **16-22**   **A** and **B,** Periapical films revealing a malignant lymphoma that has invaded the mandible. There is irregular widening of the periodontal ligament spaces *(arrows).*

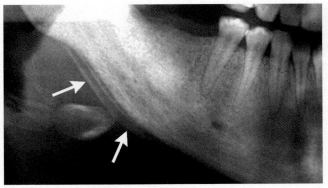

FIG. **16-23**   A panoramic image of osteomyelitis revealing at least two layers of new bone *(arrows)* produced by the periosteum at the inferior aspect of the mandible.

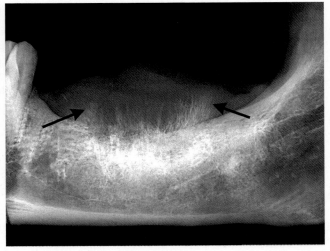

FIG. **16-24**   Specimen radiograph of a resected mandible with an osteosarcoma. Note the fine linear spicules of bone at the superior margin of the alveolar process.

a rapidly growing lesion outstrips the ability of the periosteum to respond, and the cortical plate may be missing (see Fig. 16-12). Exudate from an inflammatory lesion can lift the periosteum off the surface of the cortical bone and then stimulate the periosteum to lay down new bone (Fig. 16-23). When this process occurs more than once, an onion-skin type of pattern can be seen. This is most commonly seen in inflammatory lesions and more rarely in some malignant lesions (e.g., leukemia) and in Langerhans' cell histiocytosis. Some periosteal reactions are very specific, such as spiculated new bone formed at right angles to the outer cortical plate, which is seen

with metastatic lesions of the prostate gland or in a radiating pattern in osteogenic sarcoma (Fig. 16-24).

## STEP 5: FORMULATE A RADIOGRAPHIC INTERPRETATION

The preceding steps enable the observer to collect all the radiographic findings in an organized fashion. (Box 16-1 presents the process in

## BOX 16-1
## *Analysis of Intraosseous Lesions*

### *Step 1: Localize the Abnormality*
- Anatomic position (epicenter)
- Localized or generalized
- Unilateral or bilateral
- Single or multifocal

### *Step 2: Assess the Periphery and Shape*

PERIPHERY

*Well defined*
- Punched out
- Corticated
- Sclerotic
- Soft tissue capsule

*Ill defined*
- Blending
- Invasive

SHAPE

- Circular
- Scalloped
- Irregular

### *Step 3: Analyze the Internal Structure*
- Totally radiolucent
- Totally radiopaque
- Mixed (describe pattern)

### *Step 4: Analyze the Effects of the Lesion on Surrounding Structures*
- Teeth, lamina dura, periodontal membrane space
- Inferior alveolar nerve canal and mental foramen
- Maxillary antrum
- Surrounding bone density and trabecular pattern
- Outer cortical bone and periosteal reactions

### *Step 5: Formulate a Radiographic Interpretation*

---

abbreviated form.) Now the significance of each observation must be determined. The algorithm shown in Figure 16-25 should be used as a dynamic guide to accommodate new observations and change incorrect concepts. The ability to give more significance to some observations over others comes with experience. For instance, in the analysis of a hypothetical lesion, the observations of tooth movement, tooth resorption, and an invasive destructive border are made. The effects on the teeth in this example may indicate a benign process; however, the invasive border and bone destruction are more important characteristics and indicate a malignant process. The clinician should avoid making an interpretation from a single observation. In the analysis, all the accumulated characteristics point the way to the diagnosis. Also, occasionally any algorithm may fail because lesions sometimes do not behave as expected.

### Decision 1: Normal or Abnormal
The practitioner should determine whether the structure of interest is a variation of normal or represents an abnormality. This is a crucial decision because variations of normal do not require treatment or further investigation. However, as previously stated, to be proficient in the interpretation of diagnostic images, the practitioner needs an in-depth knowledge of the various appearances of normal anatomy.

### Decision 2: Developmental or Acquired
If the area of interest is abnormal, the next step is to decide whether the radiographic characteristics (location, periphery, shape, internal structure, and effects on surrounding structures) indicate that the region of interest represents a developmental abnormality or an acquired change. For instance, the observation that a tooth has an abnormally short root leads to the pertinent question, "Did the tooth develop a short root, or was the root at one time of normal length?" If the answer is the latter, then the process must be external root resorption and hence an acquired abnormality. If the tooth merely developed a short root, the pulp canal should not be visible to the very end of the root because of normal apexification. In contrast, external root resorption may shorten the root, but the canal remains visible to the end of the root (Fig. 16-26).

### Decision 3: Classification
If the abnormality is acquired, the next step is to select the most likely category of acquired abnormality: cysts, benign tumors, malignant tumors, inflammatory lesions, bone dysplasias (fibro-osseous lesions), vascular abnormalities, metabolic diseases, or physical changes such as fractures. Other chapters describe the characteristic radiographic findings of these abnormalities. The analysis should strive at least to narrow the interpretation to one of these groups because this directs the next course of action for continued investigation and treatment. This is a good time to bring the clinical information such as patient history and clinical signs and symptoms into the decision-making process. Introducing this information at the end helps avoid the problem of trying to make the radiographic characteristics fit a preconceived diagnosis.

### Decision 4: Ways to Proceed
After analyzing the images, the clinician must decide in what way to proceed. This may require further imaging, treatment, biopsy, or observation of the abnormality (watchful waiting). For example, if the lesion fits in the malignant category, the patient first should be referred to an oral and maxillofacial radiologist to complete the diagnostic imaging to stage the lesion and select the biopsy site and then should be referred to a surgeon for biopsy and treatment. Cemental dysplasia may not require any further investigation or treatment. In other cases a period of watchful waiting, followed by re-examination in a few months, may be indicated if the abnormality appears benign and no clear need for treatment exists.

With advanced training or experience in diagnostic imaging, the practitioner may be able to name one specific abnormality or at least make a short list of entities from one of the divisions of acquired abnormalities. It may be necessary to create a radiographic report for the purposes of documentation and communication with other clinicians.

### Radiographic Report
The radiographic report can be subdivided into the following subsections.

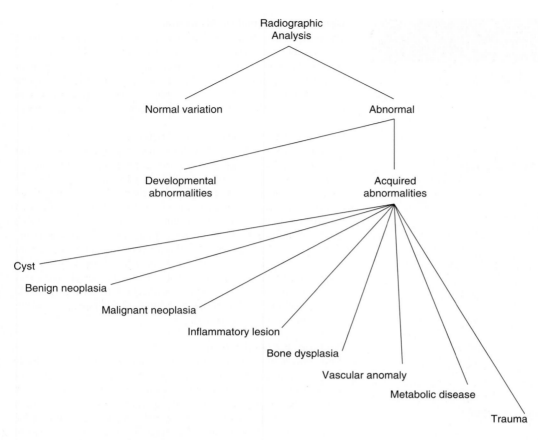

FIG. **16-25** An algorithm representing the diagnostic process that follows evaluation of the radiographic features of an abnormality.

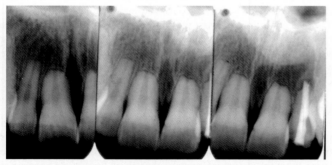

FIG. **16-26** Periapical films revealing external resorption of the maxillary incisors, which is an acquired abnormality because of the presence of the wide pulp chambers at the apex of the roots of the teeth.

*Patient and General Information.* This section appears at the beginning and contains the following information: address of the radiology clinic, the date of the dictation, the referring clinician's name, clinic or address, the patient's name, age, sex, and any numeric identification such as a clinic or medical registration number.

*Imaging Procedure.* This section provides a list of the imaging procedures provided along with the date of the examination. An example could be the following: panoramic and intraoral maxillary standard occlusal films plus axial and coronal computed tomographic (CT) images of the mandible with administration of contrast made on February 20, 2008.

*Clinical Information.* This is an optional section that includes pertinent clinical information regarding the patient provided by the referring clinician or the clinician dictating the report if a clinical examination was made before the radiologic examination. The clinical information should remain short and to the point and summarize the information, for example, mass in floor of mouth, possible ranula, and patient has a history of lymphoma.

*Findings (Observations).* This section is composed of an objective detailed list of observations, without interpretation, made from the diagnostic images. Using the step-by-step analysis of the extent of the lesion, periphery and shape, internal structure, and effects on surrounding structures will ensure completeness.

*Radiographic Interpretation (or Impression).* This section should be shorter and provides an interpretation for the preceding observations. The clinician should endeavor to provide a definitive interpretation, but when this is not possible a short list of conditions (in order of likelihood) is acceptable. In some situations advice regarding additional studies, when required, and treatment may be included.

Last, the name and signature of the clinician composing the report is included.

## SELF-TEST

The analytic technique can be practiced by looking at Figure 16-5, *A* and *B*, and writing down all observations and the results of the diagnostic algorithm before the following section is read.

### Description

*Location.* The abnormality is singular and unilateral, and the epicenter lies coronal to the mandibular first molar.

***Periphery and Shape.*** The lesion has a well-defined cortical boundary and a spherical or round shape. The periphery also attaches to the cementoenamel junction.

***Internal Structure.*** The internal structure is totally radiolucent.

***Effects.*** This lesion has displaced the first molar in an apical direction, which reinforces the decision that the origin was coronal to this tooth. Also, the lesion has displaced the second molar distally and the second premolar in an anterior direction. Apical resorption of the distal root of the second deciduous molar has occurred. The occlusal radiograph reveals that the buccal cortical plate has expanded in a smooth, curved shape, and a thin cortical boundary still exists.

***Analysis.*** Making all the observations is an important first step; the following is an analysis built on these observations. To accomplish this next step, further knowledge of pathologic conditions and a certain amount of practice are required. The first objective is to select the correct category of diseases (e.g., inflammatory, benign tumor, cyst); at this point, the clinician should try not to let all the names of specific diseases be overwhelming.

These images reveal an abnormal appearance. The coronal location of the lesion suggests that the tissue making up this abnormality probably is derived from a component of the dental follicle. The effects on the surrounding structures indicate that this abnormality is acquired. The displacement and resorption of teeth, intact peripheral cortex, curved shape, and radiolucent internal structure all indicate a slow-growing, benign, space-occupying lesion, most likely in the cyst category. Odontogenic tumors such as an ameloblastic fibroma may be considered but are less likely because of the shape. The most common type of cyst in a follicular location is a dentigerous cyst. Odontogenic keratocysts occasionally are seen in this location, but the tooth resorption and degree of expansion are not characteristic of that pathologic condition. Therefore the final interpretation is a follicular cyst, with odontogenic keratocyst and ameloblastic fibroma as possibilities in the differential diagnosis but less likely. Treatment usually is indicated for follicular cysts; therefore the patient is referred for surgical consultation.

## BIBLIOGRAPHY

Worth HM: *Principles and practice of oral radiologic interpretation,* Chicago, 1972, Mosby.

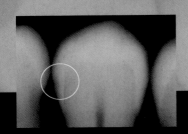

# CHAPTER 17

# Dental Caries

Ann Wenzel

Dental caries is a multifactorial disease with interaction between three factors, the tooth, the microflora, and the diet. If not disturbed, bacteria accumulate at specific tooth sites to form what is known as bacterial plaque (biofilm). The development of caries requires both the presence of bacteria and a diet containing fermentable carbohydrates. Caries is an infectious disease because it is the lactic acid produced by bacteria from the fermentation of carbohydrates that causes the dissolution, or demineralization, of the dental hard tissues. The *Streptococcus mutans* group plays a central role in the demineralization. In the initial stages of the disease bacteria are located on the tooth surface. It is only after severe demineralization or cavity formation has occurred that bacteria penetrate into the hard tissues. The demineralized tooth surface, called the *carious lesion*, is thus not the disease but a reflection of continuing or past microbial activity in the plaque.

The initial carious lesion is a subsurface loss of mineral in the outer tooth surface. It appears clinically as a chalky white (indicating present activity) or an opaque or dark, brownish spot (indicating past activity). A lesion beneath active bacterial plaque will progress, slowly or fast, but if the biofilm is removed or disturbed, the lesion will arrest. An arrested lesion may become reactive, however, and progress any time there is activity in the biofilm. Alternatively, remineralization in the outer parts of an arrested lesion can occur, for example, after the use of fluorides. Caries is therefore an ever-dynamic process.

The rate and extent of mineral loss depends on many factors. Mineral loss occurs faster in an active lesion when intercrystalline voids form. Demineralization may extend well into dentin before a breakdown of the outer surface (cavitation) occurs, resulting in a clinically visible cavity. With lesion progression and no intervention, demineralization may progress through the enamel, the dentin, and eventually into the pulp and may destroy the tooth (Fig. 17-1).

## Radiologic Examination to Detect Caries

Radiography is useful for detecting carious lesions because the caries process causes demineralization of enamel and dentin. The lesion is seen in the radiograph as a radiolucent (darker) zone because the demineralized area of the tooth does not absorb as many x-ray photons as the unaffected portion. It is important to keep in mind, though, that the lesion detected in the radiograph is merely a result of the bacterial activity on the tooth surface and radiography cannot reveal whether the lesion is active or arrested. An old inactive lesion will still appear as a demineralized "scar" in the hard tissues (Fig. 17-2). The reason is that remineralization takes place only in its outermost surface because mineral-containing solutions from saliva cannot diffuse into the body of the lesion. Because the radiograph only mirrors the current extent of demineralization, one radiograph alone cannot distinguish between an active and an arrested lesion. Only a second radiograph taken at a later time can reveal whether the disease is active. When a decision is made to monitor a lesion, factors such as oral hygiene, fluoride exposure, saliva flow, diet, caries history, extent of restorative care, and age should be considered in determining the time interval between the radiologic examinations (Chapter 15).

Radiography is a valuable supplement to a thorough clinical examination of the teeth for detecting caries. A careful clinical examination assessing the carious activity on the tooth surface may be possible for smooth surfaces and to some extent for occlusal surfaces. However, when the surface is clinically intact (i.e., no breakdown leading to cavitation has occurred), even the most meticulous examination may fail to reveal demineralizations beneath the surface, including occlusal surfaces. Clinical access to proximal tooth surfaces in contact is limited. Indeed, numerous clinical studies have shown that a radiologic examination can reveal carious lesions that would otherwise remain undetected both in occlusal and proximal surfaces.

## EXAMINATION WITH CONVENTIONAL INTRAORAL FILM

The bitewing projection is the most useful radiologic examination for detecting caries (Chapter 9). The use of a film holder with a beam-aiming device reduces the number of overlapping contact points and improves image quality, thus minimizing interpretation errors. Periapical radiographs are useful primarily for detecting changes in the periapical bone. Use of a paralleling technique for obtaining periapical radiographs increases the value of this projection in detecting caries of both anterior and posterior teeth, especially with heavily restored teeth.

Traditionally, size-2 "adult" films are used for a bitewing examination from the age of approximately 7 to 8 years onward. When it is necessary to examine all the contact surfaces from the cuspid to the most distal molar, one or two bitewing films per side are required, depending on the number of teeth that are present (Fig. 17-3). The use of a single size-3 film often results in overlapping contact points and "cone-cut" images and is not recommended. In small children

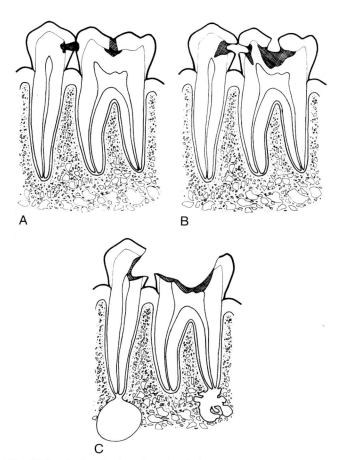

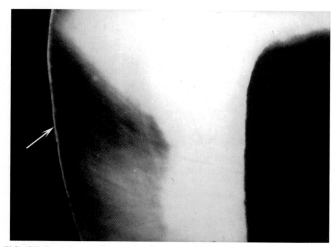

the size-0 or "child" film may be used instead of a size-2 film (Fig. 17-4).

In recent decades there has been a dramatic decline in the prevalence of caries in all Western countries, leaving a smaller fraction of the population with rapidly progressing carious lesions. Accordingly, the interval between examinations should be customized for each patient on the basis of the perceived caries activity and susceptibility. For caries-free individuals the interval may be lengthened, whereas for caries-active individuals the interval should be shorter.

Radiographs used to detect carious lesions should be mounted in frames with dark borders and interpreted with use of a light box with sufficient luminance and a magnifying viewer. Figure 17-5 is a series of radiographs showing early lesions with and without magnification.

FIG. **17-1**  **A,** Proximal and occlusal demineralization penetrating through tooth enamel and into the dentin. **B,** Proximal and occlusal tissue demineralization and cavitation nearing the pulp chamber of two vital teeth. **C,** Severe demineralization and cavitation reaching the pulp chamber resulting in two nonvital pulps and periapical inflammatory disease.

FIG. **17-2**  Microradiograph of an inactive carious lesion *(dark region)* halfway through enamel with an intact, well mineralized surface *(arrow)*. The inner dark area represents dentin.

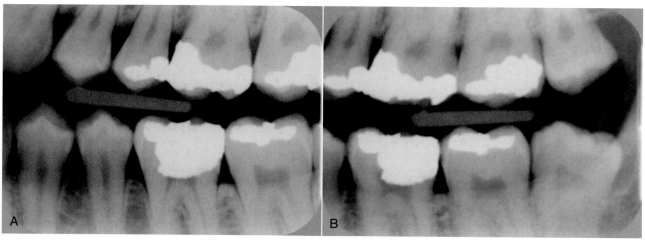

FIG. **17-3**  Two bitewing images from the patient's left side covering the surfaces from the distal surface of the canine to the distal surface of the most posterior molar.

## EXAMINATION WITH DIGITAL IMAGING

Digital image receptors may replace film for intraoral radiography. There are two different methods available: (1) solid-state sensors (charge-coupled device [CCD] and complementary metal oxide semiconductor technology [CMOS]) with a cord that connects the receptor to the computer or without a cord (signal is transferred by radio wave) and (2) storage phosphors (PSP plates) that use a filmlike plate that is processed (scanned) after exposure (Chapter 7). The holders available for bitewing examinations with phosphor plates appear like those for film, and universal sensor holders are also available. However, there may be some problems when solid-state sensors are used for

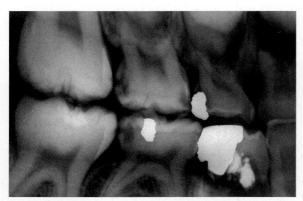

FIG. **17-4** This bitewing image of the mixed dentition demonstrates dentinal carious lesions involving the mesial and distal surfaces of the second deciduous molars and small enamel lesions in the mesial surfaces of the first permanent molars. An extensive lesion involves the crown and root structure of the mandibular first deciduous molar.

bitewing examination. First, the surface area of the sensor is smaller than the surface area of a size-2 film, resulting in the display of fewer interproximal tooth surfaces per bitewing image than with film. Further, the stiffness and increased thickness of these sensors may result in more projection errors and retakes. When digital bitewing images are used, they should be displayed on a monitor in their full resolution for interpretation and viewed in a room with subdued light.

## Radiographic Detection of Lesions

### PROXIMAL SURFACES

#### Typical Radiographic Appearance

The shape of the early radiolucent lesion in the enamel is classically a triangle with its broad base at the tooth surface (Fig. 17-5) spreading along the enamel rods, but other appearances are common, such as a "notch," a dot, a band, or a thin line (Fig. 17-6). When the demineralizing front reaches the dentinoenamel junction (DEJ), it spreads along the junction, frequently forming the base of a second triangle with apex directed toward the pulp chamber (Fig. 17-7). This triangle typically has a wider base than in the enamel and progresses toward the pulp along the direction of the dentinal tubules. Again, more irregular shapes of decalcification may be seen.

Lesions involving proximal surfaces most commonly are found in the area between the contact point and the free gingival margin (Fig. 17-8). The fact that this type of lesion does not start below the gingival margin helps distinguish a carious lesion from cervical burnout. Close attention should be paid to intact proximal surfaces adjacent to a tooth surface with a restoration because occasionally this surface is inadvertently damaged during the restorative procedure and is thus at greater risk for caries (Fig. 17-9).

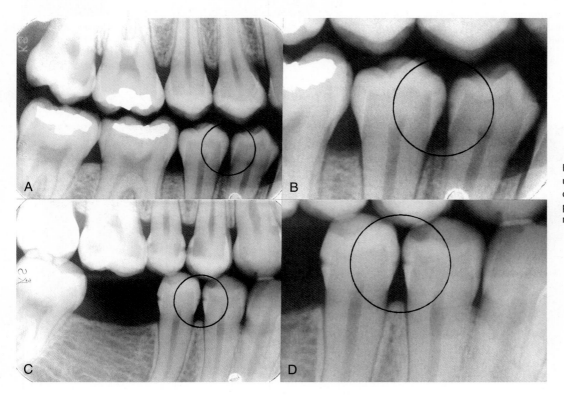

FIG. **17-5** An example of the use of image magnification to detect enamel carious lesions in premolars. **A** and **C** are not magnified. **B** and **D** are magnified.

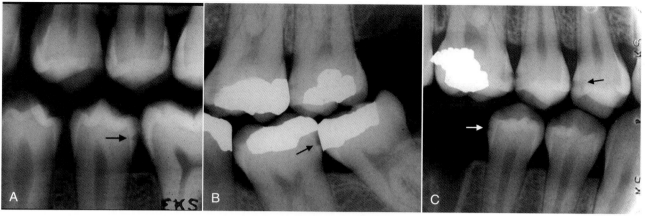

FIG. **17-6**   **A,** This bitewing image demonstrates bandlike lesions involving the enamel of the maxillary premolars and a triangular lesion *(arrow)* in the mandibular second premolar. **B,** This bitewing image shows an enamel lesion *(arrow)* and a lesion extending into the dentin involving the mesial surface of the maxillary second molar. **C,** This bitewing image reveals lesions involving the enamel of the mandibular second premolar *(white arrow)* and the distal surface of the maxillary second premolar and lesions extending into the dentin of the mesial surface of the maxillary first molar and the distal surface of the first premolar *(black arrow).*

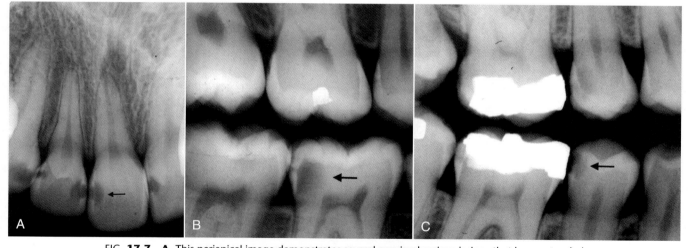

FIG. **17-7**   **A,** This periapical image demonstrates several proximal carious lesions that have extended into the dentin. Note that the lesions extend along the dentinoenamel junction to involve a greater amount of dentin than enamel *(arrow).* **B,** This bitewing image demonstrates an extensive proximal carious lesion involving the distal aspect of the mandibular first molar *(arrow).* Note that the pulp horn has been reduced as a result of the formation of tertiary (irritation) dentin. **C,** This bitewing image shows two lesions involving the dentin in the distal surfaces of the second premolars, and one lesion has resulted in cavitation *(arrow).*

Because the proximal surfaces of posterior teeth are often broad, the loss of small amounts of mineral from incipient lesions and the advancing front of active lesions are often difficult to detect in the radiographic image. Lesions confined to enamel may not be evident radiographically until approximately 30% to 40% demineralization has occurred. For this reason, the actual depth of penetration of a carious lesion is often deeper than seen radiographically.

### False Interpretations

Even experienced dentists often do not agree on the presence or absence of carious lesions when examining the same set of radio-graphs, especially when the lesions are limited to the enamel. On occasion a carious lesion may be incorrectly detected when the tooth surface is actually unaffected (a false-positive outcome). Various morphologic phenomena, such as pits and fissures, cervical burnout, and Mach band effect, and dental anomalies, such as hypoplastic pits and concavities produced by wear, can mimic the appearance of a carious lesion (Fig. 17-10). In cases where the demineralization is not yet radiographically visible, failure to detect the lesion is a false-negative outcome (Fig. 17-11). Also, overlapping contact points in the radiographic image may obscure a lesion (Fig. 17-12). Approximately half of all proximal lesions in enamel cannot be detected by radiography.

The possibility of false-positive diagnoses of small lesions, combined with the knowledge that caries progresses slowly in most individuals, argues for a conservative approach to caries diagnosis and treatment. A lesion extending into the dentin in the radiograph may be easier to detect with greater agreement among experienced observers. Occasionally demineralization in the enamel is not obvious and a dentinal lesion is overlooked (see Fig. 17-6, *A*, distal surface of the maxillary second premolar and, *B*, mesial surface of the maxillary first molar).

### Lesions with and Without Clinical Cavitation

Potentially a progressing proximal lesion may be arrested if cavitation has not developed. If cavitation has occurred, the lesion will always be active because the bacteria that colonize within the cavity cannot be removed. Unfortunately, the presence of cavitation cannot be accurately determined radiographically, although the greater the radiographic depth of the lesion the greater the likelihood of cavitation. Because extensive demineralization must occur before the surface breaks down, the percentage of enamel lesions with surface cavitation is very small. Approximately half of lesions that are just into dentin have surface cavitation. The deeper the lesion has penetrated into dentin, the more likely it is cavitated, and dentinal lesions extending more than halfway to the pulp are always cavitated. Temporarily separating proximal surfaces with orthodontic elastics or springs may allow direct inspection to determine whether there is cavitation. This method is easier in children than adults.

### Treatment Considerations

These considerations mean that operative treatment is usually not indicated for lesions detected in enamel and the dentist and the patient may arrest lesion progression with conservative intervention. Cavitated lesions, on the other hand, will need operative treatment. For dentinal lesions, the decision whether to provide operative treatment is individualized for each patient. In cases where it is decided to monitor the lesion, a follow-up radiograph should be taken to evaluate whether the lesion has arrested or is progressing. The interval between the radiologic examinations should be determined individually, taking into account previous caries history, age and, not least, the site of the lesion because the progression rate differs highly among the various tooth surfaces. Care should be taken to reproduce the same image geometry in the follow-up radiographs by using standardized film holders to provide a means of accurate comparison of depth of the lesion. When digital images are made with reproducible geometry, they can be superimposed and the information in the one image can be subtracted from the other, resulting in a subtraction image, which displays the changes that have occurred between the two examinations (Fig. 17-13).

Progression of a lesion indicates the need for operative therapy. With highly motivated patients who clean the surface and with topical fluoride treatment, more than half of shallow dentinal lesions can be arrested, thus avoiding restorative therapy.

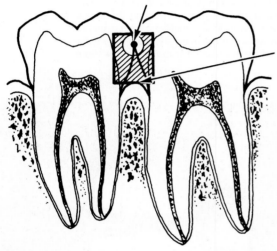

FIG. **17-8**  Proximal caries-susceptible zone. This region extends from the contact point down to the height of the free gingival margin. It increases with recession of the alveolar bone and gingival tissues.

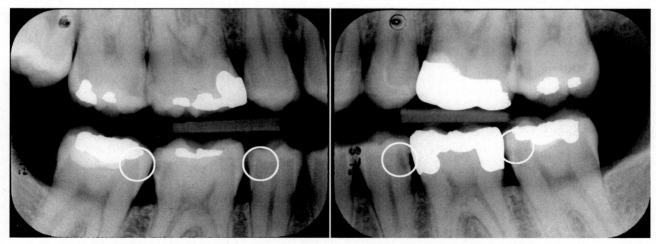

FIG. **17-9**  A pair of bitewing images. Note *(circles)* that dentinal lesions have developed in surfaces adjacent to a restored surface in the patient's left side, but not in the same surfaces of the teeth in the right side.

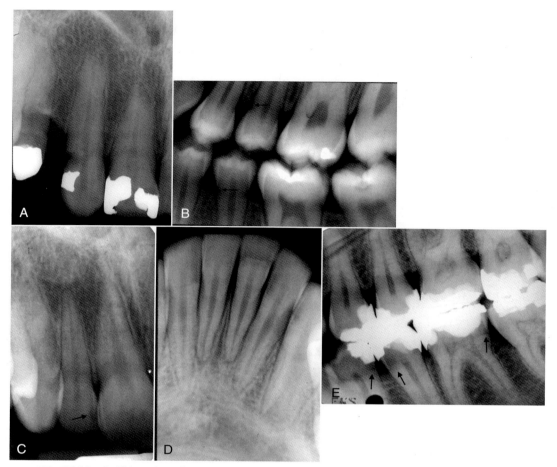

FIG. **17-10   A,** This periapical image reveals a radiolucent region similar in appearance to a carious lesion in the distal cervical aspect of the maxillary cuspid, which is caused by abrasion from a clasp from a partial denture. **B,** In this bitewing image cervical burnout *(arrows)* can mimic carious lesions. **C,** In this periapical image a small concavity in the mesial surface of the lateral incisor creates a radiolucent region similar in appearance to a carious lesion *(arrow).* **D,** In this periapical image a band of enamel hypoplasia involving the left central incisor produces a linear radiolucent region that may be misinterpreted as carious lesion. **E,** In this bitewing image the overlapping shadow of the alveolar process creates a Mach band effect *(arrows)* resulting in apparent radiolucent regions in the crowns of the premolars and first molar that may mimic carious lesions.

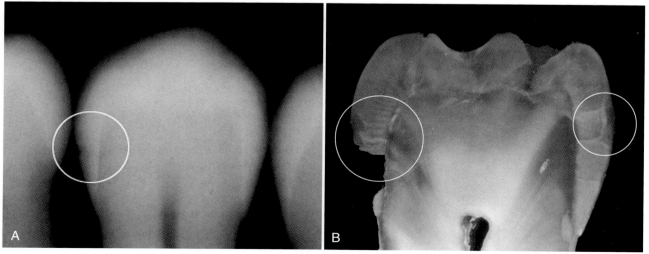

FIG. **17-11   A,** A radiograph of an extracted tooth with a lesion just into dentin in the left side *(circle)* but no visible lesion in the right side. **B,** The same tooth after sectioning assessed under a microscope reveals lesions in both sides; the lesion in the right side is only in enamel. Note that enamel in the left side has broken off during sectioning.

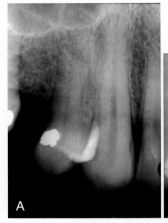

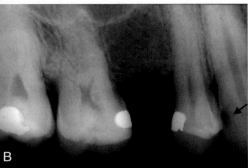

FIG. **17-12 A,** In this periapical image a proximal carious lesion involving the distal surface of the cuspid is not apparent. However, in the periapical image **(B)**, the change in the horizontal orientation of the x-ray beam has separated the overlapping images of the opposing surfaces of the premolar and cuspid, revealing the presence of the lesion *(arrow).*

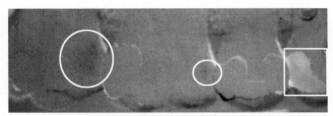

FIG. **17-13** A subtraction image made from two bitewing images taken with a 2-year interval. The contours of four maxillary teeth can be seen. Between the two examinations a filling was placed *(rectangle),* a new deep dentinal lesion has developed *(large circle),* and a lesion has progressed from enamel into dentin *(small circle).*

## OCCLUSAL SURFACES

### Typical Radiographic Appearance

Carious lesions in children and adolescents most often occur on occlusal surfaces of posterior teeth. The demineralization process originates in enamel pits and fissures where bacterial plaque can gather. The lesion spreads along the enamel rods and, if undisturbed, penetrates to the DEJ, where it may be seen as a thin radiolucent line between enamel and dentin.

Occlusal lesions commonly start in the sides of a fissure wall rather than at the base and then tend to penetrate nearly perpendicularly toward the DEJ. Early lesions appear clinically as chalky white, yellow, brown, or black discolorations of the occlusal fissures. Finding such discolored fissures in a clinically intact occlusal surface suggests that a radiologic examination is indicated to determine whether a carious lesion has penetrated beyond the DEJ. If the lesion has not crossed the DEJ, it may not be visible in the radiograph.

The classic radiographic appearance of lesions extending into the dentin is a broad-based, radiolucent zone, often beneath a fissure, with little or no apparent changes in the enamel. The deeper the occlusal lesion, the easier it is to detect on the radiograph (Fig. 17-14).

### False Interpretations

Pitfalls in the interpretation of dentinal occlusal lesions include superimposition of the image of the buccal pit with or without an associated carious lesion or a composite restoration, which may simulate an occlusal lesion or a deep occlusal fissure. Direct clinical inspection of the tooth most often eliminates any such confusion.

When an occlusal lesion is confined to enamel, the surrounding enamel often obscures the lesion. As the carious process progresses, a radiolucent line extends along the DEJ. As the lesion extends into the dentin, the margin between the carious and noncarious dentin is diffuse and may obscure the fine radiolucent line at the DEJ. Therefore false-positive detection rates may be as high as false-negative ones for shallow lesions. A false-negative outcome may not represent a severe mistake because in most cases the process progresses slowly and the lesion is detected at a later time. A false-positive outcome may result in a sound surface being irreversibly damaged. Also, when there is a sharply defined density difference, such as between enamel and dentin, there may appear to be a more radiolucent region immediately adjacent to the enamel. This is an optical illusion referred to as the Mach band (see Fig. 17-10, *E*). This can contribute to the number of false-positive interpretations; therefore when there are no clinical signs of a lesion, it would be reasonable to observe these cases and withhold operative treatment.

### Cavitation and Treatment Considerations

As an occlusal lesion spreads through the dentin, it undermines the enamel, and eventually masticatory forces cause cavitation. When the cavitation is visible on clinical inspection, it is usually an indication that the lesion is already well into dentin and if information regarding extent relative to the pulp chamber is needed, then a radiologic examination is required. Without cavitation, fissure discoloration may indicate the need for radiologic examination. Dentinal lesions without clinically apparent cavitation but with a radiolucent change indicate that the carious lesions have passed the DEJ (see Fig. 17-14) and require operative treatment.

## RAMPANT CARIES

Severe, rapidly progressing carious destruction of teeth is usually termed *rampant* caries and is usually seen in children with poor dietary and oral hygiene habits (see Fig. 17-4). This condition, however, is becoming increasingly rare because of widespread availability of fluoride in water supplements and topical application and enlightened practices of good nutrition and hygiene. Rampant caries may also be seen in people with xerostomia. Radiographs of individuals with

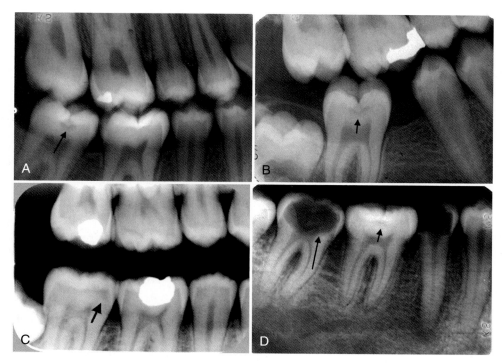

FIG. **17-14**  **A** and **B,** These bitewing images demonstrate a classic appearance of an occlusal carious lesion with a triangular shape in the enamel with the base oriented to the dentinoenamel junction *(arrows)*. The bitewing image **(C)** is not as clear, but there is an ill-defined radiolucent region under the occlusal enamel surface *(arrow)*. In the periapical image **(D)** there is a subtle occlusal lesion in the first molar *(short arrow)* and an extensive cavitated lesion in the second molar *(long arrow)*.

rampant caries demonstrate severe (advanced) carious destructions, especially of the mandibular anterior teeth.

## BUCCAL AND LINGUAL SURFACES

Buccal and lingual carious lesions often occur in enamel pits and fissures of teeth. When small, these lesions are usually round; as they enlarge, they become elliptic or semilunar. They demonstrate sharp, well-defined borders.

It may be difficult to differentiate between buccal and lingual carious lesions on a radiograph. When viewing buccal or lingual lesions, the clinician should look for a uniform noncarious region of enamel surrounding the apparent radiolucency (Fig. 17-15). This well-defined circular area represents parallel noncarious enamel rods surrounding the buccal or palatal lesion. Occlusal lesions, however, ordinarily are more extensive than lingual or buccal caries, and their outline is not as well defined. Clinical evaluation with visual and tactile methods is usually the definitive method of detecting buccal or lingual lesions.

## ROOT SURFACES

Root surface lesions involve both cementum and dentin and are associated with gingival recession. The exposed cementum is relatively soft and usually only 20 to 50 μm thick near the cementoenamel junction, so it rapidly degrades by attrition, abrasion, and erosion. Root surface caries should be detected clinically, and most often radiographs are not needed for diagnosis. In proximal root surfaces radiologic examination may reveal lesions that have gone undetected (Fig. 17-16).

A pitfall in the detection of root lesions is that a surface may appear to be carious as a result of the cervical burnout phenomenon (see Figs. 17-10, *B,* and 17-16, *C*). The true carious lesion may be distinguished from the intact surface primarily by the absence of an image of the

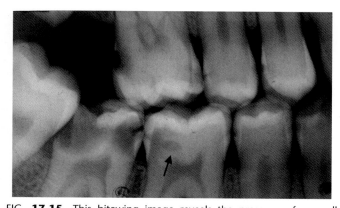

FIG. **17-15** This bitewing image reveals the presence of a small buccal lesion *(arrow)* involving the mandibular first molar. Note the presence of 12 proximal carious lesions. Also, the abnormal position of the mandibular third molar created an enhanced site for plaque accumulation resulting in an extensive carious lesion involving the second molar.

root edge and by the appearance of a diffuse rounded inner border where the tooth substance has been lost.

## ASSOCIATED WITH DENTAL RESTORATIONS

A carious lesion developing at the margin of an existing restoration may be termed *secondary* or *recurrent* caries. It should be noted, though, that a lesion developing in a restored surface is most frequently a new primary demineralization, either because of faulty shaping or inadequate extension of the restoration leading to plaque accumulation (Fig. 17-17). These lesions (secondary caries) should be treated as any new carious lesion. It is important not to confuse secondary (primary) caries with *residual* caries, which is caries that

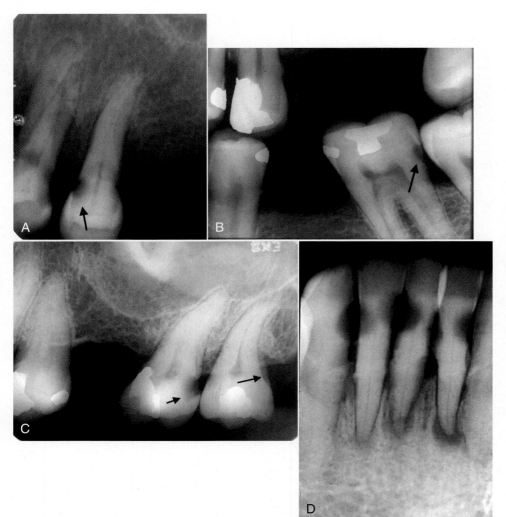

FIG. **17-16 A,** This periapical image shows root surface carious lesions involving the distal aspect of the first premolar and the mesial and distal aspect of the second premolar. Note that the lesion undermines the enamel surface *(arrow).* **B,** This bitewing image reveals a root surface lesion involving the distal cervical region of the second molar *(arrow);* this location is in part due to the low third molar contact point on the distal surface, the result of abnormal mesial tipping of both molars. **C,** This periapical image shows a carious lesion in the distal root surface of the maxillary second molar *(short arrow)* and an example of cervical burnout *(long arrow).* Note the sharp line from overlapping roots that delineates the radiolucent cervical burnout. **D,** This periapical image demonstrates multiple root lesions involving the mandibular incisors. Note the associated periapical inflammatory lesions.

remain if the original lesion is not completely removed. In situations where the radiographic lesion is very close to the pulp, carious dentin may be left on purpose during operative treatment. Medication that stimulates the development of tertiary dentin is placed in the cavity (indirect pulp capping). After some months the remaining carious dentin is removed and a permanent filling placed.

A lesion next to a restoration may be obscured by the radiopaque image of the restoration. Thus two radiographic views made at different horizontal or vertical angulations of the central ray can be an aid where there are multiple radiopaque restorations. Also, the detection of secondary carious lesions depends on a careful clinical examination. Recurrent lesions at the mesiogingival and distogingival margins are most frequently detected radiographically.

Restorative materials vary in their radiographic appearance depending on thickness, density, atomic number, and the x-ray beam energy used to make the radiograph. Some materials can be confused with caries. Older calcium hydroxide liners without barium, lead, or zinc (added to lend radiopacity) appear radiolucent and may resemble recurrent or residual caries. Despite the calcium present, the relatively large proportion of low atomic number material in calcium hydroxide causes its radiodensity to be similar to a carious lesion. Composite, plastic, or silicate restorations also may simulate lesions. It is often possible, however, to identify and differentiate these radiolucent materials from caries by their well-defined and smooth outline reflecting the preparation or from their radiopaque liners (Fig. 17-18).

## THERAPY AFTER RADIATION

Patients who have received therapeutic radiation to the head and neck may have a loss of salivary gland function, leading to xerostomia (dry mouth) and a change in the bacterial flora and possibly intrinsic change to the tooth structure. Untreated, this induces rampant destruction of the teeth, termed *radiation* caries (Chapter 2). Typically, the destruction begins at the cervical region and may aggressively encircle the tooth, causing the entire crown to be lost, with only root fragments remaining in the jaws. The radiographic appearance of radiation caries is characteristic: radiolucent shadows appearing at the necks of teeth, most obvious on the mesial and distal aspects. Variations in the depth of destruction may be present, but generally there is uniformity within a given region of the mouth. Figure 17-19

FIG. **17-17 A,** This bitewing image reveals several interproximal carious lesions; three are recurrent caries *(arrows).* **B,** This bitewing image demonstrates a recurrent carious lesion in the distal surface of the maxillary second premolar *(arrow).* Note the overhang to the restoration placed on the mesial surface of the first molar. **C,** This periapical image reveals a recurrent carious lesion *(arrow)* involving the distal surface of the second premolar. **D,** Note that there is an overhang to the restoration on the distal aspect of this maxillary second molar and an associated recurrent carious lesion *(arrow).*

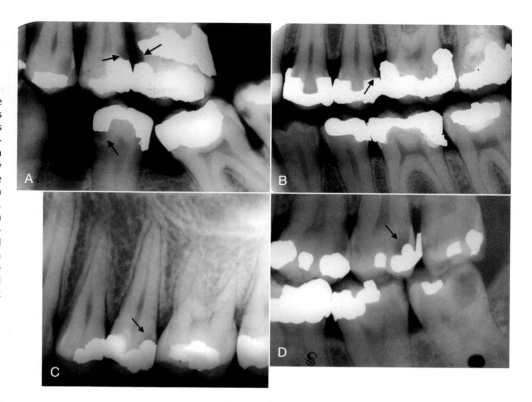

FIG. **17-18 A,** This periapical image shows radiolucent restorations placed in the mesial and distal surfaces of the lateral incisor and mesial surface of the cuspid. Note the well-defined margins, useful to differentiate from carious lesions. **B,** In this periapical image the radiopaque liner on the internal aspect of the restoration placed on the distal surface of the central incisor is useful to differentiate from a carious lesion. Note the sharp margins of the restoration placed in the mesial surface of the lateral incisor. **C,** In this periapical image there are four radiolucent restorations and one carious lesion. The carious lesion involves the distal surface of the lateral incisor. Note the diffuse margin of the lesion in contrast to the well-defined margins of the restorations. **D,** This periapical image shows a recurrent carious lesion *(arrow)* involving the distal surface of the central incisor in contact with the radiolucent restoration. Note the diffuse ill-defined margin of the lesion compared with the well-defined margin of the restoration.

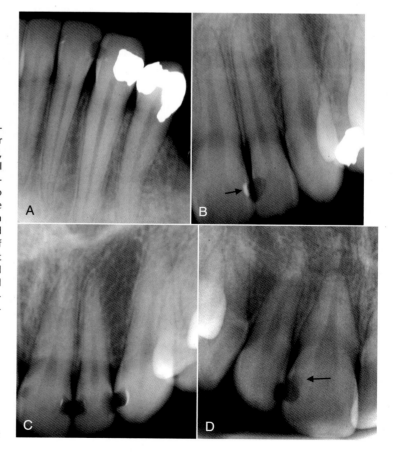

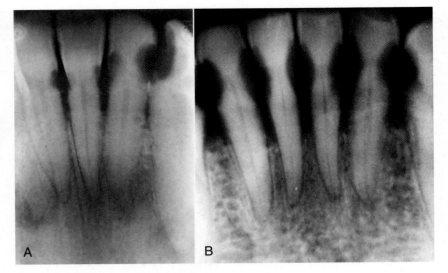

FIG. **17-19 A** and **B,** These two periapical images reveal multiple carious lesions that occurred after therapeutic radiation exposure. Note that the lesions start in the region of the cementoenamel junction.

shows examples of radiation caries in patients with xerostomia after therapeutic radiation for cancer of the head and neck. Use of topical fluorides as remineralizing solutions and meticulous oral hygiene can markedly reduce the radiation damage to teeth resulting from xerostomia.

## Alternative Diagnostic Tools to Detect Dental Caries

Other methods have been developed in addition to clinical inspection and radiography to detect carious lesions. These include light fluorescence (QLF), "Diagnodent" laser-light fiberoptic transillumination (FOTI), electrical conductance measurements (ECM), and ultrasonography. QLF may be used to quantify mineral loss on smooth surfaces, whereas Diagnodent and ECM have been applied on occlusal surfaces. These two methods operate by displaying a value that provides quantitative information on the depth of the lesion. None of the methods can unequivocally distinguish between enamel and dentin lesions or between shallow and deep dentin lesions. FOTI has been used primarily for proximal surfaces but may also be applied to occlusal surfaces. FOTI is less sensitive than radiography for distinguishing shallow and deep lesions. ECM is better than FOTI in identifying occlusal caries in young children. There is little evidence yet that these methods can substitute traditional diagnostic methods in the clinic.

## Treatment Considerations

Carious lesions in enamel require interceptive treatment but rarely operative treatment. The radiographic detection of small areas of demineralization requires a decision as to whether these represent active or inactive arrested lesions. When the radiograph shows a lesion limited to enamel, the probability of cavitation is low and the prospect of arresting or reversing the caries process is good. Also, if the radiograph shows a lesion just into the dentin, treatment should include a means to stop the microbiologic activity and possibly reverse the demineralization process. Treatment of such lesions may include reductions in sugar intake, proper oral hygiene to reduce bacteria, and use of topical fluorides to inhibit microbiologic activity, retard demin-

eralization, and promote remineralization of the outermost parts of the lesion. This may be successful if the surface of the tooth is not cavitated and a follow-up radiograph shows no progression of the lesion. However, when the surface of a lesion is cavitated or follow-up radiographs reveal progression of the lesion in dentin, a restoration is required. Cavitated carious lesions require removal of the infected tissues, possibly stepwise over a period for extensive lesions, and restoration of the tooth to form and function.

## BIBLIOGRAPHY

Fejerskov O, Kidd EAM: *Dental caries: the disease and its clinical management,* ed 1, Munksgaard, 2003, Blackwell.

Newbrun E: *Cariology,* ed 3, Baltimore, 1989, Williams & Wilkins.

NIH Consensus Development Conference on Diagnosis and Management of Dental Caries Throughout Life. Bethesda, MD, March 26-28, 2001. Conference papers. *J Dent Educ* 65:935-1179, 2001.

Pitts NB, Stamm JW: International Consensus Workshop on Caries Clinical Trials (ICW-CCT)—final consensus statements: agreeing where the evidence leads. *J Dent Res* 83(Spec No. C):C125-C128, 2004.

Selwitz RH, Ismail AI, Pitts NB: Dental caries, *Lancet* 369:51-59, 2007.

## SUGGESTED READINGS

### *RADIOGRAPHIC CARIES DETECTION*

De Araujo FB, Rosito DB, Toigo E et al: Diagnosis of approximal caries: radiographic versus clinical examination using tooth separation, *Am J Dent* 5:245-248, 1992.

Hintze H, Wenzel A: A two-film versus a four-film bite-wing examination for caries diagnosis in adults, *Caries Res* 33:380-396, 1999.

Hintze H, Wenzel A, Danielsen B: Behaviour of approximal carious lesions assessed by clinical examination after tooth separation and radiography: a 2.5-year longitudinal study in young adults, *Caries Res* 33:415-422, 1999.

Mejáre I: Bitewing examination to detect caries in children and adolescents—when and how often? *Dent Update* 32:588-590, 593-594, 596-597, 2005.

Mejáre I, Stenlund H, Zelezny-Holmlund C: Caries incidence and lesions progression from adolescence to young adulthood: a prospective 15-year cohort study in Sweden, *Caries Res* 38:130-141, 2004.

Mjör IA, Toffenetti F: Secondary caries: a literature review with case reports, *Quintessence Int* 31:165-179, 2000.

Nielsen LL, Hoernoe M, Wenzel A: Radiographic detection of cavitation in approximal surfaces of primary teeth using a digital storage phosphor system and conventional film, and the relationship between cavitation and radiographic lesion depth: an in vitro study, *Int J Paediatr Dent* 6:167-172, 1996.

Nyvad B, Fejerskov O: Assessing the stage of caries lesion activity on the basis of clinical and microbiological examination, *Community Dent Oral Epidemiol* 25:69-75, 1997.

Nyvad B, Machiulskiene V, Baelum V: Reliability of a new caries diagnostic system differentiating between active and inactive caries lesions, *Caries Res* 33:252-260, 1999.

Petersson GH, Bratthall D: The caries decline: a review of reviews, *Eur J Oral Sci* 104:436-443, 1996.

Poorterman JHG, Weerheijm KL, Groen HJ et al: Clinical and radiographic judgement of occlusal caries in adolescents, *Eur J Oral Sci* 108:93-98, 2000.

Qvist V, Johannesen L, Bruun M: Progression of approximal caries in relation to iatrogenic preparation damage, *J Dent Res* 71:1370-1373, 1992.

Ratledge DK, Kidd EA, Beighton D: A clinical and microbiological study of approximal carious lesions, 1: the relationship between cavitation, radiographic lesion depth, the site specific gingival index and the level of infection of the dentine, *Caries Res* 35:3-7, 2001.

Wenzel A: A review of dentists' use of digital radiography and caries diagnosis with digital systems, *Dentomaxillofac Radiol* 35:307-314, 2006.

Wenzel A, Anthonisen PN, Juul MB: Reproducibility in the assessment of caries lesion behaviour: a comparison between conventional film and subtraction radiography, *Caries Res* 34:214-218, 2000.

Wenzel A, Haiter-Neto F, Gotfredsen E: Risk factors for a false positive test outcome in diagnosis of caries in approximal surfaces: impact of radiographic modality and observer characteristics, *Caries Res* 41:170-176, 2007.

White SC, Yoon DC: Comparative performance of digital and conventional images for detecting proximal surface caries, *Dentomaxillofac Radiol* 26:32-38, 1997.

### TREATMENT DECISION

Bader JD, Shugars DA: What do we know about how dentists make caries-related treatment decisions? *Community Dent Oral Epidemiol* 25:97-103, 1997.

Bader JD, Shugars DA: The evidence supporting alternative management strategies for early occlusal caries and suspected occlusal dentinal caries, *J Evid Based Dent Pract* 6:91-100, 2006.

Bjorndal L, Kidd EA: The treatment of deep dentine caries lesions, *Dent Update* 32:402-404, 407-410, 413, 2005.

Pitts NB: Diagnostic tools and measurements—impact on appropriate care, *Community Dent Oral Epidemiol* 25:24-35, 1997.

Pitts NB: Are we ready to move from operative to non-operative/preventive treatment of dental caries in clinical practice? *Caries Res* 38:294-304, 2004.

Ricketts DN, Kidd EA, Innes N et al: Complete or ultraconservative removal of decayed tissue in unfilled teeth, *Cochrane Database Syst Rev* 3:CD003808, 2006.

Rimmer PA, Pitts NB: Temporary elective tooth separation as a diagnostic aid in general dental practice, *Br Dent J* 169:87-92, 1990.

Verdonschot EH, Angmar-Månsson B, ten Bosch JJ et al: Developments in caries diagnosis and their relationship to treatment decisions and quality of care. ORCA Saturday Afternoon Symposium 1997. *Caries Res* 33:32-40, 1999.

Woodward GL, Leake JL: The use of dental radiographs to estimate the probability of cavitation of carious interproximal lesions, I: evidence from the literature, *J Can Dent Assoc* 62:731-736, 1996.

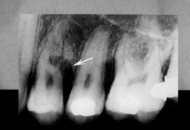

# CHAPTER 18

# Periodontal Diseases

Susanne Perschbacher

Several distinct yet related disorders of the periodontium are collectively known as periodontal diseases. They are a set of conditions characterized by an inflammatory host response in the periodontal tissues that may lead to localized or generalized alterations in the soft tissues around the teeth, loss of supporting bone, and ultimately, loss of the teeth. Periodontal diseases are broadly classified as gingival diseases and periodontitis. Gingival diseases may be dental plaque-induced or non–plaque-induced. Bacterial plaque-associated gingivitis is much more common than non–plaque-induced inflammatory diseases affecting the gingiva such as viral or fungal infections, mucocutaneous and allergic conditions, and traumatic injuries. Gingivitis presents as inflammation of the soft tissue surrounding the teeth with gingival swelling, edema, and erythema.

Periodontitis is classified, primarily by the clinical presentation, as chronic, aggressive, and periodontitis as a manifestation of a systemic disease. Other subtypes of periodontal conditions include necrotizing periodontal diseases, periodontal abscesses, and periodontitis associated with endodontic lesions. Periodontitis is distinguished from gingivitis by the clinically detectable destruction of host tissues seen as the loss of soft tissue attachment and supporting bone of the involved teeth. Although periodontitis is always preceded by gingivitis, gingivitis does not always progress to periodontitis.

Dental plaque, which may vary greatly in its bacterial composition, plays a primary role in the initiation of periodontitis. Periodontitis-implicated plaque bacteria species, predominantly gram-negative rods and spirochetes, have the ability to colonize on the tooth and root surfaces, spread into the region between the root and the gingival margin, and in some cases invade the surrounding tissue. These bacteria are capable of causing damage to the host tissue either directly, through the release of toxins, or more significantly, indirectly, by stimulating a host inflammatory reaction. As part of the host response, the release of inflammatory mediators, especially from neutrophils, is responsible for much of the injury to the surrounding soft tissue and stimulation of osteoclastic bone resorption. The resulting inflammatory response causes loss of, and apical migration of, the epithelial attachment, resulting in pocket formation and thus further enhancing bacterial colonization.

The clinical manifestation of this interplay between bacterial plaque and the host tissues are clinical signs of inflammation. Gingivitis seen as gingival swelling, edema, and erythema is the most common first clinical sign. Progression to periodontitis is manifested with pocket formation, the universal presentation of this disease. Other clinical signs include bleeding, purulent exudate, edema, resorption of the alveolar crest, and tooth mobility. Rather than progressing smoothly from mild to moderate to severe, periodontitis often progresses in bursts. There are active periods of inflammation and tissue destruction followed by healing and quiescent periods (often years) of no appreciable change. The extent of disease activity is best measured by longitudinal probing of periodontal attachment level. This cycle of disease activity may repeat. The relative duration of the destructive and quiescent phases depends on the form of periodontitis, the nature of the bacterial pathogens, and the host response. Host factors such as systemic disease, age, genetic predisposition, immune system status, occlusal trauma, and stress influence the onset and progression of the disease. Spontaneous remission of the destructive process may even occur. The disease usually is painless, and most patients are unaware of its presence. Various forms of therapy are effective, including oral hygiene, scaling, and surgical treatment.

Those more prone to periodontal disease include smokers, older individuals, and people with poor education, neglected dental care, previous periodontal destruction, and systemic diseases such as diabetes or infection with human immunodeficiency virus.

The prevalence of periodontal disease in the American population depends on the method of assessment and the threshold used. If loss of attachment by the formation of pockets measuring greater than 4 mm is used, then the prevalence is about 23%. The incidence of adult periodontitis increases with age. The prevalence of aggressive periodontitis is less than 1%. It also appears that the prevalence of periodontal disease in the United States has declined in the last 30 years, but this may change with an increasing elderly population and an increase in retention of teeth.

## Assessment of Periodontal Disease

### CONTRIBUTIONS OF RADIOGRAPHS

Radiographs play an integral role in the assessment of periodontal disease. They provide unique information about the status of the periodontium and a permanent record of the condition of the bone throughout the course of the disease. Radiographs aid the clinician in identifying the extent of destruction of alveolar bone, local contributing factors, and features of the periodontium that influence the prognosis. Important features related to periodontal status that may be identified radiographically are listed in Box 18-1.

It is important to emphasize that the clinical and radiographic examinations are complementary. The clinical examination should include periodontal probing, a gingival index, mobility charting, and an evaluation of the amount of attached gingiva. Features that are not well delineated by the radiograph are most apparent clinically, and those that the radiograph best demonstrates are difficult to identify and evaluate clinically. Radiographs are an adjunct to the diagnostic process. Although a radiograph demonstrates advanced periodontal lesions well, other equally important changes in the periodontium may not be seen radiographically. Therefore a complete diagnosis of periodontal disease requires insight from a clinical examination of the patient combined with radiographic evidence.

## LIMITATIONS OF RADIOGRAPHS

Radiographs may provide an incomplete presentation of the status of the periodontium. They have the following limitations:

1. Radiographs provide a two-dimensional view of a three-dimensional situation. Because the radiographic image fails to reveal the three-dimensional structure, bony defects overlapped by higher bony walls may be hidden. Also, because of overlapping tooth structure, only the interproximal bone is seen clearly. However, subtle changes in the density of the root structure (which is more radiolucent) may indicate bone loss on the buccal or lingual aspect of the tooth. Furthermore, use of multiple images made at different angulations, as in a full-mouth set, allows the viewer to use the buccal object rule to obtain three-dimensional information such as whether cortical plate loss has occurred on the buccal or lingual aspects.

2. Radiographs typically show less severe bone destruction than is actually present. The earliest (incipient) mild destructive lesions in bone do not cause a sufficient change in density to be detectable.

3. Radiographs do not demonstrate the soft-tissue-to-hard-tissue relationships and thus provide no information about the depth of soft tissue pockets.

4. Bone level is often measured from the cementoenamel junction; however, this reference point is not valid in situations where there is overeruption or where there is severe attrition with passive eruption.

   For these reasons, although radiographs play an invaluable role in treatment planning, their use must be supplemented by careful clinical examination.

## Technical Procedures

The usefulness of radiographs in the evaluation of periodontal disease can be improved by making radiographs with high technical quality. Interproximal (bitewing), in some cases vertical bitewings, and periapical radiographs are useful for evaluating the periodontium. This material is covered in greater detail in the chapters on projection geometry and intraoral radiographic technique (Chapters 4 and 9, respectively), but the features that are particularly important for imaging the alveolar bone are emphasized here.

## FILM PLACEMENT AND BEAM ALIGNMENT

The film should be placed parallel with the long axis of the teeth or as near to this ideal position as the size and structure of the mouth permit. The x-ray beam is directed perpendicular to the long axis of the tooth and the plane of the film. These measures result in the best undistorted images of the teeth and periodontal tissues. Interproximal (bitewing) images more accurately record the distance between the cementoenamel junction (CEJ) and the crest of the interradicular alveolar bone because with interproximal views the beam is oriented

---

### BOX 18-1
### *Radiographic Assessment of Periodontal Conditions*

Radiographs are especially helpful in the evaluation of the following features:
- Amount of bone present
- Condition of the alveolar crests
- Bone loss in the furcation areas
- Width of the periodontal ligament space
- Local irritating factors that increase the risk of periodontal disease
  - Calculus
  - Poorly contoured or overextended restorations
- Root length and morphology and the crown-to-root ratio
- Open interproximal contacts, which may be sites for food impaction
- Anatomic considerations
  - Position of the maxillary sinus in relation to a periodontal deformity
  - Missing, supernumerary, impacted, and tipped teeth
- Pathologic considerations
  - Caries
  - Periapical lesions
  - Root resorption

---

at right angles to the long axis of the teeth, thus providing an accurate view of the relationship of the height of the alveolar bone to the roots. Periapical views, especially in the posterior maxilla, may present a distorted view of the relationship between the teeth and the height of the alveolar bone because the presence of the hard palate often requires the x-ray tube to be oriented slightly downward toward the posterior teeth to see the apices of these teeth. In this circumstance, the level of the buccal alveolar bone may be projected near or even above the level of the lingual CEJ, thus making the bone height appear greater than it actually is.

The teeth will be depicted in their correct positions relative to the alveolar process when there is (1) no overlapping of the proximal contacts between crowns, (2) no overlapping of roots of adjacent teeth, and (3) overlapping of the buccal and lingual cusps of molars.

In recent years some periodontists have recommended the use of vertical interproximal radiographs for patients with periodontal disease. This method uses seven No. 2 films as vertical interproximal radiographs to cover the molar, premolar, canine, and midline regions. These views have the advantageous orientation of the interproximal views yet show the alveolar bone level even when bone loss has been considerable. Panoramic radiographs are not recommended for evaluation of periodontal disease because the distortion and poor image detail of panoramic views tend to lead the clinician to underestimate minor marginal bone destruction and overestimate major destruction.

For radiography of the alveolar bone, a beam energy of 80 kVp should be used. Films that are slightly light are more useful for

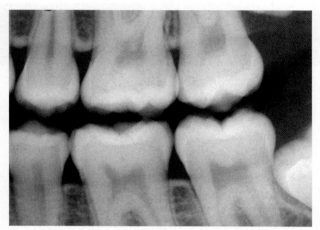

FIG. **18-1**  The normal alveolar crest lies 0.5 to 2.0 mm below the adjacent cementoenamel junctions and forms a sharp angle with the lamina dura of the adjacent tooth. Note that the crests may not always appear with a well-defined outer cortex.

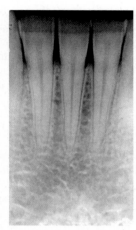

FIG. **18-2**  Between the anterior teeth, the normal alveolar crest is pointed and well corticated, coming to within 0.5 to 2.0 mm of the adjacent cementoenamel junctions.

examining cortical margins of bone. A properly collimated beam reduces scattered radiation and improves image definition.

## SPECIAL CONSIDERATIONS AND TECHNIQUES

The dentist must determine the optimal frequency of radiographic examination for patients with periodontal disease. Certainly, radiographs of all diseased areas must be available at the beginning of periodontal therapy to allow treatment planning and provide a baseline for later comparisons. The extent of continued disease activity, which can be determined clinically, should dictate the frequency of subsequent radiographic examinations.

Some clinicians have found it useful to superimpose fine wire grids when exposing radiographs to aid the measurement of relative bone height. Typically the grids form 1-mm squares (which show as fine, radiopaque lines on the resultant radiograph) that allow quantitative measurement of the position of the alveolar bone with respect to the dentition. This procedure can be useful in evaluating osseous changes over time but may be limited by difficulties in maintaining the same film position at subsequent examinations, resulting in variations in image geometry.

In recent years computers and image-processing techniques have been used to enhance radiographs to achieve improved detection of alveolar bone loss associated with periodontal disease. The most widely used of these techniques is subtraction radiography (see Chapters 7 and 14). The advantage of this method is that it allows better detection of small amounts of bone loss between radiographs made at different times than may be achieved by visual inspection. However, radiographic subtraction is difficult to use because the images must be made with the same orientation of the primary x-ray beam, bone, and film at each examination, which is impractical and difficult to accomplish in general practice. The more recent introduction of software programs that can correct for discrepancies in positioning and alignment in sequential digital images makes subtraction radiography more forgiving. Nonetheless, this diagnostic technique remains primarily a research tool.

## Normal Anatomy

The normal alveolar bone that supports the dentition has a characteristic radiographic appearance. A thin layer of opaque cortical bone often covers the alveolar crest. The height of the crest lies at a level approximately 0.5 to 2.0 mm below the level of the CEJs of adjacent teeth. Between posterior teeth the alveolar crest also is parallel to a line connecting adjacent CEJs (Fig. 18-1). Between anterior teeth the alveolar crest usually is pointed and may have a well-defined cortex (Fig. 18-2). A well-mineralized cortical outline of the alveolar crest indicates the absence of periodontitis activity. However, lack of a well-mineralized alveolar crest may be found in patients with or without periodontitis.

The alveolar crest is continuous with the lamina dura of adjacent teeth. In the absence of disease, this bony junction between the alveolar crest and lamina dura of posterior teeth forms a sharp angle next to the tooth root. The periodontal ligament (PDL) space is often slightly wider around the cervical portion of the tooth root, especially in adolescents with erupting teeth. In this situation, if the lamina dura still forms a sharp, well-defined angle with the alveolar crest, the condition is a variant of normal and is not an indication of disease. The thickness of alveolar crests varies widely, and it may be very thin coronally. This may appear radiographically as an increase in radiolucency toward the crest. These sorts of variations in density alone are not an indication of disease and may be a variation of normal.

Because gingivitis is an inflammatory condition confined to the gingiva, there are no significant changes to the underlying bone and therefore the radiographic appearance of the bone is normal.

## General Radiographic Features of Periodontal Disease

No matter the type of periodontal disease, the changes seen radiographically reflect changes seen with inflammatory lesions of bone. These changes can be divided into changes in the morphology of the supporting alveolar bone and changes to the internal density and trabecular pattern. Changes in morphology become apparent as a result of loss of the interproximal crestal bone and bone overlapping the buccal or lingual aspects of the tooth roots. Changes to the internal aspect of the alveolar bone reflect either a reduction or an increase in bone structure or a mixture of both. A reduction is seen as an increase in radiolucency because of a decrease in number and density of existing trabeculae. An increase in bone is seen as an increase in radiopacity (sclerosis) as the result of an increase primarily in the thickness, density, and number of trabeculae. Similar to all inflammatory lesions of bone, periodontal disease usually has a combination of bone loss and bone formation or sclerosis. However, acute early lesions display predominantly bone loss, whereas chronic lesions have a greater component of bone sclerosis.

The following patterns of bone loss may be seen radiographically in the assessment of periodontitis.

## CHANGES IN MORPHOLOGY OF THE ALVEOLAR BONE

### Early Bone Changes

The early lesions of chronic periodontitis appear as areas of localized erosion of the interproximal alveolar bone crest (Fig. 18-3). The anterior regions show blunting of the alveolar crests and slight loss of alveolar bone height. The posterior regions may also show a loss of the normally sharp angle between the lamina dura and alveolar crest. In early periodontal disease, this angle may lose its normal cortical surface (margin) and appear rounded off, having an irregular and diffuse border. Even if only slight radiographic changes are apparent, the disease process may not be of recent onset because significant loss of attachment must be present for 6 to 8 months before radiographic evidence of bone loss appears. Also, variations in angle of projection of the x-ray beam can cause a slight change in the apparent height of the alveolar bone. Small regions of bone loss on the buccal or lingual aspects of the teeth are much more difficult to detect.

A mild lesion does not necessarily develop into a more severe lesion later; however, if the periodontitis progresses, the destruction of alveolar bone extends beyond early changes in the alveolar crest and may induce a variety of defects in the morphology of the alveolar crest. These patterns of bone loss have been divided into horizontal bone loss, vertical (angular) defects, interdental craters, buccal or lingual cortical plate loss, and furcation involvement of multirooted teeth. The presence and severity of these bone defects may vary between patients and even within a patient. A radiograph is valuable in showing the extent and morphology of residual bone, but complete assessment of bone loss and the diagnosis and staging of periodontitis requires integration of the radiologic information with the results of a clinical examination.

### Horizontal Bone Loss

Horizontal bone loss is a term used to describe the radiographic appearance of loss in height of the alveolar bone where the crest is still horizontal (i.e., parallel to an imagined line joining the CEJs of adjacent teeth) but is positioned apically more than a couple of millimeters from the CEJs. Horizontal bone loss may be mild, moderate, or severe, depending on its extent. Mild bone loss may be defined as approximately a 1- to 2-mm loss of the supporting bone, and moderate loss is anything greater than 2 mm up to loss of half the supporting bone height. Severe loss is anything beyond this point. Care must be taken in using the CEJ as a reference point in cases of overeruption and severe attrition (Fig. 18-4). With overeruption the alveolar bone will not necessarily remodel to keep a normal relationship to the CEJ and similarly in passive eruption, which may accompany severe attrition. Although in this case bone loss is not due to periodontitis,

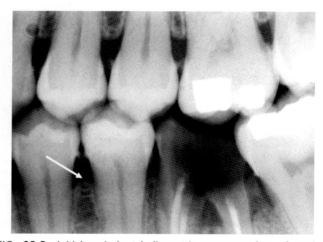

FIG. **18-3** Initial periodontal disease is seen as a loss of cortical density and a rounding of the junction between the alveolar crest and the lamina dura *(arrow)*. Note also the more pronounced bone loss around the mandibular first molar and the generalized interproximal calculus.

FIG. **18-4 A,** This maxillary second bicuspid is overerupted; the etiology of the low bone level *(arrow)* relative to the cemento-enamel junction (CEJ) is not necessarily the result of periodontal disease. Similarly, **B** is an example of passive eruption related to severe attrition, and the apparent increase in the distance from the CEJ to the bone height *(arrows)* cannot be attributed to periodontal disease. However, the resultant change in bone level relative to the CEJ may still be clinically significant.

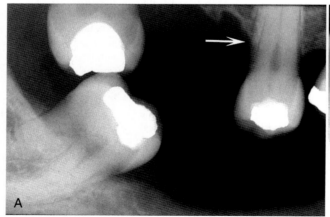

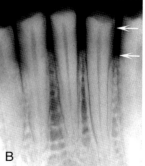

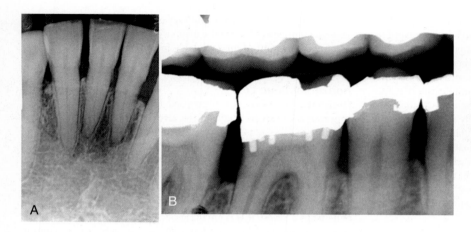

FIG. **18-5** Horizontal bone loss is seen in the anterior region **(A)** and the posterior region **(B)** as a loss of the buccal and lingual cortical plates and interdental alveolar bone.

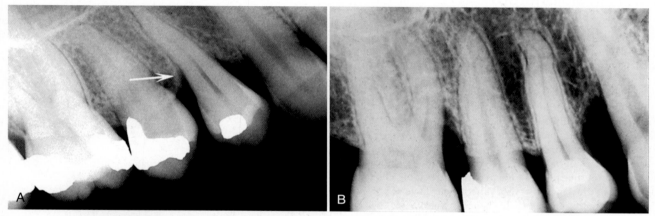

FIG. **18-6**　**A,** Example of a developing vertical defect; note the abnormal widening of the periodontal ligament space *(arrow)*. **B,** Maxillary periapical film reveals two examples of more severe vertical defects affecting the mesial surface of the first molar and the distal surface of the canine.

there may be still loss of attachment, which could be of clinical significance.

In horizontal bone loss, the crest of the buccal and lingual cortical plates and the intervening interdental bone have been resorbed (Fig. 18-5). The extent of bone loss evident at a single examination does not indicate the current activity of the disease. For example, a patient who previously had generalized periodontal disease and subsequent successful therapy will likely always show bone loss, but the bone level may remain stable.

## Vertical Bone Defects

The term *vertical* (or angular) *osseous defect* describes a bony lesion that is localized to a single tooth, although an individual may have multiple vertical osseous defects. These defects develop when bone loss progresses down the root of the tooth, resulting in deepening of the clinical periodontal pocket. The radiographic presentation is a vertical deformity within the alveolus that extends apically along the root of the affected tooth from the alveolar crest. The outline of the remaining alveolar bone typically displays an oblique angulation to an imaginary line connecting the CEJ of the affected tooth to the neighboring tooth. In its early form, a vertical defect appears as abnormal widening of the PDL space at the alveolar crest (Fig. 18-6, *A*). The vertical defect is

described as three walled (surrounded by three bony walls) when both buccal and lingual cortical plates remain; it is described as two walled when one of these plates has been resorbed and as one walled when both plates have been lost (Fig. 18-6, *B*). The distinctions among these groups are important in designing the treatment plan.

Often vertical defects are difficult or impossible to recognize on a radiograph because one or both of the cortical bony plates remain superimposed over the defect. Clinical and surgical inspections are the best means of determining the number of remaining bony walls. Visualization of the depth of pockets may be aided by inserting a gutta-percha point. The point follows the defect and appears on the radiograph because gutta-percha is relatively inflexible and radiopaque (Fig. 18-7).

## Interdental Craters

The interproximal crater is a two-walled, troughlike depression that forms in the crest of the interdental bone between adjacent teeth. The buccal and lingual outer cortical walls of the interproximal bone extend further coronally than does the cancellous bone between them, which has been resorbed. Radiographically this presents as a bandlike or irregular region of bone with less density at the crest, immediately adjacent to the more dense normal bone apical to the base of the crater (Fig. 18-8). These defects are more common in the posterior

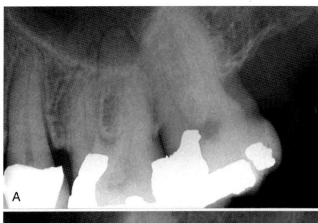

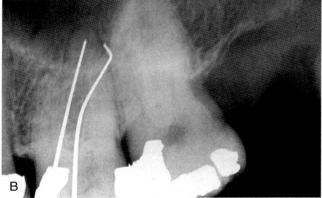

FIG. **18-7** Gutta-percha may be used to visualize the depth of infrabony defects. **A,** Radiograph fails to show the osseous defect without the use of the gutta-percha points. **B,** Radiograph reveals an osseous defect extending to the region of the apex. (Courtesy H. Takei, DDS, Los Angeles, Calif.)

segments, likely as a result of the broader buccal-lingual dimension of the alveolar crest in these regions.

### Buccal or Lingual Cortical Plate Loss

The buccal or lingual cortical plate adjacent to the teeth may resorb. Loss of a cortical plate may occur alone or with another type of bone loss such as horizontal bone loss. This type of loss is indicated by an increase in the radiolucency of the root of the tooth near the alveolar crest. The shape seen usually is a semicircular shadow with the apex of the radiolucency directed apically in relation to the tooth (Fig. 18-9). Lack of bone loss at the interproximal region of the tooth may make this kind of defect difficult to detect.

### Osseous Deformities in the Furcations of Multirooted Teeth

Progressive periodontal disease and its associated bone loss may extend into the furcations of multirooted teeth. As bone resorption

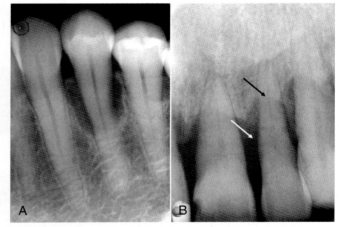

FIG. **18-9**  **A,** Loss of the lingual alveolar crest adjacent to this mandibular first bicuspid without associated interproximal bone loss. **B,** Loss of the buccal cortical bone adjacent to the maxillary central and lateral incisors. The black arrow indicates the level of the buccal alveolar crest, which demonstrates more profound loss relative to the lingual alveolar crest *(white arrow)*.

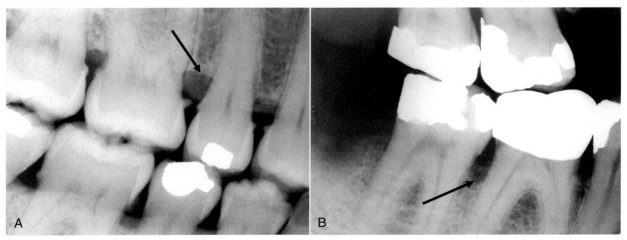

FIG. **18-8**  Interproximal craters, existing as defects between the buccal and lingual cortical plates, seen as a radiolucent band **(A)** or trough **(B)** apical to the level of the crestal edges. The arrows indicate the base of the craters.

extends down the side of a multirooted tooth, eliminating the bone covering the root, it can reach the level of the furcation and beyond. Widening of the PDL space at the apex of the interradicular bony crest of the furcation is strong evidence that the periodontal disease process involves the furcation (Fig. 18-10, *A*). If sufficient bone loss has occurred on the lingual and buccal aspects of a mandibular molar furcation, the radiolucent image of the lesion becomes prominent (Fig. 18-10, *B*). The bony defect may also involve only the buccal or lingual cortical plate and extend under the roof of the furcation. In such a case, if the defect does not extend through to the other cortical plate, it appears more irregular and radiolucent than does the adjacent normal bone. By use of the buccal object rule with films of different angulations, it may be possible to determine whether the buccal or the lingual cortical plate has been resorbed.

If the crestal bone is below the furcation but the disease process has not extended into the interradicular bone, the width of the periodontal membrane space appears normal. Also, the septal bone may appear more radiolucent but otherwise be normal. In the mandible, the external oblique ridge may mask furcation involvement of the third molars. Convergent roots may also obscure furcation defects in maxillary and mandibular second and third molars.

The loss of interradicular bone in the furcation of a maxillary molar may originate from the buccal, mesial, or distal surface of the tooth. The most common route for furcation involvement of the maxillary permanent first molar is from the mesial side. The image of furcation involvement is not as sharply defined around maxillary molars as around mandibular molars because the palatal root is superimposed on the defect (see Fig. 18-10, *C*). However, occasionally this pattern of bone destruction is prominent and appears as an inverted "J" shadow with the hook of the J extending into the trifurcation (see Fig. 18-10, *D*) or as a radiolucent triangle superimposed over the roots of the involved tooth with its apex pointing toward the furcation.

Definitive diagnosis of complex furcation deformities requires careful clinical examination and sometimes surgical exploration. Radiographs, though, are an important tool in identifying potentially involved sites as well as providing important information about root morphology and length, which is of significance to treatment planning and prognosis.

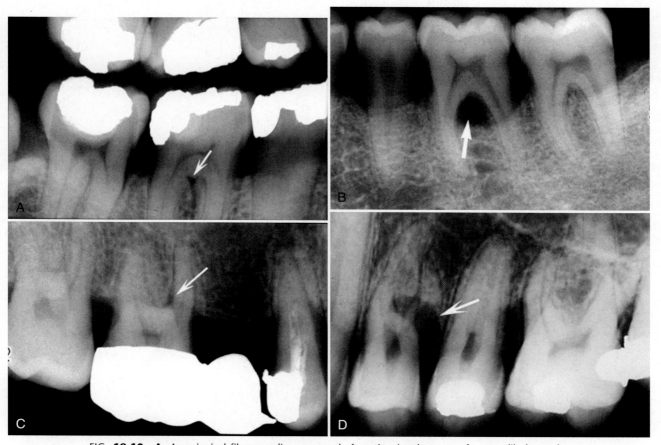

FIG. **18-10** **A,** A periapical film revealing very early furcation involvement of a mandibular molar characterized by slight widening of the periodontal ligament space in the furcation region *(arrow)*. **B,** A periapical film revealing a profound radiolucent lesion within the furcation region *(arrow)* resulting from loss of bone in the furcation region and the buccal and lingual cortical plates. **C,** The angulation of this periapical view of a maxillary first molar projected the palatal root away from the trifurcation region revealing early widening of the furcation periodontal ligament space *(arrow)*. **D,** Example of an inverted "J" shadow *(arrow)* resulting from bone destruction extending into the trifurcation region of a three-rooted maxillary first bicuspid.

FIG. **18-11 A,** Example of a primarily radiolucent reaction around this maxillary lateral incisor. Note that the trabeculae toward the alveolar crest on the mesial and distal aspect of the tooth are barely perceptible and the marrow spaces are enlarged. **B,** A periapical film revealing a predominantly sclerotic bone reaction resulting from the periodontal disease involving the mandibular molars. Note that the trabeculae are thickened and the marrow spaces are barely perceptible.

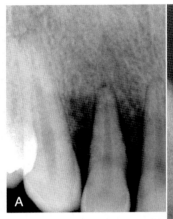
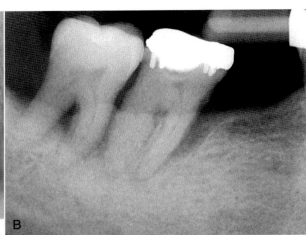

## CHANGES TO INTERNAL DENSITY AND TRABECULAR PATTERN OF BONE

As with all other inflammatory lesions, the periodontal lesion may stimulate a reaction in the surrounding bone. The peripheral bone may appear more radiolucent, or more sclerotic (radiopaque), or more commonly with a mixture of these patterns. Very rarely no apparent change will be seen in the surrounding bone. A radiolucent change reflects loss of density and number of trabeculae. The trabeculae appear very faint, which is more commonly seen in early or acute lesions (Fig. 18-11, *A*). If the trabeculae are sufficiently decalcified, they may not appear in the radiographic image although they are still present. This accounts for the apparent reformation of bone in some cases where the acute inflammation resolves with successful treatment and the trabeculae remineralize. The sclerotic bone reaction appears radiopaque because of deposition of bone on existing trabeculae at the expense of the marrow, resulting in thicker trabeculae that may eventually be so dense as to appear as an amorphous radiopaque mass (Fig. 18-11, *B*). This sclerotic reaction may extend some distance from the periodontal lesion, sometimes to the inferior aspect of the mandible. Usually the surrounding bone reaction is a mixture of both bone loss and sclerosis.

Inflammatory products from a periodontal lesion can even extend through the cortex of the floor of the maxillary sinus to cause a regional mucositis (Fig. 18-12). In rare cases a periosteal reaction might be seen on the buccal or lingual aspect of the alveolar process.

### Other Patterns of Periodontal Bone Loss

#### PERIODONTAL ABSCESS

A periodontal abscess is a rapidly progressing, destructive lesion that usually originates in a deep soft tissue pocket. It occurs when the coronal portion of the pocket becomes occluded or when foreign material becomes lodged between a tooth and the gingiva. Clinically, pain and swelling and sometimes a draining sinus are present in the region. If the lesion is acute, there may be no visible radiographic changes. If the lesion persists, a radiolucent region appears, often superimposed over the root of a tooth. The radiolucency may be a rounded area of rarefaction and a bridge of bone may be present over

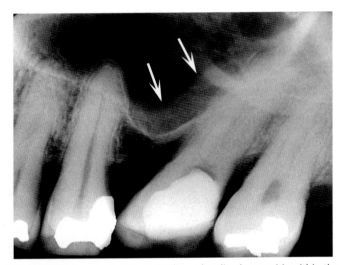

FIG. **18-12** A periapical film revealing a localized mucositis within the maxillary sinus *(arrows)* immediately adjacent to a vertical periodontal defect.

the coronal aspect of the lesion, separating it from the crest of the alveolar ridge (Fig. 18-13). After treatment, some of the lost bone may regenerate.

## AGGRESSIVE PERIODONTITIS

Aggressive periodontitis refers to periodontal disease of an aggressive and rapid nature that usually occurs in patients younger than 30 years. The severity of the disease appears to be an exuberant reaction to a minimum amount of plaque accumulation and may result in early tooth loss. The term *aggressive periodontitis* has replaced the term *early-onset periodontitis,* which included three former classifications: localized juvenile periodontitis, generalized juvenile periodontitis, and rapidly progressing periodontitis. Aggressive periodontitis is now subclassified into localized aggressive periodontitis and generalized aggressive periodontitis. The cause of aggressive periodontitis is not known; however, specific bacterial pathogens, especially *Actinobacillus actinomycetemcomitans,* functional defects of polymorphonuclear leukocytes, exuberant immune responses, and inheritable genetic factors have been implicated.

## Clinical Presentation

Localized aggressive periodontitis is associated with attachment loss involving the incisors and first molars. In this form, the amount of bone loss correlates with the time of tooth eruption, in that the teeth that erupt first (incisors and first molars) have the most bone loss. This disease usually commences around puberty and the bone loss is rapid; up to three to four times the rate seen in chronic periodontitis. Of interest is the fact that there are usually very few signs of soft tissue inflammation or plaque accumulation despite the presence of deep bony pockets. Often the patient will present with drifting and mobile incisors and early loss of first molars.

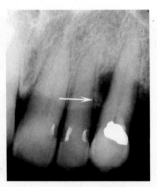

FIG. **18-13** Example of a periodontal abscess related to the maxillary canine; note the well-defined area of bone loss over the midroot region of the tooth and extending in a mesial direction toward the lateral incisor. There appears to be a layer of bone *(arrow)* separating the area of bone destruction from the crest of the alveolar process.

Generalized aggressive periodontitis can involve a variable number of teeth, from at least three to all of the dentition, and by definition is not confined to the first molars and incisors. This rapidly progressing disease usually affects individuals younger than 30 years. The gingiva may appear normal as in the localized form or may have an exuberant inflammatory response. If there is a history of premature loss of deciduous teeth and the permanent teeth are rapidly lost soon after erupting, a possible diagnosis of Papillon-Lefèvre syndrome might be considered. This syndrome is usually seen with an associated hyperkeratosis of palmar and plantar surfaces.

Estimates of prevalence of aggressive periodontitis are 0.53% and 0.13% for the localized and generalized forms, respectively, in the United States. Black individuals are affected more commonly than whites are with both the localized and generalized forms. Black male patients are more commonly affected with localized disease than are black female patients, whereas white female patients are more likely than white men to have localized disease.

## Radiographic Appearance

The radiographic appearance of the bone loss in localized aggressive periodontitis typically consists of deep vertical defects (Fig. 18-14). Maxillary teeth are involved slightly more often than mandibular teeth, and strong left-right symmetry is common. The generalized form of aggressive periodontitis can involve several teeth or all the dentition and the rapid bone loss may be of the vertical or horizontal pattern.

## Treatment

Early identification and treatment of aggressive periodontitis is important because of the rapid progression of this condition and the associated tooth loss. Response to conventional periodontal therapy is not predictable but is more likely to be successful when initiated earlier. Treatment often consists of scaling, curettage, and administration of antibiotics and may also include surgical and regenerative therapies.

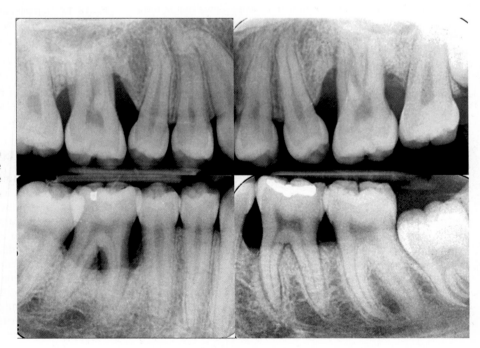

FIG. **18-14** Typical vertical bone loss in localized aggressive periodontitis. Note the bone loss is confined to the region of the first molars. (Courtesy T. D. Charbeneau, DDS, Dallas, Tex.)

## Dental Conditions Associated with Periodontal Diseases

Various changes in the dentition and its supporting structures that have been associated with and potentially can exacerbate periodontal disease may be evident in the radiographic examination. These conditions, including occlusal trauma and tooth mobility, open contacts, and local irritating factors such as overhanging and faulty restorations and calculus, should be identified as part of a complete clinical and radiologic assessment.

### OCCLUSAL TRAUMA

Traumatic occlusion causes degenerative changes in response to occlusal pressures that are greater than the physiologic tolerances of the tooth's supporting tissues. These changes occur either as a result of maladaptation in response to excessive occlusal force on teeth or by normal occlusal forces on a periodontium already compromised by bone loss. In addition to clinical signs and symptoms such as increased mobility, wear facets, unusual response to percussion, and a history of contributing habits, there are associated radiographic findings that include widening of the PDL space, thickening of the lamina dura, bone loss, and an increase in the number and size of trabeculae. Other sequelae of traumatic occlusion include hypercementosis and root fractures. Traumatic occlusion alone does not cause gingivitis or periodontitis, affect the epithelial attachment, nor lead to pocket formation, but in the presence of preexisting periodontitis bone loss may be accelerated. Traumatic occlusion can be definitively diagnosed only by clinical evaluation and not by the radiographic findings alone.

### TOOTH MOBILITY

Widening of the PDL space suggests tooth mobility, which may result from occlusal trauma or a lack of bone support arising from advanced bone loss. If the affected tooth has a single root, the socket may develop an hourglass shape. If the tooth is multirooted, it may show widening of the PDL space at the apices and in the region of the furcation. These changes result when the tooth moves about an axis of rotation at some midpoint on the roots. In addition, the radiographic image of the lamina dura may appear broad and hazy and show increased density.

### OPEN CONTACTS

When the mesial and distal surfaces of adjacent teeth do not touch, the patient has an open contact. This condition may be dangerous to the periodontium because of the potential for food debris to become trapped in the region. Trapped food particles may damage the soft tissue and induce an inflammatory response and contribute to the development of localized periodontal disease. Open contacts are associated with periodontal disease more than closed contacts are. Similar potential situations where periodontal disease may develop are discrepancies in the height of two adjacent marginal ridges or tipped teeth (Fig. 18-15). Abnormal tooth alignment does not cause periodontal disease but provides an environment where the disease may develop as a result of difficulty in maintaining adequate oral hygiene.

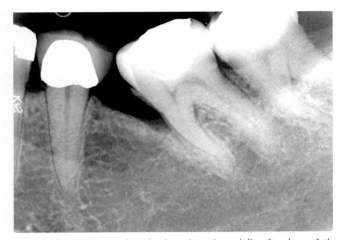

**FIG. 18-15** The second molar has tipped mesially after loss of the first molar, creating an abnormal tooth alignment that was difficult for the patient to maintain and leading to localized periodontal disease. Note the calculus on the mesial surface of the second molar. The crown on the second premolar was constructed with an enlarged distal contour to stop further tipping of the molar.

### LOCAL IRRITATING FACTORS

Other local factors that are radiographically apparent may provide an environment where periodontal disease may develop or may aggravate existing periodontal disease. For instance, calculus deposits (Fig. 18-16) can prevent effective cleansing of a sulcus and lead to enhanced plaque formation and the progression of periodontal disease. Calculus is most commonly seen on the mandibular incisors but may be localized to any surface or generalized throughout the dentition. Defective restorations with overhanging or poorly contoured margins can also lead to the accumulation of plaque, thus providing an environment where periodontal disease may develop (Fig. 18-17). Radiographs often reveal these conditions.

## Evaluation of Periodontal Therapy

Radiographs may show signs of successful treatment of periodontal disease. In some cases there may be reformation of the interproximal cortex (Fig. 18-18) and the sharp line angle between the cortex and lamina dura. The relatively radiolucent margins of bone that were undergoing active resorption before treatment may become more sclerotic (radiopaque) after successful therapy. In some cases there may have been considerable mineral loss of the cancellous bone (appearing radiolucent) so that the bone is not radiographically apparent. Successful treatment may then result in remineralization, causing the bone to become visible in the radiographic image, giving the false impression that bone has actually grown into periodontal defects. In many cases there will be no apparent radiographic changes after successful treatment. Also, radiographs do not disclose the therapeutic elimination of (radiolucent) soft tissue periodontal pockets; healing therefore is best assessed by clinical evaluation.

Sequential radiographs made with different beam angulations may give the false impression that bone has grown into the periodontal defects. Therefore in a longitudinal study effort should be given to duplicate the image geometry as well as using ideal exposure and

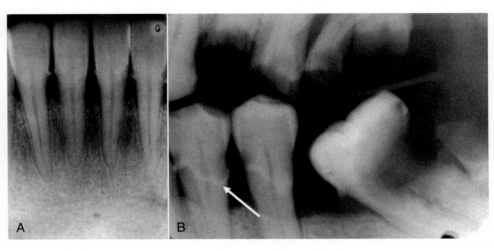

FIG. **18-16** Calculus may be seen as small angular radiopaque deposits projecting between interproximal surfaces of the teeth (**A**) or as radiopaque bands across the roots representing circumferential accumulation (**B**, *arrow*).

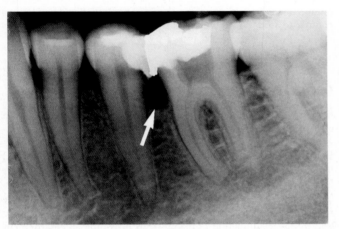

FIG. **18-17**    These overhanging restorations provided an environment suitable for plaque accumulation and subsequent localized periodontal bone loss *(arrow)*.

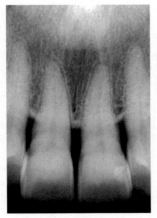

FIG. **18-18**    An example of a case where the interproximal cortex of the alveolar crest has reformed after successful periodontal therapy.

processing variables. For instance, too high an x-ray exposure or too long a developing time increases the density of the image (more radiolucent) and thin bone such as the alveolar crest may not be apparent, giving the false impression that the bone has been resorbed. Alternatively, underexposed or underdeveloped films may give the false impression of bone growth.

The clinical crown-to-tooth ratio is a useful criterion not only for determining the nature of the restorative treatment to be performed on a tooth but also for deciding on the prognosis of an individual tooth. It is a measure of the tooth's bony support, relating the proportion of tooth length that is beyond the level of bone (clinical crown) to that supported by the lowest level of bone (bony investment). Teeth have an unfavorable crown-to-root ratio when the length of the tooth out of bone exceeds the length of root supported by bone.

## DIFFERENTIAL DIAGNOSIS

The majority of cases of bone loss around teeth are caused by periodontal diseases. This fact can make the clinician less sensitive to other diseases with similar manifestations that should always be considered in the differential diagnosis. Occasionally, more serious diseases are missed or recognized late. The most likely clinical sign of disease other than periodontal disease is the presence of one or a few adjacent loose teeth when the rest of the mouth shows no signs of periodontal disease. Radiographically, suspicion should be heightened if the bone destruction does not have the pattern or morphology normally associated with periodontal disease. Squamous cell carcinoma of the alveolar process occasionally is treated as periodontal disease, resulting in an unfortunate delay in diagnosis and treatment (Fig. 18-19, *A*). This malignancy may display characteristics that suggest its true nature, such as extensive bone destruction of a localized region or invasive characteristics (see Chapter 23), or it may mimic periodontal disease. In some cases only the clinical characteristics of the lesion and the failure to respond to treatment indicate the presence of malignancy.

Any lesion of bone destruction that has ill-defined borders and a lack of peripheral bone response (sclerosis) should be viewed with suspicion. Another disease to be considered is Langerhans' cell histiocytosis (Fig. 18-19, *B*). Often this disease may manifest as single or multiple regions of bone destruction around the roots of teeth, similar to periodontal disease. The condition may appear similar to localized

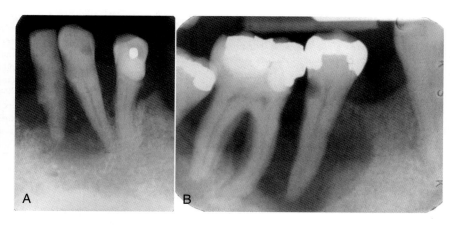

FIG. **18-19  A,** A periapical film of a case of squamous cell carcinoma of the alveolar process of the mandible; note the irregular bone destruction. **B,** A periapical film of Langerhans' cell histiocytosis demonstrating an alveolar lesion with bone destruction; note that the epicenter would be at the midroot region instead of the alveolar crest, as seen in periodontal disease.

aggressive periodontitis except that the bone destruction does not correlate with the time of tooth eruption, as is seen in periodontitis. Also, in histiocytosis the midroot region is the epicenter of bone destruction, which gives early lesions an "ice cream scoop" appearance (see Chapter 24). The alveolar crest may remain intact.

## Effect of Systemic Diseases on Periodontal Disease

Although systemic diseases do not cause periodontal disease, they do influence its course by interfering with the body's natural defenses against irritants or limiting its capacity to repair. Although any systemic disease may have some influence on other body systems, only a few appear to influence the periodontium and periodontal treatment. These include diabetes mellitus, hematologic disorders (e.g., monocytic conditions and, less often, myelogenous leukemia, neutropenia, hemophilia and nonhemophilic polycythemia vera), genetic and hereditary disturbances (e.g., Papillon-Lefèvre syndrome, Down syndrome, hypophosphatemia, Chédiak-Higashi syndrome), hormonal changes (e.g., puberty, pregnancy, menopause), and stress.

## ACQUIRED IMMUNODEFICIENCY SYNDROME

The incidence and severity of periodontal disease is high in patients with acquired immunodeficiency syndrome. In these individuals the disease process is characterized by a rapid progression that leads to bone sequestration and loss of several teeth. These patients may not respond to standard periodontal therapy.

## DIABETES MELLITUS

Diabetes mellitus is the most common and important systemic disease to influence the onset and course of periodontal disease. Uncontrolled, it may result in protein breakdown, degenerative vascular changes, lowered resistance to infection, and increased severity of infections. Consequently, patients with uncontrolled diabetes are more disposed to the development of periodontal disease than are those with normal glucose metabolism. Patients with uncontrolled diabetes and periodontal disease also show more severe and rapid alveolar bone resorption and are more prone to the development of periodontal abscesses. In patients whose diabetes is under control, periodontal disease responds normally to traditional treatment.

## RADIATION THERAPY

Although not a systemic disease, high-dose irradiation to the oral tissues as a treatment for malignant conditions may have a detrimental effect on the periodontium. Radiation therapy to the jaws results in bone that is hypovascular, hypocellular, and hypoxic. This bone may be less able to remodel and be more susceptible to infections, resulting in rapid bone loss that is indistinguishable from the radiographic characteristics of periodontal disease. Teeth that have been exposed to high-dose radiation fields have been shown to demonstrate greater recession, attachment loss, and mobility than do teeth in the same mouth that were not within the field.

## BIBLIOGRAPHY

### CLINICAL CHARACTERISTICS OF PERIODONTAL DISEASES

Armitage GC: Periodontal diseases: diagnosis, *Ann Periodontol* 1:37-215, 1996.
Herrera C, González I, Sanz M: The periodontal abscess (I): clinical and microbiological findings, *J Clin Periodontol* 27:387-394, 2000.
Newman MG, Takei HH, Klokkevold PR et al: *Carranza's clinical periodontology,* Philadelphia, 2006, WB Saunders.
Walsh TF, al-Kohail OS, Fosam EB: The relationship of bone loss observed on panoramic radiographs with clinical periodontal screening, *J Clin Periodontol* 24:153-157, 1997.

### EPIDEMIOLOGY

Melvin WL, Sandifer JB, Gray JL: The prevalence and sex ratio of juvenile periodontitis in a young racially mixed population, *J Periodontol* 62:330-334, 1991.
Papapanou PN: Periodontal diseases: epidemiology, *Ann Periodontol* 1:1-36, 1996.
Position paper: epidemiology of periodontal diseases. American Academy of Periodontology, *J Periodontol* 67:935-945, 1996.

### ETIOLOGY

Bimstein E, Garcia-Godoy F: The significance of age, proximal caries, gingival inflammation, probing depths, and the loss of lamina dura in the diagnosis of alveolar bone loss in the primary molars, *ASDC J Dent Child* 61:125-128, 1994.
Page RC, Offenbacher S, Schroeder HE et al: Advances in the pathogenesis of periodontitis: summary of developments, clinical implications and future directions, *Periodontol 2000* 14:216-248, 1997.
Salvi GE, Lawrence HP, Offenbacher S et al: Influence of risk factors on the pathogenesis of periodontitis, *Periodontol 2000* 14:173, 1997.

Schwartz Z, Goultschin J, Dean DD et al: Mechanisms of alveolar bone destruction in periodontitis, *Periodontol 2000* 14:158, 1997.

Van Dyke TE, Serhan CN: Resolution of inflammation: a new paradigm for the pathogenesis of periodontal diseases, *J Dent Res* 82:82-90, 2003.

## RADIOGRAPHIC MANIFESTATIONS

Gutteridge DL: The use of radiographic techniques in the diagnosis and management of periodontal diseases, *Dentomaxillofac Radiol* 24:107-113, 1995.

Jeffcoat MK, Wang IC, Reddy MS: Radiographic diagnosis in periodontics, *Periodontol 2000* 7:54-68, 1995.

Khocht A, Zohn H, Deasy M et al: Screening for periodontal disease: radiographs vs PSR, *J Am Dent Assoc* 127:749-756, 1996.

Koral SM, Howell TH, Jeffcoat MK: Alveolar bone loss due to open interproximal contacts in periodontal disease, *J Periodontol* 52:447-450, 1981.

Mann J, Pettigrew J, Beideman R et al: Investigation of the relationship between clinically detected loss of attachment and radiographic changes in early periodontal disease, *J Clin Periodontol* 12:247-253, 1985.

Nielsen IM, Glavind L, Karring T: Interproximal periodontal intrabony defects: prevalence, localization, and etiological factors, *J Clin Periodontol* 7:187-198, 1980.

Rams TE, Listgarten MA, Slots J: Utility of radiographic crestal lamina dura for predicting periodontitis disease activity, *J Clin Periodontol* 21:571-576, 1994.

Waite IM, Furniss JS, Wong WM: Relationship between clinical periodontal condition and the radiological appearance at first molar sites in adolescents: a 3-year study, *J Clin Periodontol* 21:155-160, 1994.

## AGGRESSIVE PERIODONTITIS

Albandar JM, Brown LJ, Löe H: Dental caries and tooth loss in adolescents with early onset periodontitis, *J Periodontol* 67:960-967, 1996.

Albandar JM, Brown LJ, Löe H: Clinical features of early onset periodontitis, *J Am Dent Assoc* 128:1393-1399, 1997.

Brown LJ, Albandar JM, Brunelle JA et al: Early onset periodontitis: progression of attachment loss during 6 years, *J Periodontol* 67:968-975, 1996.

Loe H, Brown LJ: Early onset periodontitis in the United States of America, *J Periodontol* 62:608-616, 1991,

Page RC, Altman LC, Ebersole JL et al: Rapidly progressive periodontitis: a distinct clinical condition, *J Periodontol* 54:197-209, 1983.

## RADIOGRAPHIC TECHNIQUE

Bragger I: Radiographic diagnosis of periodontal disease progression, *Curr Opin Periodontol* 3:59-67, 1996.

Gröndahl K, Gröndahl HG, Webber RL et al: Influence of variations in projection geometry on the detectability of periodontal bone lesions: a comparison between subtraction radiography and conventional radiographic technique, *J Clin Periodontol* 11:411-420, 1984.

Pepelassi EA, Diamanti-Kipioti A: Selection of the most accurate method of conventional radiography for the assessment of periodontal osseous destruction, *J Clin Periodontol* 24:557-567, 1997.

Reed B, Polson A: Relationships between bitewing and periapical radiographs in assessing crestal alveolar bone levels, *J Periodontol* 55:22-27, 1984.

## SUBTRACTION RADIOGRAPHY

Eickholz P, Hausmann E: Evidence for healing of periodontal defects 5 years after conventional and regenerative therapy: digital subtraction and bone level measurements, *J Clin Periodontol* 29:922-928, 2002.

## OCCLUSAL TRAUMA

Burgett FG: Trauma from occlusion: periodontal concerns, *Dent Clin North Am* 39:301-311, 1995.

Wank GS, Kroll YJ: Occlusal trauma: an evaluation of its relationship to periodontal prostheses, *Dent Clin North Am* 25:511-532, 1981.

## SYSTEMIC DISEASE

Emrich LJ, Shlossman M, Genco RJ: Periodontal disease in non-insulin-dependent diabetes mellitus, *J Periodontol* 62:123-131, 1991.

Epstein JB, Lunn R, Le N et al: Periodontal attachment loss in patients after head and neck radiation therapy, *Oral Surg Oral Med Oral Path Oral Radiol Endod* 86:673-677, 1998.

Farzim I, Edalat M: Periodontosis with hyperkeratosis palmaris and plantaris (the Papillon-Lefèvre syndrome): a case report, *J Periodontol* 45:316-318, 1974.

Nelson RG, Schlossman M, Budding LM et al: Periodontal diseases and NIDDM in Pima Indians, *Diabetes Care* 13:836-840, 1990.

Rateitschak-Plüss EM, Schroeder HE: History of periodontitis in a child with Papillon-Lèfèvre syndrome. A case report, *J Periodontol* 55:35-46, 1984.

Winkler JR, Grassi M, Murray PA: Clinical description and etiology of HIV-associated periodontal disease. In Robinson PB, Greenspan JS, editors: *Prospectus on oral manifestations of AIDS*, Littleton, MA, 1988, PSG Publishing.

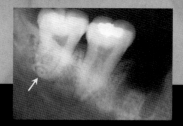

# CHAPTER 19

# Dental Anomalies

Ernest W.N. Lam

Dental anomalies may be congenital, developmental, or acquired and may include variations in the normal number, size, morphology, or eruptive pattern of the teeth. Congenital abnormalities are typically genetically inherited anomalies and developmental anomalies occur during the formation of a tooth or teeth. In contrast, acquired abnormalities result from changes to teeth after normal formation. Teeth that form abnormally short roots may represent congenital or developmental anomalies, whereas the shortening of normal tooth roots by external resorption represents an acquired change.

## Developmental Abnormalities

### NUMBER OF TEETH

#### Supernumerary Teeth

##### Synonyms

Hyperdontia, distodens, mesiodens, peridens, parateeth, and supplemental teeth

##### Definition

Supernumerary teeth are those that develop in addition to the normal complement as a result of excess dental lamina in the jaws, and the tooth or teeth that develop may be morphologically normal or abnormal. When supernumerary teeth have normal morphologic features, the term *supplemental* is sometimes used. Supernumerary teeth that occur between the maxillary central incisors are termed *mesiodens*. Those that occur in the premolar area are peridens, and those found in the molar area are distodens.

##### Clinical Features

Supernumerary teeth occur in 1% to 4% of the population, may have a greater incidence in Asians and Native Americans, and occur twice as often in males. Although supernumerary teeth can arise in either the deciduous or permanent dentitions, they are more common in the permanent dentition and can arise anywhere in either jaw. Single supernumerary teeth are most common in the anterior maxilla, where they are referred to as mesiodens (Figs. 19-1 to 19-3), and in the maxillary molar region (Fig. 19-4), whereas multiple supernumerary teeth occur most frequently in the premolar regions, usually in the mandible (Figs. 19-5 and 19-6).

Supernumerary teeth are usually discovered radiographically because they may interfere with normal tooth eruption (Fig. 19-7).

When a supernumerary tooth does erupt, it commonly does so outside the normal arch form because of space restrictions.

##### Radiographic Features

The radiographic features of supernumerary teeth are variable. They may appear entirely normal in both size and shape, but they may also be smaller in size compared with the adjacent normal dentition or have a conical shape with the appearance of a canine tooth. In extreme cases, the supernumerary teeth may appear grossly deformed. Supernumerary teeth are easily identified by counting and identifying all the teeth in the jaws.

Radiographs may reveal supernumerary teeth in the deciduous dentition (Fig. 19-8) after 3 or 4 years of age when the deciduous teeth have formed or in the permanent dentition of children older than 9 to 12 years.

In addition to periapical radiography, occlusal radiographs may aid in determining the location and number of unerupted supernumerary teeth. Care should be taken to review panoramic radiographs for supernumerary teeth. In some cases, the distorted image of a supernumerary tooth lying outside the focal trough (i.e., in the hard palate) may be easily missed.

##### Differential Diagnosis

Multiple supernumerary teeth have been associated with a number of genetically inherited syndromes including cleidocranial dysplasia (see Chapter 30), Gardner's syndrome (see Chapter 22), and pykodysostosis.

##### Management

The management of supernumerary teeth depends on many factors, including their potential effect on the developing normal dentition, their position and number, and the potential complications that may result from surgical intervention. If supernumerary teeth erupt, they can cause malalignment of the normal dentition. Those that remain in the jaws may cause root resorption and their follicles develop into dentigerous cysts or interfere with the normal eruption sequence. All the preceding factors influence the decision to either remove a supernumerary tooth or keep it under observation.

#### Missing Teeth

##### Synonyms

Hypodontia, oligodontia, and anodontia

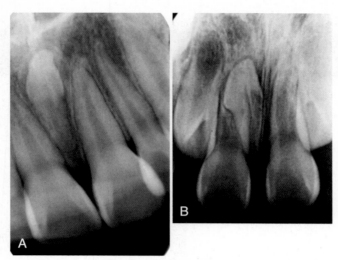

FIG. **19-1**   Periapical radiographs of inverted mesiodens.

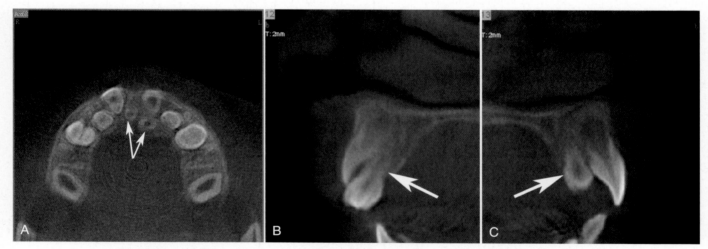

FIG. **19-2**   Axial **(A)** and cross-sectional **(B** and **C)** cone-beam computed tomographic views of two mesiodens erupting to the palatal aspect of the adjacent permanent central incisors.

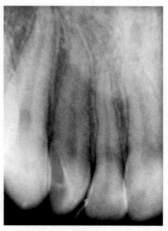

FIG. **19-3**   Periapical radiograph of a supplemental lateral incisor.

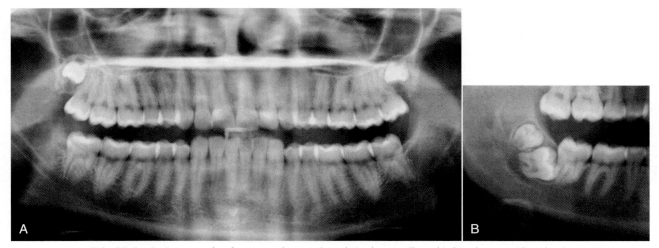

FIG. **19-4** **A,** An example of two supplemental teeth in the maxillary third molar area (distodens). **B,** An example in the mandibular third molar region. (**A** courtesy Dr. H. Grubisa, Oakville, Ontario, Canada).

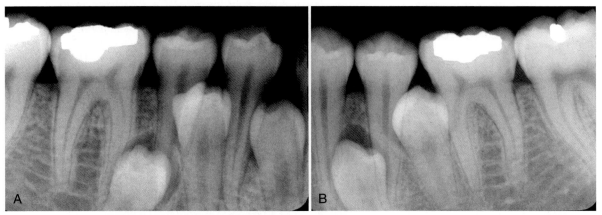

FIG. **19-5** Periapical radiographs show bilateral supplemental premolar teeth (peridens).

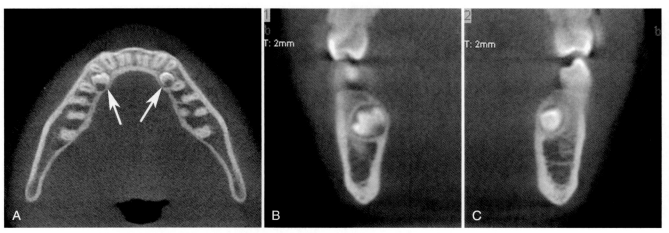

FIG. **19-6** Axial **(A),** right cross-sectional **(B),** and left cross-sectional **(C)** cone-beam computed tomographic views of peridens developing to the lingual of the adjacent mandibular first premolars.

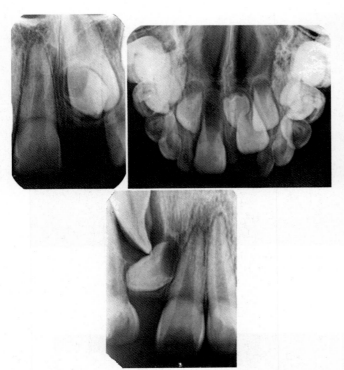

FIG. **19-7** Examples of mesiodens interfering with eruption of adjacent permanent teeth.

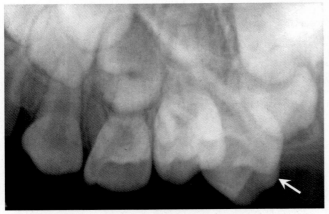

FIG. **19-8** Supplemental deciduous molar (arrow).

## Definition

The expression of developmentally missing teeth may range from the absence of one or a few teeth (hypodontia), to the absence of numerous teeth (oligodontia), to the failure of all teeth to develop (anodontia). Developmentally missing teeth may also be the result of numerous independent pathologic mechanisms that can affect the orderly formation of the dental lamina (e.g., orofaciodigital syndrome), failure of a tooth germ to develop at the optimal time, lack of necessary space imposed by a malformed jaw, or disproportion between tooth mass and jaw size.

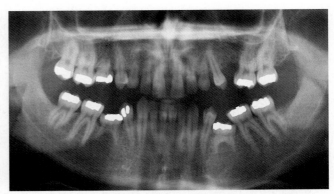

FIG. **19-9** Developmental absence of maxillary and mandibular second premolars and maxillary canines. Note the apically positioned deciduous mandibular second molars. This appearance is suggestive of ankylosis of the teeth.

### Clinical Features

Hypodontia in the permanent dentition, excluding third molars, is found in 3% to 10% of the population. Hypodontia is more frequently found in Asians and Native Americans. Although missing primary teeth are relatively uncommon, when one tooth is missing, it is usually a maxillary incisor. The most commonly missing teeth are third molars, followed by second premolars (Fig. 19-9), and maxillary lateral and mandibular central incisors. The absence may be either unilateral or bilateral. Children who have developmentally missing teeth tend to have more than one absent and more than one morphologic group (incisors, premolars, and molars) involved.

### Radiographic Features

The development of teeth may vary markedly between individuals. Missing teeth may be recognized by identifying and counting the teeth present. For some individuals, however, the eruption of some teeth may be delayed by a number of years after the established time (especially mandibular second premolars), whereas others may erupt as late as a year after the contralateral tooth.

### Differential Diagnosis

A tooth may be considered to be developmentally missing when it cannot be discerned clinically or radiographically, and no history exists of its extraction. Anodontia or oligodontia may occur in patients with ectodermal dysplasia (Fig. 19-10). This genetically inherited autosomal dominant disorder results in the absence of at least two ectodermally derived structures such as sweat glands, hair, skin, nails, and teeth. When the teeth are involved, the condition may present with multiple missing and/or malformed teeth that often have a conical or canine shape or a notable decrease in tooth size.

### Management

Missing teeth, abnormal occlusion, or altered facial appearance may cause some patients psychologic distress. If the extent of hypodontia is mild, the associated changes may likewise be slight and manageable by orthodontics. In more severe cases restorative, implant, and prosthetic procedures can be undertaken.

## SIZE OF TEETH

A positive correlation exists between tooth size (mesiodistal or buccolingual dimension) and body height. Males also have larger primary

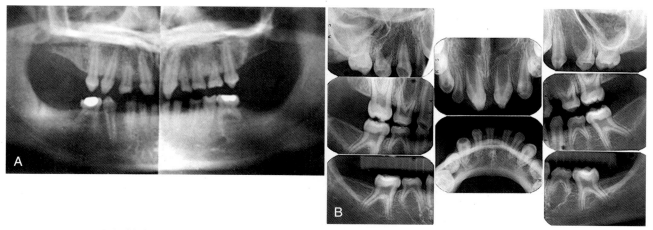

FIG. **19-10**  Two examples of multiple missing and malformed teeth in ectodermal dysplasia.

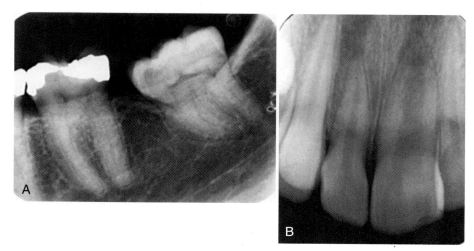

FIG. **19-11**  A large macrodont molar shows an increased mesiodistal dimension **(A)**. The macrodont central incisor shows enlarged mesiodistal and coronal-apical dimensions **(B)**. (**A** courtesy Dr. B. Gratt, Los Angeles, Calif.)

and permanent teeth than do females. Beyond these normal variations, however, individuals may occasionally have unusually large or small teeth.

## Macrodontia

### Definition
In macrodontia, the teeth are larger than normal. Macrodontia rarely affects the entire dentition. Often a single tooth, individual contralateral teeth, or a group of teeth may be involved (Fig. 19-11). Macrodontia may occur sporadically, and its cause is unknown. Vascular abnormalities such as a hemangioma (arising from within the bone or the soft tissues) can result in an increase in the size and accelerate the development of adjacent teeth. Macrodontia can also occur in hemihypertrophy of the face or in pituitary gigantism.

### Clinical Features
Clinically, macrodont teeth appear large and may be associated with crowding, malocclusion, or impaction.

### Radiographic Features
Radiographs reveal the increased size of both unerupted and erupted macrodont teeth. The shape of the tooth is usually normal, but some cases may exhibit mildly distorted morphology. Crowding may cause impaction of adjacent teeth.

### Differential Diagnosis
The differential diagnosis of a sporadic macrodont tooth includes gemination and fusion. When fusion occurs, a count of the teeth present will reveal a missing tooth. In gemination all the teeth may be present and often evidence exists of a division or cleft of the crown or root of the tooth. The differentiation between these three conditions may not influence the treatment provided.

### Management
In most cases macrodontia does not require treatment. Orthodontic treatment may be necessary if a malocclusion is present.

## Microdontia

### Definition
In microdontia, the teeth are smaller than normal. As with macrodontia, microdontia may involve all the teeth or be limited to a single tooth or group of teeth. Often the lateral incisors and third molars may be small. Generalized microdontia is extremely rare, although it does occur in some patients with pituitary dwarfism. Supernumerary teeth may also be microdonts.

### Clinical Features
The involved teeth are noticeably small and may have altered morphology. Microdont molars may have an altered shape. For example,

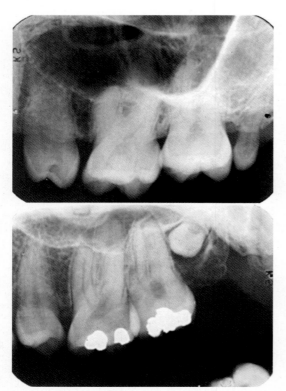

FIG. **19-12**   Periapical radiographs show a reduction in both the size and number of cusps in microdontia of the maxillary third molars.

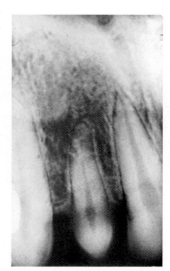

FIG. **19-13**   The "peg-shaped" deformity in microdontia of a maxillary lateral incisor.

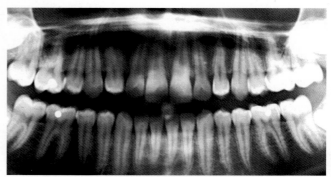

FIG. **19-14**   A cropped panoramic image demonstrating bilateral transposition of the maxillary canines and first premolars.

mandibular molars may have four cusps rather than five, and maxillary molars may have four cusps rather than three (Fig. 19-12). Microdont lateral incisors may be peg shaped (Fig. 19-13).

### Radiographic Features
These small teeth are frequently malformed.

### Differential Diagnosis
The recognition of small teeth indicates the diagnosis. The number and distribution of microdonts may also suggest consideration of syndromes (e.g., congenital heart disease, progeria).

### Management
Restorative or prosthetic treatment may be considered to create a more normal-appearing tooth, especially when considering esthetic concerns in the anterior dentition.

## ERUPTION OF TEETH

### Transposition

#### Definition

Transposition is the condition in which two typically adjacent teeth have exchanged positions in the dental arch.

#### Clinical Features
The most frequently transposed teeth are the permanent canine and the first premolar. Second premolars infrequently lie between the first

and second molars. The transposition of central and lateral incisors is rare. Transposition can occur with hypodontia, supernumerary teeth, or the persistence of a deciduous predecessor. Transposition in the primary dentition has not been reported.

### Radiographic Features
Radiographs reveal transposition when the teeth are not in their usual sequence in the dental arch (Fig. 19-14).

### Differential Diagnosis
Transposed teeth are usually easily recognized.

### Management
Transposed teeth are frequently altered prosthetically for function and/or esthetics.

## ALTERED MORPHOLOGY OF TEETH

### Fusion

#### Synonym

Synodontia

## Definition

Fusion of teeth results from the union of adjacent tooth germs of developing teeth. Some authors think that fusion results when two tooth germs develop so close together that, as they grow, they contact and fuse before calcification. Others contend that a physical force or pressure produced during development causes contact of adjacent tooth buds. Males and females experience fusion in equal numbers, and the incidence is higher in Asians and Native Americans.

## Clinical Features

Fusion results in a reduced number of teeth in the arch. Although more common between deciduous teeth, fusion may also occur in the permanent dentition. When a deciduous canine and lateral incisor fuse, the corresponding permanent lateral incisor may be absent. Fusion is more common in anterior teeth of both the permanent and deciduous dentition (Fig. 19-15). Fusion may be total or partial, depending on the stage of odontogenesis and the proximity of the developing teeth. The result can vary from a single tooth of about normal size to a tooth of nearly twice the normal size. The crowns of fused teeth usually appear to be large and single, although incisal clefts of varying depth or a bifid crown can sometimes occur.

## Radiographic Features

Radiographs disclose the unusual shape or size of the fused teeth. The true nature and extent of the union are frequently more evident on the radiograph than can be determined by clinical examination. Fused teeth may also show an unusual configuration of the pulp chamber or root canal.

## Differential Diagnosis

The differential diagnosis for fused teeth includes gemination and macrodontia. Fusion may be differentiated from gemination when the number of teeth is reduced by one, except in the unusual case in which a normal tooth and a supernumerary tooth have fused. The differentiation is usually academic because little difference exists in the treatment provided.

## Management

The management of a case of fusion depends on which teeth are involved, the degree of fusion, and the morphologic result. If the affected teeth are deciduous, they may be retained as they are. If the clinician contemplates extraction, it is important first to determine whether the permanent teeth are present. In the case of fused permanent teeth, the fused crowns may be reshaped with a restoration that mimics two independent crowns. The morphology of fused teeth require radiographic evaluation before the teeth are reshaped. Endodontic therapy may be necessary and perhaps may be difficult or impossible if the root canals are of unusual shape. In some cases it is most prudent to leave the teeth as they are.

## Concrescence

### Definition

Concrescence occurs when the roots of two or more primary or permanent teeth are fused by cementum. Although its cause is unknown, many authorities suspect that space restriction during development, local trauma, excessive occlusal force, or local infection after development plays an important role. If the condition occurs during development, it is sometimes referred to as true concrescence. If the condition occurs later, it is acquired concrescence.

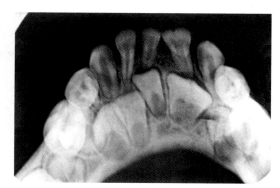

FIG. **19-15** Fusion of the central and lateral incisors in both the primary and the permanent dentitions. Note the reduction in number of teeth and the increased width of the fused tooth mass.

## Clinical Features

Maxillary molars are the teeth most frequently involved, especially a third molar and a supernumerary tooth. Involved teeth may fail to erupt or may erupt incompletely. The sexes are equally affected.

## Radiographic Features

A radiographic examination may not always distinguish between concrescence and teeth that are in close contact or that are simply superimposed (Fig. 19-16). When the condition is suspected on a radiograph and extraction of one of the teeth is being considered, additional projections at different angles may be obtained to better delineate the condition.

## Differential Diagnosis

It is usually impossible to determine radiographically with certainty whether the teeth whose root images are superimposed are actually joined. If the roots are joined, it may not be possible to tell whether the union is by cementum or by dentin (fusion). In this regard, the absence of a periodontal ligament (PDL) space between the roots may be helpful.

## Management

Concrescence affects treatment only when the decision is made to remove one or both of the involved teeth because this condition complicates the extraction. The clinician should warn the patient that an effort to remove one might result in the unintended and simultaneous removal of the other.

## Gemination

### Synonym

Twinning

### Definition

Gemination is a rare anomaly that arises when a single tooth bud attempts to divide. The result may be an invagination of the crown with partial division or, in rare cases, complete division through the crown and root, producing identical structures. Complete twinning results in a normal tooth plus a supernumerary tooth in the arch. The cause of gemination is unknown, but some evidence suggests that it is familial.

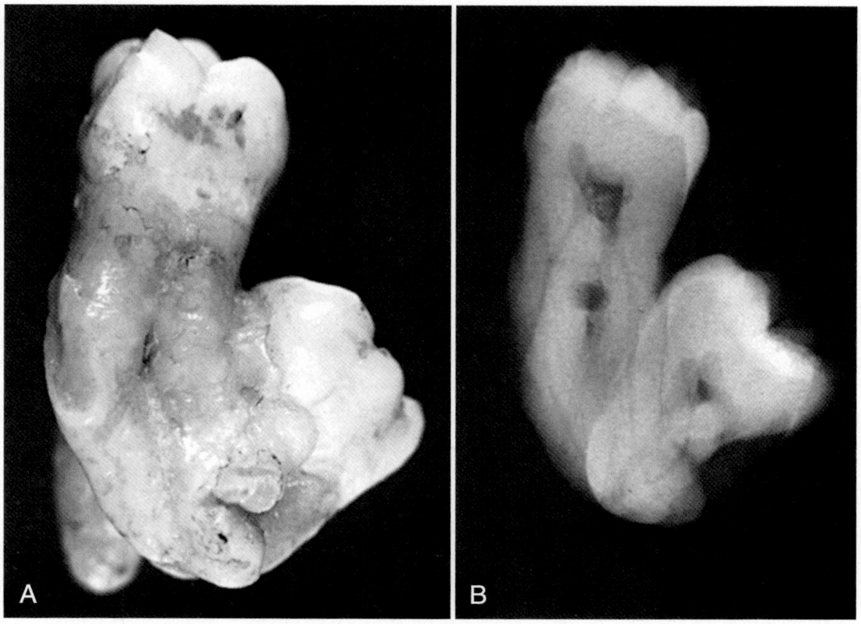

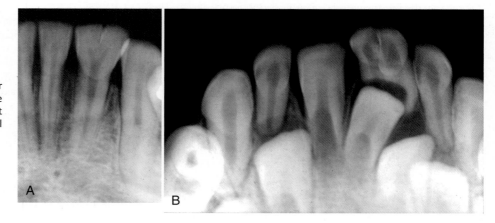

FIG. **19-16 A,** Concrescence occurs when two teeth are joined by cementum. **B,** Extraction of one tooth may result in the unintended removal of the second because the cementum bridge may not be well visualized radiographically. (Courtesy Dr. R. Kienholz, Dallas, Tex.)

FIG. **19-17** Gemination of a mandibular lateral incisor showing bifurcation of the crown and pulp chamber **(A).** Almost complete gemination of a deciduous lateral incisor **(B).**

## Clinical Features

Although gemination may occur in both the deciduous and permanent dentitions, it more frequently affects the primary teeth, usually in the incisor region. It can be detected clinically after the anomalous tooth erupts. The occurrence in males and females is about equal. The enamel or dentin of geminated teeth may be hypoplastic or hypocalcified.

## Radiographic Features

Radiographs reveal the altered shape of the hard tissue and pulp chamber of the geminated tooth. Radiopaque enamel outlines the clefts in the crowns and invaginations and thus accentuates them. The pulp chamber is usually single and enlarged and may be partially divided (Fig. 19-17). In the rare case of premolar gemination, the tooth image suggests a molar with an enlarged crown and two roots.

## Differential Diagnosis

The differential diagnosis of gemination includes fusion. If the malformed tooth is counted as one, individuals with gemination have a normal tooth count, whereas those with fusion are seen to be missing a tooth.

## Management

A geminated tooth in the anterior region may compromise arch esthetics and arch length. Areas of hypoplasia and invagination lines or areas of coronal separation represent caries-susceptible sites that may in time result in pulpal inflammation. Affected teeth can cause malocclusion and lead to periodontal disease. Consequently, the affected tooth may be removed (especially if it is deciduous), the crown(s) may be restored or reshaped, or the tooth may be left untreated and periodically examined to preclude the development of complications. Before treatment is initiated on a primary tooth, the status of the permanent succedaneous tooth and configuration of its root canals should be determined radiographically.

## Taurodontism

### Definition

The body of taurodont teeth appears elongated and the roots short. The pulp chamber extends from a normal position in the crown throughout the length of the elongated body, leading to a more apically positioned pulpal floor.

Taurodontism may occur in any tooth in either the permanent or primary dentition; however, it is usually fully expressed in the molars and less often in the premolars. Single or multiple teeth may show taurodont features.

## Clinical Features

Because the body and roots of taurodont teeth lie below the alveolar margin, the distinguishing features of these teeth are not recognizable clinically.

## Radiographic Features

The distinctive morphology of taurodont teeth are quite apparent on radiographs. The peculiar feature is the elongated pulp chamber and the more apically positioned furcation (Fig. 19-18). The shortened roots and root canals are a function of the long body and normal length of the tooth. The dimensions of the crown are normal.

## Differential Diagnosis

The image of the taurodont tooth is characteristic and easily recognized radiographically. The developing molar may appear similar; however, the identification of the wide apical foramina and incompletely formed roots aids in the differential diagnosis. Taurodontism has been reported with greater frequency in trisomy 21 syndrome.

## Management

Taurodont teeth do not require treatment.

## Dilaceration

### Definition

Dilaceration is a disturbance in tooth formation that produces a sharp bend or curve in the tooth anywhere in the crown or the root. Although this anomaly is likely developmental in nature, one of the oldest concepts is that dilaceration is the result of mechanical trauma to the calcified portion of a partially formed tooth.

### Clinical Features

Most cases of radicular dilaceration are not recognized clinically. If the dilaceration is so pronounced that the tooth does not erupt, the only clinical indication of the defect is a missing tooth. If the defect is in the crown of an erupted tooth, it may be readily recognized as an angular distortion (Fig. 19-19).

### Radiographic Features

Radiographs provide the best means of detecting a radicular dilaceration. The condition occurs most often in maxillary premolars. One or more teeth may be affected. If the roots dilacerate mesially or distally, the condition is clearly apparent on a periapical radiograph (Fig. 19-20). However, when the roots are dilacerated buccally (labially) or lingually, the central x ray passes approximately parallel with the deflected portion of the root and the apical end of the root may have

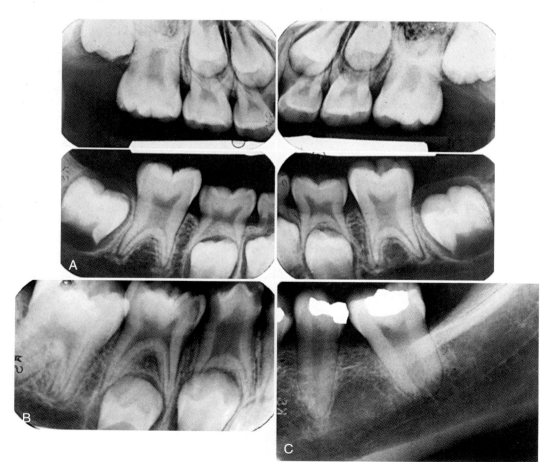

FIG. **19-18** Periapical radiographs reveal enlarged pulp chambers and apically positioned furcations in permanent first molars **(A)**, a primary first molar **(B)**, and a permanent molar **(C)**.

the appearance of a circular or oval radiopaque area with a central radiolucency (the apical foramen and root canal), giving the appearance of a bull's eye. The PDL space around this dilacerated portion may be seen as a radiolucent halo encircling the radiopaque area (Fig. 19-21). In some cases, especially in the maxilla, the geometry of the projections may preclude the recognition of a dilaceration.

### Differential Diagnosis

Occasionally dilacerated roots may be difficult to differentiate from fused roots, sclerosing osteitis, or a dense bone island. These can usually be discerned, however, by radiographs made at different angles.

### Management

The dilacerated root generally does not require treatment because it provides adequate support. If the tooth is to be extracted for some other reason, its removal can be complicated, especially if the surgeon

is not prepared with a preoperative radiograph. In contrast, dilacerated crowns are frequently restored with a prosthetic crown to improve esthetics and function.

## Dens Invaginatus, Dens in Dente, and Dilated Odontome

### Synonyms
Gestant odontome and "tooth within a tooth"

### Definition
The three entities all result from varying degrees of invagination or infolding of the enamel surface into the interior of a tooth. The least severe form of this infolding is dens invaginatus, and the most severe form is the dilated odontome. The invagination can occur in either the cingulum area (dens invaginatus) or incisal edge (dens in dente) of the crown or in the root during tooth development. It may also

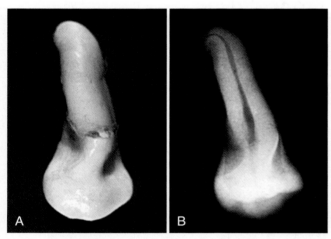

FIG. **19-19**   **A,** Dilaceration of the crown may be recognized clinically. **B,** Radiograph of the specimen in **A.** (Courtesy Dr. R. Kienholz, Dallas, Tex.)

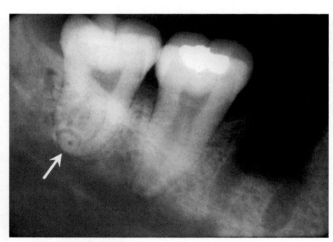

FIG. **19-21**   The most apical portion of this third molar root is dilacerated in the buccal-lingual direction so that its long axis lies along the path of the x-ray beam. Note the "bull's eye" appearance of the root apex produced by the root canal, tooth root, and PDL space *(arrow).*

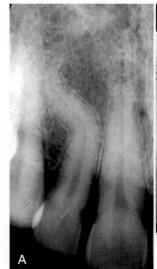
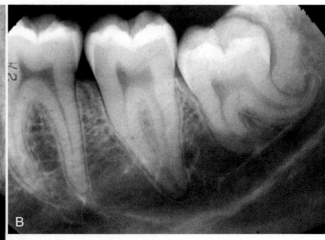

FIG. **19-20**   Dilaceration of the root of a maxillary lateral incisor **(A)** and mandibular third molar **(B).**

involve the pulp chamber or root canal system. This may result in a deformity of either the crown or the root, although these anomalies are seen most often in tooth crowns. Coronal invaginations usually originate from an anomalous infolding of the enamel organ into the dental papilla. In a mature tooth the result is a fold of hard tissue within the tooth characterized by enamel lining the fold (Fig. 19-22). When the abnormality involves the root, it may be the result of an invagination of Hertwig's epithelial root sheath and produce an accentuation of the normal longitudinal root groove.

In contrast to the coronal type, which is lined with enamel, the radicular type defect is lined with cementum. If the invagination retracts and is cut off, it leaves a longitudinal structure of cementum, bone, and remnants of PDL within the pulp canal. The structure often extends for most of the root length. In other cases the root sheath may bud off a saclike invagination that produces a circumscribed cementum defect in the root. Mandibular first premolars and second molars are especially prone to develop the radicular variety of this invagination anomaly.

Little difference in the frequency of occurrence exists among Caucasian and Asian people. If all grades of expression of invagination, mild to severe, are included, the condition is found in approximately 5% of these two ethnic groups. The condition appears to be rare in individuals of African descent. No sexual predilection exists. Although no specific mode of inheritance seems to fit all the data, a high degree of inheritability seems to exist.

## Clinical Features

Dens invaginatus may appear as nothing more than a small pit between the cingulum and the lingual surface of an incisor tooth (Fig. 19-23). In dens in dente, the pit is located at the incisal edge of the tooth and crown morphology may appear abnormal, having the appearance of a microdont (Fig. 19-24).

Dens invaginatus and dens in dente occur most frequently in the permanent maxillary lateral incisors, followed by (in decreasing frequency) the maxillary central incisors, premolars, and canines and less often in the posterior teeth. Invagination is rare in the crowns of mandibular teeth and in deciduous teeth. The abnormality occurs symmetrically in about half the cases, and concomitant involvement of the central and lateral incisors may occur.

The clinical importance of dens invaginatus and dens in dente is the risk of pulpal inflammation. Although enamel lines the coronal defect, it is frequently thin, often of poor quality, and even missing in some areas. Furthermore, the cavity is usually separated from the pulp

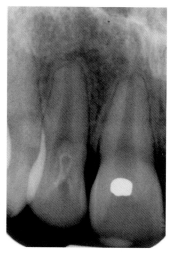

FIG. **19-23** The radiopaque, inverted tear-drop outline of dens invaginatus in a maxillary lateral incisor. Note the position of the invagination in the cingulum area of the tooth crown.

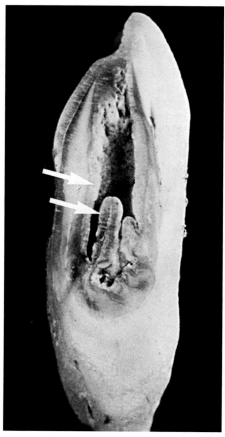

FIG. **19-22** Dens in dente is characterized by an infolding of enamel into the tooth. This sectioned canine with a dens in dente shows enamel *(arrows)* folded into the tooth's interior.

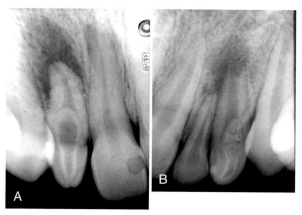

FIG. **19-24** **A** and **B**, The infolding of enamel is more severe in dens in dente as seen in these two periapical radiographs. Notice that the invagination begins near the incisal edge of these abnormally "peg-shaped" lateral incisors.

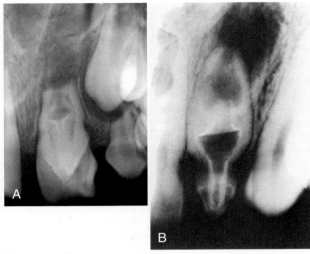

FIG. **19-25   A** and **B,** Severe forms of dens in dente usually result in necrosis of the pulp, open apices, and rarefying osteitis at the tooth apices.

chamber by a relatively thin wall that opens into the oral environment through a narrow constriction. The pit is often difficult if not impossible to keep clean, and consequently it offers conditions favorable for the development of caries. Such carious lesions are difficult to detect clinically and rapidly involve the pulp. In addition, sometimes fine canals extend between the invagination and the pulp chamber, resulting in pulpal disease even in the absence of caries.

## Radiographic Features
Most cases of dens invaginatus or dens in dente are discovered radiographically and can be identified in the radiographic image even before the tooth erupts. The infolding of the enamel lining is more radiopaque than the surrounding tooth structure and can easily be identified as an inverted teardrop-shaped radiolucency with a radiopaque border (Figs. 19-23 and 19-24). Less frequently the radicular invaginations appear as poorly defined, slightly radiolucent structures running longitudinally within the root. The defects, especially the coronal variety, may vary in size and shape from small and superficial to large and deep. If a coronal invagination is extensive, the crown is almost invariably malformed and the apical foramen is usually wide (Fig. 19-25). A frequent cause of an open apical foramen is the cessation of root development that occurs as a result of death of the pulpal tissue.

In the most severe form (dilated odontome) the tooth is severely deformed, having a circular or oval shape with a radiolucent interior (Fig. 19-26).

## Differential Diagnosis
The appearance and usual occurrence in incisors are so characteristic that, once recognized, little probability exists that the anomaly will be confused with another condition.

## Management
Although it is important to evaluate every case individually, the placement of a prophylactic restoration in the defect is typically the treatment of choice and should ensure a normal life span for the tooth.

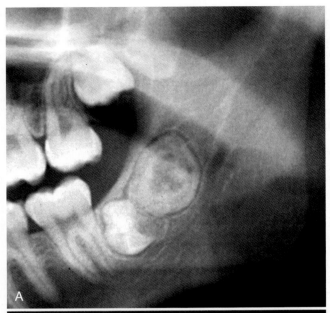

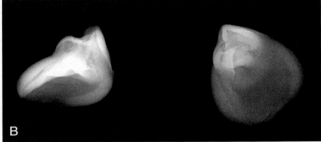

FIG. **19-26   A,** A dilated odontome, the most severe of the enamel invaginations, is positioned just posterior to the developing mandibular third molar in this panoramic image. **B,** Radiographs of the extracted dilated odontome from two different angulations.

Failure of early identification and hence treatment may result in premature tooth loss or the requirement for root canal therapy.

### Dens Evaginatus

#### Synonym
Leong's premolar

#### Definition
In contrast to dens invaginatus or dens in dente, dens evaginatus is the result of an outpouching of the enamel organ. The resultant enamel-covered tubercle usually occurs in or near the middle of the occlusal surface of a premolar or occasionally a molar (Fig. 19-27). Lateral incisors are most commonly involved, whereas canines are rarely affected. The frequency of occurrence of dens evaginatus is highest in Asians and Native Americans.

#### Clinical Features
Clinically, dens evaginatus appears as a tubercle of enamel on the occlusal surface of the affected tooth. A hard, polyplike protuberance predominantly exists in the central groove or lingual ridge of a buccal cusp of posterior teeth and in the cingulum fossa of anterior teeth. Dens evaginatus may occur bilaterally and usually in the mandible.

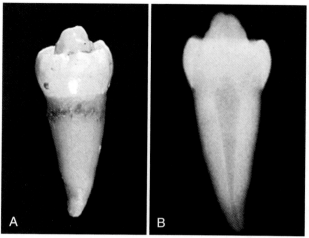

FIG. **19-27** The occlusal tubercle of dens evaginatus as seen in a mandibular premolar **(A).** A periapical radiograph of the specimen **(B).** (Courtesy Dr. R. Kienholz, Dallas, Tex.)

The tubercle often has a dentin core, and a very slender pulp horn frequently extends into the evagination. After the tubercle is worn down by the opposing teeth, it appears as a small circular facet with a small black pit in the center (Fig. 19-28). Wear, fracture, or indiscriminate surgical removal of this tubercle may precipitate a pulpal infection because of the exposure of the pulp horn. In rare cases a microscopic direct communication may occur between the pulp and the oral cavity through this tubercle. In these instances the pulp may become infected shortly after eruption.

### Radiographic Features

The radiographic image shows an extension of a dentin tubercle on the occlusal surface unless the tubercle is already worn down. The dentin core is usually covered with opaque enamel. A fine pulp horn may extend into the tubercle, but this may not be visible radiographically. If the tubercle has been worn to the point of pulpal exposure or has fractured, pulpal necrosis may result (Fig. 19-28). This is indicated by an open apical foramen and periapical radiolucency. Multiple root formation is often associated with dens evaginatus, especially in mandibular premolars.

### Differential Diagnosis

The clinical and radiographic appearance may be characteristic or may be difficult to visualize if the tubercle has been worn down to the occlusal surface.

### Management

If the tubercle causes any occlusal interference or shows evidence of marked abrasion, it should probably be removed under aseptic conditions and the pulp capped, if necessary. Such a precaution may preclude pulpal exposure and infection as the result of accidental fracture or advanced abrasion.

### Amelogenesis Imperfecta

### Definition

Amelogenesis imperfecta is a genetic anomaly arising from mutations that may have occurred in one of four different genes that play some role in enamel formation. The mutation may be inherited in an autosomal dominant or recessive manner, or it may be inherited in an

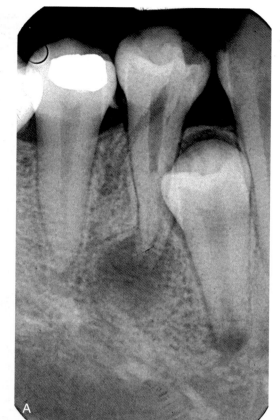

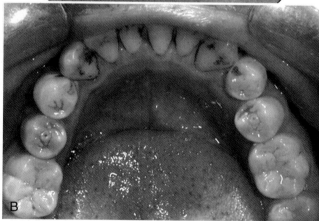

FIG. **19-28** A periapical radiograph of a mandibular first premolar with a dens evaginatus and apical rarefying osteitis **(A).** A clinical photograph of another case of dens evaginatus involving both mandibular second premolars **(B).** Note the worn tubercles located in the center of the occlusal surfaces, now seen as black pits representing communication with the pulp chamber.

X-linked pattern. The mutation leads to marked changes in the enamel of all or nearly all the teeth in both dentitions and is not related to any time or period of enamel development or any clinically demonstrable alteration (disease or dietary abnormality) in other tissues. The enamel may lack the normal prismatic structure and be laminated throughout its thickness or at the periphery. As a result, these teeth are more resistant to decay. The dentin and root form are usually normal. Eruption of the affected teeth is often delayed, and a tendency for tooth impaction exists. Although at least 14 variants of the condition have been described, four general types have been delineated on the basis of their clinical or radiographic appearances: a hypoplastic type, a hypomaturation type, a hypocalcified type, and a hypomaturation/hypoplastic type associated with taurodontism.

### Clinical Features

*Hypoplastic Type.* The enamel of the affected teeth fails to develop to its normal thickness. Consequently, the color of the underlying dentin imparts a yellowish-brown color to the tooth. As well, the enamel may be abnormal: rough, pitted, smooth, or glossy. The crowns of the teeth may appear undersized with a roughly square shape. The reduced enamel thickness also causes a loss of contact between adjacent teeth (Fig. 19-29). The occlusal surfaces of the pos-

terior teeth are relatively flat with low cusps. This is a result of the attrition of cusp tips that were initially low and not fully formed.

*Hypomaturation.* In the hypomaturation form of amelogenesis imperfecta, the enamel has a mottled appearance but is of normal thickness. The enamel is softer than normal, its density comparable to dentin, and it may break away from the crown. Its color may range from clear to cloudy white, yellow, or brown. In one form of hypomaturation amelogenesis imperfecta, the teeth may be capped with white, opaque enamel. This appearance has been referred to as "snow-capped" teeth.

*Hypocalcification.* The hypocalcific form of amelogenesis imperfecta is more common than the hypoplastic variety. The crowns of the teeth are normal in size and shape when they erupt because the enamel is of regular thickness (Fig. 19-30). However, because the enamel is poorly mineralized (it is less dense than dentin), it starts to fracture away shortly after it comes into function. This creates clinically recognizable defects. The soft enamel abrades rapidly and the softer dentin also wears down rapidly, resulting in a grossly worn tooth, sometimes to the level of the gingiva. An explorer point under pressure can penetrate the soft enamel, yet caries in these worn teeth is unusual. The hypocalcified enamel has increased permeability and becomes stained and darkened. The teeth of a young person with generalized hypomineralization of the enamel are frequently dark brown from food stains.

*Hypomaturation/Hypocalcification.* This classification indicates a combination of hypomaturation and hypocalcification that involves both the permanent and deciduous dentition. If the dominant defect is hypomaturation, then the term *hypomaturation-hypocalcification* is used. The enamel is usually mottled and discolored to a yellow or brown color. The enamel has the same radiopacity as the dentin. When the dominant defect is hypocalcification, the term *hypocalcification-hypomaturation* is used. The appearance of the teeth is similar, but the enamel is thin.

### Radiographic Features

Identification of amelogenesis imperfecta is made primarily by clinical examination, although the radiographic features substantiate the clinical impression. The radiographic signs of hypoplastic amelogenesis imperfecta include a square crown, a relatively thin radiopaque

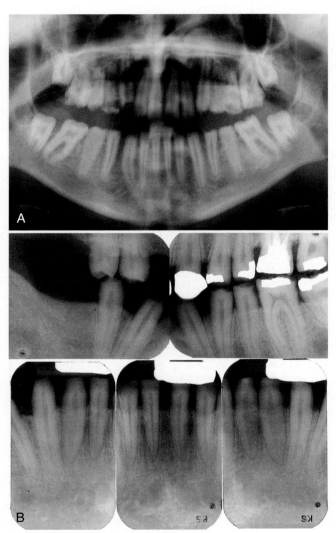

FIG. **19-29    A,** A cropped panoramic image of hypoplastic amelogenesis imperfecta. Note the absence of interproximal contacts and the "picket fence"–like appearance of the teeth. **B,** Intraoral radiographs of another case of amelogenises imperfecta. Note the very thin enamel layer. (**A** Courtesy Dr. S. Roth, Halifax, Nova Scotia, Canada.)

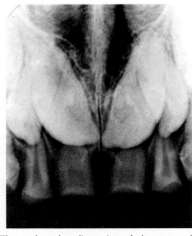

FIG. **19-30**    The reduced radiopacity of the enamel and the rapid abrasion of the crowns of the primary teeth are features of hypomineralized amelogenesis imperfecta.

layer of enamel, low or absent cusps, and multiple open contacts between the teeth. The appearance of the anterior teeth on radiographs is said to have a "picket fence"–type of appearance. The density of the enamel is normal. Pitted enamel appears as sharply localized areas of mottled density, quite different from the image cast by a tooth that is normal in shape and density. The hypomaturation form demonstrates a normal thickness of the enamel, but its density is the same as that of dentin. In the hypocalcified forms the enamel thickness is normal but its density is even less (more radiolucent) than that of dentin. With advanced abrasion, obliteration of the pulp chambers may complicate recognition of the radiographic picture.

### Differential Diagnosis

If advanced abrasion is present and secondary dentin obliterates the pulp chambers, the radiographic picture of amelogenesis imperfecta appears similar to that of dentinogenesis imperfecta. However, the presence of bulbous crowns and narrow roots, the relatively normal density of any remaining enamel, and the obliteration of pulp chambers and root canals, in the absence of marked attrition, are characteristic of dentinogenesis imperfecta (see the following section) and should distinguish it from amelogenesis imperfecta.

### Management

Appropriate treatment for amelogenesis imperfecta is restoration of the esthetics and function of the affected teeth.

## Dentinogenesis Imperfecta

### Synonym

Hereditary opalescent dentin

### Definition

Dentinogenesis imperfecta is a genetic anomaly involving primarily the dentin, although the enamel may be thinner than normal in this condition. Three types of dentinogenesis imperfecta exist, and each has been associated with a particular genetic defect. Type I is associated with osteogenesis imperfecta (see the following section) and is caused by mutations of one of two genes involved in synthesis of collagen type I. The tooth roots and pulp chambers of type I teeth are generally small and underdeveloped, and the primary dentition may be more severely affected than the permanent dentition. Type II dentinogenesis imperfecta is similar to type I but only affects the dentin without any skeletal

defects. The expression of type II dentinogenesis imperfecta is variable, and occasionally individuals show enlarged pulp chambers in the primary teeth. Type III dentinogenesis imperfecta, or the so-called Brandywine isolate, was described in a population of fewer than 200 persons in the Brandywine region of Maryland. There is some controversy regarding the differentiation between types II and III; however, type III teeth are said to exhibit enlarged pulp chambers, making them more susceptible to pulp exposure. Type II and III dentinogenesis imperfecta are associated with mutations of the dentin sialophosphoprotein *(DSPP)* gene located among a cluster of four other genes involved in bone and/or dentin formation on chromosome 4.

The incidence pattern of dentinogenesis imperfecta occurs with equal frequency in both sexes. Both the deciduous and permanent dentition may show this defect.

### Clinical Features

The appearance of the teeth with dentinogenesis imperfecta is characteristic. They show a high degree of amber-like translucency and a variety of colors from yellow to blue-gray. The colors change according to whether the teeth are observed by transmitted light or reflected light. The enamel easily fractures from the teeth and the crowns wear readily. In adults the teeth may frequently wear down to the gingiva. The exposed dentin becomes stained. The color of the abraded teeth may change to dark brown or even black. Some patients demonstrate an anterior open bite.

### Radiographic Features

The crowns in patients with dentinogenesis imperfecta are usually normal in size, but there is a constriction of the cervical portion of the tooth that gives the crown a bulbous appearance. Radiographs may reveal slight to marked attrition of the occlusal surface. The roots are usually short and slender. There may be partial or complete obliteration of the pulp chambers. Early in development, the teeth may appear to have large pulp chambers, but these are quickly obliterated by the formation of dentin. Ultimately the root canals may be absent or threadlike (Fig. 19-31). Occasionally, areas of rarefying osteitis may be seen in association with what appear to be sound teeth without evidence of pulpal involvement. These changes may occur as a result of microscopic communication(s) between the residual pulp and the oral cavity. These lesions do not occur as frequently as in dentin dysplasia. The architecture of the bone in the maxilla and mandible is normal.

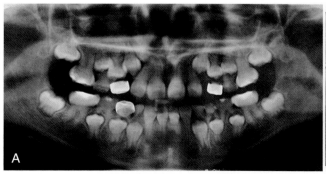
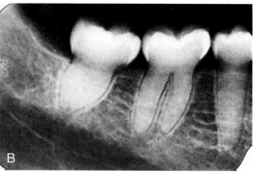

FIG. **19-31** **A** and **B,** Dentinogenesis imperfecta characteristically shows bulbous crowns, constriction of tooth at the cementoenamel junction, short roots, and a reduced size of the pulp chamber and root canals.

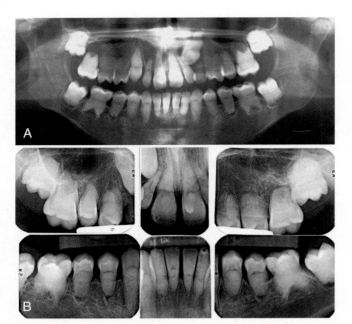

FIG. **19-32** Panoramic **(A)** and periapical images **(B)** of the same case show the short and poorly developed roots, obliterated pulp chambers and root canals, and periapical rarefying osteitis associated with type 1 (radicular) dentin dysplasia. Note the half-moon or "demilune" shape of the pulp chambers.

### Differential Diagnosis

Dentin dysplasia (see the following section)

### Management

The placement of prosthetic crowns on the affected teeth is usually unsuccessful unless the teeth have good root support. The teeth should not be extracted from patients 5 to 15 years of age. It is generally preferable to place full overdentures on the teeth to prevent alveolar resorption. In adults, extraction of the teeth and their replacement can be recommended.

## Osteogenesis Imperfecta

Osteogenesis imperfecta is a hereditary disorder characterized by osseous fractures. The pathogenesis is thought to be an inborn error in the synthesis of type I collagen, which results in brittle bones. It is usually transmitted as an autosomal dominant trait. Patients may have blue sclera, wormian bones (bones in skull sutures), skeletal deformities, and progressive osteopenia. Dentinogenesis imperfecta is found in approximately 25% of cases. In addition, oral findings may include class III malocclusions and an increased incidence of impacted first and second molars.

## Dentin Dysplasia

### Definition

Dentin dysplasia is a genetically inherited autosomal-dominant abnormality that resembles dentinogenesis imperfecta. Two types have been described: type I (radicular) and type II (coronal). In the type I form, the most marked changes are found in the appearances of the roots. In the type II form, changes in the crown are most clearly

seen in the altered shape of the pulp chambers. The genetic lesion giving rise to type I dentin dysplasia has not been identified; however, the same gene that has been implicated in dentinogenesis imperfecta type II and III has also been implicated in type II dentin dysplasia, the *DSPP* gene. Dentin dysplasia is rarer than dentinogenesis imperfecta (1:100,000 compared with 1:8,000).

### Clinical Features

Clinically, teeth with dentin dysplasia have characteristic features. Type I (the radicular form) teeth have mostly normal color and shape in both dentitions. Occasionally a slight bluish-brown translucency is apparent. The teeth are often misaligned in the arch, and patients may describe drifting and spontaneous exfoliation with little or no trauma. In type II (the coronal form), the crowns of the primary teeth appear to be of the same color, size, and contour as those in dentinogenesis imperfecta. This is interesting evidence in light of the purported close genetic linkage between the two dentin abnormalities. Although not universally accepted, reports exist that primary teeth rapidly abrade. The permanent teeth have clinically normal-appearing crowns.

### Radiographic Features

In type I dentin dysplasia, the roots of both the primary and permanent teeth are either short or abnormally shaped (Fig. 19-32). The molar roots have been described as having a shallow "W" shape. The roots of primary teeth may be only thin spicules. The pulp chambers and root canals completely fill in before eruption. The extent of obliteration of the pulp chambers and canals is variable. In addition, about 20% of type I dentin dysplasia teeth are associated with rarefying osteitis. This is likely the result of microscopic communication(s) between the residual pulp and the oral cavity. Association of these inflammatory lesions with noncarious teeth is an important feature for recognition of this particular entity. In type II dentin dysplasia, obliteration of the pulp chamber (Fig. 19-33) and reduction in the caliber of the root canals occurs after eruption (at least by 5 or 6 years). These changes are not seen before eruption. As the chambers of the molars are being filled with hypertrophic dentin, the pulp chambers may become flame or thistle shaped and may have multiple pulp stones. Occasionally the anterior teeth and premolars develop a pulp chamber that is thistle-tube in shape because of its extension into the root. The roots of the coronal variety are normal in shape and proportions.

### Differential Diagnosis

The differential diagnosis for dentin dysplasia may include only one other entity, dentinogenesis imperfecta, because the appearances of both abnormalities can appear clinically similar. Both entities can produce crowns with altered color and occluded pulp chambers. The finding of a thistle-tube–shaped pulp chamber in a single-rooted tooth strengthens the probability of dentin dysplasia. In type II dentin dysplasia, however, the pulp chambers become obliterated after eruption. Sometimes, crown size can help distinguish between the two: the teeth in dentinogenesis imperfecta typically have bulbous shaped crowns with a constriction in the cervical region, whereas the crowns in dentin dysplasia are usually of normal shape, size, and proportion. If the roots are short and narrow, the condition is likely to be dentinogenesis imperfecta. On the other hand, normal-appearing roots or practically no roots at all should suggest dentin dysplasia. Periapical rarefying osteitis in association with noncarious teeth are more commonly seen in dentin dysplasia.

## Management

Teeth with type I dentin dysplasia have such poor root support that prosthetic replacement is about the only practical treatment. On the other hand, teeth that are of normal shape, size, and support (type II) can be crowned if they seem to be rapidly abrading. At the same time the esthetics of discolored anterior teeth can be improved by prosthetic treatment.

## Regional Odontodysplasia

### Synonyms
Odontogenesis imperfecta and ghost teeth

### Definition
Regional odontodysplasia is a relatively rare condition in which both enamel and dentin are hypoplastic and hypocalcified. This localized arrest in tooth development typically affects only a few adjacent teeth in a quadrant. These teeth may be either primary or permanent. If the primary teeth are affected, their successors are usually involved. Although many theories exist regarding the etiology of this condition, its cause is unknown.

### Clinical Features
Teeth affected with regional odontodysplasia are small and mottled brown as a result of staining of the hypocalcified and hypoplastic enamel. They are especially susceptible to caries, are brittle, and are subject to fracture and pulpal infection. Central incisors are most often affected, with lateral incisors and canines also occasionally showing the defect (most often in the maxilla). Eruption of the defective teeth is often delayed and in severe cases they may not erupt.

### Radiographic Features
Because these teeth are very poorly mineralized, the radiographic images of teeth with regional odontodysplasia are have been described as having a "ghostlike" appearance. The pulp chambers are large and the root canals wide because the hypoplastic dentin is thin, just serving to outline the image of the root (Fig. 19-34). As well, the poorly outlined roots are short. The enamel is, likewise, thin and less dense than usual, sometimes so thin and poorly mineralized that it may not be evident on the radiograph. The tooth is little more than a thin shell of hypoplastic enamel and dentin. Teeth that do not erupt are so hypomineralized and hypoplastic that they appear to be resorbing.

### Differential Diagnosis
The malformed teeth occasionally seen in one of the expressions of dentinogenesis imperfecta may occasionally be confused with those in regional odontodysplasia. The fact that the dentinogenesis imperfecta trait usually carries a history of familial involvement, however, in contrast to odontodysplasia (which is not hereditary), is an important distinguishing feature. Also the enamel in regional odontodysplasia is obviously hypoplastic, which is not the case in dentinogenesis imperfecta. Finally, only a few teeth of either dentition in an isolated segment of the arch are affected in regional odontodysplasia, whereas the type of dentinogenesis imperfecta that resembles regional odontodysplasia involves all primary teeth.

### Management
With the advent of newer restorative materials, it is recommended to retain and restore the affected teeth as much as possible. Unerupted teeth should be retained during the period of skeletal growth. Severely

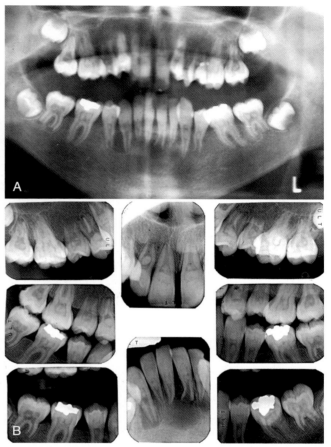

FIG. **19-33** Panoramic **(A)** and periapical **(B)** radiographs of the same case show obliteration of the pulp chamber, reduction in the caliber of root canals, and pulp stones obscuring the flame- or thistle-shaped pulp chambers associated with type II (coronal) dentin dysplasia. Note the areas of rarefying osteitis associated with some of the mandibular anterior teeth.

damaged permanent teeth that become pulpally involved may require removal and replacement.

## Enamel Pearl

### Synonyms
Enamel drop, enamel nodule, and enameloma

### Definition
The enamel pearl is a small globule of enamel 1 to 3 mm in diameter that occurs on the roots of molars (Fig. 19-35). It is found in about 3% of the population, probably formed by Hertwig's epithelial root sheath before the epithelium loses its enamel-forming potential. Usually only one pearl develops, but occasionally more develop. Enamel pearls may have a core of dentin and rarely a pulp horn extending from the chamber of the host tooth.

### Clinical Features
Most enamel pearls form below the crest of the gingiva and are not detected during a clinical examination. They typically develop in the furcal areas of molar teeth, often lying at or just apical to the cementoenamel junction. Those that form on the maxillary molars are

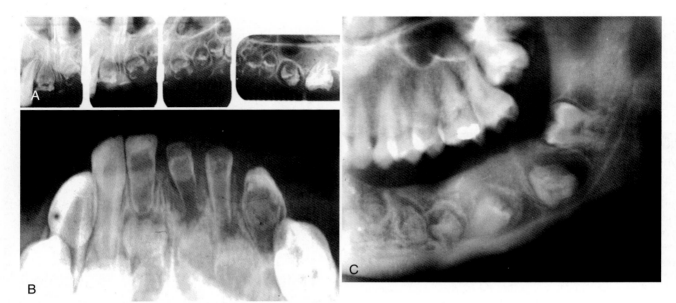

FIG. **19-34** Periapical radiographs reveal poor mineralization of all of the dental hard tissues in regional odontodysplasia. In the following cases, note how only one portion of the arch is involved. Involvement of the maxillary left dentition **(A).** Involvement of the primary incisors and canines **(B).** Involvement of the left mandibular premolars and first and second molars **(C).** Note the lack of eruption and hypoplasia of enamel and dentin expressed mainly as short roots.

usually in the mesial or distal furca and those that develop in mandibular molars are more often in the buccal or lingual furca. Usually no clinical symptoms are associated with their presence, although they may predispose to periodontal pocket formation and subsequent periodontal disease.

### Radiographic Features
The enamel pearl appears smooth, round, and comparable in degree of radiopacity to the enamel covering the crown (Fig. 19-36). Occasionally the dentine casts a small, round, radiolucent shadow in the center of the radiopaque sphere of enamel. If projected over the crown, it may be obscured.

### Differential Diagnosis
It is possible to mistake an enamel pearl for an isolated piece of calculus or a pulp stone. The differentiation between a pulp stone and an enamel pearl can be made by increasing the vertical angle of projection to move the image of the enamel pearl away from the pulp chamber. If the opacity is calculus, it is usually clinically detectable. Occasionally oblique views of maxillary or mandibular molars may cause superimposition of a portion of the roots in the region of the furcation, producing a density that appears similar to that of an enamel pearl. In this case, producing another image at a slightly different horizontal angle eliminates this radiopaque region.

### Management
As a rule, the recognition that a radiopaque mass superimposed on the tooth is an enamel pearl precludes the necessity for treatment. The clinician can remove the mass if its location at the cementoenamel junction predisposes to periodontal disease. The possibility must always be considered that it may contain a pulp horn.

## Talon Cusp

### Definition
The talon cusp is an anomalous hyperplasia of the cingulum of a maxillary or mandibular incisor. It results in the formation of a supernumerary cusp. Normal enamel covers the cusp and fuses with the lingual aspect of the tooth. Any developmental grooves that are present may become caries-susceptible areas. The cusp may or may not contain an extension (horn) of the pulp. No apparent ethnic predilection exists.

### Clinical Features
The talon cusp is infrequently encountered. It may be found in either sex and on both primary and permanent incisors. It varies in size from that of a prominent cingulum to that of a cusp-like structure extending to the level of the incisal edge. When viewed from its incisal edge, an incisor bearing the cusp is T-shaped with the top of the T representing the incisal edge. Although it usually occurs as an isolated entity, its incidence has been reported to be increased in teeth related to cleft palate syndromes and in association with other anomalies.

### Radiographic Features
The radiopaque image of a talon cusp is superimposed on that of the crown of the involved incisor (Fig. 19-37). Its outline is smooth, and a layer of normal-appearing enamel is generally distinguishable. The radiograph may not reveal a pulp horn. The cusp is often apparent radiographically before eruption and may simulate the presence of a supernumerary tooth.

### Differential Diagnosis
The appearance of a talon cusp is quite distinctive. Although it may not be distinguishable from a supernumerary tooth with a single film,

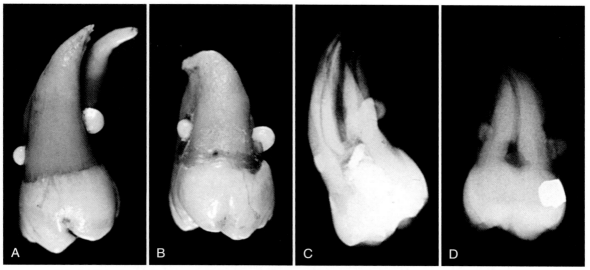

FIG. **19-35**   **A** and **B,** Enamel pearls are small outgrowths of enamel and dentin in the furcation areas of teeth. **C** and **D,** Radiographs of the teeth in **A** and **B.** (Courtesy Dr. R. Kienholz, Dallas, Tex.)

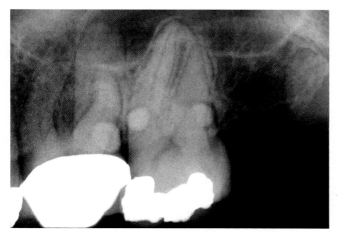

FIG. **19-36**   Three enamel pearls (one attached to the first molar and two on the second molar) are apparent in this periapical image.

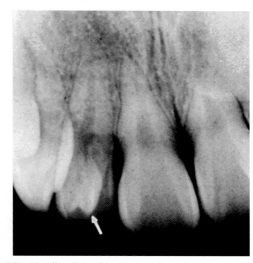

FIG. **19-37**   Maxillary lateral incisor bearing a talon cusp *(arrow).* Note that the tooth also has two enamel invaginations, one near the incisal edge and a second in the cingulum area. (Courtesy Dr. R.A. Cederberg, Dallas, Tex.)

a second image with either the parallax or the buccal object technique can demonstrate a connection to the tooth.

### Management
If developmental grooves are present where the cusp fuses with the lingual surface of the incisor, treatment may be required to prevent the development of decay. If the cusp is large, it may pose an esthetic or occlusal problem. Slowly removing the cusp over a long period may stimulate the formation of secondary dentin and prevent exposure of a pulp horn.

## Turner's Hypoplasia

### Synonym
Turner's tooth

### Definition
*Turner's hypoplasia* is a term used to describe a permanent tooth with a local hypoplastic defect in its crown. This defect may have been

caused by the extension of a periapical infection from its deciduous predecessor or by mechanical trauma transmitted through the deciduous tooth. If the trauma (whether infectious or mechanical) takes place while the crown is forming, it may adversely affect the ameloblasts of the developing tooth and result in some degree of enamel hypoplasia or hypomineralization.

### Clinical Features
Turner's hypoplasia most often affects the mandibular premolars, generally because of the relative susceptibility of the deciduous molars to caries, their proximity to the developing premolars, and their relative time of mineralization. The severity of the defect depends on the severity of the infection or mechanical trauma and on the stage of development of the permanent tooth. It may disturb matrix formation or calcification, in which case the result varies from a hypoplastic

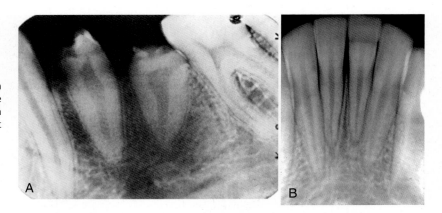

FIG. **19-38** Turner's hypoplasia, demonstrated as an extensive malformation and hypomineralization of the crowns of both premolars **(A)**. A band of hypoplasia extending across the crown of the mandibular left central incisor **(B)**.

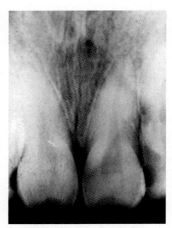

FIG. **19-39** Congenital syphilis may induce a developmental malformation of the maxillary central incisors referred to as "Hutchinson's incisors." The abnormal morphology is characterized by tapering of the mesial and distal surfaces toward the incisal edge with notching of the incisal edge.

defect to a hypomineralization spot in the enamel. The hypomineralized area may become stained, and the tooth usually shows a brownish spot on the crown. If the insult is severe enough to cause hypoplasia, the crown may show pitting or a more pronounced defect.

## Radiographic Features

The enamel irregularities associated with Turner's hypoplasia alter the normal contours of the affected tooth and are often apparent on a radiograph (Fig. 19-38). The involved region of the crown may appear as an ill-defined radiolucent region. A stained hypomineralized spot may not be apparent because a insufficient difference in the degree of radiopacity between the spot and the crown of the tooth. Also, the hypomineralized areas may become remineralized by continued contact with saliva.

## Differential Diagnosis

Other conditions that result in deformation of the tooth crown, such as the delivery of high doses of therapeutic radiation, should be con-

sidered, although usually several adjacent teeth are involved. Small defects may simulate the appearance of carious lesions but can be easily differentiated by clinical inspection.

## Management

If a radiograph of a tooth affected by Turner's hypoplasia shows that the tooth has good root support, the esthetics and function of the deformed crown can be restored.

## Congenital Syphilis

### Definition

About 30% of people with congenital syphilis have dental hypoplasia that involves the permanent incisors and first molars. Development of primary teeth is seldom disturbed. The affected incisors are called Hutchinson's incisors and the molars "mulberry molars." The changes characteristic of the condition seem to result from a direct infection of the developing tooth because the syphilitic spirochete has been identified in the tooth germ.

### Clinical Features

The affected incisor has a characteristic screwdriver-shaped crown, with the mesial and distal surfaces tapering from the middle of the crown to the incisal edge (Fig. 19-39). The effect is that the edge may be no wider than the cervical area of the tooth. The incisal edge is also frequently notched. Although maxillary central incisors usually demonstrate these syphilitic changes, the maxillary lateral and mandibular central incisors may also be involved.

As with incisor crowns, the crowns of affected first molars are quite characteristic, usually smaller than normal and maybe even smaller than second molar crowns. The most distinctive feature is the constricted occlusal third of the crown, with the occlusal surface no wider than the cervical portion of the tooth. The cusps of these molars are also reduced in size and poorly formed. The enamel over the occlusal surface is hypoplastic, unevenly formed in irregular globules, like the surface of a mulberry, a small berry having an appearance similar to a blackberry.

### Radiographic Features

The characteristic shapes of the affected incisor and molar crowns can be identified in the radiographic image. Because the crowns of these teeth form at about 1 year of age, radiographs may reveal the dental features of congenital syphilis 4 to 5 years before the teeth erupt.

## Management

Hutchinson's teeth and mulberry molars often do not require dental treatment. Esthetic restorations may be used to correct the hypoplastic defects as indicated clinically.

## Acquired Abnormalities

Acquired changes of the dentition, those that are initiated after development of the tooth, range in severity from changes that have no clinical significance to those that cause tooth loss. In the latter case early detection and treatment is required to preserve the tooth.

## ACQUIRED PATHOLOGIC CONDITIONS

### Attrition

#### Definition

Attrition is physiologic wearing of the dentition resulting from occlusal contacts between the maxillary and mandibular teeth. It occurs on the incisal, occlusal, and interproximal surfaces. Interproximal wear causes the contact points to become broad and flattened. Attrition occurs in more than 90% of young adults and is generally more severe in men than women. Its extent depends on the abrasiveness of the diet, salivary factors, mineralization of the teeth, and emotional tension. Physiologic attrition is a component of the aging process. When the loss of dental tissue becomes excessive such as from bruxism, the attrition becomes pathologic.

#### Clinical Features

The tooth wear patterns from attrition are characteristic. Wear facets first appear on cusps and marginal oblique and transverse ridges. The incisal edges of the maxillary and mandibular incisors show evidence of broadening. The wear facets on the occlusal surfaces of molars become more pronounced, with the lingual cusps of maxillary teeth and the buccal cusps of mandibular posteriors showing the most wear. When the dentin is exposed, it usually becomes stained and the color contrast between stained dentin and enamel highlights the areas of attrition. The incisal edges of mandibular incisors tend to become pitted because the dentin wears more rapidly than its surrounding enamel. In the case of pathologic attrition, the patterns of wear are generally not as uniformly progressive as those described for physiologic attrition. The wear facets develop at a faster rate. It is important to emphasize, however, that physiologic attrition is a relative term and its clinical manifestations vary with the customs (dietary and otherwise) of the population in question.

#### Radiographic Features

The radiographic appearance of attrition results in a change in the normal outline of the tooth structure, altering the normal curved surfaces into flat planes. The crown is shortened and is bereft of the incisal or occlusal surface enamel (Fig. 19-40). Often a number of adjacent teeth in each arch show this wear pattern. Reduction in the size of the pulp chambers and canals may occur because attrition stimulates the deposition of secondary dentin. This may result in complete obliteration of the pulp chamber and canals. A simultaneous widening of the PDL space frequently occurs if the tooth is mobile. Occasionally evidence of hypercementosis is present.

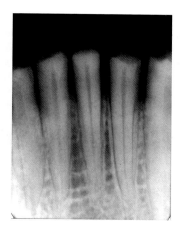

FIG. **19-40** Physiologic wear or attrition is demonstrated on this periapical radiograph of the mandibular incisors.

#### Differential Diagnosis

Recognition of physiologic attrition is usually not difficult given the characteristic history, location, and extent of wear. The general pattern is predictable and familiar.

#### Management

Physiologic attrition does not generally require treatment unless the teeth become symptomatic or there is some cosmetic concern.

### ABRASION

Abrasion is the nonphysiologic wearing of teeth in contact with foreign substances as a result of friction induced by factitious habits or occupational hazards. A history or clinical examination usually reveals the cause. Although many causes exist, two occur with moderate frequency and can usually be eliminated: that from improper tooth brushing and that from dental floss. Other causes include pipe smoking, opening hairpins with the teeth, improper use of toothpicks, denture clasps, and cutting thread with the teeth.

### Toothbrush Injury

#### Clinical Features

Toothbrush abrasion is probably the most frequently observed type of injury to the dental hard tissues. Improper "back-and-forth" movements of the toothbrush with heavy pressure cause the bristles to assume a wedge-shaped arrangement between the crowns and the gingiva. This improper brushing technique wears a V-shaped wedge or groove into the cervical area of the tooth, usually involving enamel and the softer root surface.

Abraded teeth may become sensitive as the dentin is exposed. The abraded areas are usually most severe at the cementoenamel junction on the labial and buccal surfaces of maxillary premolars, canines, and incisors, in approximately that order. The enamel generally limits the coronal extension of abrasion. The lesions are more common and more pronounced on the left side for a right-handed person, and vice versa. The deposition of secondary dentin opposite the abraded areas usually keeps pace with the destruction at the surface, so pulpal exposure is rarely a complication.

## Radiographic Features

The radiographic appearance of toothbrush abrasion is radiolucent defects at the cervical level of teeth. These defects have well-defined semicircular or semilunar shapes with borders of increasing radiopacity. The pulp chambers of the more seriously involved teeth are frequently partially or completely obliterated. The most common location of this injury is the premolar areas, usually in the upper arch.

## Dental Floss Injury

### Clinical Features

Excessive and improper use of dental floss, particularly in conjunction with toothpaste, may result in abrasion of the dentition (Fig. 19-41). The most frequent site is the cervical portion of the proximal surfaces just above the gingiva.

### Radiographic Features

The radiographic appearance of dental floss abrasion is narrow semilunar radiolucency in the interproximal surfaces of the cervical area. Most often the radiolucent grooves on the distal surfaces of the teeth are deeper than those on the mesial surfaces, probably because it is easier to exert more pressure in a forward direction by pulling than by pushing the floss backward into the mouth.

### Differential Diagnosis

Dental floss abrasion is readily identified by its clinical and radiographic appearance. Its location provides some evidence regarding the nature of the cause. This can be verified by the patient history. On occasion the radiolucencies simulate carious lesions located at the cervical region of the tooth. The differential diagnosis is accomplished with clinical inspection.

### Management

The primary treatment recommended for abrasion is elimination of the causative agents or habits. Extensively abraded areas can be restored.

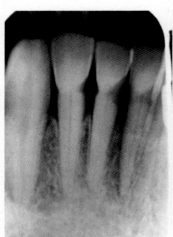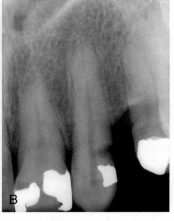

FIG. **19-41** Abrasion of the cervical areas of these incisor teeth is evident from excessive (and improper) use of dental floss **(A)**. Note the obliteration of the pulp chambers and reduction in size of the root canals. Abrasion on the distal aspect of the maxillary canine from a denture clasp **(B)**.

## Erosion

### Definition

Erosion of teeth results from a chemical action not involving bacteria. Although in many cases the cause is not apparent, in others it is obviously the contact of acid with teeth. The source of the acid may be from chronic vomiting or acid reflux from gastrointestinal disorders or from a diet rich in acidic foods, citrus fruits, or carbonated beverages. Regurgitated acids attack lingual or palatal tooth surfaces and dietary acids primarily demineralize labial surfaces. Some occupations involve contact with acids that can induce dental erosion. The location of the erosion, the pattern of eroded areas, and the appearance of the lesion usually provide clues as to the origin of the decalcifying agent.

### Clinical Features

Dental erosion is usually found on incisors, often involving multiple teeth. The lesions are generally smooth, glistening depressions in the enamel surface, frequently near the gingiva. Erosion may result in so much loss of enamel that a pink spot shows through the remaining enamel.

### Radiographic Features

Areas of erosion appear as radiolucent defects on the crown. Their margins may be either well defined or diffuse. A clinical examination usually resolves any questionable lesions.

### Differential Diagnosis

The diagnosis of erosion is based on the recognition of dished out or V-shaped defects in the buccal and labial enamel and the dentinal surfaces. The margins of a restoration may project above the remaining tooth surface. The edges of lesions caused by erosion are usually more rounded off than those caused by abrasion.

### Management

As with abrasion, erosion is managed with identification and removal of the causative agent. If the cause is chronic vomiting from a psychologic disorder, then a daily fluoride rinse should be prescribed during counseling therapy. If the cause is unknown, management depends solely on restoration of the defect. This prevents additional damage, possible pulp exposure, and objectionable esthetic appearance.

### Resorption

Resorption is the removal of tooth structure by osteoclasts, referred to as odontoclasts when they are resorbing tooth structure. Resorption is classified as internal or external on the basis of the surface of the tooth being resorbed.

External resorption affects the outer tooth surface, and internal resorption affects the inner surface of the pulp chamber and canal. These two types differ in their radiographic appearance and treatment. The resorption discussed here is not that associated with the normal physiologic loss of deciduous teeth. Although the etiology of most resorptive lesions remains unknown, at least presumptive evidence exists that some lesions are the sequelae of chronic infection (inflammation), excessive pressure and function, or factors associated with local tumors and cysts.

## Internal Resorption

### Definition

Internal resorption occurs within the pulp chamber or canal and involves resorption of the surrounding dentin. This results in enlargement of the size of the pulp space at the expense of tooth structure. This condition may be transient and self-limiting or progressive. The etiology of the recruitment and activation of odontoclasts is unknown but may be related to inflammation of the pulpal tissues. Internal resorption has been reported to be initiated by acute trauma to the tooth, direct and indirect pulp capping, pulpotomy, and enamel invagination.

## Clinical Features

Internal resorption may affect any tooth in either the primary or secondary dentitions. It occurs most frequently in permanent teeth, usually in central incisors and first and second molars. The resorptive process most commonly begins during the fourth and fifth decades and is more common in males. When the lesion is in the pulp chamber of the crown, a radiolucent area may appear to envelope the crown. If the enlarging pulp perforates the dentin and the enamel becomes

involved, the area may appear clinically as a pink spot. If the condition is not intercepted, it may perforate the crown, with hemorrhagic tissue projecting from the perforation, and lead to infectious pulpitis. When the lesion occurs in the root of a tooth, it is, for the most part, clinically silent. If the resorption is extensive, it may weaken the tooth and result in fracture. It is also possible that the pulp may expand into the periodontal ligament and communicate with a deep periodontal pocket or the gingival sulcus, also leading to pulpal infection.

## Radiographic Features

Radiographs can reveal symptomless early lesions of internal resorption. The lesions are localized, radiolucent, and round, oval, or elongated within the root or crown and continuous with the image of the pulp chamber or root canal. The outline is usually sharply defined and smooth or slightly scalloped. The result is an irregular widening of the pulp chamber or canal (Fig. 19-42). It is characteristically homo-

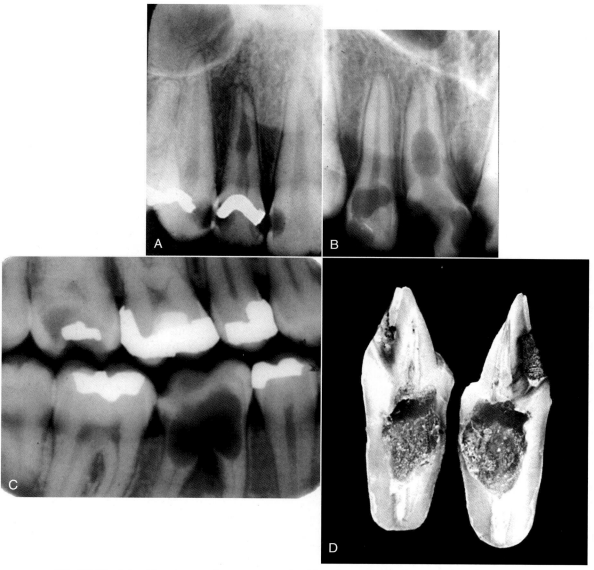

FIG. **19-42** Internal root resorption may occur in either the crown or the root of teeth. Periapical radiographs show internal resorption centered in the root canal system (**A** and **B**) and in both the crown and the roots (**C** and **D**), in a sectioned incisor (after crown reduction).

geneously radiolucent, without bony trabeculation or pulp stones. However, the internal structure may seem to be apparent if the surface of the resorbed tooth structure is very irregular and has a scalloped texture. In some cases virtually the whole pulp may enlarge within a tooth, although more commonly the lesion remains localized.

### Differential Diagnosis

The most common lesions to be confused with internal root resorption are dental caries on the buccal or lingual surface of a tooth and external root resorption. Carious lesions have more diffuse margins than do lesions caused by internal root resorption. Clinical inspection quickly reveals caries on the buccal or lingual surface of a tooth. Also, the mesial and distal surfaces of the pulp chamber and canal can usually be separated from the borders of the carious lesion. With internal root resorption, however, the image of the resorption cannot be separated from the pulp chamber or canal by altering the horizontal angulation of the x-ray beam.

### Management

The treatment for internal resorption depends on the condition of the tooth. If the process has not led to a serious weakening defect in the structure, endodontic treatment halts the resorption. If the expanding pulp has not structurally compromised the tooth but a perforation of the root has occurred, the perforated surface may be surgically exposed and retrofilled. If the tooth has been badly excavated and weakened by the resorption, extraction may be the only alternative.

## External Resorption

### Definition

In external resorption, odontoclasts resorb the outer surface of the tooth. This most commonly involves the root surface but may also involve the crown of an unerupted tooth. The resorption may involve cementum and dentin and in some cases gradually extends to the pulp. Because the recruitment of odontoclasts requires an intact blood supply, only sections of the tooth with soft tissue coverage are susceptible to this resorption. This resorption may occur to a single tooth, multiple teeth, or, in rare cases, all of the dentition. In many cases the etiology is unknown, but in others causes can be attributed to localized inflammatory lesions, reimplanted teeth, tumors and cysts, excessive mechanical and occlusal forces, and impacted teeth.

### Clinical Features

External resorption is usually not recognized because often no characteristic signs or symptoms exist. Even when considerable loss of tooth structure occurs, the tooth in question is frequently firm and immobile in the dental arch. In advanced resorption, some nonspecific pain or fracture of the resorbed root occurs.

External resorption may appear at the apex of the tooth or on the lateral root surface, although it most commonly occurs in the apical and cervical regions. It is slightly more prevalent in mandibular teeth than in maxillary teeth and involves primarily the central incisors, canines, and premolars. External root resorption is common. One study of 18- to 25-year-old men and women found that all patients exhibited some degree of external root resorption in four or more teeth.

### Radiographic Features

Common sites for external root resorption are the apical and cervical regions. When the lesion begins at the apex, it generally causes a smooth resorption of the tooth structure, resulting in blunting of the root apex (Fig. 19-43). Almost always the bone and lamina dura follow the resorbing root and present a normal appearance around this shortened structure. When external root resorption occurs as the result of a periapical inflammatory lesion, the lamina dura is lost around the apex. After normal apexification (constriction of the walls of the pulp canal at the apex) of the pulp canal, it is very difficult or impossible to see the canal exit at the apex of the tooth. However, if resorption of the apical region has occurred, the pulp canal is visible and is abnormally wide at the apex.

Occasionally external root resorption involves the lateral aspects of roots (Fig. 19-44). Such lesions tend to be irregular, may involve one side more than the other, and occur in any tooth. A common cause of external resorption on the side of a root is the presence of an unerupted adjacent tooth. Examples of such include resorption of the distal aspect of the roots of an upper second molar by the crown of the adjacent third molar and resorption of the root of a permanent central or lateral incisor, or both, by an unerupted maxillary canine. External resorption of an entire tooth can occur when the tooth is unerupted and completely embedded in bone (Fig. 19-45), usually involving the maxillary canine or third molar. In such instances the entire tooth, including the root and crown, may undergo resorption.

### Differential Diagnosis

External root resorption on the apex or lateral surface of a root is radiographically self-evident. When the lesion lies on the buccal or lingual surface of a root and above the level of the adjacent bone, the differential diagnosis includes caries and internal resorption. Internal resorption characteristically appears as an expansion of the pulp chamber or canal. In the case of external resorption, the image of the normal intact pulp chamber or canal may be traced through the radiolucent area of external resorption. Also, projections made at different angles can be compared. The location of the radiolucency caused by external root resorption moves with respect to the pulp canal, whereas the image of internal resorption remains fixed to the canal.

### Management

When the cause of external root resorption is known, the treatment is usually to remove the etiologic factors. This may mean cessation of excessive mechanical forces, removal of an adjacent impacted tooth, or eradication of a cyst, tumor, or source of inflammation. If the area of resorption is broad and on an accessible surface of the root (such as at the cervical location), curettage of the defect and the placement of a restoration usually stops the process.

## Secondary Dentin

### Definition

Secondary dentin is that deposited in the pulp chamber after the formation of primary dentin has been completed. Secondary dentin deposition may be part of physiologic aging and may result from such innocuous stimuli as chewing or slight trauma. Secondary dentin also develops after long-term trauma from such pathologic conditions as moderately progressive caries, trauma, erosion, attrition, abrasion, or a dental restorative procedure. This specific stimulus promotes a more rapid and localized coronal response than that seen as a result of normal aging. The term *tertiary dentin* has been suggested to identify dentin specifically initiated by stimuli other than the normal aging response and normal biologic function.

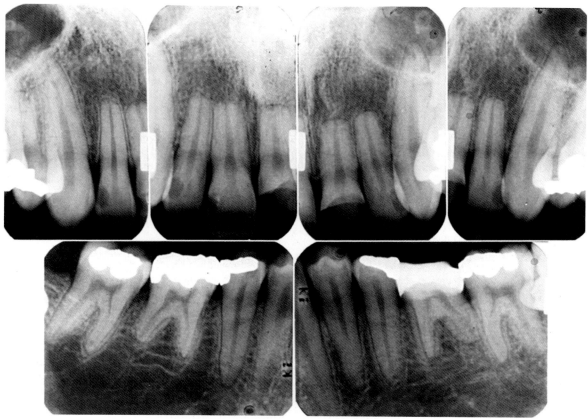

FIG. **19-43** External root resorption results in a loss of tooth structure from the apex. Note the blunted root apices, the widened pulp root canals, and the intact lamina dura.

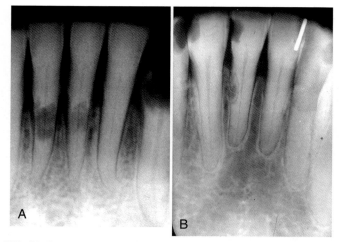

FIG. **19-44** External root resorption of the lateral surface of the root of the mandibular central incisors. These are sharply defined radiolucencies confined to the root surfaces **(A).** In **B,** the root has been replaced by an ingrowth of bone. This is sometimes referred to as inostosis.

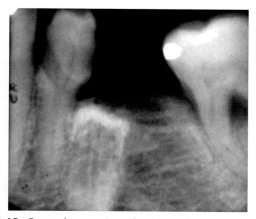

FIG. **19-45** External resorption of an impacted second premolar. Although both enamel and dentin have been resorbed, the residual enamel of the crown can still be seen as well as a hint of a pulp chamber.

## Clinical Features

The response of odontoblasts in producing secondary dentin reduces the sensitivity of teeth to stimuli from the external environment. In elderly individuals with extensive secondary dentin formation, this reduced sensitivity may be especially pronounced. Similarly, the formation of an additional layer of dentin between the pulp and a region of insult reduces the sensitivity often felt by individuals with recent dental restorations or coronal fractures.

## Radiographic Features

Secondary dentin is radiographically indistinguishable from primary dentin. Its presence is manifested as a reduction in size of the normal pulp chamber and canals (Fig. 19-46). When secondary dentin formation results from the normal aging process, the result is a generalized reduction in pulp chamber and canal size, maintaining a relatively normal shape. Often there remains only a thin, narrow pulp chamber and canal. The pulp horns usually disappear relatively early, followed by a reduction in size of the pulp chamber and narrowing of the canals. When more specific stimuli initiate secondary dentin formation, it begins in the region adjacent to the source of stimuli and alters the normal shape of the pulp chamber. Although formation of secondary dentin may continue until the pulp appears to be completely obliterated, histologic studies show that even in these extreme cases a small thread of viable pulp tissue remains.

## Differential Diagnosis

Secondary dentin is recognized indirectly by the reduction in size of the pulp chamber. This appearance differs from that of the pulp stone. The pulp stone (see the following description) simply occupies some pulp chamber or canal space, but it has a round to oval shape (conforming to the chamber).

## Management

Secondary dentin per se does not require treatment. The precipitating cause is removed if possible and the tooth restored when appropriate.

## Pulp Stones

### Definition

Pulp stones are foci of calcification in the dental pulp. They are probably apparent microscopically in more than half the teeth from young people and in almost all the teeth from people older than 50 years. Although most are microscopic, they vary in size, with some as large as 2 or 3 mm in diameter, almost filling the pulp chamber. Only these larger concretions are radiographically apparent. Although the larger masses represent only 15% to 25% of pulpal calcification, they are a common radiographic finding and may appear in a single tooth or several teeth. Their cause is unknown, and no firm evidence exists that they are associated with any systemic or pulpal disturbance.

### Clinical Features

Pulp stones are not clinically discernible.

### Radiographic Features

The radiographic appearance of pulp stones is quite variable. They may be seen as radiopaque structures within pulp chambers or root canals or they may extend from the pulp chamber into the root canals (Fig. 19-47). No uniform shape or number exists. They may occur as a single dense mass or as several small radiopacities. They may be round or oval, and some that potentially occupy most of the pulp chamber will conform to its shape. Their outline, likewise, varies from sharply defined to a more diffuse margin. They occur in all tooth types but most commonly in molars. In rare instances, the canal remodels and increases its girth to accommodate a large stone.

### Differential Diagnosis

Although pulp stones are variable in size and form, their recognition is usually not difficult. However, in some cases differentiation from pulpal sclerosis is difficult.

### Management

Pulp stones do not require treatment.

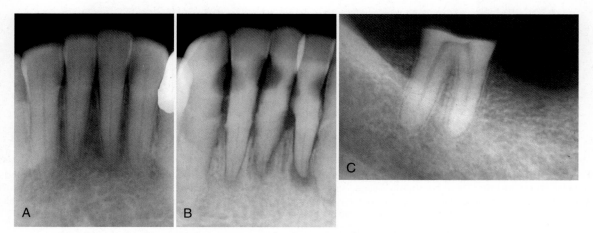

FIG. **19-46**   Normal formation of secondary dentin causes recession of the pulp chamber and narrowing of the root canals **(A)**. Secondary dentin has obliterated the pulp chambers and narrowed the root canals. This is likely a result of the carious lesions **(B)**. Secondary dentin formation has obliterated the pulp chamber stimulated by the severe attrition of the coronal aspect of this molar **(C)**.

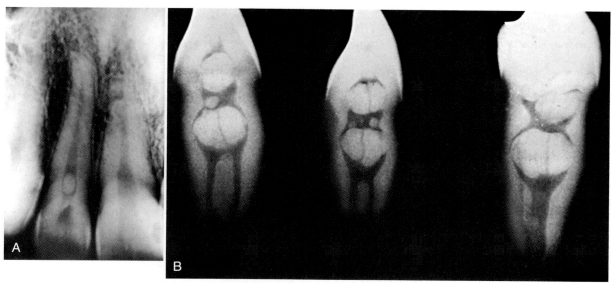

FIG. **19-47**  Pulp stones may be found as isolated calcifications in the pulp **(A)**. When large, they may cause deformation of pulp chamber and root canals **(B)**.

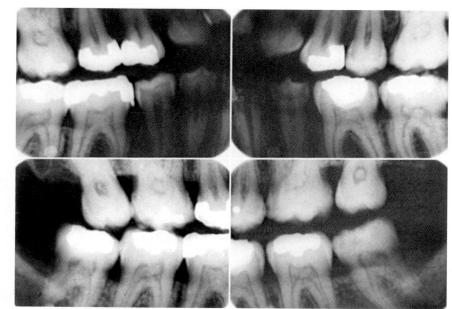

FIG. **19-48**  Pulpal sclerosis is seen as diffuse calcification of the pulp chamber and canals.

## Pulpal Sclerosis

### Definition

Pulpal sclerosis is another form of calcification in the pulp chamber and canals of teeth. In contrast to pulp stones, pulpal sclerosis is a diffuse process. Its specific cause is unknown, although its appearance correlates strongly with age. About 66% of all teeth in individuals between the ages of 10 and 20 years and 90% of all teeth in individuals between the ages of 50 and 70 years show histologic evidence of pulpal sclerosis. Histologically the pattern of calcification is amorphous and unorganized, being evident as linear strands or columns of calcified material paralleling blood vessels and nerves in the pulp.

### Clinical Features

Pulpal sclerosis is a clinically silent process without clinical manifestation.

### Radiographic Features

Early pulpal sclerosis, a degenerative process, is not radiographically demonstrable. Diffuse pulpal sclerosis produces a generalized, ill-defined collection of fine radiopacities throughout large areas of the pulp chamber and pulp canals (Fig. 19-48).

### Differential Diagnosis

The differential diagnosis includes small pulp stones, but this differentiation is academic because neither condition requires treatment.

## Management

Pulpal sclerosis does not require treatment. As with pulp stones, its only importance may be that it can cause difficulty in the performance of endodontic therapy when such a procedure is indicated for other reasons.

## Hypercementosis

### Definition

Hypercementosis is excessive deposition of cementum on the tooth roots. In most cases its cause is unknown. Occasionally it appears on a supraerupted tooth after the loss of an opposing tooth. Another cause of hypercementosis is inflammation, usually resulting from rarefying or sclerosing osteitis. In the context of inflammation, cementum is deposited on the root surface adjacent to the apex. Occasionally hypercementosis has been associated with teeth that are in hyperocclusion or that have been fractured. Finally, hypercementosis occurs in patients with Paget's disease of bone (see Chapter 24) and with hyperpituitarism (gigantism and acromegaly).

### Clinical Features

Hypercementosis does not cause any clinical signs or symptoms.

### Radiographic Features

Hypercementosis is evident radiographically as an excessive buildup of cementum around all or part of a root (Fig. 19-49). The outline is usually smooth but on occasion may be seen as an irregular but somewhat bulbous enlargement of the root. It is most evident at the apical end and is usually seen as a mildly irregular accumulation of cementum. This cementum is slightly more radiolucent than dentin. Of importance is the fact that the lamina dura and PDL space encompass the extra dentin. In the case of Paget's disease the hypercementosis is usually very exuberant and irregular in outline.

### Differential Diagnosis

The differential diagnosis may include any radiopaque structure that is seen within the vicinity of the root such as a dense bone island or mature cemento-osseous dysplasia. The differentiating characteristic is the presence of the periodontal membrane space around the hypercementosis. There may be a resemblance to a small cementoblastoma. Occasionally a severely dilacerated root may have the appearance of hypercementosis.

### Management

Hypercementosis itself requires no treatment. If a related condition such as a periapical inflammatory lesion exists, treatment may be necessary. Perhaps the primary significance of hypercementosis relates to the difficulty that the root configuration can pose if extraction is indicated.

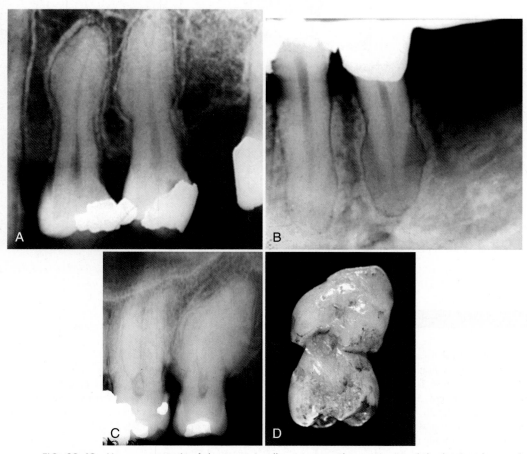

FIG. **19-49** Hypercementosis of the roots. In all cases, note the continuity of the lamina dura and the PDL space that encompasses the extra cementum **(A-C).** An extracted molar, showing extensive hypercementosis **(D).** (Courtesy Dr. R. Kienholz, Dallas, Tex.)

# SUGGESTED READINGS

## DEVELOPMENTAL ABNORMALITIES

Bergsma D, editor: *Birth defects compendium,* ed 2, New York, 1979, Alan R Liss.

Dixon GH, Stewart RE: Genetic aspects of anomalous tooth development. In Stewart RE, Prescott GH, editors: *Oral facial genetics,* St Louis, 1976, Mosby.

MacDougall M, Dong J, Acevedo AC: Molecular basis of human dentin diseases, *Am J Med Genet A* 140A:2536-2546, 2006.

Pindborg JJ: *Pathology of the dental hard tissues,* Copenhagen, 1970, Munksgaard.

Schulze C: Developmental abnormalities of the teeth and jaws. In Gorlin RJ, Goldman HM, editors: *Thoma's oral pathology,* ed 6, vol 1, St Louis, 1970, Mosby.

Witkop CJ Jr, Rao S: Inherited defects in tooth structure. In Bergsma D, editor: *Birth defects, XI: orofacial structures,* vol 7, no 7, Baltimore, 1971, Williams & Wilkins.

Witkop CJ Jr: Amelogenesis imperfecta, dentinogenesis imperfecta and dentin dysplasia revisited: problems with classification, *J Oral Pathol* 17:547-553, 1989.

Worth HM: *Principles and practice of oral radiologic interpretation,* Chicago, 1963, Year Book Medical.

Wright JT: The molecular etiologies and associated phenotypes of amelogenesis imperfecta, *Am J Med Genet A* 140A:2547-2555, 2006.

## SUPERNUMERARY TEETH

Grahnen H, Lindahl B: Supernumerary teeth in the permanent dentition: a frequency study, *Odontol Rev* 12:290-294, 1961.

Grimanis GA, Kyriakides AT, Spyropoulos ND: A survey on supernumerary molars, *Quintessence Int* 22:989-995, 1991.

Niswander JD: Effects of heredity and environment on development of the dentition, *J Dent Res* 42:1288-1296, 1963.

Rao SR: Supernumerary teeth. In Bergsma D, editor: *Birth defects compendium,* ed 2, New York, 1979, Alan R Liss.

Yusof WZ: Non-syndrome multiple supernumerary teeth: literature review, *J Can Dent Assoc* 56:147-149, 1990.

## DEVELOPMENTALLY MISSING TEETH

al-Emran S: Prevalence of hypodontia and developmental malformation of permanent teeth in Saudi Arabian school children, *Br J Orthod* 17:115-118, 1990.

Garn SM, Lewis AB: The relationship between third molar agenesis and reduction in tooth number, *Angle Orthod* 32:14-18, 1962.

Keene HJ: The relationship between third molar agenesis and the morphologic variability of the molar teeth, *Angle Orthod* 35:289-298, 1965.

Levin LS: Dental and oral abnormalities in selected ectodermal dysplasia syndromes, *Birth Defects Orig Artic Ser* 24:205-227, 1988.

O'Dowling IB, McNamara TG: Congenital absence of permanent teeth among Irish school-children, *J Ir Dent Assoc* 36:136-138, 1990.

## MACRODONTIA

Garn SM, Lewis AB, Kerewsky BS: The magnitude and implications of the relationship between tooth size and body size, *Arch Oral Biol* 13:129-131, 1968.

## TRANSPOSITION

Schacter H: A treated case of transposed upper canine, *Dent Rec (London)* 71:105-108, 1951.

## FUSION

Hagman FT: Anomalies of form and number, fused primary teeth, a correlation of the dentitions, *ASDC J Dent Child* 55:359-361, 1988.

Sperber GH: Genetic mechanisms and anomalies in odontogenesis, *J Can Dent Assoc (Tor)* 33:433-442, 1967.

## GEMINATION

Tannenbaum KA, Alling EE: Anomalous tooth development: case report of gemination and twinning, *Oral Surg Oral Med Oral Pathol* 16:883-887, 1963.

## TAURODONTISM

Bixler D: Heritable disorders affecting dentin. In Steward RE, Prescott GA, editors: *Oral facial genetics,* St Louis, 1976, Mosby.

## DENS IN DENTE

Oehlers FA: The radicular variety of dens invaginatus, *Oral Surg Oral Med Oral Pathol* 11:1251-1260, 1958.

Rushton MA: A collection of dilated composite odontomes, *Br Dent J* 63:65-86, 1937.

Soames JV, Kuyebi TA: A radicular dens invaginatus, *Br Dent J* 152:308-309, 1982.

## DENS INVAGINATUS

Oehlers FA, Lee KW, Lee EC: Dens invaginatus (invaginated odontome): its structure and responses to external stimuli, *Dent Pract Dent Rec* 17:239-244, 1967.

Sykaras SN: Occlusal anomalous tubercle on premolars of a Greek girl, *Oral Surg Oral Med Oral Pathol* 38:88-91, 1974.

Yip WK: The prevalence of dens invaginatus, *Oral Surg Oral Med Oral Pathol* 38:80-87, 1974.

## AMELOGENESIS IMPERFECTA

Crawford PJ, Aldred MJ: X-linked amelogenesis imperfecta: presentation of two kindreds and a review of the literature, *Oral Surg Oral Med Oral Pathol* 73:449-455, 1992.

Toller PA: A clinical report of six cases of amelogenesis imperfecta, *Oral Surg Oral Med Oral Pathol* 12:325-333, 1959.

Witkop CJ Jr: Amelogenesis imperfecta, dentinogenesis imperfecta and dentin dysplasia revisited: problems in classification, *J Oral Pathol* 17:547-553, 1988.

Witkop CJ Jr, Saulk JJ: Heritable defects of enamel. In Stewart RE, Prescott GA, editors: *Oral facial genetics,* St Louis, 1976, Mosby.

## DENTINOGENESIS IMPERFECTA

Schwartz S, Tsipouras P: Oral findings in osteogenesis imperfecta, *Oral Surg Oral Med Oral Pathol* 57:161-167, 1984.

Winter GB: Hereditary and idiopathic anomalies of tooth number, structure, and form, *Dent Clin North Am* 13:355-373, 1969.

Witkop CJ: Hereditary defects in enamel and dentin, *Acta Genet Stat Med* 7:236-239, 1957.

## DENTIN DYSPLASIA

O'Carroll MK, Duncan WK, Perkins TM: Dentin dysplasia: review of the literature and a proposed subclassification based on radiographic findings, *Oral Surg Oral Med Oral Pathol* 72:119-125, 1991.

Richardson AS, Fantin TD: Occlusal anomalous dysplasia of dentin: report of a case, *J Can Dent Assoc (Tor)* 36:189-191, 1970.

Shields ED, Bixler D, el-Kafrawy AM: A proposed classification for heritable human dentin defects with a description of a new entity, *Arch Oral Biol* 18:543, 1973.

Witkop CJ Jr: Hereditary defects of dentin, *Dent Clin North Am* 19:25-45, 1975.

## REGIONAL ODONTODYSPLASIA

Crawford PJ, Aldred MJ: Regional odontodysplasia: a bibliography, *J Oral Pathol Med* 18:251-263, 1989.

## ENAMEL PEARL

Moskow BS, Canut PM: Studies on root enamel, II: enamel pearls: a review of their morphology, localization, nomenclature, occurrence, classification, histogenesis, and incidence, *J Clin Periodontol* 17:275-281, 1990.

## TALON CUSP

Meskin LH, Gorlin RJ: Agenesis and peg-shaped permanent lateral incisors, *J Dent Res* 42:1476-1479, 1963.
Natkin E, Pitts DL, Worthington P: A case of talon cusp associated with other odontogenic abnormalities, *J Endod* 9:491-495, 1983.

## TURNER'S HYPOPLASIA

Via WF Jr: Enamel defects induced by trauma during tooth formation, *Oral Surg Oral Med Oral Pathol* 25:49-54, 1968.

## CONGENITAL SYPHILIS

Bradlaw RV: The dental stigmata of prenatal syphilis, *Oral Surg Oral Med Oral Pathol* 6:147-158, 1953.
Putkonen T: Dental changes in congenital syphilis: relationship to other syphilitic stigmata, *Acta Derm Venereol* 42:44-62, 1962.
Sarnat BG, Shaw NG: Dental development in congenital syphilis, *Am J Orthod* 29:270, 1943.

## ACQUIRED ABNORMALITIES

Baden E: Environmental pathology of the teeth. In Gorlin RJ, Goodman HM, editors: *Thoma's oral pathology,* ed 6, vol 1, St Louis, 1970, Mosby.
Mitchell DF, Standish SM, Fast TB: Oral diagnosis/oral medicine, Philadelphia, 1978, Lea & Febiger.
Pindborg JJ: *Pathology of the dental hard tissues,* Philadelphia, 1970, WB Saunders.
Shafer WG, Hine MK, Levy BM: *Oral pathology,* ed 4, Philadelphia, 1983, WB Saunders.

## ATTRITION

Johnson GK, Sivers JE: Attrition, abrasion, and erosion: diagnosis and therapy, *Clin Prev Dent* 9:12-16, 1987.
Murphy TR: Reduction of the dental arch by approximal attrition: quantitative assessment, *Br Dent J* 116:483-488, 1964.
Russell MD: The distinction between physiological and pathological attrition: a review, *J Ir Dent Assoc* 33:23-31, 1987.

Seligman DA, Pullinger AG, Solberg WK: The prevalence of dental attrition and its association with factors of age, gender, occlusion, and TMJ symptomatology, *J Dent Res* 67:1323-1333, 1988.

## ABRASION

Bull WH, Callender RM, Pugh BR et al: The abrasion and cleaning properties of dentifrices, *Br Dent J* 125:331, 1968.
Erwin JC, Buchner CM: Prevalence of tooth root exposure and abrasion among dental patients, *Dent Items Interest* 66:760, 1944.

## EROSION

ten Bruggen Cate HJ: Dental erosion in industry, *Br J Industr Med* 25:249, 1968.
Stafne EC, Lovestedt SA: Dissolution of tooth substance by lemon juice, acid beverages, and acid from some other sources, *J Am Dent Assoc* 34:586-592, 1947.

## RESORPTION

Bakland LK: Root resorption, *Dent Clin North Am* 36:491-507, 1992.
Bennett CG, Poleway SA: Internal resorption, postpulpotomy type, *Oral Surg* 17:228-234, 1964.
Goldman HM: Spontaneous intermittent resorption of teeth, *J Am Dent Assoc* 49:522-532, 1954.
Massler M, Perreault JG: Root resorption in the permanent teeth of young adults, *J Dent Child* 21:158-164, 1954.
Phillips JR: Apical root resorption under orthodontic therapy, *Angle Orthod* 20:1-22, 1955.
Simpson HE: Internal resorption, *J Can Dent Assoc* 30:355, 1964.
Solomon CS, Notaro PJ, Kellert M: External root resorption: fact or fancy, *J Endod* 15:219-223, 1989.
Stafne EC, Austin LT: Resorption of embedded teeth, *J Am Dent Assoc* 32:1003-1009, 1945.
Tronstad L: Root resorption: etiology, terminology, and clinical manifestations, *Endod Dent Traumatol* 4:241-252, 1988.

## SECONDARY DENTIN

Kuttler Y: Classification of dentine into primary, secondary and tertiary, *Oral Surg Oral Med Oral Pathol* 12:966-969, 1959.

## PULP STONES

Moss-Salentijn L, Hendricks-Klyvert M: Calcified structures in human dental pulps, *J Endod* 14:184-189, 1988.

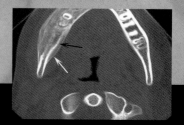

# CHAPTER 20

# Inflammatory Lesions of the Jaws

Linda Lee

Inflammatory lesions are by far the most common pathologic condition of the jaws. The jaws are unique from other bones of the body in that the presence of teeth creates a direct pathway for infectious and inflammatory agents to invade bone by means of caries and periodontal disease. The body responds to chemical, physical, or microbiologic injury with inflammation. The inflammatory response destroys or walls off the injurious stimulus and sets up an environment for repair of the damaged tissue.

Under normal conditions, bone metabolism represents a balance of osteoclastic bone resorption and osteoblastic bone production. This is a complex, interdependent relationship in which osteoblasts mediate the resorptive activity of the osteoclasts. Mediators of inflammation (cytokines, prostaglandins, and many growth factors) tip this balance to favor either bone resorption or bone formation. For the purposes of this chapter, all inflammatory conditions of bone, regardless of the specific etiology, are considered to represent a spectrum or continuum of conditions with different clinical features (e.g., site, severity, duration).

When the initial source of inflammation is a necrotic pulp and the bony lesion is restricted to the region of the tooth, the condition is called a periapical inflammatory lesion. When the infection spreads in the bone marrow and is no longer contained to the vicinity of the tooth root apex, it is called osteomyelitis. Another source of inflammatory lesion in bone is extension of inflammation into bone from the overlying soft tissues; this type of lesion includes periodontal lesions (see Chapter 18) and pericoronitis, an inflammation that arises in the tissues surrounding the crown of a partially erupted tooth. It must be emphasized that the names of the various inflammatory lesions tend to describe their clinical and radiologic presentations and behavior; however, all have the same underlying disease mechanism.

## General Clinical Features

The four cardinal signs of inflammation—*redness, swelling, heat,* and *pain*—may be observed in varying degrees with inflammation of the jaws. Acute lesions are those of recent onset. The onset typically is rapid, and these lesions cause pronounced pain, often accompanied by fever and swelling. Chronic lesions have a prolonged course with a longer insidious onset and pain that is less intense. Fever may be intermittent and low grade, and swelling may occur gradually. In fact, some chronic, low-grade infections may not produce any significant clinical symptoms.

## General Radiographic Features

### LOCATION

With periapical inflammatory lesions, which are pathologic conditions of the pulp, the epicenter typically is located at the apex of a tooth. However, lesions of pulpal origin also may be located anywhere along the root surface because of accessory canals or perforations caused by root canal therapy or root fractures. Periodontal lesions have an epicenter that is located at the alveolar crest. If periodontal bone loss is severe, the bone inflammatory changes may extend to the root furcation level or even to the root apex. Osteomyelitis, a diffuse, uncontained inflammation of the bone, most commonly is found in the posterior mandible. The maxilla rarely is involved.

### PERIPHERY

Most often the periphery is ill defined, with a gradual blending of normal trabecular pattern into a sclerotic pattern, or the normal trabecular pattern may gradually fade into a radiolucent region of bone loss.

### INTERNAL STRUCTURE

The internal structure of inflammatory lesions presents a spectrum of appearances. Cancellous bone may respond to an insult by tipping the bone metabolic balance either in favor of resorption (giving the area a radiolucent appearance) or toward bone formation (resulting in a radiopaque or sclerotic appearance). Usually there is a combination of these two reactions. The radiolucent regions may show no evidence of previous trabeculation or a very faint pattern of trabeculation. The increased radiopacity is caused by an increase in bone formation on existing trabeculae. Radiographically these trabeculae appear thicker and more numerous, replacing marrow spaces. In acute disease, resorption typically predominates; with chronic disease, excessive bone formation leads to an overall radiopaque, sclerotic appearance. In cases of osteomyelitis, careful examination of the x-ray films may reveal sequestra, which appear as ill-defined areas of radiolucency containing a radiopaque island of nonvital bone.

### EFFECTS ON SURROUNDING STRUCTURES

The effects of inflammation on surrounding cancellous bone include stimulation of bone formation, resulting in a sclerotic pattern, or bone resorption, resulting in radiolucency. The periodontal ligament space involved in the lesion will be widened; this widening is greatest at the source of the inflammation. For example, with periapical lesions the widening is greatest around the apical region of the root and in periodontal disease the widening is greatest at the alveolar crest. With chronic infections, root resorption may occur and cortical boundaries may be resorbed. The periosteal component of bone, whether on the surface of the jaws or lining the floor of the maxillary sinus, also responds to inflammation. The periosteum contains a layer of pluripotential lining cells that, under the right conditions, differentiate into osteoblasts and lay down new bone. Inflammatory exudate from infection within the bone can penetrate the cortex, lift up the periosteum from the surface of the bone, and stimulate the periosteum to produce new bone. Because inflammatory exudate is a fluid, the periosteum is lifted from the surface of bone in a manner that positions the periosteum almost parallel to the surface of the bone; thus the layer of new bone is almost parallel to the bone surface.

## PERIAPICAL INFLAMMATORY LESIONS

### Synonyms
Periapical inflammatory lesions have been called acute apical periodontitis, chronic apical periodontitis, periapical abscess, and periapical granuloma. Radiolucent presentations have been called rarefying osteitis, whereas radiopaque presentations have been called sclerosing osteitis, condensing osteitis, and focal sclerosing osteitis. Chapter 21 presents a discussion of periapical cysts of inflammatory origin (radicular cysts).

### Definition
A periapical inflammatory lesion is defined as a local response of the bone around the apex of a tooth that occurs as a result of necrosis of the pulp or through destruction of the periapical tissues by extensive periodontal disease (Fig. 20-1). The pulpal necrosis may occur as a result of pulpal invasion of bacteria through caries or trauma. In Figure 20-1, the periapical inflammatory lesion is characterized by apical periodontitis, an inflammatory process that may histologically represent either a periapical abscess or a periapical granuloma. Toxic metabolites from the necrotic pulp exit the root apex to incite an inflammatory reaction in the periapical periodontal ligament and surrounding bone (apical periodontitis). This reaction is characterized histologically by an inflammatory infiltrate composed predominantly of lymphocytes mixed with polymorphonuclear neutrophils. Depending on the severity of the response, the neutrophils may collect to form pus, resulting in an apical abscess. This result is categorized as acute inflammation. Alternatively, in an attempt to heal from apical periodontitis, the body stimulates the formation of granulation tissue mixed with a chronic inflammatory infiltrate composed predominantly of lymphocytes, plasma cells, and histiocytes, giving rise to periapical granuloma. Entrapped epithelium (the rests of Malassez)

may proliferate to form a radicular or apical cyst. Acute exacerbations of the chronic lesions may occur intermittently.

If the surrounding bone marrow becomes involved with the inflammatory reaction through the spread of pyogenic organisms, the localized periapical abscess may transform into osteomyelitis. The exact point at which a periapical inflammatory lesion becomes osteomyelitis is not easily determined or defined. The size of the area of inflammation is not as important as the severity of the reaction. However, considering the size of the lesion as one factor, periapical inflammatory lesions usually involve only the local bone adjacent to the apex of the tooth, and osteomyelitis involves a larger area of bone. Periapical lesions occasionally may be large, but the epicenter of the lesion remains in the vicinity of the tooth apex. If the periapical lesion extends farther, so that the lesion no longer is centered on the tooth apex, osteomyelitis may be considered as a possible diagnosis. The distinction between periapical inflammation and osteomyelitis can be made if sequestra are detected radiographically. Progression from periapical inflammation to osteomyelitis is relatively rare, and other factors play a role in its development, such as a decrease in the host defenses and an increase in the virulence of pathogenic microorganisms.

### Clinical Features
The symptoms of periapical inflammatory lesions can range across a broad spectrum, from being asymptomatic to an occasional toothache to severe pain with or without facial swelling, fever, and lymphadenopathy. A periapical abscess usually manifests with severe pain, mobility and sometimes elevation of the involved tooth, swelling, and tenderness to percussion. Palpation of the apical region elicits pain. Spontaneous drainage into the oral cavity through a fistula (parulis) may relieve the acute pain. In rare cases a dental abscess may manifest with systemic symptoms (e.g., fever, facial swelling, lymphadenopathy) along with the pain. The acute lesion may evolve into a chronic one (periapical granuloma or cyst), which may be asymptomatic except for intermittent flare-ups of "toothache" pain, which mark the acute exacerbation of the chronic lesion. Patients often give a history of intermittent pain. The associated tooth may be asymptomatic, or it may be sensitive to percussion and mobile. More often, however, the periapical lesion arises in the chronic form de novo; in this case it may be asymptomatic. It is important to understand that the clinical presentation does not necessarily correlate with the histologic or radiographic findings.

### Radiographic Features
The radiographic features of periapical inflammatory lesions vary depending on the time course of the lesion. Because very early lesions may not show any radiographic changes, diagnosis of these lesions relies solely on the clinical symptoms (Fig. 20-2). More chronic lesions may show lytic (radiolucent) or sclerotic (radiopaque) changes, or both.

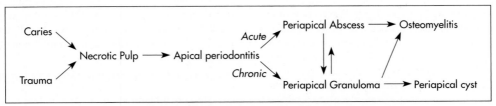

FIG. **20-1**   Interrelationship of possible results of periapical inflammation.

*Location.* In most cases the epicenter of periapical inflammatory lesions is found at the apex of the involved tooth (Fig. 20-3). The lesion usually starts within the apical portion of the periodontal ligament space. Less often, such lesions are centered about another region of the tooth root. This may occur because of accessory pulpal canals, perforation of the root structure from instrumentation of the pulp canal, and root fracture.

*Periphery.* In most instances the periphery of periapical inflammatory lesions is ill defined, showing a gradual transition from the surrounding normal trabecular pattern into the abnormal bone pattern of the lesion (Figs. 20-3, *C*, and 20-4). Rarely the periphery may be well defined, with a sharp transition zone and an appearance suggesting a cortical boundary.

*Internal Structure.* Early periapical inflammatory lesions may show no radiographic change in the normal bone pattern. The earliest detectable change is loss of bone density, which usually results in widening of the periodontal ligament space at the apex of the tooth and later involves a larger diameter of surrounding bone. At this early stage no evidence may be seen of a sclerotic bone reaction (see Fig. 20-2). Later in the evolution of the disease, a mixture of sclerosis and rarefaction (loss of bone giving a radiolucent appearance) of normal bone occurs (see Fig. 20-4). The percentage of these two bone reactions varies. When most of the lesion consists of increased bone formation, the term *periapical sclerosing osteitis* is used (Fig. 20-5), and when most of the lesion is undergoing bone resorption, the term *periapical rarefying osteitis* is used (see Fig. 20-3). The area of greatest bone destruction usually is centered on the apex of the tooth, with the sclerotic pattern located at the periphery. The radiolucent regions may be bereft of any bone structure or may have a faint outline of trabeculae. Close inspection of sclerotic regions reveals thicker than normal trabeculae and sometimes an increase in the number of trabeculae per unit area. In chronic cases the new bone formation may result in a very dense sclerotic region of bone, obscuring individual trabeculae. Occasionally the lesion may appear to be composed entirely of sclerotic bone (sclerosing osteitis), but usually some evidence exists of widening of the apical portion of the periodontal membrane space (see Fig. 20-5).

*Effects on Surrounding Structures.* As mentioned previously, periapical inflammatory lesions may stimulate either the resorption of bone or the manufacture of new bone. The lamina dura around the apex of the tooth usually is lost. The sclerotic reaction of the cancellous bone may be limited to a small region around the tooth apex or in some cases may be extensive. In rare instances in the mandible the sclerotic reaction may extend to the inferior cortex. In chronic cases external resorption of the apical region of the root may occur. If the lesion is long standing, the pulp canal may appear wider than adjacent teeth. This is a result of the death of odontoblasts and subsequent cessation of the formation of secondary dentin, which occurs naturally with time to diminish the caliber of the pulp canal slowly.

Nearby cortical boundaries may be destroyed, such as a segment of the floor of the maxillary antrum, the floor of the nasal fossa, or the buccal or lingual plates of the alveolar process immediately adjacent to the root apex. These lesions are capable of producing an inflammatory periosteal reaction, most notably in the adjacent floor of the maxillary antrum. This usually results in a thin layer of new bone produced by the inflamed periosteum within the maxillary antrum, sometimes referred to as a "halo shadow" (Fig. 20-6). A regional mucositis may be present within the adjacent segment of the

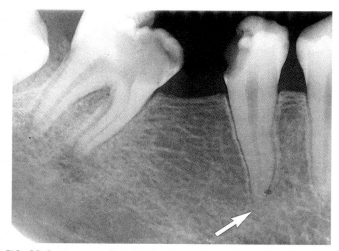

FIG. **20-2** A very early lesion involving the pulp of the second bicuspid without significant change in the periapical bone *(arrow)*. In contrast, note the loss of the lamina dura and periapical bone at the apex of the mesial root of the second molar. Also note the subtle halo of sclerotic bone reaction around this apical radiolucency.

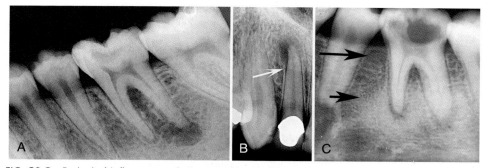

FIG. **20-3** Periapical inflammatory lesions associated with a mandibular first molar **(A)** and a maxillary lateral incisor **(B).** Note that in both cases the epicenter of bone destruction is located at the apex of the root. Also, note gradual widening of the periodontal membrane space *(arrow)* characteristic of an inflammatory lesion. **C,** This periapical image of sclerosing osteitis related to the first molar shows a gradual transition from thick and numerous trabeculae *(short arrow)* to a normal trabecular pattern *(long arrow).*

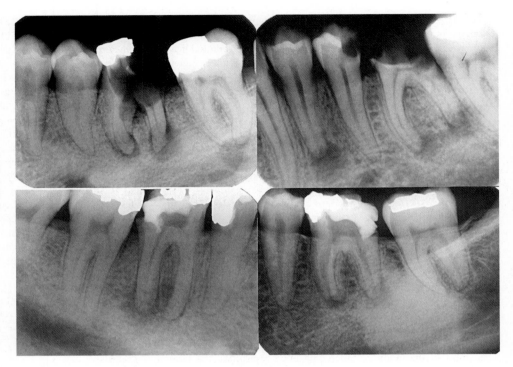

FIG. **20-4** Several examples of a mixture of rarefying and sclerosing osteitis. Note the similarity of the pattern, composed of a radiolucent region at the apex of the tooth surrounded by a radiopaque reaction of sclerotic dense bone.

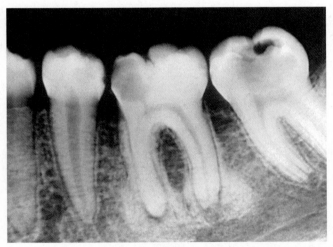

FIG. **20-5** Periapical sclerosing osteitis associated with the first molar. This is called a sclerosing lesion because most of the lesion is bone formation, resulting in a very radiopaque density. Note, however, the small region of bone loss next to the root apex and the widening of the periodontal membrane space.

maxillary antrum. Periosteal reaction may also occur on the buccal or lingual surfaces of the alveolar process and in rare cases on the inferior aspect of the mandible.

## Differential Diagnosis

The two types of lesions that most often must be differentiated from periapical inflammatory lesions are periapical cemental dysplasia (PCD) and an enostosis (dense bone island, osteosclerosis) at the apex of a tooth. In the early radiolucent phase of PCD, the radiographic characteristics may not reliably differentiate this lesion from a periapical inflammatory lesion (Fig. 20-7). The diagnosis may rely solely on the clinical examination, including a test of tooth vitality. With long-standing periapical inflammatory lesions, the pulp chamber of the involved tooth may be wider than the adjacent teeth. More mature PCD lesions may show evidence of a dense, radiopaque structure within the radiolucency, which helps in the differential diagnosis. Also, a common site for PCD is associated with the apical region of the mandibular anterior teeth. External root resorption is more common with inflammatory lesions than with PCD. When enostosis is centered on the root apex, it may mimic an inflammatory lesion. However, the periodontal ligament space around the apex of the tooth has a normal uniform width (Fig. 20-8). Also, the periphery of an enostosis usually is well defined and does not blend gradually with surrounding trabeculae.

Small, radiolucent periapical lesions with a well-defined periphery simulating a cortex may be either periapical granulomas or cysts (radicular cysts). Differentiation may not be possible unless other characteristics of a cyst, such as displacement of adjacent structures and expansion of the outer cortical boundaries of the jaw, are present. Lesions larger than 1 cm in diameter usually are radicular cysts. If the patient has had endodontic treatment or apical surgery, a periapical radiolucency may remain that may look like periapical rarefying osteitis (Fig. 20-9). In either case the destroyed bone may not be replaced with normal-appearing bone but with dense fibrous scar tissue. The differential diagnosis cannot be made on radiologic grounds alone; thus the clinical signs and symptoms must take precedence.

In rare cases metastatic lesions and malignancies such as leukemia may grow in the periapical segment of the periodontal membrane space. Close inspection of the surrounding bone may reveal other small regions of malignant bone destruction.

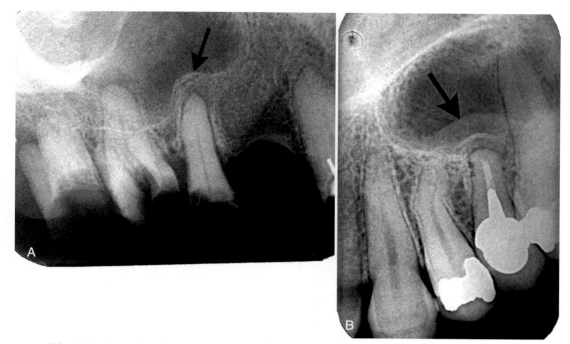

FIG. **20-6**   Periostitis resulting in bone formation emanating from the floor of the maxillary antrum that arises from apical inflammatory lesions. **A,** Laminated type of periosteal bone formation *(arrow)*. **B,** Periostitis and mucositis. The mucositis is characterized by a slight radiopaque band *(arrow)* next to the periosteal bone formation.

## Management

Standard dental treatment of periapical lesions includes root canal therapy or extraction with the intention of eliminating the necrotic material in the root canal and hence the source of inflammation. If left untreated, the tooth may become asymptomatic because of drainage established through the carious lesion or a parulis. However, the possibility always exists that the lesion will spread to involve a larger area of bone, resulting in osteomyelitis or into the surrounding soft tissue, which may result in a space infection or cellulitis.

## PERICORONITIS

### Synonym
Operculitis

### Definition
The term *pericoronitis* refers to inflammation of the tissues surrounding the crown of a partially erupted tooth. It is most often seen in association with the mandibular third molars in young adults. The gingiva surrounding the erupted portion of the crown becomes inflamed when food or microbial debris becomes trapped under the soft tissue. The gingiva subsequently becomes swollen and may become secondarily traumatized by the opposing occlusion. This inflammation may extend into the bone surrounding the crown of the tooth.

### Clinical Features
Patients with pericoronitis typically complain of pain and swelling. Trismus is a common presentation when the partially erupted tooth is a lower third molar, and usually pain is felt on occlusion. An

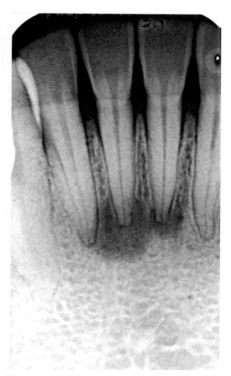

FIG. **20-7**   Two early lesions of periapical cemental dysplasia related to the apical region of the mandibular central incisors; note the similarity to apical rarefying osteitis.

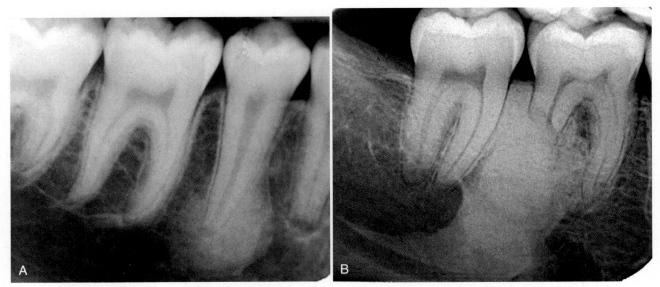

FIG. **20-8**   Enostosis (dense bone island) in periapical positions. **A,** Enostosis around the apex of a second bicuspid. Note that the periodontal membrane space is uniform in width. **B,** Enostosis associated with apical root resorption of a vital tooth. The most common site of enostosis and root resorption is the mesial or distal root of mandibular first molars.

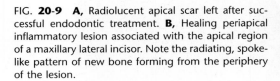

FIG. **20-9**   **A,** Radiolucent apical scar left after successful endodontic treatment. **B,** Healing periapical inflammatory lesion associated with the apical region of a maxillary lateral incisor. Note the radiating, spoke-like pattern of new bone forming from the periphery of the lesion.

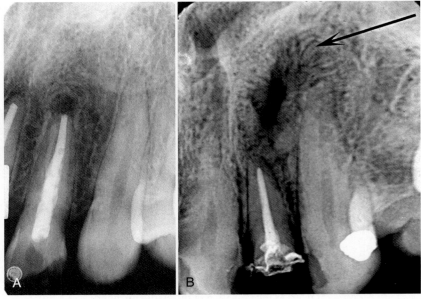

ulcerated operculum is usually the source of the pain. Pericoronitis can affect patients of any age or sex but is most commonly seen during the time of eruption of the third molars in young adults.

### Radiographic Features

The radiologic signs of pericoronitis can range from no changes when the inflammatory lesion is confined to the soft tissues to localized rarefaction and sclerosis to osteomyelitis in the most severe cases.

*Location.*   When bone changes are associated with pericoronitis, they are centered on the follicular space or the portion of the crown still embedded in bone or in close proximity to bone. The mandibular third molar region is the most common location.

*Periphery.*   The periphery of pericoronitis is ill defined, with a gradual transition of the normal trabecular pattern into a sclerotic region.

*Internal Structure.*   The internal structure of bone adjacent to the pericoronitis most often is sclerotic with thick trabeculae. An area of bone loss or radiolucency immediately adjacent to the crown that enlarges the follicular space may be seen (Fig. 20-10). If this lesion spreads considerably, the internal pattern becomes consistent with osteomyelitis (see the next section).

*Effects on Surrounding Structures.*   As with the periapical inflammatory lesions, pericoronitis may cause the typical changes of sclerosis and rarefaction of surrounding bone. In extensive cases, evidence of periosteal new bone formation may be seen at the inferior cortex, the posterior border of the ramus, and along the coronoid notch of the mandible.

## Differential Diagnosis

The differential diagnosis of pericoronitis includes other mixed density or sclerotic lesions that can exist adjacent to the crown of a partially erupted third molar. These include enostosis and fibrous dysplasia. The clinical symptoms indicative of an inflammatory lesion usually exclude these conditions. Neoplasms to be considered include the sclerotic form of osteosarcoma and, in older patients, squamous cell carcinoma. The occurrence of squamous cell carcinoma in the midst of a preexisting inflammatory lesion may be difficult to identify. Features characteristic of malignant neoplasia, such as profound cortical bone destruction and invasion, aids with the diagnosis.

## Management

The aim of treatment of pericoronitis is removal of the partially erupted tooth. However, in the acute phase, when trismus may prevent adequate access, antibiotic therapy and reduction in occlusion of the opposing tooth should relieve the symptoms until definitive treatment is provided.

# OSTEOMYELITIS

## Definition

Osteomyelitis is an inflammation of bone. The inflammatory process may spread through the bone to involve the marrow, cortex, cancellous portion, and periosteum. In the jaws pyogenic organisms that reach the bone marrow from abscessed teeth or postsurgical infection usually cause osteomyelitis. However, in some instances no source of infection can be identified, and hematogenous spread is presumed to be the origin. In some patients no infectious organisms can be identified, possibly because of previous antibiotic therapy or inadequate methods of bacterial isolation. Bacterial colonies also may be present in small, isolated pockets of bone that may be missed during sampling.

In patients with osteomyelitis, the bacteria and their products stimulate an inflammatory reaction in bone, causing destruction of the endosteal surface of the cortical bone. This destruction may progress through the cortical bone to the outer periosteum. In young patients, in whom the periosteum is more loosely attached to the outer cortex of bone than it is in adults, the periosteum is lifted up by inflammatory exudate, and new bone is laid down. This periosteal reaction is a characteristic but not pathognomonic feature of osteomyelitis. The hallmark of osteomyelitis is the development of sequestra. A sequestrum is a segment of bone that has become necrotic because of ischemic injury caused by the inflammatory process.

Numerous forms of osteomyelitis have been described. For the sake of simplicity, we group them into two major phases, acute and chronic, recognizing that these represent two ends of a continuum without a definite separating boundary in the process of bone inflammation. Other forms of osteomyelitis have been described as separate and distinct clinicopathologic entities with unique radiographic features. These are Garré's osteomyelitis and diffuse sclerosing osteomyelitis. We consider them as part of the same continuum. Garré's osteomyelitis is an exuberant periosteal response to inflammation. Diffuse sclerosing osteomyelitis is a chronic form of osteomyelitis with a pronounced sclerotic response. It is important to understand

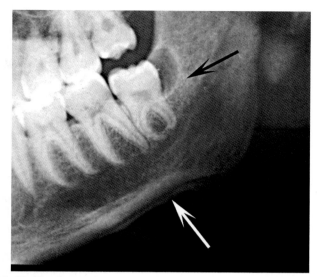

FIG. **20-10**   Cropped panoramic view of a case of pericoronitis related to a partially erupted third molar. Note the sclerotic bone reaction adjacent to the follicular cortex *(black arrow)* and the periosteal reaction *(white arrow)*.

that all these variations of osteomyelitis have the same underlying process of the bone's response to inflammation. The features expressed by each subtype represent only variations in the type and degree of bone reaction.

Osteomyelitis may resolve spontaneously or with appropriate antibiotic intervention. However, if the condition is not treated or is treated inadequately, the infection may persist and continue to spread and become chronic in about 20% of patients. Some chronic systemic diseases, immunosuppressive states, and disorders of decreased vascularity may predispose an individual to the development of osteomyelitis. For example, osteopetrosis, sickle cell anemia, and acquired immunodeficiency syndrome have been documented as underlying factors in the development of osteomyelitis.

## Acute Phase

### Synonyms

Acute suppurative osteomyelitis, pyogenic osteomyelitis, subacute suppurative osteomyelitis, Garré's osteomyelitis, proliferative periostitis, and periostitis ossificans are synonyms for the acute phase of osteomyelitis.

### Definition

The acute phase of osteomyelitis is caused by infection that has spread to the bone marrow. With this condition, the medullary spaces of the bone contain an inflammatory infiltrate consisting predominantly of neutrophils and, to a lesser extent, mononuclear cells. In the jaws the most common source of infection is a periapical lesion from a nonvital tooth. Infection also can occur as a result of trauma or hematogenous spread.

The changes described by Garré may accompany acute osteomyelitis. It is thought that the inflammatory exudate spreads subperiosteally, elevating the periosteum and stimulating formation of new bone. This condition is more common in younger people because in these individuals the periosteum is loosely attached to the bone surface and has greater osteogenic potential.

## Clinical Features

The acute phase of osteomyelitis can affect people of all ages, and it has a strong male predilection. It is much more common in the mandible than in the maxilla, possibly because of the poorer vascular supply to the mandible. The typical signs and symptoms of acute osteomyelitis are rapid onset, pain, swelling of the adjacent soft tissues, fever, lymphadenopathy, and leukocytosis. The associated teeth may be mobile and sensitive to percussion. Purulent drainage also may be present. Paresthesia of the lower lip in the third division of the fifth cranial nerve distribution is not uncommon.

## Radiologic Examination

In addition to a complete examination with plain films (panoramic, intraoral periapical and occlusal films), the following additional modalities may be used. A two-phase nuclear medicine study composed of a technetium bone scan followed by a gallium citrate scan may help to confirm the diagnosis. With inflammatory lesions, a positive result on the technetium scan indicates increased bone metabolic activity, and a positive result on the gallium scan in the same location indicates an inflammatory cell infiltrate. Computed tomography (CT) is the imaging method of choice. CT reveals more bone surface for detecting periosteal new bone and is the best imaging method for detecting sequestra (Fig. 20-11). Magnetic resonance imaging (MRI) with T2 weighted images to display abnormal bone marrow edema has been used.

## Radiographic Features

Very early in the disease, no radiographic changes may be identifiable. The bone may be filled with inflammatory exudate and inflammatory cells and may show no radiographic change.

*Location.* The most common location is the posterior body of the mandible. The maxilla is a rare site.

*Periphery.* Acute osteomyelitis most often presents an ill-defined periphery with a gradual transition to normal trabeculae.

*Internal Structure.* The first radiographic evidence of the acute form of osteomyelitis is a slight decrease in the density of the involved bone, with a loss of sharpness of the existing trabeculae. In time the bone destruction becomes more profound, resulting in an area of radiolucency in one focal area or in scattered regions throughout the involved bone (Fig. 20-12). Later, the appearance of sclerotic regions becomes apparent. Sequestra may be present but usually are more apparent and numerous in chronic forms (Fig. 20-13). Sequestra can

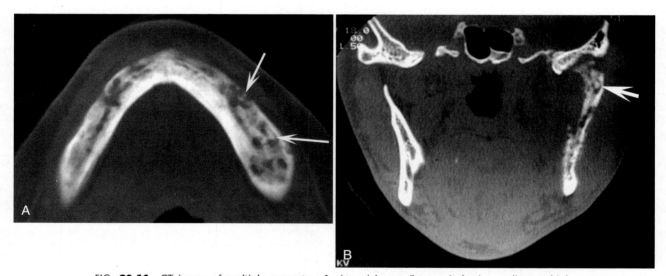

FIG. **20-11** CT image of multiple sequestra. **A,** An axial scan (bone window) revealing multiple sequestra *(arrows),* and **B,** a coronal scan (bone window) demonstrating a sequestrum *(arrow)* in two different cases of chronic osteomyelitis.

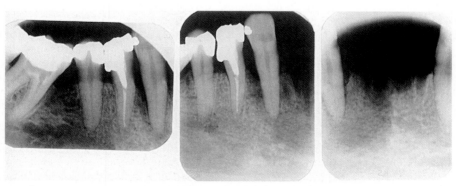

FIG. **20-12** Acute osteomyelitis involving the body of the right mandible, with initial blurring of bony trabeculae. (Courtesy Lars Hollender, DDS, PhD, Seattle, Wash.)

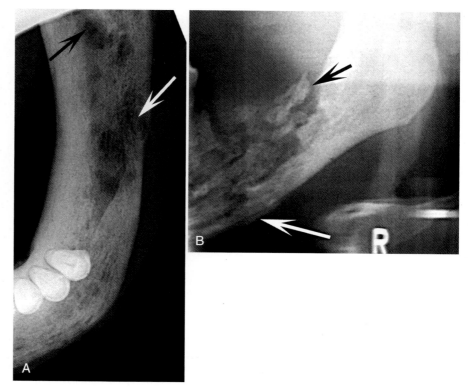

FIG. **20-13 Examples of Sequestra. A,** Occlusal film demonstrates small sequestra as radiopaque islands of bone in radiolucent regions in the chronic phase of osteomyelitis *(arrows).* **B,** Panoramic film reveals large sequestra *(black arrow)* and a periosteal reaction at the inferior border of the mandible in a case of chronic osteomyelitis *(white arrow).*

be identified by closely inspecting a region of bone destruction (radiolucency) for an island of bone. This island of nonvital bone may vary in size from a small dot (smaller sequestra usually are seen in young patients) to larger segments of radiopaque bone.

***Effects on Surrounding Structures.*** Acute osteomyelitis can stimulate either bone resorption or bone formation. Portions of cortical bone may be resorbed. An inflammatory exudate can lift the periosteum and stimulate bone formation. Radiographically, this appears as a thin, faint, radiopaque line adjacent to and almost parallel or slightly convex to the surface of the bone. A radiolucent band separates this periosteal new bone from the bone surface (Fig. 20-14). As the lesion develops into a more chronic phase, cyclic and periodic acute exacerbations may produce more inflammatory exudate, which again lifts the periosteum from the bone surface and stimulates the periosteum to form a second layer of bone. This is detected radiographically as a second radiopaque line almost parallel to the first and separated from it by a radiolucent band. This process may continue and may result in several lines (an onion-skin appearance), and eventually a massive amount of new bone may be formed. This is referred to as proliferative periostitis and is seen more often in children (Fig. 20-15). The effects on the teeth and lamina dura may be the same as those described for periapical inflammatory lesions.

### Differential Diagnosis

The differential diagnosis of the acute phase of osteomyelitis may include fibrous dysplasia, especially in children. Aside from the clinical signs of acute infection, the most useful radiographic characteristic to distinguish osteomyelitis from fibrous dysplasia is the way the enlargement of the bone occurs. The new bone that enlarges the jaws in osteomyelitis is laid down by the periosteum and therefore is on the

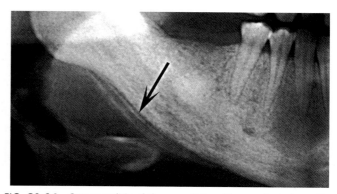

FIG. **20-14** Osteomyelitis of the mandible with a periosteal reaction located at the inferior cortex. Note the radiolucent line *(arrow)* between the inferior cortex of the mandible and the first layer of periosteal new bone. A second radiolucent line separates the second layer of new bone from the first layer.

outside of the outer cortical plate. In fibrous dysplasia the new bone is manufactured on the inside of the mandible; thus the outer cortex, which may be thinned, is on the outside and contains the lesion. This point of differentiation is important because the histologic appearance of a biopsy of new periosteal bone in osteomyelitis may be similar to that of fibrous dysplasia, and the condition may be reported as such.

Malignant neoplasia (e.g., osteosarcoma, squamous cell carcinoma) that invades the mandible at times may be difficult to differentiate from the acute phase of osteomyelitis, especially if the malignancy has been secondarily infected via an oral ulcer; this may

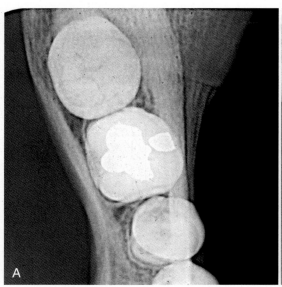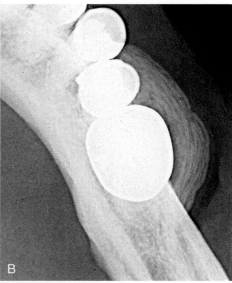

FIG. **20-15 A** and **B,** Proliferative periostitis resulting from inflammatory lesions. Note the multiple layers of new bone on the buccal aspect of the mandible, resulting in an onion-skin appearance.

result in a mixture of inflammatory and malignant radiographic characteristics. If part of the inflammatory periosteal bone has been destroyed, the possibility of a malignant neoplasm should be considered. The differential diagnosis may include other lesions that can cause bone destruction and may stimulate a periosteal reaction that is similar to that seen in inflammatory lesions. Langerhans' cell histiocytosis causes lytic ill-defined bone destruction and often results in the formation of periosteal reactive new bone. This lesion rarely stimulates a sclerotic bone reaction such as that seen in osteomyelitis. Leukemia and lymphoma may stimulate a similar periosteal reaction.

### Management

As with all inflammatory lesions of the jaws, removal of the source of inflammation is the primary goal of therapy. Antimicrobial treatment is the mainstay of treatment of acute osteomyelitis, along with establishing drainage. This may entail removal of a tooth, root canal therapy, or surgical incision and drainage.

## Chronic Phase

### Synonyms

Chronic diffuse sclerosing osteomyelitis, chronic nonsuppurative osteomyelitis, chronic osteomyelitis with proliferative periostitis, and Garré's chronic nonsuppurative sclerosing osteitis

### Definition

The chronic phase of osteomyelitis may be a sequela of inadequately treated acute osteomyelitis, or it may arise de novo. Diffuse sclerosing osteomyelitis refers to chronic osteomyelitis in which the balance in bone metabolism is tipped toward increased bone formation, producing a subsequent sclerotic radiographic appearance. The symptoms of the chronic form generally are less severe and have a longer history than those of the acute form. They include intermittent, recurrent episodes of swelling, pain, fever, and lymphadenopathy. As with the acute form, paresthesia and drainage with sinus formation also may

occur. In some cases pain may be limited to the advancing front of the osteomyelitis, or the patient may have little or no pain. Histologically, a chronic inflammatory infiltrate may be seen within the medullary spaces of bone; however, this may be quite sparse, with only fibrosis of the marrow seen with scattered regions of inflammation. At this stage of the disease, the offending etiologic agent rarely is found because culture results usually are negative. If left untreated, osteomyelitis can spread and involve both sides of the mandible. Further spread into the temporomandibular joint may cause a septic arthritis, and ear infections and infection of the mastoid air cells also may develop.

Chronic osteomyelitis as illustrated here is similar to the bone lesions described in chronic recurrent multifocal osteomyelitis (CRMO) and osteomyelitis of the SAPHO syndrome (synovitis [inflammatory arthritis], acne [pustulosa], pustulosis [psoriasis, palmoplantar pustulosis], hyperostosis [acquired], and osteitis [osteomyelitis]) with respect to the radiographic findings, lack of microbiologic findings, and clinical features such as intermittent recurrent pain and swelling of the involved bone. CRMO is a condition that often occurs symmetrically in the long bones in children. It is characterized by pain of the affected bone with or without swelling and has been described as a nonpurulent osteomyelitis with negative microbiologic cultures. The radiographic features are identical to chronic osteomyelitis as described here. Of interest is that treatment has consisted of systemic steroids, nonsteroidal anti-inflammatory drugs (NSAIDs), and bisphosphonates therapy because antibiotic and surgical therapy has not been effective treatment. It may be that chronic osteomyelitis of the jaw in children is a unifocal variant of CRMO.

The radiographic features of the bone lesions of SAPHO are similar if not identical to those of chronic osteomyelitis, and these lesions are refractory to antibiotic therapy, responding to anti-inflammatory agents such as steroids and NSAIDs.

It is possible that the pathophysiologic features of the jaw lesions of chronic osteomyelitis are identical to those of these two conditions.

## Radiologic Examination

If chronic osteomyelitis is suspected from the clinical examination, in addition to a complete series of plain films, CT is the imaging method of choice. CT is important for a correct diagnosis with the ability to demonstrate sequestra (see Fig. 20-11) and periosteal new bone and allows accurate staging of the disease, which is important for future assessment of healing. MRI is not as useful because of the lack of bone marrow edema in the chronic phase; however, it may be of use during acute exacerbation of the disease. Scintigraphy by use of bone scans, gallium, or labeled white blood cells is not particularly useful for differential diagnosis. Bone scans indicate increased bone formation, which is nonspecific, and often gallium scans (which highlight inflammatory cells) are not positive because of a very low population of inflammatory cells. The amount of bone activity assessed with bone scans with SPECT (single-photon emission CT) has been used to monitor healing. There are also reports of the use of positron emission tomography to detect a high cellular metabolic rate in tissues, but this type of imaging is nonspecific.

## Radiographic Features

*Location.* As in the acute phase of osteomyelitis, the most common site is the posterior mandible.

*Periphery.* The periphery may be better defined than in the acute phase, but it is still difficult to determine the exact extent of chronic osteomyelitis. Usually a gradual transition is seen between the normal surrounding trabecular pattern and the dense granular pattern characteristic of this disease. When the disease is active and is spreading through bone, the periphery may be more radiolucent and have poorly defined borders.

*Internal Structure.* The internal structure comprises regions of greater and lesser radiopacity compared with surrounding normal bone. Most of the lesion usually is composed of the more radiopaque or sclerotic bone pattern (Fig. 20-16). In older, more chronic lesions the internal bone density can be exceedingly radiopaque and equivalent to cortical bone. In these cases no obvious regions of radiolucency may be seen. In other cases, small regions of radiolucency may be scattered throughout the radiopaque bone. A close inspection of the radiolucent regions may reveal an island of bone or sequestrum within the center (Fig. 20-17). Often the sequestrum appears more radiopaque than the surrounding bone. Detection may require illumination of the radiolucent regions of the film with an intense light source. CT is superior for revealing the internal structure and sequestra, especially in cases with very dense sclerotic bone. The bone pattern usually is very granular, obscuring individual bone trabeculae.

*Effects on Surrounding Structures.* Chronic osteomyelitis often stimulates the formation of periosteal new bone, which is seen radiographically as a single radiopaque line or a series of radiopaque lines (similar to onion skin) parallel to the surface of the cortical bone. Over time the radiolucent strip that separates this new bone from the outer cortical bone surface may be filled in with granular sclerotic bone. When this occurs, it may not be possible to identify the original cortex, which makes it difficult to determine whether the new bone is derived from the periosteum. After a considerable amount of time the outer contour of the mandible also may be altered, assuming an abnormal shape, and the girth of the mandible may be much larger than on the unaffected side. The roots of teeth may undergo external resorption, and the lamina dura may become less apparent as it blends with the surrounding granular sclerotic bone. If a tooth is nonvital, the periodontal ligament space usually is enlarged in the apical region. In patients with extensive chronic osteomyelitis, the disease may

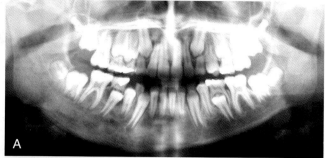

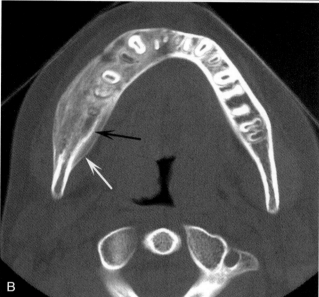

FIG. **20-16** Chronic osteomyelitis. **A,** This panoramic film demonstrates chronic osteomyelitis of the patient's right mandible; note the increase in density and size of the right mandible compared with the left side. **B,** An axial CT image using bone window of the mandible of the same case. Note the increase in bone density, width of the mandible, and the new periosteal bone formation *(white arrow)* and evidence of the original cortex *(black arrow).*

slowly spread to the mandibular condyle and into the joint, resulting in a septic arthritis. Further spread may involve the inner ear and mastoid air cells. Chronic lesions may develop a draining fistula, which may appear as a well-defined break in the outer cortex or in the periosteal new bone (Fig. 20-18).

## Differential Diagnosis

Very sclerotic, radiopaque chronic lesions of osteomyelitis may be difficult to differentiate from fibrous dysplasia, Paget's disease, and osteosarcoma. In children, osteomyelitis with a proliferative periosteal response may be misinterpreted as fibrous dysplasia (see the section Differential Diagnosis under Acute Osteomyelitis). Differentiation of the chronic form of osteomyelitis may be even more difficult if considerable remodeling and loss of a distinct original cortex have occurred. In these cases, inspection of the bone surface at the most peripheral part of the lesion may reveal subtle evidence of periosteal new bone formation. The presence of sequestra indicates osteomyelitis. Paget's disease affects the entire mandible, which is rare in

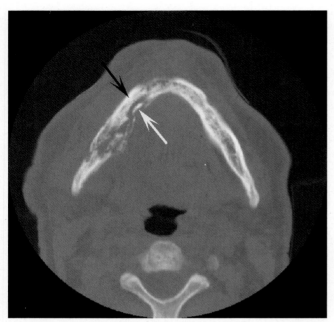

FIG. **20-17** An axial CT image using bone window of chronic osteo-myelitis with a mixture of increased bone density *(black arrow)*, areas of radiolucency, and presence of sequestra *(white arrow)*.

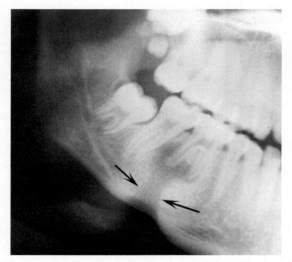

FIG. **20-18** A fistulous tract extending inferiorly from the apex of the first molar through the inferior cortex of the mandible *(arrows)*.

osteomyelitis. Periosteal new bone formation and sequestra are not seen in Paget's disease. Dense, granular bone may be seen in some forms of osteosarcoma, but usually evidence of bone destruction is found. A characteristic spiculated (sunraylike) periosteal response also may be seen. As mentioned in the section on acute osteomyelitis, other entities such as Langerhans' cell histiocytosis, leukemia, and lymphoma may stimulate a similar periosteal response, but these usually produce evidence of bone destruction characteristic of malignant tumors.

The imaging method of choice for aiding in the differential diagnosis is CT because of its ability to reveal sequestra and periosteal new bone.

### Management

Chronic osteomyelitis tends to be more difficult to eradicate than the acute form. In cases involving an extreme osteoblastic response (very sclerotic mandible), the subsequent lack of a good blood supply may work against healing. Hyperbaric oxygen therapy and creative modes of long-term antibiotic delivery have been used with limited success. Surgical intervention, which may include sequestrectomy, decortication, or resection, often is necessary. The probability of successful treatment, especially when using long-term antibiotic therapy with decortication, is greater in the first two decades of life. If cultures are negative, antibiotic therapy is not effective. It may be that the inflammatory response has become the main disease process and anti-inflammatory agents such as steroids and NSAIDs are more effective. More recently, the use of bisphosphonate therapy has provided some therapeutic success.

## Diagnostic Imaging of Soft Tissue Infections

Diagnostic imaging may be used to confirm the presence and extent of soft tissue infections. MRI and CT may be used to differentiate soft tissue neoplasia from inflammatory lesions. MRI can be used in the T2 or TI with gadolinium and fat suppression modes to detect the presence of soft tissue edema. CT usually is used with intravenous contrast. The CT image characteristics that suggest the presence of a soft tissue inflammation include abnormal fascial planes, thickening of the overlying skin and adjacent muscles, streaking of the fat planes, and abnormal collections of gas in the soft tissue (Fig. 20-19). Over time the contrast between soft tissue planes may disappear, and the presence of an abscess may become evident as a well-defined region of low density surrounded by a wide border of contrast-enhanced (more radiopaque) tissue. Lymphadenopathy resulting from infections such as tuberculosis of the head and neck may be visualized on magnetic resonance and CT images (Fig. 20-20).

### RADIATION-INDUCED CHANGES TO BONE

Therapeutic radiation damages the cellular elements of bone tissue by immediate or delayed cell death, cellular injury with recovery, arrested cellular division, or abnormal repair with neoplasia. The maturity and type of bone and the dose of radiation are factors that affect how the bone responds to this injury. When immature bone is irradiated, growth retardation occurs; the amount is related to the radiation dose and the stage of bone growth: the earlier the stage the greater the effect. Radiation damage to mature bone affects the osteoblasts, resulting in a decrease in matrix formation and damage to the fine blood vessels. The following discussion is limited to the mature bone of the maxillofacial region.

As with osteomyelitis, there is a spectrum of radiographic appearances of radiation damage to bone. These range from sclerosis with patchy radiolucency to osteoradionecrosis. When radiation damage to bone progresses to osteoradionecrosis, it is often first diagnosed clinically as an exposed bone sequestrum in the oral cavity before there are significant radiographic changes.

### OSTEORADIONECROSIS

#### Definition

Osteoradionecrosis refers to an inflammatory condition of bone (osteomyelitis) that occurs after the bone has been exposed to thera-

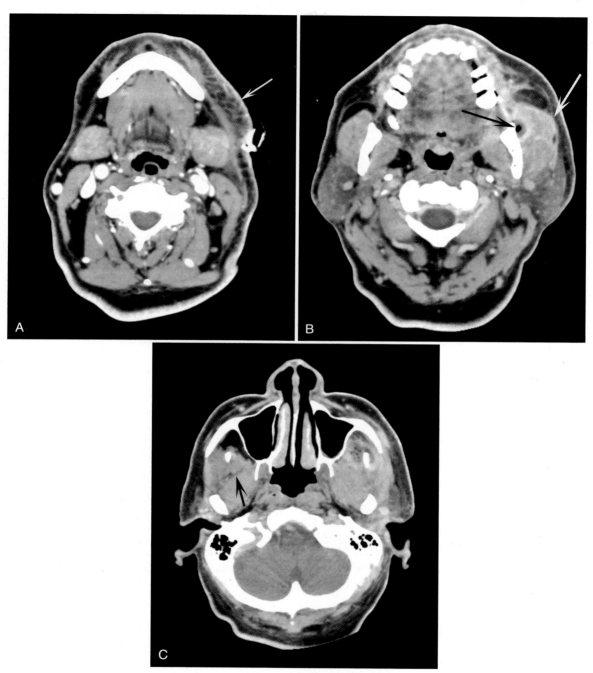

FIG. **20-19**    Three axial CT images, using a contrast medium, of a soft tissue infection demonstrating streaking (reticulation pattern) of the fat planes and thickening of the skin *(arrow)* **(A);** thickening of the masseter muscle *(white arrow)* and a radiolucent pocket of gas *(black arrow)* **(B);** and loss of distinctive soft tissue planes for example individual muscles defined by fat planes (the lateral border of the normal lateral pterygoid muscle *[arrow]* is not apparent on the opposite affected side) **(C).** (Courtesy Stuart White, DDS, Los Angeles, Calif.)

peutic doses of radiation usually given for a malignancy of the head and neck region. It is characterized by the presence of exposed bone for a period of at least 3 months occurring at any time after the delivery of the radiation therapy. Doses above 50 Gy usually are required to cause this irreversible damage. Bone that has been irradiated is hypocellular and hypovascular. The lack of sufficient vascularity results in a hypoxic environment in which adequate healing of bone is compromised. Although infection may be a contributing factor, it is not necessarily the primary insult after the radiation damage has occurred. In many cases dental extraction and denture trauma after radiation therapy have been implicated as etiologic factors. Secondary infection is common, further fomenting the inflammatory reaction.

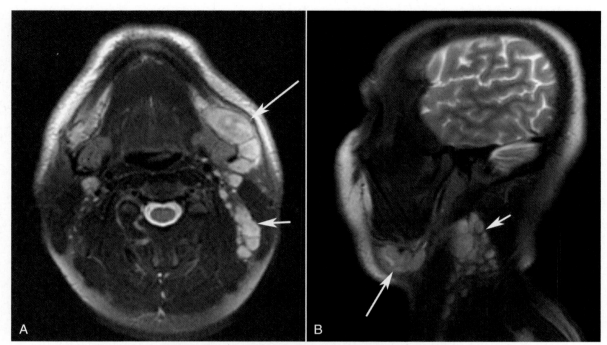

FIG. **20-20** **A,** Axial T2-weighted and **B,** sagittal T2-weighted magnetic resonance images of a case of tuberculosis with significant lymphadenopathy involving the submandibular lymph nodes *(long arrows)* and level II nodes *(short arrows).*

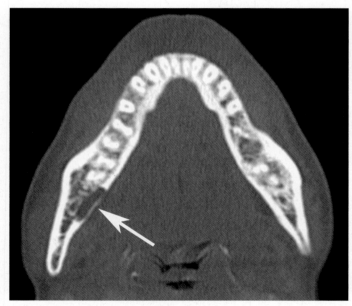

FIG. **20-21** An axial CT image showing a well-defined region of cortical bone resorption *(arrow),* an early change in therapeutic radiation exposure.

Because of the difficulty of management, this serious complication of radiation therapy carries a high morbidity rate.

## Clinical Features

The mandible is much more commonly affected than the maxilla is. This is likely due to the microanatomy and comparatively less vascu-lature of this bone. The posterior mandible is affected more often than the anterior portion. The posterior body of the mandible is more frequently in the direct field of the radiation treatment because primary tumors and metastatic lesions in lymph nodes being treated are commonly adjacent to this part of the mandible. Loss of mucosal covering and exposure of bone is the hallmark of osteoradionecrosis. Pathologic fracture also may occur. The exposed bone becomes necrotic as a result of loss of vascularity from the periosteum and subsequently sequestrates, often leading to exposure of more bone. Pain may or may not be present. Intense pain may occur, with inter-mittent swelling and drainage extraorally. However, many patients feel no pain with bone exposure.

## Radiologic Examination

The prescription of diagnostic imaging would be the same as used for chronic-phase osteomyelitis with CT being the imaging modality of choice.

## Radiographic Features

The radiographic features of osteoradionecrosis have many similari-ties to those of chronic osteomyelitis, and the reader is referred to that section for a detailed description. The following is a description of the radiographic changes seen in bone that has received a considerable amount of therapeutic radiation. An early characteristic change is a well-defined area of bone resorption within the outer cortical plate of the mandible (Fig. 20-21). Later changes are quite variable and may be predominantly lytic or sclerotic or a mixture (Fig. 20-22). However, the presence of osteoradionecrosis cannot always be diag-nosed radiographically and often clinically obvious signs of exposed necrotic bone may not be accompanied by significant radiologic changes.

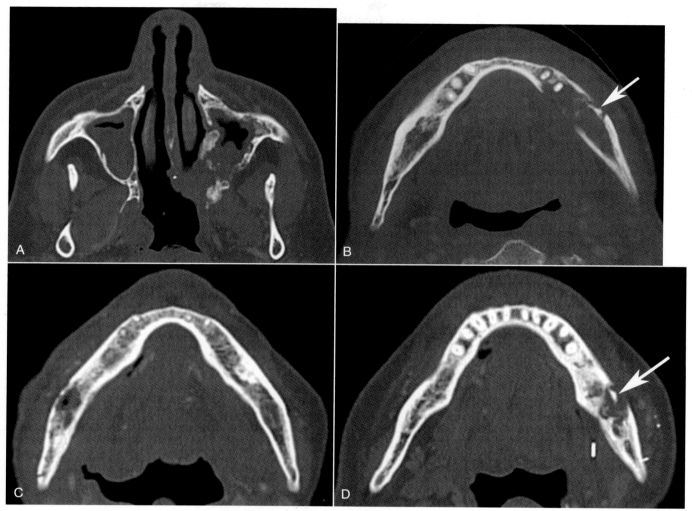

FIG. **20-22**  A series of axial CT images of different patients with various reactions to therapeutic levels of radiation exposure, including irregular resorption of the maxilla in **A**, mostly a resorptive reaction in the mandible with a sequestra *(arrow)* in **B**, a mixture of sclerosis and resorption in the mandible in **C** and **D**; note the sequestra *(arrow)* and slight periosteal response in **D**.

*Location.*  The mandible, especially the posterior mandible, is the most common location for osteoradionecrosis. The maxilla may be involved in some cases.

*Periphery.*  The periphery is ill defined and similar to that in osteomyelitis. If the lesion reaches the inferior border of the mandible, irregular resorption of this bony cortex often occurs.

*Internal Structure.*  A range of bone formation to bone destruction occurs, often with the balance heavily toward more bone formation, giving the affected bone an overall sclerotic or radiopaque appearance. This is very similar to chronic osteomyelitis. The bone pattern is granular. Scattered regions of radiolucency may be seen, with and without central sequestra. The affected maxillary bone may also be very sclerotic and have areas of bone resorption (see Fig. 20-22).

*Effects on Surrounding Structures.*  Inflammatory periosteal new bone formation is uncommon, possibly because of the deleterious effects of radiation on potential osteoblasts in the periosteum. In very rare cases the periosteum appears to have been stimulated to produce bone, resulting in new bone formation on the outer cortex in an unusual shape. Radiation exposure may also stimulate the resorption of bone, especially in the maxilla, which may be similar in appearance to bone destruction caused by a malignant neoplasm. The most common effect on the surrounding bone is the stimulation of sclerosis. In the alveolar process of the maxilla and mandible, there may be irregular widening of the periodontal membrane space similar to that seen in malignant neoplasia or it may simulate periapical rarefying osteitis. Also, there may be bone resorption, very similar to periodontal disease (Fig. 20-23).

## Differential Diagnosis

Bone resorption, stimulated by high levels of irradiation, may simulate bone destruction from a malignant neoplasm, especially in the maxilla. For this reason, the detection of a recurrence of the malignant neoplasm (usually squamous cell carcinoma) in the presence of osteoradionecrosis may be very difficult. If recurrence is suspected, CT and MRI may be used to detect an associated soft tissue mass.

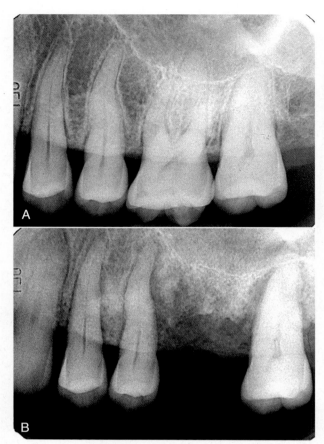

FIG. **20-23**   Osteoradionecrosis of the maxilla. These periapical films were taken before radiotherapy (**A**) and within 6 months of receiving the radiation (**B**). Note the combination of bone sclerosis and profound bone destruction around the teeth and alveolar crest and widening of the periodontal membrane space.

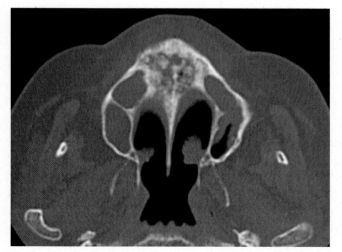

FIG. **20-24**   An axial CT image of a patient with bisphosphonate-related osteonecrosis; note the several sequestra in the anterior palate.

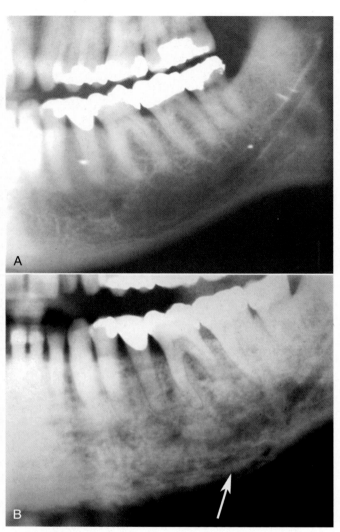

FIG. **20-25**   Two cropped panoramic images (**A** and **B**) of the same patient taken 1 year apart demonstrate a developing sclerotic bone pattern with a sequestra (*arrow*) related to bisphosphonate therapy.

Differentiation from other sclerotic lesions, as in chronic osteomyelitis, is less difficult because of the history of radiation therapy.

### Management

The treatment of osteoradionecrosis currently is unsatisfactory. Decortication with sequestrectomy and hyperbaric oxygen with antibiotics have been used with limited success because of poor healing after surgery. Conservative approaches with the aim of therapy to maintain the integrity of the lower border of the mandible, keeping the site free of infection and the patient free of pain, may in the long term prove more successful. Fortunately, the incidence of osteoradionecrosis has declined because preventive therapy has proved quite effective. Removal of teeth that have significant periodontal disease or have a poor prognosis before radiation treatment and excellent oral and denture hygiene are the mainstays of preventive treatment.

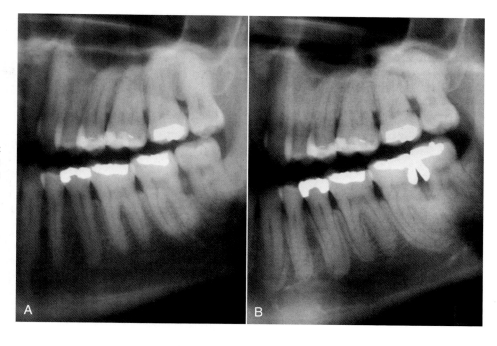

FIG. **20-26** Two cropped panoramic images (**A** and **B**) of the same patient taken 7 years apart reveal thickening of the lamina dura around the teeth.

## BISPHOSPHONATE-RELATED OSTEONECROSIS OF THE JAWS

### Definition

Bisphosphonates are potent synthetic analogs of pyrophosphates that act to inhibit osteoclasts and reduce bone metabolism. These drugs have become important in the treatment of bone lesions of multiple myeloma, hypercalcemia of malignancy, metastatic bone tumors, and osteoporosis. In recent years a complication of intraoral exposure of necrotic bone has been described in patients receiving these medications. The bone exposure occurs more commonly in patients receiving the more potent aminobisphosphonates intravenously and after an invasive dental surgical procedure such as extraction, periodontal or endodontic surgery, or implant placement. Bisphosphonate-related osteonecrosis has now been well documented, although the pathogenesis remains unclear.

### Clinical Features

Clinically, patients typically have an area of exposed bone after an invasive dental surgical procedure. However, denture trauma and spontaneous cases have been known to occur. Ulceration of palatal tori resulting in bone exposure is most likely the result of trauma. The most common areas affected are the posterior mandible (60%) and the maxilla (40%) and both (9%). The incidence of bone exposure is difficult to determine, but recent studies suggest that approximately 3% of patients receiving these drugs will have exposed bone. The areas may be asymptomatic or present with pain and swelling.

### Radiographic Features

There is a spectrum of radiographic findings that may or may not correlate well with the clinical symptoms. More often than not, there are no specific radiographic findings with the clinically exposed bone. In other cases the radiographic changes are not dissimilar to osteoradionecrosis or chronic osteomyelitis with the presence of sequestra (Fig. 20-24). Other reported findings include an increase in bone sclerosis (Fig. 20-25), widening of the periodontal membrane space, and thickening of the lamina dura (Fig. 20-26).

### Management

Unfortunately, treatment of bisphosphonate-related bone exposure is not satisfactory. Surgical intervention and hyperbaric oxygen therapy have not been consistently successful. The mainstay of therapy is preventive in nature. Patients who will be administered the potent aminobisphosphonates should have a dental examination to remove potential and real sources of infection to obviate the need for invasive dental procedures in the future. This is further complicated by the fact that the half-life of these drugs in bone can be quite lengthy (estimated at ≈12 years). Once bone is exposed, treatment is aimed at controlling the symptoms of pain and infection with antibiotic mouthrinses and systemic antibiotic therapy.

## BIBLIOGRAPHY

### PERIAPICAL INFLAMMATORY LESIONS

Heersche JNM: Bone cells and bone turnover: the basis for pathogenesis. In Tam CS, Heersche JNM, Murray TM, editors: *Metabolic bone disease: cellular and tissue mechanisms,* Boca Raton, FL, 1989, CRC Press.

Stern MH, Dreizen S, Mackler BF et al: Quantitative analysis of cellular composition of human periapical granuloma, *J Endocrinol* 7:117-122, 1981.

### PERICORONITIS

Blakey GH, White RP Jr, Offenbacher S et al: Clinical/biological outcomes of treatment for pericoronitis, *J Oral Maxillofac Surg* 54:1150-1160, 1996.

### OSTEOMYELITIS

Becker W: Imaging osteomyelitis and the diabetic foot, *Q J Nucl Med* 43:9-20, 1999.

Compeyrot-Lacassagne S, Rosenberg AM, Babyn P et al: Pamidronate treatment of chronic noninfectious inflammatory lesions of the mandible in children, *J Rheumatol* 34:1585-1589, 2007.

Guhlmann A, Brecht-Krauss D, Suger G et al: Chronic osteomyelitis: detection with FDG PET and correlation with histopathologic findings, *Radiology* 2006:749-754, 2006.

Ledermann HP, Kaim A, Bongartz G et al: Pitfalls and limitations of magnetic resonance imaging in chronic posttraumatic osteomyelitis, *Eur Radiol* 10:1815-1823, 2000.

Morrison WB, Schweitzer ME, Batte WG et al: Osteomyelitis of the foot: relative importance of primary and secondary MR imaging signs, *Radiology* 207:625-632, 1998.

Nordin U, Wannfors K, Colque-Navarro P et al: Antibody response in patients with osteomyelitis of the mandible, *Oral Surg Med Oral Pathol Oral Radiol Endod* 79:429, 1995.

Orpe EC, Lee L, Pharoah MJ: A radiological analysis of chronic sclerosing osteomyelitis of the mandible, *Dentomaxillofac Radiol* 25:125-129, 1996.

Petrikowski CG, Pharoah MJ, Lee L et al: Radiographic differentiation of osteogenic sarcoma, osteomyelitis, and fibrous dysplasia of the jaws, *Oral Surg Oral Med Oral Pathol Oral Radiol Endod* 80:744-750, 1995.

Suei Y, Taguchi A, Tanimoto K: Diagnostic points and possible origin of osteomyelitis in synovitis, acne, pustulosis, hyperostosis and osteitis (SAPHO) syndrome: a gradiographic study of 77 mandibular osteomyelitis cases, *Rheumatology* 42:1398-1403, 2003.

Suei Y, Tanimoto K, Taguchi A et al: Possible identity of diffuse sclerosing osteomyelitis and chronic recurrent multifocal osteomyelitis: one entity or two, *Oral Med Oral Pathol Oral Radiol Endod* 80:401-408, 1995.

Van Merkesteyn JP, Groot RH, Bras J et al: Diffuse sclerosing osteomyelitis of the mandible: clinical radiographic and histologic findings in twenty-seven patients, *J Oral Maxillofac Surg* 46:825-829, 1988.

Wannfors K, Hammarström L: Infectious foci in chronic osteomyelitis of the jaws, *Int J Oral Surg* 14:493-503, 1985.

Wood RE, Nortjé CJ, Grotepass F et al: Periostitis ossificans versus Garré's osteomyelitis, Part I: what did Garré really say? *Oral Surg Oral Med Oral Pathol* 65:773-777, 1988.

## RADIATION-INDUCED CHANGES TO BONE

Becker M, Schroth G, Zbären P et al: Long-term changes induced by high-dose irradiation of the head and neck region: imaging findings, *Radiographics* 17:5-26, 1997.

Williams HJ, Davies AM: The effect of x-rays on bone: a pictorial review, *Eur Radiol* 16: 619-633, 2006.

## OSTERADIONECROSIS

Curi MM, Dib LL: Osteoradionecrosis of the jaws: a retrospective study of the background factors and treatment in 104 cases, *J Oral Maxillofac Surg* 55:540-544, 1997.

Hermans R, Fossion E, Ioannides C et al: CT findings in osteoradionecrosis of the mandible, *Skeletal Radiol* 25:31-36, 1996.

Hutchison IL, Cullum ID, Langford JA et al: The investigation of osteoradionecrosis of the mandible by 99mTc-methylene diphosphonate radionuclide bone scans, *Br J Oral Maxillofac Surg* 28:143-149, 1990.

Marx RE: Osteoradionecrosis: a new concept of its pathophysiology, *J Oral Maxillofac Surg* 41:283-288, 1983.

Wong JK, Wood RE, McLean M: Conservative management of osteoradionecrosis, *Oral Surg Oral Med Oral Pathol Oral Radiol Endod* 84:16-21, 1997.

## BISPHOSPHONATE-RELATED OSTEONECROSIS

Jadu F, Lee L, Pharoah M et al: A retrospective study assessing the incidence, risk factors and comorbidities of pamidronate-related necrosis of the jaws in multiple myeloma patients, *Ann Oncol* 18:2015-2019, 2007.

Woo SB, Hellstein J, Kalmar JR: Narrative [corrected] review: bisphosphonates and osteonecrosis of the jaws, *Ann Intern Med* 144:753-761, 2006.

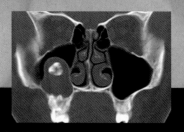

# CHAPTER 21

# Cysts and Cystlike Lesions of the Jaws

A cyst is a pathologic cavity filled with fluid, lined by epithelium, and surrounded by a definite connective tissue wall. The cystic fluid either is secreted by the cells lining the cavity or derives from the surrounding tissue fluid.

## Clinical Features

Cysts occur more often in the jaws than in any other bone because most cysts originate from the numerous rests of odontogenic epithelium that remain after tooth formation. Cysts are radiolucent lesions, and the prevalent clinical features are swelling, lack of pain (unless the cyst becomes secondarily infected or is related to a nonvital tooth), and association with unerupted teeth, especially third molars.

## Radiographic Features

### LOCATION

Cysts may occur centrally (within bone) in any location in the maxilla or mandible but are rare in the condyle and coronoid process. Odontogenic cysts are found most often in the tooth-bearing region. In the mandible, they originate above the inferior alveolar nerve canal. Odontogenic cysts may grow into the maxillary antrum. Some nonodontogenic cysts also originate within the antrum (see Chapter 27). A few cysts arise in the soft tissues of the orofacial region.

### PERIPHERY

Cysts that originate in bone usually have a periphery that is well defined and corticated (characterized by a fairly uniform, thin, radiopaque line). However, a secondary infection or a chronic state can change this appearance into a thicker, more sclerotic boundary or make the cortex less apparent.

### SHAPE

Cysts usually are round or oval, resembling a fluid-filled balloon. Some cysts may have a scalloped boundary.

### INTERNAL STRUCTURE

Cysts often are totally radiolucent. However, long-standing cysts may have dystrophic calcification, which can give the internal aspect a sparse, particulate appearance. Some cysts have septa, which produce multiple loculations separated by these bony walls or septa. Cysts that have a scalloped periphery may appear to have internal septa. Occa-

sionally the image of bony ridges produced by the peripheral scalloping are positioned so that their image overlaps the internal aspect of the cyst, giving the false impression of internal septa.

### EFFECTS ON SURROUNDING STRUCTURE

Cysts grow slowly, sometimes causing displacement and resorption of teeth. The tooth resorption often has a sharp, curved shape. Cysts can expand the mandible, usually in a smooth, curved manner, and change the buccal or lingual cortical plate into a thin cortical boundary. Cysts may displace the inferior alveolar nerve canal in an inferior direction or invaginate into the maxillary antrum, maintaining a thin layer of bone that separates the internal aspect of the cyst from the antrum.

## Odontogenic Cysts

### Radicular Cyst

**Synonyms**

Periapical cyst, apical periodontal cyst, and dental cyst

**Definition**

A radicular cyst is a cyst that most likely results when rests of epithelial cells (Malassez) in the periodontal ligament are stimulated to proliferate and undergo cystic degeneration by inflammatory products from a nonvital tooth.

**Clinical Features**

Radicular cysts are the most common type of cyst in the jaws. They arise from nonvital teeth (i.e., teeth that have lost vitality because of extensive caries, large restorations, or previous trauma). Often radicular cysts produce no symptoms unless secondary infection occurs. A cyst that becomes large may cause swelling. On palpation the swelling may feel bony and hard if the cortex is intact, crepitant as the bone thins, and rubbery and fluctuant if the outer cortex is lost. The incidence of radicular cysts is greater in the third to sixth decades and shows a slight male predominance.

**Radiographic Features**

*Location.* In most cases the epicenter of a radicular cyst is located approximately at the apex of a nonvital tooth (Fig. 21-1). Occasionally it appears on the mesial or distal surface of a tooth root, at the opening of an accessory canal, or infrequently in a deep periodontal pocket. Most radicular cysts (60%) are found in the maxilla, especially around incisors and canines. Because of the distal inclination of the root, cysts

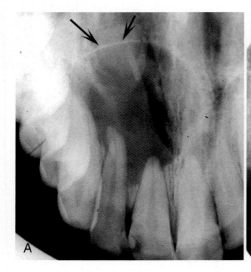

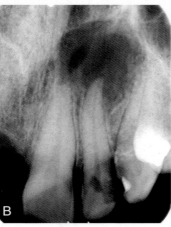

FIG. **21-1   Radicular Cysts.** In **A** note that the epicenter is apical to the lateral incisor and the presence of a peripheral cortex *(arrows)*. In **B** note the lack of a well-defined peripheral cortex because this cyst was secondarily infected and that the root canal of the lateral incisor is abnormally wide and it is visible at the root apex.

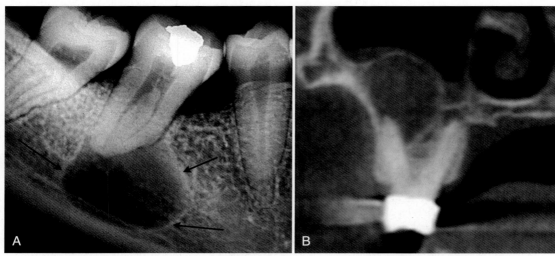

FIG. **21-2   A,** A periapical film of a radicular cyst reveals a lesion with a well-defined cortical boundary *(arrows)*. Note that the presence of the inferior cortex of the mandible has influenced the circular shape of the cyst. **B,** A coronal cone beam CT image of a radicular cyst related to the buccal root of a maxillary molar. Note the circular shape of the cyst as it invaginates the maxillary sinus. (Courtesy Dr. Bernard Friedland, Harvard University.)

that arise from the maxillary lateral incisor may invaginate the antrum. Radicular cysts may also form in relation to a nonvital deciduous molar and be positioned buccal to the developing bicuspid.

*Periphery and Shape.* The periphery usually has a well-defined cortical border (Fig. 21-2). If the cyst becomes secondarily infected, the inflammatory reaction of the surrounding bone may result in loss of this cortex (see Fig. 21-1, *B*) or alteration of the cortex into a more sclerotic border. The outline of a radicular cyst usually is curved or circular unless it is influenced by surrounding structures such as cortical boundaries.

*Internal Structure.* In most cases the internal structure of radicular cysts is radiolucent. Occasionally, dystrophic calcification may develop in long-standing cysts, appearing as sparsely distributed, small particulate radiopacities.

*Effects on Surrounding Structures.* If a radicular cyst is large, displacement and resorption of the roots of adjacent teeth may occur. The resorption pattern may have a curved outline. In rare cases the cyst may resorb the roots of the related nonvital tooth. The cyst may invaginate the antrum, but there should be evidence of a cortical boundary between the contents of the cyst and the internal structure of the antrum (Fig. 21-2, *B*). The outer cortical plates of the maxilla or mandible may expand in a curved or circular shape (Fig. 21-3). Cysts may displace the mandibular alveolar nerve canal in an inferior direction.

### Differential Diagnosis

Differentiation of a small radicular cyst from an apical granuloma may be difficult and in some cases impossible. A round shape, a well-

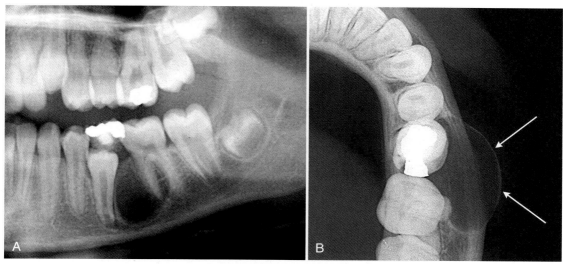

FIG. **21-3**  **A** and **B,** Two images of a radicular cyst originating from a nonvital deciduous second molar show expansion of the buccal cortical plate to a circular or hydraulic shape *(arrows)* and displacement of the adjacent permanent teeth.

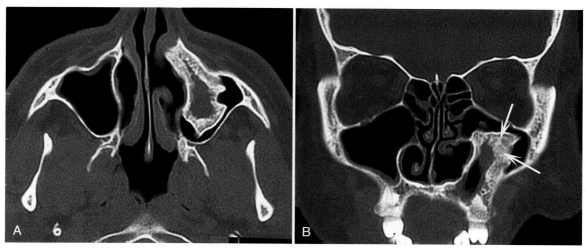

FIG. **21-4**    Axial **(A)** and coronal **(B)** CT images with use of a bone algorithm of a collapsing radicular cyst within the sinus. Note the unusual shape and the fact that new bone is being formed from the periphery *(arrows)* toward the center. (Courtesy Drs. S. Ahing and T. Blight, University of Manitoba.)

defined cortical border, and a size greater than 2 cm in diameter are more characteristic of a cyst. Other periapical radiolucencies to consider are an early stage of periapical cemental dysplasia and an apical scar or a surgical defect because in such cases, normal bone may never fill in the defect completely. The patient's history helps with the differentiation. Radicular cysts that originate from the maxillary lateral incisor and are positioned between the roots of the lateral incisor and the cuspid may be difficult to differentiate from an odontogenic keratocyst or a lateral periodontal cyst. The vitality of the involved tooth should be tested. A nonvital tooth may have a larger pulp chamber than neighboring teeth because of the lack of secondary dentin, which normally forms with time in the pulp chamber and canal of a vital tooth (see Fig. 21-1).

A large radicular cyst that has invaginated the maxillary antrum may collapse and start filling in with new bone (Fig. 21-4). With biopsy, the histologic analysis may result in an erroneous diagnosis of ossifying fibroma or a benign fibro-osseous lesion. Radiographically, the important feature is that the new bone always forms first at the periphery of the cyst wall as the cyst shrinks and not in the center of the cyst; this is a different pattern of bone formation than is seen with benign fibro-osseous lesions.

## Management
Treatment of a tooth with a radicular cyst may include extraction, endodontic therapy, and apical surgery. Treatment of a large radicular cyst usually involves surgical removal or marsupialization. The

radiographic appearance of the periapical area of an endodontically treated tooth should be checked periodically to make sure that normal healing is occurring (Fig. 21-5). Characteristically, new bone grows into the defect from the periphery, sometimes resulting in a radiating pattern resembling the spokes of a wheel. However, in a few cases normal bone may not completely fill the defect, especially if a secondary infection or a considerable amount of bone destruction, including the buccal and lingual cortical plates, has occurred. Recurrence of a radicular cyst is unlikely if it has been removed completely.

## Residual Cyst

### Definition

A residual cyst is a cyst that remains after incomplete removal of the original cyst. The term *residual* is used most often for a radicular cyst that may be left behind, most commonly after extraction of a tooth.

### Clinical Features

A residual cyst usually is asymptomatic and often is discovered on radiographic examination of an edentulous area. However, there may be some expansion of the jaw or pain in the case of secondary infection.

### Radiographic Features

*Location.* Residual cysts occur in both jaws, although they are found slightly more often in the mandible. The epicenter is positioned in the former periapical region of the involved and missing tooth. In the mandible the epicenter is always above the inferior alveolar nerve canal (Fig. 21-6).

*Periphery and Shape.* A residual cyst has a cortical margin unless it becomes secondarily infected. Its shape is oval or circular.

*Internal Structure.* The internal aspect of a residual cyst typically is radiolucent. Dystrophic calcifications may be present in long-standing cysts.

*Effects on Surrounding Structures.* Residual cysts can cause tooth displacement or resorption. The outer cortical plates of the jaws may expand. The cyst may invaginate into the maxillary antrum or depress the inferior alveolar nerve canal.

### Differential Diagnosis

Without the patient's history and previous radiographs, the clinician may have difficulty determining whether a solitary cyst in the jaws is a residual cyst. Other examples of common solitary cysts include odontogenic keratocysts. A residual cyst has greater potential for expansion compared with an odontogenic keratocyst. The epicenter of a Stafne developmental salivary gland defect is located below the mandibular canal (and thus is unlikely to be odontogenic in nature).

### Management

The treatment for residual cysts is surgical removal or marsupialization, or both, if the cyst is large.

## Dentigerous Cyst

### Synonym

Follicular cyst

### Definition

A dentigerous cyst is a cyst that forms around the crown of an unerupted tooth. It begins when fluid accumulates in the layers of reduced enamel epithelium or between the epithelium and the crown of the unerupted tooth. An eruption cyst is the soft tissue counterpart of a dentigerous cyst.

### Clinical Features

Dentigerous cysts are the second most common type of cyst in the jaws. They develop around the crown of an unerupted or supernumerary tooth. The clinical examination reveals a missing tooth or teeth and possibly a hard swelling, occasionally resulting in facial asymmetry. The patient typically has no pain or discomfort. Dentigerous cysts around supernumerary teeth account for about 5% of all dentigerous cysts, most developing around a mesiodens in the anterior maxilla.

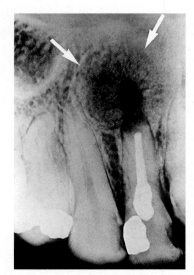

FIG. **21-5  A Radicular Cyst That Is Healing After Endodontic Treatment.** *Arrows* show the original outline of the cyst; note that the new bone grows toward the center from the periphery.

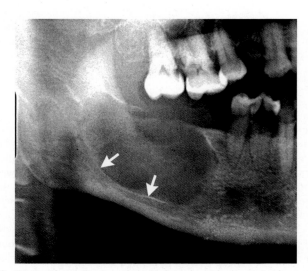

FIG. **21-6** The epicenter of this infected residual cyst is above the inferior alveolar nerve canal and has displaced the canal in an inferior direction *(arrows)*. Note that the cortical boundary is not continuous around the whole cyst.

## Radiographic Features

*Location.* The epicenter of a dentigerous cyst is found just above the crown of the involved tooth, most commonly the mandibular or maxillary third molar or the maxillary canine (Fig. 21-7). An important diagnostic point is that this cyst attaches at the cementoenamel junction. Some dentigerous cysts are eccentric, developing from the lateral aspect of the follicle so that they occupy an area beside the crown instead of above the crown (see Fig. 21-7, *D*). Cysts related to maxillary third molars often grow into the maxillary antrum and may become quite large before they are discovered. Cysts attached to the crown of mandibular molars may extend a considerable distance into the ramus.

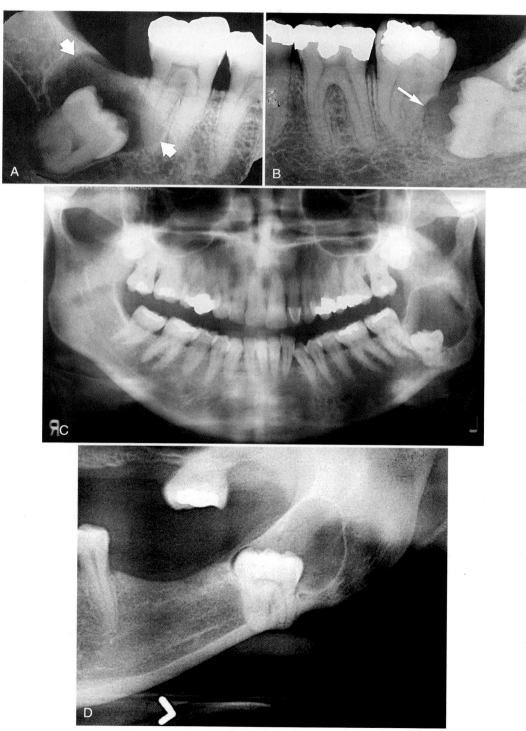

FIG. **21-7** **Dentigerous Cysts. A,** A cyst surrounds the crown of a third molar *(arrows)*. **B,** The cyst has caused resorption of the distal root of the second molar *(arrow)*. **C,** A cyst that involves the ramus of the mandible. **D,** A dentigerous cyst that is expanding distally from the involved third molar.

***Periphery and Shape.*** Dentigerous cysts typically have a well-defined cortex with a curved or circular outline. If infection is present, the cortex may be missing.

***Internal Structure.*** The internal aspect is completely radiolucent except for the crown of the involved tooth.

***Effects on Surrounding Structures.*** A dentigerous cyst has a propensity to displace and resorb adjacent teeth (Figs. 21-7 and 21-8). It commonly displaces the associated tooth in an apical direction (Fig. 21-9). The degree of displacement may be considerable. For instance, maxillary third molars or cuspids may be pushed to the floor of the orbit (see Fig. 21-8), and mandibular third molars may be moved to the condylar or coronoid regions or to the inferior cortex of the mandible. The floor of the maxillary antrum may be displaced as the cyst invaginates the antrum (Fig. 21-10), and the cyst may displace the inferior alveolar nerve canal in an inferior direction. This slow-growing cyst often expands the outer cortical boundary of the involved jaw.

## Differential Diagnosis

Because the histopathologic appearance of the lining epithelium is not specific, the diagnosis relies on the radiographic and surgical observation of the attachment of the cyst to the cementoenamel junction.

However, histopathologic examination must always be done to eliminate other possible lesions in this location.

One of the most difficult differential diagnoses to make is between a small dentigerous cyst and a hyperplastic follicle. A cyst should be considered with any evidence of tooth displacement or considerable expansion of the involved bone. The size of the normal follicular space is 2 to 3 mm. If the follicular space exceeds 5 mm, a dentigerous cyst is more likely. If uncertainty remains, the region should be reexamined in 4 to 6 months to detect any increase in size or any influence on surrounding structures characteristic of cysts.

The differential diagnosis also may include an odontogenic keratocyst, an ameloblastic fibroma, and a cystic ameloblastoma. An odontogenic keratocyst does not expand the bone to the same degree as a dentigerous cyst, is less likely to resorb teeth, and may attach further apically on the root instead of at the cementoenamel junction. It may not be possible to differentiate a small ameloblastic fibroma or cystic ameloblastoma from a dentigerous cyst if there is no internal structure. Other rare lesions that may have a similar pericoronal appearance are adenomatoid odontogenic tumors and calcified odontogenic cysts, both of which can surround the crown and root of the involved tooth. Evidence of a radiopaque internal structure should be sought in these two lesions. Occasionally a radicular cyst at the apex of a

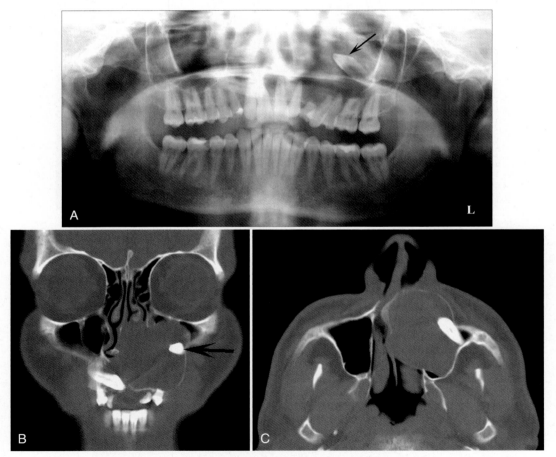

FIG. **21-8** **A,** This panoramic image reveals the presence of a large dentigerous cyst associated with the left maxillary cuspid *(arrow)*, which has been displaced. Notice the displacement and resorption of other teeth in the left maxilla. **B** and **C,** Coronal and axial CT images of the same case showing superior-lateral displacement of the cuspid, expansion of the anterior wall of the maxilla, and expansion of the cyst into the nasal fossa.

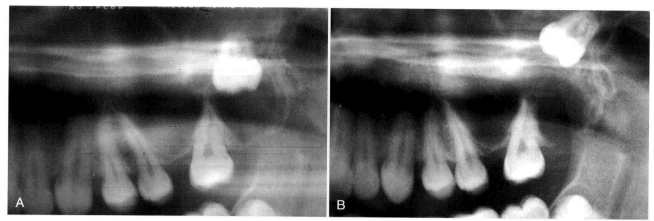

FIG. **21-9** **A** and **B,** These panoramic films of the same case taken several years apart demonstrate superior-posterior displacement of a maxillary third molar by a dentigerous cyst.

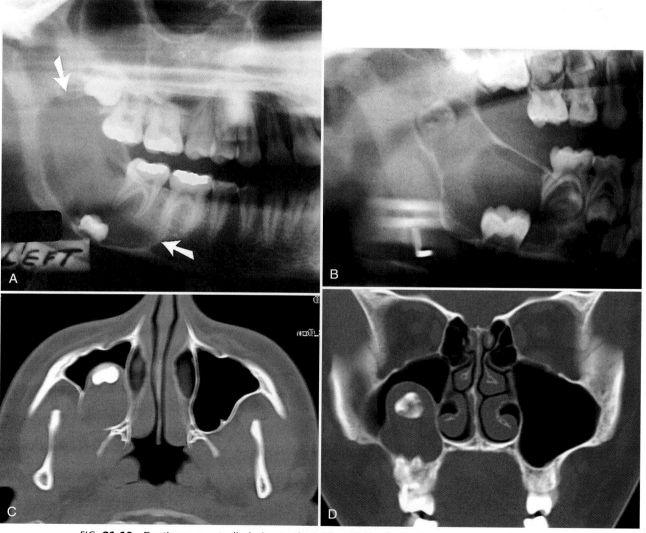

FIG. **21-10**   Dentigerous cysts displacing teeth. **A,** The third molar has been displaced to the inferior cortex. **B,** The developing second molar has been displaced into the ramus by a cyst associated with the first molar. Axial **(C)** and coronal **(D)** CT images with bone algorithm reveal a maxillary third molar displaced into the space occupied by the maxillary antrum; note the presence of a cortex between the cyst and the antrum.

primary tooth surrounds the crown of the developing permanent tooth positioned apical to it, giving the false impression of a dentigerous cyst associated with the permanent tooth. This occurs most often with the mandibular deciduous molars and the developing bicuspids. In these cases the clinician should look for extensive caries or large restorations in a primary tooth that would indicate a radicular cyst.

### Management

Dentigerous cysts are treated by surgical removal, which may include the tooth as well. Large cysts may be treated by marsupialization before removal. The cyst lining should be submitted for histologic examination because ameloblastomas have been reported to occur in the cyst lining. In addition, squamous cell carcinoma has been reported to arise from the cyst lining of chronically infected cysts. Mucoepidermoid carcinoma also has been reported.

## Buccal Bifurcation Cyst

### Synonyms

Mandibular infected buccal cyst, paradental cyst, and inflammatory paradental cyst

### Definition

The source of epithelium probably is the epithelial cell rests in the periodontal membrane of the buccal bifurcation of mandibular molars. The histopathologic characteristics of the lining are not distinctive. The etiology of proliferation is unknown; one theory holds that inflammation is the stimulus, but inflammation is not always present. The World Health Organization includes these cysts under inflammatory cysts.

It is possible that the paradental cyst of the third molar and the buccal bifurcation cyst (BBC) (associated with first and second molars) are the same entity. The BBC is certainly a distinct clinical entity. An associated enamel extension into the furcation region of third molars with paradental cysts has not been documented with molars involved in a BBC. Also, the inflammatory component associated with paradental cysts is not always present with BBCs.

### Clinical Features

A common sign is the lack of or a delay in eruption of a mandibular first or second molar. On clinical examination the molar may be missing or the lingual cusp tips may be abnormally protruding through the mucosa, higher than the position of the buccal cusps. The first molar is involved more frequently than is the second molar. The teeth are always vital. A hard swelling may occur buccal to the involved molar, and if it is secondarily infected, the patient has pain. The age of detection is younger, within the first two decades for a BBC rather than the third decade with a paradental cyst of the third molar.

### Radiographic Features

*Location.* The mandibular first molar is the most common location of a BBC, followed by the second molar. The cyst occasionally is bilateral. It is always located in the buccal furcation of the affected molar (Fig. 21-11). On periapical and panoramic films the lesion may

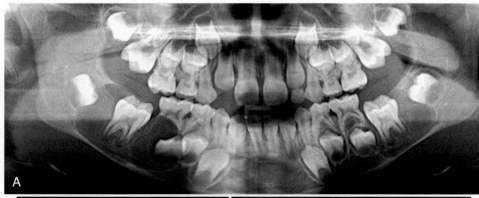

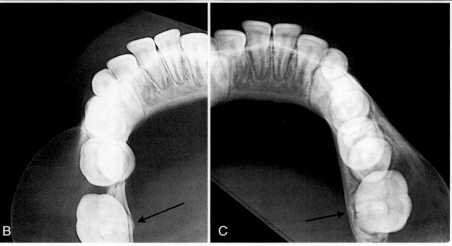

FIG. **21-11 Bilateral Buccal Bifurcation Cysts. A,** A panoramic image showing cysts related to the mandibular first molars. The occlusal surface of each tooth has been tipped in relation to the other teeth and adjacent teeth have been displaced. **B** and **C,** Occlusal films of the same case. Note the smooth curved expansion of the buccal cortex and the displacement of the roots of the first molars into the lingual cortical plate *(arrows).*

appear to be centered a little distal to the furcation of the involved tooth.

*Periphery and Shape.* In some cases the periphery is not readily apparent, and the lesion may be a very subtle radiolucent region superimposed over the image of the roots of the molar. In other cases the lesion has a circular shape with a well-defined cortical border. Some cysts can become quite large before they are detected.

*Internal Structure.* The internal structure is radiolucent.

*Effects on Surrounding Structures.* The most striking diagnostic characteristic of a BBC is the tipping of the involved molar so that the root tips are pushed into the lingual cortical plate of the mandible (see Fig. 21-11, *B* and *C*) and the occlusal surface is tipped toward the buccal aspect of the mandible (see Fig. 21-11, *A*). This accounts for the lingual cusp tips being positioned higher than the buccal tips. This tipping may be detected in a panoramic or periapical film if the image of the occlusal surface of the affected tooth is apparent whereas the unaffected teeth are not. The best diagnostic film is the cross-sectional (standard) mandibular occlusal projection, which demonstrates the abnormal position of the tooth roots. If the cyst is large enough, it may displace and resorb the adjacent teeth and cause a considerable amount of smooth expansion of the buccal cortical plate. If the cyst is secondarily infected, periosteal new bone formation is seen on the buccal cortex adjacent to the involved tooth (Fig. 21-12).

## Differential Diagnosis

Diagnosis of a BBC relies entirely on clinical and radiographic information. The major differential diagnosis includes lesions that could elicit an inflammatory periosteal response on the buccal aspect of mandibular molars, such as a periodontal abscess or Langerhans' cell histiocytosis (see Fig. 21-12). The fact that only a BBC tilts the molar as described helps to differentiate it from other lesions. Also in the differential diagnosis is the dentigerous cyst. However, the epicenter of a dentigerous cyst is different because a BBC starts near the bifurcation region of the tooth and does not surround the crown, as does a dentigerous cyst.

## Management

A BBC usually is removed by conservative curettage, although some cases have resolved without intervention. The involved molar should not be removed. BBCs do not recur.

## Keratocystic Odontogenic Tumor

### Synonyms
Odontogenic keratocyst and primordial cyst

### Definition

The World Health Organization has reclassified this cystic lesion into a unicystic or multicystic odontogenic tumor on the basis of the tumorlike characteristics of the lining epithelium. Because the gross and radiographic appearance of keratocystic odontogenic tumor (KOT) is cystic in nature, this neoplasm is presented in this chapter. Unlike most cysts, which are thought to grow solely by osmotic pressure, the epithelium in the KOT appears to have innate growth potential, consistent with a benign tumor. This difference in the mechanism of growth gives KOT a different radiographic appearance from cysts. The epithelial lining is distinctive also because it is keratinized (hence the name) and thin (four to eight cells thick). Occasionally budlike proliferations of epithelium grow from the basal layer into the adja-

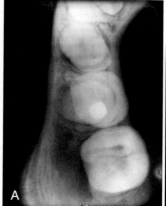
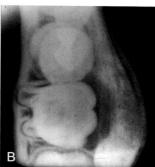

FIG. **21-12** Occlusal views of two examples of buccal bifurcation cysts that have been secondarily infected; note the laminated periosteal new bone formation on the buccal aspect of the first molars and also the abnormal position of the roots of the first molar in **B**. (Courtesy Dr. Doug Stoneman, University of Toronto.)

cent connective tissue wall. Also, islands of epithelium in the wall may give rise to satellite microcysts. The inside of the cyst often contains a viscous or cheesy material derived from the epithelial lining.

### Clinical Features

KOTs account for about one tenth of all cystic lesions in the jaws. They occur in a wide age range, but most develop during the second and third decades, with a slight male predominance. The cysts sometimes form around an unerupted tooth. KOTs usually have no symptoms, although mild swelling may occur. Pain may occur with secondary infection. Aspiration may reveal a thick, yellow, cheesy material (keratin). It is important to note that, unlike cysts, KOTs have a high propensity for recurrence, possibly because of small satellite cysts or fragments of epithelium left behind after surgical removal of the cyst.

### Radiographic Features

*Location.* The most common location of KOT is the posterior body of the mandible (90% occur posterior to the canines) and ramus (more than 50%) (Fig. 21-13). The epicenter is located superior to the inferior alveolar nerve canal. This type of cyst occasionally has the same pericoronal position as, and is indistinguishable from, a dentigerous cyst (Fig. 21-13, *B*).

*Periphery and Shape.* As with cysts, KOTs usually show evidence of a cortical border unless they have become secondarily infected. The cyst may have a smooth round or oval shape identical to that of other cysts, or it may have a scalloped outline (a series of contiguous arcs) (see Figs. 21-13 and 21-15, *C*).

*Internal Structure.* The internal structure is most commonly radiolucent. The presence of internal keratin does not increase the radiopacity. In some cases curved internal septa may be present, giving the lesion a multilocular appearance (see Figs. 21-13 and 21-14, *A*).

*Effects on Surrounding Structures.* An important characteristic of the KOT is its propensity to grow along the internal aspect of the jaws, causing minimal expansion (Fig. 21-15). This occurs throughout the mandible except for the upper ramus and coronoid process, where considerable expansion may occur (Fig. 21-14, *C*). Occasionally the

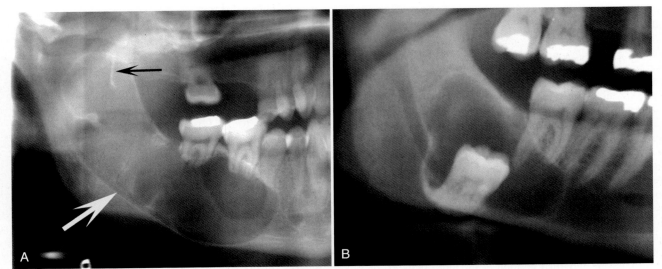

FIG. **21-13**    In panoramic image **A** a large keratocystic odontogenic tumor occupies the ramus and body of the mandible; note the septa *(black arrow),* inferiorly displaced mandibular canal *(white arrow),* and the root resorption. The keratocyst in **B** has a pericoronal position relative to the impacted third molar and the distal margin has a scalloped shape.

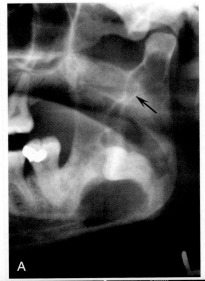

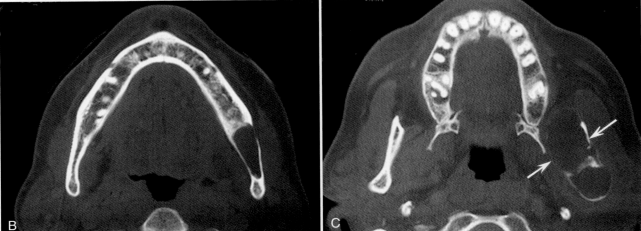

FIG. **21-14**    **A,** Cropped panoramic image of a keratocystic odontogenic tumor occupying the mandibular ramus; note the septa *(arrow).* **B** and **C,** Two axial CT images with bone algorithm of the same case demonstrating very little expansion in the body **(B)** but significant expansion in the upper ramus in **C** *(arrows).*

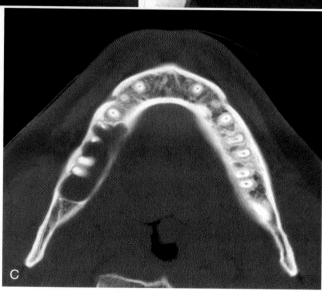

FIG. **21-15** A large keratocystic odontogenic tumor (KOT) occupying most of the right body and ramus of the mandible. **A,** Despite the large size, the buccal and lingual cortical plates of the mandible have been expanded only slightly, as can be seen in the occlusal film **(B). C,** A KOT within the body of the mandible; note the lack of expansion and the cyst scalloping between the roots of the teeth.

expansion of large lesions may exceed the ability of the periosteum to form new bone, thus allowing the cystic wall to contact soft tissue peripheral to the outer cortex of the mandible (Fig. 21-16). The relatively slight expansion common with these lesions probably contributes to their late detection, which occasionally allows them to reach a large size. KOTs can displace and resorb teeth but to a slightly lesser degree than dentigerous cysts. The inferior alveolar nerve canal may be displaced inferiorly. In the maxilla this cyst can invaginate and occupy the entire maxillary antrum.

### Differential Diagnosis

When in a pericoronal position, a KOT may be indistinguishable from a dentigerous cyst. The lesion is likely to be a KOT if the cystic outline is connected to the tooth at a point apical to the cementoenamel junction or if no expansion of the cortical plates has occurred. Also, although KOTs can develop occlusal to developing teeth, often the follicle of the involved tooth is not enlarged as in dentigerous cysts. The typical scalloped margin and multilocular appearance of the KOT may resemble an ameloblastoma, but the latter has a greater propensity to expand. A KOT may show some similarity to an odontogenic myxoma, especially in the characteristics of mild expansion and multilocular appearance. A simple bone cyst often has a scalloped margin and minimal bone expansion, as with the KOT; however, the

margins of a simple bone cyst usually are more delicate and often difficult to detect. If several KOTs are found (which occurs in 4% to 5% of cases), these tumors may constitute part of a basal cell nevus syndrome.

### Management

If a KOT is suspected, referral to a radiologist for a complete radiologic examination is advisable. Because this tumor has a propensity to recur, an accurate determination of the extent and location of any cortical perforations with soft tissue extension is best achieved with computed tomography (CT). In the case of multiple cysts and the possibility of basal cell nevus syndrome, a thorough radiologic examination that includes CT is required. This allows accurate determination of the number of cysts and other osseous characteristics that confirm the diagnosis.

Surgical treatment may vary and can include resection, curettage, or marsupialization to reduce the size of large lesions before surgical excision. More attention usually is devoted to complete removal of the cystic walls to reduce the chance of recurrence. After surgical treatment, it is important to make periodic posttreatment clinical and radiographic examinations to detect any recurrence. Recurrent lesions usually develop within the first 5 years but may be delayed as long as 10 years.

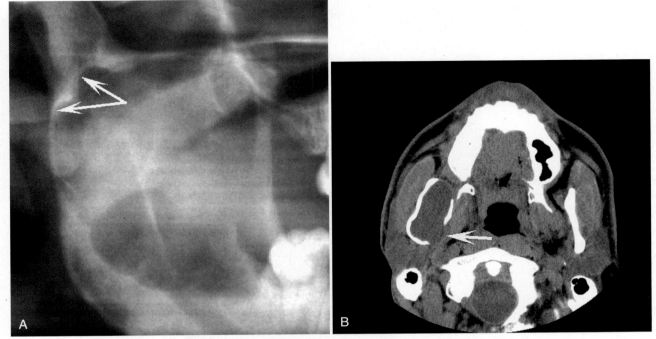

FIG. **21-16   A,** This cropped panoramic image reveals a large keratocystic odontogenic tumor occupying most of the ramus; note the scalloping margin *(arrows).* **B,** This axial CT with soft tissue window of the same case showing perforation of the medial cortex and contacting the medial pterygoid muscle *(arrow).*

## Basal Cell Nevus Syndrome

### Synonyms
Nevoid basal cell carcinoma syndrome or Gorlin-Goltz syndrome

### Definition
The term basal cell nevus syndrome comprises a number of abnormalities such as multiple nevoid basal cell carcinomas of the skin, skeletal abnormalities, central nervous system abnormalities, eye abnormalities, and multiple KOTs. It is inherited as an autosomal dominant trait with variable expressivity.

### Clinical Features
Basal cell nevus syndrome starts to appear early in life, usually after 5 years of age and before 30 years of age, with the development of KOTs within the jaws and skin basal cell carcinomas. Typically there are multiple KOTs, usually appearing in multiple quadrants and earlier in life than solitary KOTs do. The recurrence rate of KOTs in this syndrome appears to be higher than with the solitary variety. A thorough radiologic examination including CT imaging is required to detect all the jaw lesions. The skin lesions are small, flattened, flesh-colored or brown papules that can occur anywhere on the body but are especially prominent on the face, neck, and trunk. Occasionally the basal cell carcinomas will form later in life than the jaw lesions or not at all. Skeletal anomalies include bifid rib (most common) and other costal abnormalities such as agenesis, deformity, and synostosis of the ribs, kyphoscoliosis, vertebral fusion, polydactyly, shortening of the metacarpals, temporal and temporoparietal bossing, minor hyper-

telorism, and mild prognathism. Calcification of the falx cerebri and other parts of the dura occur early in life.

### Radiographic Features
*Location.* The location is the same as that of solitary KOTs, as described previously. The multiple KOTs may develop bilaterally and can vary in size from 1 mm to several centimeters in diameter (Fig. 21-17).

*Other Radiographic Features.* The reader should refer to the preceding radiographic description of KOTs. In addition, a radiopaque line of the calcified falx cerebri may be prominent on the postero-anterior skull projection. Occasionally this calcification may appear laminated.

### Differential Diagnosis
The presence of a cortical boundary and other cystic characteristics differentiate basal cell nevus syndrome from other abnormalities characterized by multiple radiolucencies (e.g., multiple myeloma). Cherubism appears as bilateral multilocular lesions but usually has significant jaw expansion, which is not characteristic of basal cell nevus syndrome. Also, cherubism pushes posterior teeth in an anterior direction, a distinctive characteristic. Occasionally patients with multiple dentigerous cysts may show some similarities, but dentigerous cysts are more expansile.

### Management
The KOTs are treated more aggressively than other solitary KOTs because there appears to be an even greater propensity for recurrence.

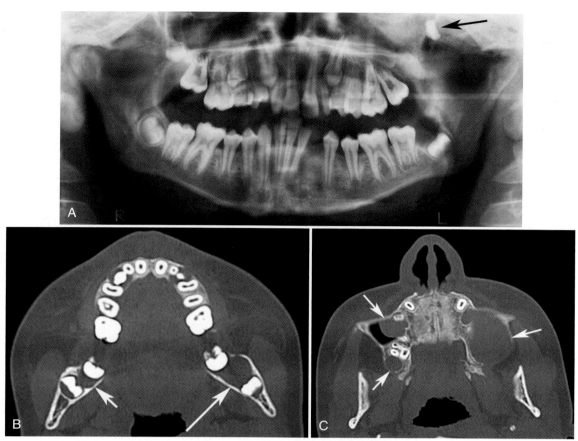

FIG. 21-17   **A,** Panoramic image of a case of basal cell nevus syndrome; note the small Keratocystic odontogenic tumor (KOT) related to the unerupted left mandibular third molar and a large KOT within the left maxilla that has displaced the left maxillary third molar *(arrow).* **B,** Axial CT of the same case; note the small mandibular KOT *(long arrow)* seen in the panoramic image and another small KOT *(short arrow)* in the right mandible not seen in the panoramic film. **C,** Another axial CT from the same case revealing the large KOT in the left maxilla and two other KOTs not readily apparent in the panoramic image.

It is reasonable to examine the patient yearly for new and recurrent cysts. A panoramic film may not be an adequate screening film (see Fig. 21-17) and therefore CT is the modality of preference. Referral for genetic counseling may be appropriate.

## Lateral Periodontal Cyst

### Definition
Lateral periodontal cysts are thought to arise from epithelial rests in periodontium lateral to the tooth root. This condition usually is unicystic, but it may appear as a cluster of small cysts, a condition referred to as botryoid odontogenic cysts. It has been postulated that the lateral periodontal cyst is the intrabony counterpart of the gingival cyst in the adult.

### Clinical Features
The lesions usually are asymptomatic and less than 1 cm in diameter. The disorder has no apparent sexual predilection, and the age distribution extends from the second to the ninth decades (the mean age is about 50 years). If these cysts become secondarily infected, they will mimic a lateral periodontal abscess.

### Radiographic Features
*Location.* A total of 50% to 75% of lateral periodontal cysts develop in the mandible, mostly in a region extending from the lateral incisor to the second premolar (Fig. 21-18). Occasionally these cysts appear in the maxilla, especially between the lateral incisor and the cuspid.

*Periphery and Shape.* A lateral periodontal cyst appears as a well-defined radiolucency with a prominent cortical boundary and a round or oval shape. Rare large cysts have a more irregular shape.

*Internal Structure.* The internal aspect usually is radiolucent. The botryoid variety may have a multilocular appearance, although this aspect is related more to the histologic appearance.

*Effects on Surrounding Structures.* Small cysts may efface the lamina dura of the adjacent root. Large cysts can displace adjacent teeth and cause expansion.

### Differential Diagnosis
Because the location and radiographic appearance of a lateral periodontal cyst are similar in other conditions, the following lesions should be included in the differential diagnosis: a small KOT, mental

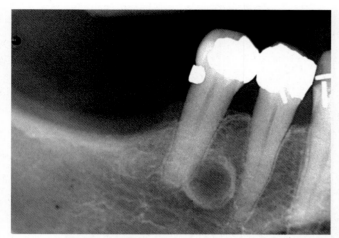

FIG. **21-18**   A lateral periodontal cyst in the mandibular premolar region; note the classic well defined cortical border.

foramen, small neurofibroma, or a radicular cyst at the foramen of a lateral (accessory) pulp canal. The multiple (botryoid) cysts with a multilocular appearance may resemble a small ameloblastoma.

### Management

Lateral periodontal cysts usually do not require sophisticated imaging because of their small size. Excisional biopsy or simple enucleation is the treatment of choice because these cysts do not tend to recur.

## Glandular Odontogenic Cyst

### Synonym
Sialo-odontogenic cyst

### Definition
The glandular odontogenic cyst is a rare cyst derived from odontogenic epithelium with a spectrum of characteristics including salivary gland features such as mucus-producing cells. Some authors hypothesize a relationship to a central mucoepidermoid carcinoma.

### Clinical Features
There is a slight female predominance with a mean age ranging from 46 to 50 years. This cyst has an aggressive behavior and a tendency to recur after surgery.

### Radiographic Features
*Location.*  This cyst occurs more commonly in the mandible and most often in the anterior mandible and in the maxilla, commonly the globulomaxillary region.

*Periphery and Shape.*  There is usually a cortical boundary that may be smooth or scalloped.

*Internal Structure.*  This cyst has been reported in both unilocular and multilocular appearances (Fig. 21-19).

*Effects on Surrounding Structures.*  Expansion of the outer cortical plates of the jaws with regions of perforation through the cortex has been reported. Displacement of teeth is a common feature.

### Differential Diagnosis
This cyst can appear identical to an ameloblastoma and in some cases may be similar to a KOT. It is interesting to note that similar multi-

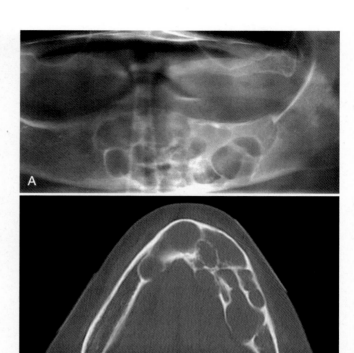

FIG. **21-19**   **A,** Cropped panoramic image of a glandular odontogenic cyst with a multilocular appearance very similar to an ameloblastoma. **B,** Axial CT image detailing the multilocular internal cystic structure.

locular appearances have been associated with central mucoepidermoid carcinomas.

### Treatment
Because of the high rate of recurrence with conservative treatments such as enucleation, more aggressive treatment including resection may be considered. Treated cases should be followed with periodic radiographic examinations to assess for recurrence.

## Calcifying Cystic Odontogenic Tumor

### Synonyms
Calcifying odontogenic cyst, calcifying epithelial odontogenic cyst, or Gorlin cyst

### Definition
The World Health Organization now categorizes this entity as a tumor. Calcifying cystic odontogenic tumors (CCOTs) are uncommon, slow-growing, benign lesions. They occupy a spectrum ranging from a cyst to an odontogenic tumor, with characteristics of a cyst alone or sometimes those of a solid neoplasm (epithelial proliferation and a tendency to continue growing). This lesion may manufacture calcified tissue identified as dysplastic dentin, and in some instances the lesion is associated with an odontoma. This lesion also sometimes contains a more solid component that gives it an appearance resembling an ameloblastoma, although it does not behave like one.

## Clinical Features

CCOTs have a wide age distribution that peaks at 10 to 19 years of age, with a mean age of 36 years. A second incidence peak occurs during the seventh decade. Clinically, the lesion usually appears as a slow-growing, painless swelling of the jaw. Occasionally the patient complains of pain. In some cases the expanding lesion may destroy the cortical plate, and the cystic mass may become palpable as it extends into the soft tissue. The patient may report a discharge from such advanced lesions. Aspiration often yields a viscous, granular, yellow fluid.

## Radiographic Features

*Location.* At least 75% of CCOTs occur in bone, with a nearly equal distribution between the jaws. Most (75%) occur anterior to the first molar, especially associated with cuspids and incisors, where the cyst sometimes manifests as a pericoronal radiolucency.

*Periphery and Shape.* The periphery can vary from well defined and corticated with a curved, cystlike shape to ill defined and irregular.

*Internal Structure.* The internal aspect can vary in appearance. It may be completely radiolucent; it may show evidence of small foci of calcified material that appear as white flecks or small smooth pebbles; or it may show even larger, solid, amorphous masses (Fig. 21-20). In rare cases the lesion may appear multilocular.

*Effects on Surrounding Structures.* Occasionally (20% to 50% of cases) this tumor is associated with a tooth (most commonly a cuspid) and impedes its eruption. Displacement of teeth and resorption of roots may occur. Perforation of the cortical plate may be seen radiographically with enlarging lesions.

## Differential Diagnosis

When no internal calcifications are evident and this lesion has a pericoronal position, it may be indistinguishable from a dentigerous cyst. Other lesions that have internal calcifications to be considered include an adenomatoid odontogenic tumor, ameloblastic fibro-odontoma, and calcifying epithelial odontogenic tumor. The common location for the CCOT is not common for either the fibro-odontoma or the calcifying epithelial odontogenic tumor. Finally, long-standing cysts may have dystrophic calcification, giving a similar appearance.

## Management

This tumor can be treated with enucleation and curettage. Because clinicians generally have little experience with the more solid neoplastic variants, it is wise to follow treatment with periodic radiographic evaluations for recurrence.

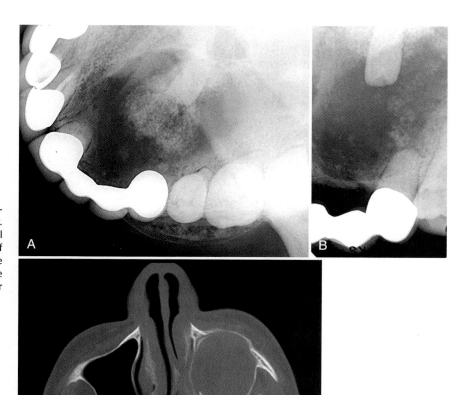

FIG. **21-20 A** and **B,** Calcifying cystic odontogenic tumor (CCOT) related to the lateral incisor. Note the well-defined corticated border, internal calcifications, and resorption of part of the root of the central incisor. **C,** Axial CT image of a large CCOT invaginating into the maxillary sinus; note the small calcifications along the posterior border (arrow).

# Nonodontogenic Cysts

## Nasopalatine Duct Cyst

### Synonyms

Nasopalatine canal cyst, incisive canal cyst, nasopalatine cyst, median palatine cyst, and median anterior maxillary cyst

### Definition

The nasopalatine canal usually contains remnants of the nasopalatine duct, a primitive organ of smell, and the nasopalatine vessels and nerves. Occasionally a cyst forms in the nasopalatine canal when these embryonic epithelial remnants of the nasopalatine duct undergo proliferation and cystic degeneration.

### Clinical Features

Nasopalatine duct cysts account for about 10% of jaw cysts. The age distribution is broad, with most cases being discovered in the fourth through sixth decades. The incidence is three times higher in males. Most of these cysts are asymptomatic or cause such minor symptoms that they are tolerated for long periods. The most frequent complaint is a small, well-defined swelling just posterior to the palatine papilla. This swelling usually is fluctuant and blue if the cyst is near the surface. The deeper nasopalatine duct cyst is covered by normal-appearing mucosa unless it is ulcerated from masticatory trauma. If the cyst expands, it may penetrate the labial plate and produce a swelling below the maxillary labial frenum or to one side. The lesion also may bulge into the nasal cavity and distort the nasal septum. Pressure from the cyst on the adjacent nasopalatine nerves that occupy the same canal may cause a burning sensation or numbness over the palatal mucosa. In some cases cystic fluid may drain into the oral cavity through a sinus tract or a remnant of the nasopalatine duct. The patient usually detects the fluid and reports a salty taste.

### Radiographic Features

*Location.* Most nasopalatine duct cysts are found in the nasopalatine foramen or canal. However, if this cyst extends posteriorly to involve the hard palate (Fig. 21-21), it often is referred to as a median palatal cyst (Fig. 21-22). If it expands anteriorly between the central incisors, destroying or expanding the labial plate of bone and causing the teeth to diverge, it sometimes is referred to as a median anterior maxillary cyst. This cyst may not always be positioned symmetrically.

*Periphery and Shape.* The periphery usually is well defined and corticated and is circular or oval in shape. The shadow of the nasal spine sometimes is superimposed on the cyst, giving it a heart shape.

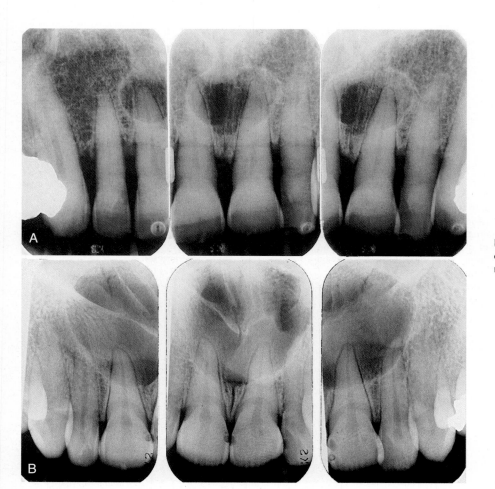

FIG. **21-21** Two examples of nasopalatine duct cysts. Note the uniform periodontal membrane space around all the apices.

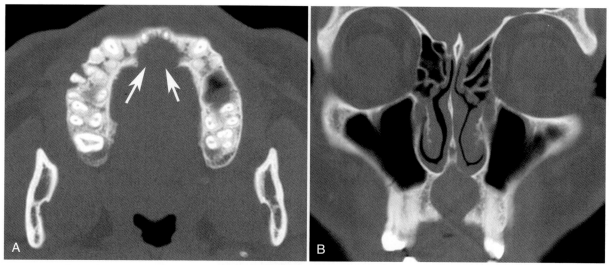

FIG. **21-22**  **A,** Axial CT image of a nasopalatine duct cyst positioned palatal to both maxillary central incisors *(arrows)*. **B,** Coronal CT image of the same case.

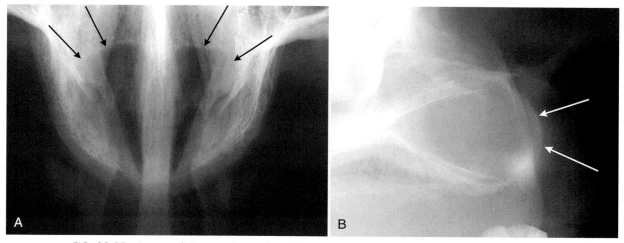

FIG. **21-23**  A nasopalatine canal cyst viewed from two perspectives: **(A)** a standard occlusal view and **(B)** from the lateral aspect, which is created by placing the film outside the mouth against the cheek and directing the x-ray beam at a tangent to the labial surface of the central incisors.

*Internal Structure.*  Most nasopalatine duct cysts are totally radiolucent. Some rare cysts may have internal dystrophic calcifications, which may appear as ill-defined, amorphous, scattered radiopacities.

*Effects on Surrounding Structures.*  Most commonly this cyst causes the roots of the central incisors to diverge, and occasionally root resorption occurs. Seen from a lateral perspective, the cyst may expand the labial cortex and the palatal cortex (Fig. 21-23). The floor of the nasal fossa may be displaced in a superior direction.

## Differential Diagnosis

The most common differential diagnosis is a large incisive foramen. A foramen larger than 6 mm may simulate the appearance of a cyst. However, a clinical examination should reveal the expansion characteristic of a cyst and other changes that occur with a space-occupying lesion, such as displacement of teeth. A lateral view of the anterior maxilla, with an occlusal film held outside the mouth and against the cheek, also can help in making the differential diagnosis, as can a cross-sectional (standard) occlusal view. If doubt still exists, comparison with previous images may be useful, or aspiration may be attempted, or another image may be made in 6 months to 1 year to assess any change in size. A radicular cyst or granuloma associated with a central incisor is similar in appearance to an asymmetric nasopalatine cyst. The presence or absence of the lamina dura and enlargement of the periodontal ligament space around the apex of the central incisor indicate an inflammatory lesion. A vitality test of the central incisor may be useful. A second periapical view taken at a different horizontal angulation should show an altered position of the image of a nasopalatine duct cyst, whereas a radicular cyst should remain centered about the apex of the central incisor.

## Management

The appropriate treatment for a nasopalatine cyst is enucleation, preferably from the palate to avoid the nasopalatine nerve. If the cyst is large and the danger exists of devitalizing the tooth or creating a naso-oral or antro-oral fistula, the surgeon may elect to marsupialize the cyst.

## Nasolabial Cyst

### Synonym
Nasoalveolar cyst

### Definition

The exact origin of nasolabial cysts is unknown. They may be fissural cysts arising from the epithelial rests in fusion lines of the globular, lateral nasal, and maxillary processes. Alternatively, the source of the epithelium may be from the embryonic nasolacrimal duct, which initially lies on the bone surface.

### Clinical Features

When this rare lesion is small, it may produce a very subtle, unilateral swelling of the nasolabial fold and may elicit pain or discomfort. When large, it may bulge into the floor of the nasal cavity, causing some obstruction, flaring of the alae, distortion of the nostrils, and fullness of the upper lip. If infected, it may drain into the nasal cavity. It usually is unilateral, but bilateral lesions have occurred. The age of detection ranges from 12 to 75 years, with a mean age of 44 years. About 75% of these lesions occur in females.

### Radiographic Features

*Location.* Nasolabial cysts are primarily soft tissue lesions located adjacent to the alveolar process above the apices of the incisors. Because this is a soft tissue lesion, plain radiographs may not show any detectable changes. The investigation could include either CT or magnetic resonance imaging (MRI), both of which can provide an image of soft tissues (Fig. 21-24).

*Periphery and Shape.* Thin axial CT images with use of the soft tissue algorithm with contrast reveal a circular or oval lesion with slight soft tissue enhancement of the periphery.

*Internal Structure.* In CT images with the soft tissue algorithm the internal aspect appears homogeneous and relatively radiolucent compared with the surrounding soft tissues.

*Effects on Surrounding Structures.* Occasionally a cyst causes erosion of the underlying bone (Fig. 21-25), producing an increased radiolucency of the alveolar process beneath the cyst and apical to the incisors. Also, the usual outline of the inferior border of the nasal fossa may become distorted, resulting in a posterior bowing of this margin.

### Differential Diagnosis

The swelling caused by an infected nasolabial cyst may simulate an acute dentoalveolar abscess. It is important to establish the vitality of the adjacent teeth. This cyst may also resemble a nasal furuncle if it pushes upward into the floor of the nasal cavity. A large mucous extravasation cyst or a cystic salivary adenoma should also be considered in the differential diagnosis of an uninfected nasolabial cyst.

### Management

The nasolabial cyst should be excised through an intraoral approach. These cysts do not tend to recur.

## Dermoid Cyst

### Definition

Dermoid cysts are a cystic form of a teratoma thought to be derived from trapped embryonic cells that are totipotential. The resulting cysts are lined with epidermis and cutaneous appendages and filled with keratin or sebaceous material (and in rare cases with bone, teeth, muscle, or hair, in which case they are properly called teratomas).

### Clinical Features

Dermoid cysts may develop in the soft tissues at any time from birth, but they usually become clinically apparent between 12 and 25 years of age, about equally distributed between the sexes. The swelling, which is slow and painless, can grow to several centimeters in diameter, and when located in the neck or tongue, it may interfere with breathing, speaking, and eating. Depending on how deep the cyst is positioned in the neck, it can deform the submental area. On palpation

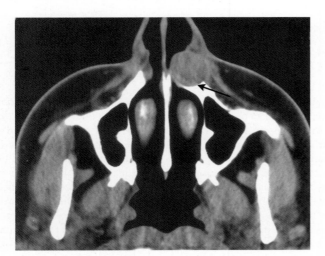

FIG. **21-24** A nasolabial cyst shown in an axial CT image with a soft tissue algorithm. Note the well-defined periphery and the erosion of the labial aspect of the alveolar process *(arrow).*

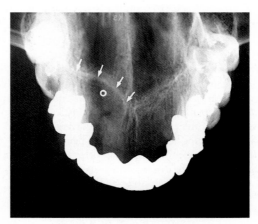

FIG. **21-25** An occlusal view of a nasolabial cyst. The radiograph shows erosion of the alveolar bone *(o)* and elevation of the floor of the nasal fossa *(arrows).* (From Chinellato LE, Damante JH: *Oral Surg Oral Med Oral Pathol* 58:729-735, 1984.)

these cysts may be fluctuant or doughy, according to their contents. Because they usually are in the midline, they do not affect the teeth.

## Radiographic Features

Because dermoid cysts are soft tissue cysts, diagnostic imaging is best accomplished by CT or MRI.

*Location.* A dermoid cyst is a rare developmental anomaly that may occur anywhere in the body. About 10% or fewer arise in the head and neck, and only 1% to 2% develop in the oral cavity. Of these, about 25% occur in the floor of the mouth and on the tongue. They may be midline or lateral in location.

*Periphery and Shape.* The periphery of the lesion usually is well defined by more radiopaque soft tissue of this cyst compared with surrounding soft tissue, as seen in CT scans.

*Internal Structure.* Dermoid cysts seldom have any internal mineralized structures when they occur in the oral cavity; therefore they are radiolucent on conventional radiographs. However, a CT scan of the area may reveal a soft tissue multilocular appearance (Fig. 21-26). If teeth or bone form in the cyst, their radiopaque images, with characteristic shapes and densities, are apparent on the radiograph.

## Differential Diagnosis

Lesions that are clinically similar to dermoid cysts are ranula (unilateral or bilateral blockage of Wharton's ducts), thyroglossal duct cysts, cystic hygromas, branchial cleft cysts, cellulitis, tumors (lipoma and liposarcoma), and normal fat masses in the submental area.

## Management

Dermoid cysts do not recur after surgical removal.

## Former Cysts

With time it has become clear that some names used to describe distinct entities are no longer valid. These names include primordial cysts (now recognized largely to be KOTs), median palatal cysts (now recognized as a variant of the nasopalatine duct cyst), and median mandibular and globulomaxillary cysts (because the entrapment of epithelium theory is no longer accepted). Globulomaxillary cysts are now recognized to be radicular or lateral periodontal cysts or KOTs.

## Cystlike Lesions

Simple bone cysts (SBCs) are included in this chapter because of their historic classification and because the characteristics and behavior seen in diagnostic imaging are cystic in nature. However, it is important to remember that these lesions are not true cysts.

## Simple Bone Cyst

### Synonyms

Traumatic bone cyst, hemorrhagic bone cyst, extravasation cyst, progressive bone cavity, solitary bone cyst, and unicameral bone cyst

### Definition

An SBC is a cavity within bone that is lined with connective tissue. It may be empty, or it may contain fluid. However, because it has no epithelial lining, it is not a true cyst. The etiology of SBCs is unknown, although they may be a localized aberration in normal bone remodeling or metabolism. This theory is supported indirectly by the fact that

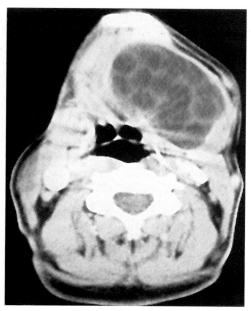

FIG. **21-26** A CT scan of a dermoid cyst showing an encapsulated mass on the left and several soft tissue loculations. (From Hunter TB, Paplanus HS, Chemin MM et al: *AJR Am J Roentgenol* 141:1239-1240, 1983.)

these bony cavities often occur inside lesions of cemento-osseous dysplasia and fibrous dysplasia. No evidence exists to support a traumatic cause.

### Clinical Features

SBCs are very common lesions. Most occur in the first two decades of life, with a mean age of 17 years. The lesion shows a male predominance of approximately 2:1. Multiple SBCs can develop, especially when the disorder occurs with cemento-osseous dysplasia. The occurrence of SBCs in cemento-osseous dysplasia is seen in an older population, with a mean age of 42 years, and with a female predominance of 4:1. SBCs are asymptomatic in most cases, but occasionally pain or tenderness may be present, especially if the cyst has become secondarily infected. Expansion of the mandible or tooth movement is possible but unusual. The teeth in the affected region usually are vital. Most SBCs are discovered only by chance, during radiographic examinations, and for this reason they can become quite large. There is no significant incidence of pathologic fractures. Aspiration usually produces only a few milliliters of straw-colored or serosanguineous fluid.

### Radiographic Features

*Location.* Almost all SBCs are found in the mandible (Fig. 21-27); in rare cases they develop in the maxilla. The lesion can occur anywhere in the mandible but is seen most often in the ramus and posterior mandible in older patients. SBCs also frequently occur with cemento-osseous and fibrous dysplasia.

*Periphery and Shape.* The margin may vary from a well-defined, delicate cortex to an ill-defined border that blends into the surrounding bone. The boundary usually is better defined in the alveolar process around the teeth than in the inferior aspect of the body of the mandible. The shape most often is smooth and curved, like a cyst, with an oval or scalloped border. The lesion often scallops between the roots of the teeth (see Fig. 21-27).

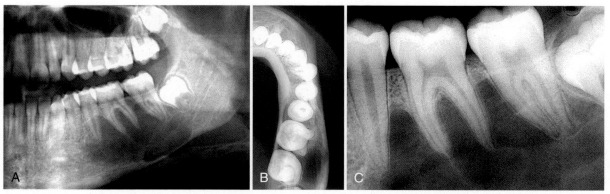

FIG. **21-27** A panoramic film demonstrating an SBC **(A)**, an occlusal film **(B)**, and a periapical film **(C).** The occlusal film shows that no expansion has occurred in the buccal or lingual cortical plates. Except for the superior border, the borders are ill defined and the lesion has scalloped around the teeth and thinned the inferior border of the mandible, but the lamina dura is still present.

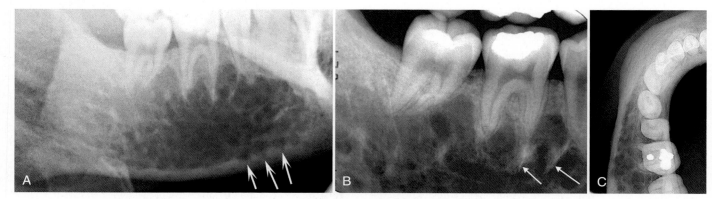

FIG. **21-28** **A,** A simple bone cyst has a multilocular appearance in this lateral oblique view of the mandible. **B,** The periapical view appears to show internal septa *(arrows)* because of the scalloping of the endosteal surface of the cortical plates, as seen in the inferior cortex *(arrows)* in **A** and of the endosteal surface of the buccal cortex in the occlusal view **(C).**

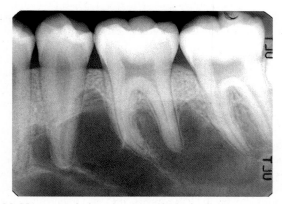

FIG. **21-29** A simple bone cyst in which the lamina dura is maintained on most root surfaces involved with the lesion except for the mesial surface of the distal root tip of the first molar.

*Internal Structure.* The internal structure is totally radiolucent, but occasionally it may appear multilocular, although the lesion does not contain true septa. This appearance is the result of pronounced scalloping of the endosteal surface of either the buccal or lingual plates (Fig. 21-28). The ridges of bone produced by the scalloping give the appearance of septa on a lateral view of the mandible.

*Effects on Surrounding Structures.* In most cases these lesions have no effect on the surrounding teeth, although rare cases of tooth displacement and resorption have been documented. Often the lesion involves all the bone around the roots of the teeth but leaves the lamina dura intact or only partly disrupted (Fig. 21-29). Similarly, the sparing of the cortical boundary of the crypt around a developing tooth is characteristic. As previously mentioned, these lesions have a propensity to scallop the endosteal surface of the outer cortex of the mandible. SBCs also have a tendency to grow along the long axis of the bone, causing minimal expansion (Fig. 21-30). However, expansion of the involved bone can occur and is more common with larger lesions (Fig. 21-31).

### Differential Diagnosis

An SBC may have an appearance similar to that of a true cyst, especially a KOT. This is because KOTs tend to grow along bone with very

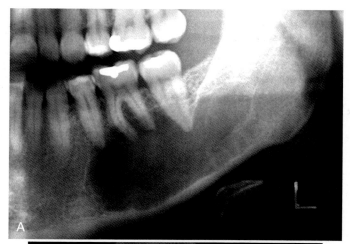

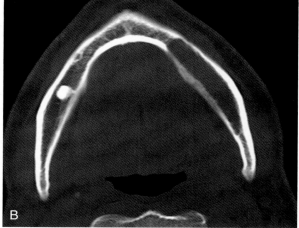

FIG. **21-30  A** and **B,** A simple bone cyst extending from the first bicuspid posteriorly to the base of the ramus and occupying most of the mandible. Considering the extent of the lesion, very little expansion of the buccal or lingual cortical plates has occurred, as can be seen in the axial CT image **(B)** with bone algorithm.

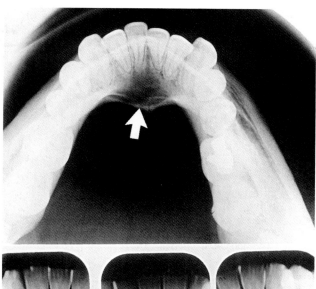

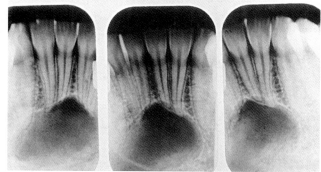

FIG. **21-31**  A simple bone cyst *(arrow)* positioned in the anterior of the mandible. Note that the superior aspect of the peripheral cortex is better defined than the inferior border and that evidence exists of some expansion of the mandible's lingual cortex, which in part may due to muscle attachment at the genial tubercles.

little expansion and often have scalloped borders similar to those of an SBC. However, KOTs usually have a more definite cortical boundary, resorb and displace teeth, and occur in an older age group. Because the SBC may remove bone around teeth without affecting the teeth, there may be a tendency to include a malignant lesion in the differential diagnosis. However, maintenance of some lamina dura and the lack of an invasive periphery and bone destruction should be enough to remove this category of diseases from consideration.

The diagnosis relies primarily on radiographic and surgical observations because the histopathologic aspects are not characteristic. These lesions occasionally heal spontaneously. A biopsy and analysis of a healing cyst may falsely indicate the presence of an ossifying fibroma or fibrous dysplasia because of the formation of new immature bone (Fig. 21-32).

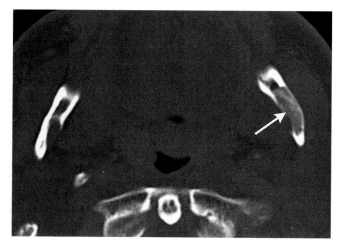

FIG. **21-32**  An axial CT image with a bone algorithm displaying a small simple bone cyst in the process of healing *(arrow)*. Note the fine internal granular bone and very slight expansion of the ramus.

## Management

The customary treatment is a conservative opening into the lesion and careful curettage of the lining; this usually initiates bleeding and subsequent healing. Spontaneous healing has been reported. Periodic follow-up radiographic examinations are advisable, especially if the patient declines treatment. These lesions can recur but it is rare.

## BIBLIOGRAPHY

Shear M: Cysts of the jaws: recent advances, *J Oral Pathol* 14:43-59, 1985.
Shear M: Developmental odontogenic cysts: an update, *J Oral Pathol Med* 23:1-11, 1994.

### ODONTOGENIC CYSTS

#### Radicular Cyst

Stockdale CR, Chandler NP: The nature of the periapical lesion: a review of 1108 cases, *J Dent* 16:123-129, 1988.
Syrjänen S, Tammisalo E, Lilja R et al: Radiological interpretation of the periapical cysts and granulomas, *Dentomaxillofac Radiol* 11:89-92, 1982.
Toller PA: Origin and growth of cysts of the jaws, *Ann R Coll Surg Engl* 40:306-336, 1967.
Wood RE, Nortjé CJ, Padayachee A et al: Radicular cysts of primary teeth mimicking premolar dentigerous cysts: report of three cases, *ASDC J Dent Child* 55:288-290, 1988.

#### Residual Cyst

High AS, Hirschmann PN: Age changes in residual cysts, *J Oral Pathol* 15:524-528, 1986.
Schwimmer AM, Aydin F, Morrison SN: Squamous cell carcinoma arising in residual odontogenic cyst: report of a case and review of literature, *Oral Surg Oral Med Oral Pathol* 72:218-221, 1991.

#### Dentigerous Cyst

Daley TD, Wysocki GP: The small dentigerous cyst, *Oral Surg Oral Med Oral Pathol Oral Radiol Endod* 79:77-81, 1995.
Lustmann J, Bodner L: Dentigerous cysts associated with supernumerary teeth, *Int J Oral Maxillofac Surg* 17:100-102, 1988.
Main DM: Follicular cysts of mandibular third molar teeth: radiological evaluation of enlargement, *Dentomaxillofac Radiol* 18:156-159, 1989.
Maxymiw WG, Wood RE: Carcinoma arising in a dentigerous cyst: a case report and review of the literature, *J Oral Maxillofac Surg* 49:639-643, 1991.

#### Buccal Bifurcation Cyst

Bohay RN, Weinberg S: The paradental cyst of the mandibular permanent first molar: report of a bilateral case, *J Dent Child* 59:361-365, 1992.
Packota GV, Hall JM, Lanigan DT et al: Paradental cysts on mandibular first molars in children: report of five cases, *Dentomaxillofac Radiol* 19:126-132, 1990.
Shear M: *Cysts of the oral regions,* Bristol, UK, 1976, John Wright & Sons.
Stoneman DW, Worth HM: The mandibular infected buccal cyst-molar area, *Dent Radiogr Photogr* 56:1-14, 1983.
Philipsen HP, Reichert PA, Ogawa I et al: The inflammatory paradental cyst: a critical review of 342 from a literature survey, including 17 new cases from the author's files, *J Oral Pathol Med* 33:147-155, 2004.

#### Keratocystic Odontogenic Tumor

Barnes L: *World Health Organization classification of tumours: pathology and genetics: head and neck tumours,* Lyon, 2005, IARC Press.
Brannon RB: The odontogenic keratocyst: a clinicopathological study of 312 cases, I: clinical features, *Oral Surg Oral Med Oral Pathol* 42:54-72, 1976.
Kakarantza-Angelopoulou E, Nicolatou O: Odontogenic keratocysts: clinicopathologic study of 87 cases, *J Oral Maxillofac Surg* 48:593-599, 1990.

Myoung H, Hong SP, Hong SD et al: Odontogenic keratocyst: review of 256 cases for recurrence and clinicopathologic parameters, *Oral Surg Oral Med Oral Pathol Oral Radiol Endod* 91:328-333, 2001.
Shear M: The aggressive nature of the odontogenic keratocyst: is it a benign cystic neoplasm, II: proliferation and genetic studies, *Oral Oncol* 38:323-331, 2002.

#### Basal Cell Nevus Syndrome

Angelopoulou E, Angelopoulos AP: Lateral periodontal cyst: review of the literature and report of a case, *J Periodontol* 61:126-131, 1990.
Donatsky O, Hjörting-Hansen E, Philipsen HP et al: Clinical, radiographic, and histologic features of the basal cell nevus syndrome, *Int J Oral Surg* 5:19-28, 1976.
Evans DC, Farndon PA, Burnell LD et al: The incidence of Gorlin syndrome in 173 consecutive cases of medulloblastoma, *Br J Cancer* 64:959-961, 1991.
Gorlin RJ: Nevoid basal cell carcinoma syndrome, *Medicine* 66:98-113, 1987.

#### Lateral Periodontal Cyst

Shear M, Pindborg JJ: Microscopic features of the lateral periodontal cyst, *Scand J Dent Res* 83:103-110, 1975.
Weathers DR, Waldron CA: Unusual multilocular cysts of the jaws (botryoid odontogenic cysts), *Oral Surg Oral Med Oral Pathol* 36:235-241, 1973.
Wysocki GP, Brannon RB, Gardner DG et al: Histogenesis of the lateral periodontal cyst and the gingival cyst of the adult, *Oral Surg Oral Med Oral Pathol* 50:327-334, 1980.

#### Glandular Odontogenic Cyst

Koppang HS, Johannessen S, Haugen LK et al: Glandular odontogenic cyst: report of two cases and literature review of 45 previously reported cases, *J Oral Pathol Med* 27:455-462, 1998.
Noffke C, Raubenheimer EJ: The glandular odontogenic cyst: clinical and radiologic features: review of the literature and report of nine cases, *Dentomaxillofac Radiol* 31:333-338, 2002.

#### Calcifying Cystic Odontogenic Tumor

Johnson A III, Fletcher M, Gold L et al: Calcifying odontogenic cyst: a clinicopathologic study of 57 cases with immunohistochemical evaluation for cytokeratin, *J Oral Maxillofac Surg* 55:679-683, 1997.
Moleri AB, Moreira LC, Carvalho JJ: Comparative morphology of 7 new cases of calcifying odontogenic cysts, *J Oral Maxillofac Surg* 60:689-696, 2002.
Yoshiura K, Tabata O, Miwa K et al: Computed tomographic features of calcifiying odontogenic cysts, *Dentomaxillofac Radiol* 27:12-16, 1998.

### NONODONTOGENIC CYSTS

#### Nasopalatine Duct Cyst

Elliott KA, Franzese CB, Pitman KT: Diagnosis and surgical management of nasopalatine duct cysts, *Laryngoscope* 114:1336-1340, 2004.
Mraiwa RJ, Jacobs R, Van Cleynenbreugel J et al: The nasopalatine duct cyst revisited using 2D and 3D CT imaging, *Dentomaxillofac Radiol* 33:396-402, 2004.
Swanson KS, Kaugars GE, Gunsolley JC: Nasopalatine duct cyst: an analysis of 334 cases, *J Oral Maxillofac Surg* 49:268-271, 1991.

#### Nasolabial Cyst

Choi JH, Cho JH, Kang HJ et al: Nasolabial cysts: a retrospective analysis of 18 cases, *Ear Nose Throat J* 81:94-96, 2002.
Yuen H, Julian CY, Samuel CL: Nasolabial cysts: clinical features, diagnosis and treatment, *Br J Oral Maxillofac Surg* 45:293-297, 2007.

#### Dermoid Cyst

Seward GR: Dermoid cysts of the floor of the mouth, *Br J Oral Surg* 3:36-47, 1965.

## CYSTLIKE LESIONS

### Simple Bone Cyst

Damante JH, Da S, Guerra EN et al: Spontaneous resolution of simple bone cysts, *Dentomaxillofac Radiol* 31:182-186, 2002.

Kaugars GE, Cale AE: Traumatic bone cyst, *Oral Surg Oral Med Oral Pathol* 63:318-324, 1987.

Perdigao AF, Silva EC, Sakurai E et al: Idiopathic bone cavity: a clinical, radiographic and histological study, *Br J Oral Maxillofac Surg* 41:407-409, 2003.

Saito Y, Hoshina Y, Nagamine T et al: Simple bone cyst: a clinical and histopathologic study of fifteen cases, *Oral Surg Oral Med Oral Pathol* 74:487-491, 1992.

Sapp PJ, Stark ML: Self-healing traumatic bone cysts, *Oral Surg Oral Med Oral Pathol* 69:597-602, 1990.

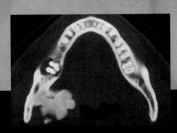

# CHAPTER 22

# Benign Tumors of the Jaws

## Definition

Benign tumors represent a new uncoordinated growth that generally has the following characteristics. Benign tumors are slowly growing and spread by direct extension and not by metastases. Histologically they tend to resemble the tissue of origin. For example, an ameloblastoma, a tumor thought to be derived from odontogenic epithelium, is often composed of cells that resemble ameloblasts. It is thought that benign tumors have unlimited growth potential. Often hamartomas are included in the category of benign tumors. However, hamartomas are overgrowths of disorganized normal tissue that have a limited growth potential. For example, an odontoma is a hamartoma of dental tissue (disorganized enamel, dentine, and pulp tissues) derived from the dental follicle that stops growing at approximately the same time as other normal dental tissues. Included in this chapter are hyperplasias. Hyperplasia refers to a growth formed by an increase in the number of cells of a tissue but differs from hamartomas in that the tissue is in a normal arrangement. Hyperplasia is generally thought to be a reaction to a stimulus such as inflammation. Therefore they have limited growth potential and tend to regress when the stimulus is removed.

## Clinical Features

Benign tumors typically have an insidious onset and grow slowly. These tumors usually are painless, do not metastasize, and are not life threatening unless they interfere with a vital organ by direct extension.

Benign tumors are usually detected clinically by enlargement of the jaws or are found during a radiographic examination. Sometimes the radiologic examination is to try to discover the reason for the lack of development of a tooth.

## Radiographic Examination

Once the clinician has made a preliminary diagnosis of the presence of a tumor, a full radiologic examination should be made to fully document the extent and characteristics of the lesion. This may entail further films such as intraoral and occlusal radiographs or a panoramic film. For central bone lesions the addition of computed tomography is essential for assessing the effects on the surrounding osseous structures. If the lesion originates in soft tissue or has extended from bone into the surrounding soft tissue, then magnetic resonance imaging may be required.

A thorough radiologic examination will provide information regarding the extent of the lesion, and sometimes the characteristics

are so specific that a preliminary diagnosis of the type of benign tumor can be made. On the other hand, the imaging characteristics of the lesion may fail to indicate the type of tumor. A thorough workup will also indicate the most favorable biopsy site. The radiologic examination should always be completed before the biopsy procedure.

## Radiographic Features

The following general features suggest the presence of a benign neoplasm.

### LOCATION

Because many tumors have a specific anatomic predilection, the location of a particular neoplasm is important in establishing the differential diagnosis. For example, odontogenic lesions occur in the alveolar processes above the inferior alveolar nerve canal, where tooth formation occurs. Vascular and neural lesions may originate inside the mandibular canal, arising from the neurovascular tissues. Cartilaginous tumors occur in jaw locations where residual cartilaginous cells lie, such as around the mandibular condyle.

### PERIPHERY AND SHAPE

Benign tumors enlarge slowly by formation of additional internal tissue. Because of this, the radiographic borders of benign tumors appear relatively smooth, well defined, and sometimes corticated. If the tumor produces a calcified product, for example, abnormal tooth material or abnormal bone, the most mature part of the tumor will be in the central region with the most immature aspect at the periphery. This sometimes results in a radiolucent band of soft tissue or capsule at the periphery where the calcified product has not yet formed; this band separates the more mature internal radiopaque portion from the surrounding normal bone.

### INTERNAL STRUCTURE

The internal structure may be completely radiolucent or radiopaque or may be a mixture of radiolucent and radiopaque tissues. If the lesion contains radiopaque elements, these structures usually represent either residual bone or a calcified material that is being produced by the tumor. For instance, curved septa that are characteristic in ameloblastoma represent residual bone trapped inside the tumor that has remodeled into curved septa. The ameloblastoma does not produce bone. On the other hand, the osteoblastoma often has an internal granular radiopaque pattern produced by the abnormal bone that is actually being manufactured by the tumor. Often the internal pattern is characteristic for specific types of tumors and may help with the diagnosis. A totally radiolucent internal structure is not as useful as an aid to the diagnosis.

## EFFECTS ON SURROUNDING STRUCTURES

The manner in which a tumor affects adjacent tissues may suggest a benign behavior. For example, a benign tumor exerts pressure on neighboring structures, resulting in the displacement of teeth or bony cortices. If the growth is slow enough, there will be adequate time for the outer cortex to remodel in response to the pressure, resulting in an appearance that the cortex has been displaced by the tumor (Fig. 22-1). This is caused by simultaneous resorption of bone along the inner surface (endosteal) of the cortex and deposition of bone along the outer cortical surface by the periosteum (Fig. 22-2). Through this remodeling process, the cortex maintains its integrity and resists perforation, although faster growing tumors may exceed this process, resulting in perforation of the cortex. Benign tumors may also cause bodily displacement of nearby teeth (Fig. 22-3). The movement of teeth adjacent to benign tumors is slow because these lesions grow slowly.

The roots of teeth may be resorbed by either benign or malignant tumors, but root resorption is more commonly associated with benign processes. The benign tumors especially likely to resorb roots are ameloblastomas, ossifying fibromas, and central giant cell granulomas. Benign tumors tend to resorb the adjacent root surfaces in a smooth fashion. Bone dysplasias such as fibrous dysplasia do not usually resorb teeth. When root resorption is associated with malignant tumors, the resorption is usually in smaller quantities, causing thinning of the root into a "spiked" shape.

## Hyperplasias

Bony hyperplasias are included in this chapter but are not considered tumors because of the normal arrangement of the tissue and the limited growth potential; in some cases this growth is in response to a stimulus. Bony hyperplasias are growths of normal new bone that sometimes occur in characteristic locations. In dentistry the terms *exostosis* and *hyperostosis* are both used to describe a bony growth that occurs on the surface of normal bone. It should be noted that in medicine the term *exostosis* often is used for a surface bony growth with a cartilage cap (osteochondroma). Therefore the term *hyperostosis* may be preferred to avoid confusion.

### Torus Palatinus

**Synonym**
Palatine torus

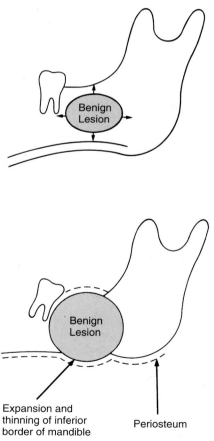

FIG. **22-1** Benign lesions growing in bone tend to be round or oval. They grow by displacing adjacent tissues. (From Matteson SR, Tyndall DA, Burkes EJ et al: The radiology of benign and malignant lesion, *Dent Radiogr Photogr* 57:35-52, 78-84, 1985.)

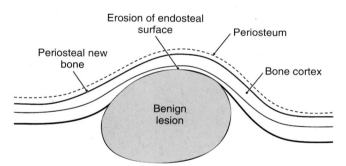

FIG. **22-2** The host bone of a benign tumor may expand as a result of outward remodeling of its cortical borders. As the benign tumor extends toward the periphery of the bone, the periosteum lays down new bone along the outer cortex, thereby maintaining the integrity of the cortex.

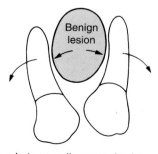

FIG. **22-3** A benign lesion usually grows slowly, causing displacement of adjacent teeth. (From Matteson SR, Tyndall DA, Burkes EJ et al: The radiology of benign and malignant lesions, *Dent Radiogr Photogr* 57:35-52, 78-84, 1985.)

## Definition

Torus palatinus is a bony protuberance (hyperostosis) that occurs in the middle third of the midline of the hard palate.

## Clinical Features

Torus palatinus, the most common exostoses, occurs in about 20% of the population, although various studies have shown marked differences in racial groups. It develops about twice as often in women as in men and more often in Native Americans, Eskimos, and Norwegians. Although it may be discovered at any age, it is rare in children. It usually begins developing in young adults before 30 years of age and is thought to arise through interplay of genetic and environmental factors. The base of the bony nodule extends along the central portion of the hard palate, and the bulk reaches downward into the oral cavity. The size and shape of a torus palatinus can vary, and these lesions have been described as flat, lobulated, nodular, or mushroomlike (Fig. 22-4, *A*). Normal mucosa covers the bony mass and may appear pale and sometimes ulcerated when traumatized. Patients often are unaware of this hyperplasia, and those who do discover it may insist that it occurred suddenly and has been growing rapidly.

## Radiographic Features

*Location.* On maxillary periapical or panoramic radiographs, a torus palatinus appears as a dense radiopaque shadow below and attached to the hard palate. It may be superimposed over the apical areas of the maxillary teeth, especially if the torus has developed in the middle or anterior regions of the palate. The image of a palatal torus may project over the roots of the maxillary molars (Fig. 22-4, *B*), but the shadow will usually move in its position relative to the roots of the teeth if another film is taken with a different horizontal or vertical angulation of the central ray (Fig. 22-5).

*Periphery and Shape.* The border of the radiopaque shadow usually is well defined and may have a convex or a lobulated outline (Fig. 22-6).

*Internal Structure.* The internal aspect is homogeneously radiopaque.

## Treatment

A torus palatinus usually does not require treatment, although removal may be necessary if a maxillary denture is to be made.

### Torus Mandibularis

## Synonym

Mandibular torus

## Definition

Torus mandibularis is a hyperostosis that protrudes from the lingual aspect of the mandibular alveolar process, usually near the premolar teeth.

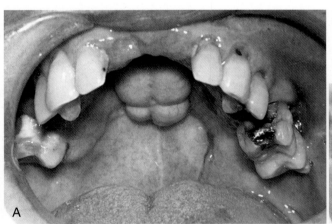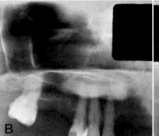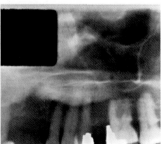

FIG. **22-4** **A,** A clinical photograph of torus palatinus. **B,** A panoramic radiograph shows the radiopaque shadow of torus palatinus above the maxillary premolars and canine. (Courtesy Ronald Baker, DDS, Chapel Hill, N.C.)

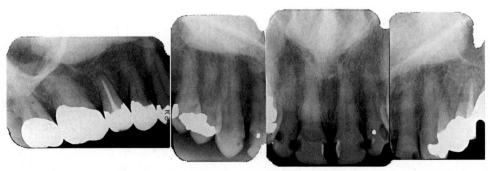

FIG. **22-5** Maxillary periapical radiographs show a radiopaque area with the well-defined borders of torus palatinus.

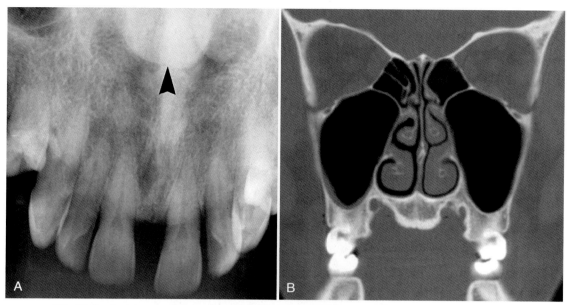

FIG. **22-6**  **A,** A torus palatinus *(arrowhead)* in an occlusal image and, **B,** in a coronal CT image.

### Clinical Features

Tori occur less often on the lingual surface of the mandible than on the palate, with the former occurring in about 8% of the population. These tori develop singly or multiply, unilaterally or bilaterally (usually bilaterally), and most often in the premolar region. The size also varies, ranging from an outgrowth that is just palpable to one that contacts a torus on the opposite side. In contrast to torus palatinus, torus mandibularis develops later, being first discovered in middle-aged adults. However, it has the same sex predilection as torus palatinus. In women the occurrence of torus mandibularis correlates with that of torus palatinus, but this apparently is not the case in men. As with torus palatinus, torus mandibularis may occur more often in those of East Asian ancestry.

Genetic and environmental factors seem to be involved in the development of torus mandibularis, but masticatory stress is reported as an essential factor underlying its formation. The high prevalence among Eskimos and other subarctic peoples who make extraordinary chewing demands on their teeth seems to support this suggestion. Also, a patient with a torus mandibularis has, on average, more teeth present than a patient without a torus.

### Radiographic Features

*Location.* Recognition of mandibular tori relies on their appearance and location. Their presence bilaterally reinforces this impression, although they can occur unilaterally. On mandibular periapical radiographs, a torus mandibularis appears as a radiopaque shadow, usually superimposed on the roots of premolars and molars and occasionally over a canine or incisor. It usually is superimposed over about three teeth.

*Periphery.* Mandibular tori are sharply demarcated anteriorly on periapical films and are less dense and less well defined as they extend posteriorly (Fig. 22-7). There is no margin between the periphery of the torus and the surface of the mandible because the torus is continuous with the mandibular cortex.

*Internal Structure.* On occlusal radiographs a mandibular torus appears as a radiopaque and homogeneous (Fig. 22-8).

### Treatment

A torus mandibularis usually does not require treatment, although removal may be necessary if a mandibular denture is planned.

## OTHER EXOSTOSES

### Synonym

Hyperostosis

### Definition

In addition to the torus, other exostoses may occur at other sites in the jaws. These are usually small regions of osseous hyperplasia of cortical bone and occasionally internal cancellous bone that usually occur on the surface of the alveolar process.

### Clinical Features

Exostoses may develop most commonly on the buccal surface of the maxillary alveolar process, usually in the canine or molar area. They may also occur on the palatal surface or crest and less commonly on the mandibular alveolar process. Occasionally they will grow on the crest under a pontic of a fixed bridge. They are less common than mandibular or palatine tori, may attain a large size, and may be solitary or multiple. They are nodular, pedunculated, or flat prominences on the surface of the bone. They are covered with a normal mucosa and are bony hard on palpation. No published data indicate their actual incidence or whether they occur more often in one sex. As with the exostoses described previously, they appear to be more prevalent in Native Americans.

### Radiographic Features

*Location.* The maxillary alveolar process is the most common location and usually the image overlaps the roots of the adjacent teeth.

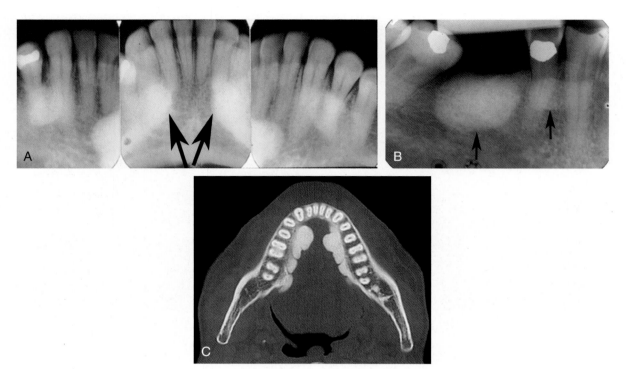

FIG. **22-7** Mandibular tori usually are seen as dense radiopacities *(arrows)* in **A** and **B. C,** An axial CT image with bilateral mandibular tori.

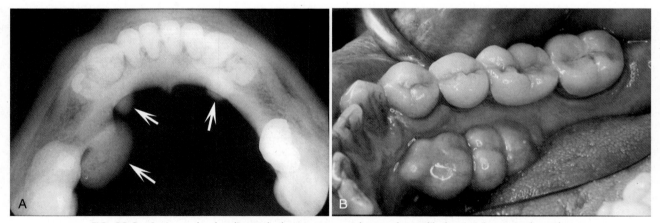

FIG. **22-8** **A,** An occlusal radiograph shows an unusual case of mandibular tori *(arrows)* where the number and size are not symmetric between the sides. **B,** Clinical picture of a different case; the tori extend from the region of the cuspid to the first molar. (**B** courtesy Dr. Bernard Friedland, Harvard University.)

**Periphery.** The periphery of an exostosis is usually well defined and smoothly contoured with a curved border (Fig. 22-9). However, some may have poorly defined borders that blend radiographically into the surrounding normal bone.

**Internal Structure.** The internal aspect of an exostosis usually is homogeneous and radiopaque. Although large exostoses can have an internal cancellous bone pattern, they most often consist only of cortical bone.

**Treatment**

Exostoses usually do not require treatment.

## Dense Bone Island

### Synonyms

Enostosis and periapical idiopathic osteosclerosis

### Definition

Dense bone islands (DBIs) are the internal counterparts of exostoses. They are localized growths of compact bone that develop within the cancellous bone.

### Clinical Features

DBIs are asymptomatic.

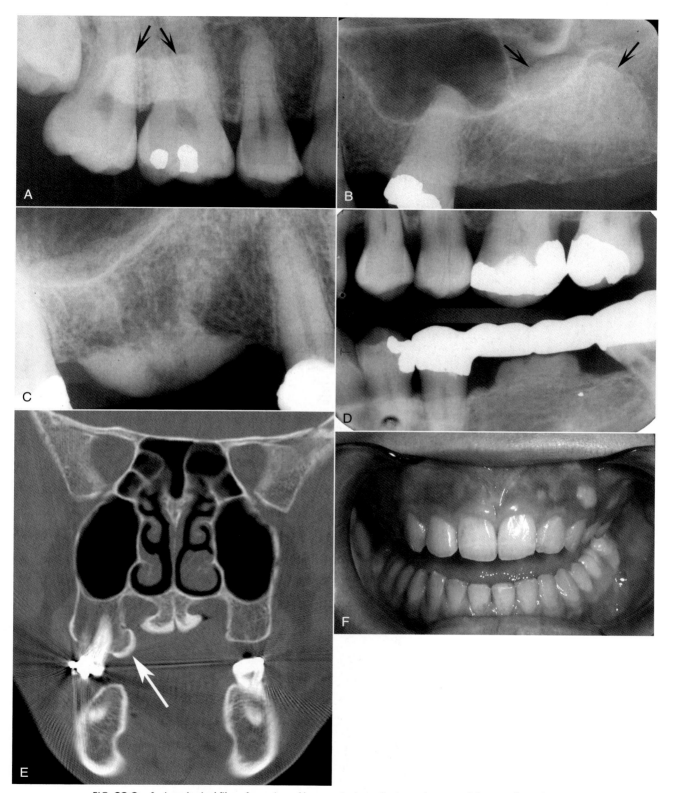

FIG. **22-9**   **A,** A periapical film of a region of hyperostosis on the buccal aspect of the maxillary alveolar process, seen as an region of slight increase in radiopacity overlapping the roots of the molars *(arrows)*. **B,** Another example overlapping an edentulous ridge. **C,** An example occurring on the crest of the alveolar ridge. **D,** An example occurring under a bridge pontic. **E,** A coronal CT image of hyperostosis located on the palatal aspect of the right maxillary alveolar process; note the presence of a maxillary torus. **F,** A clinical photograph of a small hyperostosis occurring on the labial surface of the maxillary alveolar ridge.

## Radiographic Features

*Location.* DBIs are more common in the mandible than in the maxilla. They occur most often in the premolar-molar area (Fig. 22-10), although their existence does not correlate with the presence or absence of teeth.

*Periphery.* The periphery is usually well defined but occasionally blends with the trabeculae of the surrounding bone. There is no trace of a radiolucent margin or capsule; the radiopaque dense bone island abuts directly against normal bone.

*Internal Structure.* The internal aspect of DBIs usually is uniformly radiopaque without any characteristic pattern, but sometimes, depending on its form and thickness, there may be patches of more radiolucent areas.

*Effects on Surrounding Structures.* In rare instances a DBI is located periapical to a tooth root and is associated with external root resorption (see Fig. 22-10, *C*). The tooth most often involved is the mandibular first molar. In all circumstances the tooth is vital and the

root resorption appears to be self-limiting. In very rare cases DBIs can inhibit the eruption of a tooth and even displace a tooth.

### Differential Diagnosis

Several radiopaque lesions must be considered in forming a differential diagnosis. Periapical cemental dysplasia can be differentiated by the presence of its radiolucent periphery. When a DBI is located at the root apex, it may resemble periapical sclerosing osteitis. However, in periapical osteitis there is an associated widening of the periapical portion of the periodontal membrane space. Also, periapical osteitis should be centered on the root apex of the tooth and extend in a more symmetric form in every direction. Finally, an inflammatory lesion may have an apparent etiology such as a large restoration or carious lesion. There may be some similarity to hypercementosis or a benign cementoblastoma, but in both cases there should be a soft tissue (radiolucent) capsule at the periphery. DBIs are often static but may increase in size, especially when there is active growth of the jaws. If

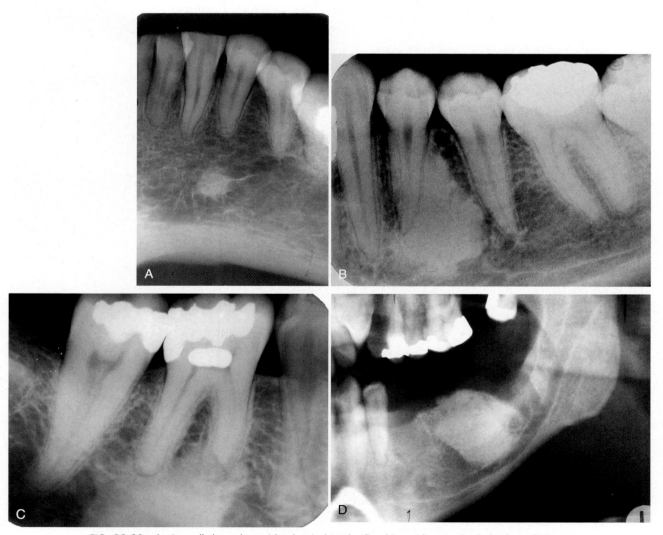

FIG. **22-10**  **A,** A small dense bone island apical to the first bicuspid; note the lack of a soft tissue capsule and that some of the surrounding trabeculae appear to merge into the radiopaque mass. **B,** A larger dense bone island between the bicuspids; note the normal-appearing periodontal membrane space. **C,** Another example apical to the first molar causing external root resorption of the mesial root. **D,** A large dense bone island occupying the body of the left mandible.

several DBIs (five or more) are present, multiple polyposis syndromes (e.g., Gardner's syndrome) should be considered.

### Treatment

Enostosis does not require treatment. If multiple, the patient's family history should be reviewed for incidences of cancer of the intestine.

## Benign Tumors

The benign neoplasias are separated into two major groups, odontogenic tumors and nonodontogenic tumors.

## ODONTOGENIC TUMORS

Odontogenic tumors arise from the tissues of the odontogenic apparatus. According to the World Health Organization (WHO), these tumors can be classified into three categories depending on the type of tissue that comprises each tumor. The categories are tumors of odontogenic epithelium, mixed tumors of both odontogenic epithelium and odontogenic ectomesenchyme (connective tissue), and tumors composed of primarily ectomesenchyme. Odontogenic tumors comprise 1.3% to 15% of all oral tumors. The following text presents benign jaw tumors according to their tissues of origin. This format should assist the reader in learning to correlate the radiographic appearance of tumors with the underlying pathologic basis of the disease process.

## ODONTOGENIC EPITHELIAL TUMORS

### Ameloblastoma

#### Synonyms

Adamantinoma, adamantoblastoma, adontomes embryolastiques, and epithelial odontoma

#### Definition

The ameloblastoma, a true neoplasm of odontogenic epithelium, is a persistent and locally invasive tumor; it has aggressive but benign growth characteristics. The ameloblastoma represents about 1% of all oral odontogenic epithelial tumors and 11% of all odontogenic tumors. It is an aggressive neoplasm that arises from remnants of the dental lamina and dental organ (odontogenic epithelium). Malignant forms of this neoplasm do exist and are discussed in Chapter 23. Ameloblastomas may be divided into the solid/multicystic type, the unicystic type, and the desmoplastic type. The unicystic variant may develop as a single entity or may form from the epithelial lining of a dentigerous cyst, called a mural (within the wall) ameloblastoma. The existence of peripheral (soft tissue location) forms of this neoplasm is well documented.

*Clinical Features.* There is a slight predilection for this lesion to occur in men, and it develops more often in blacks. Although it may be found in the young (age 3 years) and in individuals older than 80 years, most patients are between 20 and 50 years, with the average age at discovery about 40 years.

Ameloblastomas grow slowly, and few, if any, symptoms occur in the early stages. The tumor is frequently discovered during a routine dental examination. Usually the patient eventually notices gradually increasing facial asymmetry. Swelling of the cheek, gingiva, or hard palate has been reported as the chief complaint in 95% of untreated maxillary ameloblastomas. The mucosa over the mass is normal, but teeth in the involved region may be displaced and become mobile. In most cases patients with ameloblastomas do not have pain, paresthesia, fistula, ulcer formation, or tooth mobility. As the tumor enlarges, palpation may elicit a bony hard sensation or crepitus as the bone thins. If the lesion destroys overlying bone, the swelling may feel firm or fluctuant. As it grows, this tumor can cause bony expansion and sometimes erosion through the adjacent cortical plate with subsequent invasion of the adjacent soft tissues.

An untreated tumor may grow to great size and is more of a concern in the maxilla, where it can extend into vital structures and reach into the cranial base. Tumors that develop in the maxilla may extend into the paranasal sinuses, orbit, nasopharynx, or vital structures at the base of the skull. Recurrence rates are higher in older patients and in those with multilocular lesions. As seen with other jaw tumors, local recurrence, whether detected radiographically or histologically, may have a more aggressive character than the original tumor.

#### Radiographic Features

*Location.* Most ameloblastomas (80%) develop in the molar-ramus region of the mandible, but they may extend to the symphyseal area. Most lesions that occur in the maxilla are in the third molar area and extend into the maxillary sinus and nasal floor. In either jaw this tumor can originate in an occlusal position to a developing tooth (Fig. 22-11).

*Periphery.* The ameloblastoma is usually well defined and frequently delineated by a cortical border. The border is often curved, and in small lesions the border and shape may be indistinguishable from a cyst (Fig. 22-12). The periphery of lesions in the maxilla is usually more ill defined.

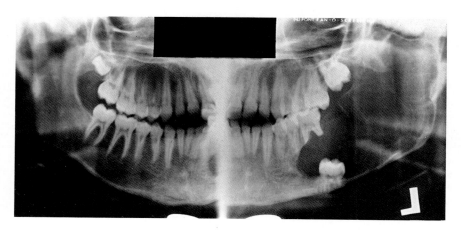

FIG. 22-11 A unicystic ameloblastoma developing occlusal to the left second mandibular molar causing expansion of the mandibular body and ramus to the sigmoid notch and condylar neck and inferior displacement of the mandibular second molar and root resorption of the alveolar left first molar. (Courtesy E. J. Burkes, DDS, Chapel Hill, N.C.)

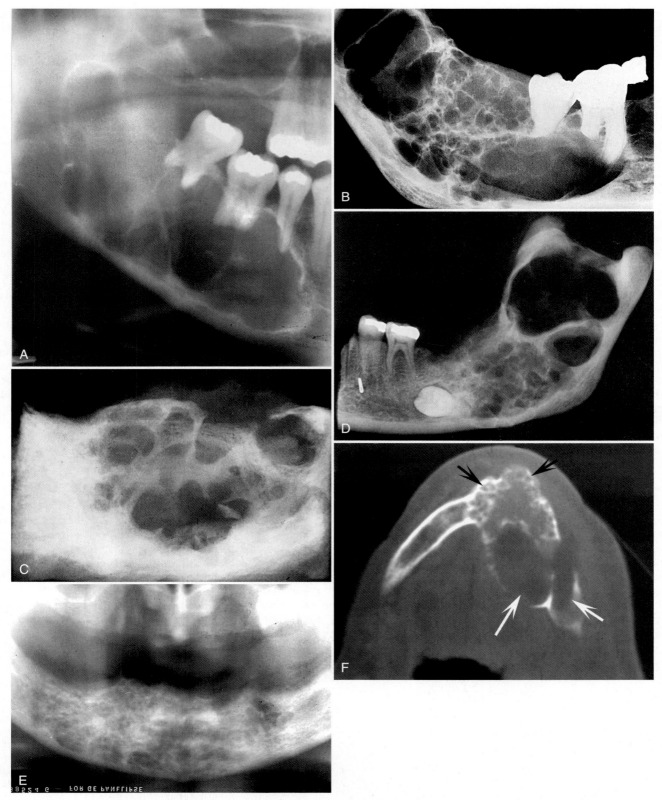

FIG. **22-12** **Multilocular Ameloblastomas. A,** A large lesion in the mandibular body and ramus shows only a few rather straight septa. **B,** Lateral radiograph of a resected mandibular specimen containing a multilocular ameloblastoma; note the coarse curved septa. **C,** Another surgical specimen of an ameloblastoma. **D,** A large multilocular lesion in the right mandibular ramus. **E,** A cropped panoramic image showing small loculations that are more common in the anterior mandible. **F,** An axial CT image with bone algorithm showing a large ameloblastoma; note the smaller loculations in the anterior mandible *(black arrows)* and the larger loculations in the posterior mandible *(white arrows).*

*Internal Structure.* The internal structure varies from totally radiolucent (see Fig. 22-11) to mixed with the presence of bony septa creating internal compartments. These septa can be straight but are more commonly coarse and curved and originate from normal bone that has been trapped within the tumor. Because this tumor frequently has internal cystic components, these septa are often remodeled into curved shapes providing a honeycomb (numerous small compartments or loculations) or soap bubble (larger compartments of variable size) patterns (see Fig. 22-12). Generally the loculations are larger in the posterior mandible and smaller in the anterior mandible. In the desmoplastic variety the internal structure can be composed of very irregular sclerotic bone resembling a bone dysplasia or bone-forming tumor (Fig. 22-13).

*Effects on Surrounding Structures.* There is a pronounced tendency for ameloblastomas to cause extensive root resorption (Fig. 22-14). Tooth displacement is common. Because a common point of origin is occlusal to a tooth, some teeth may be displaced apically. An occlusal radiograph may demonstrate cystlike expansion and thinning of an adjacent cortical plate leaving a thin "eggshell" of bone (Fig. 22-15). Computed tomographic (CT) images often reveal regions of perforation of the expanded cortical plate as a result of the inability of the production of periosteal new bone to keep up with the rate of growth of the expanding ameloblastoma (Fig. 22-16). Unicystic types of ameloblastoma may cause extreme expansion of the mandibular ramus, and often the anterior border of the ramus is no longer visible in the panoramic image (Fig. 22-17).

## RECURRENT AMELOBLASTOMA

Ameloblastomas may recur when the initial surgical procedure inadequately removes the entire tumor. Recurrent tumor has a characteristic appearance of multiple small cystlike structures with very coarse sclerotic cortical margins (Fig. 22-18) sometimes separated by normal bone.

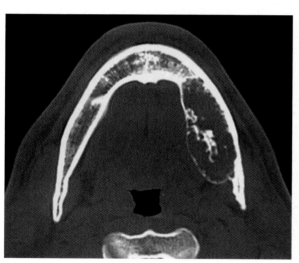

FIG. **22-13** An example of the desmoplastic type of ameloblastoma; note the internal irregular bone formation in this axial CT image.

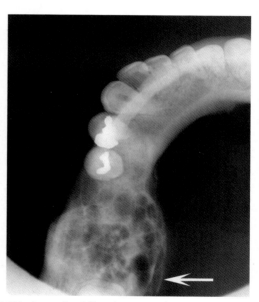

FIG. **22-15** An occlusal film demonstrating expansion of the lingual cortex with maintenance of a thin outer shell of bone *(arrow).*

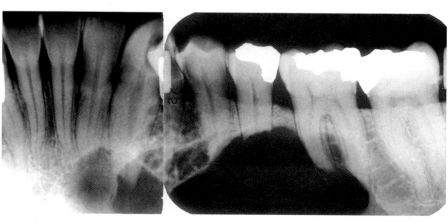

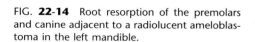

FIG. **22-14** Root resorption of the premolars and canine adjacent to a radiolucent ameloblastoma in the left mandible.

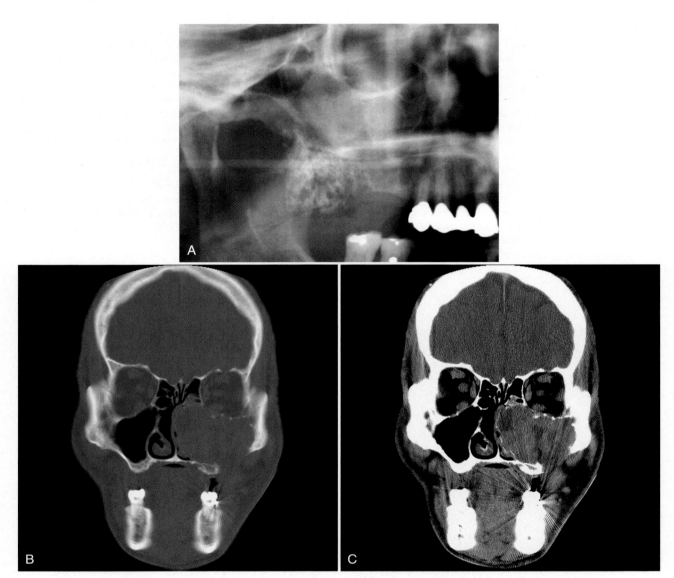

FIG. **22-16** A cropped panoramic image of an ameloblastoma involving the left maxilla; note the multilocular appearance in the tuberosity region. It is not possible to determine the extent of the lesion with the panoramic film. **B** and **C,** The same coronal CT image slices with both bone and soft tissue algorithms of the same case; note the aggressive nature of the tumor as it has grown into the sinus and nasal fossa and perforated the lateral cortical plate of the maxilla.

## Additional Imaging

If a preliminary diagnosis of ameloblastoma is made, then CT imaging is highly recommended. CT imaging cannot only confirm the diagnosis but also will accurately demonstrate the anatomic extent of the tumor (see Fig. 22-16). Of importance is the ability of CT imaging to detect perforation of the outer cortex and invasion into the surrounding soft tissues. If soft tissue invasion is extensive, magnetic resonance imaging (MRI) will provide superior images of the nature and extent of the invasion. CT examination is essential in the postsurgical follow-up assessment of ameloblastoma.

## Differential Diagnosis

Small unilocular ameloblastomas that are located around the crown of an unerupted tooth often cannot be differentiated from a dentiger-ous cyst. Because the appearance of the internal bony septa is important for the identification of ameloblastoma, other types of lesions that also have internal septa such as the odontogenic kerato-cyst, giant cell granuloma, odontogenic myxoma, and ossifying fibroma may have a similar appearance. The odontogenic keratocyst may contain curved septa, but usually the keratocyst tends to grow along the bone without marked expansion, which is characteristic of ameloblastomas. Giant cell granulomas occur in a younger age group and have more granular or wispy ill-defined septa. Odontogenic myxomas may have similar-appearing septa; however, there are usually one or two thin sharp, straight septa, which is characteristic of the myxoma. Even the presence of one such septum may indicate a myxoma. Also, myxomas are not as expansile as ameloblastomas and tend to grow along the bone. The septa in ossifying fibroma are usually wide, granular, and ill defined and often there are small irregular trabeculae.

## Treatment

The most common treatment is surgical resection. The surgical procedure should take into account the tendency of the neoplasm to invade adjacent bone beyond its apparent radiographic margins. CT and MRI are useful in determining the exact extent of the tumor. If the ameloblastoma is relatively small, it may be removed completely by an intraoral approach, but larger lesions may require resection of the jaw. The maxilla is usually treated more aggressively because of the tendency of ameloblastoma to invade adjacent vital structures. Radiation therapy may be used for inoperable tumors, especially those in the posterior maxilla.

## Calcifying Epithelial Odontogenic Tumor

### Synonyms

Pindborg tumor and ameloblastoma of unusual type with calcification

### Definition

Calcifying epithelial odontogenic tumors (CEOTs) are rare neoplasms. They account for about 1% of odontogenic tumors. These tumors usually are located within bone and produce a mineralized substance within amyloid-like material. CEOTs have a distinctive microscopic appearance with epithelium that resembles the stratum intermedium of the enamel organ.

### Clinical Features

A CEOT is less aggressive than the ameloblastoma and is found in about the same age group. Rarely this tumor may have an extraosseous location. The neoplasm is somewhat more common in men, and patients range in age from 8 to 92 years, with an average age of about 42 years (considerably younger in men and somewhat older in women). Jaw expansion is a regular feature and usually the only symptom. Palpation of the swelling reveals a hard tumor.

### Radiographic Features

*Location.* As with ameloblastomas, CEOTs have a definite predilection for the mandible, with a ratio of at least 2:1, and most develop in the premolar-molar area, with a 52% association with an unerupted or impacted tooth. In about half of cases, radiographs taken early in the development of these tumors reveal a radiolucent area around the crown of a mature, unerupted tooth.

*Periphery.* The border may have a well defined cystlike cortex. In some tumors the boundary may be irregular and ill defined.

*Internal Structure.* The internal aspect may appear unilocular or multilocular with numerous scattered, radiopaque foci of varying size and density. The most characteristic and diagnostic finding is the appearance of radiopacities close to the crown of the embedded tooth (Fig. 22-19). In addition, small, thin, opaque trabeculae may cross the radiolucency in many directions.

*Effects on Surrounding Structures.* CEOTs may displace a developing tooth or prevent its eruption. Associated expansion of the jaw with maintenance of a cortical boundary may also occur.

### Differential Diagnosis

Lesions with completely radiolucent internal structures may mimic dentigerous cysts or even ameloblastomas. Other lesions with radiopaque foci, including adenomatoid odontogenic tumor, ameloblastic

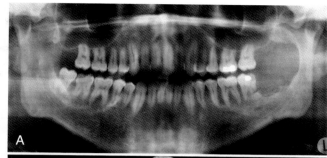

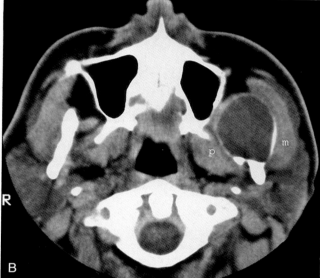

FIG. **22-17** **A,** Panoramic film of a unicystic ameloblastoma occupying the left mandibular ramus; note the absence of the anterior border of the ramus. **B,** An axial CT image with soft tissue algorithm showing significant expansion toward the masseter *(m)* and lateral pterygoid *(p)* muscles.

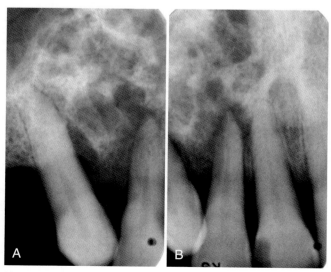

FIG. **22-18** Periapical films of a recurrent ameloblastoma of the right maxilla. Note the sclerotic margins of the small cystic lesions.

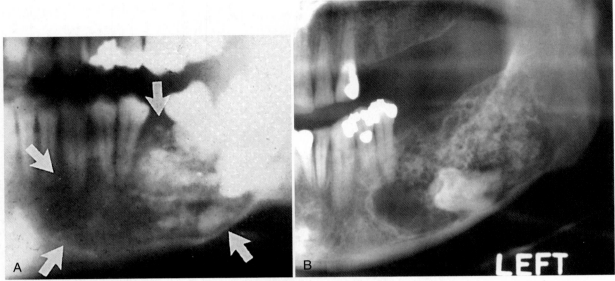

FIG. **22-19**   **A,** Calcifying odontogenic tumor, or Pindborg tumor *(arrows).* **B,** The tumor appears as a mixed radiolucent-radiopaque lesion associated with an unerupted tooth. (**A** courtesy M. Gornitsky, DDS, Montreal, Canada; **B** courtesy Dr. D. Lanigan, University of Saskatchewan.)

fibro-odontoma, and calcifying odontogenic cyst may have similar appearances. However, the prominent location of the CEOT and the age of the patient will help in the differential diagnosis.

## Treatment

The treatment of the CEOT is more conservative than the ameloblastoma, with local resection.

## MIXED TUMORS (OF ODONTOGENIC EPITHELIUM AND ODONTOGENIC ECTOMESENCHYME)

### Odontoma

#### Synonyms

Compound odontoma, compound composite odontoma, complex odontoma, complex composite odontoma, odontogenic hamartoma, calcified mixed odontoma, and cystic odontoma

#### Definition

The term *odontoma* is used to identify a tumor that is radiographically and histologically characterized by the production of mature enamel, dentin, cementum, and pulp tissue. These components are seen in various states of histodifferentiation and morphodifferentiation. Because of its limited and slow growth and well-differentiated tooth tissue, this lesion is considered to be a hamartoma and not a true tumor.

The structural relationship of the component tissues may vary from nondescript masses of dental tissue referred to as a complex odontoma to multiple well-formed teeth (denticles) of a compound odontoma. A dilated odontoma has been described as another type of odontoma; however, this is a single structure that actually may be the most severe expression of a dens in dente.

#### Clinical Features

Odontomas are the most common odontogenic tumor. They often interfere with the eruption of permanent teeth (Fig. 22-20). The lesion shows no sex predilection, and most begin forming while the normal dentition is developing. Odontomas develop and mature while the corresponding teeth are forming and cease development when the associated teeth complete development. Most odontomas occur in the second decade of life and many times are found during investigation of delayed eruption of adjacent teeth or retained primary teeth. In rare cases odontomas are associated with primary teeth. They persist if left untreated, although they do not continue to increase in size and so may be detected later in life. Compound odontomas are about twice as common as the complex type. Although the compound variety forms equally between men and women, 60% of complex odontomas occur in women. In rare circumstances a compound odontoma may erupt into the oral cavity of a child.

#### Radiographic Features

*Location.*   More of the compound type (62%) occur in the anterior maxilla in association with the crown of an unerupted canine. In contrast, 70% of complex odontomas are found in the mandibular first and second molar area.

*Periphery.*   The borders of odontomas are well defined and may be smooth or irregular. These lesions have a cortical border, and immediately inside and adjacent to the cortical border is a soft tissue capsule.

*Internal Structure.*   The contents of these lesions are largely radiopaque. Compound odontomas have a number of toothlike structures or denticles that look like deformed teeth (Fig. 22-21). Complex odontomas contain an irregular mass of calcified tissue (see Fig. 22-20). The degree of radiopacity is equivalent to or exceeds that of adjacent tooth structure and may vary in the degree of radiopacity from one region to another, reflecting variations in amount and type

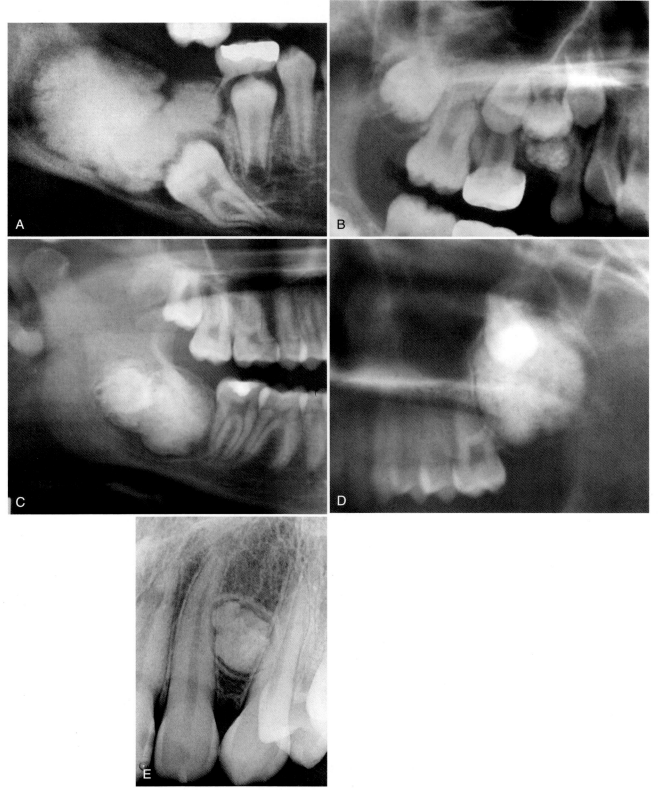

FIG. **22-20**   A series of complex odontomas; note the toothlike density of the internal structure, a thin radiolucent capsule that in many cases interfered with the eruption of associated teeth.

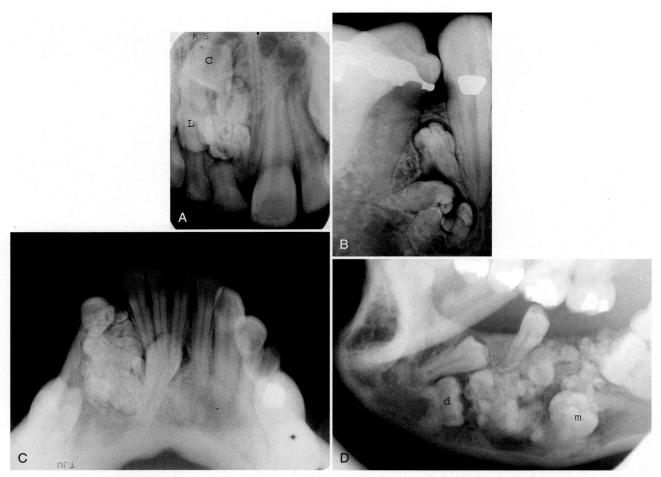

FIG. **22-21**   Several examples of compound odontomas; note the numerous internal components and the radiolucent capsule. **A,** An example in the anterior maxilla that has interfered with the eruption of the central incisor *(C)* and the lateral incisor *(L).* **B,** Within the mandible. **C,** Within the anterior mandible interfering with the eruption of the cuspid. **D,** Within the mandible interfering with the eruption of the first premolar, deciduous molar *(d),* and the first molar *(m).*

of hard tissue that has been formed. A dilated odontoma has a single calcified structure with a more radiolucent central portion that has an overall form like a donut (Fig. 22-22).

    ***Effects on Surrounding Structures.*** Odontomas can interfere with the normal eruption of teeth. Most odontomas (70%) are associated with abnormalities such as impaction, malpositioning, diastema, aplasia, malformation, and devitalization of adjacent teeth. Large complex odontomas may cause expansion of the jaw with maintenance of the cortical boundary.

## Differential Diagnosis

A toothlike appearance of the radiopaque structures within a well-defined lesion leads to easy recognition of a compound odontoma. Complex odontomas differ from cemento-ossifying fibromas by their tendency to associate with unerupted molar teeth and because they usually are more radiopaque than cemento-ossifying fibromas. Odontomas may also develop in much younger patients than do cemento-ossifying fibromas. Periapical cemental dysplasia may resemble complex odontomas but lesions are usually multiple and centered on the periapical region of teeth. However, if the cemental dysplastic lesion is solitary and located in an edentulous region of the jaws, the differential diagnosis may be more difficult. The periphery of cemental dysplasia usually has a wider uneven sclerotic border, whereas odontomas have a well-defined cortical border and usually the soft tissue capsule is more uniform and better defined with odontomas than in cemental dysplasia. Dense bone islands, although radiopaque, do not have a soft tissue capsule, as is seen with odontomas.

## Treatment

Complex and compound odontomas are usually removed by simple excision. They do not recur and are not locally invasive.

## Ameloblastic Fibroma

### Synonyms

Soft odontoma, soft mixed odontoma, mixed odontogenic tumor, fibroadamantoblastoma, and granular cell ameloblastic fibroma

### Definition

Ameloblastic fibromas are benign mixed odontogenic tumors. They are characterized by neoplastic proliferation of epithelium resembling dental lamina and the primitive mesenchymal components resem-

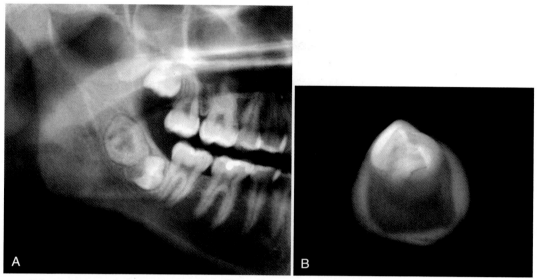

FIG. **22-22**   **A,** A cropped panoramic image demonstrating a dilated odontoma positioned immediately distal to the unerupted third molar. **B,** A radiograph of a specimen; part of the odontoma resembles a tooth crown.

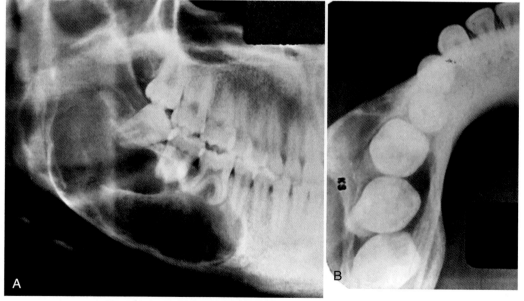

FIG. **22-23**   An ameloblastic fibroma in the body and ramus of the right mandible. **A,** A panoramic radiograph. **B,** An occlusal radiograph showing mediolateral expansion of the mandible.

bling the dental papilla. Enamel, dentin, and cementum are not formed in this tumor.

## Clinical Features
The behavior of ameloblastic fibromas is completely benign. Complete agreement has not been reached regarding sex predilection. Most of these tumors occur between 5 and 20 years of age, during the period of tooth formation, with an average age of about 15 years. They usually produce a painless, slow-growing expansion and displacement of the involved teeth (Fig. 22-23). Although the most common symptom is swelling or occlusal pain, the tumor may be discovered on a routine dental radiograph. It may be associated with a missing tooth.

## Radiographic Features
*Location.*   Ameloblastic fibromas usually develop in the premolar-molar area of the mandible. In some cases the tumor may involve the ramus and extend forward to the premolar-molar area. A common location is near the crest of the alveolar process (Fig. 22-24) or in a follicular relationship with an unerupted tooth (located occlusal

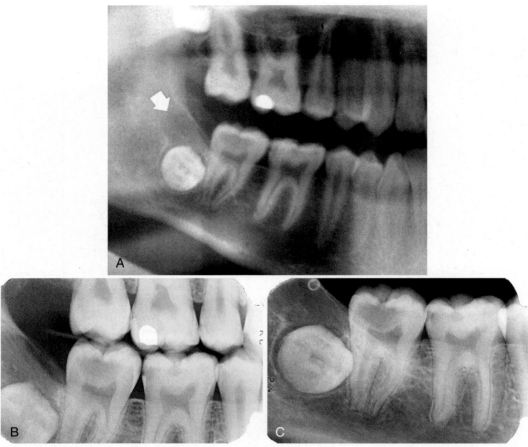

FIG. **22-24**   An ameloblastic fibroma. **A,** An ameloblastic fibroma seen as a radiolucency above the unerupted third molar *(arrow).* **B,** A bitewing radiograph of the same lesion. **C,** A periapical radiograph. (Courtesy G. Sanders, DDS, LaCrosse, Wis.)

to the tooth), or it may arise in an area where a tooth failed to develop.

*Periphery.* The borders of an ameloblastic fibroma are well defined and often corticated in a manner similar to that of a cyst.

*Internal Structure.* An ameloblastic fibroma is more commonly unilocular (totally radiolucent) (Fig. 22-25) but may be multilocular with indistinct curved septa (see Fig. 22-23).

*Effects on Surrounding Structures.* If the lesion is large, there may be expansion with an intact cortical plate. The associated tooth or teeth may be inhibited from normal eruption or may be displaced in an apical direction.

### Differential Diagnosis

A common difficulty will occur in differentiating a small tumor with a follicular relationship to an unerupted tooth from a small dentigerous cyst or a hyperplastic follicle. In fact, the radiologic features may not allow differentiation among these three entities. This tumor may have similar features to an ameloblastoma; however, the ameloblastic fibroma occurs at an earlier age and the septa in an ameloblastoma are more defined and coarse. The septa in ameloblastic fibroma are infrequent and often very fine. Giant cell granulomas may appear multilocular, but these tumors usually have an epicenter anterior to the first molar in young patients and the septa are characteristically granular and ill defined. Odontogenic myxomas can appear multilocular, but usually a few sharp straight septa can be identified, which are not characteristic of ameloblastic fibromas and myxomas, and usually occur in an older age group.

### Treatment

Ameloblastic fibromas are benign, and the rate of recurrence is low. A conservative surgical approach, including enucleation and mechanical curettage of the surrounding bone, is reported to be successful for these cases.

## Ameloblastic Fibro-odontoma

### Definition

An ameloblastic fibro-odontoma is a mixed tumor with all the elements of an ameloblastic fibroma but with scattered collections of enamel and dentine. Some authorities consider the ameloblastic fibro-odontoma to be an early stage of a developing odontoma; however, there is compelling evidence that the ameloblastic fibro-odontoma is a separate entity that has a more neoplastic behavior than does the odontoma. On the other hand, there are probably some lesions that are incorrectly identified as an ameloblastic fibro-odontoma that are really developing odontomas.

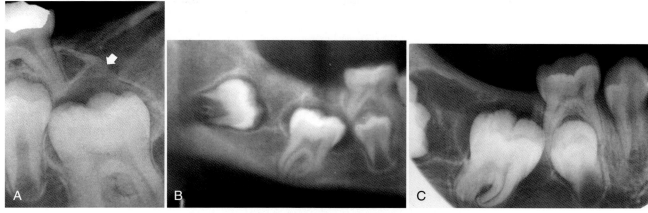

FIG. **22-25** **A,** An ameloblastic fibroma appearing as a unilocular outgrowth of the follicle of the unerupted first permanent molar. **B,** A cropped panoramic image. **C,** A periapical film illustrating an ameloblastic fibroma associated with the crowns of the first and second molars.

## Clinical Features

The clinical features are similar to those of odontomas, often associated with a missing tooth or a tooth that has failed to erupt. Occasionally, this tumor takes the position of a missing tooth. This tumor appears during the same age as odontomas and ameloblastic fibromas with no particular sex predilection.

## Radiographic Features

*Location.* Most cases occur in the posterior aspect of the mandible. The epicenter of the lesion is usually occlusal to a developing tooth or toward the alveolar crest.

*Periphery.* This tumor is usually well defined and sometimes corticated.

*Internal Structure.* The internal structure is mixed, with the majority of the lesion being radiolucent. Small lesions may appear as enlarged follicles with only one or two small discrete radiopacities. Larger lesions may have a more extensive calcified internal structure (Fig. 22-26). In some cases these small calcifications have a round shape with a radiopaque enamel-like margin, giving a shape similar to that of a small doughnut. Most often an associated impacted tooth is present.

## Differential Diagnosis

If calcification is not detected, this tumor cannot be differentiated from an ameloblastic fibroma. Differentiation from a developing odontoma may be difficult, but generally these tumors have a greater soft tissue component (radiolucent) than does an odontoma. It may be argued that, given time, the amount of hard tissue will increase; however, the distribution of hard tissue is different. A complex odontoma, which shares a common location, usually has one mass of disorganized tissue in the center, whereas the ameloblastic fibro-odontoma will usually have multiple scattered mature small pieces of dental hard tissue. Although the compound odontoma has multiple denticles, the posterior mandible is a rare location and the organization of the tooth material in ameloblastic fibro-odontomes is never organized enough to resemble a tooth. Last, the ameloblastic fibro-odontomas do not occur early enough, compared with odontomas, to be considered a precursor.

## Treatment

Usually conservative enucleation is used, although recurrence has been reported.

### Adenomatoid Odontogenic Tumor

## Synonyms

Adenoameloblastoma and ameloblastic adenomatoid tumor

## Definition

Adenomatoid odontogenic tumors are uncommon nonaggressive tumors of odontogenic epithelium in variety of patterns mixed with mature connective tissue stroma. The origin of adenomatoid odontogenic tumors may be from enamel organ epithelium, and it is classified as a mixed tumor because it contains connective tissue stroma and sometimes dentinoid material. Adenomatoid odontogenic tumors comprise 3% of all oral tumors. Both central and peripheral tumors occur. The central tumors are divided into the follicular type (those associated with the crown of an embedded tooth) and the extrafollicular type (those with no embedded tooth). Approximately 73% of central lesions are of the follicular type.

## Clinical Features

Adenomatoid odontogenic tumors appear in the age range of 5 to 50 years; however, about 70% occur in the second decade, with an average age of 16 years. The tumor has a 2:1 female predilection. The follicular type is diagnosed somewhat earlier than the extrafollicular type, probably because the failure of the associated tooth to erupt is noted. The tumor is slow growing and presents as a gradually enlarging, painless swelling or asymmetry, often associated with a missing tooth.

## Radiographic Features

*Location.* At least 75% of adenomatoid odontogenic tumors occur in the maxilla (Fig. 22-27). The incisor-canine-premolar region, especially the cuspid region, is the usual area involved in both jaws. It occurs more commonly in the maxilla. This tumor may have a follicular relationship with an impacted tooth; however, often it does not

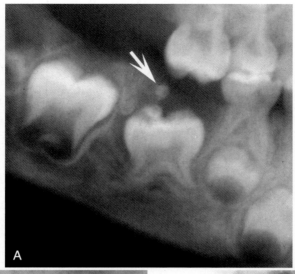

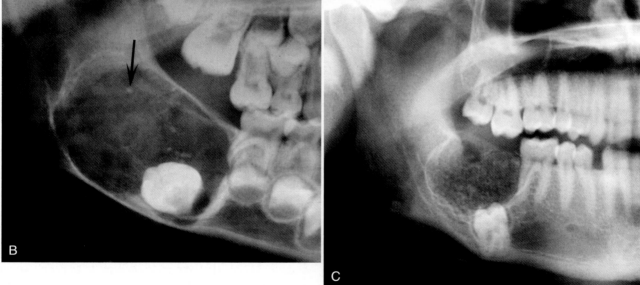

FIG. **22-26**  Three examples of ameloblastic fibro-odontoma. **A,** A cropped panoramic film with a lesion occlusal to a second deciduous molar. The lesion is ill defined and radiolucent except for two small radiopacities *(arrow).* **B,** A cropped panoramic image of a well-defined radiolucent lesion with only a few scattered radiopacities. **C,** A cropped panoramic image of a lesion with a larger number of radiopacities.

attach at the cementoenamel junction but surrounds a greater part of the tooth, most often a canine (Fig. 22-28).

*Periphery.*  The usual radiographic appearance is a well-defined corticated or sclerotic border.

*Internal Structure.*  Radiographically, radiopacities develop in about two thirds of cases. One tumor may be completely radiolucent, another may contain faint radiopaque foci (Fig. 22-28), and some may show dense clusters of ill-defined radiopacities; occasionally the calcifications are small with well-defined borders, like a cluster of small pebbles (see Fig. 22-28, *B*). Intraoral radiographs may be required to demonstrate the calcifications within the lesion, which may not be seen on panoramic radiographs. Microscopic studies have verified that the size, number, and density of small radiopacities in the central

radiolucency of the lesion vary from tumor to tumor and seem to increase with age.

*Effects on Surrounding Structures.*  As the tumor enlarges, adjacent teeth are displaced. Root resorption is rare. This lesion also may inhibit eruption of an involved tooth. Although some expansion of the jaw may occur, the outer cortex is maintained.

### Differential Diagnosis

When this tumor is completely radiolucent and has a follicular relationship with an impacted tooth, differentiation from a follicular cyst or a pericoronal odontogenic keratocyst may be difficult. If the attachment of the radiolucent lesion is more apical than the cementoenamel junction, a follicular cyst can be discounted. However, this would not exclude an odontogenic keratocyst. If there is a calcified product (radiopacities) in this tumor, then other lesions with calcifications might be entertained in the differential diagnosis. The maxillary and mandibular anterior regions are also common sites for calcifying odontogenic cysts. It may not be possible to differentiate the extrafollicular type of adenomatoid odontogenic tumor from the calcifying odontogenic cyst. The ameloblastic fibro-odontoma and the CEOT occur more commonly in the posterior mandible.

### Treatment

Conservative surgical excision is adequate because the tumor is not locally invasive, is well encapsulated, and is separated easily from the bone. The theory that adenomatoid odontogenic tumors are hamartomas is supported by the innocuous behavior of the lesion because, as with odontomas, adenomatoid odontogenic tumors stop developing about the time tooth structures complete their growth. The recurrence rate is 0.2%.

## MESENCHYMAL TUMORS (ODONTOGENIC ECTOMESENCHYME)

### Odontogenic Myxoma

### Synonyms

Myxoma, myxofibroma, and fibromyxoma

### Definition

Odontogenic myxomas are uncommon, accounting for only 3% to 6% of odontogenic tumors. They are benign, intraosseous neoplasms that arise from odontogenic ectomesenchyme and resemble the mesenchymal portion of the dental papilla. These myxomas are not encapsulated and tend to infiltrate the surrounding cancellous bone but do not metastasize. They have a loose, gelatinous consistency and show microscopic characteristics similar to those of soft tissue myxomas of the extremities. Odontogenic myxomas develop only in the bones of the facial skeleton. The theory that this lesion develops from odontogenic rather than nonodontogenic ectomesenchyme is supported by the fact that it appears only in the jaws, it affects young

people, it occasionally is related to a tooth that failed to erupt or is missing, and in some cases odontogenic epithelium can be detected microscopically.

### Clinical Features

If odontogenic myxomas have a sex predilection, they slightly favor females. Although the lesion can occur at any age, more than half arise in individuals between 10 and 30 years old; it rarely occurs before age

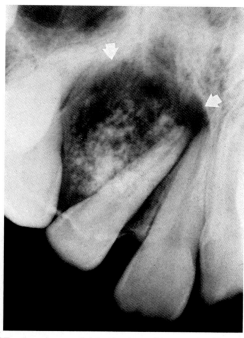

FIG. **22-27** An adenomatoid odontogenic tumor in the region of the right maxillary canine and lateral incisor. Calcification is present within the tumor mass, and the canine and lateral incisor have been displaced by the lesion. (Courtesy R. Howell, DDS, Morgantown, W.V.)

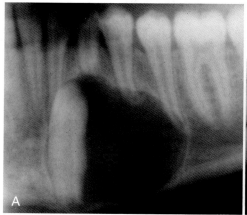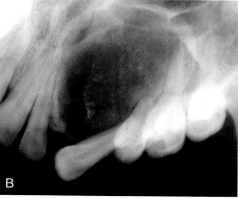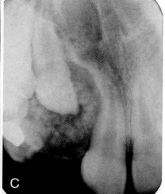

FIG. **22-28** Examples of adenomatoid odontogenic tumor with various amount of internal calcification. **A,** A cropped panoramic film with a totally radiolucent lesion associated with a mandibular cuspid. **B,** A lesion with sparse pebblelike calcifications associated with a maxillary cuspid. **C,** A lesion related to a maxillary lateral incisor with abundant calcification.

10 years or after age 50 years. It grows slowly and may or may not cause pain. Eventually it causes swelling and may grow quite large if left untreated. It may also invade the maxillary sinus. Recurrence rates as high as 25% have been reported. This high rate may be explained by the lack of encapsulation of the tumor, its poorly defined boundaries, and the extension of nests or pockets of myxoid (jellylike) tumor into trabecular spaces, where they are difficult to detect and remove surgically.

### Radiographic Features

*Location.* Myxomas more commonly affect the mandible by a margin of 3:1. In the mandible these tumors occur in the premolar and molar areas and only rarely in the ramus and condyle (non–tooth-bearing areas). Myxomas in the maxilla usually involve the alveolar process in the premolar and molar regions and the zygomatic process.

*Periphery.* The lesion usually is well defined, and it may have a corticated margin but most often is poorly defined, especially in the maxilla.

*Internal Structure.* When it occurs pericoronally with an impacted tooth, an odontogenic myxoma may have a cystlike unilocular outline, although the majority has a mixed radiolucent-radiopaque internal pattern. Residual bone trapped within the tumor will remodel into curved and straight, coarse or fine septa. The presence of these septa gives the tumor a multilocular appearance. A characteristic septa identified with this tumor is a straight, thin-etched septa (Fig. 22-29). These have been described as making a tennis racket–like or stepladder-like pattern, but this pattern is rarely seen. In reality, the majority of the septa are curved and coarse but the finding of one or two of these straight septa will help in the identification of this tumor (Fig. 22-30).

*Effects on Surrounding Structures.* When growing in a tooth-bearing area, the tumor displaces and loosens teeth but rarely causes resorption of teeth. The lesion also frequently scallops between the roots of adjacent teeth, similar to a simple bone cyst. This tumor has a tendency to grow along the involved bone without the same amount of expansion seen with other benign tumors; however, when a large size is achieved, there may be considerable expansion.

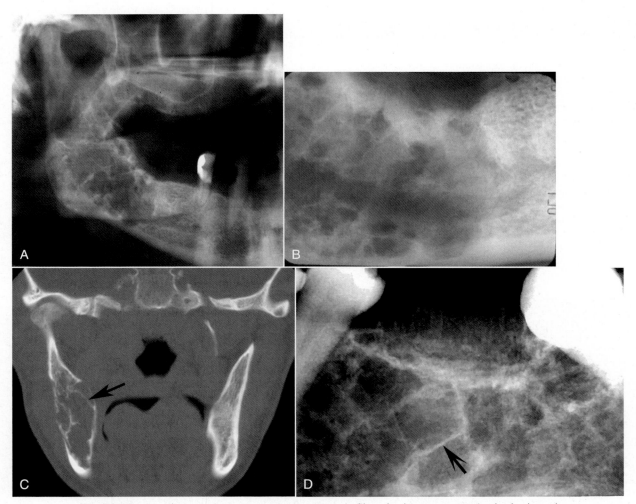

FIG. **22-29**  An odontogenic myxoma. **A,** A panoramic film of a large myxoma in the body and ramus of the right mandible. **B,** A periapical view. **C,** A coronal CT image of the same case; note the presence of a few straight septa, especially visible in the CT image *(arrow)*. The CT image also shows some modest expansion considering the overall size of the tumor. **D,** A periapical view of a different lesion; note the one straight sharp septa *(arrow)*.

*Additional Imaging.* CT and in particular MRI can help in establishing the intraosseous extent of the tumor and thus guide the surgeon in planning the resection margins. The high tissue signal characteristic of this tumor in T2-weighted magnetic resonance images is particularly useful in establishing tumor extent and the presence of a recurrent tumor (Fig. 22-31).

### Differential Diagnosis

Because odontogenic myxomas most often have a multilocular internal pattern, the differential diagnosis should include other multilocular lesions such as ameloblastomas, central giant cell granulomas, and central hemangiomas. The finding of characteristic thin straight septa with less-than-expected bone expansion is very useful in the differential diagnosis. On occasion, a small area of expansion with straight septa may be projected over an intact outer bony cortex and give a spiculated appearance seen in osteogenic sarcomas (see Fig. 22-29, *D*). Careful inspection of this area of expansion will reveal a thin but intact outer cortex that would not be seen in osteogenic sarcoma. On occasion, the odontogenic fibroma will have the same radiographic characteristics as, and cannot be reliably differentiated from, the myxoma.

### Treatment

Odontogenic myxomas are treated by resection with a generous amount of surrounding bone to ensure removal of myxomatous tumor that infiltrates the adjacent marrow spaces. With appropriate treatment, the prognosis is good.

### Benign Cementoblastoma

#### Synonyms
Cementoblastoma and true cementoma

#### Definition
Benign cementoblastomas are slow-growing mesenchymal neoplasms composed principally of cementum-like tissue. The tumor manifests as a bulbous growth around and attached to the apex of a tooth root. Its histologic characteristics are similar to those of osteoblastomas, and some authors consider cementoblastomas to be osteoblastomas. Putative cementoblasts that compose this tumor produce cementum-like material and abnormal bone. The tumor most often develops with permanent teeth but in rare cases occurs with primary teeth.

#### Clinical Features
Although statistical data suggest that benign cementoblastomas are uncommon, many believe that they occur more often than published accounts indicate. The lesion is more common in males than in females, and the ages of reported patients range from 12 to 65 years, although most patients are relatively young. There is no racial predilection. The tumor usually is a solitary lesion that is slow growing but that may eventually displace teeth. The involved tooth is vital and often painful. The pain seems to vary from patient to patient and can be relieved by anti-inflammatory drugs.

#### Radiographic Features
*Location.* Benign cementoblastomas occur more often in the mandible (78%) and form most commonly on a premolar or first molar (90%).

*Periphery.* The lesion is a well-defined radiopacity with a cortical border and then a well-defined radiolucent band just inside the cortical border.

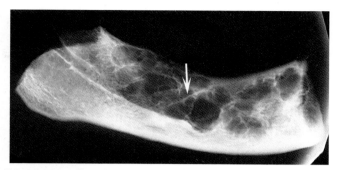

FIG. **22-30** A film of a surgical specimen of an odontogenic myxoma; note the sharp straight septa *(arrow).*

*Internal Structure.* Benign cementoblastomas are mixed radiolucent-radiopaque lesions where the majority of the internal structure is radiopaque. The resulting pattern may be amorphous or may have a wheel spoke pattern (Fig. 22-32). The density of the cemental mass usually obscures the outline of the enveloped root. This central radiopaque mass as mentioned is surrounded by a radiolucent band, indicating that the tumor is maturing from the central aspect to the periphery.

*Effects on Surrounding Structures.* If the root outline is apparent, in most cases various amounts of external resorption can be seen. If large enough, this tumor can cause expansion of the mandible but with an intact outer cortex.

### Differential Diagnosis

The most common lesion to simulate this appearance is a solitary lesion of periapical cemental dysplasia. The differential diagnosis may be difficult in some cases and the presence or absence of symptoms or observation of the lesion over a period of time may be required. In general, the radiolucent band around the benign cementoblastoma is usually better defined and uniform than with cemental dysplasia. Also, the pattern of growth of the cementoblastoma results in a more uniform circular shape than the more irregular undulating outline of cemental dysplasia. Other lesions that may be included in the differential diagnosis would be periapical sclerosing osteitis, dense bone island, and hypercementosis. However, periapical sclerosing osteitis and dense bone islands do not have a soft tissue capsule, as does the benign cementoblastoma. Hypercementosis should be surrounded by a periodontal membrane space, which is usually thinner than the soft tissue capsule of the benign cementoblastoma, and there is no root resorption or jaw expansion with hypercementosis.

*Treatment.* Benign cementoblastomas are apparently self-limiting and rarely recur after enucleation. Simple excision and extraction of the associated tooth are sufficient treatment. In some cases the tumor may be amputated from the tooth, which is then treated endodontically.

### Central Odontogenic Fibroma

#### Synonyms
Simple odontogenic fibroma and odontogenic fibroma (WHO type)

#### Definition
Central odontogenic fibromas are rare neoplasms that sometimes are divided into two types according to histologic appearance: the simple type contains mature fibrous tissue with sparsely scattered

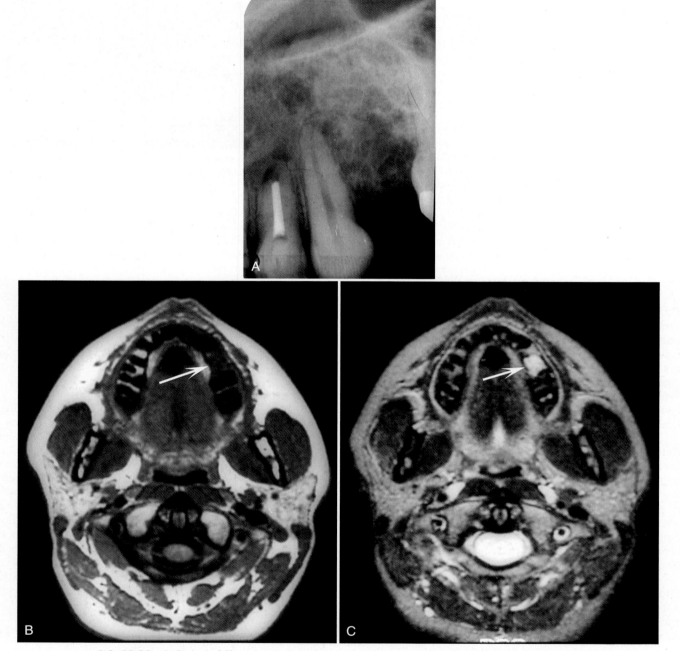

FIG. **22-31   A,** Periapical film taken to investigate a possible recurrence of an odontogenic myxoma in the alveolar process between the cuspid and the first molar after treatment by surgical curettage. **B,** Magnetic resonance axial image with T1 weighting showing a low signal *(black)* from the segment of the alveolar process between the cuspid and molar. **C,** Magnetic resonance axial image of the same image slice as **B** but with T2 weighting resulting in a high signal *(white)* from the same alveolar segment, which is characteristic of an odontogenic myxoma and confirming the presence of a recurrence.

odontogenic epithelial rests and the WHO type, which is more cellular, has more epithelial rests and may contain calcifications that resemble dysplastic dentin, cementum, or osteoid. One theory is that these types merely represent a spectrum and that odontogenic myxoma may be a part of this range.

## Clinical Features

Most cases of central odontogenic fibromas occur between the ages of 11 and 39 years. The neoplasm shows a definite female preponderance, with a reported ratio of 2.2 : 1. Affected patients may be asymptomatic or may have swelling and mobility of the teeth.

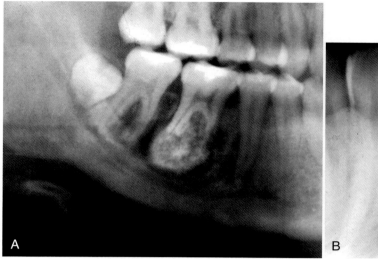
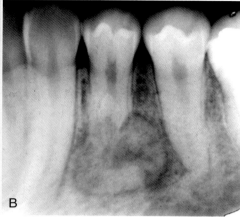

FIG. 22-32 Cementoblastoma. **A,** A portion of a panoramic radiograph showing a large, bulbous, radiopaque mass attached to the roots of the mandibular right first molar. A radiolucent band can be seen surrounding the mass, and root resorption of the molar roots has occurred. **B,** A periapical radiograph of a lesion associated with a bicuspid. (Courtesy B. Pynn, Canada.)

## Radiographic Features

*Location.* Central odontogenic fibromas occur slightly more often in the mandible. The prevalent site in the mandible is the molar-premolar region and in the maxilla anterior to the first molar.

*Periphery.* The periphery usually is well defined.

*Internal Structure.* Smaller lesions usually are unilocular, and larger lesions have a multilocular pattern. The internal septa may be fine and straight, as in odontogenic myxomas, or it may be granular, resembling those seen in giant cell granulomas. Some lesions are totally radiolucent, whereas unorganized internal calcification has been reported in others.

*Effects on Surrounding Structures.* A central odontogenic fibroma may cause expansion with maintenance of a thin cortical boundary or on occasion can grow along the bone with minimum expansion, similar to an odontogenic myxoma. Tooth displacement is common, and root resorption has been reported.

## Differential Diagnosis

The histologic features may resemble those of a central (originating in bone) desmoplastic fibroma if no epithelial rests are apparent. Desmoplastic fibromas are more aggressive and tend to break through the peripheral cortex and invade surrounding soft tissue. The septa in desmoplastic fibroma will be very thick, straight, and angular. If thin, straight septa are present in the odontogenic fibroma, it may not be possible to differentiate this neoplasm from an odontogenic myxoma on radiographic criteria alone. If granular septa are present, the radiographic appearance may be identical to that of a giant cell granuloma.

## Treatment

Central odontogenic fibromas are treated with simple excision. These lesions have a very low recurrence rate.

## Nonodontogenic Tumors

### BENIGN TUMORS OF NEURAL ORIGIN

#### Neurilemmoma

**Synonym**

Schwannoma

**Definition**

A central neurilemmoma is a tumor of neuroectodermal origin, arising from the Schwann cells that make up the inner layer covering the peripheral nerves. Although rare, it is the most common intraosseous nerve tumor. This tumor has practically no potential for malignant transformation.

**Clinical Features**

Neurilemmomas grow slowly, can occur at any age (but most commonly arise in the second and third decades), and occur with equal frequency in both males and females. The mandible and sacrum are the most common sites. These lesions cause few symptoms other than those related to the location and size of the tumor. The usual complaint is a swelling. Although pain is uncommon unless the tumor encroaches on adjacent nerves, paresthesia may arise, especially with lesions originating in the inferior alveolar canal. Pain, when present, usually develops at the site of the tumor; if paresthesia occurs, it is felt anterior to the tumor.

**Radiographic Features**

*Location.* Neurilemmomas most often involve the mandible, with fewer than 1 in 10 cases occurring in the maxilla. The tumor most often is located within an expanded inferior alveolar nerve canal posterior to the mental foramen (Fig. 22-33).

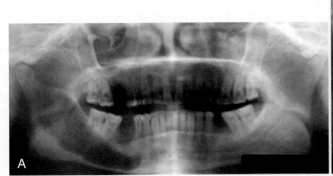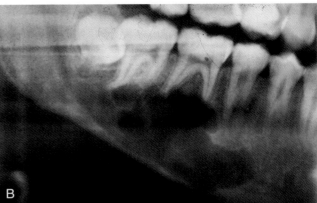

FIG. **22-33** **A,** A panoramic film of a large neurilemoma expanding all of the inferior alveolar nerve canal from the mandibular to the mental foramen. **B,** A cropped panoramic image of a smaller tumor.

*Periphery.* In keeping with its slow growth rate, the margins of this tumor are well defined and usually corticated as it expands the cortical walls of the inferior alveolar canal. Small lesions may appear cystlike but more commonly are fusiform in shape as the tumor expands the canal.

*Internal Structure.* The internal structure is uniformly radiolucent. When lesions have a scalloping outline, this may give a false impression of a multilocular pattern.

*Effects on Surrounding Structures.* If the tumor reaches either the mandibular foramen or mental foramen, it can cause enlargement of the foramen. Expansion of the inferior alveolar canal is slow and thus the outer cortex of the canal is maintained; the expansion of the canal is usually localized with a definite epicenter, unless the lesion is large. The expanding tumor may cause root resorption of adjacent teeth (see Fig. 22-33).

### Differential Diagnosis

Because neurilemmomas most commonly originate within the inferior alveolar canal, vascular lesions such as a hemangioma or arteriovenous fistula should be considered. However, neurilemmomas have a distinct epicenter, whereas vascular lesions will usually cause a more uniform widening of the whole canal; they do not have an obvious epicenter and usually change the course of the canal, most commonly to a serpiginous shape. Only neural tumors and vascular lesions originate within the inferior alveolar canal, but malignant lesions that grow down and enlarge the canal should be in the differential diagnosis. When this happens, the appearance is different, with an irregular widening and destruction of the cortical boundaries of the canal.

### Treatment

Excision is usually the treatment of choice. These lesions generally do not recur if they are completely removed. A capsule usually is present, facilitating surgical removal, although occasionally preservation of the nerve may not be possible. However, periodic examination is indicated to check for recurrence.

## Neuroma

### Synonyms
Amputation neuroma and traumatic neuroma

### Definition

Despite its name, a neuroma is not a neoplasm. Rather, it is an overgrowth of severed nerve fibers attempting to regenerate with abnormal proliferation of scar tissue after a fracture involving a peripheral nerve. As a result, the proliferating nerve forms a disorganized collection of nerve fibers composed of varying proportions of axons, perineural connective tissue, Schwann cells, and scar tissue. The original nerve damage may be the result of mechanical or chemical irritation of the nerve caused by fracture, orthognathic surgery, removal of a tumor or cyst, extrusion of endodontic cement, dental implants, or tooth extraction.

### Clinical Features

Central neuromas are slow-growing reactive hyperplasias that seldom become large, rarely exceeding 1 cm in diameter. They may cause a variety of symptoms, including severe pain resulting from pressure applied as the tangled mass enlarges in its bony cavity or as the result of external trauma. The patient may have reflex neuralgia, with pain referred to the eyes, face, and head.

### Radiographic Features

The radiographic features of a neuroma relate to the extent and shape of the proliferating mass of neural tissue.

*Location.* The most common location is the mental foramen, then the anterior maxilla and the posterior mandible.

*Periphery.* Neuromas usually have well-defined, corticated borders. They may occur in various shapes, depending on the amount of resistance to expansion offered by the surrounding bone. In the mandible the tumor usually forms in the mandibular canal.

*Internal Structure.* The internal structure is totally radiolucent.

*Effects on Surrounding Structures.* Some expansion of the inferior alveolar nerve canal may occur.

### Differential Diagnosis

It is not possible to differentiate this lesion from other benign neural tumors.

### Treatment

Treatment is recommended because neuromas tend to continue to enlarge. They also may cause pain. Regardless of the type of injury that precipitates development of the neuroma, recurrence is uncommon after simple excision.

## Neurofibroma

### Synonym
Neurinoma

### Definition
Neurofibromas are moderately firm, benign, well-circumscribed tumors caused by proliferation of Schwann cells in a disorderly pattern that includes portions of nerve fibers, such as peripheral nerves, axons, and connective tissue of the sheath of Schwann. As neurofibromas grow, they incorporate axons. In contrast, neurilemomas are composed entirely of Schwann cells and grow by displacing axons.

### Clinical Features
The central lesion of a neurofibroma may be the same as the multiple lesions that develop in von Recklinghausen disease. Central lesions also may occur in that syndrome but are rare. Neurofibromas can occur at any age but usually are found in young patients. Neurofibromas associated with the mandibular nerve may produce pain or paresthesia. Neurofibromas also may expand and perforate the cortex; causing swelling that is hard or firm to palpation.

### Radiographic Features
*Location.* Central neurofibromas may occur in the mandibular canal, in the cancellous bone, and below the periosteum.

*Periphery.* As with neurilemomas, the margins of the radiolucency in neurofibromas usually are sharply defined and may be corticated. However, despite the benign nature and slow growth of the neurofibroma, some of these lesions have indistinct margins.

*Internal Structure.* The tumors usually appear unilocular but on occasion may have a multilocular appearance.

*Effects on Surrounding Structures.* A neurofibroma of the inferior dental nerve shows a fusiform enlargement of the canal (Fig. 22-34).

### Differential Diagnosis
Differentiation from other types of neural lesions may not be possible. This tumor can be differentiated from vascular lesions because the expansion of the canal is in a fusiform shape, whereas vascular lesions enlarge the whole canal and alter its path.

### Treatment
Solitary central lesions that have been excised seldom recur. However, it is wise to re-examine the area periodically because these tumors are not encapsulated and some undergo malignant change.

## Neurofibromatosis

### Synonym
von Recklinghausen disease

### Definition
Neurofibromatosis is a syndrome consisting of café-au-lait spots on the skin, multiple peripheral nerve tumors, and a variety of other dysplastic abnormalities of the skin, nervous system, bones, endocrine organs, and blood vessels. The two major classifications are NF-1, a generalized form, and NF-2, a central form. Oral lesions may occur as part of NF-1 or may be solitary and are called segmental or forme fruste manifestations (Fig. 22-35). Recent observations of abnormal fat tissue in close association with changes in the osseous structure of the mandible support the theory that a mesodermal dysplasia is part of the spectrum of changes that may be observed in NF-1 lesions.

### Clinical Features
Neurofibromatosis is one of the most common genetic diseases, occurring in 1 in every 3000 births and present in about 30 people per 10,000 population. The peripheral nerve tumors are of two types, schwannomas and neurofibromas. Some manifestations are congenital, but most appear gradually during childhood and adult life. Café-au-lait spots become larger and more numerous with age; most

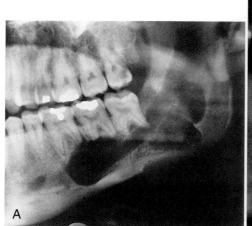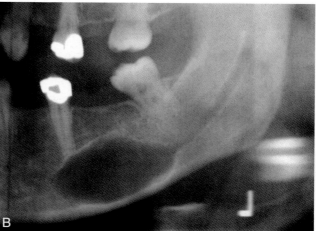

FIG. **22-34** Neurofibroma. **A,** A portion of a panoramic radiograph showing a neurofibroma forming in the mandibular body along the path of the mandibular canal. **B,** A cropped panoramic image of a neurofibroma within the body of the left mandible; note the fusiform shape as the tumor expands the canal.

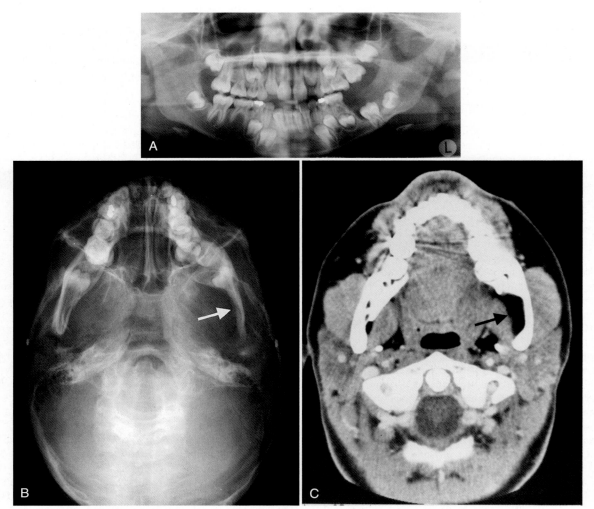

FIG. **22-35** An example of segmental neurofibromatosis involving the mandible. **A,** Panoramic film demonstrating enlargement of the left coronoid notch, enlargement of the mandibular foramen, and interference of the eruption of the first and second molars. **B,** Basal skull view of the same case revealing thinning and bowing of the ramus in a lateral direction *(arrow).* **C,** CT axial image with soft tissue algorithm showing fatty tissue adjacent to the abnormal ramus *(arrow).*

patients eventually have more than six spots larger than 1.5 cm in diameter. Other skin lesions include freckles, soft pedunculated cutaneous neurofibromas, and firm subcutaneous neurofibromas.

### Radiographic Features

The radiographic changes in the jaws with neurofibromatosis can be characteristic. These changes include the following alterations in the shape of the mandible: enlargement of the coronoid notch in either or both the horizontal and vertical dimensions, an obtuse angle between the body and the ramus, deformity of the condylar head, lengthening of the condylar neck, and lateral bowing and thinning of the ramus, as seen in basal skull views (see Fig. 22-35). Changes in mandibular morphology can continue to increase in severity through the second decade. Other radiographic changes include enlargement of the mandibular canal and mental and mandibular foramina and an increased incidence of branched mandibular canal. Erosive changes to the outer contour of the mandible and interference with normal eruption of the molars also may occur. Abnormal accumulations of fatty tissue within deformities of the mandible have been observed in images produced by CT (see Fig. 22-35, *C*).

### Treatment

Most patients live a normal life with few or no symptoms. Small cutaneous and subcutaneous neurofibromas can be removed if they are painful, but large plexiform neurofibromas should be left alone. Malignant conversion of these lesions has occurred in rare cases.

## MESODERMAL TUMORS

### Osteoma

### Definition

Osteomas can form from membranous bones of the skull and face. The cause of the slowly growing osteoma is obscure, but the tumor may arise from cartilage or embryonal periosteum. It is not clear whether osteomas are benign neoplasms or hamartomas. This lesion may be solitary or multiple, occurring on a single bone or on numerous bones. Osteomas originate from the periosteum and may occur either externally or within the paranasal sinuses (Fig. 22-36). It is more common in the frontal and ethmoid sinuses than in the maxillary sinuses (see Chapter 27). Structurally, osteomas can be divided into three types: those composed of compact bone (ivory), those composed of cancellous bone, and those composed of a combination of compact and cancellous bone.

## Clinical Features

Osteomas can occur at any age but most frequently are found in individuals older than 40 years. The only symptom of a developing osteoma is the asymmetry caused by a bony, hard swelling on the jaw. The swelling is painless until its size or position interferes with function. Osteomas are attached to the cortex of the jaw by a pedicle or along a wide base. The mucosa covering the tumor is normal in color and freely movable. Cortical-type osteomas develop more often in men, whereas women have the highest incidence of the cancellous type. Although most osteomas are small, some may become large enough to cause severe damage, especially those that develop in the frontoethmoid region.

## Radiographic Features

*Location.* The mandible is more commonly involved than the maxilla. Osteomas are found most frequently on the posterior aspect of the mandible commonly on the lingual side of the ramus or on the inferior mandibular border below the molars (Fig. 22-37). Other locations include the condylar and coronoid regions. The mandibular lesion may be exophytic, extending outward into adjacent soft tissues (Fig. 22-38). The lesions also occur in the paranasal sinuses, especially the frontal sinus.

*Periphery.* Osteomas have well-defined borders.

*Internal Structure.* Osteomas composed solely of compact bone are uniformly radiopaque; those containing cancellous bone show evidence of internal trabecular structure.

*Effects on Surrounding Structures.* Large lesions can displace adjacent soft tissues, such as muscles, and cause dysfunction.

## Differential Diagnosis

Usually the appearance is characteristic and does not present a problem with diagnosis. However, osteomas involving the condylar head can be difficult to differentiate from osteochondromas, osteophytes, or condylar hyperplasia; those involving the coronoid process may be similar to osteochondromas. A small osteoma may be similar in appearance to a torus or a large hyperostosis (exostosis).

## Treatment

Unless the osteoma interferes with normal function or presents a cosmetic problem, this lesion may not require treatment. In such cases the osteoma should be kept under observation. Resection of osteomas is possible and may be difficult if the osteoma is of the cortical (ivory) type.

## Gardner's Syndrome

### Synonym
Familial multiple polyposis

### Definition
Gardner's syndrome is a type of familial multiple polyposis where there is an associated neoplasm. This syndrome is a hereditary condition characterized by multiple osteomas, multiple dense bone islands (enostosis), epidermoid cysts, subcutaneous desmoid tumors, and multiple polyps of the small and large intestine. The associated osteomas appear during the second decade. They are most common in the frontal bone, mandible, maxilla, and sphenoid bones (Fig. 22-39). A significant feature of familial multiple polyposis is the strong predilection of the intestinal polyps to undergo malignant conversion, making early detection of the syndrome important. Because the osteomas and enostosis often develop before the intestinal polyps, early recognition of the syndrome may be a lifesaving event. Occasionally osteomas may not be present, but the presence of five or more dense bone islands may indicate the presence of a familial multiple polyposis syndrome (Fig. 22-40). Multiple unerupted supernumerary and permanent teeth in both jaws also occur with Gardner's syndrome. Multiple osteomas may occur as isolated findings in the absence of the diseases associated with Gardner's syndrome.

FIG. 22-36 An osteoma in the frontal sinus. **A,** A Caldwell view shows a large amorphous mass in the frontal sinus *(arrows).* **B,** A lateral view shows an osteoma occupying most of the space in the sinus *(arrow).* (Courtesy G. Himadi, DDS, Chapel Hill, N.C.)

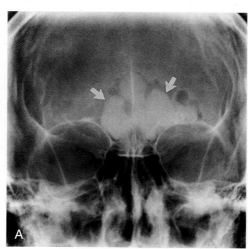
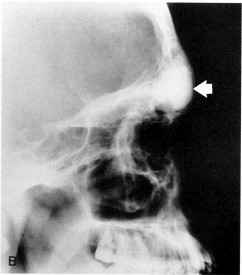

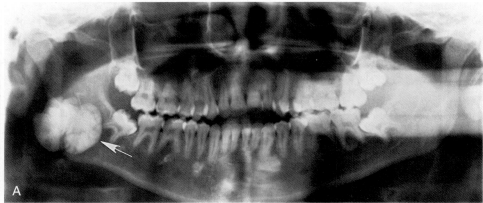

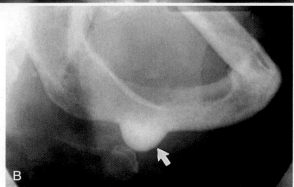

FIG. **22-37** An osteoma. **A,** A panoramic radiograph shows an osteoma in the right mandibular angle region *(arrow).* **B,** An oblique lateral jaw radiograph shows a solid radiopaque osteoma attached to the inferior border of the mandible *(arrow).* (**A** from Matteson SR et al: *Semin Adv Oral Radiol Dent Radiol Photogr* 57:1, 1985.)

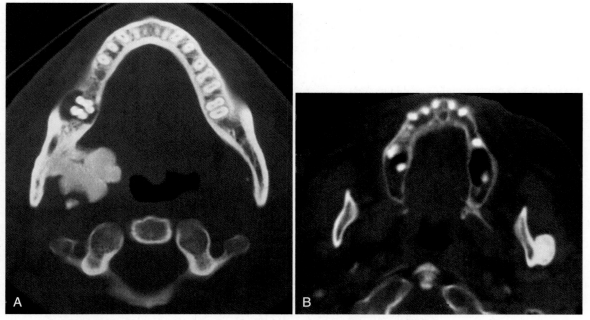

FIG. **22-38** CT scans of osteomas. **A,** An osteoma on the lingual side of the mandibular ramus. **B,** An osteoma on the lateral side of the mandibular ramus.

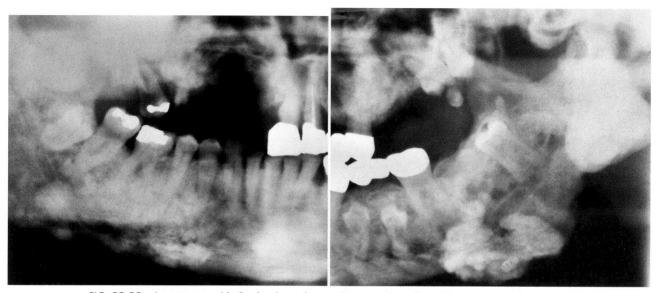

FIG. **22-39**  An osteoma with Gardner's syndrome. A panoramic radiograph shows several osteomas and dense bone islands throughout both jaws. Note the impacted mandibular left second premolars.

FIG. **22-40** A panoramic film of a patient with familial multiple polyposis syndrome; note the multiple dense bone islands throughout the jaws, one of which has interfered with the eruption of the maxillary right first bicuspid.

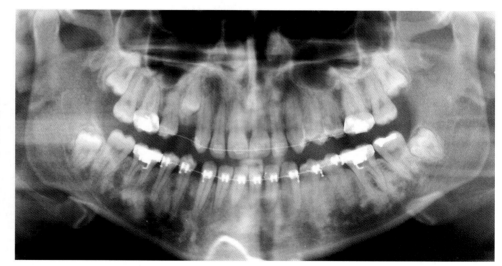

## Treatment

The removal of osteomas is not generally necessary unless the tumors interfere with normal function or present a cosmetic concern. It is most important to recognize the relationship of multiple osteomas and multiple dense bone islands with familial multiple polyposis syndromes for early diagnosis. A family history of intestinal cancer may also help. These patients should be referred to their family physicians for examination for intestinal polyposis and treatment.

## Central Hemangioma

### Definition

A hemangioma is a proliferation of blood vessels creating a mass that resembles a neoplasm, although in many cases it is actually a hamartoma. Hemangiomas can occur anywhere in the body but are most frequently noticed in the skin and subcutaneous tissues. The central (intraosseous) type most often is found in the vertebrae and skull. It rarely develops in the jaws, and an even smaller number of maxillary lesions have been reported. The lesions may be developmental or traumatic in origin.

### Clinical Features

Hemangiomas are more prevalent in females than males, at a ratio of 2:1. This tumor occurs most commonly in the first decade but may occur later in life. Enlargement is slow, producing a nontender expansion of the jaw that occurs over several months or years. The swelling may or may not be painful, is not tender, and usually is bony hard. Pain, if present, probably is the throbbing type. Some tumors may be compressible or pulsate, and a bruit may be detected on auscultation.

Anesthesia of the skin supplied by the mental nerve may occur. The lesion may cause loosening and migration of teeth in the affected area. Bleeding may occur from the gingiva around the neck of the affected teeth. These teeth may demonstrate rebound mobility; that is, when depressed into their sockets, they rebound to their original position within several minutes because of the pressure of the vascular network around the tooth. Aspiration with a syringe produces arterial blood that may be under considerable pressure.

### Radiographic Features

*Location.* Hemangiomas affect the mandible about twice as often as the maxilla. In the mandible the most common site is the posterior body and ramus and within the inferior alveolar canal.

*Periphery.* In some instances the periphery is well defined and corticated, and in other cases it may be ill defined and even simulate the appearance of a malignant tumor. This variation probably is related to the amount of residual bone present around the blood vessels. The formation of linear spicules of bone emanating from the surface of the bone in a sunraylike appearance can occur when the

hemangioma breaks through the outer cortex and displaces the periosteum (Fig. 22-41).

*Internal Structure.* When residual bone is trapped around the blood vessels, the result may be a multilocular appearance. Small radiolucent locules may resemble enlarged marrow spaces surrounded by coarse, dense, and well-defined trabeculae (Fig. 22-42). These internal trabeculae may produce a honeycomb pattern composed of small circular radiolucent spaces that represent blood vessels that are oriented in the same direction of the x-ray beam. When the inferior alveolar canal is involved, the whole canal is increased in width, and often the normal path of the canal is altered into a serpiginous shape sometimes creating a multilocular appearance (Fig. 22-43). Some lesions may be totally radiolucent. When the hemangioma involves soft tissue, the formation of phlebolith (small areas of calcification or

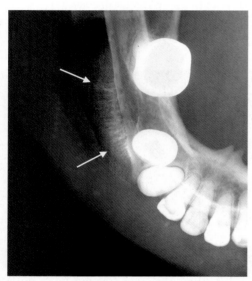

FIG. **22-41**   An occlusal film of a case of a central hemangioma of the mandible with adjacent spiculation *(arrows),* which has a very similar appearance to the spiculation seen in osteogenic sarcoma.

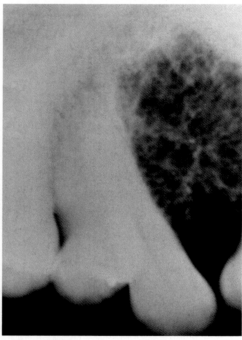

FIG. **22-42**   A hemangioma in the anterior maxilla shows a coarse trabecular pattern. (Courtesy E. J. Burkes, DDS, Chapel Hill, N.C.)

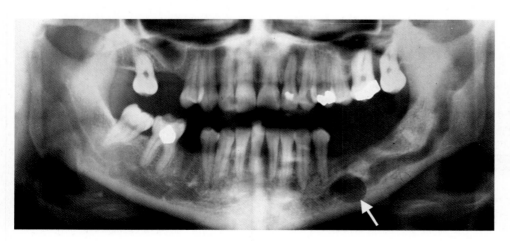

FIG. **22-43**   A panoramic film of a vascular lesion; the whole width of the left inferior alveolar canal is enlarged and it has an irregular abnormal path and the mental foramen has been enlarged *(arrow).*

concretions found in a vein with slow blood flow) may occur within surrounding soft tissues (Fig. 22-44). They develop from thrombi that become organized and mineralized and consist of calcium phosphate and calcium carbonate.

**Effects on Surrounding Structures.** The roots of teeth in the region of the vascular lesion are often resorbed or displaced. When the lesion involves the inferior alveolar nerve canal, the canal can be enlarged along its entire length and its shape may be changed to a serpiginous path. The mandibular and mental foramen may be enlarged. Hemangiomas can influence the growth of bone and teeth. The involved bone may be enlarged and have coarse internal trabeculae. Also, developing teeth may be larger and erupt earlier when in intimate relationship with a hemangioma (Fig. 22-45).

Further diagnostic imaging to better document the distribution and degree of involvement of the osseous and soft tissues of the maxillofacial region should include modalities such as conventional angiography and magnetic resonance angiography.

### Differential Diagnosis

Hemangiomas should be considered in the differential diagnosis of multilocular lesions involving the body of the ramus and body of the

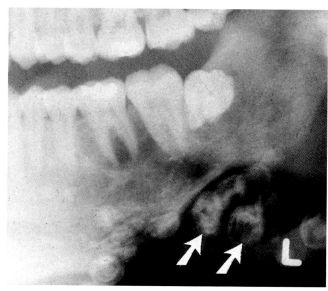

FIG. **22-44**  A soft tissue hemangioma with phleboliths *(arrows)*.

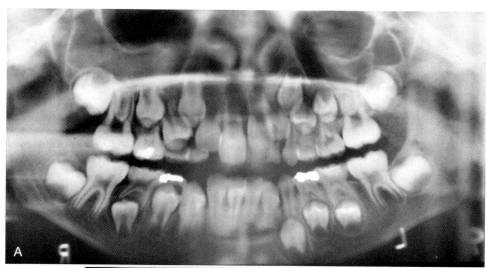

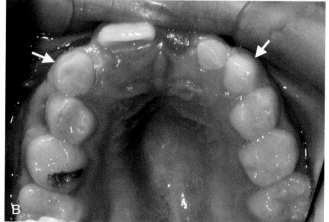

FIG. **22-45**  **A,** A panoramic film demonstrating the effect of a soft tissue hemangioma on the developing dentition. The root development and eruption of the right cuspids and bicuspids are significantly advanced compared with the left side. **B,** An occlusal photograph from the same case; note the difference in size of the maxillary deciduous cuspids.

mandible. Demonstration of involvement of the inferior alveolar canal is an important indicator of a vascular lesion. In most cases soft tissue changes suggest a vascular lesion. When a hemangioma produces a sunray spiculated bone pattern at its periphery, the appearance may be difficult to differentiate from an osteogenic sarcoma (see Fig. 22-41).

## Treatment

Central hemangiomas should be treated without delay because trauma that disrupts the integrity of the affected jaw may result in lethal exsanguination. Specifically, embolization (introduction of inert materials into the lesion by a vascular route), surgery (en bloc resection with ligation of the external carotid artery), and sclerosing techniques have been used singly or together.

## Arteriovenous Fistula

### Synonyms

Arteriovenous (A-V) defect, A-V shunt, A-V aneurysm, and A-V malformation

### Definition

An A-V fistula, an uncommon lesion, is a direct communication between an artery and a vein that bypasses the intervening capillary bed. It usually results from trauma but in rare instances may be a developmental anomaly. An A-V fistula can occur anywhere in the body, in soft tissue, in the alveolar process, and centrally in the jaw. The head and neck are the most common sites.

### Clinical Features

The clinical appearance of a central A-V aneurysm can vary considerably, depending on the extent of bone or soft tissue involvement. The lesion may expand bone, and a mass may be present in the extraosseous soft tissue. The soft tissue swelling may have a purple discoloration. Palpation or auscultation of the swelling may reveal a pulse. On the other hand, neither the bone nor the soft tissue may be expanded, and no pulse may be clinically apparent. Aspiration produces blood. Recognition of the hemorrhagic nature of these lesions is of utmost importance because extraction of an associated tooth may be immediately followed by life-threatening bleeding.

### Radiographic Features

*Location.* These lesions most commonly develop in the ramus and retromolar area of the mandible and involve the mandibular canal.

*Periphery.* The margins usually are well defined and corticated.

*Internal Structure.* A tortuous path of an enlarged vessel in bone may give a multilocular appearance. Otherwise the lesion is radiolucent.

*Effects on Surrounding Structures.* Both central lesions and those in adjacent soft tissue can erode bone resulting in well-defined (cyst like) lesions in the bone. Changes in the inferior alveolar canal may occur, as described in the preceding section on hemangiomas.

*Additional Imaging.* CT with contrast injection is a useful method for aiding the differential diagnosis of any vascular lesion and other neoplasms of the jaws (Fig. 22-46). An imaging modality called magnetic resonance angiography is now being used routinely to document the size and extent and the vessels involved with the vascular lesion. Angiography, a radiographic procedure performed by injecting a radiopaque contrast agent into the blood vessels and making radio-

graphs, will provide the same information and is usually used when interventional therapy is planned in conjunction with the angiography (Fig. 22-47).

### Differential Diagnosis

Occasionally the radiographic appearance is not specific for the A-V aneurysm. The differential diagnosis is similar to that for hemangiomas and includes multilocular lesions. However, association with the inferior alveolar canal is important in the differentiation.

### Treatment

An A-V aneurysm is treated surgically.

## Osteoblastoma

### Synonym

Giant osteoid osteoma

### Definition

An osteoblastoma is an uncommon, benign tumor of osteoblasts with areas of osteoid and calcific tissue. This tumor occurs most often in the spine of a young person. Agreement apparently is increasing that, if osteoblastomas and osteoid osteomas are different lesions, they differ only in size and morphologic and histologic features. For example, the osteoid trabeculae in an osteoblastoma generally are larger (broader and longer, with wider trabecular spaces than those in an osteoid osteoma). An osteoblastoma is usually less painful, and it has more osteoclasts. In addition, benign osteoblastomas are considered more aggressive lesions. On the level of their ultrastructures, the two lesions essentially are similar or at least closely related.

### Clinical Features

Both osteoblastomas and osteoid osteomas are rare in the jaws. The male-to-female ratio is 2:1, although some studies indicate a higher female occurrence and the average age is 17 years, with most lesions occurring in the second and third decades of life. Clinically, patients often report pain and swelling of the affected region; however, the pain is more severe in osteoid osteomas and is often relieved by salicylates.

### Radiographic Features

*Location.* Osteoblastomas are found both in the tooth-bearing regions and commonly around the temporomandibular joint (within the condyle or the temporal bone).

*Periphery.* The borders may be diffuse or may show some sign of a cortex. Lesions often have a soft tissue capsule around the periphery, indicating that this tumor is more mature in the central regions where there is evidence of abnormal bone (Fig. 22-48).

*Internal Structure.* The internal structure may be entirely radiolucent in early developing tumors or may show varying degrees of calcific material. The internal calcification may take the form of a sunray pattern or fine granular bone trabeculae.

*Effects on Surrounding Structures.* Osteoblastomas can expand bone, but usually a thin outer cortex is maintained. This lesion may invaginate the maxillary sinus or the middle cranial fossa.

### Differential Diagnosis

An important differential diagnosis may be a well-defined osteogenic sarcoma because the histologic appearance may be very similar. The differentiation may rely on the benign features of the osteoblastoma

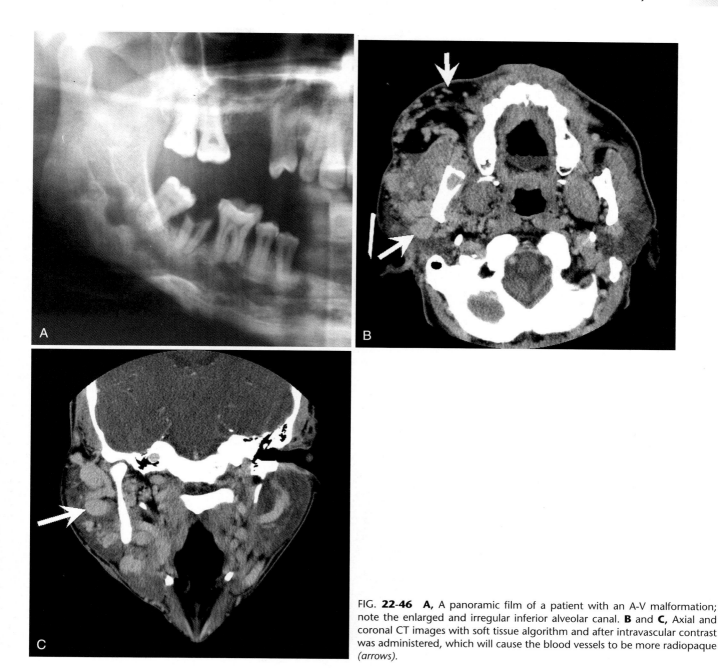

FIG. **22-46** **A,** A panoramic film of a patient with an A-V malformation; note the enlarged and irregular inferior alveolar canal. **B** and **C,** Axial and coronal CT images with soft tissue algorithm and after intravascular contrast was administered, which will cause the blood vessels to be more radiopaque *(arrows).*

as revealed in the radiographic images. Osteoblastomas do not normally break through cortical boundaries and invade surrounding soft tissue. Osteoid osteomas are usually smaller and have an associated sclerotic bone reaction at the periphery. Sometimes the appearance of an osteoblastoma may be similar to a large area of cemental dysplasia. Both have a soft tissue capsule, but the osteoblastoma behaves more aggressively, like a tumor.

## Treatment

Osteoblastomas are treated with curettage or local excision. Recurrences have been described, and in a few cases the differentiation from a low-grade osteosarcoma may be difficult.

## Osteoid Osteoma

### Definition

An osteoid osteoma is a benign tumor that is extremely rare in the jaws. Its true nature is not known, but some investigators think it is a variant of osteoblastoma. The tumor has an oval or round, tumorlike core usually only about 1 cm in diameter, although some may reach 5 or 6 cm. This core consists of osteoid and newly formed trabeculae within highly vascularized, osteogenic connective tissue. The tumor usually develops within the outer cortex but may form within the cancellous bone. There is a sclerotic bone reaction around the periphery, often thinner in lesions within the cancellous bone.

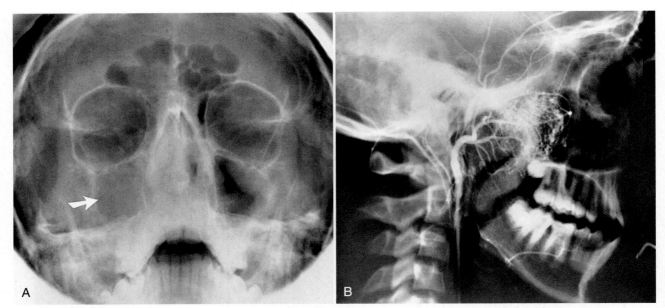

FIG. **22-47**  A vascular lesion in the right maxillary sinus. **A,** A Waters' radiograph shows the opacified maxillary antrum *(arrow)*. **B,** Note the tumor vascularization in this angiogram. A radiopaque dye has been injected into the vasculature to enhance visualization. (Courtesy G. Himadi, DDS, Chapel Hill, N.C.)

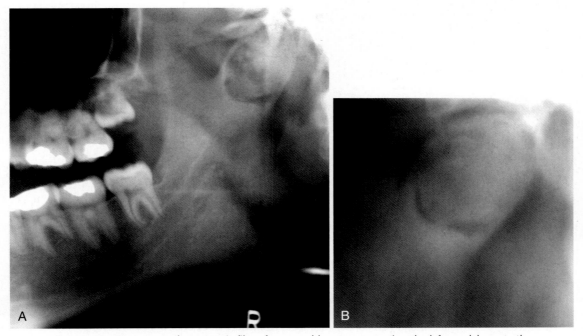

FIG. **22-48**  **A,** A cropped panoramic film of an osteoblastoma occupying the left condyle; note the enlargement of the condyle and the presence of a soft tissue capsule surrounding an internal structure of granular bone. **B,** A tomograph of the left condyle.

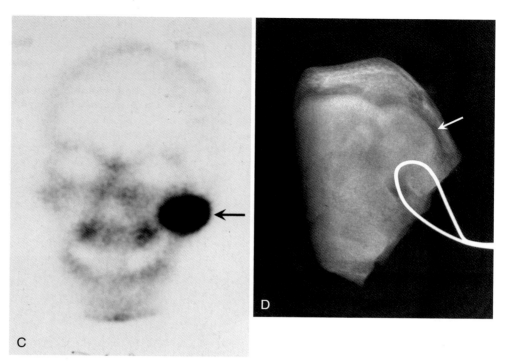

FIG. **22-48, cont'd  C,** A technetium bone scan demonstrating increased bone activity in the left condyle *(arrow).* **D,** A radiograph of the surgical specimen; note the internal granular bone surrounded by a soft tissue capsule *(arrow).*

## Clinical Features

Osteoid osteomas occur most often in young people, usually males between the ages of 10 and 25 years. They seldom occur before 4 years or after 40 years. This condition affects at least twice as many males as females. Most of the lesions occur in the femur and tibia; the jaws are rarely involved. Severe pain in the bone that can be relieved by anti-inflammatory drugs is characteristic. In addition, the soft tissue over the involved bony area may be swollen and tender.

## Radiographic Features

*Location.* The lesion is most common in the cortex of the limb bones. In those that do occur in the jaws, somewhat more develop in the body of the mandible.

*Periphery.* The margins are well defined by a rim of sclerotic bone (Fig. 22-49).

*Internal Structure.* The internal aspect of young lesions is composed of a small ovoid or round radiolucent area (core). In more mature lesions the central radiolucency may have a radiopaque foci representing abnormal bone.

*Effects on Surrounding Structures.* As previously mentioned, this tumor can stimulate a sclerotic bone reaction and cause thickening of the outer cortex by stimulating periosteal new bone formation.

## Differential Diagnosis

Osteoid osteomas are extremely rare in the jaws. A clinician who suspects that a sclerotic lesion is an osteoid osteoma should also consider sclerosing osteitis, cemento-ossifying fibroma, benign cementoblastoma, and cemental dysplasia. The presence of a central radiolucency usually eliminates enostosis or osteosclerosis. Scintigraphy by a bone scan will help in the differential diagnosis by revealing considerable vascularity in the blood pool phase and a very high comparative bone metabolism.

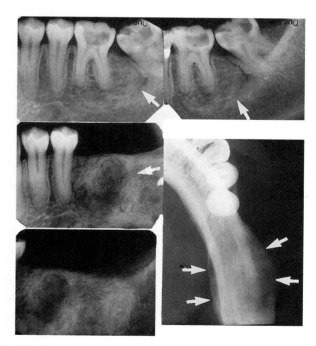

FIG. **22-49** An osteoid osteoma *(arrow)* appears as a mixed radiolucent-radiopaque lesion in the molar region; the lesion has caused expansion of the buccal and lingual cortex of the mandible *(arrows).* (Courtesy A. Shawkat, DDS, Radcliff, Ky.)

## Treatment

Complete excision is currently the recommended treatment because it often relieves the pain and cures the disease. Although spontaneous remission can occur in some cases, the data are insufficient for identifying such cases in advance.

## Desmoplastic Fibroma of Bone

### Synonym
Aggressive fibromatosis (usually reserved for tumors that originate in soft tissue)

### Definition
A desmoplastic fibroma of bone is an aggressive, infiltrative neoplasm that produces abundant collagen fibers. It is composed of fibroblast-like cells that have ovoid or elongated nuclei in abundant collagen fibers. The lack of pleomorphism of the cells is important.

### Clinical Features
Patients usually complain of facial swelling, pain (in rare cases), and sometimes dysfunction, especially when the neoplasm is close to the joint. The lesion occurs most often in the first two decades of life, with a mean reported age of 14 years. Although it originates in bone, the tumor may invade the surrounding soft tissue extensively. It also may occur as part of Gardner's syndrome.

### Radiographic Features
*Location.* Desmoplastic fibromas of bone may occur in the mandible or maxilla, but the most common site is the ramus and posterior mandible.

*Periphery.* The periphery is most often ill defined and has an invasive characteristic commonly seen in malignant tumors.

*Internal Structure.* The internal aspect may be totally radiolucent, especially when the lesion is small. Larger lesions appear to be multilocular with very coarse, thick septa. These wide septa may be straight or have an irregular shape (Fig. 22-50). In T1-weighted MRI

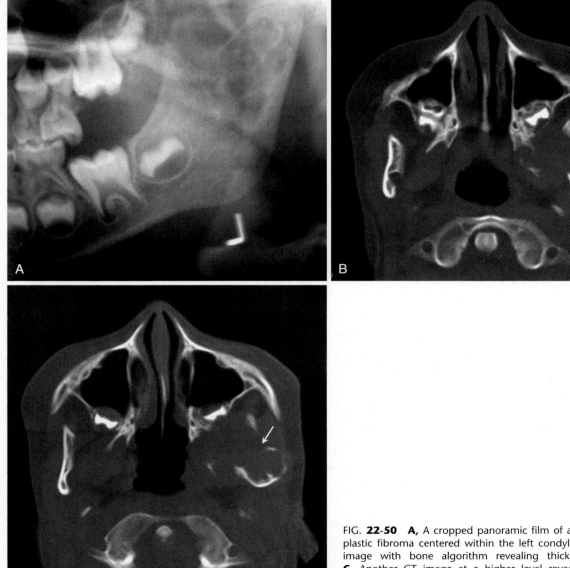

FIG. **22-50** **A,** A cropped panoramic film of a case of a central desmoplastic fibroma centered within the left condyle and ramus. **B,** Axial CT image with bone algorithm revealing thick, straight septa *(arrow).* **C,** Another CT image at a higher level revealing that the tumor has broken through the anterior cortex of the condylar head.

scans the internal structure has a low signal, which helps in determining intraosseous extent because of the contrast with the high signal from the bone marrow.

*Effects on Surrounding Structures.* Desmoplastic fibromas of bone can expand bone and often break through the outer cortex, invading the surrounding soft tissue. Usually CT or MRI is required to determine the exact soft tissue extent of the lesion.

## Differential Diagnosis

Distinguishing this neoplasm from a fibrosarcoma may be difficult during the histologic examination. The radiographic appearance may not be helpful because a desmoplastic fibroma often has the appearance of a malignant neoplasm. However, the presence of coarse, irregular, and sometimes straight septa may help support the correct diagnosis. The appearance of these septa also helps differentiate the lesion from other multilocular tumors. Very small lesions may resemble simple bone cysts.

## Treatment

Resection of this neoplasm with adequate margins is recommended because of its high recurrence rate. Patients who have been treated for the condition should be closely followed up with frequent radiologic examinations.

## BIBLIOGRAPHY

Barnes L, Eveson JW, Reichart P et al: Odontogenic tumors. In *Pathology and genetics of head and neck tumours,* World Health Organization Classification of Tumours, Lyon, 2005, IARC Press.

Daley TD, Wysocki GP, Pringle GA: Relative incidence of odontogenic tumors and oral and jaw cysts in a Canadian population, *Oral Surg Oral Med Oral Pathol* 77:276-280, 1994.

Hoffman S, Jacoway JR, Krolls SO: *Intraosseous and parosteal tumors of the jaws, atlas of tumor pathology,* series 2, fascicle 24, Washington, DC, 1987, Armed Forces Institute of Pathology.

Krishnan Unni K: *Dahlin's bone tumors: general aspects and data on 11,087 cases,* ed 5, Philadelphia, 1996, Lippincott-Raven.

Regezi JA, Kerr DA, Courtney RM: Odontogenic tumors: an analysis of 706 cases, *J Oral Surg* 36:771-778, 1978.

### TORUS PALATINUS

Eggan S, Natvig B, Gåsemyr J: Variation in torus palatinus prevalence in Norway, *Scand J Dent Res* 102:54-59, 1994.

Gorsky M, Raviv M, Kfir E et al: Prevalence of torus palatinus in a population of young and old Israelis, *Arch Oral Biol* 41:623-625, 1996.

Haugen LK: Palatine and mandibular tori; a morphologic study in the current Norwegian population, *Acta Odontol Scand* 50:65-77, 1992.

### TORUS MANDIBULARIS

Eggen S, Natvig B: Concurrence of torus mandibularis and torus palatinus, *Scand J Dent Res* 102:60-63, 1994.

### ENOSTOSIS

McDonnel D: Dense bone island: a review of 107 patients, *Oral Surg Oral Med Oral Pathol* 76:124-128, 1993.

Petrikowski GC, Peters E: Longitudinal radiographic assessment of dense bone islands of the jaws, *Oral Surg Oral Med Oral Pathol Oral Radiol Endod* 83:627-634, 1997.

### AMELOBLASTOMA

Atkinson CH, Harwood AR, Cummings BJ: Ameloblastoma of the jaw: a reappraisal of the role of megavoltage irradiation, *Cancer* 53:869-873, 1984.

Heffez L, Mafee MF, Vaiana J: The role of magnetic resonance imaging in the diagnosis and management of ameloblastoma, *Oral Surg Oral Med Oral Pathol* 65:2-12, 1988.

Ueta E, Yoneda K, Ohno A et al: Intraosseous carcinoma arising from mandibular ameloblastoma with progressive invasion and pulmonary metastasis, *Int J Oral Maxillofac Surg* 25:370-372, 1996.

Weissman JL, Snyderman CH, Yousem SA et al: Ameloblastoma of the maxilla: CT and MR appearance, *AJNR Am J Neuroradiol* 14:223-226, 1993.

### ADENOMATOID ODONTOGENIC TUMOR

Dare A, Yamaguchi A, Yoshiki S et al: Limitation of panoramic radiography in diagnosing adenomatoid odontogenic tumors, *Oral Surg Oral Med Oral Pathol* 77:662-668, 1994.

Hicks MJ, Flaitz CM, Batsakis JG: Pathology consultation: adenomatoid and calcifying epithelial odontogenic tumors, *Ann Otol Rhinol Laryngol* 102:159, 1993.

Philipsen HP, Reichart PA, Zhang KH et al: Adenomatoid odontogenic tumor: biologic profile based on 499 cases, *J Oral Pathol Med* 20:149-158, 1991.

### CALCIFYING EPITHELIAL ODONTOGENIC TUMOR

Franklin CD, Pindborg JJ: The calcifying epithelial odontogenic tumor: a review and analysis of 113 cases, *Oral Surg Oral Med Oral Pathol* 42:753-765, 1976.

Kaplan I, Buckner A, Calderon S et al: Radiological and clinical features of calcifying epithelial odontogenic tumor, *Dentomaxillofac Radiol* 30:22-28, 2001.

Patiño B, Fernández-Alba J, Garcia-Rosado A et al: Calcifying epithelial odontogenic (Pindborg) tumor: a series of 4 distinctive cases and review of the literature, *J Oral Maxillofac Surg* 63:1361-1368, 2005.

### COMPOUND ODONTOMA

Haishima K, Haishima H, Yamada Y et al: Compound odontomes associated with impacted maxillary primary central incisors: report of 2 cases, *Int J Paediatr Dent* 4:251-256, 1994.

Kaugars GE, Miller ME, Abbey LM: Odontomas, *Oral Surg Oral Med Oral Pathol* 67:172-176, 1989.

Nik-Hussein NN, Majid ZA: Erupted compound odontoma, *Ann Dent* 52:9-11, 1993.

### AMELOBLASTIC FIBROMA

Dallera P, Bertoni F, Marchetti C et al: Ameloblastic fibroma: a follow-up of six cases, *Int J Oral Maxillofac Surg* 25:199-202, 1996.

Trodahl JN: Ameloblastic fibroma: a survey of cases from the Armed Forces Institute of Pathology, *Oral Surg Oral Med Oral Pathol* 33:547-558, 1972.

### ODONTOGENIC MYXOMA

Cohen MA, Mendelsohn DB: CT and MR imaging of myxofibroma of the jaws, *J Comput Assist Tomogr* 14:281-285, 1990.

Peltola J, Magnusson B, Happonen RP et al: Odontogenic myxoma: a radiographic study of 21 tumours, *Br J Oral Maxillofac Surg* 32:298-302, 1994.

Simon ENM, Merkx MA, Vuhahula E et al: Odontogenic myxoma: a clinicopathological study of 33 cases, *Int J Oral Maxillofac Surg* 33:333-337, 2004.

Sumi Y, Miyaishi O, Ito K et al: Magnetic resonance imaging of myxoma in the mandible: a case report, *Oral Surg Oral Med Oral Pathol Oral Radiol Endod* 90:671-676, 2000.

### BENIGN CEMENTOBLASTOMA

Brannon RB, Fowler CB, Carpenter WM et al: Cementoblastoma: An innocuous neoplasm? A clinicopathologic study of 44 cases and review of the literature with special emphasis on recurrence, *Oral Surg Oral Med Oral Pathol Oral Radiol Endod* 93:311-320, 2002.

Jelic JS, Loftus MJ, Miller AS et al: Benign cementoblastoma: report of an unusual case and analysis of 14 additional cases, *J Oral Maxillofac Surg* 51:1033-1037, 1993.

Ruprecht A, Ross AS: Benign cementoblastoma (true cementoblastoma), *Dentomaxillofac Radiol* 12:31-33, 1983.

## CENTRAL ODONTOGENIC FIBROMA

Gardner DG: Central odontogenic fibroma: current concepts, *J Oral Pathol Med* 25:556-561, 1996.

Handlers JP, Abrams AM, Melrose RJ et al: Central odontogenic fibroma: clinicopathologic features of 19 cases and review of the literature, *J Oral Maxillofac Surg* 49:46-54, 1991.

Kaffe I, Buchner A: Radiologic features of central odontogenic fibroma, *Oral Surg Oral Med Oral Pathol* 78:811-818, 1994.

## NEURILEMMOMA

Chi AC, Carey J, Muller S et al: Intraosseous schwannoma of the mandible; case report and review of the literature, *Oral Surg Oral Med Oral Pathol Oral Radiol Endod* 96:54, 2003.

Minowa K, Sakakibara N, Yoshikawa K et al: CT and MRI findings of intraosseous schwannoma of the mandible: a case report, *Dentomaxillofac Radiol* 36:113-116, 2007.

## HEMANGIOMA

Fan X, Qiu W, Zhang Z et al: Comparative study of clinical manifestation, plain-film radiography and computed tomographic scan in arteriovenous malformations of the jaws, *Oral Surg Oral Med Oral Pathol Oral Radiol Endod* 94:503-509, 2002.

Lund BA, Dahlin DC: Hemangiomas of the mandible and maxilla, *J Oral Surg* 22:234-242, 1964.

Zlotogorski A, Buchner A, Kaffe I et al: Radiological features of central haemangioma of the jaws, *Dentomaxillofac Radiol* 34:292-296, 2005.

## OSTEOMA

Bilkay U, Erdem O, Ozek C et al: Benign osteoma with Gardner syndrome: review of the literature and report of a case, *J Craniofac Surg* 15:506-509, 2004.

Earwaker J: Paranasal osteomas: a review of 46 cases, *Skeletal Radiol* 22:417-423, 1993.

Matteson S, Deahl ST, Alder ME et al: Advanced imaging methods, *Crit Rev Oral Biol Med* 7:346-395, 1996.

Thakker NS, Evans DG, Horner K et al: Florid oral manifestations in an atypical familial adenomatous polyposis family with late presentation of colorectal polyps, *J Oral Pathol Med* 25:459-462, 1996.

## NEUROFIBROMATOSIS

D'Ambrosio JA, Langlais RP, Young RS: Jaw and skull changes in neurofibromatosis, *Oral Surg Oral Med Oral Pathol* 66:391, 1988.

Lee L, Yan YH, Pharaoah MJ: Radiographic features of the mandible in neurofibromatosis: a report of 10 cases and review of the literature, *Oral Surg Oral Med Oral Pathol Oral Radiol Endod* 81:361-367, 1996.

## OSTEOBLASTOMA

Alvares Capelozza AL, Gião Dezotti MS, Casati Alvares L et al: Osteoblastoma of the mandible: systematic review of the literature and report of a case, *Dentomaxillofac Radiol* 34:1-8, 2005.

Jones AC, Prihoda TJ, Kacher JE et al: Osteoblastoma of the maxilla and mandible: a report of 24 cases, review of the literature, and discussion of its relationship to osteoid osteoma of the jaws, *Oral Surg Oral Med Oral Pathol Oral Radiol Endod* 102:639-650, 2006.

Lucas DR, Unni KK, McLeod RA et al: Osteoblastoma: clinicopathologic study of 306 cases, *Hum Pathol* 25:117-134, 1994.

## DESMOPLASTIC FIBROMA OF BONE

Hopkins KM, Huttula CS, Kahn MA et al: Desmoplastic fibroma of the mandible: review and report of two cases, *J Oral Maxillofac Surg* 54:1249-1254, 1996.

Said-Al-Naief N, Fernandes R, Louis P et al: Desmoplastic fibroma of the jaw: a case report and review of literature, *Oral Surg Oral Med Oral Pathol Oral Radiol Endod* 101:82-94, 2006.

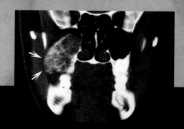

# CHAPTER 23

# Malignant Diseases of the Jaws

Robert E. Wood

## Definition

Malignant tumors represent an uncontrolled growth of tissue. Unlike benign neoplasms, they are more locally invasive, have a greater degree of cellular anaplasia, and have the ability to metastasize regionally to lymph nodes or distantly to other sites. Malignant tumors that arise de novo are termed primary tumors, and those that originate from distant primary tumors are termed secondary or metastatic malignancy. Cancers may be caused by viruses, significant radiation exposure, genetic defects, or exposure to carcinogenic chemicals. For instance, using tobacco is strongly associated with oral carcinoma.

The most convenient method of classification of cancers is on the basis of histopathologic characteristics. In the following text the malignancies that commonly affect the jaws have been divided into four categories: carcinomas (lesions of epithelial origin), metastatic lesions from distant sites, sarcomas (lesions of mesenchymal origin), and malignancies of the hematopoietic system. Of these four categories, carcinomas are by far the most commonly encountered in dental practice. Unusual malignant tumors have been omitted to concentrate on those lesions that a general practitioner may encounter.

## Clinical Features

The following are clinical signs and symptoms that suggest that a lesion may be malignant: displaced teeth, loosened teeth over a short time, foul smell, ulceration, presence of an indurated or rolled border, exposure of underlying bone, sensory or motor neural deficits, lymphadenopathy, weight loss, dysgeusia, dysphagia, dysphonia, hemorrhage, lack of normal healing after oral surgery, and pain or rapid swelling with no demonstrable dental cause. Most oral cancers occur in men aged 50 years and older; however, malignant tumors may occur at any age in either sex.

Dentists must watch vigilantly for the possibility of malignancy in their patients. Because the prevalence of oral malignancy is low, many general practitioners practice years without encountering a patient with a malignant tumor. This rarity may make a dentist less likely to recognize a malignant condition when it is present. The risks of lack of attention to this possibility are delayed diagnosis, delayed treatment, increased need for aggressive treatment with added morbidity, and, in the worst case, premature death.

## Radiographic Examination

Radiology has a number of important roles in the management of the patient with cancer. First, diagnostic images may aid in the establish-

ment of an initial diagnosis of a tumor. Diagnostic imaging also aids in the appropriate staging of disease from early small cancers to large cancers that have spread. Appropriate radiologic investigations assist the surgeon or radiation oncologist to determine the anatomic spread of the tumor so that it can be excised or irradiated adequately. Radiologic investigation has the potential to determine the presence of osseous involvement from soft tissue tumors and allow the practitioner to assess the involvement of lymph nodes and treatment outcome. Finally, a thorough radiographic dental examination plays a part in the management of the cancer survivor, who often is rendered xerostomic, neutropenic, and susceptible to dental caries, periodontal disease, and systemic infection.

There are various diagnostic imaging modalities available to aid in the diagnosis. Intraoral radiographs still provide the best image resolution and are able to reveal subtle malignant changes such as irregular widening of the periodontal membrane space. Panoramic radiographs provide an overall assessment of the maxillofacial osseous structures and can reveal relevant changes such as destruction of the boundaries of the maxillary sinus. Either cone beam computed tomography (CT) or medical CT images can provide a superior three-dimensional analysis of the osseous structures and better determine the position and extent of the tumor. Positron emission tomographic (PET) scans, a technique capable of detecting abnormal cellular metabolic activity associated with malignant tumors, have been fused with CT images to provide an accurate location of the tumor in preparation for radiotherapy. Finally, magnetic resonance imaging (MRI) has provided three-dimensional soft tissue images of tumors and information regarding perineural spread and involvement of lymph nodes.

## RADIOGRAPHIC FEATURES

The following features may suggest the presence of a malignant tumor. The absence of visible radiologic signs as described does not preclude malignancy. It only implies that no visible radiographic signs exist.

### Location

Primary and metastatic malignant tumors may occur anywhere in the oral and maxillofacial region. Primary carcinomas are more commonly seen in the tongue, floor of mouth, tonsillar area, lip, soft palate, or gingiva and may invade the jaws from any of these sites. Sarcomas are more common in the mandible and in posterior regions of both jaws. Metastatic tumors are most common in the posterior mandible and maxilla. Some metastatic lesions grow at the apices of teeth or in the follicles of developing teeth (Fig. 23-1, *D*).

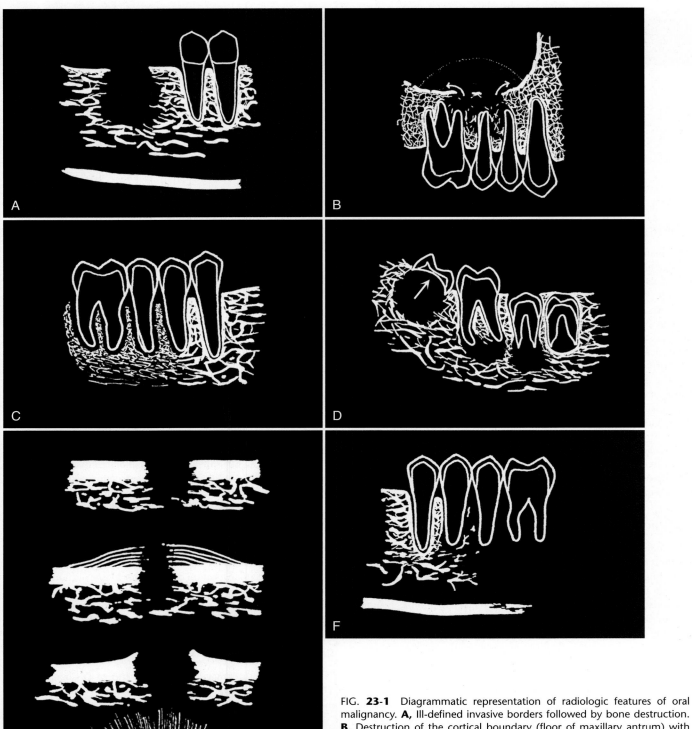

FIG. **23-1** Diagrammatic representation of radiologic features of oral malignancy. **A,** Ill-defined invasive borders followed by bone destruction. **B,** Destruction of the cortical boundary (floor of maxillary antrum) with an adjacent soft tissue mass *(arrows)*. **C,** Tumor invasion along the periodontal membrane space causing irregular thickening of this space. **D,** Multifocal lesions located at root apices and in the papilla of a developing tooth destroying the crypt cortex and displacing the developing tooth in an occlusal direction *(arrow)*. **E,** Four types of effects on cortical bone and periosteal reaction, from top to the bottom: cortical bone destruction without periosteal reaction, laminated periosteal reaction with destruction of the cortical bone and the new periosteal bone, destruction of cortical bone with periosteal reaction at the periphery forming Codman's triangles, and a spiculated or sunray type of periosteal reaction. **F,** Bone destruction around existing teeth, producing an appearance of teeth floating in space.

## Periphery and Shape

The typical appearance of the periphery (border) of a malignant lesion is an ill-defined border with lack of cortication and absence of encapsulation (a soft tissue or radiolucent periphery). This infiltrative border has uneven extensions of bone destruction. Fingerlike extension of the tumor occurs in many directions; this extension is followed by osseous destruction producing a region of radiolucency (Fig. 23-1, *A*). Evidence of destruction of a cortical boundary with adjacent soft tissue mass is highly suggestive of malignancy (Fig. 23-1, *B*). Such a mass may exhibit a smooth or ulcerated peripheral border if cast against a radiolucent background such as the air within the maxillary sinus. The shape of a malignant tumor of the jaw is commonly irregular.

## Internal Structure

Because most malignancies do not produce bone nor do they stimulate the formation of reactive bone, the internal aspect is typically radiolucent in most instances. Occasionally residual islands of bone are present, resulting in a pattern of patchy destruction with some scattered residual internal osseous structure. Some tumors, such as metastatic prostate or breast lesions, can induce bone formation, resulting in an abnormal-appearing internal sclerotic osseous architecture, whereas others, such as osteogenic sarcomas, can produce abnormal bone, giving the involved bone a sclerotic (radiopaque) appearance.

## Effects on Surrounding Structures

Malignancy is destructive, often rapidly so. The effect on surrounding structures mirrors this behavior. Slower-growing benign tumors or cysts may resorb tooth roots or displace teeth in a bodily fashion without causing loose teeth. In contrast, rapidly growing malignant lesions generally destroy supporting alveolar bone so that teeth may appear to be floating in space (Fig. 23-1, *F*).

Occasionally root resorption is present, more commonly in sarcomas. Internal trabecular bone is destroyed, as are cortical boundaries such as the sinus floor (Fig. 23-1, *B*), the inferior border of the mandible, the follicular cortices of developing teeth, and the cortex of the inferior alveolar neurovascular canal. Because malignant tumors tend to grow rapidly, they invade by means of the easiest routes, such as through the maxillary antrum or through the periodontal ligament space around teeth, resulting in irregular widening with destruction of the lamina dura (Fig. 23-1, *C*); they also may spread through the inferior alveolar neurovascular canal, causing similar widening. Where the tumor has destroyed the outer cortex of bone, usually no periosteal reaction occurs; however, some tumors stimulate unusual periosteal new bone formation (Fig. 23-1, *E*). Lesions such as osteosarcoma and metastatic prostate lesions and other tumors can stimulate the formation of thin straight spicules of bone, giving a hair-on-end or sunburst appearance. If there is a secondary inflammatory lesion coexisting with the malignancy, a periosteal reaction normally associated with an inflammatory lesion (e.g., "onion skin" like) may be seen.

## Carcinomas

### Squamous Cell Carcinoma Arising in Soft Tissue

#### Synonym

Epidermoid carcinoma

## Definition

Squamous cell carcinoma, the most common oral malignancy, may be defined as a malignant tumor originating from surface epithelium. It is characterized initially by invasion of malignant epithelial cells into the underlying connective tissue with subsequent spread into deeper soft tissues and occasionally into adjacent bone, local-regional lymph nodes, and ultimately to distant sites such as the lung, liver, and skeleton.

## Clinical Features

Squamous cell carcinoma appears initially as white or red (sometimes mixed) irregular patchy lesions of the affected epithelium. With time these lesions exhibit central ulceration; a rolled or indurated border, which represents invasion of malignant cells; and palpable infiltration into adjacent muscle or bone. Pain may be variable, and regional lymphadenopathy with hard lymph nodes that may or may not be tethered to underlying structures may be present. Other clinical features include a soft tissue mass, paresthesia, anesthesia, dysesthesia, pain, foul smell, trismus, grossly loosened teeth, or hemorrhage. Large lesions can obstruct the airway, the opening of the eustachian tube (leading to diminished hearing), or the nasopharynx. Patients often report a significant weight loss and feel unwell. Males are more commonly affected than females. The condition is often fatal, if untreated. Most squamous cell carcinomas occur in persons older than 50 years.

## Radiographic Features

*Location.* Squamous cell carcinoma commonly involves the lateral border of the tongue. Therefore a common site to observe bone invasion is the posterior lingual aspect of the mandible. Lesions of the lip and floor of the mouth may similarly invade the anterior mandible. Lesions involving attached gingiva and underlying alveolar bone may mimic inflammatory disease such as periodontal disease. This malignancy is also seen on the tonsils, soft palate, and buccal vestibule. It is uncommon on the hard palate.

*Periphery and Shape.* Squamous cell carcinoma may erode into underlying bone from any direction, producing a radiolucency that is polymorphous and irregular in outline. Invasion occurs in half of cases and is characterized most commonly by an ill-defined, noncorticated border (Fig. 23-2). Rarely, the border may appear smooth without a cortex, indicating underlying erosion rather than invasion. If bone involvement is extensive, the periphery appears to have fingerlike extensions preceding a zone of impressive osseous destruction. If pathologic fracture occurs, the borders show sharpened thinned bone ends with displacement of segments and an adjacent soft tissue mass. Sclerosis in underlying osseous structures (likely from secondary inflammatory disease) may be seen in association with erosions from surface carcinomas.

*Internal Structure.* The internal structure of squamous cell carcinoma in jaw lesions is totally radiolucent; the original osseous structure can be completely lost. Occasionally small islands of residual normal trabecular bone are visible within this central radiolucency.

*Effects on Surrounding Structures.* Evidence of invasion of bone around teeth may first appear as widening of the periodontal ligament space with loss of adjacent lamina dura. Teeth may appear to float in a mass of radiolucent soft tissue bereft of any bony support. In extensive tumors this soft tissue mass may grow with the teeth in it as "passengers," so teeth are grossly displaced from their former position. Tumors may grow along the inferior neurovascular canal and through the mental foramen, resulting in an increase in the width

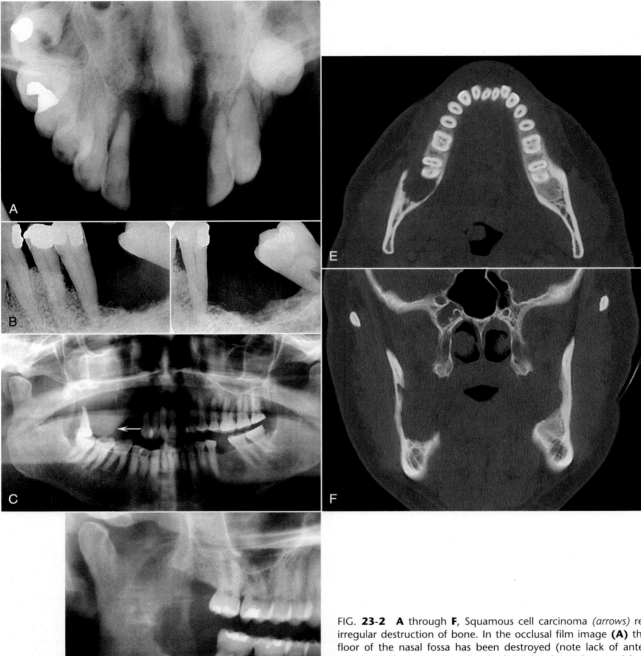

**FIG. 23-2** **A** through **F,** Squamous cell carcinoma *(arrows)* resulting in irregular destruction of bone. In the occlusal film image **(A)** the anterior floor of the nasal fossa has been destroyed (note lack of anterior nasal spine). **B,** The supporting alveolar bone has been destroyed from around the teeth. **C,** There is destruction of the right alveolar process and floor of maxillary sinus and the soft tissue mass *(arrow).* **D,** Destruction of bone in the mandibular retromolar area by a squamous cell carcinoma. **E** and **F,** Axial and coronal CT images of the tumor displayed in **D.** Note destruction of lateral cortical plate in the axial image and medial cortical plate in the coronal image and lack of bone reaction at the margins of the tumor.

and loss of the cortical boundary. Destruction of adjacent normal cortical boundaries such as the floor of the nose, maxillary sinus, or buccal or lingual mandibular plate may occur. The posterior aspect of the maxilla may also be effaced. The inferior border of the mandible may be thinned or destroyed. If the tumor is extensive, pathologic fracture may occur.

## Differential Diagnosis

Squamous cell carcinoma is discernible from other malignancies by its clinical and histologic features. Occasionally it is difficult to differentiate inflammatory lesions such as osteomyelitis from squamous cell carcinoma, especially when oral bacteria secondarily infect the tumor. Both osteomyelitis and squamous cell carcinoma are destructive, leaving islands of osseous structure that may appear to be consistent with sequestra. Evidence of profound bone destruction or invasive characteristics helps to identify the presence of a malignancy when a mixture of inflammatory changes and carcinoma exists. Osteomyelitis usually produces some periosteal reaction, whereas squamous cell carcinoma does not. In cases of osteoradionecrosis, where the patient has had prior malignancy, periosteal new bone is absent. If osseous destruction is present, the differentiation of this condition from squamous cell carcinoma requires advanced imaging and biopsy. The bone loss from squamous cell carcinoma originating in the soft tissues of the alveolar process may appear very similar to that from periodontal disease (Fig. 23-3, *A*). Enlargement of a recent extraction socket instead of evidence of healing new bone formation can indicate the presence of an alveolar squamous cell carcinoma (Fig. 23-3, *B*).

## Management

Oral squamous cell carcinoma is usually managed with a combination of surgery and radiation therapy. The choice of which modality to use depends on the protocol of the treating center and the location and severity of the tumor. Generally, if an adequate margin of normal tissue can be obtained, surgery is the usual treatment, followed by radiation treatment. Alternately, radiation may be used as the primary treatment followed by surgical salvage. Currently, the trend is to add concomitant chemotherapy as an adjunct to either radiation or surgi-

cal treatment, which requires the dental practitioner to be aware of changes in the patient's circulating blood count.

### Squamous Cell Carcinoma Originating in Bone

#### Synonyms
Primary intraosseous carcinoma, intra-alveolar carcinoma, primary intra-alveolar epidermoid carcinoma, primary epithelial tumor of the jaw, central squamous cell carcinoma, primary odontogenic carcinoma, intramandibular carcinoma, and central mandibular carcinoma

#### Definition
Primary intraosseous carcinoma is a squamous cell carcinoma that arises within the jaw and has no original connection with the surface epithelium of the oral mucosa. Primary intraosseous carcinomas are presumed to arise from intraosseous remnants of odontogenic epithelium. Carcinoma from surface epithelium, odontogenic cysts, or distant sites (metastases) must be excluded.

#### Clinical Features
These neoplasms are rare and may remain silent until they have reached a fairly large size. Pain, pathologic fracture, and sensory nerve abnormalities such as lip paresthesia and lymphadenopathy may occur with this tumor. It is more common in men and in patients in the fourth to eighth decade of life. The surface epithelium is invariably normal in appearance.

#### Radiographic Features
*Location.* The mandible is far more commonly involved than the maxilla, with most cases being present in the molar region (Fig. 23-4) and less frequently in the anterior aspect of the jaws. Because the lesion is by definition associated with remnants of the dental lamina, it originates only in tooth-bearing parts of the jaw.

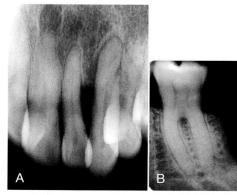
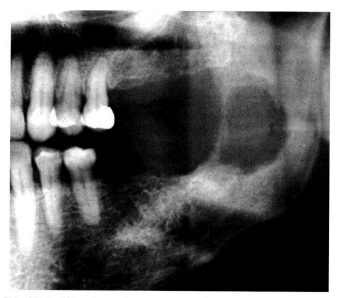

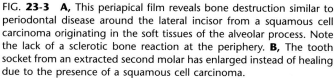
FIG. **23-3**  **A,** This periapical film reveals bone destruction similar to periodontal disease around the lateral incisor from a squamous cell carcinoma originating in the soft tissues of the alveolar process. Note the lack of a sclerotic bone reaction at the periphery. **B,** The tooth socket from an extracted second molar has enlarged instead of healing due to the presence of a squamous cell carcinoma.

FIG. **23-4**  This primary intraosseous carcinoma in the left mandible exhibits no internal structure, a poorly defined periphery, and thinning of the overlying mandibular bone.

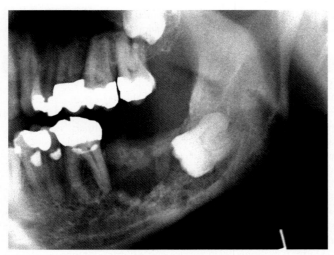

FIG. **23-5** Carcinoma arising in a preexisting dentigerous cyst related to the mandibular left third molar shows absence of a cyst cortex, invasion into adjacent bone, and ill-defined borders.

***Periphery and Shape.*** The periphery of the majority of lesions is ill defined, although some have been described as well defined. They are most often rounded or irregular in shape and have a border that demonstrates osseous destruction and varying degrees of extension at the periphery. The degree of raggedness of the border may reflect the aggressiveness of the lesion. If the lesion is of sufficient size, pathologic fracture occurs, with its associated step defects, thinned cortical borders, and subsequent soft tissue mass.

***Internal Structure.*** The internal structure is wholly radiolucent with no evidence of bone production and very little residual bone left within the center of the lesion. If the lesion is small, overlying buccal or lingual plates may cast a shadow that may mimic the appearance of internal trabecular bone.

***Effects on Surrounding Structures.*** These lesions are capable of causing destruction of the antral or nasal floors, loss of the cortical outline of the mandibular neurovascular canal, and effacement of the lamina dura. Root resorption is unusual. Teeth that lose both lamina dura and supporting bone appear to be floating in space.

## Differential Diagnosis

If the lesions are not aggressive and have a smooth border and radiolucent area, they may be mistaken for periapical cysts or granulomas. Alternately, if lesions are not centered about the apex of a tooth, occasionally it is difficult to differentiate this condition from odontogenic cysts or tumors. If the border is obviously infiltrative with extensive bone destruction, a metastatic lesion must be excluded, as well as multiple myeloma, fibrosarcoma, and carcinoma arising in a dental cyst. Examination of the oral cavity and especially the surface epithelium assists in differentiating this condition from surface squamous cell carcinoma.

## Management

Generally these tumors are excised with their surrounding osseous structure in an en bloc resection. Radiation and chemotherapy may be used as adjunctive therapies.

### Synonyms
Epidermoid cell carcinoma and carcinoma ex odontogenic cyst

### Definition
Squamous cell carcinoma arising in a preexisting dental cyst is uncommon and excludes invasion from surface epithelial carcinomas, metastatic tumors, and primary intraosseous carcinoma. They may arise from inflammatory periapical, residual, dentigerous, and odontogenic keratocysts. Histologically the lining squamous epithelium of the cyst gives rise to the malignant neoplasm.

### Clinical Features
The most common presenting sign or symptom associated with this condition is pain. The pain may be characterized as dull and of several months' duration. Swelling is occasionally reported. Pathologic fracture may occur, as may fistula formation and regional lymphadenopathy. If the upper jaw is involved, sinus pain or swelling may be present.

### Radiographic Features
***Location.*** This tumor may occur anywhere an odontogenic cyst is found, namely, the tooth-bearing portions of the jaws. Most cases occur in the mandible (Fig. 23-5), with a few cases reported in the anterior maxilla.

***Periphery and Shape.*** The radiologic picture of squamous cell carcinoma originating in a cyst mirrors the histologic findings. Because the lesion arises from a cyst, the shape is often round or ovoid. If it is a small lesion in a cyst wall, the periphery may be mostly well defined and even corticated. In this case the radiographic differentiation from a normal cyst is impossible. As the malignant tissue progressively replaces cyst lining, the smooth border is lost or becomes ill defined. The advanced lesion has an ill-defined, infiltrative periphery that lacks any cortication. Its shape becomes less "hydraulic" looking and more diffuse.

***Internal Structure.*** This lesion lacks any ability to produce bone. It is wholly radiolucent, perhaps more so than invasive surface carcinoma, owing to prior osteolysis from the cyst.

***Effects on Surrounding Structures.*** Carcinoma arising in dental cysts is capable of thinning and destroying the lamina dura of adjacent teeth or adjacent cortical boundaries, such as the inferior border of the jaw or the floor of the nose. It can produce complete destruction of the alveolar process.

### Differential Diagnosis
If a dental cyst is infected, it may lose its normal cortical boundary and appear ragged and identical to a malignant lesion arising in a preexisting cyst. However, inflamed cysts usually show a reactive peripheral sclerosis because of inflammatory products present in the cyst lumen. This is not normally present in a cyst, which has undergone malignant transformation. Nevertheless, the two may be difficult to differentiate radiologically, and therefore cysts should always be submitted for histologic examination. Multiple myeloma may appear as a solitary lesion and may be difficult to distinguish, especially if it has a cystic well-defined shape. Metastatic disease may be similar, although it is commonly multifocal.

### Management
The treatment of squamous cell carcinoma originating in a cyst is identical to that described with primary intraosseous carcinoma.

## Central Mucoepidermoid Carcinoma

### Synonym
Mucoepidermoid carcinoma

### Definition
Central mucoepidermoid carcinoma is an epithelial tumor arising in bone, likely originating from pluripotential odontogenic epithelium or from a cyst lining. It is histologically indistinguishable from its soft tissue counterpart. The criteria for diagnosis of a central mucoepidermoid tumor are the presence of intact cortical plates, radiographic evidence of bone destruction, and typical histologic findings consistent with mucoepidermoid tumor. Additionally, the practitioner must exclude the possibility of an invasive overlying mucoepidermoid tumor or odontogenic tumor.

### Clinical Features
Unlike other malignant tumors of the jaws, the central mucoepidermoid tumor is more likely to mimic a benign tumor or cyst. The most common complaint is of a painless swelling. The swelling may have been present for months or even years and has been reported to cause facial asymmetry. Occasionally it may feel as if teeth have been moved or a denture may no longer fit. Tenderness rather than severe pain may also be present. Paresthesia of the inferior alveolar nerve and spreading of the lesion to regional lymph nodes has been reported. Central mucoepidermoid tumor, unlike other oral malignancies, is more common in females than males.

### Radiographic Features
*Location.* The lesion is twice as common in the mandible as the in maxilla, usually in the premolar and molar region with a few cases reported in the anterior mandible. The lesion most commonly occurs above the mandibular canal, similar to odontogenic tumors.

*Periphery and Shape.* Mucoepidermoid tumor presents as a unilocular or multilocular expansile mass (Fig. 23-6). The border is most often well defined and well corticated and often crenated or undulating in nature, which is similar to benign odontogenic tumors. The peripheral cortication may be impressively thick, which belies its malignant nature. Rarely, the periphery is not corticated and has a more malignant appearance.

*Internal Structure.* The internal structure has features like those of a benign odontogenic tumor such as an ameloblastoma. Lesions are often described as being multilocular or having either a soap bubble or honeycomb internal structure, implying the presence of compartments separated by thin or thick cortical septa. This bone is not produced by the tumor but is merely remodeled residual bone taking the form of septa.

*Effects on Surrounding Structures.* Mucoepidermoid tumor is capable of causing expansion of adjacent normal bony walls. The buccal and lingual cortical plates, inferior border of the mandible, and alveolar crest are usually intact; however, they may be thinned and grossly displaced. The mandibular canal may be depressed or pushed laterally or medially. These characteristics are more similar to benign tumors than to malignant tumors. Teeth remain largely unaffected by this disease, although adjacent lamina dura may be lost.

### Differential Diagnosis
The differential diagnosis of this lesion reflects its lack of features commonly associated with oral malignancy. The chief differential diagnosis is ameloblastoma and glandular odontogenic cyst, with which it shares similarities in its peripheral and internal features. It may not be possible to differentiate the two. Odontogenic myxoma and central giant cell granuloma also may be confused with mucoepidermoid tumor, as may other odontogenic cysts or tumors.

### Management
Mucoepidermoid carcinoma is treated surgically with en bloc resection encompassing a margin of adjacent normal bone. Neck dissection and postoperative radiation therapy may be required to control spread to lymph nodes.

## Malignant Ameloblastoma and Ameloblastic Carcinoma

### Definition
Malignant ameloblastoma is defined as an ameloblastoma with typical benign histologic features that is deemed malignant because of its biologic behavior, namely, metastasis. The histologic features may not correlate with the clinical behavior. On the other hand, ameloblastic carcinoma is an ameloblastoma exhibiting the histologic criteria of a malignant neoplasm such as increased and abnormal mitosis and large hyperchromatic, pleomorphic nuclei.

### Clinical Features
Clinically these lesions may behave as benign ameloblastomas, exhibiting a hard expansile mass of the jaw with displaced and perhaps loosened teeth and normal overlying mucosa. Tenderness of the overlying soft tissue has been reported. Metastatic spread may be to the cervical lymph nodes, lung or other viscera, and the skeleton, especially the spine. Local extension may occur into adjacent bones, connective tissue, or salivary glands. These tumors occur most commonly between the first and sixth decades of life and are more common in males than in females.

### Radiographic Features
*Location.* These lesions are more common in the mandible than in the maxilla, with most occurring in the premolar and molar region, where ameloblastoma is typically found.

*Periphery and Shape.* Similar to ameloblastoma, a well-defined border occurs with cortication, presence of crenations, or scalloping of the border. Malignant ameloblastoma may show some of the signs more commonly seen in malignant neoplasms, namely, loss of and

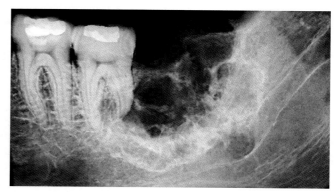

FIG. 23-6 The multilocular radiolucency in this radiograph is characteristic of central mucoepidermoid carcinoma; this lesion has displaced the mandibular canal and destroyed the superior crest of the alveolar process and the distal supporting bone of the second molar.

subsequent breaching of the cortical boundary invading into the surrounding soft tissue.

*Internal Structure.* The lesions are either unilocular or, more commonly, multilocular, giving the appearance of a honeycomb or soap-bubble pattern as seen in benign ameloblastomas. Most of the septa are robust and thick.

*Effects on Surrounding Structures.* Teeth may be moved bodily by the tumor and may exhibit root resorption similar to a benign tumor. Bony borders may be effaced or breached, and, as in benign ameloblastoma, the lesions may erode the lamina dura and displace normal anatomic boundaries such as the floor of the nose and maxillary sinus. The mandibular neurovascular canal may be displaced or eroded.

## Differential Diagnosis

The differential diagnosis of this lesion should include benign ameloblastoma, odontogenic keratocyst, odontogenic myxoma, and central mucoepidermoid tumor, from which it may not be distinguishable radiologically. If the lesion is locally invasive and this is apparent radiologically, a diagnosis of carcinoma arising in a dental cyst should be entertained. If the patient is young and the location of the lesion is anterior to the second permanent molar, central giant cell granuloma may mimic some of its radiologic features. Often the final diagnosis is the result of histologic evaluation or the detection of metastatic lesions.

## Management

These lesions are most often treated with en bloc surgical resection. However, many may not be discovered to be malignant until the time of the first surgery or even later. Because the histologic appearance of these lesions may mimic benign ameloblastoma, the initial treatment often is inadequate. In addition, the metastatic lesions may not appear for many months or years after treatment of the primary tumor, adding another reason for treatment failure.

## Metastatic Tumors

### Synonym
Secondary malignancy

### Definition
Metastatic tumors represent the establishment of new foci of malignant disease from a distant malignant tumor, usually by way of the blood vessels. An interesting feature of these lesions is that metastatic lesions in the jaws usually arise from sites that are anatomically inferior to the clavicle. Metastatic lesions of the jaws usually occur when the distant primary lesion is already known, although on occasion the presence of a metastatic tumor may reveal the presence of a silent primary lesion. Jaw involvement accounts for fewer than 1% of metastatic malignancies found elsewhere, with most affecting the spine, pelvis, skull, ribs, and humerus. Most frequently the tumor is a type of carcinoma; the most common primary sites are the breast, kidney, lung, colon and rectum, prostate, thyroid, stomach, melanoma, testes, bladder, ovary, and cervix. In children the tumors include neuroblastoma, retinoblastoma, and Wilms' tumor. Metastatic carcinoma must be differentiated from the more common locally invading squamous carcinoma.

### Clinical Features
Metastatic disease is more common in patients in their fifth to seventh decades of life. Patients may complain of dental pain, numbness or paresthesia of the third branch of the trigeminal nerve, pathologic fracture of the jaw, or hemorrhage from the tumor site.

### Radiographic Features

*Location.* The posterior areas of the jaws are more commonly affected (Fig. 23-7), with the mandible favored over the maxilla. The maxillary sinus may be the next most common site, followed by the anterior hard palate and mandibular condyle. Frequently metastatic lesions of the mandible are bilateral (Fig. 23-7, *B* and *C*). Also, lesions may be located in the periodontal ligament space (sometimes at the root apex), mimicking periapical and periodontal inflammatory disease, or in the papilla of a developing tooth.

*Periphery and Shape.* Metastatic lesions may be moderately well demarcated but have no cortication or encapsulation at their tumor margins; they may also have ill-defined invasive margins (see Fig. 23-7, *A*). The lesions are not usually round but polymorphous in shape. Both prostate and breast lesions may stimulate bone formation of the adjacent bone, which will be sclerotic. The tumor may begin as a few zones of osseous destruction separated by normal bone. After a time these small areas coalesce into a larger, ill-defined mass and the jaw may become enlarged.

*Internal Structure.* Lesions are generally radiolucent, in which case the internal structure is a combination of residual normal trabecular bone in association with areas of bone lysis. If sclerotic metastases are present (i.e., prostate and breast), the normally ragged radiolucent area may appear as an area of patchy sclerosis, the result of new bone formation (Fig. 23-8). The origin of this new bone is not the tumor but stimulation of surrounding normal bone. If the tumor is seeded in multiple regions of the jaw, the result is a multifocal appearance (multiple small radiolucent lesions) with normal bone between the foci. Significant dissemination of metastatic tumor may give the jaws a general radiolucent appearance or even that of osteopenia.

*Effects on Surrounding Structures.* Metastatic carcinomas may stimulate a periosteal reaction that usually takes the form of a spiculated pattern (prostate and neuroblastoma) (Fig. 23-8). Typical of malignancy, the lesion effaces the lamina dura and can cause an irregular increase in the width of the periodontal ligament space. If the tumor has seeded in the papilla of a developing tooth, the cortices of the crypt may be totally or partially destroyed. Teeth may seem to be floating in a soft tissue mass and may be in an altered position because of loss of bony support. Extraction sockets may fail to heal and may increase in size. Resorption of teeth is rare (sometimes associated with multiple myeloma and chondrosarcoma); this is more common in benign lesions. The cortical bone of adjacent structures such as the neurovascular canal, sinus, and nasal fossa is destroyed. On occasion the tumor breaches the outer cortical plate of the jaws and extends into surrounding soft tissues or presents as an intraoral mass (see Fig. 23-7, *E*).

### Differential Diagnosis

In most cases a known primary malignancy is present, and the diagnosis of metastasis is straightforward. Multiple myeloma may be confused with metastatic tumors; however, the border of multiple myeloma is usually better circumscribed than in metastatic disease. When a lesion starts within the periodontal ligament space of a tooth, the appearance may be identical to that of a periapical inflammatory lesion. A point of differentiation is that the periodontal ligament space widening from inflammation is at its greatest width and centered about the apex of the root. In contrast, the malignant tumor usually

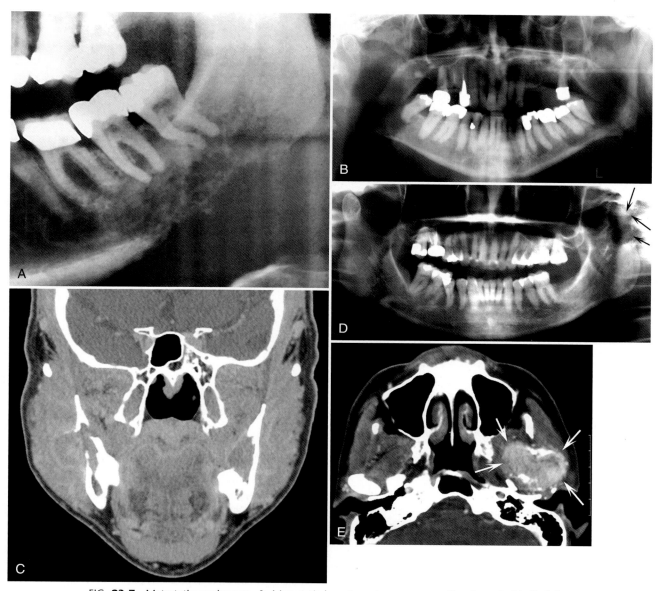

FIG. **23-7**   Metastatic carcinomas. **A,** Metastatic breast carcinoma surrounding the apical half of the second and third molar roots and extending inferiorly. It has destroyed the inferior border of the mandible. **B,** Bilateral metastatic lesions from the lung destroying the mandibular rami. **C,** Coronal CT image with soft tissue algorithm of the same case. **D,** Destruction of the left mandibular condyle *(arrows)* from a thyroid metastatic lesion. **E,** Axial CT image with soft tissue algorithm of the same case showing invasion into surrounding soft tissue *(arrows)*.

causes irregular widening, which may extend up the side of the root. Odontogenic cysts, if secondarily infected, may have an ill-defined border giving a similar appearance to a metastatic lesion. Invasion of the jaws by primary tumors of the overlying epithelium such as squamous cell carcinoma may be indistinguishable from metastatic disease but can be differentiated by clinical examination.

## Management

The presence of a metastatic tumor in the jaw indicates a poor prognosis. If metastatic disease is present, the patient will usually die within 1 to 2 years. If the radiographic appearance is suspicious, an opinion from a dental radiologist should be sought and tissue submitted for histologic analysis. Nuclear medicine may be used to detect other metastatic lesions. Isolated malignant deposits, if symptomatic, may be treated with localized high-dose radiation. In the rare occasion that the jaw is the first diagnosed site of malignant spread, it is imperative that the patient be referred quickly to an oncologist so that anticancer treatment can be delivered promptly. This treatment may take the form of chemotherapy, radiation therapy, surgery, immunotherapy, or hormone treatment.

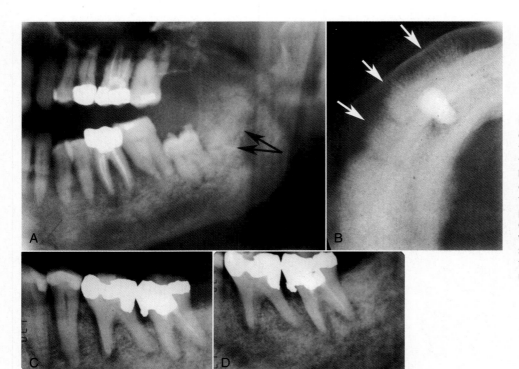

FIG. **23-8 A,** Partial panoramic image of prostate metastatic lesions involving the body and ramus of the body; note the sclerotic bone reaction *(arrows).* **B,** Occlusal image of prostate lesions causing sclerosis and spiculated periosteal reaction *(arrows).* **C** and **D,** Two periapical images of a metastatic lesion of breast carcinoma; note the irregular widening of the periodontal membrane spaces and patchy sclerotic bone reaction, especially around the roots of the molars.

# Sarcomas

## Osteosarcoma

### Synonym
Osteogenic sarcoma

### Definition
Osteosarcoma is a malignant neoplasm of bone in which osteoid is produced directly by malignant stroma as opposed to adjacent reactive bone formation. The three major histologic types are chondroblastic, osteoblastic, and fibroblastic osteosarcoma. The cause of osteosarcoma is unknown, but genetic mutation and viral causes have been suggested. It is also known to occur in association with Paget's disease and fibrous dysplasia after therapeutic irradiation.

### Clinical Features
Osteosarcoma of the jaws is quite rare and accounts for approximately 7% of all osteosarcomas. Despite its rarity, the dentist may be the first health professional who observes tumors involving the jaws. The lesion occurs in all racial groups worldwide and in males twice as frequently as females. Jaw lesions typically occur with a peak in the fourth decade, about 10 years later on average than long bone lesions occur. The most commonly reported symptom or sign is swelling, which may be present as long as 6 months before diagnosis; the swelling is usually rapid. Other indicators are pain, tenderness, erythema of overlying mucosa, ulceration, loose teeth, epistaxis, hemorrhage, nasal obstruction, exophthalmos, trismus, and blindness. Hypoesthesia has also been reported in cases involving neurovascular canals.

### Radiographic Features
*Location.* The mandible is more commonly affected than the maxilla is. Although the lesion can occur in any part of either jaw, the posterior mandible, including the tooth-bearing region, angle, and vertical ramus, is most commonly affected. The posterior areas are also more commonly affected in the maxilla, with the most frequent sites being the alveolar ridge, antrum, and palate. The lesion may cross the midline.

*Periphery and Shape.* Osteosarcoma has an ill-defined border in most instances. When viewed against normal bone, the lesion is usually radiolucent with no peripheral sclerosis or encapsulation. If the lesion involves the periosteum directly or by extension, the typical sunray spicules or "hair-on-end" trabeculae may be seen (Fig. 23-9). This occurs when the periosteum is displaced, partially destroyed, and disorganized. If the periosteum is elevated and maintains its osteogenic potential but is breached in the center, a Codman's triangle at the edges is formed (see Fig. 23-1, *E*). Even more rarely, laminar periosteal new bone may be present. In many cases, extension is even more prominent, and a soft tissue mass is visible radiographically.

*Internal Structure.* Osteosarcoma may be entirely radiolucent, mixed radiolucent-radiopaque, or quite radiopaque. The internal osseous structure may take the appearance of granular- or sclerotic-appearing bone, cotton balls, wisps, or honeycombed internal structures in areas with adjacent destruction of the preexisting osseous architecture. Whatever the resultant internal structure, the normal trabecular structure of the jaws is lost.

*Effects on Surrounding Structures.* Widening of the periodontal membrane is associated with osteosarcoma but is also seen in other malignancies (Fig. 23-10). The antral or nasal wall cortices may be lost in maxillary lesions. Mandibular lesions may destroy the cortex of the neurovascular canal and adjacent lamina dura. Alternatively, the neurovascular canal may be symmetrically widened and enlarged. Effects on the periosteum are discussed under the discussion on periphery.

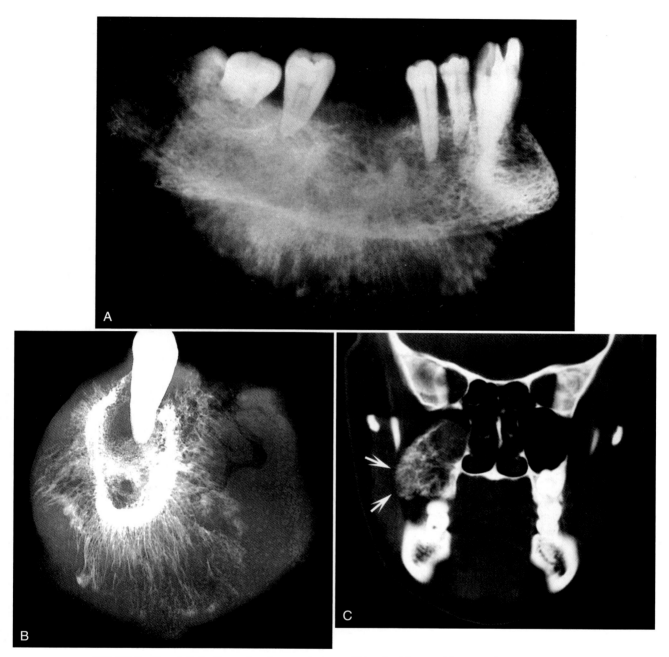

FIG. **23-9**  **A** and **B,** Radiographs of a resected mandible of a 25-year-old man with osteosarcoma, showing sunray spicules. **C,** Coronal CT image of an osteosarcoma of the maxilla; spiculated bone formation extends laterally from the maxilla *(arrows).*

## Differential Diagnosis

If internal structure is minimal or absent, fibrosarcoma or metastatic carcinoma may appear similar to osteosarcoma. If osseous structure is visible, the practitioner should also consider chondrosarcoma. If spiculated periosteal new bone is present, prostate and breast metastases should be considered. Comprehensive physical examination and laboratory tests assist in determining whether the lesion is primary or metastatic. Benign tumors such as ossifying fibroma and benign conditions such as fibrous dysplasia may mimic osteosarcoma radiographically. The former conditions, however, are usually better demarcated and have a more uniform internal structure. The histo-

pathologic features of osteosarcoma may be interpreted as a benign fibro-osseous lesion, and in these cases, the correct diagnosis may rely on the radiographic characteristics alone. Ewing's sarcoma, solitary plasmacytoma, and even osteomyelitis share some of the radiographic characteristics of osteosarcoma. Osteosarcoma is generally not associated with signs of infection.

## Management

The management of osteosarcoma is resection with a large border of adjacent normal bone. This may be possible in orthopedic cases but may be complicated by the presence of important adjacent anatomic

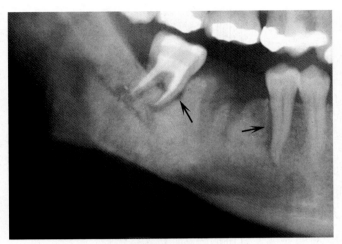

FIG. **23-10** Cropped panoramic image of an osteosarcoma occupying the body of the right mandible. Note the widened ligament spaces *(arrows)* and that the density of the mandible in the first molar region is greater than normal due to abnormal bone formation from the tumor.

structures in the head and neck. Generally, radiation therapy and chemotherapy are used only for controlling metastatic spread or for palliation.

## Chondrosarcoma

### Synonym
Chondrogenic sarcoma

### Definition
Chondrosarcoma is a malignant tumor of cartilaginous origin. The four histologic subtypes, which develop most commonly in the craniofacial region, are the clear cell, dedifferentiated, myxoid, and mesenchymal forms. They may occur centrally within bone, on the periphery of bone, or less commonly in soft tissue. They can arise directly from cartilage or may occur within benign cartilaginous tumors. In the case of the latter, they are termed *secondary chondrosarcomas*.

### Clinical Features
Generally these tumors occur at any age, although they are more common in adults (mean age 47 years). They affect males and females equally. A patient with chondrosarcoma may have a firm or hard mass of relatively long duration. Enlargement of these lesions may cause pain, headache, and deformity. Less frequent signs and symptoms include hemorrhage from tumor or from the necks of the teeth, sensory nerve deficits, proptosis, and visual disturbances. Invariably the tumors are covered with normal overlying skin or mucosa unless secondarily ulcerated. If chondrosarcoma occurs in or near the temporomandibular joint region, trismus or abnormal joint function may result.

### Radiographic Features
*Location.* Chondrosarcomas are unusual in the facial bones, accounting for about 10% of all cases. They occur in the mandible and maxilla with equal frequency. Maxillary lesions typically occur in the anterior region in areas where cartilaginous tissues may be present in the maxilla. Mandibular lesions occur in the coronoid process, condylar head and neck (Fig. 23-11, *B* and *C*), and occasionally the symphyseal region.

*Periphery and Shape.* Chondrosarcomas are slow-growing tumors, and their radiologic signs may be misleading and benign in nature. The lesions are generally round, ovoid, or lobulated. Generally their borders are well defined and at times corticated, whereas at other times melding with adjacent normal bone occurs. Occasionally peripheral periosteal new bone may be present perpendicular to the original cortex, giving the so-called sunray or hair-on-end appearance. Uncommonly these lesions are ill defined and invasive. Aggressive lesions such as these have infiltrative, ill-defined, and noncorticated borders.

*Internal Structure.* Chondrosarcomas usually exhibit some form of calcification within their center, giving them a mixed radiolucent-radiopaque appearance. At times this mixture takes the form of moth-eaten bone alternating with islands of residual bone unaffected by tumor. Lesions are rarely completely radiolucent. The central radiopaque structure has been described as "flocculent," implying snow-like features. This diffuse calcification may be superimposed on a bony background that resembles granular or ground-glass–appearing abnormal bone (Fig. 23-11, *A*). Careful examination of these areas of flocculence may reveal a central radiolucent nidus, which is probably cartilage surrounded by calcification. The result is rounded or speckled areas of calcification.

*Effects on Surrounding Structures.* Chondrosarcoma, because it is relatively slow growing, often expands normal cortical boundaries rather than rapidly destroying them. In mandibular cases the inferior border or alveolar process may be grossly expanded while still maintaining its cortical covering. Maxillary lesions may push the walls of the maxillary sinus or nasal fossa and impinge on the infratemporal fossa. Lesions of the condyle cause its expansion and perhaps remodeling of the corresponding articular fossa and eminence. If lesions occur in the articular disk region, a widened joint space may be present with corresponding remodeling of the condylar neck. Erosion of the articular fossa may also occur. If lesions occur near teeth, root resorption and tooth displacement may occur, as may widening of the periodontal membrane space.

### Differential Diagnosis
Osteosarcoma is often indistinguishable radiographically from chondrosarcoma. Although the typical calcifications of chondrosarcoma may be absent from osteosarcoma, the two share many other radiologic features. Fibrous dysplasia may also be difficult to differentiate from chondrosarcoma because similarities in the internal pattern. (The radiopaque portion of fibrous dysplasia is abnormal bone, not calcification. The calcifications in chondrosarcoma represent calcified cartilage.) Generally, the periphery of fibrous dysplasia is better defined and its margin with adjacent teeth differs from that of chondrosarcoma. For instance, fibrous dysplasia alters the bone pattern up to and including the lamina dura, leaving a normal or thin periodontal ligament space. The greatest danger results from the misleading benign characteristics of chondrosarcoma, which may delay correct diagnosis.

*Management.* The management of chondrosarcoma is surgical. Radiation therapy and chemotherapy generally have no role to play. Patients with chondrosarcomas have a relatively good 5-year survival rate but a poor 10-year survival rate.

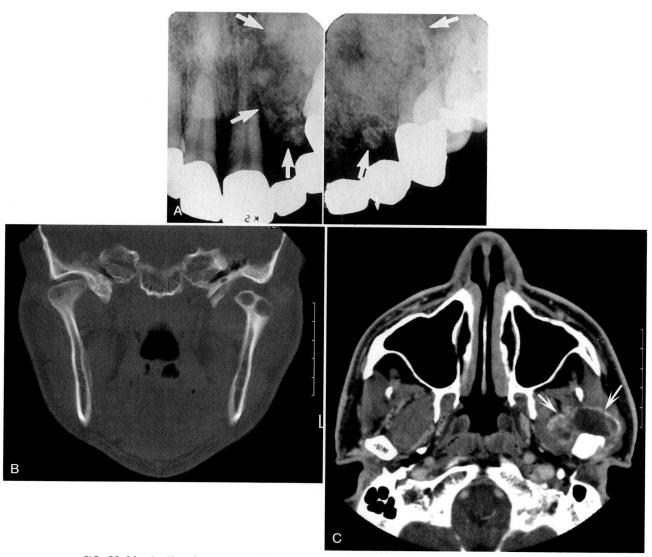

FIG. **23-11**  **A,** Chondrosarcoma of the anterior maxilla, with irregular calcification in the internal structure of the tumor *(arrows).* **B,** Coronal CT image with bone algorithm of a chondrosarcoma involving the mandibular condyle (note the two areas of bone destruction). **C,** Axial CT scan with soft tissue algorithm demonstrating the soft tissue extent of the lesion *(arrows)* and sparse calcifications. (**A** courtesy L. Hollender, DDS, Seattle, Wash.)

## Ewing's Sarcoma

### Synonyms
Endothelial myeloma and round cell sarcoma

### Definition
Ewing's sarcoma is of indeterminate histogenesis. It is a tumor of long bones that is relatively rare in the jaws. Lesions arise in the medullary portion of the bone and spread to the endosteal and later to the periosteal surfaces.

### Clinical Features
Ewing's sarcoma is most common in the second decade of life; most patients are between the ages of 5 and 30 years. Males are twice as likely to manifest the disease as females. In addition, multicentric lesions have been reported. Other reported findings at the time of presentation include, in descending frequency, swelling, pain, loose teeth, paresthesia, exophthalmos, ptosis, epistaxis, ulceration, shifted teeth, trismus, and sinusitis. Cervical lymphadenopathy has also been reported.

### Radiographic Features
*Location.*  Mandibular cases outnumber maxillary cases by about two to one, with the highest frequency found in posterior areas in both jaws. Generally the lesions develop within the marrow space first and then extend to involve overlying cortical plates. This neoplasm rarely occurs in the jaws.

*Periphery and Shape.*  Ewing's sarcoma is a radiolucency that is poorly demarcated and never corticated. Its advancing edge destroys

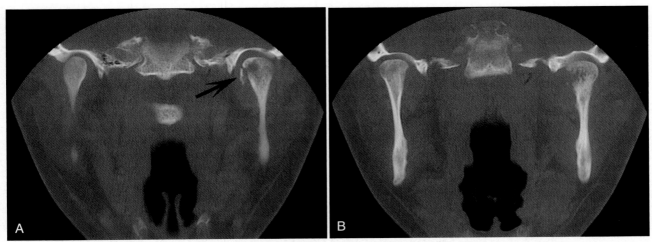

FIG. **23-12** **A** and **B,** Coronal CT images with bone algorithm demonstrating Ewing's sarcoma involving the left mandibular condyle; note the irregular margins, destruction of the medial cortex of the condyle, and a small pathologic fracture *(arrow).*

bone in an uneven fashion, resulting in a ragged border. The lesions are usually solitary and may cause pathologic fracture with adjacent radiographically visible soft tissue masses (Fig. 23-12). They may be round or ovoid but generally have no typical shape.

*Internal Structure.* Ewing's sarcoma is a destructive process with little induction of bone formation. Because it commences on the internal aspect of the bone and involves the endosteal and periosteal surfaces later in its course, it is usually entirely radiolucent.

*Effects on Surrounding Structures.* Ewing's sarcoma may stimulate the periosteum to produce new bone. This is usually the result of gross disturbances to the overlying periosteum and takes the form of Codman's triangle or sunray or hair-on-end spiculation. Laminar periosteal new bone formation has been reported to occur but is not a common feature of active Ewing's sarcoma lesions. Adjacent normal structures such as the mandibular neurovascular canal, inferior border of the mandible, and alveolar cortical plates may be effaced. If the lesion abuts teeth or tooth follicles, the cortices of these structures are destroyed. This tumor does not characteristically cause root resorption, although it does destroy the supporting bone of adjacent teeth.

### Differential Diagnosis

Inflammatory or infectious lesions such as osteomyelitis of the jaw may share some of the radiographic features of Ewing's sarcoma. Although both are radiolucent, osteomyelitis is likely to have demonstrable sequestra present within the confines of the lesion, whereas Ewing's sarcoma does not. Inflammatory lesions contain some sign of reactive bone formation, resulting in some sclerosis internally or at the periphery, and differ in the associated periosteal bone formation.

Eosinophilic granuloma of the jaw is also a destructive process that occurs in the same part of the bone. It is associated with laminar periosteal bone reaction, whereas, in the jaws, Ewing's sarcoma is not. The other central primary malignancies of bone such as osteosarcoma, chondrosarcoma, and fibrosarcoma may be difficult to differentiate from this condition.

### Management

Too few cases of maxillofacial Ewing's sarcoma are available at any single treatment center for any specific treatment policy to have been adopted. Surgery, radiation therapy, and chemotherapy may be used alone or in combination.

## Fibrosarcoma

### Definition

Fibrosarcoma is a neoplasm composed of malignant fibroblasts that produce collagen and elastin. The etiology is unknown, although it may arise secondarily in tissues that have received therapeutic levels of radiation.

### Clinical Features

These lesions occur equally in males and females with a mean age in the fourth decade. A slowly to rapidly enlarging mass is the usual presenting symptom. The mass may be within bone, in which case it usually is accompanied by pain. Peripheral lesions or those exiting from bone may invade local soft tissues, causing a bulky, clinically obvious lesion. If central or peripheral lesions reach a large size, pathologic fracture may occur. If fibrosarcomas involve the course of peripheral nerves, sensory-neural abnormalities may occur. Overlying mucosa, although initially normal, may become erythematous or ulcerated. Involvement of the temporomandibular joint or paramandibular musculature is often accompanied by trismus.

### Radiographic Features

*Location.* Most cases of fibrosarcoma of the jaws occur in the mandible, with the greatest number of these occurring in the premolar/molar region.

*Periphery and Shape.* Fibrosarcomas have ill-defined borders that are best described as ragged (Fig. 23-13). They are poorly demarcated, noncorticated, and lack any semblance of a capsule. These tumors are generally shaped in a fashion that suggests that they have grown along a bone, so they tend to be elongated through the marrow space. The radiographic border may underestimate the extent of the tumor because these lesions typically are infiltrative. If soft tissue lesions occur adjacent to bone, they may cause a saucerlike depression in the underlying bone or invade it as would a squamous cell carcinoma. Finally, sclerosis may occur in the adjacent normal bone whether the fibrosarcoma is peripheral to bone or central.

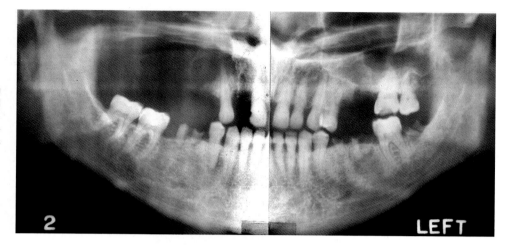

FIG. 23-13 A fibrosarcoma involving the right maxillary sinus has destroyed the cortical boundaries of the sinus, zygomatic process, hard palate and posterior maxilla, and the alveolar process in this panoramic film.

*Internal Structure.* Fibrosarcomas have little internal structure. In most cases the lesions are entirely radiolucent. If the lesions have been present for some time and are not overly aggressive, either residual jawbone or reactive osseous bone formation occurs.

*Effects on Surrounding Structures.* The most common effect on adjacent structures is destruction. In the mandible, the alveolar process, inferior border of the jaw, and cortices of the neurovascular canal are lost. In the maxilla, the inferior floor of the maxillary sinus, posterior wall of the maxilla, and nasal floor can be destroyed. In either jaw, lamina dura and follicular cortices are obliterated. Destruction of the outer cortical plate is usually accompanied by a protruding soft tissue mass. Root resorption is uncommon. Teeth are more likely to be grossly displaced and lose their support bone so that they appear to be floating in space. In addition, widening of the periodontal membrane space occurs with this tumor, as in other malignancies. Periosteal reaction is uncommon; however, if the lesion disrupts the periosteum, a Codman's triangle or sunray spiculation may be evident.

### Differential Diagnosis

This solitary, ragged radiolucency with little internal structure is difficult to differentiate from other central malignancies. If the lesion does not cause enlargement of the jaw, the practitioner must rule out metastatic carcinoma, multiple myeloma, and primary or secondary intraosseous carcinoma. Another possibility is a grossly infected dental cyst, although these usually show some degree of induced peripheral sclerosis in adjacent bone. If a fibrosarcoma exhibits enlargement of the affected jaw with an associated soft tissue mass, other sarcomas such as chondrosarcoma and osteosarcoma (both usually have internal structure) should be ruled out. Ewing's sarcoma and radiolucent osteosarcomas may not be distinguishable from this tumor. Finally, peripheral invasive squamous cell carcinoma shares some of these radiologic features, but its ulcerative surface features differentiate it from fibrosarcoma, which usually lacks these.

### Management

The management of fibrosarcoma is chiefly surgical. A wide margin of adjacent normal bone is taken if anatomically possible. Radiation therapy and chemotherapy are usually reserved for palliation.

## Malignancies of the Hematopoietic System

### Multiple Myeloma

#### Synonyms

Myeloma, plasma cell myeloma, and plasmacytoma

#### Definition

Multiple myeloma is a malignant neoplasm of plasma cells. It is the most common malignancy of bone in adults. Single lesions are called plasmacytoma, and multiple lesions are termed multiple myeloma.

#### Clinical Features

Multiple myeloma is a fatal systemic malignancy. A patient with multiple myeloma is usually between the ages of 35 and 70 years (mean age 60 years). The patient may complain of fatigue, weight loss, fever, bone pain, and anemia, although the typical presenting feature is low back pain. Secondary signs include amyloidosis and hypercalcemia; in half of all patients, characteristic Bence Jones protein is present in the urine, which causes the urine to be foamy. The disease is more common in men. When this clonal cellular proliferation occurs, these cells occupy first cancellous and later cortical bone, replacing the normally radiopaque bone with areas of radiolucency.

Orally, patients may complain of dental pain, swelling, hemorrhage, paresthesia, and dysesthesia, or they may have no complaints. The number of patients with demonstrable radiologic findings in the jaws at the time of diagnosis is relatively small.

#### Radiographic Features

*Location.* Multiple myeloma (Fig. 23-14) is seen more frequently in the mandible than the maxilla but is uncommon in either. The incidence of jaw involvement has been reported to vary from 2% to 78%. In the mandible the posterior body and ramus is favored. Maxillary lesions usually appear in posterior sites.

*Periphery and Shape.* The periphery of multiple myeloma lesions is well defined but not corticated; it lacks any sign of bone reaction (Fig. 23-15). The lesions have been described as appearing "punched out." However, many appear ragged and even infiltrative. Some lesions have an oval or cystic shape. Untreated or aggressive areas of destruction may become confluent, giving the appearance of multilocularity. If the lesion is located in the periapical periodontal

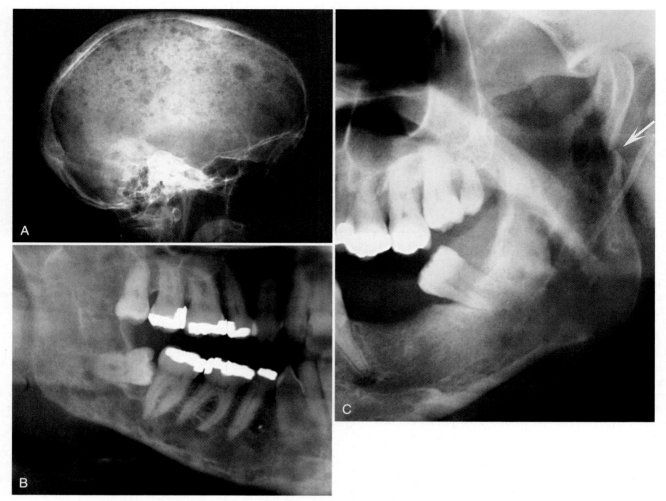

FIG. **23-14**  Multiple myeloma, seen as multiple circular radiolucent lesions in the skull **(A).** In a different case **(B)** multiple small lesions of multiple myeloma are present through the body and ramus of the mandible in this cropped panoramic image. **C,** Cropped panoramic image shows a solitary lesion in the condylar neck region and a pathologic fracture *(arrow).*

ligament space, it may have a border similar to that seen in inflammatory or infectious periapical disease. Soft tissue lesions have been reported in the jaws and nasopharynx. When visible on radiographs, they appear as smooth-bordered soft tissue masses, possibly with underlying bone destruction.

*Internal Structure.* No internal structure is radiographically visible. Occasionally islands of residual bone, yet unaffected by tumor, give the appearance of the presence of new trabecular bone within the mass. Very rarely the lesions appear radiopaque internally.

*Effects on Surrounding Structures.* If a good deal of bone mineral is lost, teeth may appear to be "too opaque" and may stand out conspicuously from their osteopenic background. Lamina dura and follicles of impacted teeth may lose their typical corticated surrounding bone in a manner analogous to that seen in hyperparathyroidism. The same may be said of the mandibular neurovascular canal, which, although usually visible, loses its cortical boundary in whole or in part. These changes are profound when there is associated renal disease. Mandibular lesions may cause thinning of the lower border of the mandible or endosteal scalloping. Any cortical boundary may be effaced if lesions involve them. Periosteal reaction is uncommon, but if it is present takes the form of a single radiopaque line or more rarely a sunray appearance.

**Differential Diagnosis**
The most likely disease to be mistaken for multiple myeloma is the radiolucent form of metastatic carcinoma. Knowledge of a prior malignancy in a patient may help differentiate multiple myeloma from metastatic carcinoma. Osteomyelitis, if severe, may yield a radiologic picture similar to that of multiple myeloma; however, a visible cause for it usually exists. In addition, inflammatory lesions and infections in general cause sclerosis in adjacent bone, which multiple myeloma does not. Simple bone cysts may be bilateral in the mandible and therefore may be mistaken for multiple myeloma. They are usually corticated in part and characteristically interdigitate between the roots of the teeth in a much younger population. Generalized radiolucency of the jaws may be caused by hyperparathyroidism but is differenti-

ated on the basis of abnormal blood chemistry. However, brown tumors of hyperparathyroidism, if present with generalized radiolucency of the jaws and similar symptoms, can readily be confused with multiple myeloma radiographically. Other metabolic diseases such as Gaucher's disease or oxalosis may cause many of the changes similar to multiple myeloma that are observed on dental radiographs.

## Management

The management of multiple myeloma is usually chemotherapeutic with or without autologous or allogeneic bone marrow transplantation. Radiation therapy may be used for treatment of symptomatic osseous lesions when palliation is required.

## Non-Hodgkin's Lymphoma

### Synonyms

Malignant lymphoma and lymphosarcoma

### Definition

Non-Hodgkin's lymphoma is a malignant tumor of cells normally resident in the lymphatic system. In general, lymphomas occur within lymph nodes; however, extranodal sites such as bone, skin, gastrointestinal mucosa, tonsils, and Waldeyer's ring can be involved. The term *non-Hodgkin's lymphoma* describes a family of heterogeneous tumors of varying type and severity. The classification of these diseases is difficult, and numerous means exist of subdividing these tumors. Currently the working formulation for clinical usage classifies tumors on the basis of their histologic appearance into low grade, intermediate grade, or high grade tumors, with the last being the most aggressive.

### Clinical Features

Non-Hodgkin's lymphoma occurs in all age groups but is rare in patients in the first decade. The maxillary sinus, palate, tonsillar area, and bone may be sites of primary or secondary lymphoma spread. Lesions occurring outside lymph nodes in the head and neck are present in as much as one out of five cases. Patients may feel unwell, experiencing night sweats, pruritus, and weight loss. Palpable painless swelling, lymphadenopathy, and sensorineural deficits may accompany isolated lesions of the jaws. Lesions present for some time may cause pain and ulceration. Teeth resident in a lymphoma may become mobile as the supporting bone is lost.

### Radiographic Features

*Location.* Most non-Hodgkin's lymphomas of the head and neck occur in the lymph nodes. Those that are extranodal are likely to affect the maxillary sinus, posterior mandible, and maxillary regions.

*Periphery and Shape.* Most non-Hodgkin's lymphomas initially take the shape and form of the host bone. If untreated, however, they are capable of causing destruction of the overlying cortex (Fig. 23-16). They may appear rounded or multiloculated and lack a defining outer cortex. Generally the borders are ill defined and invasive. Occasionally, lymphoma appears as multiple areas of destruction, which likely appear as fingerlike extensions of malignant tumor cells in a buccal or lingual direction. Visible lesions occurring in the maxillary sinus or nasopharynx have a smooth periphery.

*Internal Structure.* The internal structure of lymphoma is almost always entirely radiolucent. It is rare to see reactive bone formation. Occasionally patchy radiopacity may be present, but this is rare.

*Effects on Surrounding Structures.* In maxillary sinus lesions the antral walls may be effaced and a soft tissue mass may be

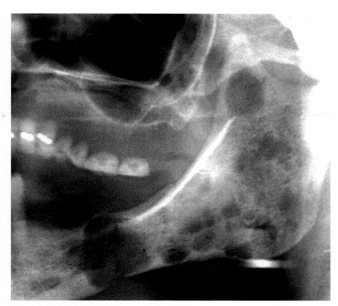

FIG. **23-15** Cropped panoramic image depicting multiple areas of well-defined bone destruction lacking any cortical boundary. The lesions are multiple, separate, and appear to be "punched out," typical of changes seen in multiple myeloma. (Courtesy G. Petrikowski, DDS, Toronto, Ontario, Canada.)

visible radiographically, either internally within the sinus or external to the maxillary sinus. Lesions involving the mandible destroy the cortex of the neurovascular canal. This tumor has a propensity to grow in the periodontal ligament space of mature teeth (Fig. 23-17). The cortex of the crypts of developing teeth may be lost when the lymphoma is located in the developing papilla, and the involved teeth may be displaced in an occlusal direction and exfoliated. Periosteal reaction is not common but may take the form of laminated or spiculated bone formation. With the advent of soft tissue imaging with MRI, it has become apparent that this tumor has a habit of growing along soft tissue spaces (fat layers) and along the surface of bone.

### Differential Diagnosis

Multiple myeloma and metastatic carcinoma are easily confused with non-Hodgkin's lymphoma of the jaws. However, Ewing's sarcoma and Langerhans' histiocytosis, although also capable of producing the same effects, occur in a slightly younger age group. Osteolytic osteosarcoma and any of the central squamous cell carcinomas may not be distinguishable radiographically from non-Hodgkin's lymphoma. Squamous cell carcinoma arising in the maxillary sinus may be difficult to differentiate from lymphoma of the maxillary sinus. Other lesions that can displace developing teeth in an occlusal direction include leukemia and Langerhans' histiocytosis. Differentiation from apical rarefying osteitis may be difficult; however, careful inspection of the radiographic film may reveal the presence of an infiltrative border and adjacent bone destruction.

### Management

The management of extranodal or isolated nodal disease is radiation therapy with or without concomitant chemotherapy. Treatment depends on histologic variants and the location and extent of disease.

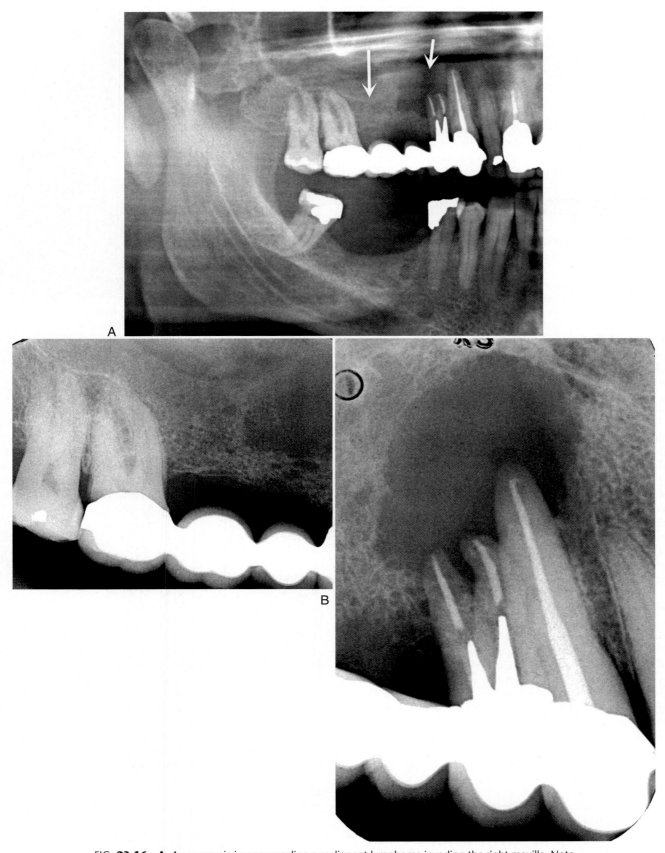

FIG. **23-16    A,** A panoramic image revealing a malignant lymphoma invading the right maxilla. Note the ill-defined bone destruction and loss of the anterior aspect of the floor of the maxillary antrum *(arrows).* The intraoral radiographs **(B)** also show ill-defined bone destruction and the lack of any bone reaction or formation.

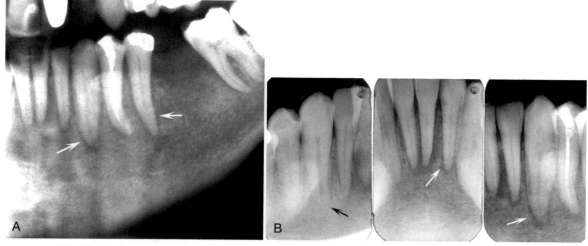

FIG. **23-17** A cropped panoramic image **(A)** revealing an ill-defined lymphoma invading the left body of the mandible; note the irregular widening of the periodontal ligament spaces *(arrows)*. Intra-oral films of the same case **(B)** and the widened periodontal ligament spaces *(white arrows)* compared with the normal periodontal ligament space of the right mandibular cuspid *(black arrow)*.

## Burkitt's Lymphoma

### Synonym
African jaw lymphoma

### Definition
Burkitt's lymphoma is a high-grade B-cell lymphoma that differs from other B-cell lymphomas with respect to its histologic appearance and clinical behavior. It was first described by Denis Burkitt in East Africa as an African jaw lymphoma.

Two separate forms of the disease have been described: the endemic African Burkitt's lymphoma and the American form. The latter is not characterized by jaw involvement (although it occurs), but by involvement of abdominal viscera. African Burkitt's lymphoma affects young children, whereas American Burkitt's lymphoma affects adolescents and young adults. Cases of endemic and nonendemic Burkitt's tumor have been described throughout the world.

### Clinical Features
The disease affects more males than females. Clinically the hallmark of this tumor is rapidity of growth with a tumor doubling time of less than 24 hours. It may involve children as young as 2 years and adults in the seventh decade, although it is primarily a disease of youth. Jaw tumors are rapidly growing and cause facial deformity very early in their course. They are capable of blocking nasal passages, displacing orbital contents, causing gross facial swelling, and eroding through skin. These rapidly growing tumors are more characteristic of African Burkitt's lymphoma than the American form and cause pain and paresthesia. Teeth may become loosened rapidly and alveolar bone grossly distended. Paresthesia of the inferior alveolar nerve or other sensory facial nerves is common.

### Radiographic Features
*Location.* Extranodal disease is the norm in Burkitt's tumor. African cases may involve one jaw or both the maxilla and mandible and affect the posterior parts of the jaws. By contrast, American cases

may not involve the facial bones but are more likely to affect the abdominal viscera and testes.

*Periphery and Shape.* The lesions may begin as multiple ill-defined noncorticated radiolucencies that later coalesce into larger ill-defined radiolucencies with an expansile periphery. They are of no specific shape, although they expand rapidly and have been likened to a balloon. This expansion breaches its outer cortical limits, causing gross balloonlike expansion with thinning of adjacent structures and production of a soft tissue tumor mass adjacent to the osseous lesion. Lesions that abut the orbital contents or the maxillary sinus may show a smooth surface soft tissue mass radiologically.

*Internal Structure.* Burkitt's lymphoma does not produce bone and rarely induces production of reactive bone within its center. For this reason, the lesions are radiolucent in almost all cases. It is particularly radiolucent in the jaw of a child.

*Effects on Surrounding Structures.* Erupted teeth in the area of Burkitt's tumor are grossly displaced, as are developing tooth crypts. Tumor cells within the crypt may displace the developing tooth bud to one side of its crypt. A tumor that is located apical to a developing tooth may cause it to be displaced such that it appears to erupt with little if any root formation. After tumor involvement of the developing dental structures occurs, root development ceases. Lamina dura of teeth in the area is destroyed, and cortical boundaries such as the maxillary sinus, nasal floor, orbital walls, and inferior border of the mandible are thinned and later destroyed. The cortex of the inferior alveolar canal is lost, although it is difficult to see in the radiographs of a normal pediatric patient in any case. If periosteum is involved, the border may show sunray spiculation, although this is rare. Cases that involve the orbit displace the orbital contents, seen both clinically and radiologically.

### Differential Diagnosis
Metastatic neuroblastoma may give similar changes clinically and radiologically, as may Ewing's tumor. Osteolytic osteosarcoma can grow rapidly and may be indistinguishable from Burkitt's tumor on

clinical and radiologic grounds. Cherubism has more internal structure, does not breach bony borders, is bilateral, and grows much more slowly. Finally, non-Hodgkin's lymphoma must be considered, although it occurs in a much older age group in most cases.

### Management

The management of Burkitt's tumor is chemotherapeutic. Chemotherapy regimens vary from geographic locales, but the tumor is exquisitely sensitive to combinations of chemotherapeutic agents.

## Leukemia

### Synonyms

Acute myelogenous leukemia, acute lymphoblastic leukemia, chronic myelogenous leukemia, and chronic lymphocytic leukemia are types of leukemia.

### Definition

Leukemia is a malignant tumor of hematopoietic stem cells. These malignant cells displace normal bone marrow constituents and spill out into the peripheral blood. They are subdivided into acute leukemias and chronic leukemias and further subdivided by the cell of origin. The acute leukemias occur with a bimodal age distribution, with very young patients and very old patients being the most commonly affected. Most cases of leukemia are associated with nonrandom chromosomal abnormalities.

### Clinical Features

The patient with chronic leukemia may have no presenting signs or complaints. Acute leukemia patients generally feel unwell with weakness and bone pain. They may exhibit pallor, spontaneous hemorrhage, hepatomegaly, splenomegaly, lymphadenopathy, and fever. Oral symptoms are generally absent but, if present, include loose teeth, petechiae, ulceration, and boggy enlarged gingiva.

### Radiographic Features

Radiologic signs associated with chronic leukemia are comparatively rare.

*Location.* Leukemia affects the entire body because it is a malignancy of bone marrow, which discharges malignant cells into circulating blood. Its manifestations in the jaws may be seen more often in areas of developing teeth. Frequently, leukemia may be localized around the periapical region of a tooth, giving the appearance of a rarefying osteitis.

*Periphery and Shape.* Leukemia must be considered a systemic malignancy, and as such its oral radiologic features may be present bilaterally as ill-defined patchy radiolucent areas. With time and lack of treatment, these patchy areas may coalesce to form larger areas of ill-defined radiolucent regions of bone (Fig. 23-18). The teeth may appear to stand out conspicuously from their surrounding, osteopenic bone.

*Internal Structure.* The internal structure of leukemia is characterized by patchy areas of radiolucency and generalized radiolucency of the bone. Rarely, granular bone may be seen within these lesions. Occasionally, foci of leukemic cells may be present as a mass that may behave like a localized malignant tumor. These lesions, called chloromas, are rare in the jaws.

*Effects on Surrounding Structures.* Leukemia does not cause expansion of bone, although occasionally a single layer of periosteal new bone may be seen in association with this disease, which is uncommon in chronic leukemia. Developing teeth in their crypts and teeth undergoing eruption may be displaced in an occlusal direction (Fig. 23-19) or into the oral cavity before root development. Less commonly, developing teeth may be displaced from their normal positions. The result of this is premature loss of teeth. The lamina dura and cortical outlines of follicles may be effaced. If lesions affect the periodontal structures, the crestal bone may be lost.

### Differential Diagnosis

Generally, by the time oral radiologic signs of leukemia are present, a medical diagnosis has been reached. However, the development of radiologic changes may be the first indication of the relapse of treatment. Occasionally, lymphoma or neuroblastoma may mimic some of the features of destruction seen in leukemia. Metabolic disorders may be considered in those cases in which generalized rarefaction of bone

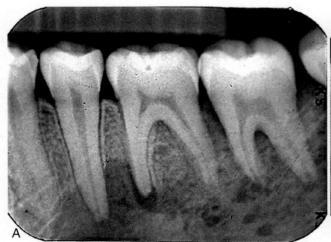
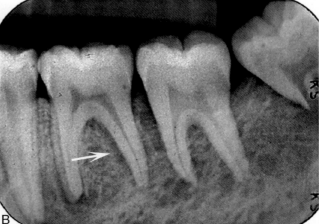

FIG. **23-18** Periapical radiographs of the left mandible illustrating multifocal areas of bone destruction and widening of portions of the periodontal ligament space *(arrow)* characteristic of infiltration of the mandible with leukemia.

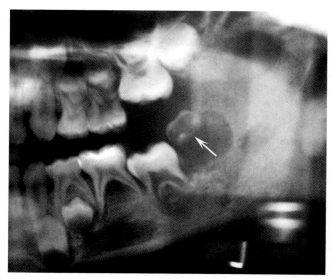

FIG. **23-19** A cropped panoramic film demonstrating occlusal displacement of the developing mandibular second molar out of its follicle (arrow).

is seen. These conditions are all excluded on the basis of blood testing. With apical lesions, careful examination of the involved tooth clinically and radiologically typically shows no apparent cause for rarefying osteitis.

### Management

The management of leukemia is primarily through a combination of chemotherapy with or without allogeneic or autologous bone marrow transplantation. Some chronic leukemias are managed with low-dose chemotherapy.

## Dental Radiology for the Cancer Survivor

The cancer survivor requires dental treatment just as any other patient. For the cancer survivor, dental radiologic examination may be more important than for a healthy patient receiving a routine examination. Some patients who have received a full course of radiation therapy are concerned about the additional exposure from a dental radiographic examination. However, this is not a valid concern because the small dose associated with dental radiographic examinations is negligible compared with the radiation dose received from cancer therapy.

The patient treated for head and neck malignancy with radiation therapy, even with today's advanced radiotherapeutic methods, is prone to development of postradiation dental caries and osteoradionecrosis. Careful clinical examination and a thorough dental radiologic examination may be required periodically to ensure that the remaining dentition and periodontal apparatus is in good shape. Radiation caries occur in many patients and appears clinically different from typical dental caries. If untreated, these carious teeth become nonvital and may cause infection in the underlying jaw. If they require extraction, healing can be expected to be slow and occasionally osteoradionecrosis may result.

The role of radiology in these patients, however, is not restricted to examination of the teeth and supporting structures. Equally important is the monitoring of the outcome of treatment, specifically the examination of dental radiographs for evidence of tumor recurrence, development of metastases, and osteoradionecrosis.

## SUGGESTED READINGS

### SQUAMOUS CELL CARCINOMA

Carter RL: Patterns and mechanisms of spread of squamous carcinomas of the oral cavity, *Clin Otolaryngol Allied Sci* 15:185-191, 1990.

Casiglia J, Woo SB: A comprehensive review of oral cancer, *Gen Dent* 49:72-82, 2001.

Marchetta FC, Sako K, Murphy JB: The periosteum of the mandible and intraoral carcinoma, *Am J Surg* 122:711-713, 1971.

McGregor AD, MacDonald DG: Routes of entry of squamous cell carcinoma to the mandible, *Head Neck Surg* 10:294-301, 1988.

Noyek AM, Wortzman G, Holgate RC et al: The radiologic diagnosis of malignant tumors of the paranasal sinuses and related structures, *J Otolaryngol* 6:399-406, 1977.

O'Brien CJ, Carter RL, Soo KC et al: Invasions of the mandible by squamous carcinomas of the oral cavity and oropharynx, *Head Neck Surg* 8:247-256, 1986.

Rao LP, Das SR, Mathews A et al: Mandibular invasion in oral squamous cell carcinoma: investigation by clinical examination and orthopantomogram, *Int J Oral Maxillofac Surg* 33:454-457, 2004.

Stambuk HE, Karimi S, Lee N et al: Oral cavity and oropharynx tumors, *Radiol Clin North Am* 45:1-20, 2007.

### SQUAMOUS CELL CARCINOMA ORIGINATING IN BONE

Ariji E, Ozeki S, Yonetsu K et al: Central squamous cell carcinoma of the mandible: computed tomographic findings, *Oral Surg Oral Med Oral Pathol* 77:541-548, 1994.

Elzay RP: Primary intraosseous carcinoma of the jaws. Review and update of odontogenic carcinomas, *Oral Surg Oral Med Oral Pathol* 54:299-303, 1982.

Lin YJ, Chen CH, Wang WC et al : Primary intraosseous carcinoma of the mandible, *Dentomaxillofacial Radiol* 34:112-116, 2005.

Suei Y, Tanimoto K, Taguchi A et al: Primary intra-osseous carcinoma: review of the literature and diagnostic criteria, *J OralMaxillofac Surg* 52:580, 1994.

### SQUAMOUS CELL CARCINOMA ORGINATING IN A CYST

Cavalcanti MG, Veltrini VC, Ruprecht A et al: Squamous-cell carcinoma arising from an odontogenic cyst—the importance of computed tomography in the diagnosis of malignancy, *Oral Surg Oral Med Oral Pathol Oral Radiol Endod* 100:365-368, 2005.

Dabbs DJ, Schweitzer RJ, Schweitzer LE et al: Squamous cell carcinoma arising in recurrent odontogenic keratocyst, *Head Neck* 16:375-378, 1994.

Eversole LR, Sabes WR, Rovin S: Aggressive growth and neoplastic potential of odontogenic cysts: with special reference to central epidermoid and mucoepidermoid carcinomas, *Cancer* 35:270-282, 1975.

Kaffe I, Ardekian L, Peled M et al: Radiological features of primary intra-osseous carcinoma of the jaws: analysis of the literature and report of a new case, *Dentomaxillofac Radiol* 27:209-214, 1998.

van der Wal KG, de Visscher JG, Eggink HF: Squamous cell carcinoma arising in a residual cyst. A case report, *Int J Oral Maxillofac Surg* 23:350-352, 1993.

### MUCOEPIDERMOID CARCINOMA

Bilge OM, Dayi E: Central mucoepidermoid carcinoma of the jaws: review of the literature and case report, *Ann Dent* 51:36-39, 1992.

Browand BC, Waldron CA: Central mucoepidermoid tumors of the jaws: report of nine cases and review of the literature, *Oral Surg Oral Med Oral Pathol* 40:631-643, 1975.

Freije JE, Campbell BH, Yousif NJ et al: Central mucoepidermoid carcinoma of the mandible, *Otolaryngol Head Neck Surg* 112:453-456, 1995.

Inagaki M, Yuasa K, Nakayama E et al: Mucoepidermoid carcinoma in the mandible: findings of panoramic radiography and computed tomography, *Oral Surg Oral Med Oral Pathol Oral Radiol Endod:*85: 613-618, 1998.

Lopez JI, Elizalde JM, Landa S: Central mucoepidermoid carcinoma: report of a case and review of the literature, *Pathol Res Pract* 189:365, 368, 1993.

Sidoni A, D'Errico P, Simoncelli C et al: Central mucoepidermoid carcinoma of the mandible, *J Oral Maxillofac Surg* 54:1242-1245, 1996.

Strick MJ, Kelly C, Soames JV et al: Malignant tumours of the minor salivary glands—a 20 year review, *Br J Plas Surg* 57:624-631, 2004.

## MALIGNANT AMELOBLASTOMA AND AMELOBLASTIC CARCINOMA

Ameerally P, McGurk M, Shaheen O: Atypical ameloblastoma: report of 3 cases and review of the literature, *Br J Oral Maxillofac Surg* 34:235-239, 1996.

Buff SJ, Chen JT, Ravin CC et al: Pulmonary metastasis from ameloblastoma of the mandible: report of a case and review of the literature, *J Oral Surg* 38:374-376, 1980.

Slootweg PJ, Müller H: Malignant ameloblastoma or amelo-blastic carcinoma, *Oral Surg Oral Med Oral Pathol* 57:168-176, 1984.

Suomalainen A, Hietanen J, Robinson S et al: Ameloblastic carcinoma of the mandible resembling odontogenic cyst in a panoramic radiograph, *Oral Surg Oral Med Oral Pathol Oral Radiol Endod* 101: 638-642, 2006.

## METASTATIC TUMORS

Ciola B: Oral radiographic manifestations of a metastatic prostatic carcinoma, *Oral Surg Oral Med Oral Pathol* 52:105-108, 1981.

Mast HL, Nissenblatt MJ: Metastatic colon carcinoma to the jaw: a case report and review of the literature, *J Surg Oncol* 34:202-207, 1987.

Mucitelli DR, Zuna RE, Archard HO: Hepatocellular carcinoma presenting as an oral cavity lesion, *Oral Surg Oral Med Oral Pathol* 66:701-705, 1988.

Nevins A, Ruden S, Pruden P et al: Metastatic carcinoma of the mandible mimicking periapical lesion of endodontic origin, *Endod Dent Traumatol* 4:238-239, 1988.

Redman RS, Behrens AS, Calhoun NR: Carcinoma of the lung presenting as a mandibular metastasis, *J Oral Maxillofac Surg* 40:745-750, 1982.

Vigneul JC, Nouel O, Klap P et al: Metastatic hepatocellular carcinoma of the mandible, *J Oral Maxillofac Surg* 40:745-749, 1982.

## OSTEOGENIC SARCOMA

Bainchi SD, Boccardi A: Radiological aspects of osteosarcoma of the jaws, *Dentomaxillofac Radiol* 28:42-47, 1999.

Batsakis JG: Osteogenic and chondrogenic sarcomas of the jaws, *Ann Otol Rhinol Laryngol* 96:474-475, 1987.

Chindia ML: Osteosarcoma of the jaw bones, *Oral Oncol.* 37:545-547, 2001.

Clark JL, Unni KK, Dahlin DC et al: Osteosarcoma of the jaw, *Cancer* 51:2311-2316, 1983.

Gardner DG, Mills DM: The widened periodontal ligament of osteosarcoma of the jaws, *Oral Surg Oral Med Oral Pathol* 41:652-656, 1976.

Givol N, Buchner A, Taicher S et al: Radiological features of osteogenic sarcoma of the jaws: a comparative study of different radiographic modalities, *Dentomaxillofac Radiol* 27:313-320, 1998.

Seeger LL, Gold RH, Chandnani VP: Diagnostic imaging of osteosarcoma, *Clin Orthop Rel Res* 270:254-263, 1991.

Vener J, Rice DH, Newman AN: Osteosarcoma and chondrosarcoma of the head and neck, *Laryngoscope* 94:240-242, 1984.

## CHONDROSARCOMA

Garrington GE, Collett WK: Chondrosarcoma, I: a selected literature review, *J Oral Pathol* 17:1-11, 1988.

Garrington GE, Collett WK: Chondrosarcoma, II: Chondrosarcoma of the jaws: analysis of 37 cases, *J Oral Pathol* 17:12-20, 1988.

Gorsky M, Epstein JB: Craniofacial osseous and chondromatous sarcomas in British Columbia—a review of 34 cases, *Oral Oncol* 36:27-31, 2000.

Hayt MW Becker L Katz DS: Chondrosarcoma of the maxilla: panoramic radiographic and computed tomographic with multiplanar reconstruction findings, *Dentomaxillofac Radiol* 27:113-116, 1998.

Hertzanu Y, Mendelsohn DB, Davidge-Pitts K et al: Chondrosarcoma of the head and neck-the value of computed tomography, *J Surg Oncol* 28:97-102, 1985.

## EWING'S SARCOMA

Dahlin DC, Coventry MB, Scanlon PW: Ewing's sarcoma. A critical analysis of 165 cases, *J Bone Joint Surg Am* 2:185-192, 1961.

Greer RO, Mierau GW, Favara BE: *Tumors of the head and neck in children,* New York, 1983, Praeger.

Wood RE, Nortje CJ, Hesseling P et al: Ewing's tumor of the jaw, *Oral Surg Oral Med Oral Pathol* 69:120-127, 1990.

## FIBROSARCOMA

Dahlin DC: *Bone tumors,* Springfield, IL, 1981, Charles C Thomas.

Huvos AG: *Bone tumors,* Philadelphia, 1979, WB Saunders.

O'Day RA, Soule EH, Goresg RJ: Soft tissue sarcomas of the oral cavity, *Mayo Clin Proc* 39:169-181, 1964.

Slootweg PJ, Müller H: Fibrosarcoma of the jaws. A study of 7 cases, *J Maxillofac Surg* 12:157-162, 1984.

Taconis WK, van Rijssel TG: Fibrosarcoma of the jaws, *Skeletal Radiol* 15: 10-13, 1986.

van Blarcom CW, Masson JMK, Dahlin DC: Fibrosarcoma of the mandible. A clinicopathologic study, *Oral Surg Oral Med Oral Pathol* 32:428-439, 1971.

## RHABDOMYOSARCOMA

Bras J, Batsakis JG, Luna MA: Rhabdomyosarcoma of the oral soft tissues, *Oral Surg Oral Med Oral Pathol* 64:585-596, 1987.

Grieman RB, Katsikeris NK, Symington JM: Rhabdomyosarcoma of the maxillary sinus: review of the literature and report of a case, *J Oral Maxillofac Surg* 46:1090, 1988.

Masson JK, Soule EH: Embryonal rhabdomyosarcoma of the head and neck: report of 88 cases, *Am J Surg* 110:585, 1965.

Sekhar MS, Desai S, Kumar GS: Alveolar rhabdomyosarcoma involving the jaws: a case report, *J Oral Maxillofac Surg* 58:1062-1065, 2000.

Stobbe GD, Dargeon HW: Embryonal rhabdomyosarcoma of the head and neck in children and adolescents, *Cancer* 3:826-836, 1950.

## MULTIPLE MYELOMA

Furutani M, Ohnishi M, Tanaka Y: Mandibular involvement in patients with multiple myeloma, *J Oral Maxillofac Surg* 52:23-25, 1994.

Huvos AG: Bone tumors, Philadelphia, 1979, WB Saunders.

Kaffe I, Ramon Y, Hertz M: Radiographic manifestations of multiple myeloma in the mandible, *Dentomaxillofac Radiol* 15:31-35, 1986.

Witt C, Borges AC, Klein K et al: Radiographic manifestations of multiple myeloma in the mandible: a retrospective study of 77 patients, *J Oral Maxillofac Surg* 55:450-453, 1997.

## NON-HODGKIN'S LYMPHOMA

Dahlin DC: Bone tumors, ed 3, Springfield, IL, 1981, Charles C Thomas.

Daramola JO, Ajagbe HA: Presentation and behaviour of primary malignant lymphoma of the oral cavity in adult Africans, *J Oral Med* 38:177-179, 1983.

Maxymiw WG, Goldstein M, Wood RE: Extranodal non-Hodgkin's lymphoma of the maxillofacial region: analysis of 88 consecutive cases, *SADJ* 56:524-527, 2001.

Pazoki A, Jansisyanont P, Ord RA: Primary non-Hodgkin's lymphoma of the jaws: report of 4 cases and review of the literature, *J Oral Maxillofac Surg* 61:112-117, 2003.

Yamada T, Kitagawa Y, Ogasawara T et al: Enlargement of the mandibular canal without hypesthesia caused by extranodal non-Hodgkin's lymphoma: a case report, *Oral Surg Oral Med Oral Pathol Oral Radiol Endod* 89:388-392, 2000.

*BURKITT'S LYMPHOMA*

Adatia AK: Significance of jaw lesions in Burkitt's lymphoma, *Br Dent J* 145:263-266, 1978.

Adatia AK: Radiology of Burkitt's tumour in the jaws, *East Afr Med J* 43:290-297, 1966.

Burkitt D: A sarcoma involving the jaws in African children, *Br J Surg* 46:218-223, 1958.

Jan A, Vora K, Sandor GKB: Sporadic Burkitt's lymphoma of the jaws: the essentials of prompt life-saving referral and management, *J Can Dent Assoc* 71:165-168, 2005.

Levine PH, Kamaraju LS, Connelly RR et al: The American Burkitt's lymphoma registry: eight years' experience, *Cancer* 49:1016, 1982.

Sariban E, Donahue A, Magrath IT: Jaw involvement in American Burkitt's Lymphoma, *Cancer* 53:1777-1782, 1984.

*LEUKEMIA*

Curtis AB: Childhood leukemias: initial oral manifestations, *J Am Dent Assoc* 83:159-164, 1971.

Ficarra G, Silverman S Jr, Quivey JM et al: Granulocytic sarcoma (chloroma) of the oral cavity: a case with a leukemic presentation, *Oral Surg* 53:709-714, 1987.

Greer RO, Mierau GW, Favara BE: *Tumors of the head and neck in children,* New York, 1983, Praeger Scientific.

Nortjé CJ: General practitioner's radiology case 16. Acute leukemia, *SADJ* 58:393, 2001.

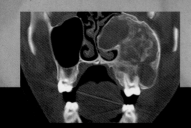

# CHAPTER 24

# Diseases of Bone Manifested in the Jaws

This chapter discusses disorders of bone that do not easily fit into well-defined categories of disease.

## Bone Dysplasias

Bone dysplasias constitute a group of conditions in which normal bone is replaced with fibrous tissue containing abnormal bone or cementum. These lesions must be differentiated from tumors because the treatment is very different. *Fibro-osseous lesion,* originally a histo-pathologic term, is a commonly used term that includes the following bone dysplasias and neoplasms and other lesions of bone.

### FIBROUS DYSPLASIA

#### Definition

Fibrous dysplasia results from a localized change in normal bone metabolism that results in the replacement of all the components of cancellous bone by fibrous tissue containing varying amounts of abnormal-appearing bone. This may be the result of a sporadic gene mutation. At the histologic level, the result is the appearance of numerous short, irregularly shaped trabeculae of woven bone. These trabeculae are not aligned in response to stress, but rather have a random orientation. This histologic appearance is responsible for the abnormal internal trabecular pattern seen in radiographs. Fibrous dysplasias may be solitary or multiple (Jaffe type) or may occur in another multiple form associated with McCune-Albright syndrome, which usually comprises polyostotic fibrous dysplasia, cutaneous pigmentation (café au lait spots), and hyperfunction of one or more of the endocrine glands.

#### Clinical Features

The solitary (monostotic) form of fibrous dysplasia, which accounts for 70% of all cases, is the type that most often involves the jaws. The most common sites (in order) are the ribs, femur, tibia, maxilla, and mandible. The multiple (polyostotic) form usually is found in children younger than 10 years, whereas monostotic disease typically is discovered in a slightly older age group. The lesions usually become static when skeletal growth stops, but proliferation may continue, particularly in the polyostotic form. The lesions may become active in pregnant women or with the use of oral contraceptives; and abnormal growth may occur after surgical intervention in young patients. Studies of the sex distribution of fibrous dysplasia show no sexual predilection except for McCune-Albright syndrome, which affects females almost exclusively. Symptoms of the disease may be mild or absent. Monostotic fibrous dysplasia often is discovered as an incidental radiographic finding. Patients with jaw involvement first may complain of unilateral facial swelling or an enlarging deformity of the alveolar process. Pain and pathologic fractures are rare. If extensive craniofacial lesions have impinged on nerve foramina, neurologic symptoms such as anosmia (loss of the sense of smell), deafness, or blindness may develop.

#### Radiographic Features

*Location.* Fibrous dysplasia involves the maxilla almost twice as often as the mandible and occurs more frequently in the posterior aspect. Lesions more commonly are unilateral (Fig. 24-1) except for very rare extensive lesions of the maxillofacial region that are bilateral.

*Periphery.* The periphery of fibrous dysplasia lesions most commonly is ill defined, with a gradual blending of normal trabecular bone into an abnormal trabecular pattern. Occasionally the boundary between normal bone and the lesion can appear sharp and even corticated, especially in young lesions (Fig. 24-2).

*Internal Structure.* The density and trabecular pattern of fibrous dysplasia lesions vary considerably. The variation is more pronounced in the mandible and more homogeneous in the maxilla. The internal aspect of bone may be more radiolucent, more radiopaque, or a mixture of these two variations compared with normal bone (see Fig. 24-1). The internal density is more radiopaque in the maxilla and the base of the skull. Early lesions may be more radiolucent (Fig. 24-3) than are mature lesions and in rare cases may appear to have granular internal septa, giving the internal aspect a multilocular appearance.

The abnormal trabeculae usually are shorter, thinner, irregularly shaped, and more numerous than normal trabeculae are. This creates a radiopaque pattern that can vary; it may have a granular appearance (or "ground-glass" appearance, resembling the small fragments of a shattered windshield), a pattern resembling the surface of an orange (peau d'orange), a wispy arrangement (cotton wool), or an amorphous, dense pattern (Fig. 24-4). A distinctive characteristic is the organization of the abnormal trabeculae into a swirling pattern similar to a fingerprint (Fig. 24-5). Occasionally, radiolucent regions resembling cysts may occur in mature lesions of fibrous dysplasia. These are bone cavities that are analogous to simple bone cysts (Fig. 24-6).

*Effects on Surrounding Structures.* If the fibrous dysplasia lesion is small, it may have no effect on surrounding structures (subclinical variety). The effects on the involved bone may include expansion with maintenance of a thinned outer cortex (Fig. 24-7). Fibrous

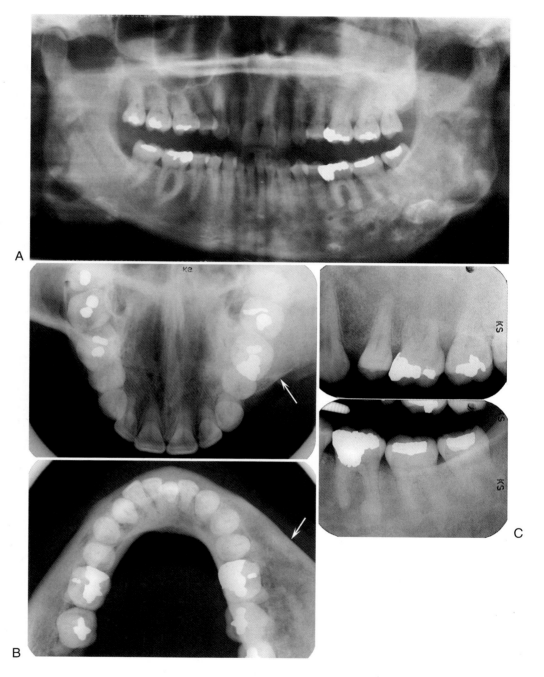

FIG. **24-1 A,** Unilateral fibrous dysplasia involving the left maxilla and mandible. **B,** Note the expansion of the lateral aspect of the maxilla and mandible *(arrow)* and the increased bone density caused by an increase in the number of internal trabeculae. **C,** Periapical films show a mixed radiolucent-radiopaque internal structure; however, the overall radiopacity is greater than on the right side of the jaws.

dysplasia may expand into the antrum by displacing its cortical boundary and subsequently occupying part or most of the maxillary sinus. Extension into the maxillary antrum usually occurs from the lateral wall, and the last section of the sinus to be involved usually is the most posterosuperior portion. Often the extension into the sinuses appears as a parallel thickening of the outer cortical border, resulting in a residual antral air space that still has approximately the normal anatomic shape of a an antrum (Fig. 24-8). Cortical boundaries such as the floor of the antrum may be changed into the abnormal bone pattern. Often the bone surrounding the teeth is altered without affecting the dentition, and a distinct lamina dura disappears because this bone also is changed into the abnormal bone pattern (see Fig. 24-5). If the fibrous dysplasia increases the bone density, the periodontal ligament space may appear to be very narrow. Fibrous dysplasia can displace teeth or interfere with normal eruption, complicating orthodontic therapy. In rare cases, some root resorption may occur. Involved teeth may have hypercementosis. Fibrous dysplasia appears to be unique in its ability to displace the inferior alveolar nerve canal in a superior direction (Fig. 24-8).

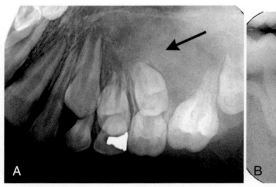
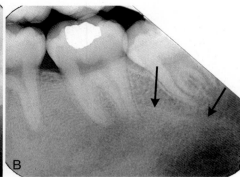

FIG. **24-2** **A,** Fibrous dysplasia in the posterior maxilla, with an ill-defined anterior margin that blends into the normal bone pattern in the region of the unerupted cuspid. The internal pattern is granular *(arrow).* **B,** In contrast, the margin of this case of mandibular fibrous dysplasia has a well-defined, almost corticated margin *(arrows).*

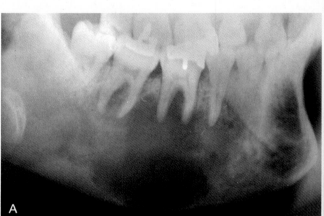
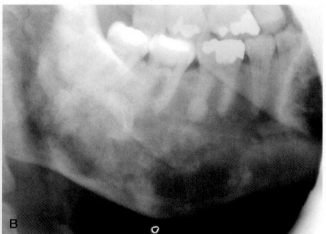

FIG. **24-3** Fibrous dysplasia in the mandible. **A,** An early radiolucent stage. **B,** The same case 18 years later shows a more mature radiopaque appearance.

## Differential Diagnosis

Other diseases can alter the bone pattern in a similar fashion. Metabolic bone diseases such as hyperparathyroidism may produce a similar pattern. However, these diseases are polyostotic; bilateral; and, unlike fibrous dysplasia, do not cause bone expansion. Paget's disease may produce a similar pattern and may cause expansion, but it occurs in an older age group, and when it involves the mandible, the whole mandible is involved, unlike the unilateral tendency of fibrous dysplasia. Occasionally periapical cemental dysplasia may show a similar bone pattern, but the distribution is different in that it often is bilateral, with an epicenter in the periapical region. Furthermore, periapical cemental dysplasia also occurs in an older age group. With spontaneous healing of a simple bone cyst, the radiographic and histologic appearance of the new bone may be very similar to that of fibrous dysplasia.

Of paramount importance is the differentiation of osteomyelitis and osteogenic sarcoma because of both radiologic and histologic similarities. Osteomyelitis may result in enlargement of the jaws, but the additional bone is generated by the periosteum; therefore the new bone is laid down on the surface of the outer cortex, and close examination may reveal evidence of the original cortex within the expanded portion of the jaw. Fibrous dysplasia, in contrast, expands the internal aspect of bone, displacing and thinning the outer cortex so that the remaining cortex maintains its position at the outer surface of the bone. The identification of sequestra aids in the identification of osteomyelitis. Osteogenic sarcoma may produce a similar pattern but should show malignant radiologic features (see Chapter 23).

Some difficulty may arise in differentiating cemento-ossifying fibroma of the maxilla, especially the juvenile ossifying fibroma type. If the bone pattern is altered around the teeth without displacement of the teeth from one specific epicenter, the lesion probably is fibrous dysplasia. The shape of the bone expansion of fibrous dysplasia into the antrum reflects the original outer contour of the antral wall, which is different from the more convex extension of a neoplasm.

## Management

In most cases the radiographic characteristics of fibrous dysplasia and the clinical information are sufficient to allow the practitioner to make a diagnosis without a biopsy. There are reports of exaggerated growth from stimulation of a lesion during surgical intervention in young patients. A consultation with a dental radiologist is advisable. The radiologist may supplement the examination with computed tomography (CT), which can give a more accurate, three-dimensional representation of the extent of the lesion and can serve as a precise baseline study for future comparisons. It is reasonable to continue occasional monitoring of the lesion or ask the patient to report any

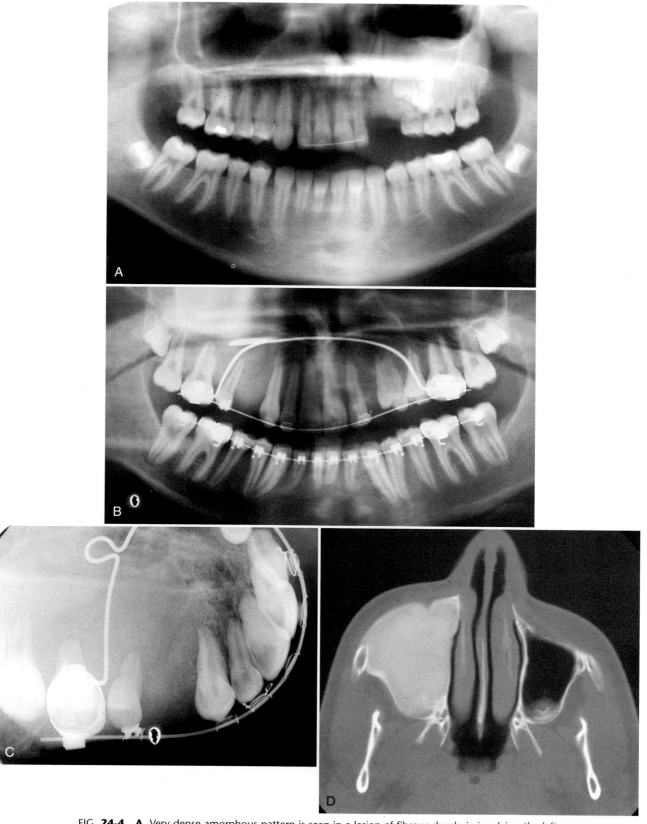

FIG. 24-4 **A,** Very dense amorphous pattern is seen in a lesion of fibrous dysplasia involving the left maxilla and preventing the normal eruption of the cuspid and the bicuspids. **B** through **E,** Panoramic, occlusal, axial, and coronal computed tomographic images of an example of fibrous dysplasia with a homogeneous, dense pattern that occupies most of the right maxillary sinus.

*Continued*

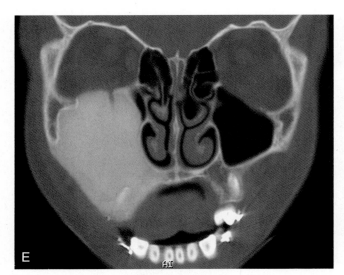

FIG. **24-4, cont'd**   For legend see p. 431.

changes. With most lesions, growth is complete at skeletal maturation; therefore orthodontic treatment and cosmetic surgery may be delayed until this time. Sarcomatous changes are unusual but have been reported, especially if therapeutic radiation has been given. In the case of female patients, hormonal changes from pregnancy or the use of oral contraceptives may stimulate growth or result in the development of lesions within the area of fibrous dysplasia, such as aneurysmal bone cysts or giant cell granulomas.

## CEMENTO-OSSEOUS DYSPLASIAS

Periapical cemental dysplasia and florid osseous dysplasia are essentially the same process but are separated on the basis of the extent of involvement of the jaws.

### Periapical Cemental Dysplasia

#### Synonyms
Cementoma, fibrocementoma, sclerosing cementoma, periapical osteofibrosis, periapical fibrous dysplasia, and periapical fibro-osteoma

#### Definition
Periapical cemental dysplasia (PCD) is a localized change in normal bone metabolism that results in the replacement of the components

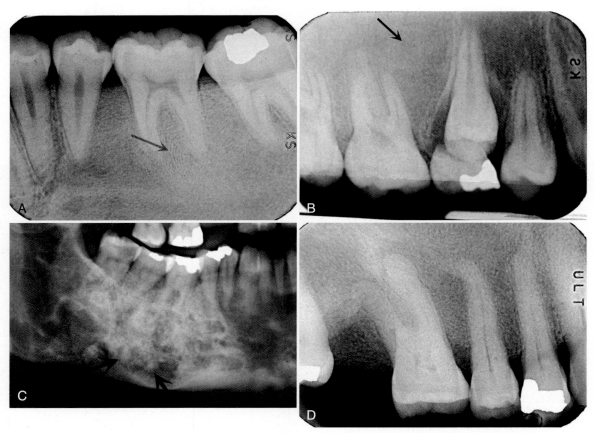

FIG. **24-5**   A series of films showing a variety of internal patterns of fibrous dysplasia. **A,** A fingerprint pattern around the roots of the first molar *(arrow)*. Note the change in the lamina dura around the molars into the abnormal bone pattern. **B,** A granular, or ground-glass, pattern *(arrow)*. **C,** A cotton wool pattern. Note the almost circular radiopaque regions *(arrows)*. **D,** An orange-peel pattern.

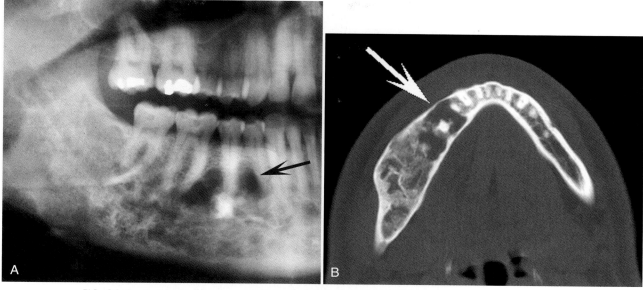

FIG. **24-6**  **A,** A cropped panoramic image of fibrous dysplasia of the mandible. There is a cystlike radiolucent lesion in the region of the bicuspids *(arrow)*. **B,** An axial computed tomographic scan with bone algorithm of the same case also revealing the same simple bonelike cyst *(arrow)*.

of normal cancellous bone with fibrous tissue and cementum-like material, abnormal bone (similar to that seen in fibrous dysplasia), or a mixture of the two. By definition the lesion is located near the apex of a tooth.

## Clinical Features

PCD is a common bone dysplasia that typically occurs in middle age; the mean age is 39 years. It occurs nine times more often in females than in males and almost three times more often in blacks than in whites. It also frequently is seen in Asians. The involved teeth are vital, and the patient usually has no history of pain or sensitivity. The lesions usually come to light as an incidental finding during a periapical or panoramic radiographic examination made for other purposes. The lesions can become quite large, causing a notable expansion of the alveolar process, and may continue to enlarge slowly.

## Radiographic Features

*Location.* The epicenter of a PCD lesion usually lies at the apex of a tooth (Fig. 24-9). In rare cases the epicenter is slightly higher and over the apical third of the root. The condition has a predilection for the periapical bone of the mandibular anterior teeth, although any tooth can be involved, and in rare cases the maxillary teeth may be involved (Fig. 24-10). In most cases the lesion is multiple and bilateral, but occasionally a solitary lesion arises. If the involved teeth have been extracted, this lesion can still develop but the periapical location is less evident (Fig. 24-11). In these cases the term *cemental dysplasia* may be more appropriate.

*Periphery and Shape.* In most cases the periphery of a PCD lesion is well defined. Often a radiolucent border of varying width is present, surrounded by a band of sclerotic bone that also can vary in width (Fig. 24-12). The sclerotic bone represents a reaction of the immediate surrounding bone. The lesion may be irregularly shaped or may have an overall round or oval shape centered over the apex of the tooth.

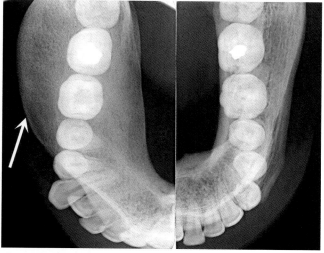

FIG. **24-7**  Occlusal views of both sides of the mandible of the same patient. Note the expansion of the right side of the mandible caused by fibrous dysplasia. The outer cortical plates have been displaced and thinned but are still intact *(arrow)*.

*Internal Structure.* The internal structure varies, depending on the maturity of the lesion. In the early stage, normal bone is resorbed and replaced with fibrous tissue that usually is continuous with the periodontal ligament (causing loss of the lamina dura). Radiographically, this appears as a radiolucency at the apex of the involved tooth (see Fig. 24-9).

In the mixed stage, radiopaque tissue appears in the radiolucent structure. This material usually is amorphous; has a round, oval, or irregular shape; and is composed of cementum or abnormal bone (Fig. 24-12). Sometimes the cementum-like material forms a swirling pattern (Fig. 24-13). These structures sometimes are called cementi-

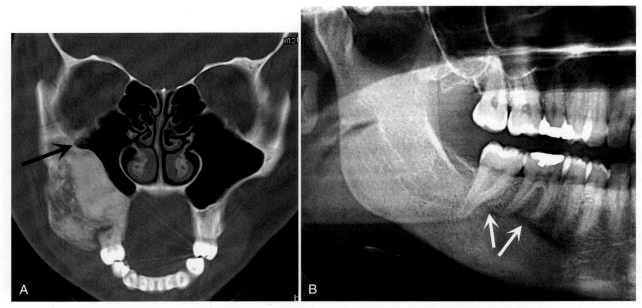

**FIG. 24-8** **A,** A coronal CT scan with bone algorithm of a maxillary lesion of fibrous dysplasia. The lesion has caused the lateral wall of the maxilla to expand into the maxillary antrum. The shape of the lateral wall of the sinus has maintained the zygomatic recess *(arrow)*. **B,** Mandibular fibrous dysplasia that has displaced the inferior alveolar nerve canal in a superior direction *(arrows)*.

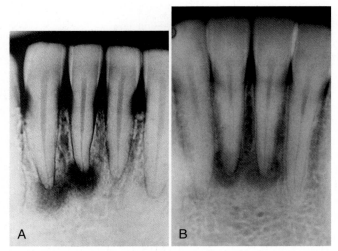

**FIG. 24-9 Periapical Cemental Dysplasia: Radiolucent Stage.** Two periapical films showing loss of lamina dura; however, the periodontal membrane space can still be seen around some of the teeth.

cles; however, this is a radiographic term that does not necessarily represent the histologic appearance. In rare cases the radiopaque material resembles the abnormal trabecular patterns seen in fibrous dysplasia (Fig. 24-13).

In the mature stage, the internal aspect may be totally radiopaque without any obvious pattern. Usually, a thin radiolucent margin can be seen at the periphery because this lesion matures from the center outward (Fig. 24-14). Occasionally, this radiolucent margin is not apparent, which makes the differential diagnosis more difficult. The

internal structure may appear dramatically radiolucent if cavities resembling simple bone cysts form within the cemental lesions (Fig. 24-15). In some cases the simple bone cyst extends beyond the original margin of the cemental lesion.

*Effects on Surrounding Structures.* The normal lamina dura of the teeth involved with the lesion is lost, making the periodontal ligament space either less apparent or giving it a wider appearance (see Fig. 24-9). The tooth structure usually is not affected, although in rare cases some root resorption may occur. Also, occasionally hypercementosis occurs on the root of a tooth positioned within the lesion. Some lesions stimulate a sclerotic bone reaction from the surrounding bone. Small lesions do not cause expansion of the involved jaw. However, larger lesions may cause expansion of the jaw, an area that is always bordered by a thin, intact outer cortex similar to that seen in fibrous dysplasia. The expansion is usually undulating in shape. This lesion may elevate the floor of the maxillary antrum.

### Differential Diagnosis

In early (radiolucent) PCD lesions, the most important differential diagnosis is periapical rarefying osteitis. Occasionally PCD cannot be distinguished from this inflammatory lesion by radiographic characteristics alone. In these cases the final diagnosis must rely on clinical information such as testing of the vitality of the involved tooth.

In the case of a solitary mature form of PCD, the differential diagnosis may include a benign cementoblastoma, especially when the lesion is periapical to the mandibular first molar. This tumor is usually is attached to the surface of the root, which may be partly resorbed. Also, the peripheral soft tissue capsule is better defined and there may be a unique pattern to the internal structure, such as a radiating pattern. Expansion caused by the tumor is more concentric and less undulating than in PCD. The presence or absence of clinical symptoms may help distinguish PCD from benign cementoblastoma.

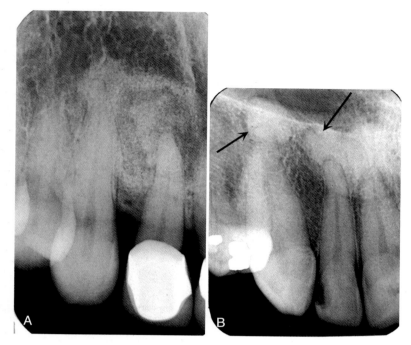

FIG. **24-10** Examples of periapical cemental dysplasia in the maxilla. **A,** A mixed lesion. **B,** Mature lesions *(arrows).*

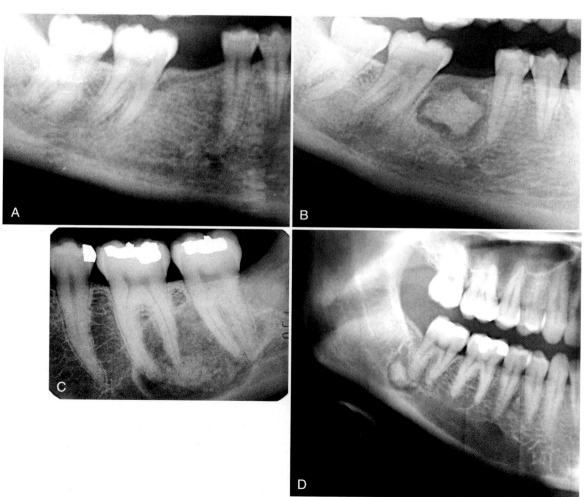

FIG. **24-11**    **A** and **B,** Portions of panoramic views of the same patient taken 3 years apart. Note the development of a solitary lesion of periapical cemental dysplasia in the apical region of the first molar extraction site. **C** and **D,** Solitary lesions in the posterior mandible.

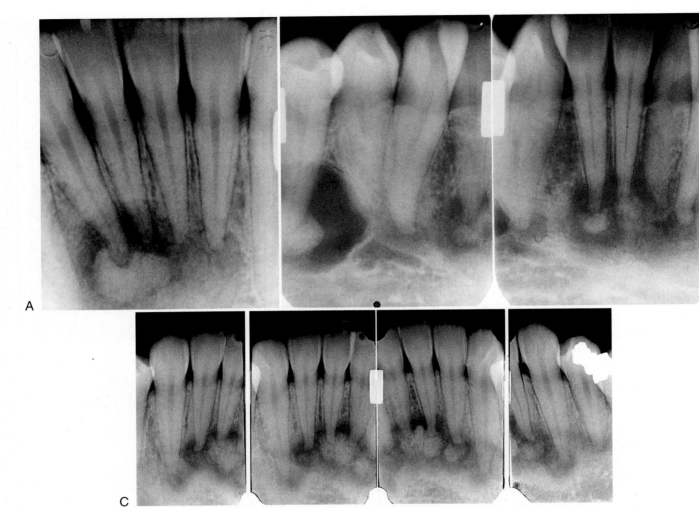

FIG. **24-12**   **Periapical Cemental Dysplasia: Mixed Stage.  A** and **B,** Radiopacity in the center of a radiolucent area. **C,** Multiple lesions. Note the band of sclerotic bone reaction at the periphery of the lesion.

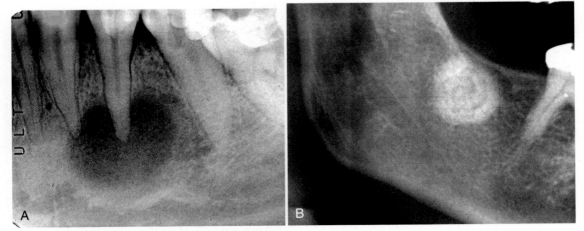

FIG. **24-13   A,** Periapical cemental dysplasia with a fibrous dysplasia type of internal bone pattern. **B,** A swirling internal pattern of cemental dysplasia.

Another lesion to consider is an odontoma. Odontomas often start occlusal to a tooth and prevent its eruption, but some odontomas may have a periapical position. The organization of the internal aspect into toothlike structures and the identification of enamel (very radiopaque) can help in the differential diagnosis. Also, the peripheral cortex and soft tissue capsule of an odontoma are more uniform in width and better defined than is the periphery of PCD. In mature PCD lesions, the appearance may resemble that of a dense bone island. The finding of a radiolucent periphery, even if very slight, indicates a diagnosis of PCD. Solitary lesions may be difficult to differentiate from a cemento-ossifying fibroma. Cases that have been quiescent and then suddenly start to grow aggressively suggest that there may be a continuum between the category of cemento-osseous dysplasia and cemento-osseous tumors.

## Management

The diagnosis of PCD can be made on the basis of the appropriate radiologic and clinical characteristics. In fact, a possible complication of biopsy is secondary infection, which may occur in lesions that have abundant cementum formation and poor vascularity. Normally treatment is not required. However, if the teeth have been removed and if considerable atrophy of the alveolar ridge has occurred, these segments of cementum may reach the mucosal surface, much in the same way as stones become exposed in old, worn concrete. These pieces of cementum can perforate the mucosa when positioned under a denture, and the result is secondary infection. If this occurs, the pieces of cementum may have to be removed surgically because they can act as sequestra in osteomyelitis.

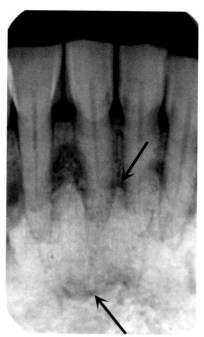

**FIG. 24-14**  The mature stage of periapical cemental dysplasia. Note the thin radiolucent periphery *(arrows)*.

## Florid Osseous Dysplasia

### Synonyms

Florid cemento-osseous dysplasia, gigantiform cementoma, and familial multiple cementomas

### Definition

Florid osseous dysplasia (FOD) is a widespread form of PCD. Normal cancellous bone is replaced with dense acellular cemento-osseous tissue in a background of fibrous connective tissue. The lesion has a poor vascular supply, a condition that likely contributes to its susceptibility to infection. In some cases a familial trend can be seen. No clear definition indicates when multiple regions of PCD should be termed FOD. However, if PCD is identified in three or four quadrants or is extensive throughout one jaw, it usually is considered to be FOD.

### Clinical Features

Several key similarities exist between FOD and PCD, including the age, sex, and racial profiles of patients and comparable radiographic and histologic appearances. Most patients with FOD are female and middle aged (mean age, 42 years), although the age range is broad. The condition shows a marked predilection for blacks and Asians. A few documented cases appear to have a familial pattern. Often FOD produces no symptoms and is found incidentally during a radiographic examination. Occasionally patients complain of low-grade, intermittent, poorly localized pain in the affected bone, especially when a simple bone cyst has developed within the lesion. Extensive lesions often have an associated bony swelling. If the lesions become secondarily infected, features of osteomyelitis may develop, including mucosal ulceration, fistulous tracts with suppuration, and pain. In fact, historically, FOD that was secondarily infected was diagnosed as

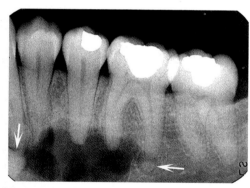

**FIG. 24-15**  A simple bone cyst within an area of periapical cemental dysplasia. Only a few regions of cementum-like tissue remain *(arrows)*.

chronic sclerosing osteomyelitis without the identification of the underlying bone dysplasia. A CT examination should be ordered to determine the extent of involvement with osteomyelitis. Teeth in the involved bone are vital unless other dental disease coincidentally affects them.

### Radiographic Features

*Location.*  FOD lesions usually are bilateral and present in both jaws (Fig. 24-16). However, when they are present in only one jaw, the mandible is the more common location. The epicenter is apical to the teeth, within the alveolar process and usually posterior to the cuspid. In the mandible, lesions occur above the inferior alveolar canal.

*Periphery.*  The periphery usually is well defined and has a sclerotic border that can vary in width, very similar to PCD. The soft tissue capsule may not be apparent in mature lesions.

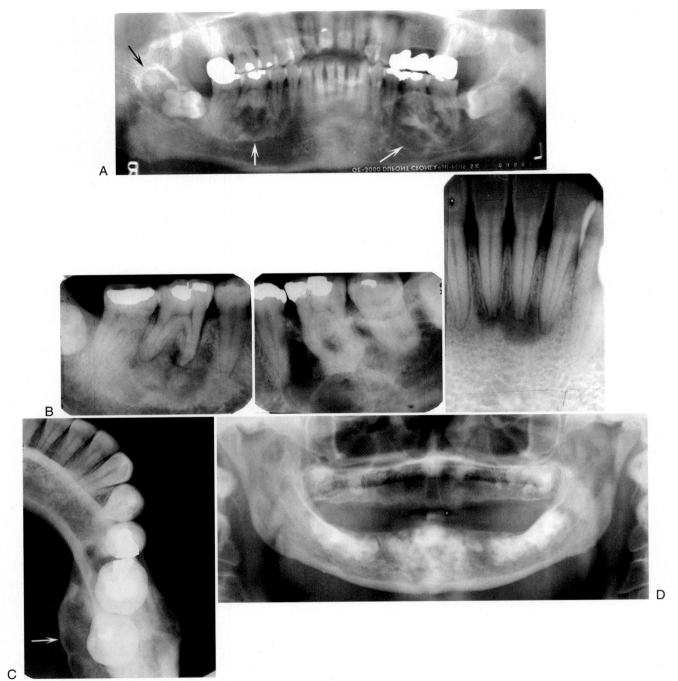

FIG. **24-16** **Florid Osseous Dysplasia. A,** Three mixed radiopaque-radiolucent lesions in the periapical regions throughout the jaws *(arrows);* although the right third molar is horizontally impacted, the lesion still has a periapical relationship *(black arrow).* **B,** Composite of periapical films of the same case; note the appearance of the lesions involving the mandibular incisors (not apparent in the panoramic film), which are identical to periapical cemental dysplasia. **C,** Occlusal film of the left mandibular lesion showing undulating expansion of the medial cortical plate *(arrow).* **D,** Panoramic film of a different case showing multiple, very mature, almost totally radiopaque lesions in edentulous jaws. The epicenter of all lesions is above the inferior alveolar canal.

***Internal Structure.*** The density of the internal structure can vary from an equal mixture of radiolucent and radiopaque regions to almost complete radiopacity. Some prominent radiolucent regions, which usually represent the development of a simple bone cyst, may be present (Fig. 24-17). These cysts may enlarge with time, even beyond the boundary of the lesion into the surrounding normal bone, or may fill in with abnormal dysplastic cemento-osseous tissue. The radiopaque regions can vary from small oval and circular regions (cotton-wool appearance) to large, irregular, amorphous areas of calcification. These calcified masses are similar in appearance to those seen in mature PCD lesions.

***Effects on Surrounding Structures.*** Large FOD lesions can displace the inferior alveolar nerve canal in an inferior direction. FOD also can displace the floor of the antrum in a superior direction and can cause enlargement of the alveolar bone by displacement of the buccal and lingual cortical plates. The roots of associated teeth may have a considerable amount of hypercementosis, which may fuse with the abnormal surrounding cemental tissue of the lesion. Extraction of these teeth may be difficult.

## Differential Diagnosis

The fact that FOD is bilateral and centered in the alveolar process helps in the differentiation from other lesions. Paget's disease of bone may also show cotton wool–type radiopaque regions with associated hypercementosis. However, Paget's disease affects the bone of the entire mandible, whereas FOD is centered above the inferior alveolar canal. Furthermore, Paget's disease often is polyostotic, involving other bones as well as the jaws. The well-defined nature of FOD, with its radiolucent periphery and surrounding sclerotic border, also is useful in making the differential diagnosis.

Another disease that may resemble FOD is chronic sclerosing osteomyelitis. Regions of cementum-like masses may appear similar to the sequestrum seen in osteomyelitis. This is not to be confused with a situation where FOD has become secondarily infected, resulting in osteomyelitis. The cemental-like masses that are secondarily infected have a wider and more profound radiolucent border (Fig. 24-18). CT imaging is essential for the diagnosis and to determine the extent of the osteomyelitis within the FOD.

## Management

Under normal circumstances, FOD does not require treatment, although there is value in obtaining a panoramic film to establish the extent of the disease. Unlike with fibrous dysplasia, no age limit is apparent for the cessation of growth of FOD. Because of the propensity for development of secondary infections in FOD, the patient should be encouraged to maintain an effective oral hygiene program to avoid odontogenic infections. Also, if the teeth are extracted and severe atrophy of the alveolar process occurs, as in PCD, the cementum-like masses emerge and the pressure of the overlying denture may cause dehiscence in the mucosa, resulting in osteomyelitis. If this occurs, the avascular cementum-like masses become large sequestra. The osteomyelitis may spread slowly throughout the jaw from one region of FOD to another. It may be necessary to remove large areas of cementum-like tissue, leaving very little residual bone for prosthetic treatment.

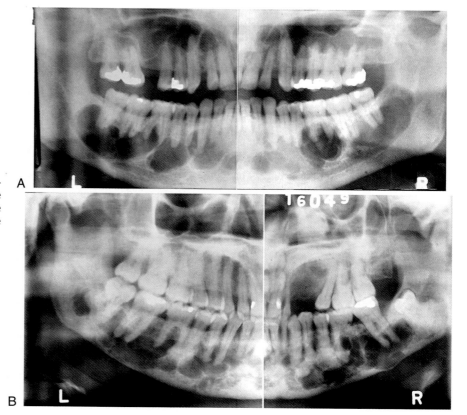

FIG. **24-17** Two examples of florid osseous dysplasia (FOD) associated with multiple simple bone cysts. **A**, Large cysts occupy most of the bone involved with the FOD lesions. **B**, Another example of multiple simple bone cysts in lesions of FOD.

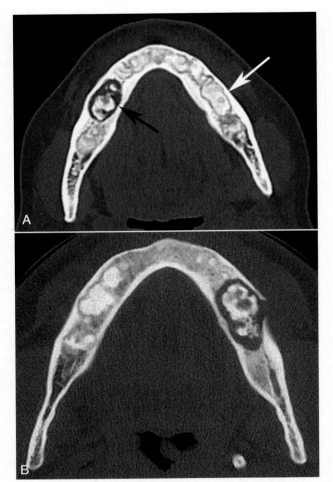

**FIG. 24-18  A,** Axial CT image with bone algorithm of a case of florid osseous dysplasia (FOD); multiple foci of cemental dysplasia are bordered by a soft tissue capsule *(white arrow)* and a cemental mass has become secondarily infected with a wider and more pronounced radiolucent border *(black arrow)*. **B,** Axial CT image of a different case of osteomyelitis from secondarily infected FOD; note the break in the outer cortex where the lesion is draining into the surrounding soft

## Other Lesions of Bone

### Cemento-Ossifying Fibroma

#### Synonyms
Ossifying fibroma and cementifying fibroma

#### Definition
Cemento-ossifying fibroma (COF) is classified as and behaves like a benign bone neoplasm. However, it appears in this chapter because it often is considered to be a type of fibro-osseous lesion. This bone tumor consists of highly cellular, fibrous tissue that contains varying amounts of abnormal bone or cementum-like tissue. In the past this lesion was classified as two different entities depending on whether bone or cementum was the predominant calcified product. When the histologic appearance of most of the calcified tissue was of irregular trabeculae of woven bone, the term *ossifying fibroma* was used. The resulting internal pattern may be very similar to or indistinguishable from that of fibrous dysplasia. One distinguishing feature that may be

present is a soft tissue capsule at the periphery, not seen in fibrous dysplasia. When the predominant calcified component was cementum, the term cementifying fibroma was used. However, the microscopic appearance of an ossifying fibroma and a cementifying fibroma can be very similar, and the two are now thought to represent a spectrum of one disease and are combined under the name cemento-ossifying fibroma.

Juvenile ossifying fibroma is a very aggressive form of COF that occurs in the first two decades of life. Although the histopathologic definition of this entity is controversial, the radiologic appearance has similarities to that of COF.

#### Clinical Features
The clinical features of COF can vary from indolent to aggressive behavior. The characteristics are more like those of a tumor than a bone dysplasia. COF can occur at any age but usually is found in young adults. Females are affected more often than males. The disease usually is asymptomatic at the time of discovery. Occasionally facial asymmetry develops. Displacement of the teeth may be an early clinical feature, although most lesions are discovered during routine dental examinations. In cases of juvenile ossifying fibroma, rapid growth may occur in a young patient, resulting in deformity of the involved jaw.

#### Radiographic Features
*Location.* COF appears almost exclusively in the facial bones and most commonly in the mandible, typically inferior to the premolars and molars and superior to the inferior alveolar canal. In the maxilla it occurs most often in the canine fossa and zygomatic arch area.

*Periphery.* The borders of COF lesions usually are well defined. A thin, radiolucent line, representing a fibrous capsule, may separate it from surrounding bone (Fig. 24-19). Sometimes the bone next to the lesion develops a sclerotic border.

*Internal Structure.* The internal structure of a COF lesion is a mixed radiolucent-radiopaque density with a pattern that depends on the amount and form of the manufactured calcified material. In some instances the internal structure may appear almost totally radiolucent with just a hint of calcified material. In the type that contains mainly abnormal bone, the pattern may be similar to that seen in fibrous dysplasia, or a wispy (similar to stretched tufts of cotton) or flocculent pattern (similar to large, heavy snowflakes) may be seen (Fig. 24-20). Lesions that produce more cementum-like material may contain solid, amorphous radiopacities (cementicles) similar to those seen in cemental dysplasia (see Fig. 24-19).

*Effects on Surrounding Structures.* COF can be distinguished from the previously mentioned bone dysplasias by its tumorlike behavior. This is reflected in the growth of the lesion, which tends to be concentric within the medullary part of the bone with outward expansion approximately equal in all directions. This can result in displacement of teeth or of the inferior alveolar canal and expansion of the outer cortical plates of bone. A significant point is that the outer cortical plate, although displaced and thinned, remains intact. The COF lesion can grow into and occupy the entire maxillary sinus (Fig. 24-21), expanding its walls outward; however, a bony partition always exists between the internal aspect of the remaining sinus and the tumor. The lamina dura of involved teeth usually is missing, and resorption of teeth may occur.

#### Differential Diagnosis
The differential diagnosis of COF includes lesions with a mixed radiolucent-radiopaque internal structure. The differentiation from

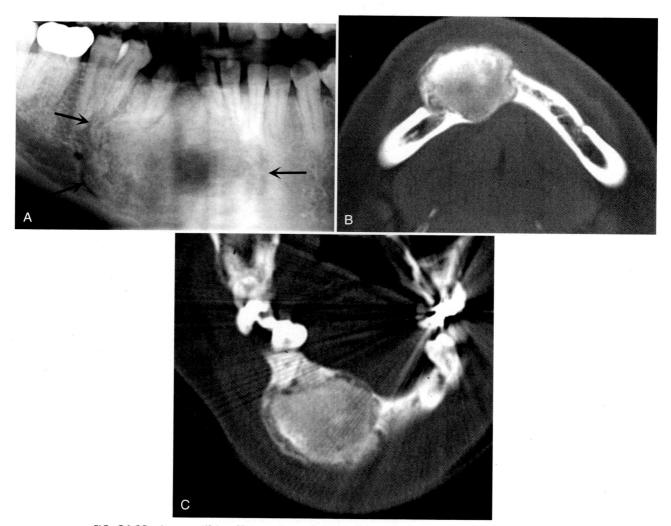

FIG. **24-19**   A cementifying fibroma *(arrows)* depicted in a panoramic film **(A)**, an axial CT scan **(B)**, and a coronal CT scan **(C)**. Note the homogeneous, radiopaque internal structure and the radiolucent band at the periphery.

fibrous dysplasia can be very difficult. The boundaries of a COF lesion usually are better defined, and these lesions occasionally have a soft tissue capsule and cortex, whereas fibrous dysplasia usually blends in with surrounding bone. The internal structure of fibrous dysplasia lesions in the maxilla may be more homogeneous and may show less variation. Both types of lesions can displace teeth, but COF displaces from a specific point or epicenter. Fibrous dysplasia rarely resorbs teeth. The expansion of the jaws associated with COF is more concentric about a definite epicenter but fibrous dysplasia enlarges the bone while distorting the overall shape to a smaller degree; in other words, the expanded bone still resembles normal morphology.

Great difficulty may arise in differentiating ossifying fibroma from fibrous dysplasia when the lesion involves the maxillary antrum. Fibrous dysplasia usually displaces the lateral wall of the maxilla into the maxillary antrum, maintaining the outer shape of the wall, whereas an ossifying fibroma has a more convex shape because it extends into the maxillary antrum (see Figs. 24-8 and 24-21). Also, fibrous dysplasia may change the bone around the teeth without displacing them

from an obvious epicenter of a concentrically growing benign tumor. The importance of this differentiation lies in the treatment, which is resection for an ossifying fibroma and observation for fibrous dysplasia.

The differential diagnosis of the type of COF that produces mainly cementum-like material from PCD may be difficult, especially with large single lesions of PCD. However, cemental dysplasia usually is multifocal where as COF is not. Also, the presence of a simple bone cyst is a characteristic of cemental dysplasia. COF behaves in a more tumorlike fashion, with the displacement of teeth and concentric expansion. A wide sclerotic border and undulating expansion are more characteristic of the slow-growing cemental dysplasia.

Other lesions to be considered include those that may have internal calcifications similar to the pattern seen in COF. These include giant cell granuloma, calcifying odontogenic cysts, calcifying epithelial odontogenic (Pindborg) tumors, and adenomatoid odontogenic tumors.

Occasionally, the diagnosis of osteogenic sarcoma is considered. However, characteristics suggesting a malignant lesion should be seen,

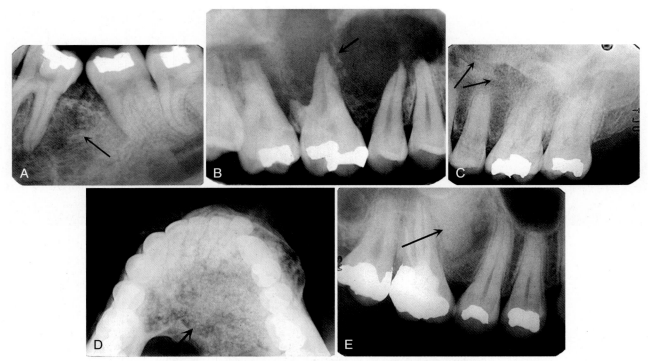

FIG. **24-20** **Various Bone Patterns Seen in Cemento-Ossifying Fibromas. A,** A wispy trabecular pattern *(arrow).* **B,** Most of this pattern is radiolucent with a few wispy trabeculae *(arrow).* **C,** A fibrous dysplasia, granular-like pattern *(arrows).* **D,** A flocculent pattern with larger tufts of bone formation *(arrow).* **E,** A solid, radiopaque, cementum-like pattern *(arrow).*

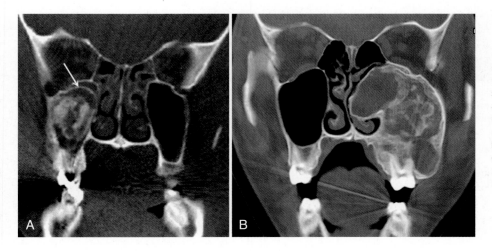

FIG. **24-21** Large cemento-ossifying fibromas involving the maxilla. **A,** A coronal CT scan of a lesion invaginating the maxillary antrum. Unlike in fibrous dysplasia, the peripheral border of the lesion *(arrow)* does not parallel the original shape of the antrum. **B,** A coronal CT scan of a larger lesion expanding the maxilla, occupying all the maxillary antrum and extending into the nasal fossa.

such as cortical bone destruction and invasion into the surrounding soft tissues and along the periodontal ligament space.

### Management
The prognosis of COF is favorable with surgical enucleation or resection. Large lesions require a detailed determination of the extent of the lesion, which can be obtained with CT imaging. Even if the lesion has reached appreciable size, it usually can be separated from the surrounding tissue and completely removed. Recurrence after removal is unlikely.

## Central Giant Cell Granuloma

### Synonyms
Giant cell reparative granuloma, giant cell lesion, and giant cell tumor

### Definition
Central giant cell granuloma (CGCG) is thought to be a reactive lesion to an as-yet-unknown stimulus and not a neoplastic lesion. However, radiographically the characteristics of the lesion are similar to those of a benign tumor and occasionally maxillary lesions may have some

malignant-type characteristics. The histologic appearance consists primarily of fibroblasts, numerous vascular channels, multinucleated giant cells, and macrophages. The relationship of the benign giant cell tumor to the giant cell granuloma is controversial and unclear.

### Clinical Features

CGCG is a common lesion in the jaws that affects mostly adolescents and young adults; at least 60% of cases occur in individuals younger than 20 years. The most common presenting sign of CGCG is painless swelling. Palpation of the suspect bone area may elicit tenderness, although in a minority of cases the patient may complain of pain. The overlying mucosa may have a purple color. Some of these lesions cause no symptoms and are found only on routine examination. The lesion usually grows slowly, although it may grow rapidly, creating the suspicion of a malignancy.

### Radiographic Features

*Location.* Lesions develop in the mandible twice as often as in the maxilla. In the fist two decades there is a tendency for the epicenter of the lesion to be anterior to the first molar in the mandible and anterior to the cuspid in the maxilla. However, in older individuals this lesion can occur in greater frequency in the posterior aspect of the jaws.

*Periphery.* Because this neoplasm grows relatively slowly, it usually produces a well-defined radiographic margin in the mandible. In most cases the periphery shows no evidence of cortication. Lesions in the maxilla may have ill-defined, almost malignant-appearing, borders.

*Internal Structure.* Some CGCG lesions show no evidence of internal structure (Fig. 24-22), especially small lesions. Other cases have a subtle granular pattern of calcification that may require a bright light source behind the film to enable visualization. Occasionally this granular bone is organized into ill-defined, wispy septa (Fig. 24-23). If present, these granular septa are characteristic of this lesion, especially if they emanate at right angles from the periphery of the lesion. This characteristic is even stronger if a small indentation of the expanded cortical margin is seen at the point where this right-angle

septum originates (Fig. 24-24). In some instances the septa are better defined and divide the internal aspect into compartments, creating a multilocular appearance.

*Effects on Surrounding Structures.* Giant cell granulomas often displace and resorb teeth. The resorption of tooth roots is not a constant feature, but when it occurs, it may be profound and irregular in outline. The lamina dura of teeth within the lesion usually is missing. The inferior alveolar canal may be displaced in an inferior direction. This lesion has a strong propensity to expand the cortical boundaries of the mandible and maxilla. The expansion usually is uneven or undulating in nature, which may give the appearance of a double

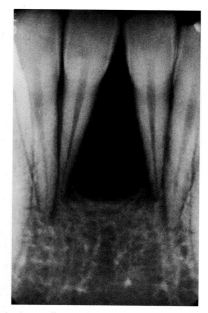

FIG. **24-22** A giant cell granuloma in the anterior mandible with no evidence of internal structure.

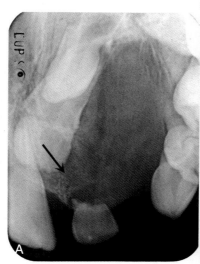

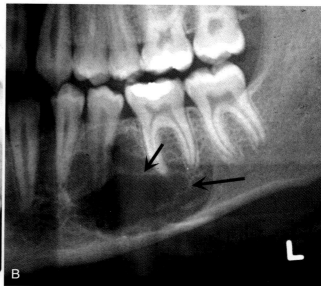

FIG. **24-23** Various internal patterns seen in giant cell granulomas. **A,** A lesion in the anterior maxilla with a very fine granular pattern *(arrow).* **B,** A portion of a panoramic film showing wispy, ill-defined internal septa *(arrows).*

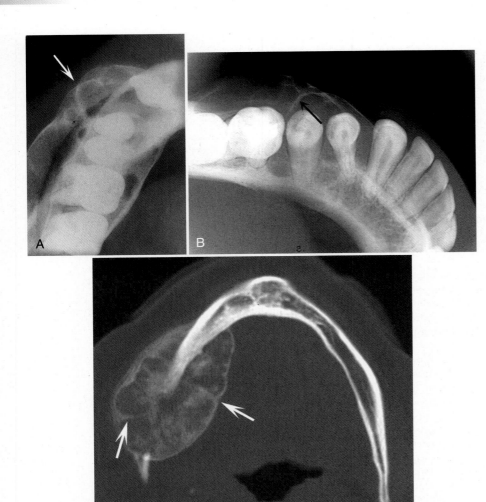

FIG. **24-24** Characteristic expansion of the outer cortical plates caused by giant cell granulomas. Note the uneven expansion in **A** *(arrow)* and the indentation of the expansion with a right-angled septum in **B** *(arrow)*. **C,** Axial CT scan with bone algorithm revealing a giant cell granuloma within the mandible causing undulating expansion and containing two right-angled septa *(arrows)*.

boundary when the expansion is viewed by use of occlusal film. The bone forming the border of the expanded mandible often has a granular texture compared with cortical bone (see Fig. 24-23, C). In some instances the outer cortical plate of bone is destroyed instead of expanded; this occurs more often in the maxilla, where the cortical bone destruction may give the lesion a malignant appearance.

## Differential Diagnosis

If the internal structure of the CGCG contains septa, the differential diagnosis may include ameloblastoma, odontogenic myxoma, and aneurysmal bone cyst. If a granular internal structure is present, COF may be considered. Useful characteristics for differentiating an ameloblastoma include the following: ameloblastomas tend to occur in an older age group and more often in the posterior mandible, and ameloblastomas have coarse, curved, well-defined trabeculae, whereas giant cell granulomas have wispy, ill-defined trabeculae, some of which are at right angles to the periphery. Odontogenic myxomas occur in an older age group, may have sharper and straighter septa, and do not have the same propensity to expand as do giant cell granulomas. Interestingly, aneurysmal bone cysts can appear identical radiographically to giant cell granulomas, especially in the appearance of the internal septa. However, aneurysmal bone cysts are comparatively rare lesions that occur more often in the posterior aspect of the jaws and usually cause profound expansion.

A small CGCG lesion with a totally radiolucent internal structure may be similar in appearance to a cyst, especially a simple bone cyst. Evidence of displacement or resorption of the adjacent teeth or expansion of the outer cortical bone is more characteristic of a giant cell granuloma. The radiographic image and histologic appearance of brown tumors of hyperparathyroidism may be identical to those of CGCG. Also, the appearance may be identical to that seen in cherubism; however, the lesions in cherubism or multiple and have epicenters that are located in the most posterior aspect of the mandible and maxilla.

## Management

If the lesion is in the maxilla, CT scans can be used to establish the exact extent and involvement of surrounding structures, such as the maxillary antrum or nasal cavity. Also, CT imaging is required for large lesions, which pose the possibility of destruction of the outer cortical bone, to determine whether the adjacent soft tissue has been invaded. Occasionally this lesion behaves very aggressively. If CGCG occurs after the second decade of life, hyperparathyroidism should be considered and serum testing for elevated calcium or parathormone levels or full-body technetium bone scans can be ordered.

Treatment may include enucleation and curettage and in some instances resection of the jaw. The patient should be followed up carefully to rule out recurrence, especially if conservative treatment is used. Recurrences are rare and are more common in the maxilla.

## Aneurysmal Bone Cyst

### Definition

An aneurysmal bone cyst (ABC) usually is considered to be a reactive lesion of bone rather than a cyst or true neoplasm. Some believe that it represents an exaggerated localized proliferative response of vascular tissue in bone. This lesion may be related to the CGCG because of similarities in both the radiographic and histologic appearance (presence of giant cells). ABCs occasionally develop in association with other primary lesions such as fibrous dysplasia, central hemangioma, giant cell granuloma, and osteosarcoma. Its etiology remains unclear.

### Clinical Features

More than 90% of reported jaw lesions have occurred in individuals younger than 30 years. The condition appears to have a predilection for females. An ABC in the jaw usually manifests as a fairly rapid bony swelling (usually buccal or labial). Pain is an occasional complaint, and the involved area may be tender on palpation.

### Radiographic Features

*Location.* The mandible is involved more often than the maxilla (ratio of 3:2), and the molar and ramus regions are more involved than the anterior region (Fig. 24-25).

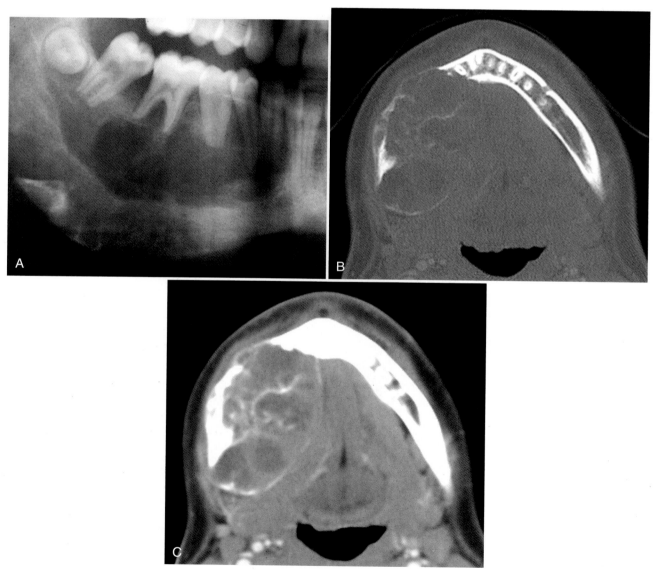

FIG. **24-25** **A,** A cropped panoramic image of aneurysmal bone cyst occupying the body of the right mandible. Two axial CT images at the same level of this case with bone algorithm **(B);** note the wispy, faint septa and soft tissue algorithm **(C)** and the low-attenuation regions of the internal structure representing fluid density.

*Periphery and Shape.* The periphery usually is well defined, and the shape is circular or "hydraulic."

*Internal Structure.* Small initial lesions may show no evidence of an internal structure. Often the internal aspect has a multilocular appearance. The septa bear a striking resemblance to the wispy, ill-defined septa seen in giant cell granulomas (Figs. 24-25 and 24-26). Another similar finding is septa positioned at right angles to the outer expanded border. In CT soft tissue algorithm images, there may be more radiolucent regions, some of which have a roughly circular shape. These likely represent large vascular spaces.

*Effects on Surrounding Structures.* After an ABC becomes large, there is a strong propensity for extreme expansion of the outer cortical plates (see Figs. 24-25 and 24-26). This characteristic is more dramatic in these cysts than in most other lesions. ABCs can displace and resorb teeth.

## Differential Diagnosis

The multilocular appearance of ABCs most resembles that of giant cell granulomas; in fact, the radiographic appearance of the two lesions may be identical. However, ABCs may expand to a greater degree, and they are more common in the posterior parts of the mandible. Ameloblastoma may be considered, but this lesion usually occurs in an older age group. ABCs may show a similarity to cherubism, which interestingly has giant cell–like features, but cherubism is a multifocal bilateral disease.

The diagnosis is based on biopsy results. A hemorrhagic aspirate favors the diagnosis of ABC. A CT scan also is recommended to better determine the extent of the lesion.

## Management

Surgical curettage and partial resection are the primary means of treatment. The recurrence rate is fairly high, ranging from 19% to about 50% after curettage and approximately 11% after resection. This indicates a need for careful follow-up.

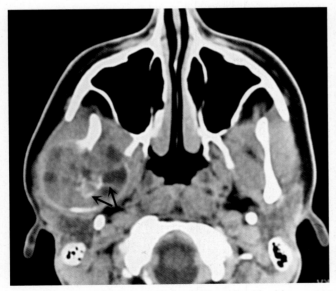

FIG. **24-26** An axial CT scan with a soft tissue algorithm demonstrating the presence of an aneurysmal bone cyst of the left mandibular condyle. Note the severe expansion and the wispy ill-defined septa *(arrows).*

## Cherubism

### Synonym
Familial fibrous dysplasia

### Definition
Cherubism is a rare inherited autosomal dominant disease that causes bilateral enlargement of the jaws, giving the child a cherubic facial appearance. Rare unilateral lesions have been reported. The term *familial fibrous dysplasia* was an unfortunate choice of early terminology because this lesion is not a bone dysplasia. It is composed of giant cell granuloma–like tissue and does not form a bone matrix. These lesions regress with age.

### Clinical Features
Cherubism develops in early childhood between 2 and 6 years of age. The most common presenting sign is a painless, firm, bilateral enlargement of the lower face. Enlargement of the submandibular lymph nodes may occur, but no systemic abnormalities are involved. Because children's faces are rather chubby, mild cases may go undetected until the second decade. Profound swelling of the maxilla may result in stretching of the skin of the cheeks, which depresses the lower eyelids, exposing a thin line of sclera and causing an "eyes raised to heaven" appearance.

### Radiographic Features
*Location.* This lesion is bilateral and often affects both jaws. When it is present in only one jaw, the mandible is the most common location. The epicenter is always in the posterior aspect of the jaws, in the ramus of the mandible or the tuberosity of the maxilla (Fig. 24-27). The lesion grows in an anterior direction and in severe cases can extend almost to the midline.

*Periphery.* The periphery usually is well defined and in some instances corticated.

*Internal Structure.* The internal structure resembles that of CGCG, with fine, granular bone and wispy trabeculae forming a prominent multilocular pattern.

*Effects on Surrounding Structures.* Expansion of the cortical boundaries of the maxilla and mandible by cherubism can result in severe enlargement of the jaws. Maxillary lesions enlarge into the maxillary sinuses. Because the epicenter is in the posterior aspect of the jaws, the teeth are displaced in an anterior direction. The degree of displacement can be severe, and with some lesions the tooth buds are destroyed.

### Differential Diagnosis
Although the radiographic appearance of cherubism may be similar to that of giant cell granuloma, the fact that cherubism is bilateral with an epicenter in the ramus should provide a clear differentiation. The differentiation of cherubism from fibrous dysplasia should not present any difficulties because fibrous dysplasia is more commonly a unilateral disease; also, the multilocular appearance and anterior displacement of teeth are more characteristic of cherubism. Cherubism may bear some similarity to multiple odontogenic keratocysts in basal cell nevus syndrome. The bilateral symmetry of cherubism, along with the anterior displacement of teeth and multilocular appearance, are characteristics that will help with the differential diagnosis.

### Management
The distinctive radiographic features of cherubism may be more diagnostic than the histopathologic findings; therefore the diagnosis can

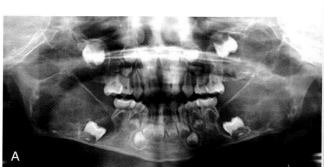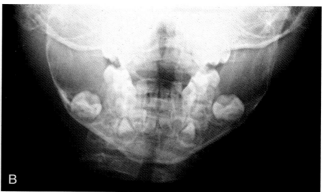

FIG. **24-27**  A case of cherubism. **A,** A panoramic image showing four lesions in the maxilla and mandible. The epicenters of the lesions are in the maxillary tuberosity and mandibular ramus; note the anterior displacement of the unerupted maxillary first molars. The internal structure contains ill-defined septa. **B,** A portion of the posteroanterior skull view showing expansion of the mandible.

rely on the radiologic findings alone. Treatment can be delayed because the cystlike lesions usually become static and fill in with granular bone during adolescence and at the end of skeletal growth. After skeletal growth has stopped, conservative surgical procedures, if required, may be done for cosmetic problems. Surgery also may be required to uncover displaced teeth, and orthodontic treatment may be needed.

## Paget's Disease

### Synonym
Osteitis deformans

### Definition
Paget's disease is a skeletal disorder and essentially a disease involving osteoclasts, resulting in abnormal resorption and apposition of osseous tissue in one or more bones. The disease may involve many bones simultaneously, but it is not a generalized skeletal disease. It is initiated by an intense wave of osteoclastic activity, with resorption of normal bone resulting in irregularly shaped resorption cavities. After a period of time, vigorous osteoblastic activity ensues, forming woven bone. Paget's disease is seen most frequently in Britain and Australia and somewhat less often in North America.

### Clinical Features
Paget's disease is primarily a disease of later middle and old age, having an incidence of about 3.5% in individuals older than 40 years. The incidence of involvement in males is approximately twice that of females at age 65 years.

Affected bone is enlarged and commonly deformed, resulting in bowing of the legs, curvature of the spine, and enlargement of the skull. The jaws also enlarge when affected. Separation and movement of teeth may occur, causing malocclusion. Dentures may be tight or may fit poorly in edentulous patients.

Bone pain is an inconsistent symptom, most often directed toward the weight-bearing bones; facial or jaw pain is uncommon. Patients with Paget's disease may also have ill-defined neurologic pain as the result of bone impingement on foramina and nerve canals. Patients with Paget's disease often have severely elevated levels of serum alkaline phosphatase (greater than with any other disorder) during osteo-

blastic phases of the disease. These patients also often have high levels of hydroxyproline in the urine.

### Radiographic Features
*Location.* Paget's disease occurs most often in the pelvis, femur, skull, and vertebrae and infrequently in the jaws (Fig. 24-28). It affects the maxilla about twice as often as the mandible. Whenever the jaws are involved, it is important to note that the entire mandible or maxilla is affected. Although this disease is bilateral, occasionally it affects only one maxilla or the involvement may be significantly greater on one side.

*Internal Structure.* Generally the appearance of the internal structure depends on the developmental stage of the disease. Paget's disease has three radiographic stages, although these often overlap in the clinical setting: an early radiolucent resorptive stage, a granular or ground glass–appearing second stage, and a denser, more radiopaque appositional late stage. These stages are less apparent in the jaws.

The trabeculae are altered in number and shape. Most often they increase in number, but in the early stage they may decrease. The trabeculae may be long and may align themselves in a linear pattern (Fig. 24-29), which is more common in the mandible. They also may be short, with random orientation, and may have a granular pattern similar to that of fibrous dysplasia. A third pattern occurs when the trabeculae may be organized into rounded, radiopaque patches of abnormal bone, creating a cotton-wool appearance (Fig. 24-30).

The overall density of the jaws may decrease or increase, depending on the number of trabeculae. Often the disease produces areas of bone that appear radiolucent (commonly the alveolar process) and regions of increased density in one bone.

*Effects on Surrounding Structures.* Paget's disease always enlarges an affected bone to some extent, even in the early stage. Often the bone enlargement is impressive. Prominent pagetoid skull bones may swell to three or four times their normal thickness. In enlarged jaws the outer cortex may be thinned but remains intact. The outer cortex may appear to be laminated in occlusal projections (see Fig. 24-29). When the maxilla is involved, the disease invariably involves the sinus floor. However, the air space usually is not diminished to a great extent. Cortical boundaries such as the sinus floor may be more granular and less apparent

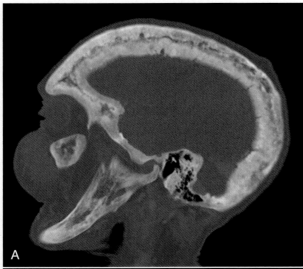

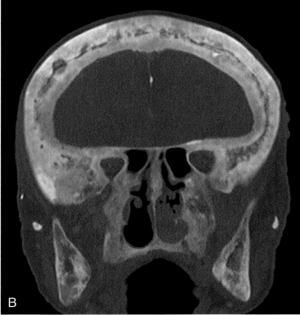

FIG. **24-28** **A,** Sagittal and, **B,** coronal bone algorithm CT images of a case of Paget's disease involving all the cranial bones and the maxilla and mandible; note the increase in bone density and dimension between the internal and outer cortex of the skull. The coronal CT image demonstrates enlargement of the mandibular ramus.

as sharp boundaries. The lamina dura may become less evident and may be altered into the abnormal bone pattern. Often hypercementosis develops on a few or most of the teeth in the involved jaw. This hypercementosis may be exuberant and irregular, which is characteristic of Paget's disease (Fig. 24-31). As previously mentioned, the teeth may become spaced or displaced in the enlarging jaw.

## Differential Diagnosis

Paget's disease may appear similar to fibrous dysplasia. However, Paget's disease occurs in an older age group and is almost always bilateral. In the maxilla, fibrous dysplasia has a tendency to encroach on the antral air space, whereas Paget's disease does not. The linear trabeculae and cotton-wool appearance of Paget's disease are distinctive. FOD may have a cotton-wool pattern, but these lesions are centered above the inferior alveolar nerve canal and most commonly have a radiolucent capsule. The changes seen in FOD do not affect all of the jaw, unlike with Paget's disease. The bone pattern in Paget's disease may show some similarities to the bone pattern in metabolic bone diseases, and both conditions may be bilateral. However, Paget's disease enlarges bone, and metabolic diseases do not.

The specific bone pattern changes, the late age of onset, the enlargement of the involved bone, and the extreme elevation of serum alkaline phosphatase aid in the differential diagnosis.

## Management

Currently Paget's disease usually is managed medically, with calcitonin, sodium etidronate, or lately bisphosophonates. Medication relieves pain and reduces the serum alkaline phosphatase levels and osteoclastic activity. Surgery may be required to correct deformities of the long bones and to treat fractures.

There are complications of this disease that are of concern. Extraction sites heal slowly. The incidence of jaw osteomyelitis is higher than for nonaffected individuals. Osteogenic sarcoma develops in about 10% of patients with polyostotic disease. Characteristics such as invasion and bone destruction, as described in Chapter 22, indicate the presence of a malignant neoplasm.

## Langerhans' Cell Histiocytosis

### Synonyms
Histiocytosis X, idiopathic histiocytosis, and Langerhans' cell disease

### Definition
The disorders included in the category of Langerhans' cell histiocytosis (LCH) are abnormalities that result from the abnormal proliferation of Langerhans' cells or their precursors. Langerhans' cells are specialized cells of the histiocytic cell line that normally are found in the skin. The abnormal proliferation of Langerhans' cells and eosinophils results in a spectrum of clinical diseases. Historically, histiocytosis X was classified into three distinct clinical forms: eosinophilic granuloma (solitary), Hand-Schüller-Christian disease (chronic disseminated), and Letterer-Siwe disease (acute disseminated).

A newly proposed LCH classification creates two categories: nonmalignant disorders, such as unifocal or multifocal eosinophilic granuloma, and malignant disorders, including Letterer-Siwe disease and variants of histiocytic lymphoma. Research has shown that all forms of LCH are clonal and therefore have a neoplastic nature.

### Clinical Features
Head and neck lesions are common at initial presentation, and approximately 10% of all patients with LCH have oral lesions. Often the oral changes are the first clinical signs of the disease.

Eosinophilic granuloma (EG) usually appears in the skeleton (ribs, pelvis, long bones, skull, and jaws) and in rare cases in soft tissue. This condition occurs most often in older children and young adults but may develop later in life. The lesions often form quickly and may cause a dull, steady pain. In the jaws the disease may cause bony swelling, a soft tissue mass, gingivitis, bleeding gingiva, pain, and ulceration. Loosening or sloughing of the teeth often occurs after destruction of alveolar bone by one or more foci of EG. The sockets of teeth lost to

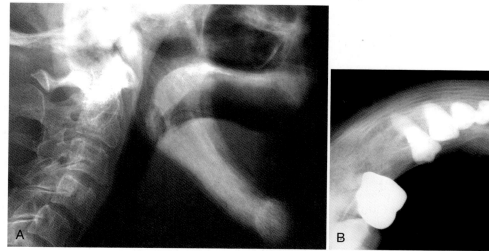

FIG. **24-29**  **A,** An edentulous mandible involved with Paget's disease. **B,** An occlusal film of another case; note the loss of normal outer cortex and the linear alignment of trabeculae. (**B** courtesy Dr. Ross Macdonald, Adelaide, Australia.)

FIG. **24-30**  **Paget's Disease. A,** Multiple radiopaque masses in the mandible that have a cotton-wool appearance. **B,** Note the expansion of the mandible and the maintenance of a thin outer cortical plate.

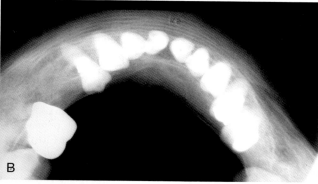

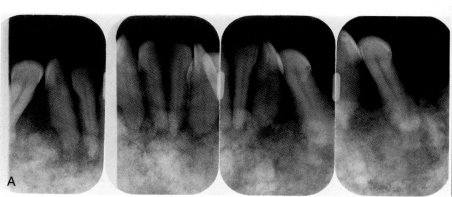

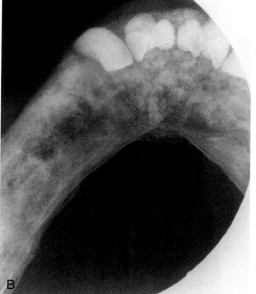

the disease generally do not heal normally. EG may have a single focus or may develop into a multifocal, aggressive disease. The disseminated form may involve multiple bone lesions, diabetes insipidus, and exophthalmos, a condition previously defined as Hand-Schüller-Christian disease.

Letterer-Siwe disease is a malignant form of LCH that most often occurs in infants less than 3 years of age. Soft tissue and bony granulomatous reactions disseminate throughout the body, and the condition is marked by intermittent fever, hepatosplenomegaly, anemia, lymphadenopathy, hemorrhage, and failure to thrive. Lesions in bone are rare. Death usually occurs within several weeks of the onset of the disease.

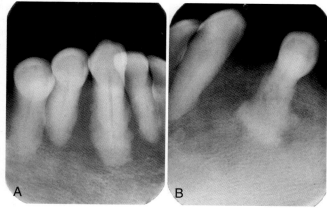

FIG. **24-31**  Two periapical films of Paget's disease showing exuberant irregular hypercementosis of the roots.

## Radiographic Features

For ease of discussion, this chapter divides LCH jaw lesions into two groups: those that occur in the alveolar process and intraosseous lesions that occur elsewhere in the jaws. The radiographic features of this condition generally are similar to those of malignant neoplasms.

*Location.* The alveolar type of LCH lesions are commonly multiple, whereas the intraosseous type usually is solitary. The mandible is a more common site than the maxilla, and the posterior regions are more involved than are the anterior regions (Fig. 24-32). The mandibular ramus is a common site of intraosseous lesions. Solitary lesions of the jaws may be accompanied by lesions in other bones.

*Periphery and Shape.* The periphery of EG lesions varies from moderately to well defined but without cortication; the periphery sometimes appears punched out (Fig. 24-33). The margins may be smooth or somewhat irregular. The alveolar lesions commonly start in the midroot region of the teeth. The bone destruction progresses in a circular shape, and after it includes a portion of the superior border of the alveolar process, it may give the impression that a section of the alveolar process has been scooped out (see Figs. 24-32 and 24-34). The shape of intraosseous lesions may be irregular, oval, or round.

*Internal Structure.* The internal structure usually is totally radiolucent.

*Effects on Surrounding Structures.* LCH destroys bone. In alveolar lesions the bone around teeth, including the lamina dura, is destroyed, and as a result the teeth appear to be standing in space. The lesion does not displace teeth, although teeth may move because they are bereft of bone support (Fig. 24-35). Only minor root resorption has been reported. Of note is the ability of these lesions to stimulate periosteal new bone formation; this occurs more commonly with the intraosseous type of lesion (Fig. 24-36). The periosteal new bone formation is indistinguishable from the appearance seen in inflammatory lesions of the jaws. This lesion can destroy the outer cortical plate and in rare cases it extends into the surrounding soft tissues on CT examination.

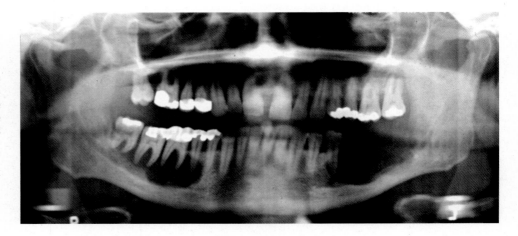

FIG. **24-32** A panoramic film of multiple lesions of Langerhans' cell histiocytosis. Note the scooped out shape of the bone destruction in the mandible. The floor of the right maxillary antrum has been destroyed.

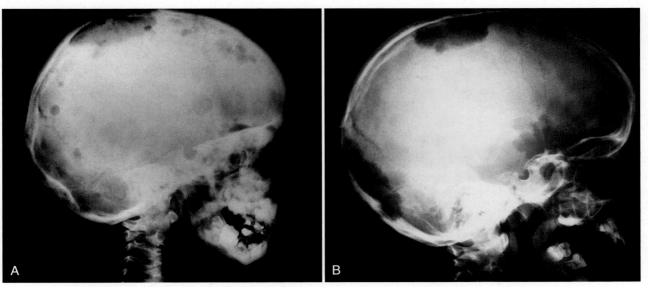

FIG. **24-33** Two lateral skull films of lesions of Langerhans' cell histiocytosis showing well-defined, punched-out lesions. (Courtesy Dr. H. G. Poyton, Toronto, Ontario.)

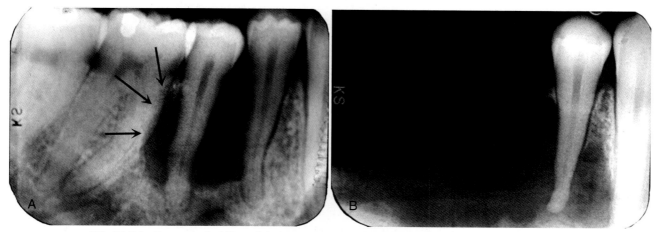

FIG. **24-34**  Two periapical films of the same area of the mandible taken approximately 1 year apart in a patient with Langerhans' cell histiocytosis. **A,** The earlier phase of the disease produces a scooped out shape *(arrows)* that shows that the epicenter of the lesion is in the midroot area of the involved teeth, unlike in periodontal disease. **B,** One year later, bone destruction is extensive, resulting in loss of teeth. (Courtesy Dr. D. Stoneman, Toronto, Ontario, Canada.)

FIG. **24-35**  A panoramic film showing the bone destruction that can occur with Langerhans' cell histiocytosis. The bone around many of the remaining mandibular teeth has been destroyed, leaving the teeth apparently unsupported. (Courtesy Dr. D. Stoneman, Toronto, Ontario, Canada.)

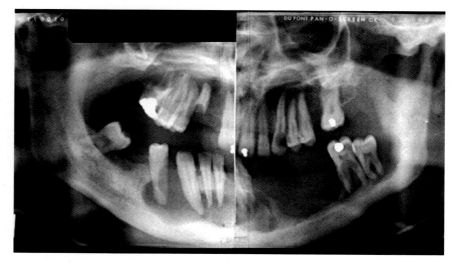

## Differential Diagnosis

The major differential diagnosis of alveolar type lesions is periodontal disease and squamous cell carcinoma. An important characteristic in differentiation of periodontal disease is the fact that the epicenter of the bone destruction in LCH is approximately in the midroot region, resulting in a scooped out appearance. In contrast, the bone destruction in periodontal disease starts at the alveolar crest and extends apically down the root surface. Differentiation of a squamous cell carcinoma may not be possible by radiographic characteristics alone, although the borders of an LCH lesion typically are better defined. Multiple lesions in a younger age group (usually in the first three decades) are more likely to be LCH than squamous cell carcinoma, which typically appears as a single lesion in middle or old age. LCH may bear a superficial resemblance to simple bone cysts, but the alveolar crest is maintained in simple bone cysts and a partial cortex may be present.

The differential diagnosis of solitary intraosseous lesions includes metastatic malignant neoplasia and malignant tumors from adjacent soft tissues. However, the well-defined borders and the periosteal reaction seen in histiocytosis help in the differential diagnosis.

Patients suspected of having LCH should be referred to an oral and maxillofacial radiologist for a complete workup; this may include nuclear imaging to detect other possible bone lesions. The radiologic workup should be followed by a biopsy. The histologic appearance of histiocytosis may be hidden by changes caused by secondary infection from the oral cavity in alveolar lesions. Therefore it is important to correlate the radiographic findings with the histologic appearance of the biopsy.

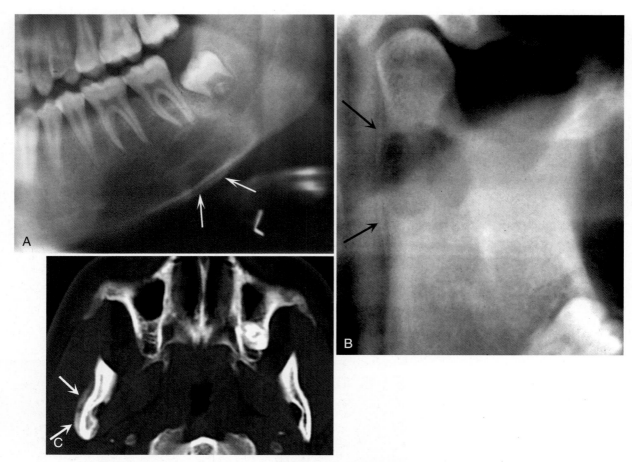

FIG. **24-36** Examples of Langerhans' cell histiocytosis with periosteal reaction. **A,** A large region of bone destruction in the body of the mandible with periosteal reaction along the inferior border *(arrows)*. **B,** A lesion in the condylar neck with a faint periosteal reaction along the posterior border of the ramus *(arrows)*. **C,** An axial CT scan of the lesion in **B** showing a periosteal reaction *(arrows)* that extends beyond the area of bone destruction.

## Management

Treatment of localized lesions usually consists of surgical curettage or limited radiation therapy. Surgical management of jaw lesions usually is preferable because it has a low recurrence rate. The earlier EG of the mandible is diagnosed and controlled, the fewer teeth are lost to bone destruction. Disseminated disease is treated with chemotherapy.

## SUGGESTED READINGS

### FIBROUS DYSPLASIA

Cohen MM, Howell RE: Etiology of fibrous dysplasia and McCune-Albright syndrome, *Int J Oral Maxillofac Surg* 28:366-371, 1999.

Ebata K, Usami T, Tohnai I et al: Chondrosarcoma and osteosarcoma arising in polyostotic fibrous dysplasia, *J Oral Maxillofac Surg* 50:761-764, 1992.

MacDonald-Jankowski DS, Yeung R, Li TK et al: Computed tomography of fibrous dysplasia, *Dentomaxillofac Radiol* 33:114-118, 2004.

Ozek C, Gundogan H, Bilkay U et al: Craniomaxillofacial fibrous dysplasia, *J Craniofac Surg* 13:382-389, 2002.

Petrikowski CG, Pharoah MJ, Lee L et al: Radiographic differentiation of osteogenic sarcoma, osteomyelitis and fibrous dysplasia of the jaws, *Oral Surg Oral Med Oral Pathol Oral Radiol Endod* 80:744-750, 1995.

Tokano H, Sugimoto T, Noguchi Y et al: Sequential computed tomography images demonstrating characteristic changes in fibrous dysplasia, *J Laryngol Otol* 115:757-759, 2001.

Waldron C, Giansanti J: Benign fibroosseous lesions of the jaws: a clinical-radiologic-histologic review of sixty-five cases, *Oral Surg Oral Med Oral Pathol* 35:190-201, 1973.

### PERIAPICAL CEMENTAL DYSPLASIA

Waldron C, Giansanti J: Benign fibro-osseous lesions of the jaws: a clinical-radiologic-histologic review of sixty-five cases, II: benign fibro-osseous lesions of periodontal ligament origin, *Oral Surg Oral Med Oral Pathol* 35:340-350, 1973.

### FLORID OSSEOUS DYSPLASIA

Loh FL, Yeo JF: Florid osseous dysplasia in Orientals, *Oral Surg Oral Med Oral Pathol* 68:748-753, 1989.

MacDonald-Jankowski DS: Florid cemento-osseous dysplasia: a systematic review, *Dentomaxillofac Radiol* 32:141-149, 2003.

Mahomed F, Altini M, Meer S et al: Cemento-osseous dysplasia with associated simple bone cysts, *J Oral Maxillofac Surg* 63:1549-1554, 2005.

Melrose RJ, Abrams AM, Mills BG: Florid osseous dysplasia: a clinical-pathologic study of 34 cases, *Oral Surg* 41:62-82, 1976.

Toffanin A, Bennett R, Manconi R: Familial florid cemento-osseous dysplasia: a case report, *J Oral Maxillofac Surg* 58:1440-1446, 2000.

## CEMENTOOSSIFYING FIBROMA

Eversole L, Merrell PW, Strub D: Radiographic characteristics of central ossifying fibroma, *Oral Surg* 59:522-527, 1985.

Sciubba JJ, Younai F: Ossifying fibroma of the mandible and maxilla: review of 18 cases, *J Oral Pathol Med* 18:315-321, 1989.

Williams HK, Mangham C, Speight PM: Juvenile ossifying fibroma: an analysis of eight cases and a comparison with other fibro-osseous lesions, *J Oral Pathol Med* 29:13-18, 2000.

## GIANT CELL GRANULOMA

De Lange J, Van den Akker HP: Clinical and radiological features of central giant-cell lesions of the jaw, *Oral Surg Oral Med Oral Pathol Oral Radiol Endod* 99:464-470, 2005.

Kaffe I, Ardekian L, Taicher S et al: Radiologic features of central giant cell granuloma of the jaws, *Oral Surg Oral Med Oral Pathol Oral Radiol Endod* 81:720-726, 1996.

Waldron CA, Shafer WG: The central giant cell reparative granuloma of the jaws. An analysis of 38 cases, *Am J Clin Pathol* 45:437-447, 1966.

## ANEURYSMAL BONE CYST

Buraczewski J, Dabska M: Pathogenesis of aneurysmal bone cyst. Relationship between the aneurysmal bone cyst and fibrous dysplasia of bone, *Cancer* 28:597-604, 1971.

Kaffe I, Naor H, Calderon S et al: Radiological and clinical features of aneurysmal bone cyst of the jaws, *Dentomaxillofac Radiol* 28:167-172, 1999.

Struthers P, Shear M: Aneurysmal bone cyst of the jaws, I: clinicopathological features, *Int J Oral Surg* 13:85-91, 1984.

Struthers P, Shear M: Aneurysmal bone cyst of the jaws, II: pathogenesis, *Int J Oral Surg* 13:92-100, 1984.

## CHERUBISM

Bianchi SD, Boccardi A, Mela F et al: The computed tomographic appearances of cherubism, *Skeletal Radiol* 16:6-10, 1987.

Hyckel P, Berndt A, Schleier P et al: Cherubism—new hypotheses on pathogenesis and therapeutic consequences, *J Craniomaxillofac Surg* 33:61-68, 2005.

Von Wowern N: Cherubism: a 36-year long-term follow-up of 2 generations in different families and review of the literature, *Oral Surg Oral Med Oral Pathol Oral Radiol Endod* 90:765-772, 2000.

## PAGET'S DISEASE

Rao VM, Karasick D: Hypercementosis—an important clue to Paget disease of the maxilla, *Skeletal Radiol* 9:126-128, 1982.

Reddy SV: Etiology of Paget's disease and osteoclast abnormalities, *J Cell Biochem* 93:688-696, 2004.

Sofaer J: Dental extractions in Paget's disease of bone, *Int J Oral Surg* 13:79-84, 1984.

Van Staa TP, Selby P, Leufkens FG et al: Incidence and natural history of Paget's disease in bone in England and Wales, *J Bone Miner Res* 17:465-471, 2002.

## LANGERHANS' CELL HISTIOCYTOSIS

Cline MJ: Histiocytes and histiocytosis, *Blood* 84:2840-2853, 1996.

Coppes-Zantinga A, Egeler RM: The Langerhans cell histiocystosis X files revealed, *Br J Haematol* 116:3-9, 2002.

Dagenais M, Pharoah MJ, Sikorski PA: The radiographic characteristics of histiocytosis X. A study of 29 cases that involve the jaws, *Oral Surg Oral Med Oral Pathol* 74:230-236, 1992.

Hicks J, Flaitz CM: Langerhans cell histiocytosis: current insights in a molecular age with emphasis on clinical oral and maxillofacial pathology practice, *Oral Surg Oral Med Oral Pathol Oral Radiol Endod* 100(2 suppl):S42-S66, 2005.

Wong GB, Pharoah MJ, Weinberg S et al: Eosinophilic granuloma of the mandibular condyle: report of three cases and review of the literature, *J Oral Maxillofac Surg* 55:870-878, 1997.

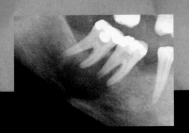
# Systemic Diseases Manifested in the Jaws

## Definition

Disorders of the endocrine system, bone metabolism, and other systemic diseases may have an effect on the form and function of bone and teeth. The function of bone not only includes support, protection, and an environment for hemopoiesis but also serves as a major reserve of calcium for the body. More than 99% of the total body calcium is contained within the skeletal structure. When the influence of systemic conditions on the jaws is considered, it is important to bear in mind that bone is constantly remodeling. Approximately 5% to 10% of the total bone mass is replaced each year. The turnover rate of trabecular bone is higher than for cortical bone; 20% of its mass is replaced per year compared with 5% for cortical bone. The effects of systemic diseases of bone are brought about by changes in the number and activity of osteoclasts, osteoblasts, and osteocytes.

## Radiographic Features

Because systemic disorders affect the entire body, the radiographic changes manifested in the jaws are generalized (Table 25-1). In most cases it is not possible to identify diseases on the basis of radiographic characteristics. The general changes include the following:
1. A change in size and shape of the bone
2. A change in the number, size, and orientation of trabeculae
3. Altered thickness and density of cortical structures
4. An increase or decrease in overall bone density
Changes in the first three elements can result in a decrease or increase in bone density.

Because many parameters in the production of a radiograph influence the density of the image, it may be difficult to detect genuine changes in the density of bone. Systemic conditions that result in a decrease in bone density do not affect mature teeth; therefore the image of the teeth may stand out with normal density against a generally radiolucent jaw. In severe cases the teeth may appear to be bereft of any bony support. Also, cortical structures appear thin, less defined, and occasionally disappear. On the other hand, a true increase in bone density may be detected by a loss of contrast of the inferior cortex of the mandible as the radiopacity of the cancellous bone approaches that of cortical bone. Often the inferior alveolar nerve canal appears more distinct in contrast to the surrounding dense bone.

Some systemic diseases that occur during tooth formation may result in dental alterations. Lamina dura is part of the bone structure of the alveolar process, but because it is usually examined in conjunction with the periodontal membrane space and roots of teeth, it is

included with the description of the dental structures (Table 25-2). Changes to teeth and associated structures include the following:
1. Accelerated or delayed eruption
2. Hypoplasia
3. Hypocalcification
4. Loss of a distinct lamina dura

Often bone and teeth exhibit no detectable radiographic changes associated with systemic diseases. However, on occasion the first symptoms of a disease may present as a dental problem.

## Endocrine Disorders

### HYPERPARATHYROIDISM

#### Definition

Hyperparathyroidism is an endocrine abnormality in which there is an excess of circulating parathyroid hormone (PTH). An excess of serum PTH increases bone remodeling in preference of osteoclastic resorption, which mobilizes calcium from the skeleton. In addition, PTH increases renal tubular reabsorption of calcium and renal production of the active vitamin D metabolite 1,25(OH)2D. The net result of these functions is in an increase in serum calcium levels.

Primary hyperparathyroidism usually results from a benign tumor (adenoma) of one of the four parathyroid glands, resulting in the production of excess PTH. An abnormality named hyperparathyroidism–jaw tumor syndrome, which involves tumors of parathyroid glands, jaws, and kidneys, has been shown to have genetic basis. Less frequently, individuals may have hyperplastic parathyroid glands that secrete excess PTH. The combination of hypercalcemia and an elevated serum level of PTH is diagnostic of primary hyperparathyroidism. The incidence of primary hyperparathyroidism is about 0.1%.

Secondary hyperparathyroidism results from a compensatory increase in the output of PTH in response to hypocalcemia. The underlying hypocalcemia may result from an inadequate dietary intake or poor intestinal absorption of vitamin D or from deficient metabolism of vitamin D in the liver or kidney. This condition produces clinical and radiographic effects similar to those of primary hyperparathyroidism.

#### Clinical Features

Women are two to three times more commonly affected than men by primary hyperparathyroidism. The condition occurs mainly in those 30 to 60 years of age. Clinical manifestations of the disease cover a broad range, but most patients have renal calculi, peptic ulcers,

## TABLE 25-1
## *Radiographic Changes in Bone Observed in Systemic Disease**

| SYSTEMIC DISEASE | DENSITY | SIZE OF JAWS | BONES TRABECULAE INCREASE | DECREASE | GRANULAR |
|---|---|---|---|---|---|
| Hyperparathyroidism | Decrease | No | Yes | Yes | Yes |
| Hypoparathyroidism | Rare increase | No | No | No | No |
| Hyperpituitarism | No | Large | No | No | No |
| Hypopituitarism | No | Small | No | No | No |
| Hypothyroidism | Decrease | No | No | No | No |
| Hyperthyroidism | No | Small | No | No | No |
| Cushing's syndrome | Decrease | No | No | Yes | Yes |
| Osteoporosis | Decrease | No | No | Yes | No |
| Rickets | Decrease | No | No | Yes | No |
| Osteomalacia | Rare decrease | No | No | Rare decrease | No |
| Hypophosphatasia | Decrease | No | No | Yes | No |
| Renal osteodystrophy | Decrease; rare increase | No | Rare | Yes | Yes |
| Hypophosphatemia | Decrease | No | No | Yes | Yes |

*This table summarizes the major radiographic changes to bone with endocrine and metabolic bone diseases. It does not include all the possible variable appearances.

## TABLE 25-2
## *Effects on Teeth and Associated Structures**

| SYSTEMIC DISEASE | HYPOCALCIFICATION | HYPOPLASIA | LARGE PULP CHAMBER | LOSS OF LAMINA DURA | LOSS OF TEETH | ERUPTION |
|---|---|---|---|---|---|---|
| Hyperparathyroidism | No | No | No | Yes | Rare | No |
| Hypoparathyroidism | No | Yes | No | No | No | Delayed |
| Hyperpituitarism | No | No | No | No | No | Supereruption |
| Hypopituitarism | No | No | No | No | No | Delayed |
| Hypothyroidism | No | No | No | No | Yes | Early |
| Hyperthyroidism | No | No | No | Thin | Yes | Delayed |
| Cushing's syndrome | No | No | No | Partial | No | Premature |
| Osteoporosis | No | No | No | Thin | No | No |
| Rickets | Yes, enamel | Yes, enamel | No | Thin | No | Delayed |
| Osteomalacia | No | No | No | No | No | No |
| Hypophosphatasia | Yes | Yes | Yes | Yes | Yes | No |
| Renal osteodystrophy | Yes | Yes | No | Yes | Yes | No |
| Hypophosphatemia | Yes | Yes | Yes | Yes | Yes | No |
| Osteopetrosis | No | Rare | No | No | No | delayed |

*This table summarizes the major radiographic changes that can occur to teeth and associated structures with endocrine and metabolic bone diseases. It does not include all the possible variable appearances.

psychiatric problems, or bone and joint pain. These clinical symptoms are mainly related to hypercalcemia. Gradual loosening, drifting, and loss of teeth may occur. Definite consistent hypercalcemia is virtually pathognomonic of primary hyperparathyroidism. (Rarely, multiple myeloma and metastatic tumors may produce the same serum alterations.) Because of daily fluctuations, the serum calcium level should be tested at different intervals. The serum alkaline phosphatase level, a reliable indicator of bone turnover, may also be elevated in hyperparathyroidism.

### Radiographic Features
Only about one in five patients with hyperparathyroidism has radiographically observable bone changes.

*General Radiographic Features.* The following are the major manifestations of hyperparathyroidism:

1. The earliest and most reliable changes of hyperparathyroidism are subtle erosions of bone from the subperiosteal surfaces of the phalanges of the hands.
2. Demineralization of the skeleton results in an unusual radiolucent appearance.
3. Osteitis fibrosa cystica are localized regions of bone loss produced by osteoclastic activity resulting in a loss of all apparent bone structure.
4. Brown tumors occur late in the disease and in about 10% of cases. These peripheral or central tumors of bone are radiolucent. The gross specimen has a brown or reddish-brown color.
5. Pathologic calcifications in soft tissues have a punctate or nodular appearance and occur in the kidneys and joints.

6. In prominent hyperparathyroidism, the entire calvarium has a granular appearance caused by the loss of central (diploic) trabeculae and thinning of the cortical tables (Fig. 25-1).

*Radiographic Features of the Jaws.* Demineralization and thinning of cortical boundaries often occur in the jaws in cortical boundaries such as the inferior border, mandibular canal, and the cortical outlines of the maxillary sinuses. The density of the jaws is decreased, resulting in a radiolucent appearance that contrasts with the density of the teeth. The teeth stand out in contrast to the radiolucent jaws (Fig. 25-2). A change in the normal trabecular pattern may occur, resulting in a ground-glass appearance of numerous, small, randomly oriented trabeculae.

Brown tumors of hyperparathyroidism may appear in any bone but are frequently found in the facial bones and jaws, particularly in long-standing cases of the disease. These lesions may be multiple within a single bone. They have variably defined margins and may produce cortical expansion. If solitary, the tumor may resemble a central giant cell granuloma or an aneurysmal bone cyst (Fig. 25-3). It is interesting to note that the histologic appearance of the brown tumor is identical to that of the giant cell granuloma. Therefore if a giant cell granuloma occurs later than the second decade, the patient should be screened for an increase in serum calcium, PTH, and alkaline phosphatase levels.

*Radiographic Features of the Teeth and Associated Structures.* Occasionally periapical radiographs reveal loss of the lamina dura in patients (only about 10%) with hyperparathyroidism. Depending on the duration and severity of the disease, loss of the lamina dura may occur around one tooth or all the remaining teeth

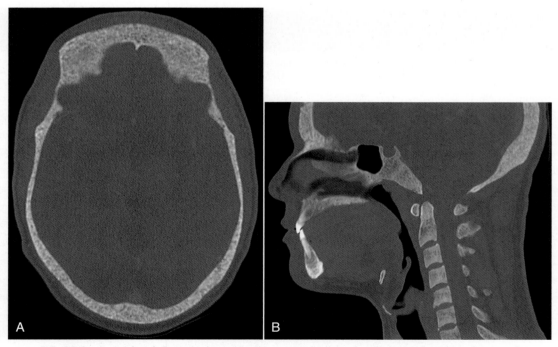

FIG. 25-1　**A,** Axial and, **B,** sagittal computed tomographic images with bone algorithm of a case of secondary hyperparathyroidism. Note the lack of normal cortical bone at the inner and outer tables of the skull, internal granular bone pattern, and generalized lack of defined outer cortical boundary of the osseous structures.

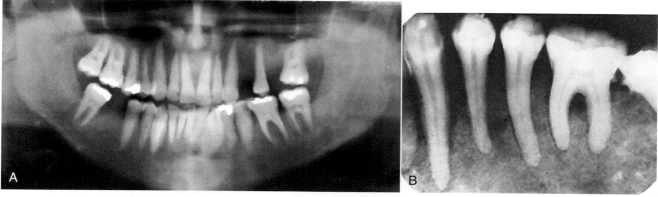

FIG. **25-2  A,** Panoramic image. The loss of bone in hyperparathyroidism results in the radiopaque teeth standing out in contrast to the radiolucent jaws. **B,** Note the loss of a distinct lamina dura and the granular texture of the bone pattern in this periapical film of a different case. (**B** courtesy H. G. Poyton, DDS, Toronto, Ontario, Canada.)

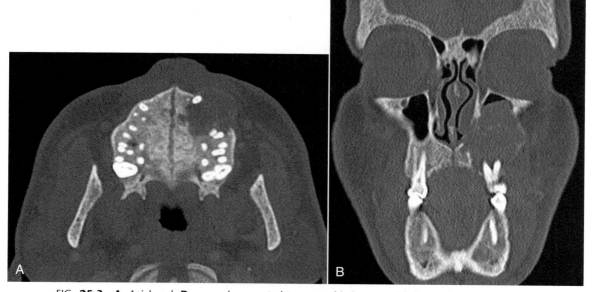

FIG. **25-3  A,** Axial and, **B,** coronal computed tomographic images with bone algorithm of a case of secondary hyperparathyroidism with a brown tumor involving the maxilla. This tumor has features of a central giant cell granuloma with a granular expanded cortex of the maxilla and very subtle and ill-defined internal septa.

(Fig. 25-4). The loss may be either complete or partial around a particular tooth. The result of lamina dura loss may give the root a tapered appearance because of loss of image contrast. Although PTH mobilizes minerals from the skeleton, mature teeth are immune to this systemic demineralizing process.

## Management

After successful surgical removal of the causative parathyroid adenoma, almost all radiographic changes revert to normal. The only exception may be the site of a brown tumor, which often heals with bone that is radiographically more sclerotic than normal. Many people with this disease are being diagnosed earlier, resulting in fewer severe cases.

## HYPOPARATHYROIDISM AND PSEUDOHYPOPARATHYROIDISM

### Definition

Hypoparathyroidism is an uncommon condition in which insufficient secretion of PTH occurs. Several causes exist, but the most common is damage or removal of the parathyroid glands during thyroid surgery. In pseudohypoparathyroidism there is a defect in the response of the tissue target cells to normal levels of PTH.

### Clinical Features

Both hypoparathyroidism and pseudohypoparathyroidism produce hypocalcemia, which has a variety of clinical manifestations. Most

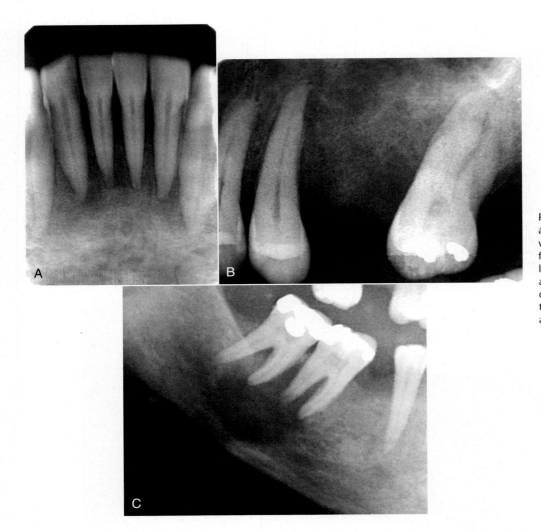

FIG. **25-4** Hyperparathyroidism. **A** and **B**, Granular bone pattern that was characteristic in all intraoral films. Note the loss of a distinct lamina dura and floor of the maxillary antrum. **C**, This view of the same case reveals a brown tumor related to the apical region of the second and third molars.

often this includes sharp flexion (tetany) of the wrist and ankle joints (carpopedal spasm). Some patients have sensory abnormalities consisting of paresthesia of the hands, feet, or the area around the mouth. Neurologic changes may include anxiety and depression, epilepsy, parkinsonism, and chorea. Chronic forms may produce a reduction in intellectual capacity. Some patients show no changes at all. Patients with pseudohypoparathyroidism often have early closure of certain bony epiphyses and thus manifest short stature or extremity disproportions.

### Radiographic Features

The principal radiographic change is calcification of the basal ganglia. On skull radiographs this calcification appears flocculent and paired within the cerebral hemispheres on the posteroanterior view. Radiographic examination of the jaws may reveal dental enamel hypoplasia, external root resorption, delayed eruption, or root dilaceration (Fig. 25-5).

### Treatment

These conditions are managed with orally administered supplemental calcium and vitamin D.

## HYPERPITUITARISM

### Synonyms

Acromegaly and giantism

### Definition

Hyperpituitarism results from hyperfunction of the anterior lobe of the pituitary gland, which increases the production of growth hormone. An excess of growth hormone causes overgrowth of all tissues in the body still capable of growth. The usual cause of this problem is a benign functioning tumor of the acidophilic cells in the anterior lobe of the pituitary gland.

### Clinical Features

Hyperpituitarism in children involves generalized overgrowth of most hard and soft tissues, a condition termed giantism. Active growth occurs in those bones in which the epiphyses have not united with the bone shafts. Throughout adolescence, generalized skeletal growth is excessive and may be prolonged. Those affected may ultimately attain heights of 7 to 8 feet or more, yet exhibit remarkably normal proportions. The eyes and other parts of the central nervous system do not

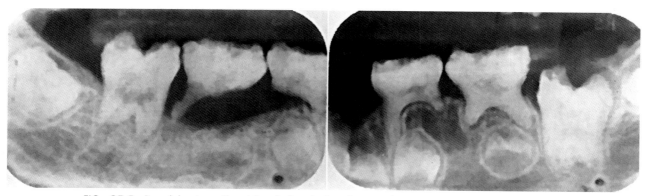

FIG. **25-5**  Pseudohypoparathyroidism-induced dental anomalies. (Courtesy Dr. S. Bricker, San Antonio, Tex.)

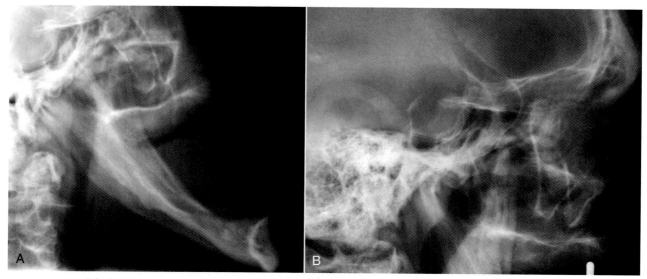

FIG. **25-6**  **A,** An example of acromegaly manifesting as excessive growth of the mandible, resulting in a class III skeletal relationship of the jaws. **B,** A portion of a lateral skull view of the same patient demonstrating enlargement of the sella turcica.

enlarge, except in rare cases in which the condition is manifested in infancy.

Adult hyperpituitarism, called acromegaly, has an insidious clinical course, quite different from the clinical profile seen in the childhood disease. In adults the clinical effects of a pituitary adenoma develop quite slowly because many types of tissues have lost the capacity for growth. This is true of much of the skeleton; however, an excess of growth hormone can stimulate the mandible and the phalanges of the hand. Mandibular condylar growth may be very prominent. Also, the supraorbital ridges and the underlying frontal sinus may be enlarged. Excess growth hormone in adults may also produce hypertrophy of some soft tissues. The lips, tongue, nose, and soft tissues of the hands and feet typically overgrow in adults with acromegaly, sometimes to a striking degree.

## Radiographic Features
*General Radiographic Features.* The pituitary tumor responsible for hyperpituitarism often produces enlargement ("ballooning")

of the sella turcica (Fig 25-6, *B*). It is important to note that in some examples the sella may not expand at all. Skull radiographs characteristically reveal enlargement of the paranasal sinuses (especially the frontal sinus). These air sinuses are more prominent in acromegaly than in pituitary giantism because sinus growth in giantism tends to be more in step with the generalized enlargement of the facial bones. Hyperpituitarism in adults also produces diffuse thickening of the outer table of the skull.

*Radiographic Features of the Jaws.* Hyperpituitarism causes enlargement of the jaws, most notably the mandible (Fig. 25-6, *A*). The increase in the length of the dental arches results in spacing of the teeth. In acromegaly the angle between the ramus and body of the mandible may increase. This, in combination with enlargement of the tongue (macroglossia), may result in anterior flaring of the teeth and the development of an anterior open bite. The sign of incisor flaring is a helpful point of differentiation between acromegalic prognathism and inherited prognathism. In acromegaly the most profound growth occurs in the condyle and ramus, often resulting in a class III skeletal relationship between the jaws. The thickness and height of the alveolar processes may also increase.

***Radiographic Changes Associated with the Teeth.*** The tooth crowns are usually normal in size, although the roots of posterior teeth often enlarge as a result of hypercementosis. This hypercementosis may be the result of functional and structural demands on teeth instead of a secondary hormonal effect. Supereruption of the posterior teeth may occur in an attempt to compensate for the growth of the mandible.

## HYPOPITUITARISM

### Definition
Hypopituitarism results from reduced secretion of pituitary hormones.

### Clinical Features
Individuals with this condition show dwarfism but have relatively well-proportioned bodies. One study reported a marked failure of development of the maxilla and the mandible. The dimensions of these bones in adults with this disorder were approximately those of normal children 5 to 7 years of age.

### Radiographic Features
Eruption of the primary dentition occurs at the normal time, but exfoliation is delayed by several years. The crowns of the permanent teeth form normally, but their eruption is delayed several years. The third molar buds may be completely absent. In hypopituitarism the jaws, especially the mandible, are small, which results in crowding and malocclusion.

### Treatment
Treatment is usually directed toward removal of the cause or replacement of the pituitary hormones or those of its target gland. The response of the dentition to treatment with growth hormone is variable but seems to parallel the skeletal response.

## HYPERTHYROIDISM

### Synonyms
Thyrotoxicosis and Graves' disease

### Definition
Hyperthyroidism is a syndrome that involves excessive production of thyroxin in the thyroid gland. This condition occurs most commonly with diffuse toxic goiter (Graves' disease) and less frequently with toxic nodular goiter or toxic adenoma, a benign tumor of the thyroid gland. Each of these conditions results in increased levels of circulating thyroxine. Excessive thyroxine causes a generalized increase in the metabolic rate of all body tissues, resulting in tachycardia, increased blood pressure, sensitivity to heat, and irritability. Hyperthyroidism is more common in females.

### Radiographic Features
Hyperthyroidism results in an advanced rate of dental development and early eruption, with premature loss of the primary teeth. Adults may show a generalized decrease in bone density or loss of some areas of edentulous alveolar bone.

## HYPOTHYROIDISM

### Synonyms
Myxedema and cretinism

### Definition
Hypothyroidism usually results from insufficient secretion of thyroxine by the thyroid glands despite the presence of thyroid-stimulating hormone.

### Clinical Features
In children, hypothyroidism may result in retarded mental and physical development. The base of the skull shows delayed ossification, and the paranasal sinuses only partially pneumatize. Dental development is delayed, and the primary teeth are slow to exfoliate.

Hypothyroidism in the adult results in myxedematous swelling but not the dental or skeletal changes seen in children. Adult symptoms may range from lethargy, poor memory, inability to concentrate, constipation, and cold intolerance to the more florid clinical picture of dull and expressionless face, periorbital edema, large tongue, sparse hair, and skin that feels "doughy" to the touch.

### Radiographic Features
Radiographic features in children include delayed closing of the epiphyses and skull sutures with the production of numerous wormian bones (accessory bones in the sutures). Effects on the teeth include delayed eruption, short roots, and thinning of the lamina dura. The maxilla and mandible are relatively small. Patients with adult hypothyroidism may show periodontal disease, loss of teeth, separation of teeth as a result of enlargement of the tongue, and external root resorption.

## DIABETES MELLITUS

### Definition
Diabetes mellitus is a metabolic disorder that has two primary forms. Type I, insulin-dependent diabetes mellitus (previously known as juvenile-onset diabetes), results from an absence or insufficiency of insulin, a hormone normally produced by the beta cells of the islets of Langerhans in the pancreas. Type II, non–insulin-dependent diabetes mellitus, results from insulin resistance. Patients with type I diabetes have virtually no β cells (in the islets), whereas patients with type II diabetes have approximately half the normal number. A shortage of insulin adversely affects carbohydrate metabolism. The principal clinical laboratory signs of the disease are hyperglycemia and glycosuria, both reflecting a complex biochemical imbalance between tissue demand for glucose and the release of this nutrient by the liver.

### Clinical Features
Untreated diabetes may manifest classic symptoms and signs such as polydipsia (excessive intake of fluids), polyuria (excessive urination), and, in more severe cases, acetone present in the urine and on the breath. This metabolic disorder, if not adequately treated, lowers the resistance of the body to infection. Diabetes may demonstrate a number of adverse effects in the oral cavity. Most prominently, uncontrolled diabetes acts as a continuing factor that predisposes to, aggravates, and accelerates periodontal disease. Patients with controlled diabetes do not appear to have more periodontal problems than do

persons without diabetes. Some children with uncontrolled diabetes have an increased likelihood of caries activity because of a high-carbohydrate diet. Another occasional oral complication of diabetes mellitus is xerostomia resulting from a reduced salivary flow (about one third of normal). Recently diabetes has been documented as a risk factor in the development of bisphosphonate-related osteonecrosis.

### Radiographic Features

Diabetes mellitus exhibits no characteristic radiographic features of the jaws or teeth. Periodontal disease associated with diabetes is indistinguishable radiographically from periodontal disease in patients without diabetes.

## CUSHING'S SYNDROME

### Definition

Cushing's syndrome arises from an excess of secretion of glucocorticoids by the adrenal glands. This may result from any of the following:

1. An adrenal adenoma
2. An adrenal carcinoma
3. Adrenal hyperplasia (usually bilateral)
4. A basophilic adenoma of the anterior lobe of the pituitary gland (Cushing's disease), producing excess adrenocorticotropic hormone
5. Medical therapy with exogenous corticosteroids

The increased level of glucocorticoid results in a loss of bone mass from reduced osteoblastic function and either directly or indirectly increased osteoclastic function.

### Clinical Features

Patients with Cushing's syndrome often show obesity (which spares the extremities), kyphosis of the thoracic spine ("buffalo hump"), weakness, hypertension, striae, or concurrent diabetes. This condition affects females three to five times as frequently as males. Onset may occur at any age but is usually seen in the third or fourth decade.

### Radiographic Features

The primary radiographic feature of Cushing's syndrome is generalized osteoporosis, which may have a granular bone pattern. This demineralization may result in pathologic fractures. The skull can show diffuse thinning accompanied by a mottled appearance. The teeth may erupt prematurely, and partial loss of the lamina dura may occur (Fig. 25-7).

## Metabolic Bone Diseases

## OSTEOPOROSIS

### Definition

Osteoporosis is a generalized decrease in bone mass in which the histologic appearance of bone is normal. An imbalance occurs in bone resorption and formation. Decrease in bone formation results in changes in trabecular architecture, the volume of trabecular bone, and the size and thickness of individual trabeculae.

Osteoporosis occurs with the aging process of bone and can be considered a variation of normal (primary osteoporosis). Bone mass normally increases from infancy to about 30 years of age. At this time there begins a gradual and progressive decline, occurring at the rate

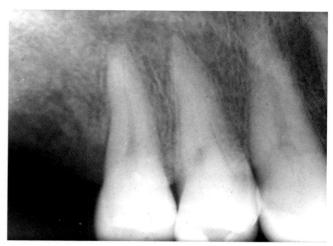

FIG. **25-7** Cushing's syndrome manifested in the jaws as thinning of the lamina dura. (Courtesy H. G. Poyton, DDS, Toronto, Ontario, Canada.)

of about 8% per decade in women and 3% per decade in men. The loss of bone mass with age is so gradual that it is virtually imperceptible until it reaches significant proportions.

Secondary osteoporosis may result from nutritional deficiencies, hormonal imbalance, inactivity, or corticosteroid or heparin therapy.

### Clinical Features

The most important clinical manifestation of osteoporosis is fracture. The most common locations are the distal radius, proximal femur, ribs, and vertebrae. Patients may have bone pain. The population most at risk is postmenopausal women.

### Radiographic Features

Osteoporosis results in an overall reduction in the density of bone. This reduction may be observed in the jaws by using the unaltered density of teeth as a comparison. There may be evidence of a reduced density and thinning of cortical boundaries such as the inferior mandibular cortex (Fig. 25-8). Reduction in the volume of cancellous bone is more difficult to assess, although new techniques to analyze the trabecular pattern in intraoral films are being developed. Reduction in the number of trabeculae is least evident in the alveolar process, possibly because of the constant stress applied to this region of bone by the teeth. On occasion the lamina dura may appear thinner than normal. In other regions of the mandible a reduction in the number of trabeculae may be evident. Accurate assessment of bone mass loss is difficult but may be done with sophisticated techniques such as dual-energy photon absorption or quantitative computed tomography programs.

### Treatment

The administration of estrogens and calcium and vitamin D supplements after menopause helps to reduce the rate of cortical and trabecular bone loss. Weight-bearing exercise programs are also effective (not swimming, for instance).

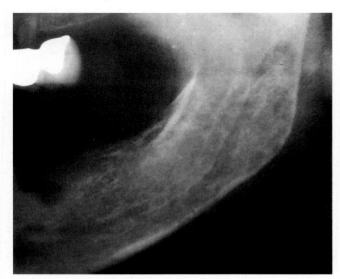

FIG. **25-8** Osteoporosis evident as a loss of the normal thickness and density of the inferior cortex of the mandible.

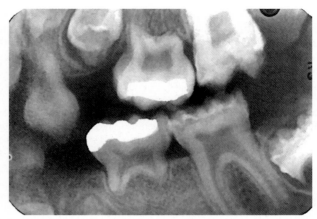

FIG. **25-9** Rickets may cause thinning (hypoplasia) or decreased mineralization (hypocalcification) of the enamel as seen in this bitewing view. (Courtesy H. G. Poyton, DDS, Toronto, Ontario, Canada.)

## RICKETS AND OSTEOMALACIA

### Definition

Rickets and osteomalacia result from inadequate serum and extracellular levels of calcium and phosphate, minerals required for the normal calcification of bone and teeth. Both abnormalities result from a defect in the normal activity of the metabolites of vitamin D, especially 1,25(OH)$_2$D, required for resorption of calcium in the intestine. Failure of normal mineralization is seen histologically as wide uncalcified osteoid (new bone matrix) seams. The term *rickets* is usually applied when the disease affects the growing skeleton in infants and children. The term *osteomalacia* is used when this disease affects the mature skeleton in adults.

Failure of normal activity of vitamin D may occur as a result of the following:
1. Lack of vitamin D in the diet
2. Lack of absorption of vitamin D resulting from various gastrointestinal malabsorption problems
3. Lack of metabolism of the active metabolite 1,25(OH)$_2$D, which is required for intestinal absorption of calcium

Interference may occur anywhere along the metabolic pathway for 1,25(OH)$_2$D:
1. Lack of exposure to ultraviolet light required for conversion of provitamin D$_3$
2. Lack of conversion of vitamin D$_3$ to 25(OH)D in the liver because of liver disease
3. Lack of metabolism of 25(OH)D$_2$ to 1,25(OH)$_2$D by the kidney because of kidney diseases
4. A defect in the intestinal target cell response to 1,25(OH)$_2$D or inadequate calcium supply

### Clinical Features

*Rickets.* In the first 6 months of life, tetany or convulsions are the most common clinical problems resulting from the hypocalcemia of rickets. Later in infancy the skeletal effects of the disease may be more clinically prominent. Craniotabes, a softening of the posterior of the parietal bones, may be the initial sign of the disease. The wrists and ankles typically swell. Children with rickets usually have short stature and deformity of the extremities. Development of the dentition is delayed, and the eruption rate of the teeth is retarded.

*Osteomalacia.* Most patients with osteomalacia have some degree of bone pain. The majority of patients with osteomalacia have muscle weakness of varying severity. Other clinical features include a peculiar waddling or "penguin" gait, tetany, and greenstick bone fractures.

### Radiographic Features

*General Radiographic Features.* In rickets the earliest and most prominent radiographic manifestation is a widening and fraying of the epiphyses of the long bones. The soft weight-bearing bones such as the femur and tibia undergo a characteristic bowing. Greenstick fractures (an incomplete fracture) occur in many patients with rickets.

In osteomalacia the cortex of bone may be thin. Pseudofractures, which are poorly calcified ribbonlike zones extending into bone at approximate right angles to the margin of the bone, may also be present. Pseudofractures occur most commonly in the ribs, pelvis, and weight-bearing bones and rarely in the mandible.

*Radiographic Features of the Jaws.* In rickets, jaw cortical structures such as the inferior mandibular border or the walls of the mandibular canal may thin. Changes in the jaws generally occur after changes in the ribs and long bones. Within the cancellous portion of the jaws, the trabeculae become reduced in density, number, and thickness. In severe cases, the jaws appear so radiolucent that the teeth appear to be bereft of bony support.

Most cases of osteomalacia produce no radiographic manifestations in the jaws. However, when radiographic manifestations are present, there may be an overall radiolucent appearance and sparse trabeculae.

*Radiographic Changes Associated with the Teeth.* Rickets in infancy or early childhood may result in hypoplasia of developing dental enamel (Fig. 25-9). If the disease occurs before the age of 3 years, such enamel hypoplasia is fairly common. Radiographs may reveal this early manifestation of rickets in unerupted and erupted teeth. Radiographs may also document retarded tooth eruption in early rickets. The lamina dura and the cortical boundary of tooth follicles may be thin or missing.

Osteomalacia does not alter the teeth because they are fully developed before the onset of the disease. The lamina dura may be especially thin in individuals with long-standing or severe osteomalacia.

## HYPOPHOSPHATASIA

### Definition

Hypophosphatasia is a rare inherited disorder that is caused by either a reduced production or a defective function of alkaline phosphatase. This enzyme is required for normal mineralization of osteoid. Patients have a low level of serum alkaline phosphatase activity and elevated urinary excretion of phosphoethanolamine. The usual pattern of inheritance is an autosomal dominant mode of disease transmission, although an autosomal recessive pattern exists.

### Clinical Features

The disease in individuals with homozygous involvement usually begins in utero, and affected patients often die within the first year. These infants demonstrate bowed limb bones and a marked deficiency of skull ossification. Individuals with heterozygous disease show the biochemical defects but a milder disease clinically. These children show poor growth, fractures, and deformities similar to those of rickets. A history may exist of fractures, delayed walking, or ricketslike deformities that heal spontaneously. About 85% of these children show premature loss of the primary teeth, particularly the incisors, and delayed eruption of the permanent dentition. This is often the first clinical sign of hypophosphatasia.

### Radiographic Features

*General Radiographic Features.* In young children with hypophosphatasia, the long bones show irregular defects in the epiphysis, and the skull is poorly calcified. In older children with premature closure of the skull sutures, multiple lucent areas of the calvarium may exist, called gyral or convolutional markings. These markings resemble hammered copper. The skull may assume a brachycephalic shape. A generalized reduction in bone density may occur in adults.

*Radiographic Features of the Jaws.* A generalized radiolucency of the mandible and maxilla is evident. The cortical bone and lamina dura are thin, and the alveolar bone is poorly calcified and may appear deficient.

*Radiographic Changes Associated with the Teeth.* Both primary and permanent teeth have a thin enamel layer and large pulp chambers and root canals (Fig. 25-10). The teeth may also be hypoplastic and may be lost prematurely.

## RENAL OSTEODYSTROPHY

### Synonym
Renal rickets

### Definition

In renal osteodystrophy, bone changes result from chronic renal failure. The kidney disease interferes with the hydroxylation of 25(OH)D into 1,25(OH)$_2$D, which normally occurs in the kidney. The vitamin D metabolite 1,25(OH)$_2$D is responsible for the active transport of calcium in the duodenum and upper jejunum. Affected patients often have hypocalcemia as a result of impaired calcium absorption and hyperphosphatemia resulting from reduction in renal phosphorus excretion. A prolonged low serum level of calcium stimulates the parathyroid glands to produce PTH. The result is a secondary hyperparathyroidism.

### Clinical Features

The clinical features of renal osteodystrophy are those of chronic renal failure. In children, growth retardation and frequent bone fractures may occur. Adults may have a gradual softening and bowing of the bones.

### Radiographic Features

*General Radiographic Features.* The radiographic features of renal osteodystrophy are quite variable. Some changes of the skeleton resemble those seen in rickets, and other changes are consistent with hyperparathyroidism, including generalized loss of bone density and thinning of bony cortices. Of interest is the occasional finding of an increase in bone density (Fig. 25-11). There may be brown tumors, similar to those seen in primary hyperthyroidism, but these are less frequent. Also, jaw enlargement has been reported in patients with renal disease who were treated with renal dialysis. The size increase is due to enlargement of the cancellous bone component that has a dense granular trabecular pattern.

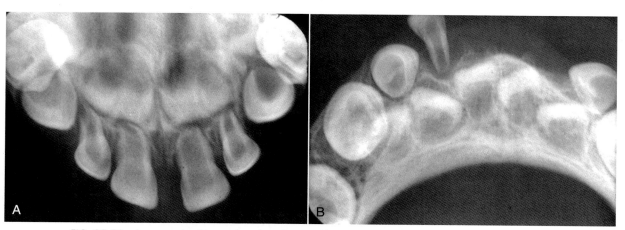

FIG. **25-10**  An example of hypophosphatasia; note the large pulp chambers in the deciduous dentition and the premature loss of the mandibular incisors. (Courtesy H. G. Poyton, DDS, Toronto, Ontario, Canada.)

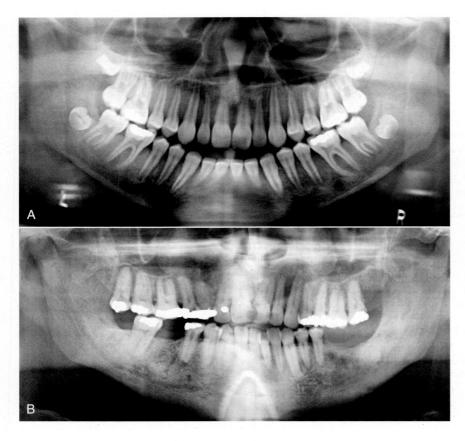

FIG. **25-11** Two cases of renal osteodystrophy. **A,** This panoramic image reveals areas of radiolucency corresponding to loss of bone mass, loss of distinct lamina dura, and a sclerotic bone pattern around the roots of the teeth. **B,** This panoramic image reveals a diffuse sclerotic (radiopaque) bone pattern throughout the jaws. Note the loss of a distinct inferior cortex of the mandible resulting from an increase in the radiopacity of the internal aspect of the bone.

*Radiographic Features of the Jaws.* In renal osteodystrophy the density of the mandible and maxilla may be less than normal and occasionally may be greater than normal. Manifestations include a decrease or an increase in the number of internal trabeculae, and the trabecular bone pattern may be granular. The cortical boundaries may be thinner or less apparent. It is important to note that these bone changes may persist after a successful renal transplant because of hyperplasia of the parathyroid glands, resulting in a continued elevation of PTH.

*Radiographic Changes Associated with the Teeth.* Hypoplasia and hypocalcification of the teeth are possible, sometimes resulting in loss of any radiographic evidence of enamel. The lamina dura may be absent or less apparent in instances of bone sclerosis.

## HYPOPHOSPHATEMIA

### Synonym

Vitamin D–resistant rickets and hypophosphatemic rickets

### Definition

Hypophosphatemia represents a group of inherited conditions that produce renal tubular disorders resulting in excessive loss of phosphorus. There is a failure to reabsorb phosphorus in the distal renal tubules, resulting in a decrease in serum phosphorus (hypophosphatemia). Normal calcification of the osseous structures requires the correct amount and ratio of serum calcium and phosphorus. Multiple

myeloma may induce hypophosphatemia as a result of secondary damage to the kidneys.

### Clinical Features

Children with hypophosphatemia show reduced growth and rickets-like bony changes. These include bowing of the legs, enlarged epiphyses, and skull changes. Adults have bone pain, muscle weakness, and vertebral fractures.

### Radiographic Features

*General Radiographic Features.* In children with hypophosphatemia, radiographic findings are indistinguishable from those of rickets. In adults the long bones may show persistent deformity, fractures, or pseudofractures.

*Radiographic Features of the Jaws.* The jaws are usually osteoporotic and in extreme cases are remarkably radiolucent. Cortical boundaries may be unusually radiolucent or not apparent (Fig. 25-12).

Other possibilities include fewer visible trabeculae and a granular trabecular pattern.

*Radiographic Features Associated with the Teeth.* The teeth may be poorly formed, with thin enamel caps and large pulp chambers and root canals (Fig. 25-12, *B* and *C*). In addition, periapical and periodontal abscesses occur frequently. The occurrence of periapical rarefying osteitis without an etiology may be a result of large pulp chambers and defects in the formation of dentin. This may allow for the ingress of oral microorganisms and subsequent pulp necrosis. If

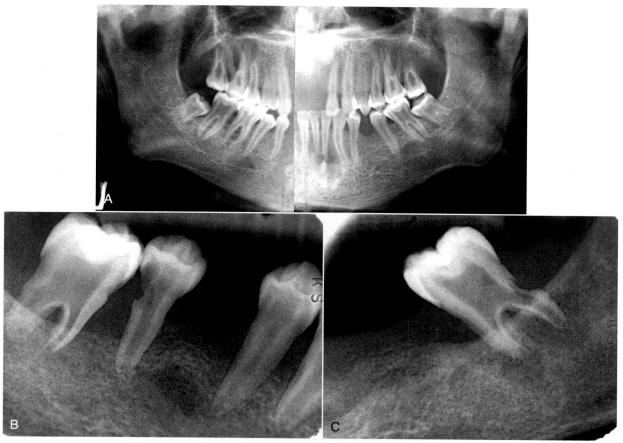

FIG. 25-12  **A,** A panoramic image of hypophosphatemia. Note the radiolucent appearance of the jaws and hence the lack of bone density and the large pulp chambers. **B** and **C,** These periapical films of a different case of hypophosphatemia demonstrate apparent bone loss around the teeth, a granular bone pattern, large pulp chambers, and external root resorption.

the disease is severe, the patient has premature loss of the teeth. The lamina dura may become sparse, and cortical boundaries around tooth crypts may be thin or entirely absent.

## OSTEOPETROSIS

### Synonyms
Albers-Schönberg and marble bone disease

### Definition
Osteopetrosis is a disorder of bone that results from a defect in the differentiation and function of osteoclasts. The lack of normally functioning osteoclasts results in abnormal formation of the primary skeleton and a generalized increase in bone mass. The failure of normal bone remodeling results in dense, fragile bones that are susceptible to fracture and infection. Obliteration of the marrow compromises hematopoiesis and compresses cranial nerves. This disorder is inherited as an autosomal recessive type (osteopetrosis congenita) and autosomal dominant type (osteopetrosis tarda).

### Clinical Features
The more severe, recessive form of osteopetrosis is seen in infants and young children, and the more benign, dominant form appears later. The severe form is invariably fatal early in life. The patient has progressive loss of the bone marrow and its cellular products and a severe increase in bone density. The narrowing of bony canals results in hydrocephalus, blindness, deafness, vestibular nerve dysfunction, and facial nerve paralysis. The benign dominant form is milder and may be entirely asymptomatic. It may be discovered any time from childhood into adulthood. The disease may be found as an incidental finding or appear as a pathologic fracture of a bone. In some of the more chronic cases, bone pain and cranial nerve palsies caused by neural compression may be clinical problems. Osteomyelitis may complicate this disease because of the relative lack of vascularity of the dense bone. This problem is more common in the mandible, whereas osteomyelitis is usually a result of dental or periodontal disease.

### Radiographic Features
*General Radiographic Features.* In the classic radiographic presentation of osteopetrosis, all bones show greatly increased density,

which is bilaterally symmetric. The increased density throughout the skeleton is homogeneous and diffuse (Fig. 25-13). The internal aspect of the involved bone may be so dense or radiopaque that the trabecular patterns of the medullary cavity may not be visible. The internal radiopacity also reduces the contrast between the outer cortical border and the cancellous portion of the bone. The entire bone may be mildly enlarged.

*Radiographic Features of the Jaws.* The increased radiopacity of the jaws may be so great that the radiographic image may fail to reveal any internal structure and even the roots of the teeth may not be apparent. The increased bone density and relatively poor vascularity results in a susceptibility of the mandible to osteomyelitis, usually from odontogenic inflammatory lesions (Fig. 25-14).

*Radiographic Features Associated with the Teeth.* Effects on teeth may include delayed eruption, early tooth loss, missing teeth, malformed roots and crowns, and teeth that are poorly calcified and prone to caries. The normal eruption pattern of the primary and secondary dentition may be delayed as a result of bone density or ankylosis. The lamina dura and cortical borders may appear thicker than normal.

### Differential Diagnosis

The differential diagnosis includes other sclerosing bone dysplasias such as sclerosteosis, infantile cortical hyperostosis, pyknodysostosis, craniometaphyseal dysplasia, diaphyseal dysplasia, melorheostosis, and osteopathia striata. Osteosclerosis from fluoride poisoning and secondary hyperparathyroidism from renal disease also may have a general sclerotic appearance.

### Treatment

Treatment of osteopetrosis consists of bone marrow transplants to attempt to stimulate the formation of functional osteoclasts and sys-

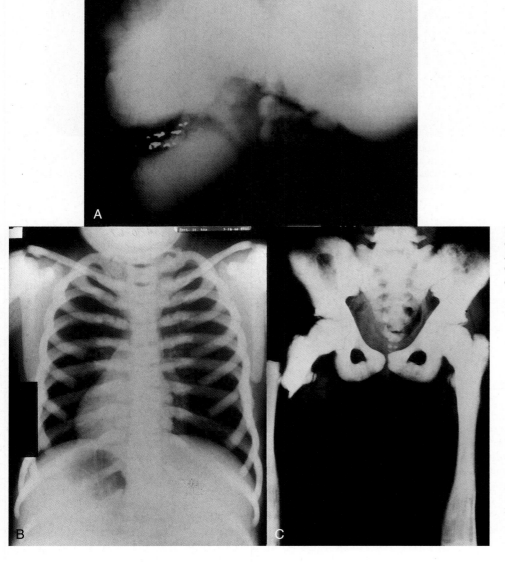

FIG. **25-13** Osteopetrosis, showing dense calcification of all the bones. **A,** Skull and facial bones. **B,** Chest. **C,** Pelvis and femurs (note the fracture of the proximal right femur).

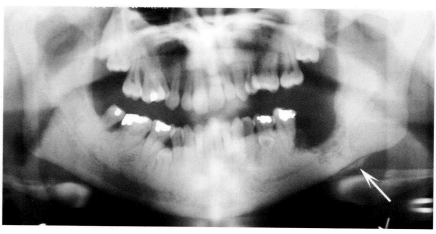

FIG. **25-14** A panoramic film of a patient with osteopetrosis; note the increased density of the jaws, lack of eruption of the mandibular second bicuspids, narrow inferior alveolar nerve canal, and development of osteomyelitis in the body of the left mandible with periostitis *(arrow)*.

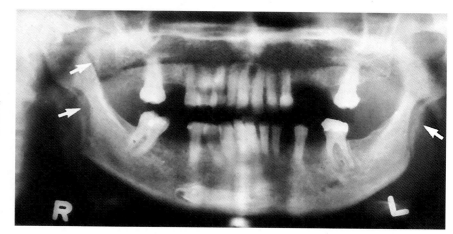

FIG. **25-15** Progressive systemic sclerosis demonstrating a loss of bone in the region of the angle of the mandible *(arrows)* and at the right coronoid process *(arrow)*, which are locations of muscle attachments.

temic steroids for the hematologic component. The osteomyelitis is difficult to treat, and a combination of antibiotics and hyperbaric oxygen therapy is used. It is imperative that affected patients avoid odontogenic inflammatory disease.

## Other Systemic Diseases
### PROGRESSIVE SYSTEMIC SCLEROSIS

#### Synonym
Scleroderma

#### Definition
Progressive systemic sclerosis (PSS) is a generalized connective tissue disease that causes excessive collagen deposition resulting in hardening (sclerosis) of the skin and other tissues. The involvement of the gastrointestinal tract, heart, lungs, and kidneys usually results in more serious complications. The cause of the disease is unknown.

#### Clinical Features
PSS is a disease of middle age, with the greatest incidence between the ages of 30 and 50 years. It is seen rarely in adolescence or in the elderly. Women are affected about three times as often as men.

In most patients with moderate to severe PSS, the involved skin has a thickened, leathery quality. The skin is not mobile over the underlying soft tissues, and involvement of the facial region may inhibit normal mandibular opening. Patients with diffuse disease are also likely to have xerostomia; increased numbers of decayed, missing, or filled teeth; and carious lesions. Further, patients with systemic disease are more likely to have deeper periodontal pockets and higher gingivitis scores. Patients with cardiac and pulmonary problems may have varying degrees of heart failure and respiratory insufficiencies. Renal involvement usually leads to some degree of uremia, with or without hypertension.

#### Radiographic Features
*Radiographic Features of the Jaws.* A radiographic feature in some cases of PSS is an unusual pattern of mandibular erosions at regions of muscle attachment such as the angles, coronoid process, digastric region, or condyles (Fig. 25-15). This type of resorption is typically bilateral and fairly symmetric. Most of these erosive borders are smooth and sharply defined. This resorption may be progressive with the disease.

*Radiographic Changes Associated with the Teeth.* The most common oral radiographic manifestation of PSS is an increase in the width of the periodontal ligament (PDL) spaces around the teeth (Fig.

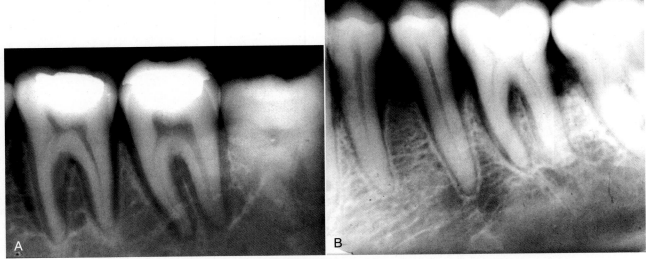

FIG. **25-16**  Two periapical films of two different patients with PSS; note the widening of the periodontal membrane space around some of the teeth.

25-16). Approximately two thirds of patients with PSS show this change. The PDL spaces affected by PSS usually are at least twice as thick as normal and both anterior and posterior teeth are affected, although it is more pronounced around the posterior teeth. The lamina dura remains normal. Despite the widening of the PDL spaces, the clinician finds that involved teeth are often not mobile and their gingival attachments are usually intact. Almost half the patients with PDL space thickening also have some mandibular erosive bone changes.

### Differential Diagnosis

Other causes of widening of the periodontal membrane space include tooth mobility, orthodontic tooth movement, intermaxillary fixation with arch bars, and invasion of the PDL by malignant neoplasms. Widening of the PDL space with malignant neoplasia differs in destruction of the lamina dura and irregular widening.

### Management

The aforementioned thickening of PDL spaces does not seem to present any clinical difficulties. The progressive loss of bone in the region of the mandibular angle, however, is more serious because of potential fracture. It is reasonable to obtain initial and periodic panoramic radiographs in all patients with PSS to assess mandibular integrity.

## SICKLE CELL ANEMIA

### Definition

Sickle cell anemia is an autosomal recessive, chronic hemolytic blood disorder. Patients with this disorder have abnormal hemoglobin (deoxygenated hemoglobins), which under low oxygen tension results in sickling of the red blood cells. These blood cells have a reduced capacity to carry oxygen to the tissues and, because of damage to their membrane lipids and proteins, adhere to vascular endothelium and obstruct capillaries. The spleen traps and readily destroys these abnormal red blood cells. The hematopoietic system responds to the resultant anemia by increasing the production of red blood cells, which requires compensatory hyperplasia of the bone marrow.

### Clinical Features

The homozygous form of sickle cell anemia occurs in approximately one in every 400 African-Americans. Although the gene is present in the heterozygous state in about 6% to 8% of African-Americans, those who manifest this form of the sickle cell trait do not show related clinical findings.

Although symptoms and signs vary considerably, most patients with the disease normally manifest mild, chronic features. Long quiet spells of hemolytic latency occur, occasionally punctuated by exacerbations known as sickle cell crises. During the crisis state, patients often have severe abdominal, muscle, and joint pain and a high temperature and may even undergo circulatory collapse. During milder periods the patient may complain of fatigability, weakness, shortness of breath, and muscle and joint pain. As in the other chronic anemias, the heart is usually enlarged and a murmur may be present. The disease occurs mostly in children and adolescents. It is compatible with a normal life span, although many patients die of complications of the disease before the age of 40 years.

### Radiographic Features

The hyperplasia of the bone marrow at the expense of cancellous bone is the primary reason for the radiographic manifestations of sickle cell anemia. The extent of bone changes in sickle cell anemia relates to the degree of this hyperplasia.

*General Radiographic Features.* The thinning of individual cancellous trabeculae and cortices is most common in the vertebral bodies, long bones, skull, and jaws. The skull may have widening of the diploic space and thinning of the inner and outer tables (Fig. 25-17). In extreme cases (5%) the outer table of the skull will not be apparent and a hair-on-end appearance may occur. Small areas of infarction may be present within bones after blockage of the microvasculature; these are seen radiographically as areas of localized bone sclerosis.

Osteomyelitis may complicate sickle cell anemia if infection begins in an area of pronounced hypovascularity. There may also be retardation of generalized bone growth.

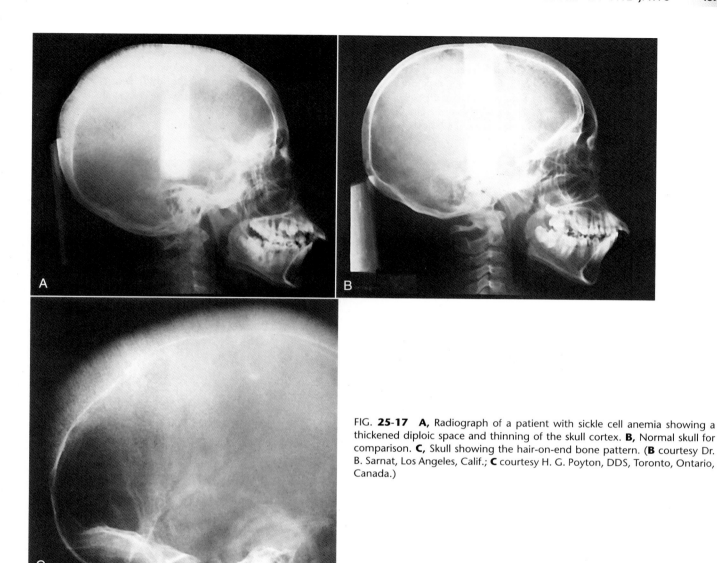

FIG. **25-17  A,** Radiograph of a patient with sickle cell anemia showing a thickened diploic space and thinning of the skull cortex. **B,** Normal skull for comparison. **C,** Skull showing the hair-on-end bone pattern. (**B** courtesy Dr. B. Sarnat, Los Angeles, Calif.; **C** courtesy H. G. Poyton, DDS, Toronto, Ontario, Canada.)

***Radiographic Features of the Jaws.*** The radiographic manifestations of sickle cell anemia in the jaws include general osteoporosis. This occurs because of a decrease in the volume of trabecular bone and, to a lesser extent, thinning of the cortical plates. In most cases the change is mild or moderate, with extreme radiographic manifestations being unusual. The bone pattern may be altered to one with fewer but coarser trabeculae. Radiographs of the jaws of children with sickle cell anemia have been reported to show a high frequency of severe osteoporosis. Rarely, bone marrow hyperplasia may cause enlargement and protrusion of the maxillary alveolar ridge.

## THALASSEMIA

### Synonyms
Cooley's anemia, Mediterranean anemia, and erythroblastic anemia

### Definition
Thalassemia is a hereditary disorder that results in a defect in hemoglobin synthesis. This defect may involve either the a α- or β-globulin genes. The resultant red blood cells have reduced hemoglobin content, are thin, and have a shortened life span. The heterozygous form of the disease (thalassemia minor) is mild. The homozygous form (thalassemia major) may be severe. A less severe form, thalassemia intermedia, also occurs.

### Clinical Features
In the severe form of the disease, the onset is in infancy and the survival time may be short. The face develops prominent cheekbones and a protrusive premaxilla, resulting in a "rodentlike" face. The milder form of the disease occurs in adults.

## Radiographic Features

*General Radiographic Features.* Similar to sickle cell anemia, the radiographic features of thalassemia generally result from hyperplasia of the ineffective bone marrow and its subsequent failure to produce normal red blood cells. However, these changes are usually more severe than with other anemias. There is a generalized radiolucency of the long bones with cortical thinning. In the skull the diploic space exhibits marked thickening, especially in the frontal region. The skull shows a generalized granular appearance (Fig. 25-18), and occasionally a hair-on-end effect may develop.

*Radiographic Appearance of the Jaws.* Severe bone marrow hyperplasia prevents pneumatization of the paranasal sinuses, especially the maxillary sinus, and causes an expansion of the maxilla that results in malocclusion (Fig. 25-19, *A*). The jaws appear radiolucent,

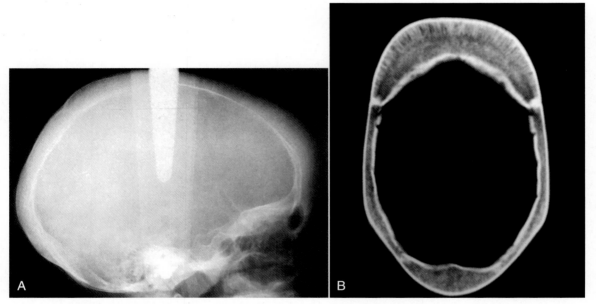

FIG. **25-18** **A,** A skull radiograph of a patient with thalassemia showing a granular appearance of the skull and thickening of the diploic space. **B,** An axial CT image of the skull of a patient with thalassemia; note the thickened diploic space and that there is hint linear orientation of the trabeculae, especially in the frontal bone. (**A** courtesy H. G. Poyton, DDS, Toronto, Ontario, Canada.)

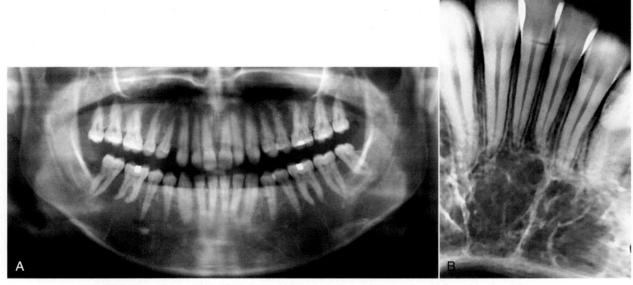

FIG. **25-19** **A,** A panoramic film of a patient with thalassemia; note the thickened body of the mandible and the sparse trabeculae and lack of maxillary antra. **B,** Radiograph of a different patient with thalassemia with thick trabeculae and large bone marrow spaces. (Courtesy H. G. Poyton, DDS, Toronto, Ontario, Canada.)

with thinning of the cortical borders and enlargement of the marrow spaces. The trabeculae are large and coarse (Fig. 25-19, *B*). The lamina dura is thin, and the roots of the teeth may be short.

# SUGGESTED READINGS

Adler C: *Bone diseases: macroscopic, histological and radiological diagnosis of structural changes in the skeleton*, Berlin, 2000, Springer-Verlag.
Paterson CR: *Metabolic disorders of bone*, Oxford, 1974, Blackwell Scientific.
Trapnell DH, Boweman JE: *Dental manifestation of systemic disease*, London, 1973, Butterworth.

## DIABETES MELLITUS

Collin HL, Niskanen L, Uusitupa M et al: Oral symptoms and signs in elderly patients with type 2 diabetes mellitus. A focus on diabetic neuropathy, *Oral Surg Oral Med Oral Pathol Oral Radiol Endod* 90:299-305, 2000.
Lamey PJ, Darwazeh AM, Frier BM: Oral disorders associated with diabetes mellitus, *Diabetes Med* 9:410-416, 1992.
Murrah VA: Diabetes mellitus and associated oral manifestations: a review, *J Oral Pathol* 14:271-281, 1985.

## HYPERPARATHYROIDISM

Aldred MJ, Talacko AA, Savarirayan R et al: Dental findings in a family with hyperparathyroidism-jaw tumor syndrome and a novel HRPT2 gene mutation, *Oral Surg Oral Med Oral Pathol Oral Radiol Endod* 101:212-218, 2006.
Bilezikian JP: Hyper- and hypoparathyroidism. In Rakel R, editor: *Conn's current therapy*, Philadelphia, 1985, WB Saunders.
Daniels JM: Primary hyperparathryroidism presenting as a palatal brown tumor, *Oral Surg Oral Med Oral Pathol Oral Radiol Endod* 98:409-413, 2004.
Rosenberg EH, Guralnick W: Hyperparathyroidism: a review of 220 proved cases with special emphasis on findings in the jaws, *Oral Surg Oral Med Oral Pathol* 15(2 Suppl):84-94, 1962.

## HYPOPARATHYROIDISM

Frensilli J, Stoner R, Hinrichs E: Dental changes of idiopathic hypoparathyroidism: report of three cases, *J Oral Surg* 29:727-731, 1971.
Glynne A, Hunter I, Thomson J: Pseudohypoparathyroidism with paradoxical increase in hypocalcemic seizures due to long-term anticonvulsant therapy, *Postgrad Med J* 48:632, 1972.

## HYPOPHOSPHATASIA

Eastman JR, Bixler D: Clinical, laboratory, and genetic investigations of hypophosphatasia: support for autosomal dominant inheritance with homozygous lethality, *J Craniofac Genet Dev Biol* 3:213-234, 1983.
Jedrychowski JR, Duperon D: Childhood hypophosphatasia with oral manifestations, *J Oral Med* 34:18-22, 1979.
Macfarlane JD, Swart JGN: Dental aspects of hypophosphatasia: a case report, family study, and literature review, *Oral Surg Oral Med Oral Pathol* 67:521-526, 1989.

## HYPOPITUITARISM

Conley H, Steflik DE, Singh B et al: Clinical and histologic findings of the dentition in a hypopituitary patient: report of case, *ASDC J Dent Child* 57:376-379, 1990.
Edler RJ: Dental and skeletal ages in hypopituitary patients, *J Dent Res* 56:1145-1153, 1977.
Kosowicz J, Rzymski K: Abnormalities of tooth development in pituitary dwarfism, *Oral Surg Oral Med Oral Pathol* 44:853-863, 1977.
Myllarniemi S, Lenko HL, Perheentupa J: Dental maturity in hypopituitarism, and dental response to substitution treatment, *Scand J Dent Res* 86:307-312, 1978.

## OSTEOPOROSIS

Lee BD, White SC: Age and trabecular features of alveolar bone associated with osteoporosis, *Oral Surg Oral Med Oral Pathol Oral Radiol Endod* 100:92-98, 2005.
Mohammad AR, Alder M, McNally MA: A pilot study of panoramic film density at selected sites in the mandible to predict osteoporosis, *Int J Prosthodont* 9:290-294, 1996.
Taguchi A, Suei Y, Ohtsuka M et al: Usefulness of panoramic radiography in the diagnosis of postmenopausal osteoporosis in women: width and morphology of inferior cortex of the mandible, *Dentomaxillofac Radiol* 25:263-267, 1996.
White SC: Oral radiographic predictors of osteoporosis, *Dentomaxillofac Radiol* 31:84-92, 2002.

## OSTEOPETROSIS

Barry CP, Ryan CD, Stassen LF: Osteomyelitis of the maxilla secondary to osteopetrosis: a report of 2 cases in sisters, *J Oral Maxillofac Surg* 65:144-147, 2007.
Ruprecht A, Wagner H, Engel H: Osteopetrosis: report of a case and discussion of the differential diagnosis, *Oral Surg Oral Med Oral Pathol* 66:674-679, 1988.
Waguespack SG, Hui SL, Dimeglio LA et al: Autosomal dominant osteopetrosis: clinical severity and natural history of 94 subjects with a chloride channel 7 gene mutation, *J Clin Endocrinol Metab* 92:771-778, 2007.
Younai F, Eisenbud L, Sciubba JJ: Osteopetrosis: a case report including gross and microscopic findings in the mandible at autopsy, *Oral Surg Oral Med Oral Pathol* 65:214-221, 1988.

## PROGRESSIVE SYSTEMIC SCLEROSIS

Alexandridis C, White SC: Periodontal ligament changes in patients with progressive systemic sclerosis, *Oral Surg Oral Med Oral Pathol* 58:113-118, 1984.
Auluck A, Pai KM, Shetty C et al: Mandibular resorption in progressive systemic sclerosis: a report of three cases, *Dentomaxillofac Radiol* 34:384-386, 2005.
Rout PG, Hamburger J, Potts AJ: Orofacial radiological manifestations of systemic sclerosis, *Dentomaxillofac Radiol* 25:193-196, 1996.
Wood RE, Lee P: Analysis of the oral manifestations of systemic sclerosis (scleroderma), *Oral Surg Oral Med Oral Pathol* 65:172-178, 1988.

## RENAL OSTEODYSTROPHY

Damm DD, Neville BW, McKenna S et al: Macrognathia of renal osteodystrophy in dialysis patients, *Oral Surg Oral Med Oral Pathol Oral Radiol Endod* 83:489-495, 1997.
Hata T, Irei I, Tanaka K et al: Macrognathia secondary to dialysis-related renal osteodystrophy treated successfully by parathyroidectomy, *Int J Oral Maxillofac Surg* 35:378-382, 2006.
Proctor R, Kumar N, Stein A et al: Oral and dental aspects of chronic renal failure, *J Dent Res* 84:199-208, 2005.
Scutellari PN, Orzincolo C, Bedani PL et al: Radiographic manifestations in teeth and jaws in chronic kidney insufficiency, *Radiol Med (Torino)* 92:415-420, 1996.

## RICKETS

Harris R, Sullivan HR: Dental sequelae in deciduous dentition in vitamin-D resistant rickets: case report, *Aust Dent J* 5:200-203, 1960.
Marks SC, Lindahl RL, Bawden JW: Dental and cephalometric findings in vitamin D resistant rickets, *J Dent Child* 32:259, 1965.

## SICKLE CELL ANEMIA

Brown DL, Sebes JI: Sickle cell gnathopathy: radiologic assessment, *Oral Surg Oral Med Oral Pathol* 61:653-656, 1986.

Ejindu VC, Hine AL, Mashayeckhi M et al: Musculoskeletal manifestations of sickle cell disease. *Radiographics* 27:1005-1021, 2007.

Lawrenz DR: Sickle cell disease: a review and update of current therapy. *J Oral Maxillofac Surg* 57:171-178, 1999.

Sears RS, Nazif MM, Zullo T: The effects of sickle-cell disease on dental and skeletal maturation, *ASDC J Dent Child* 48:275-277, 1981.

White SC, Cohen JM, Mourshed FA: Digital analysis of trabecular pattern in jaws of patients with sickle cell anemia, *Dentomaxillofac Radiol* 29: 119-124, 2000.

## THALASSEMIA

Hazza'a AM, Al-Jamal G: Radiographic features of the jaws and teeth in thalassaemia major, *Dentomaxillofac Radiol* 35:283-288, 2006.

Poyton HG, Davey KW: Thalassemia: changes visible in radiographs used in dentistry, *Oral Surg Oral Med Oral Pathol* 25:564-576, 1968.

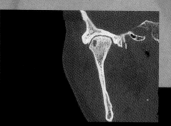

# CHAPTER 26

# Diagnostic Imaging of the Temporomandibular Joint

C. Grace Petrikowski

Disorders of the temporomandibular joint are abnormalities that interfere with the normal form or function of the joint. These disorders include dysfunction of the articular disk and associated ligaments and muscles, joint arthritides, inflammatory lesions, neoplasms, and growth or developmental abnormalities.

## Clinical Features

Temporomandibular joint (TMJ) dysfunction is the most common jaw disorder, with 28% to 86% of adults and adolescents showing one or more clinical signs or symptoms. A higher incidence of the disorder has been reported in females, although the reason for this preponderance is not clear. Signs and symptoms of dysfunction may include one or more of the following: pain in the TMJ or ear or both, headache, muscle tenderness, joint stiffness, clicking or other joint noises, reduced range of motion, locking, and subluxation. In most cases the clinical signs and symptoms are transitory, and treatment is not indicated. A small group of patients (5%) has severe dysfunction (e.g., severe pain, marked functional impairment, or both), which requires a thorough diagnostic workup, including diagnostic imaging, before treatment is begun.

The clinical signs and symptoms of other disorders of the TMJ may include swelling in and around the joint, an elevated temperature, and redness of the overlying skin.

## Application of Diagnostic Imaging

TMJ imaging may be necessary to supplement information obtained from the clinical examination, particularly when an osseous abnormality or infection is suspected, conservative treatment has failed, or symptoms are worsening. Diagnostic imaging also should be considered for patients with a history of trauma, significant dysfunction, alteration in range of motion, sensory or motor abnormalities, or significant changes in occlusion. TMJ imaging is not indicated for joint sounds if other signs or symptoms are absent or for asymptomatic children and adolescents before orthodontic treatment. The purposes of TMJ imaging are to evaluate the integrity and relationships of the hard and soft tissues, confirm the extent or stage of progression of known disease, and evaluate the effects of treatment. The clinician must correlate the radiographic information with the patient's history and clinical findings to arrive at a final diagnosis and plan the management of the underlying disease process.

## Radiographic Anatomy of the Temporomandibular Joint

A thorough understanding of the anatomy and morphology of the TMJ is essential so that a normal variant is not mistaken for an abnormality. The TMJs are unique in that, although they constitute two separate joints anatomically, they function together as a single unit. Each condyle articulates with the mandibular fossa of the temporal bone. A disk composed of fibrocartilage is interposed between the condyle and mandibular fossa. A fibrous capsule lined with synovial membrane surrounds and encloses the joint. Ligaments and muscles restrict or allow movement of the condyle.

### CONDYLE

The condyle is a bony ellipsoid structure connected to the mandibular ramus by a narrow neck (Fig. 26-1). The condyle is approximately 20 mm long mediolaterally and 8 to 10 mm thick anteroposteriorly. The shape of the condyle varies considerably; the superior aspect may be flattened, rounded, or markedly convex, whereas the mediolateral contour usually is slightly convex. These variations in shape may cause difficulty with radiographic interpretation; this underlines the importance of understanding the range of normal appearance. The extreme aspects of the condyle are called the medial pole and lateral pole. The long axis of the condyle is slightly rotated on the condylar neck so that the medial pole is angled posteriorly, forming an angle of 15 to 33 degrees with the sagittal plane. The two condylar axes typically intersect near the anterior border of the foramen magnum in the axial or horizontal plane of the skull.

Most condyles have a pronounced ridge oriented mediolaterally on the anterior surface, marking the anteroinferior limit of the articulating area. This ridge is the upper limit of the pterygoid fovea, a small depression on the anterior surface at the junction of the condyle and neck. It is the attachment site of the superior head of the lateral pterygoid muscle and should not be mistaken for an osteophyte (spur), which indicates degenerative joint disease.

Although the mandibular and temporal components of the TMJ are calcified by 6 months of age, complete calcification of cortical borders may not be completed until 20 years of age. As a result, radiographs of condyles in children may show little or no evidence of a cortical border. In the absence of disease, the cortical borders in adults

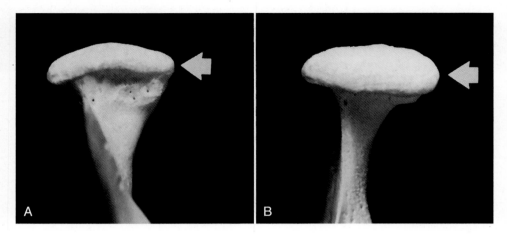

FIG. **26-1 Mandibular Condyle.** The medial pole *(arrow)* is on the right in each case. **A,** Anterior aspect. **B,** Superior aspect.

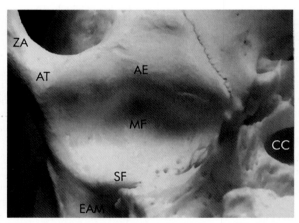

FIG. **26-2** Basal view of the skull showing the mandibular fossa. *AE,* Articular eminence; *AT,* articular tubercle; *CC,* carotid canal; *EAM,* external auditory meatus; *MF,* mandibular fossa; *SF,* squamotympanic fissure; *ZA,* zygomatic arch.

are visible radiographically. A layer of fibrocartilage covers the condyle but is not visible radiographically.

## MANDIBULAR FOSSA

The glenoid (mandibular) fossa, located at the inferior aspect of the squamous part of the temporal bone, is composed of the glenoid fossa and articular eminence of the temporal bone (Fig. 26-2). It is sometimes described as the temporal component of the TMJ. The articular eminence forms the anterior limit of the glenoid fossa and is convex in shape. Its most inferior aspect is called the summit or apex of the eminence. In a normal TMJ, the roof of the fossa, the posterior slope of the articular eminence, and the eminence itself form an S shape when viewed in the sagittal plane. The most lateral aspect of the eminence consists of a protuberance, called the articular tubercle, which is a ligamentous attachment. The squamotympanic fissure and its medial extension, the petrotympanic fissure, form the posterior limit of the fossa. The middle portion of the roof of the fossa forms a small portion of the floor of the middle cranial fossa, and only a thin layer of cortical bone separates the joint cavity from the intracranial sub-

dural space. The spine of the sphenoid forms the medial limit of the fossa. Fossa depth varies, and the development of the articular eminence relies on functional stimulus from the condyle. For example, the mandibular fossa is very flat and underdeveloped in patients with micrognathia or condylar agenesis. The fossa and articular eminence develop during the first 3 years and reach mature shape by the age of 4 years; young infants lack a definite fossa and articular eminence (Fig. 26-3).

All aspects of the temporal component may be pneumatized with small air cells derived from the mastoid air cell complex (see Fig. 26-3, *E*). Pneumatization of the articular eminence is seen radiographically in approximately 2% of patients. Like the condyle, the mandibular fossa is covered with a thin layer of fibrocartilage.

## INTERARTICULAR DISK

The interarticular disk (meniscus), composed of fibrous connective tissue, is located between the condylar head and mandibular fossa. The disk divides the joint cavity into two compartments, called the inferior (lower) and superior (upper) joint spaces, which are located below and above the disk, respectively (Fig. 26-4). A normal disk has a biconcave shape with a thick anterior band, thicker posterior band, and a thin middle part. The disk also is thicker medially than laterally. The medial and lateral margins of the disk blend with the capsule. The thin central portion normally serves as an articulating cushion between the condyle and articular eminence. The anterior band is thought to be attached to the superior head of the lateral pterygoid muscle, and the posterior band attaches to the posterior retrodiskal tissues (also called the posterior attachment). The junction between the posterior band and posterior attachment usually lies within 10 degrees of vertical above the condylar head. The disk and posterior attachment are collectively called the soft tissue components of the TMJ.

During mandibular opening, as the condyle rotates and translates downward and forward, the disk also moves forward and rotates so that its thin central portion remains between the articulating convexities of the condylar head and articular eminence. At maximum opening, the condyle is usually positioned beneath the anterior band of the disk. Laterally and medially the disk attaches to the condylar poles, helping to ensure passive movement of the disk with the condyle so that the condyle and disk translate forward together to the summit of the articular eminence. As the mandible opens, the condyle also

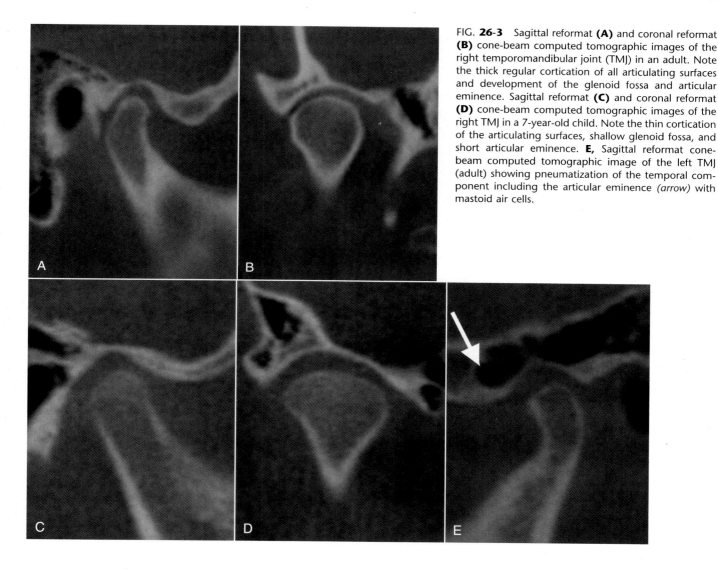

FIG. **26-3** Sagittal reformat **(A)** and coronal reformat **(B)** cone-beam computed tomographic images of the right temporomandibular joint (TMJ) in an adult. Note the thick regular cortication of all articulating surfaces and development of the glenoid fossa and articular eminence. Sagittal reformat **(C)** and coronal reformat **(D)** cone-beam computed tomographic images of the right TMJ in a 7-year-old child. Note the thin cortication of the articulating surfaces, shallow glenoid fossa, and short articular eminence. **E,** Sagittal reformat cone-beam computed tomographic image of the left TMJ (adult) showing pneumatization of the temporal component including the articular eminence *(arrow)* with mastoid air cells.

rotates against the lower surface of the disk in the inferior joint space. On mandibular closing, this process reverses, with the disk moving back with the condyle into the mandibular fossa.

## POSTERIOR ATTACHMENT (RETRODISKAL TISSUES)

The posterior attachment consists of a bilaminar zone of vascularized and innervated loose fibroelastic tissue. The superior lamina, which is rich in elastin, inserts into the posterior wall of the mandibular fossa. The superior lamina stretches and allows the disk to move forward with condylar translation. The inferior lamina attaches to the posterior surface of the condyle. The posterior attachment is covered with a synovial membrane that secretes synovial fluid, which lubricates the joint. As the condyle moves forward, tissues of the posterior attachment expand in volume, primarily as a result of venous distention, and as the disk moves forward, tension is produced in the elastic posterior attachment. This tension is thought to be responsible for the smooth recoil of the disk posteriorly as the mandible closes.

## TEMPOROMANDIBULAR JOINT BONY RELATIONSHIPS

Radiographic joint space is a general term used to describe the radiolucent area between the condyle and temporal component (see Fig. 26-4). This general term should not be confused with the terms superior joint space and inferior joint space described earlier, which refer to soft tissue spaces above and below the disk. The radiographic joint space contains the soft tissue components of the joint. The left and right condylar positions within the fossa can be determined and compared by the dimensions of the radiographic joint space viewed on corrected lateral images. A condyle is positioned concentrically when the anterior and posterior aspects of the radiolucent joint space are uniform in width. The condyle is retruded when the posterior joint space width is less than the anterior and protruded when the posterior joint space is wider than the anterior. However, because the radiographic outline of the glenoid fossa and the condyle do not match like a smooth ball-and-socket

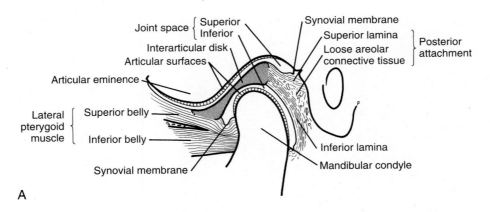

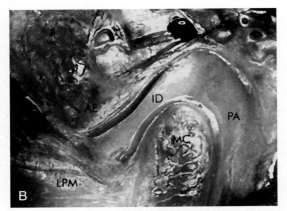

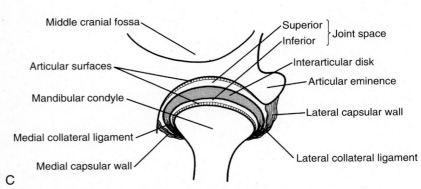

FIG. **26-4**   Temporomandibular Joint Anatomy. **A,** Lateral view. **B,** Sectioned cadaver specimen in the same orientation. *AE,* Articular eminence; *ID,* interarticular disk; *LPM,* lateral pterygoid muscle; *MC,* mandibular condyle; *PA,* posterior attachment. **C,** Coronal view. (Courtesy Dr. W.K. Solberg, Los Angeles, Calif.)

joint, the joint space often varies from medial to lateral aspects of the joint (Fig. 26-5).

The diagnostic significance of mild or moderate condylar eccentricity is not clear; condylar eccentricity is seen in one third to one half of asymptomatic individuals and is not a reliable indicator of the soft tissue status of the joint, particularly because the shape of the condylar head is not concentric to the shape of the fossa. Markedly eccentric condylar positioning usually represents an abnormality. For example, inferior condylar positioning (widened joint space) may be seen in cases involving fluid or blood within the joint, and superior condylar positioning (decreased joint space or no joint space, with osseous contact of joint components) may indicate loss, displacement, or perforation of intracapsular soft tissue components. Marked posterior condylar positioning is seen in some cases of disk displacement, and marked anterior condylar positioning may be seen in juvenile rheumatoid arthritis.

## CONDYLAR MOVEMENT

The condyle undergoes complex movement during mandibular opening. Downward and forward translation (sliding) of the condyle occurs where the superior surface of the disk slides against the articular eminence; at the same time a hingelike, rotatory movement occurs with the superior surface of the condyle against the inferior surface of the disk. The extent of normal condylar translation varies consider-

ably. In most individuals, at maximal opening the condyle moves down and forward to the summit of the articular eminence or slightly anterior to it (see Fig. 26-5). The condyle typically is found within a range of 2 to 5 mm posterior and 5 to 8 mm anterior to the crest of the eminence. Reduced condylar translation, in which the condyle has little or no downward and forward movement and does not leave the mandibular fossa, is seen in patients who clinically have a reduced degree of mouth opening. Hypermobility of the joint may be suspected if the condyle translates more than 5 mm anterior to the eminence. This may permit anterior locking or dislocation of the condyle if a superior movement also occurs above and anterior to the summit of the articular eminence.

## Diagnostic Imaging of the Temporomandibular Joint

The type of imaging technique selected depends on the specific clinical problem, whether imaging of hard or soft tissues is desired, the amount of diagnostic information available from a particular imaging modality, the cost of the examination, and the radiation dose. Both joints should be imaged during the examination, for comparison. When selecting the imaging modality the strengths and weakness of each imaging modality should be considered. The following not only outlines the imaging modalities that can be applied but also the best modalities for displaying osseous or soft tissue structures.

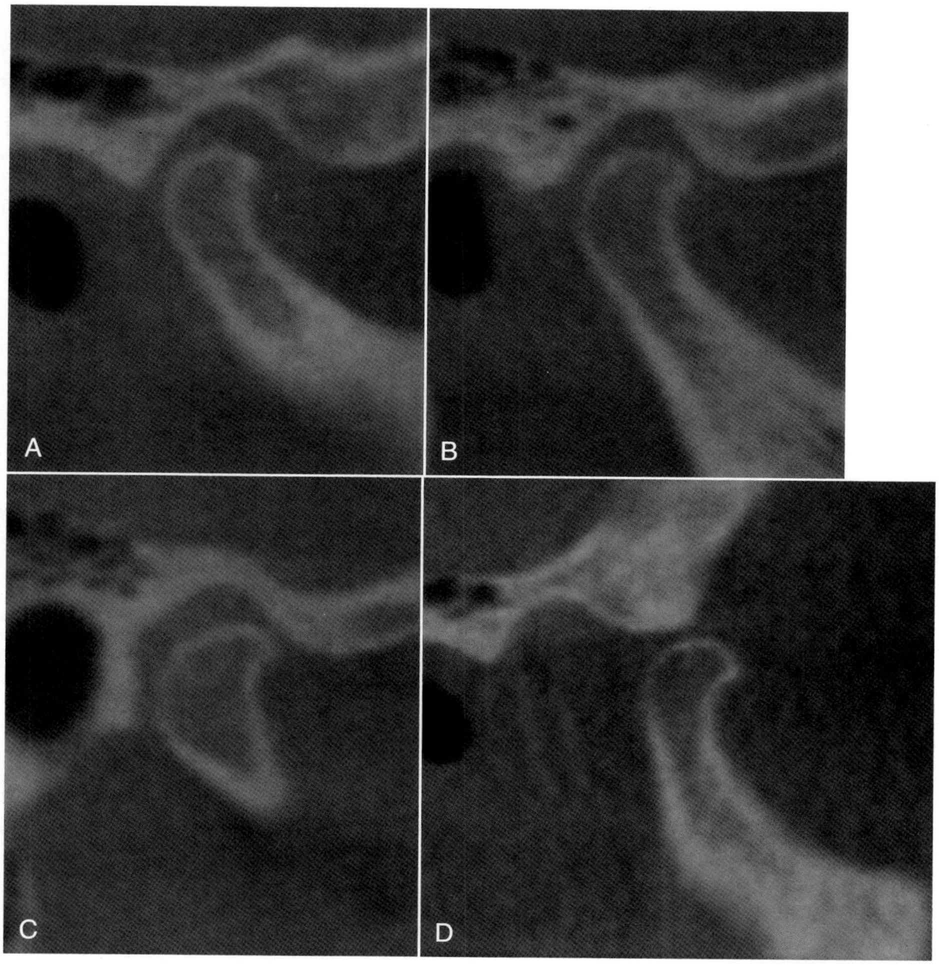

FIG. **26-5** **Sagittal Reformat Cone-Beam Computed Tomographic Image. A to C,** Closed position. **A,** Lateral image slice. **B,** Central image slice. **C,** Medial image slice of the same joint. Notice that the condyle appears retruded in the lateral slice, centered in the central slice, and anteriorly positioned in the medial slice. **D,** Open view showing the degree of condyle translation during mandibular opening.

## OSSEOUS STRUCTURES

### Panoramic Projection

The panoramic projection is often included as part of the examination because it provides an overall view of the teeth and jaws, provides a means of comparing left and right sides of the mandible, and serves as a screening projection to identify odontogenic diseases and other disorders that may be the source of TMJ symptoms. Some panoramic machines have specific TMJ programs, but these are of limited usefulness because of thick image layers and the oblique, distorted view of the joint they provide, which severely limits image quality. Gross osseous changes in the condyles may be identified, such as asymmetries, extensive erosions, large osteophytes, tumors or fractures (Fig. 26-6). However, no information about condylar position or function is provided because the mandible is partly opened and protruded when this radiograph is exposed. Also, mild osseous changes may be obscured, and only marked changes in articular eminence morphology can be seen as a result of superimposition by the skull base and zygomatic arch. For these reasons, the panoramic view should not be used as the sole imaging modality and should be supplemented.

### Plain Film Imaging Modalities

Plain films, usually consisting of a combination of transcranial, transpharyngeal (Parma), transorbital, and submentovertex (basal) projections allow visualization of the TMJs in various planes (Fig. 26-7). Transcranial and transpharyngeal projections provide lateral views. The transcranial view is taken in the closed and open mouth positions and depicts the lateral aspect of the TMJ, whereas the transpharyngeal projection is taken in the mouth open position only and depicts the medial aspect of the condyle. The transorbital projection is taken in the open or protruded position and depicts the entire medial-lateral aspect of the condyle in the frontal plane and is very useful in detecting condylar neck fractures. A submentovertex projection provides a view of the skull base and condyles in the horizontal plane; it is often used to determine the angulation of the long axes of the condylar heads for corrected tomography. These imaging techniques are gradually being replaced with more advanced imaging such as cone-beam computed tomography (CT).

### Conventional Tomography

Tomography is a radiographic technique that produces multiple thin image slices, permitting visualization of the osseous structures

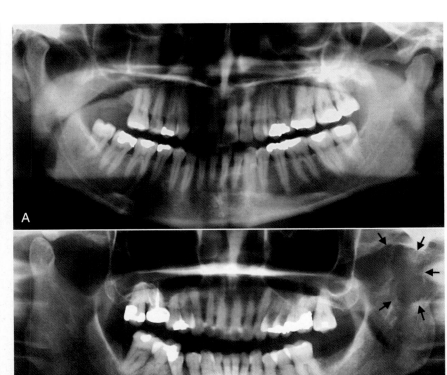

FIG. **26-6** Panoramic images that revealed right condylar hyperplasia **(A)** and destruction of the condyle by a malignant tumor **(B)** *(arrows).*

essentially free of superimpositions of overlapping structures (see Chapter 14). This technique can provide multiple image slices at right angles through the joint, depicting true condylar position and revealing osseous changes. Conventional tomography is gradually being replaced by cone-beam CT (CBCT) as the imaging technique of choice for assessing the osseous structures of the TMJ. Tomographs typically are exposed in the sagittal (lateral) plane, corrected to the condylar long axis, with several image slices in the closed (maximal intercuspation) position and usually only one image in the maximal open position. It is desirable to supplement the sagittal images with coronal (frontal) tomographs (Fig. 26-8), particularly when morphologic abnormalities or erosive changes of the condylar head are suspected. The entire condylar head is visible in the mediolateral plane.

### Computed Tomography

CT provides more information about the three-dimensional shape and internal structure of the osseous components of the joint by providing detailed image slices and three-dimensional images. There are two CT devices available, conventional CT (sometimes referred to as medical CT, see Chapter 14) and CBCT. Both modalities can give excellent images of the osseous structures, but only conventional CT provides images of the surrounding soft tissues; however, this is only required in a minimal number of specific situations. CBCT has the advantage of reduced patient dose compared with medical CT and is likely to replace conventional tomography. In CBCT the patient is usually scanned in the closed position and low-resolution scans can be done in the open or other positions (see Chapter 13). Data from

the axial slices can be manipulated to produce (reformat) corrected lateral and frontal images of the TMJs (see Fig. 26-3). Panoramic and three-dimensional reformatted images also can be produced. These are useful for assessing osseous deformities of the jaws or surrounding structures. Conventional and CBCT cannot produce accurate images of the articular disk.

CT is also useful for determining the presence and extent of ankylosis and neoplasms and the degree of bone involvement in some arthritides, for imaging complex fractures, and for evaluating complications from the use of polytetrafluoroethylene or silicon sheet implants, such as erosions into the middle cranial fossa and heterotopic bone growth.

### SOFT TISSUE STRUCTURES

Soft tissue imaging is indicated when TMJ pain and dysfunction are present and when the clinical findings suggest disk displacement along with symptoms that are unresponsive to conservative therapy. Imaging should be prescribed only when the anticipated results are expected to influence the treatment plan. Historically, arthrography was the first imaging modality used to image the soft tissues of the joint.

Arthrography is a technique in which an indirect image of the disk is obtained by injecting a radiopaque contrast agent into the joint spaces under fluoroscopic guidance. Magnetic resonance imaging (MRI) has replaced arthrography and is now the imaging technique of choice for the soft tissues of the TMJ. MRI can not only display the articular disk but also the surrounding soft tissue structures and also

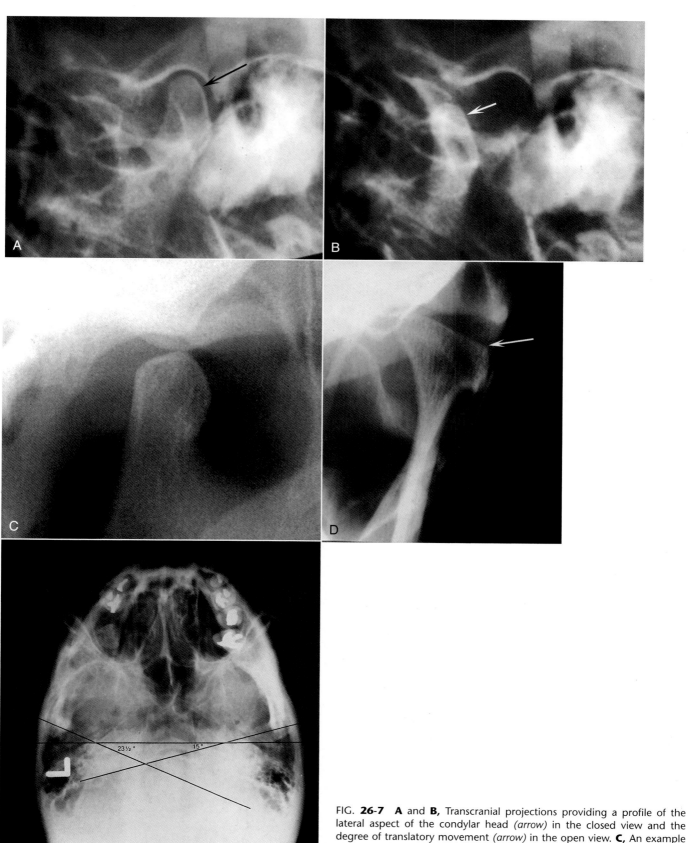

FIG. **26-7** **A** and **B,** Transcranial projections providing a profile of the lateral aspect of the condylar head *(arrow)* in the closed view and the degree of translatory movement *(arrow)* in the open view. **C,** An example of a transpharyngeal projection showing a medial profile of the condyle. **D,** An example of a transorbital projection showing a frontal view of the condyle. The lateral pole is indicated with an *arrow.* This submentovertex projection **(E)** shows the measurement of the angle of the long axis of the condylar heads used for tomography.

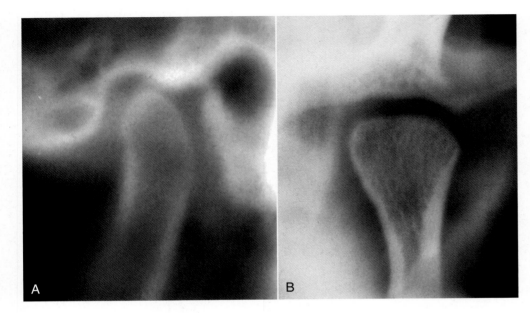

FIG. **26-8 A,** Sagittal tomograph through the mid region of the joint. **B,** Frontal tomographic image of the mandibular condyle.

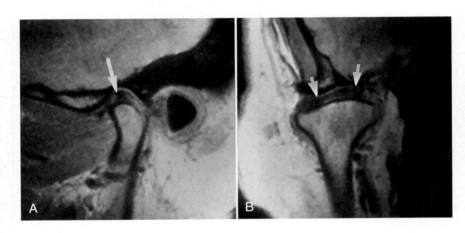

FIG. **26-9 MRI of a Normal Temporomandibular Joint. A,** Closed sagittal view showing the condyle and temporal component. The biconcave disk is located with its posterior band *(arrow)* over the condyle. **B,** Closed coronal view showing the osseous components and disk *(arrows)* superior to the condyle. (Courtesy Dr. Per-Lennart Westesson, Rochester, N.Y.)

can reveal the presence of joint effusion. MRI displays the osseous structures of the TMJ but not in the comparable detail seen in CT imaging. The technique is noninvasive and does not use ionizing radiation.

### Magnetic Resonance Imaging

MRI uses a magnetic field and radiofrequency pulses rather than ionizing radiation to produce multiple digital image slices (see Chapter 14). Because MRI can provide superb images of soft tissues, this technique can be used for imaging the articular disk. MRI allows construction of images in the sagittal and coronal planes without repositioning the patient (Fig. 26-9). These images usually are acquired in open and closed mandibular positions with use of surface coils to improve image resolution. Sagittal slices should be oriented perpendicular to the condylar long axis. The examinations usually are performed with use of T1-weighted, proton-weighted, or T2-weighted pulse sequences. T1-weighted and proton-weighted images best demonstrate osseous and diskal tissues, whereas T2-weighted images demonstrate inflammation and joint effusion. Motion MRI studies during opening and closing can be obtained by having the patient open in a series of

stepped distances and with use of rapid image acquisition ("fast scan") techniques.

MRI is contraindicated in patients who are pregnant or who have pacemakers, intracranial vascular clips, or metal particles in vital structures. Some patients may not be able to tolerate the procedure because of claustrophobia or an inability to remain motionless.

## Radiographic Abnormalities of the Temporomandibular Joint

### DEVELOPMENTAL ABNORMALITIES

Developmental abnormalities may be broadly categorized as anomalies in the form and size of joint components. The most striking radiographic changes usually are seen in the condyle, although the temporal component also may be deformed, often remodeling to accommodate the abnormal condyle. Condylar articular cartilage is a mandibular growth site, and, as a result, developmental abnormalities at this location may manifest as altered growth on the affected side of the condyle, mandibular ramus, mandibular body, and alveolar process on the affected side(s).

## Condylar Hyperplasia

### Definition

Condylar hyperplasia is a developmental abnormality that results in enlargement and occasionally deformity of the condylar head; this may have a secondary effect on the mandibular fossa as it remodels to accommodate the abnormal condyle. Some proposed etiologic factors include hormonal influences, trauma, infection, heredity, intrauterine factors, and hypervascularity. The mechanism may be overactive cartilage or persistent cartilaginous rests, which increases the thickness of the entire cartilaginous and precartilaginous layers. This condition usually is unilateral and may be accompanied by varying degrees of hyperplasia of the ipsilateral mandible.

### Clinical Features

Condylar hyperplasia is more common in males, and it usually is discovered before the age of 20 years. The condition is self-limiting and tends to arrest with termination of skeletal growth, although in a small number of cases continued growth and adult onset have been reported. The condition may progress slowly or rapidly. Patients have a mandibular asymmetry that varies in severity, depending on the degree of condylar enlargement. The chin may be deviated to the unaffected side, or it may remain unchanged but with an increase in the vertical dimension of the ramus, mandibular body, or alveolar process of the affected side. As a result of this growth pattern, patients may have a posterior open bite on the affected side. Patients may also have symptoms related to TMJ dysfunction and may complain of limited or deviated mandibular opening, or both, caused by restricted mobility of the enlarged condyle.

### Radiographic Features

The condyle may appear relatively normal but symmetrically enlarged, or it may be altered in shape (e.g., conical, spherical, elongated, lobulated) or irregular in outline. It may be more radiopaque because of the additional bone present. A morphologic variation manifesting as elongation of the condylar head and neck with a compensating forward bend, forming an inverted L, may be seen. Also, the condylar neck may be elongated and thickened and may bend laterally when viewed in the coronal (anteroposterior) plane (Fig. 26-10). The cortical thickness and trabecular pattern of the enlarged condyle usually are normal, which helps to distinguish this condition from a condylar neoplasm. The glenoid fossa may be enlarged, usually at the expense of the posterior slope of the articular eminence. The ramus and mandibular body on the affected side also may be enlarged, resulting in a characteristic depression of the inferior mandibular border at the midline, where the enlarged side joins the contralateral normal mandible. The affected ramus may have increased vertical depth and may be thicker in the anteroposterior dimension.

### Differential Diagnosis

A condylar tumor, most notably an osteochondroma, is included in the differential diagnosis. An osteochondroma usually is irregular in shape compared with a hyperplastic condyle. Surface irregularities and continued growth after cessation of skeletal growth should increase suspicion of this tumor. Occasionally a condylar osteoma or large osteophyte that occurs in chronic degenerative joint disease may simulate condylar hyperplasia.

### Treatment

Treatment consists of orthodontics combined with orthognathic surgery and it may be initiated before condylar growth is complete to avoid functional problems (mastication and speech) and worsening esthetic disfigurement. If treatment is delayed, severe mandibular deformation and compensatory changes in the maxilla, dentoalveolar structures, and associated soft tissues may result, which may compromise treatment outcome. On the other hand, treatment before condylar growth is completed may result in relapse of occlusal and esthetic problems. Cessation of growth of the condyle may be determined with technetium bone scans.

## Condylar Hypoplasia

### Definition

Condylar hypoplasia is failure of the condyle to attain normal size because of congenital and developmental abnormalities or acquired diseases that affect condylar growth. The condyle is small, but condylar morphology usually is normal (Fig. 26-11). The condition may be inherited or may appear spontaneously. Some cases have been attributed to early injury or injury to the articular cartilage by birth trauma or intra-articular inflammatory lesions.

### Clinical Features

Condylar hypoplasia usually is a component of a mandibular growth deficiency and therefore is often associated with an underdeveloped ramus and (occasionally) mandibular body. Congenital abnormalities may be unilateral or bilateral and usually are a manifestation of a more generalized condition (e.g., micrognathia, Treacher Collins syndrome); they also may be associated with congenital defects of the ear and zygomatic arch. Developmental abnormalities that manifest during growth usually are unilateral. Acquired abnormalities are the result of damage during the growth period from sources, such as therapeutic radiation or infection, that diminish or prevent further condylar growth and development. Patients with condylar hypoplasia have mandibular asymmetry and may have symptoms of TMJ dysfunction. The chin commonly is deviated to the affected side, and the mandible deviates to the affected side during mandibular opening. Degenerative joint disease is a common long-term sequela.

### Radiographic Features

The condyle may be normal in shape and structure but is diminished in size, and the mandibular fossa also is proportionally small (Fig. 26-12). The condylar neck and coronoid process usually are very slender and are shortened or elongated in some cases. The posterior border of the ramus and condylar neck may have a dorsal (posterior) inclination. The ramus and mandibular body on the affected side may also be small, resulting in a mandibular asymmetry and occasional dental crowding, depending on the severity of mandibular underdevelopment. The antegonial notch is deepened. The associated mandibular hypoplasia is more pronounced if the effect takes place early in life.

### Differential Diagnosis

Condylar destruction from juvenile rheumatoid arthritis may appear similar to that of hypoplasia. A survey of other joints or testing for rheumatoid factor may be helpful. Changes in condylar morphology in severe degenerative joint disease or other arthritic conditions may have a similar appearance, although arthritic disease does not cause mandibular hypoplasia of the affected side unless it occurs during

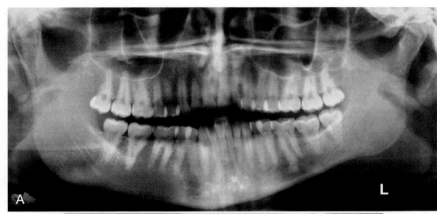

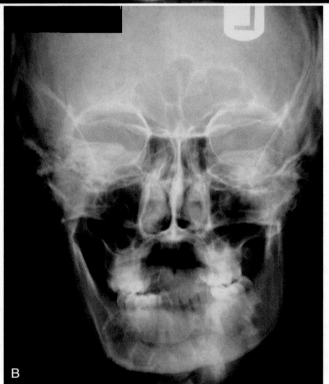

FIG. **26-10** **A,** A panoramic image of condylar hyperplasia involving the right condyle; the resulting asymmetry of the mandible is apparent in the posterior-anterior skull view **(B).**

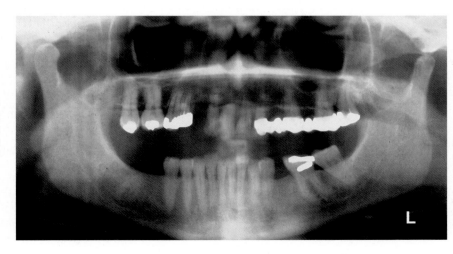

FIG. **26-11** A panoramic image revealing hypoplasia of the left condyle. In this case the hypoplasia is restricted to the condylar head and neck with minimum involvement of the mandibular ramus and body.

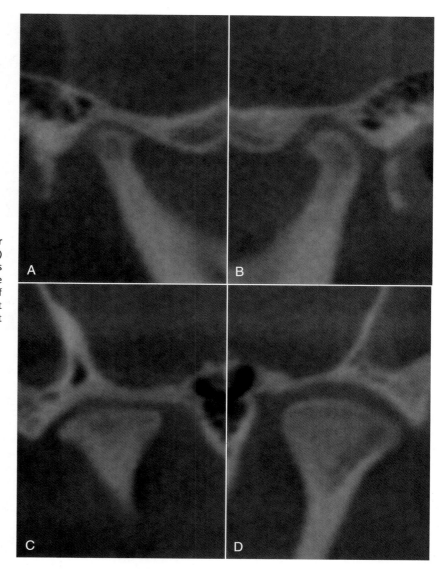

FIG. **26-12** Cone-beam CT of unilateral condylar hypoplasia, sagittal (**A** and **B**) and coronal (**C** and **D**) reformatted images. **A** and **C,** The right condyle is hypoplastic and there is secondary remodeling. The articular surfaces of the condyle and anterior aspect of the glenoid fossa are flattened and the superior joint space is thinner compared with the left. **B** and **D,** Left side of same patient showing normal condyle.

growth, and other signs of arthritis are usually visible in the affected joint.

## Treatment
Orthognathic surgery, bone grafts, and orthodontic therapy may be required.

### Juvenile Arthrosis

## Synonyms
Boering's arthrosis and arthrosis deformans juvenilis

## Definition
Juvenile arthrosis, a condylar growth disturbance first described by Boering, manifests as hypoplasia and characteristic morphologic abnormalities. This condition may be a form of condylar hypoplasia but is thought to differ in that the affected condyle at one time was normal, becoming abnormal during growth. Juvenile arthrosis may be unilateral or bilateral, and it predisposes the TMJ to secondary degenerative changes.

## Clinical Features
Juvenile arthrosis affects children and adolescents during the period of mandibular growth. It is more common in females. It may be an incidental finding in a panoramic projection, or the patient may have mandibular asymmetry, signs and symptoms of TMJ dysfunction, or both.

## Radiographic Features
The condylar head develops a characteristic "toadstool" appearance, with marked flattening and apparent elongation of the articulating condylar surface and dorsal (posterior) inclination of the condyle and neck. The condylar neck is shortened or even absent in some cases, with the condyle resting on the upper margin of the ramus (Fig. 26-13). The articulating surface of the temporal component often is flattened. Progressive shortening of the ramus occurs on the affected

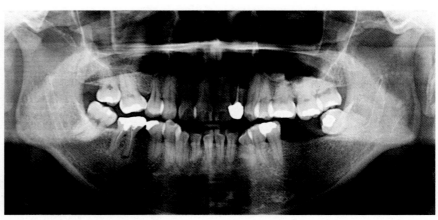

FIG. **26-13** Panoramic Image of Juvenile Arthrosis. The condylar heads have a "toadstool" appearance and are posteriorly inclined. The condylar necks are absent.

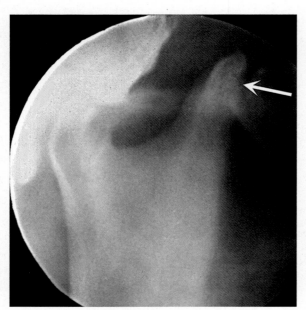

FIG. **26-14** Sagittal Tomogram of Coronoid Hyperplasia. The coronoid process is elongated and extends above the inferior rim of the zygomatic arch *(arrow)* but otherwise is shaped normally.

side, and the antegonial notch may be deepened, indicating mandibular hypoplasia. In long-standing cases, superimposed degenerative changes may be present.

### Differential Diagnosis

The radiographic appearance of juvenile arthrosis may be very similar to, and in some cases is indistinguishable from, developmental hypoplasia of the condyle. Destruction of the anterior aspect of the condylar head from rheumatoid arthritis and severe degenerative joint disease or severe condylar degeneration after orthognathic surgery or joint surgery also may simulate juvenile arthrosis.

### Treatment

Orthognathic surgery and orthodontic therapy may be required to correct the mandibular asymmetry. Caution should be exercised in undertaking orthodontic therapy because stress on the joint may result in further degeneration and orthodontic relapse.

### Coronoid Hyperplasia

#### Definition

Coronoid process hyperplasia may be acquired or developmental, resulting in elongation of the coronoid process. In the developmental variant, the condition usually is bilateral. Acquired types may be unilateral or bilateral and usually are a response to restricted condylar movement caused by abnormalities such as ankylosis.

#### Clinical Features

Bilateral developmental coronoid hyperplasia is more common in males, often commencing at the onset of puberty, although the condition was reported in a 3-year-old child. Patients complain of a progressive inability to open the mouth and may have an apparent closed lock. The condition is painless.

#### Radiographic Features

Coronoid hyperplasia is best seen in panoramic, Waters, and lateral tomographic views and on CT scans. The coronoid processes are elongated, and the tips extend at least 1 cm above the inferior rim of the zygomatic arch (Fig. 26-14). As a result, the coronoid processes may impinge on the medial surface of the zygomatic arch during opening, restricting condylar translation. This can be confirmed by using CT imaging (Fig. 26-15). The coronoid processes may have a large but normal shape or may curve anteriorly and may appear very radiopaque. The posterior surface of the zygomatic process of the maxilla may be remodeled to accommodate the enlarged coronoid process during function. The radiographic appearance of the TMJs usually is normal.

#### Differential Diagnosis

Unilateral cases should be differentiated from a tumor of the coronoid process such as an osteochondroma or osteoma. Unlike coronoid hyperplasia, tumors usually have an irregular shape. The differential diagnosis also includes any cause of inability to open, such as soft tissue abnormalities and ankylosis, emphasizing the importance of including the coronoid process in images of the TMJs. An axial CT image with the patient in a wide open position is useful in establishing coronoid interference to opening.

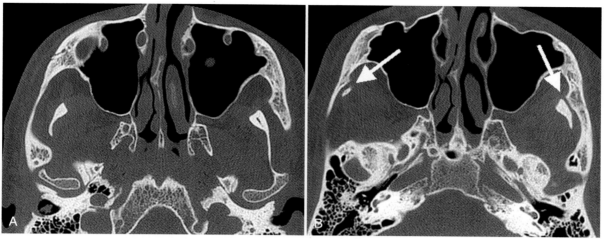

FIG. **26-15** Two axial CT images taken in the closed mouth **(A)** and open mouth **(B)** positions showing impingement of hyperplastic coronoid processes with the medial aspect of the zygomatic arch *(arrows).* Note the hyperostosis on the medial surface of the zygomatic process at the point of impingement.

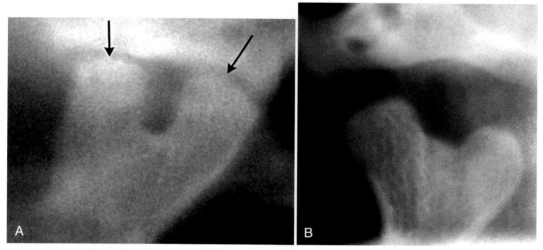

FIG. **26-16** **Bifid Condyle. A,** Sagittal tomogram showing a deep central notch with duplication of the condylar head *(arrows).* The glenoid fossa has remodeled (enlarged) to accommodate the abnormal condyle. **B,** Coronal tomogram showing a depression in the center of the condylar head.

### Treatment

Treatment consists of surgical removal of the coronoid process and postoperative physiotherapy. Regrowth of the coronoid process after surgery has been reported.

### Bifid Condyle

#### Definition

A bifid condyle has a vertical depression, notch, or deep cleft in the center of the condylar head, seen in the frontal or sagittal plane, or actual duplication of the condyle, resulting in the appearance of a "double" or "bifid" condylar head. This condition is rare and is more often unilateral, although it may be bilateral. It may result from an obstructed blood supply or other embryopathy, although a traumatic cause has been postulated as a result of a longitudinal linear fracture of the condyle.

#### Clinical Features

Bifid condyle usually is an incidental finding in panoramic views or anteroposterior projections. Some patients have signs and symptoms of temporomandibular dysfunction, including joint noises and pain.

#### Radiographic Features

A depression or notch is present on the superior condylar surface, giving the anteroposterior silhouette a heart shape; in more severe cases a duplicate condylar head is present in the mediolateral plane (Fig. 26-16). The orientation of the bifid condyle may be anteroposterior or mediolateral. The mandibular fossa may remodel to accommodate the altered condylar morphology.

## Differential Diagnosis

A slight medial depression on the superior condylar surface may be considered a normal variation; the point at which the depth of the depression signifies a bifid condyle is unclear. The differential diagnosis also includes a vertical fracture through the condylar head.

## Treatment

Treatment is not indicated unless pain or functional impairment is present.

## SOFT TISSUE ABNORMALITIES

### Internal Derangements

#### Definition

An internal derangement is an abnormality in the position and sometimes the morphology of the articular disk that may interfere with normal function. The disk most often is displaced in an anterior direction, but it may be displaced anteromedially, medially, or anterolaterally. Lateral and posterior displacements are extremely rare. Some hypothesize that disk displacements may be considered a normal variation on the basis of the frequency of this finding in asymptomatic patients. The cause of internal derangements is unknown, although parafunction, jaw injuries (e.g., direct trauma), whiplash injury, and forced opening beyond the normal range have been implicated.

Internal derangements can be diagnosed by MRI. In some instances the disk may resume a normal position with respect to the condyle (called reduction of the disk) during mandibular opening; when the disk remains displaced throughout the entire range of mandibular movement, the term nonreduction is used (Fig. 26-17). A long-standing displaced disk may become deformed, losing its normal biconcave shape, and it may become thickened and fibrotic. Possible complications are degenerative joint disease and perforation through the disk or (more commonly) the posterior attachment.

#### Clinical Features

Disk displacement has been found both in symptomatic patients and in healthy volunteers, suggesting that it may be a normal variant and not necessarily a predisposing factor in TMJ dysfunction. It is not known why some disks remain displaced or why symptoms of pain and dysfunction are not found in all affected patients. Symptomatic patients may have a decreased range of mandibular motion. Internal derangements can be unilateral or bilateral; unilateral cases may manifest clinically as mandibular deviation to the affected side on opening. Joint noises are common and may manifest as a click as the disk reduces to a normal position during mandibular opening and occasionally as a softer click as the disk becomes displaced again during mandibular closing. Noises may be absent in long-term displaced, nonreducing disks, or crepitus may be heard. Patients may complain of pain in the preauricular region or headaches and may have episodes of closed or open locking of the joint. Patients may have to manipulate the mandible to open it fully past an apparent closed lock by applying medially directed pressure to the affected joint or mandible with the hand.

#### Radiographic Features

The disk cannot be visualized with conventional radiography or tomography; MRI is the technique of choice. Although a retruded

FIG. **26-17** Position and movement of the disk during jaw opening. Normal position **(A)**, mildly displaced anteriorly (with reduction, **B**), and severely displaced anteriorly (without reduction, **C**). (Courtesy Dr. W. K. Solberg, Los Angeles, Calif.)

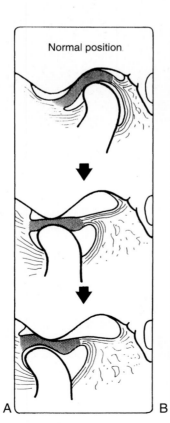
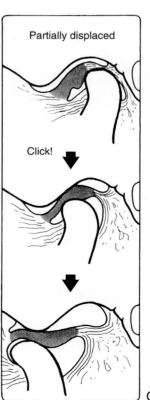
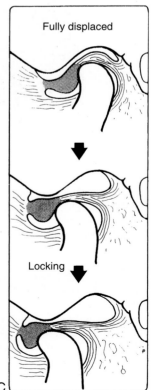

condylar position has been associated with disk displacement, condylar position in maximal intercuspation is not a reliable indicator of disk displacement. Likewise, diminished range of motion at maximal opening is not a reliable indication of a nonreducing disk. In MRI the normal disk has a low signal intensity (is dark between bone and muscle), and the signal intensity of the bilaminar zone is usually higher (i.e., lighter). In the closed-mouth position, the normal disk is positioned with the posterior band directly superior to the condylar head and the thin intermediate part between the anterosuperior surface of the condyle and the posteroinferior surface of the articular eminence (see Fig. 26-9). It is important to note that in all positions of mouth opening the thin intermediate part remains the articulating surface of the disk between condyle and articular eminence.

## Disk Displacement

Identifying the disk may be difficult in cases of gross deformation of the disk and other soft tissue components. Anterior displacement is the most common disk displacement. When the mandible is in maximal intercuspation, partial or full anterior disk displacement is indicated by anterior location of the posterior band of the disk from the normal position, which is directly superior to the condylar head. An indication of anterior displacement is positioning of the posterior band forward so that it sits between the anterosuperior surface of the condyle and the eminence (Fig. 26-18). However, correct identification of the posterior band may be impossible if the tissue signal of the bilaminar zone approximates the posterior band, which occurs in chronic disk displacements. Therefore it is also important to evaluate

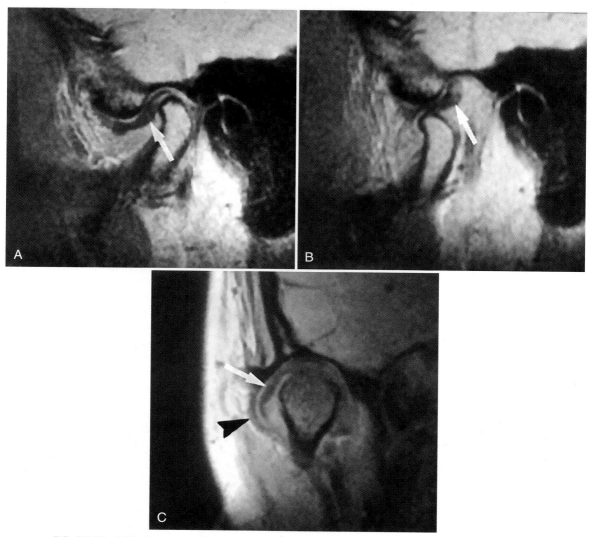

FIG. **26-18**  MRI of anterior disk displacement with reduction. **A,** Closed sagittal view showing the disk with its posterior band *(arrow)* anterior to the condyle; note the anterior position of the thin intermediate section of the disk. **B,** Open view showing the normal relationship of the disk and condyle and the posterior band of the disk *(arrow)*. **C,** Coronal view showing the disk *(white arrow)* laterally displaced. The joint capsule *(black arrowhead)* bulges laterally. (**B** courtesy Dr. Per-Lennart Westesson, Rochester, NY.)

the position of the thin intermediate part of the disk, which should be adjacent to the anterosuperior part of the condyle. Anteromedial displacement is indicated in sagittal image slices when the disk is in a normal position in the medial images of the joint but anteriorly positioned in the lateral images of the same joint. Medial or lateral displacement is indicated in MRI coronal images when the body of the disk is positioned at the medial aspect of the condyle (Fig. 26-18). Posterior disk displacement is rare.

### Disk Reduction and Nonreduction

During mouth opening, an anteriorly displaced disk may reduce to a normal relationship with the condylar head during any part of the opening movement. In motion studies, this is usually a rapid posterior movement of the disk and it is often accompanied by an audible click. This is referred to as disk reduction and can be diagnosed if the disk is in a normal position in the open mouth magnetic resonance images (see Fig. 26-18).

If the disk remains anteriorly displaced (nonreduction) on opening, it may bend or deform as the condyle pushes against it (Fig. 26-19). If the disk remains displaced, it will undergo permanent deformation, losing its biconcave shape. The nonreduced disk is readily seen on MRI scans, although fibrotic changes of the bilaminar zone may alter its tissue signal to approximate the signal of the disk and thus make identification of the disk itself difficult. In such cases the disk may be erroneously interpreted as occupying a normal position at maximal opening.

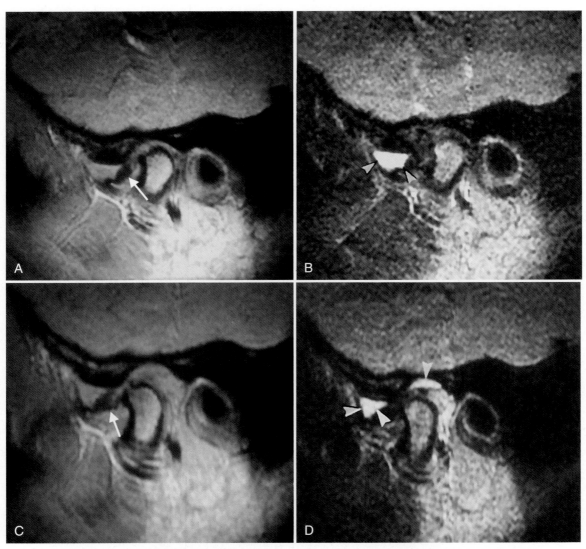

FIG. **26-19** MRI of disk displacement without reduction in the presence of joint effusion. **A,** The disk *(arrow)* is anteriorly displaced in this closed T1-weighted image. **B,** A T2-weighted image of the same section shows the collection of joint effusion *(arrowheads)* in the anterior recess of the upper joint space. **C,** Open T1-weighted image showing the disk remains anterior to the condyle. The posterior band of the disk is indicated with an arrow. **D,** This T2-weighted image is at the same level as **C.** Note the joint effusion *(arrowheads)* in the anterior and posterior recesses of the upper joint space. (Courtesy Dr. Per-Lennart Westesson, Rochester, N.Y.)

## Perforation and Deformities

Perforations between the superior and inferior joint spaces most commonly occur in the retrodiskal tissue, just behind the posterior band of the disk (Fig. 26-20, *C*) and can be detected in arthrographic investigations but are not reliably detected with MRI. MRI can indicate alteration in the normal biconcave outline of the disk, which may vary from enlargement of the posterior band to a bilinear or biconvex disk outline. Disk deformities may be accompanied by changes in its signal intensity, sometimes an increase in signal. Changes to the condyle and temporal component of the joint consistent with degenerative joint disease often accompany cases with long-standing displaced disks (Fig. 26-20).

## Fibrous Adhesions and Effusion

Fibrous adhesions are masses of fibrous tissue or scar tissue that form in the joint space, particularly after TMJ surgery. Adhesions are best identified with arthrography by resistance to injection of contrast agent or they may be detected in MRI studies as tissue with low signal intensity. The pressure of injected contrast agent may tear some of these adhesions, resulting in increased joint mobility after the procedure. Joint effusion (fluid in the joint) is considered to be an early change that may precede degenerative joint disease. MRI can detect joint effusion, which presents as an area of high-signal intensity in the joint spaces in T2-weighted images (see Fig. 26-19).

## Remodeling and Arthritic Conditions

### Remodeling

#### Definition

Remodeling is an adaptive response of cartilage and osseous tissue to forces applied to the joint that may be excessive, resulting in alteration of the shape of the condyle and articular eminence. This adaptive response may result in flattening of curved joint surfaces, which effectively distributes forces over a greater surface area. The number of trabeculae also increases, increasing the density of subchondral cancellous bone (sclerosis) to better resist applied forces. No destruction or degeneration of articular soft tissues occurs. TMJ remodeling occurs throughout adult life and is considered abnormal only if it is accompanied by clinical signs and symptoms of pain or dysfunction or if the degree of remodeling seen radiographically is judged to be severe. Remodeling may be unilateral and does not invariably serve as a precursor to degenerative joint disease.

#### Clinical Features

Remodeling may be asymptomatic, or patients may have signs and symptoms of temporomandibular dysfunction that may be related to the soft tissue components, associated muscles, or ligaments. Accompanying internal derangement of the disk may be a factor.

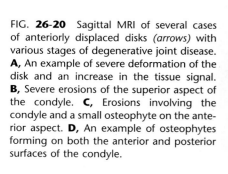

FIG. **26-20** Sagittal MRI of several cases of anteriorly displaced disks *(arrows)* with various stages of degenerative joint disease. **A,** An example of severe deformation of the disk and an increase in the tissue signal. **B,** Severe erosions of the superior aspect of the condyle. **C,** Erosions involving the condyle and a small osteophyte on the anterior aspect. **D,** An example of osteophytes forming on both the anterior and posterior surfaces of the condyle.

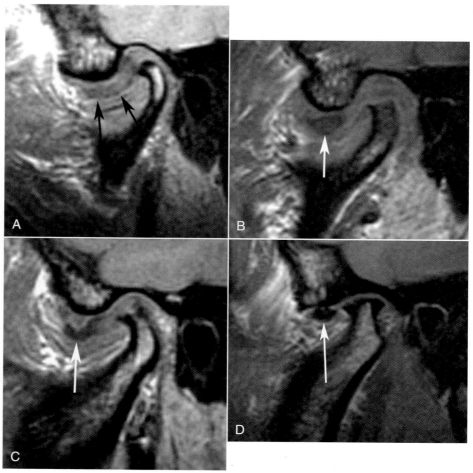

## Radiographic Features

Radiographic changes may affect the condyle, temporal component, or both; they first occur on the anterosuperior surface of the condyle and the posterior slope of the articular eminence. The lateral aspect of the joint is affected in early stages, and the central and medial aspects become involved as remodeling progresses. The radiographic appearance may include one or a combination of the following: flattening, cortical thickening of articulating surfaces, and subchondral sclerosis (Fig. 26-21).

## Differential Diagnosis

Severe joint flattening and subchondral sclerosis may be difficult to differentiate from early degenerative joint disease. It is known that the microscopic changes of degeneration occur before they can be detected radiographically. The radiographic appearance of bone erosions, osteophytes, and loss of joint space are signs signifying degenerative joint disease.

## Treatment

When no clinical signs or symptoms are present, treatment is not indicated. Otherwise, treatment directed to relieve stress on the joint, such as splint therapy, may be considered. This should be preceded by an attempt to discover the cause of the joint stress.

### Degenerative Joint Disease

## Synonym

Osteoarthritis

## Definition

Degenerative joint disease (DJD) is a noninflammatory disorder of joints characterized by joint deterioration and proliferation. Joint deterioration is characterized by loss of articular cartilage and bone erosion. The proliferative component is characterized by new bone formation at the articular surface and in the subchondral region. Usually a variable combination of deterioration and proliferation occurs, but occasionally one aspect predominates; deterioration is more common in acute disease, and proliferation predominates in chronic disease. DJD is thought to occur when the ability of the joint to adapt to excessive forces (remodel) is exceeded. The etiology of DJD is unknown, although a number of factors may be important, including acute trauma, hypermobility, and loading of the joint such as occurs in parafunction. Internal disk derangements may be contributing etiologic factors, but this theory is controversial.

## Clinical Features

DJD can occur at any age, although the incidence increases with age. DJD has a female preponderance. The disease may be asymptomatic, or patients may complain of signs and symptoms of TMJ dysfunction, including pain on palpation and movement, joint noises (crepitus), limited range of motion, and muscle spasm. The onset of symptoms may be sudden or gradual, and symptoms may disappear spontaneously, only to return in recurring cycles. Some studies report that the disease eventually "burns out" and symptoms disappear or markedly decrease in severity in long-standing cases.

## Radiographic Features

Osseous changes in DJD are more accurately depicted in CT images, but gross osseous changes may be evident in MRI studies, particularly in T1-weighted images. When the patient is in maximal intercuspation, the joint space may be narrow or absent, which often correlates with an internal derangement and frequently with a perforation of the disk or posterior attachment, resulting in bone-to-bone contact of the joint components. Signs of previous remodeling, such as flattening and subchondral sclerosis, may be evident, although degenerative changes may obscure these findings. Loss of cortex or erosions of the articulating surfaces of the condyle or temporal component (or both) are characteristic of this disease (Fig. 26-22). In some cases small, round, radiolucent areas with irregular margins surrounded by a varying area of increased density are visible deep to the articulating surfaces. These lesions are called "Ely" or subchondral bone cysts but are not true cysts; they are areas of degeneration that contain fibrous tissue, granulation tissue, and osteoid (Fig. 26-22).

Later in the course of the disease, bony proliferation occurs at the periphery of the articulating surface, increasing the articulating surface area. This new bone is called an osteophyte, which typically appears on the anterosuperior surface of the condyle, the lateral aspect

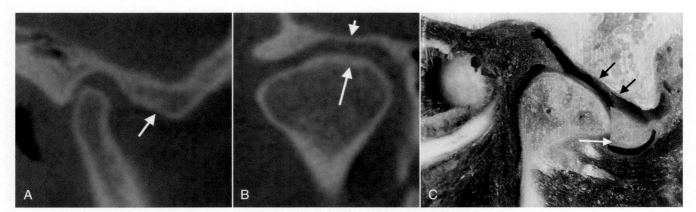

FIG. **26-21**   Cone-beam CT, sagittal **(A)** and coronal **(B)** reformat images of the right TMJ showing remodeling. **A,** The right temporal component shows subchondral sclerosis and flattening *(arrow)*. **B,** The right condyle shows mild flattening of the lateral aspect and subchondral sclerosis of the medial aspect *(arrow)*. The right temporal component is also flattened *(arrowhead)*. **C,** A cadaver specimen. Note the flattening of the temporal component *(black arrows)* and large perforation posterior to a residual deformed disk *(white arrow)*.

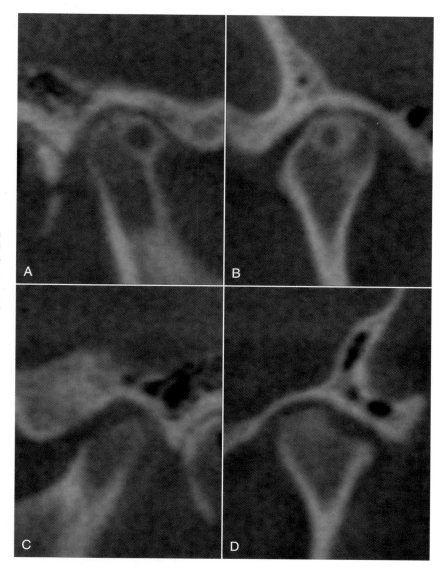

FIG. **26-22**  Cone-beam CT, closed position depicting various erosions in degenerative joint disease. **A** and **B,** Same patient, right side. Large subchondral cystlike erosion ("Ely cyst") of the condyle surrounded by a broad zone of sclerosis. Note also the thin joint space. **C** and **D,** Same patient, left side. Broad erosion of the anterolateral condylar surface. Note also the lack of cortication of the remaining condylar surface and flattening of the temporal component.

of the temporal component, or both (Fig. 26-23). Osteophytes also may form on the lateral, medial, and posterosuperior aspects of the condyle. In severe cases, osteophyte formation originating in the glenoid fossa extends from the articular eminence to almost encase the condylar head. Osteophytes may break off and lie free within the joint space (these fragments are known as "joint mice"), and these must be differentiated from other conditions that cause joint space radiopacities (Figs. 26-23 and 26-24). It has been reported that joints with long-term nonreducing disk displacement have a higher incidence of progressive radiographic changes of DJD than in joints with no disk displacement or reducing disks.

In severe DJD, the glenoid fossa may appear grossly enlarged because of erosion of the posterior slope of the articular eminence, and the condyle may be markedly diminished in size and altered in shape because of destruction and erosion of the condylar head. This in turn may allow the condylar head to move forward and superiorly into an abnormal anterior position that may result in an anterior open bite.

### Differential Diagnosis

DJD can have a spectrum of appearances ranging from substantial subchondral sclerosis and osteophyte formation (proliferative component) to extensive erosions (degenerative component). A more erosive appearance may simulate inflammatory arthritides such as rheumatoid arthritis, whereas a more proliferative appearance with extensive osteophyte formation may simulate a benign tumor such as osteoma or osteochondroma.

### Treatment

Treatment is directed toward relieving joint stress (e.g., splint therapy), relieving secondary inflammation with anti-inflammatory drugs, and increasing joint mobility and function (e.g., physiotherapy).

## Rheumatoid Arthritis

### Definition

Rheumatoid arthritis (RA) is a heterogeneous group of systemic disorders that manifests mainly as synovial membrane inflammation in several joints. The TMJ becomes involved in approximately half of affected patients. The characteristic radiographic findings are a result of villous synovitis, which leads to formation of synovial granulomatous tissue (pannus) that grows into fibrocartilage and bone, releasing enzymes that destroy articular surfaces and underlying bone.

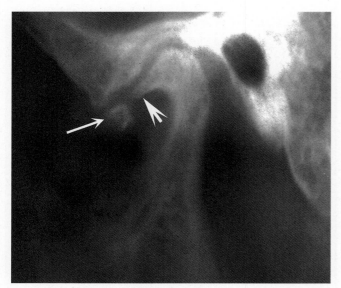

FIG. **26-23**  Sagittal tomogram of the left temporomandibular joint. A large osteophyte emanating from the anterior aspect of the condyle *(short arrow)* and a "joint mouse" *(long arrow)* positioned anterior to the condyle in the joint space.

## Clinical Features

RA is more common in females and can occur at any age but increases in incidence with increasing age. A juvenile variant is discussed separately. Usually the small joints of the hands, wrists, knees, and feet are affected in a bilateral, symmetric fashion, whereas TMJ involvement varies. Patients with TMJ involvement complain of swelling, pain, tenderness, stiffness on opening, limited range of motion, and crepitus. The chin appears receded, and an anterior open bite is a common finding because of the bilateral destruction and anterosuperior positioning of the condyles. TMJ involvement usually is bilateral and symmetric.

## Radiographic Features

The initial changes may be generalized osteopenia (decreased density) of the condyle and temporal component. The pannus may destroy the disk, resulting in diminished width of the joint space. Bone erosions by the pannus most often involve the articular eminence and the anterior aspect of the condylar head, which permits anterosuperior positioning of the condyle when the teeth are in maximal intercuspation and results in an anterior open bite (Fig. 26-25). Erosion of the anterior and posterior condylar surfaces at the attachment of the synovial lining may result in a "sharpened pencil" appearance of the condyle. Erosive changes may be so severe that the entire condylar head is destroyed, with only the neck remaining as the articulating surface. Similarly, the articular eminence may be destroyed to the extent that a concavity replaces the normally convex eminence. Joint destruction eventually leads to secondary DJD. Subchondral sclerosis and flattening of articulating surfaces may occur, as well as subchondral "cyst" and osteophyte formation. Fibrous ankylosis or, in rare cases, osseous ankylosis, may occur (Fig. 26-26); reduced mobility is related to the duration and severity of the disease.

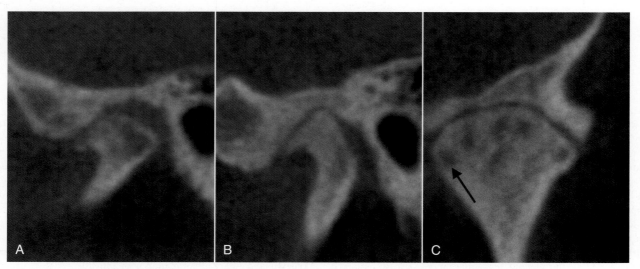

FIG. **26-24**  Cone-beam CT, closed position displaying two cases of degenerative joint disease (different patients). **A,** Sagittal reformat. Surface erosions of the condyle with osteophyte formation at the anterior aspect. Subchondral sclerosis, flattening and erosions of the temporal component. The condyle is also anteriorly positioned in the glenoid fossa. **B,** Sagittal reformat. Prominent osteophyte formation at the anterior aspect of the condyle, flattening and subchondral sclerosis of all joint components, with decreased width of the joint space. **C,** Coronal reformat, same patient as **B.** Multiple subchondral erosions not visible in the sagittal reformat *(arrow,* one example).

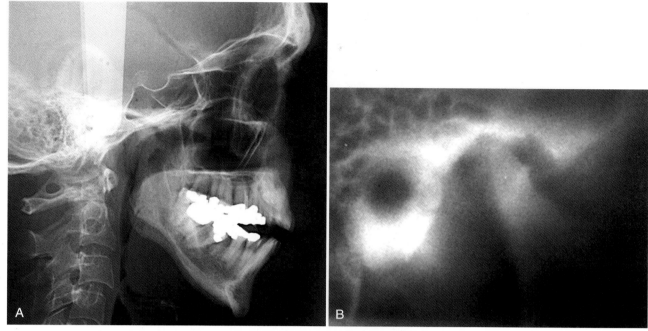

**FIG. 26-25** Rheumatoid arthritis. **A,** Lateral cephalometric view illustrating a steep mandibular plane and anterior open bite. **B,** Lateral tomogram (closed position) illustrating a large erosion of the antero-superior condylar head accompanied by severe erosions of the temporal component, including the articular eminence.

## Differential Diagnosis

The differential diagnosis includes severe DJD and psoriatic arthritis. Osteopenia and severe erosions, particularly of the articular eminence, are more characteristic of RA. Psoriatic arthritis may be ruled out by the patient's history.

## Treatment

Treatment is directed toward pain relief (analgesics), reduction or suppression of inflammation (nonsteroidal anti-inflammatory drugs, gold salts, corticosteroids), and preservation of muscle and joint function (physiotherapy). Joint replacement surgery may be necessary in patients with severe joint destruction.

## Juvenile Arthritis

### Synonyms

Juvenile rheumatoid arthritis, juvenile chronic arthritis, and Still's disease

### Definition

Juvenile arthritis (JA), formerly called juvenile rheumatoid arthritis and juvenile chronic arthritis, is a chronic inflammatory disease that appears before the age of 16 years (the mean age is 5 years). It is characterized by chronic, intermittent synovial inflammation that results in synovial hypertrophy, joint effusion, and swollen, painful joints. As the disease progresses, cartilage and bone are destroyed. Rheumatoid factor may be absent, hence the preferred terminology of JA rather than juvenile rheumatoid arthritis. JA differs from adult RA in that it has an earlier onset, and systemic involvement usually is more severe. TMJ involvement occurs in approximately 40% of patients and may be unilateral or bilateral.

## Clinical Features

The patient usually has pain and tenderness in the affected joint or joints, although the disease can be asymptomatic. Unilateral onset is common, but contralateral involvement may occur as the disease progresses. Severe TMJ involvement results in inhibition of mandibular growth. Affected patients may have micrognathia and posteroinferior chin rotation, resulting in a facial appearance known as "bird face," which may also be accompanied by an anterior open bite. The degree of micrognathia is proportional to the severity of joint involvement and the early onset of disease. Additionally, when only one TMJ is involved or if one side is more severely affected, the patient may have a mandibular asymmetry with the chin deviated to the affected side.

## Radiographic Features

Osteopenia (decreased density) of the affected TMJ components may be the only initial radiographic finding. Radiographic findings are similar to those for the adult form except for the addition of impaired mandibular growth. Erosions may extend to the mandibular fossa, and the articular eminence may be destroyed. Similarly, erosion of the anterior or superior aspect of the condyle may occur, and in more severe cases only a pencil-shaped small condyle remains; the condyle may be destroyed. Because the inflammation is intermittent, during quiescent periods the cortex of the joint surfaces may reappear, and the surfaces will appear flattened. As a result of bone destruction, the condylar head typically is positioned anterosuperiorly in the mandibular fossa (Fig. 26-27). Hypomobility at maximal opening is common, and fibrous ankylosis may occur in some cases. Secondary degenerative changes manifesting as sclerosis and osteophyte formation may be superimposed on the rheumatoid changes, and ankylosis may occur. An abnormal disk shape is often observed in patients with long-term TMJ involvement. Manifestations of inhibited mandibular

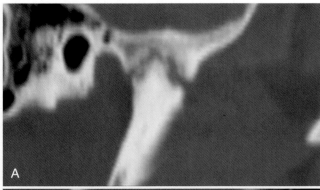

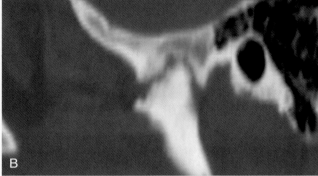

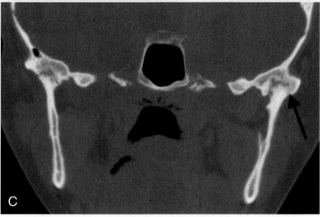

FIG. **26-26**   Sagittal reformat (**A** and **B**) CT images with bone algorithm of the right and left joints of a case of RA. Note the irregular surface of the condyle and articular eminence and that the shapes are similar to opposing pieces of a puzzle, suggesting the possibility of fibrous ankylosis. Because of erosion of the articular eminentia, the condyles have an abnormal anterior position near the residual articular eminentia. **C,** A coronal CT image of the same case. Note the osseous ankylosis on the lateral aspect of the left joint *(arrow).*

growth, such as deepening of the antegonial notch, diminished height of the ramus, and dorsal bending of the ramus and condylar neck, also may occur unilaterally or bilaterally, resulting in an obtuse angle between the mandibular body and the ascending ramus.

## Psoriatic Arthritis and Ankylosing Spondylitis

Psoriatic arthritis and ankylosing spondylitis are seronegative, systemic arthritides that may affect the TMJs. Psoriatic arthritis occurs

in patients with psoriasis of the skin, with inflammatory joint disease occurring in 7% of patients. Ankylosing spondylitis occurs predominantly in males, progressing to spinal fusion. TMJ radiographic changes seen in these disorders may be indistinguishable from those caused by RA, although occasionally a profound sclerotic change is seen in psoriatic arthritis.

### Septic Arthritis

#### Synonym
Infectious arthritis

#### Definition
Septic arthritis is infection and inflammation of a joint that can result in joint destruction. It is rare in comparison to the incidence of DJD and RA in the TMJ. Septic arthritis may be caused by direct spread of organisms from an adjacent cellulitis or from parotid, otic, or mastoid infections. It also may occur by direct extension of osteomyelitis of the mandibular body and ramus or spread from a middle ear infection, although hematogenous spread from a distant nidus has also been reported. Other causes include systemic and autoimmune diseases (e.g., RA, diabetes, immunosuppression, hypogammaglobulinemia), prolonged use of systemic steroids, and sexually transmitted diseases. Septic arthritis has also been reported in children after blunt trauma, as a result of hyperemia and increased exposure to microorganisms, damage to local structure allowing bacterial access, or hematoma formation providing a favorable growth medium.

#### Clinical Features
Individuals can be affected at any age, and the condition shows no sex predilection. It usually occurs unilaterally. The patient may have redness and swelling over the joint; trismus; severe pain on opening; inability to occlude the teeth; large, tender cervical lymph nodes; fever; and malaise. The mandible may be deviated to the unaffected side as a result of joint effusion.

#### Radiographic Features
No radiographic signs may be present in early stages of the disease, although the space between the condyle and the roof of the mandibular fossa may be widened because of inflammatory exudate in the joint spaces. Osteopenic (radiolucent) changes of the joint components and mandibular ramus may be evident. More obvious bony changes are seen approximately 7 to 10 days after the onset of clinical symptoms. As a result of the osteolytic effects of inflammation, the condylar articular cortex may become slightly radiolucent, erosions of the surface of the condyle and articular eminence may be seen, sequestra may become apparent, and there may be periosteal new bone formation (Fig. 26-28). As the disease progresses, the condyle and articular eminence, including the disk, may be destroyed. Osseous ankylosis may occur after the infection subsides. If the disease occurs during the period of mandibular growth, radiographic manifestations of inhibited mandibular growth may be evident.

#### Differential Diagnosis
The diagnosis of septic arthritis is ideally made by identification of organisms in joint aspirate, although cultures occasionally remain negative. The radiographic changes caused by septic arthritis may mimic those of severe DJD or RA, although septic arthritis usually occurs unilaterally, and the patient often has clinical signs and symptoms of infection. Inflammatory changes that may accompany septic arthritis may be seen in CT images, such as involvement of mastoid

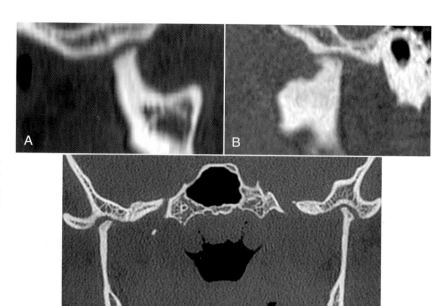

FIG. **26-27**  **A** and **B,** Sagittal CT reformat images of a case of juvenile arthritis. Note the severe erosion of the articular eminence and the condyles and the abnormal anterior positioning of both condyles. **C,** This coronal CT image of the same case shows small remnants of the condylar heads after severe erosion.

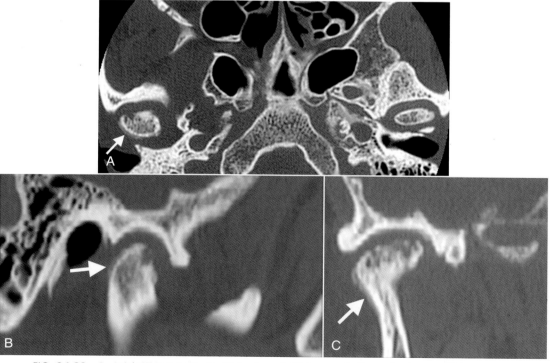

FIG. **26-28**  **A,** Axial CT image. **B,** Sagittal reformat CT image. **C,** Coronal reformat CT image of a case of septic arthritis involving the right joint. Note the erosions, sclerosis and periosteal reaction that extends along the back of the condyle and lateral neck of the condyle (arrows).

air cells, osteomyelitis of the mandible, and inflammation of surrounding soft tissue. MRI, with T2-weighted images, may show muscle enlargement, joint effusion, or abscess. Scintigraphy by use of a technetium bone scan will show increased bone metabolism within the osseous components, especially the condyle, and gallium confirms the presence of infection.

## Treatment

Treatment includes antimicrobial therapy, drainage of effusion, and joint rest. Physiotherapy to re-establish joint mobility is initiated after the acute phase of infection has passed.

## Articular Loose Bodies

Articular loose bodies are radiopacities of varying origin located in the synovium, within the capsule in the joint spaces, or outside the capsule in soft tissue. They appear radiographically as soft tissue calcifications positioned around the condylar head. The loose bodies may represent bone that has separated from joint components, as in DJD (joint mice), hyaline cartilage metaplasia (calcification) that occurs in synovial chondromatosis, crystals deposited in the joint space in crystal-associated arthropathy (pseudogout), or tumoral calcinosis associated with renal disease. In rare cases chondrosarcoma also may mimic the appearance of articular loose bodies.

## Synovial Chondromatosis

### Synonyms
Synovial chondrometaplasia and osteochondromatosis

### Definition
Synovial chondromatosis is an uncommon disorder characterized by metaplastic formation of multiple cartilaginous and osteocartilaginous nodules within connective tissue of the synovial membrane of joints. Some of these nodules may detach and form loose bodies in the joint space, where they persist and may increase in size, being nourished by synovial fluid. This condition is more common in the axial skeleton than in the TMJ. When the cartilaginous nodules ossify, the term *synovial osteochondromatosis* may be used.

### Clinical Features
Patients may be asymptomatic or may complain of preauricular swelling, pain, and decreased range of motion. Some patients have crepitus or other joint noises. The condition usually occurs unilaterally.

### Radiographic Features
The osseous components may appear normal or may exhibit osseous changes similar to those in DJD. The joint space may be widened, and if ossification of the cartilaginous nodules has occurred, a radiopaque mass or several radiopaque loose bodies may be seen surrounding the condylar head (Fig. 26-29). CT imaging can identify the location of the calcifications. Sclerosis of the glenoid fossa and condyle may be seen, which is considered to be a chronic bone reaction to an active lesion. Occasionally, erosion through the glenoid fossa into the middle cranial fossa may occur, which is best detected with CT. MRI may be useful in defining the tissue planes between the synovial chondromatosis mass and surrounding soft tissue.

### Differential Diagnosis
The appearance of synovial osteochondromatosis cannot always be differentiated from chondrocalcinosis; however, often the soft tissue calcifications in osteochondromatosis are larger and may have a peripheral cortex that identifies their bony nature. Conditions that appear similar include DJD with joint mice or chondrosarcoma or osteosarcoma. Either sarcoma may be accompanied by severe bone destruction, which may help in differentiating the condition from synovial chondromatosis.

### Treatment
Treatment consists of removal of the loose bodies and resection of abnormal synovial tissue in the joint by arthroscopic or open joint surgery.

## Chondrocalcinosis

### Synonyms
Pseudogout and calcium pyrophosphate dihydrate deposition disease

### Definition
Chondrocalcinosis is characterized by acute or chronic synovitis and precipitation of calcium pyrophosphate dihydrate crystals in the joint space. It differs from gout, in which urate crystals are precipitated, hence the term *pseudogout*.

### Clinical Features
The joints more commonly affected are the knee, wrist, hip, shoulder, and elbow; TMJ involvement is uncommon. The condition occurs unilaterally and is more common in males. Patients may be asymptomatic or may complain of pain and joint swelling.

### Radiographic Features
The radiographic appearance of chondrocalcinosis may simulate synovial chondromatosis, described previously. Often the radiopacities within the joint space are finer and have a more even distribution than in osteochondromatosis (Fig. 26-30). Bone erosions and a severe increase in condylar bone density also have been described. Erosions of the glenoid fossa may be present, which require CT for detection. Soft tissue swelling and edema of the surrounding muscles may be seen with MRI.

### Differential Diagnosis
The differential diagnosis is the same as for synovial chondromatosis.

### Treatment
Treatment consists of surgical removal of the crystalline deposits. Steroids, aspirin, and nonsteroidal anti-inflammatory agents may provide relief. Colchicine may be used to alleviate acute symptoms and for prophylaxis.

## Trauma

### Effusion

#### Definition
Effusion is an influx of fluid into the joint, usually as a result of trauma (hemorrhage) or inflammation (exudate). Inflammation may result from an internal derangement, traumatic injuries, arthritis, or rheumatic diseases.

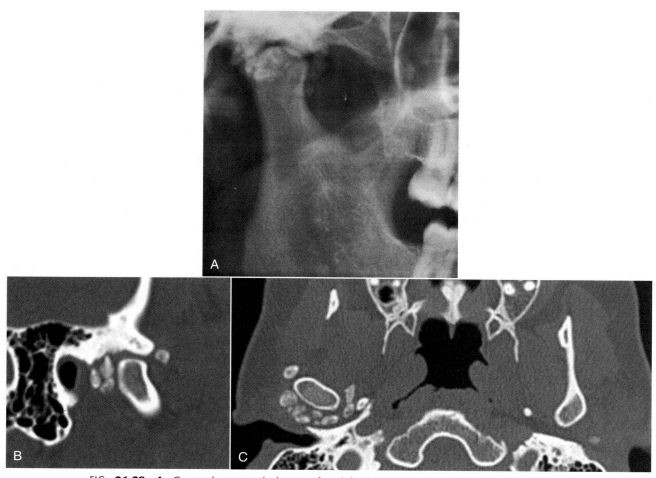

FIG. **26-29**  **A,** Cropped panoramic image of a right joint involved with osteochondromatosis. **B,** Sagittal CT reformat image. **C,** Axial CT image revealing multiple ossified bodies surrounding the condyle and within the joint capsule.

## Clinical Features

The patient may have swelling over the affected joint; pain in the TMJ, preauricular region, or ear; and limited range of motion. Patients may also complain of the sensation of fluid in the ear, tinnitus, hearing difficulties, and difficulty occluding the posterior teeth.

## Radiographic Features

Joint effusion is more commonly seen in conjunction with internal derangements, although it has been described in normal joints. The joint space is widened, and T2-weighted MRI studies may show a bright signal (white), indicating fluid adjacent to the disk or posterior to the condyle (see Fig. 26-19).

## Differential Diagnosis

Effusion must be differentiated from septic arthritis; in the latter case the accompanying signs and symptoms of infection are present.

## Treatment

Treatment may include anti-inflammatory drugs, although surgical drainage of the effusion occasionally is necessary.

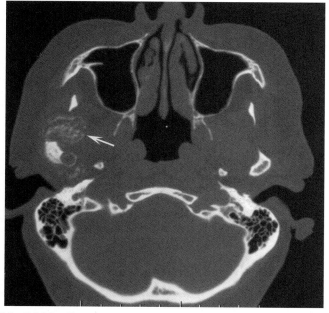

FIG. **26-30**  Chondrocalcinosis (CT, axial image, bone algorithm). Note the calcifications anterior to the right condyle *(arrow)* and the large erosion involving the medial pole of the condyle.

## Dislocation

### Definition

Dislocation is abnormal positioning of the condyle out of the mandibular fossa but within the joint capsule. It usually occurs bilaterally and most commonly in an anterior direction. Dislocation may be caused by a failure of muscular coordination, subluxation, or external trauma and may be associated with a condylar fracture. Dislocation may occur into the middle cranial fossa as a result of trauma, but this is rare.

### Clinical Features

In anterior dislocation, patients are unable to close the mandible to maximal intercuspation; some patients cannot reduce the dislocation, whereas others may be able to reduce the mandible by manipulation. In the former case associated pain and muscle spasm often are present.

### Radiographic Features

In bilateral cases both condyles are located anterior and superior to the summits of the articular eminentia. Clinical information is important because the normal range of motion may extend anterior to the summit of the articular eminence.

### Differential Diagnosis

The diagnosis is confirmed by the radiographic findings, although some fracture dislocations may be difficult to visualize, particularly if the dislocation is very slight. For this reason, CT or tomography is essential for diagnosis because routine plain film views may not show the dislocation because of anatomic superimpositions.

### Treatment

Treatment consists of manual manipulation of the mandible to reduce the dislocation. Surgery occasionally is necessary to reduce the condyle in the case of a fracture dislocation, although treatment may not be indicated for this type of dislocation if mandibular function is adequate.

## Fracture

### Definition

Fractures of the TMJ usually occur at the condylar neck and often are accompanied by dislocation of the condylar head. Fractures may be classified according to the anatomic location of the fracture: condylar head, condylar neck, and subchondral region. Occasionally more than one anatomic location is involved. On rare occasions the fracture may involve the temporal component.

### Clinical Features

Unilateral fractures, which are more common than bilateral fractures, may be accompanied by a parasymphyseal or mandibular body fracture on the contralateral side. The patient may have swelling over the TMJ, pain, limited range of motion, and an anterior open bite. Some TMJ fractures are relatively asymptomatic and may not be discovered at the time of trauma; instead, these come to light as incidental findings at a later time when radiographs are taken for other reasons. Condylar fractures should be ruled out if the patient has a history of a blow to the mandible, especially to the anterior aspect.

If a condylar fracture occurs during the period of mandibular growth, growth may be inhibited because of damage to the condylar growth center. The degree of subsequent hypoplasia is related to the stage of mandibular development at the time of injury (younger patients have more profound hypoplasia) and the severity of the injury. Patients younger than 10 years old have a higher remodeling potential and may have less deformity compared with older patients, although injuries in patients younger than 3 years old tend to produce severe asymmetries. Injury to the joint may result in hemorrhage or effusion into the joint spaces that eventually may form bone during the healing process, which in turn may result in severe hypoplasia and limited joint function.

### Radiographic Features

In relatively recent condylar neck fractures, a radiolucent line limited to the outline of the neck is visible. This line may vary in width, depending on whether the bone fragments are still aligned (narrow line) or displacement/dislocation has occurred (wider line). If the bone fragments overlap, an area of apparent increase in radiopacity may be seen instead of a radiolucent line (Fig. 26-31). Also, the outer cortical boundary may have an irregular outline or a step defect. Approximately 60% of condylar fractures show evidence of fragment angulation and a variable degree of displacement (dislocation) of the fracture ends. Fractures of the condylar head are less common and may be of the vertical (responsible for the traumatic type of bifid condyle) or compressive type (Fig. 26-32). CT is the preferred imaging modality to evaluate condylar fractures because there is no superimposition of adjacent structures and TMJ reformats provide images in several different planes. Two- and three-dimensional reformatted images are useful to accurately locate a fractured fragment. Alterna-

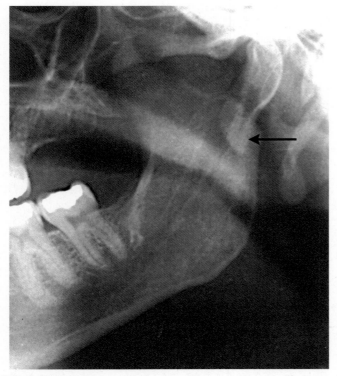

FIG. **26-31** Condylar neck fracture (panoramic image). The arrow points to overlapped fragments, as evidenced by increased radiopacity.

tively, if CT is not available, multiple right-angle radiographic projections from the lateral, frontal, and basilar aspects may be used to detect a fracture.

The amount of remodeling seen in the TMJ after a condylar fracture with medial displacement varies considerably. In some cases the condyle remodels to a form that is essentially normal, whereas in other cases the condyle and mandibular fossa become flattened, with loss of vertical height on the affected side. The condyle eventually may show degenerative changes, including flattening, erosion, osteophyte formation, and ankylosis. These changes are more severe if the condyle is displaced. Condylar fractures can also be associated with damage of the intracapsular soft tissues, including the disk, joint capsule and retrodiskal tissues, and with hemarthrosis and joint effusion.

### Differential Diagnosis

Occasionally old fractures that have remodeled may be difficult to differentiate from developmental abnormalities of the condyle. The most common difficulty is in determining whether a fracture is indeed present. Panoramic views taken as an initial examination must be supplemented with a Towne's view, especially if there is suspected medial displacement of the condylar head.

### Treatment

Treatment may not be indicated if mandibular mobility is adequate; otherwise, the fracture is reduced surgically.

### Neonatal Fractures

The use of forceps during delivery of neonates may result in fracture and displacement of the rudimentary condyle, which later manifests as severe mandibular hypoplasia and lack of development of the glenoid fossa and articular eminence. Such cases have a characteristic radiographic appearance in the panoramic image, having the appearance of a partly opened pair of scissors in place of a normal condyle

(Fig. 26-33). This presentation results from the overlapping images of the medially displaced carrot-shaped condyle and remnants of the condylar neck.

### Differential Diagnosis

This condition often is not diagnosed until later in life, at which time a diagnosis of fracture may be made without a history that the fracture occurred at the time of birth. The condition must be differentiated from a developmental hypoplasia of the mandible, which is unrelated to birth injury.

### Treatment

The fracture usually is not treated, but the mandibular asymmetry may be corrected with a combination of orthodontics and orthognathic surgery.

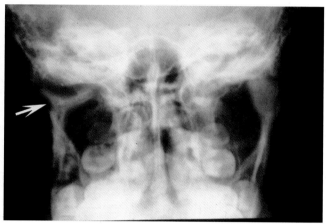

FIG. **26-32** Open Towne's view of a compression fracture of the right condylar head *(arrow).*

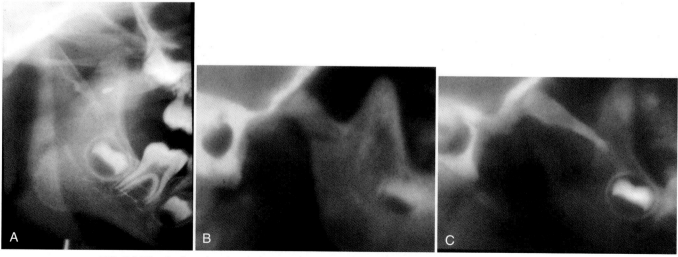

FIG. **26-33** **A,** A cropped panoramic image of a neonatal fracture of the right condyle. Note the unusual shape of the coronoid notch, similar to a partially opened pair of scissors. **B,** Tomographic image slice of the lateral aspect of the same joint. Note the normal-appearing coronoid notch but a lack of formation of the glenoid fossa and eminence and the abnormal anterior position of the condyle. **C,** Medial tomographic slice of the same case disclosing the fractured segment.

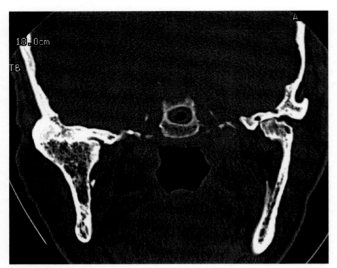

FIG. **26-34**   Bony ankylosis (CT, coronal image slice, bone algorithm). The right condyle and ramus are markedly enlarged. The articulating surface is irregular, and the central and lateral aspects are fused to the roof of the glenoid fossa, as evidenced by a lack of joint space. Note that the left condylar articulating surface is eroded, and the joint space is decreased on the medial aspect; these changes are consistent with degenerative joint disease.

## Ankylosis

### Definition
Ankylosis is a condition in which condylar movement is limited by a mechanical problem in the joint ("true" ankylosis) or by a mechanical cause not related to joint components ("false" ankylosis). True ankylosis may be bony or fibrous. In bony ankylosis the condyle or ramus is attached to the temporal or zygomatic bone by an osseous bridge. In fibrous ankylosis a soft tissue (fibrous) union of joint components occurs; the bone components appear normal. False ankylosis may result from conditions that inhibit condylar movement, such as muscle spasm, myositis ossificans, or coronoid process hyperplasia.

### Clinical Features
Most unilateral cases are caused by mandibular trauma or infection. The most common cause of bilateral TMJ ankylosis is rheumatoid arthritis, although in rare cases bilateral fractures may be the cause. Most if not all cases of TMJ ankylosis in infancy occur as a result of birth injury. Patients have a history of progressively restricted jaw opening, or they may have a long-standing history of limited opening. Some degree of mandibular opening usually is possible through flexing of the mandible, although opening may be restricted to only a few millimeters, particularly in the case of bony ankylosis.

### Radiographic Features
In fibrous ankylosis the articulating surfaces are usually irregular because of erosions. The joint space is usually very narrow and the two irregular surfaces may appear to fit one another like a jigsaw puzzle (see Fig. 26-26). Little or no condylar movement is seen. Radiographic signs of remodeling occasionally are visible as the joint components adapt to repeated attempts at mandibular opening. In bony ankylosis the joint space may be partly or completely obliterated by

the osseous bridge, which can vary from a slender segment of bone, which may be difficult to locate, to a large bony mass. This extensive new bone may fuse the condyle to the cranial base (Fig. 26-34). Secondary degenerative changes of the joint components are common. Often morphologic changes occur, such as compensatory progressive elongation of the coronoid processes and deepening of the antegonial notch in the mandibular ramus on the affected side as a result of muscle function during attempted mandibular opening. If ankylosis occurs before mandibular growth is complete, growth of the affected side of the mandible is inhibited. Coronal CT images are the best diagnostic imaging method to evaluate ankylosis.

### Differential Diagnosis
The major differential diagnosis is a condylar tumor. However, a history of trauma, infection, or other joint diseases should help rule out neoplastic disease. Detection of fibrous ankylosis is difficult because fibrous tissue is not visible in the radiographic image and therefore may be difficult to differentiate from false ankylosis.

### Treatment
Joint mobility is improved by surgical removal of the osseous bridge or creation of a pseudarthrosis.

## Tumors

Benign and malignant tumors originating in or involving the TMJ are rare. Tumors may be intrinsic or extrinsic (adjacent) to the TMJ. Intrinsic tumors may develop in the condyle, temporal bone, or coronoid process. Extrinsic tumors may affect the morphology, structure, or function of the joint without invading the joint itself. They may cause indirect effects on growth, such as those seen with vascular lesions or from pressure, or may influence mandibular positioning.

## Benign Tumors

The most common benign intrinsic tumors affecting the TMJ are osteomas, osteochondromas, Langerhans histiocytosis, and osteoblastomas. Chondroblastomas, fibromyxomas, benign giant cell lesions, and aneurysmal bone cysts also occur. Benign tumors and cysts of the mandible (e.g., ameloblastomas, odontogenic keratocysts, simple bone cysts) may involve the entire ramus and in rare cases the condyle. In cases of false ankylosis in which the TMJs appear radiographically normal, hyperplasia or a tumor of the coronoid process must be ruled out.

### Clinical Features
Condylar tumors grow slowly and may attain considerable size before becoming clinically noticeable. Patients may complain of TMJ swelling, which may be accompanied by pain and decreased range of motion; the symptoms often mimic TMJ dysfunction. The clinical examination may reveal facial asymmetry, malocclusion, and deviation of the mandible to the unaffected side; these may be accompanied by symptoms of TMJ dysfunction. Tumors of the coronoid process typically are painless, but patients may complain of progressive limitation of motion.

### Radiographic Features
Condylar tumors cause condylar enlargement that often is irregular in outline. The trabecular pattern may be altered, resulting in regions of destruction seen as radiolucencies or new abnormal bone forma-

tion, which may increase the radiopacity of the condyle with abnormal trabeculae. An osteoma or osteochondroma appears as an abnormal, pedunculated mass attached to the condyle (Fig. 26-35). Osteochondromas often extend from the anterior or superior surface of the condyle. Tumors of the coronoid process may affect TMJ function, which emphasizes the need to image and evaluate the coronoid process when evaluating joint abnormalities. The most common benign tumor is the osteochondroma. This tumor may interfere with joint function and erode adjacent osseous structures.

## Differential Diagnosis

Condylar neoplasms may simulate unilateral condylar hyperplasia because of condylar enlargement, although osteomas and osteochondromas give an irregular appearance, such as bulbous or globular expansion of the condyle or, more commonly, a pedunculated growth. Also, the characteristic condylar shape and proportions are better preserved in condylar hyperplasia. Coronoid tumors must be differentiated from coronoid hyperplasia, which differs from a condylar tumor in that the coronoid process remains regular in shape.

## Treatment

Treatment consists of surgical excision of the tumor and occasionally excision of the condylar head or coronoid process.

## Malignant Tumors

Malignant tumors of the jaws may be primary or, more commonly, metastatic. Primary intrinsic malignant tumors of the condyle are extremely rare and include chondrosarcoma, osteogenic sarcoma, synovial sarcoma, and fibrosarcoma of the joint capsule. Extrinsic malignant tumors may represent direct extension of adjacent parotid salivary gland malignancies, rhabdomyosarcoma (particularly in children), or other regional carcinomas from the skin, ear, and nasopharynx. The most common metastatic lesions include neoplasms originating in the breast, kidney, lung, colon, prostate, and thyroid gland.

## Clinical Features

Malignant tumors (primary or metastatic) may be asymptomatic or patients may have symptoms of TMJ dysfunction such as pain, limited mandibular opening, mandibular deviation, and swelling. Unfortunately, a patient occasionally is treated for TMJ dysfunction without recognition that the underlying condition is a malignancy.

## Radiographic Features

Malignant primary and metastatic TMJ tumors appear as a variable degree of bone destruction with ill-defined, irregular margins. Most lack tumor bone formation, with the exception of osteogenic sarcoma. Chondrosarcoma may appear as an indistinct, essentially radiolucent destructive lesion of the condyle with surrounding discrete soft tissue calcifications that may simulate the appearance of the articular loose bodies seen in chondrocalcinosis or pseudogout (Fig. 26-36). In the case of metastatic tumors, the radiographic appearance usually is nonspecific condylar destruction (with a few exceptions, such as metastatic prostate carcinoma) and does not indicate the site of origin (Fig. 26-37). CT is the imaging modality of choice to view bone involvement and MRI is useful for displaying the extent of involvement into the surrounding soft tissues.

## Differential Diagnosis

Joint destruction caused by a malignant tumor must be differentiated from the osseous destruction seen in severe DJD. Malignant tumors cause profound central bone destruction, whereas DJD causes more

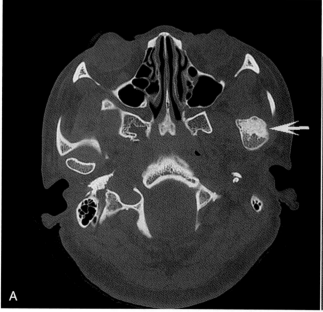
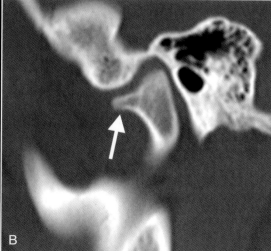

FIG. 26-35  **A,** Axial bone algorithm CT image of an osteochondroma extending from the anterior surface of the left condylar head (arrow). **B,** Sagittal reformat CT image of a different case; the internal aspect of the osteochondroma (arrow) is continuous with the cancellous portion of the condylar head.

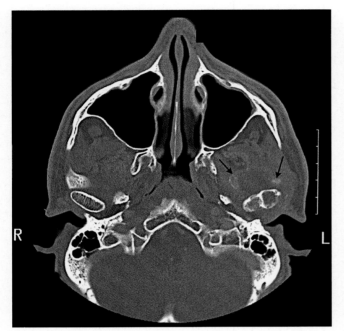

FIG. **26-36** Chondrosarcoma (CT, axial section, bone algorithm). A radiolucent destructive lesion is present in the left condylar head, and faint radiopacities (soft tissue calcifications) are visible anterior to the condylar head (arrows).

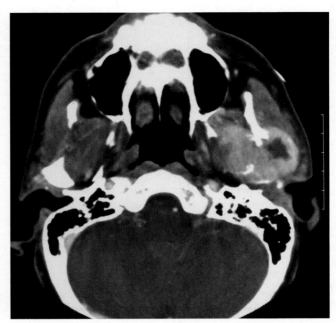

FIG. **26-37** An axial, soft tissue algorithm, CT image of a metastatic lesion from a carcinoma of the thyroid gland that has destroyed all of the left mandibular condyle.

peripheral bone destruction. Proliferative changes such as osteophyte formation may be seen in DJD, but unlike with a malignant tumor, no soft tissue mass or swelling is evident. Chondrosarcoma may simulate joint space calcifications (discussed earlier), but in the case of malignancy, severe bone destruction also occurs.

## Treatment

In the case of primary malignant tumors, treatment consists of wide surgical removal of the tumor. Tumor extension to vital anatomic structures may compromise survival. Metastatic tumors of the TMJ rarely are treated surgically; treatment mainly is palliative and may include radiotherapy and chemotherapy.

## SUGGESTED READINGS

### DISORDERS OF THE TEMPOROMANDIBULAR JOINT

Brooks SL, Brand JW, Gibbs SJ et al: Imaging of the temporomandibular joint, position paper of the American Academy of Oral and Maxillofacial Radiology [review], *Oral Surg Oral Med Oral Pathol Oral Radiol Endod* 83:609-618, 1997.

Helkimo M: Studies on function and dysfunction of the masticatory system, II: index for anamnestic and clinical dysfunction and occlusal state, *Sven Tandlak Tidskr* 67:101-121, 1974.

McNeill C, Mohl ND, Rugh JD et al: Temporomandibular disorders: diagnosis, management, education, and research, *J Am Dent Assoc* 120:253, 255, 257, 1990.

Petrikowski CG, Grace MG: Temporomandibular joint radiographic findings in adolescents, *Cranio* 14:30-36, 1996.

Rugh JD, Solberg WK: Oral health status in the United States: temporomandibular disorders, *J Dent Educ* 49:398-406, 1985.

Wänman A, Agerberg G: Mandibular dysfunction in adolescents, I: prevalence of symptoms, *Acta Odontol Scand* 44:47-54, 1986.

### ANATOMY OF THE TEMPOROMANDIBULAR JOINT

Blaschke DD, Blaschke TJ: A method for quantitatively determining temporomandibular joint bony relationships, *J Dent Res* 60:35-43, 1981.

Drace JE, Enzmann DR: Defining the normal temporomandibular joint: closed, partially open, and open mouth MR imaging of asymptomatic subjects, *Radiology* 177:67-76, 1990.

Hansson LG, Hansson T, Petersson A: A comparison between clinical and radiologic findings in 259 temporomandibular joint patients, *J Prosthet Dent* 50:89-94, 1983.

Ingervall B, Carlsson GE, Thilander B: Postnatal development of the human temporomandibular joint. II. A microradiographic study, *Acta Odont Scand* 34:133-139, 1976.

Larheim TA: Radiographic appearance of the normal temporomandibular joint in newborns and small children, *Acta Radiol Diagn (Stockh)* 22:593-599, 1981.

Pullinger AG, Hollender L, Solberg WK et al: A tomographic study of mandibular condyle position in an asymptomatic population, *J Prosthet Dent* 53:706-713, 1985.

Taylor RC, Ware WH, Fowler D et al: A study of temporomandibular joint morphology and its relationship to the dentition, *Oral Surg* 33:1002-1013, 1972.

Ten Cate AR: Gross and micro anatomy. In Zarb GA, Carlsson BJ, Mohl ND, editors: *Temporomandibular joint and masticatory muscle disorders*, ed 2, Copenhagen, 1994, Munksgaard.

Westesson P-L, Kurita K, Eriksson L et al: Cryosectional observations of functional anatomy of the temporomandibular joint, *Oral Surg Oral Med Oral Pathol* 68:247-251, 1989.

Yale SH, Allison BD, Hauptfuehrer JD: An epidemiological assessment of mandibular condyle morphology, *Oral Surg* 21:169-177, 1966.

### DIAGNOSTIC IMAGING OF THE TEMPOROMANDIBULAR JOINT

Brooks SL, Brand AW, Gibbs SJ et al: Imaging of the temporomandibular joint, position paper of the American Academy of Oral and Maxillofacial

Radiology, *Oral Surg Oral Med Oral Pathol Oral Radiol Endod* 83:609-618, 1997.

Helms CA, Kaplan P: Diagnostic imaging of the temporomandibular joint: recommendations for use of the various techniques, *AJR Am J Roentgenol* 154:319-322, 1990.

Katzberg RW: Temporomandibular joint imaging, *Radiology* 170:297-307, 1989.

## Hard Tissue Imaging

Christiansen EL, Chan TT, Thompson JR et al: Computed tomography of the normal temporomandibular joint, *Scand J Dent Res* 95:499-509, 1987.

Coin CG: Tomography of the temporomandibular joint, *Med Radiogr Photogr* 50:26-39, 1974.

Tsiklakis K, Syriopoulos K, Stamatakis HC: Radiographic examination of the temporomandibular joint using cone beam computed tomography, *Dentomaxillofac Radiol* 33:196-201, 2004.

## Soft Tissue Imaging

Conway WF, Hayes CW, Campbell RL: Dynamic magnetic resonance imaging of the temporomandibular joint using FLASH sequences, *J Oral Maxillofac Surg* 46:930-938, 1988.

Hansson LG, Westesson PL, Eriksson L: Comparison of tomography and midfield magnetic resonance imaging for osseous changes of the temporomandibular joint, *Oral Surg Oral Med Oral Pathol Oral Radiol Endod* 82:698-703, 1996.

Moses JJ, Salinas E, Goergen T et al: Magnetic resonance imaging or arthrographic diagnosis of internal derangement of the temporomandibular joint, *Oral Surg Oral Med Oral Pathol* 75:268-272, 1993.

Tomas X, Pomes J, Berenquer J et al: MR Imaging of temporomandibular joint dysfunction: a pictorial review, *Radiographics* 26:765-781, 2006.

# RADIOGRAPHIC ABNORMALITIES OF THE TEMPOROMANDIBULAR JOINT

## Condylar Hyperplasia

Gray RJM, Sloan P, Quayle AA et al: Histopathological and scintigraphic features of condylar hyperplasia, *Int J Oral Maxillofac Surg* 19:65-71, 1990.

Rubenstein LK, Campbell RL: Acquired unilateral condylar hyperplasia and facial asymmetry: report of a case, *ASDC J Dent Child* 52:114-120, 1985.

Shira RB: Facial asymmetry and condylar hyperplasia, *Oral Surg* 40:567, 1975.

Wolford LM, Mehra P, Reiche-Fischel O et al: Efficacy of high condylectomy for management of condylar hyperplasia, *Am J Orthod Dentofacial Orthop* 121:136-151, 2002.

## Condylar Hypoplasia

Jerell RG, Fuselier B, Mahan P: Acquired condylar hypoplasia: report of a case, *ASDC J Dent Child* 58:147-153, 1991.

Worth HM: Radiology of the temporomandibular joint. In Zarb GA, Carlsson BJ, Mohl ND, editors: *Temporomandibular joint function and dysfunction*, Copenhagen, 1979, Munksgaard.

## Juvenile Arthrosis

Boering G: Temporomandibular joint arthrosis and facial deformity, *Trans Int Conf Oral Surg* 258-260, 1967.

Worth HM: Radiology of the temporomandibular joint. In Zarb GA, Carlsson BJ, Mohl ND, editors: *Temporomandibular joint function and dysfunction*, Copenhagen, 1979, Munksgaard.

## Coronoid Hyperplasia

McLoughlin PM, Hopper C, Bowley NB: Hyperplasia of the mandibular coronoid process: an analysis of 31 cases and a review of the literature, *J Oral Maxillofac Surg* 53:250-255, 1995.

Satoh K, Ohno S, Aizawa T et al: Bilateral coronoid hyperplasia in an adolescent: report of a case and review of the literature, *J Oral Maxillofac Surg* 64:334-338, 2006.

## Bifid Condyle

Daniels JSM, Ali I: Post-traumatic bifid condyle associated with temporomandibular joint ankylosis: report of a case and review of the literature, *Oral Surg Oral Med Oral Pathol Oral Radiol Endod* 99:682-688. 2005.

Loh FC, Yeo JF: Bifid mandibular condyle, *Oral Surg Oral Med Oral Pathol* 69:24-27, 1990.

# SOFT TISSUE ABNORMALITIES

Dolwick MF, Sanders B: TMJ internal derangement and arthrosis. In *Surgical atlas*, St. Louis, 1985, Mosby.

Helms CA, Kaban LB, McNeill C et al: Temporomandibular joint: morphology and signal intensity characteristics of the disk at MR imaging, *Radiology* 172:817-820, 1989.

Katzberg RW: Temporomandibular joint imaging, *Radiology* 170:297, 1989.

Katzberg RW, Tallents RH, Hayakawa K et al: Internal derangements of the temporomandibular joint: findings in the pediatric age group, *Radiology* 154:125-127, 1985.

Larheim TA: Current trends in temporomandibular joint imaging, *Oral Surg Oral Med Oral Pathol Oral Radiol Endod* 80:555-576, 1995.

Nuelle DG, Alpern MC, Ufema JW: Arthroscopic surgery of the temporomandibular joint, *Angle Orthod* 56:118-142, 1986.

Rammelsberg P, Pospiech PR, Jäger L et al: Variability of disk position in asymptomatic volunteers and patients with internal derangements of the TMJ, *Oral Surg Oral Med Oral Pathol Oral Radiol Endod* 83:393-399, 1997.

Sano T, Westesson P-L: Magnetic resonance imaging of the temporomandibular joint: increased T2 signal in the retro-diskal tissue of painful joints, *Oral Surg Oral Med Oral Pathol Oral Radiol Endod* 79:511-516, 1995.

Wilkes CH: Internal derangements of the temporomandibular joint: pathological variations, *Arch Otolaryngol Head Neck Surg* 115:469-477, 1989.

# REMODELING AND ARTHRITIC CONDITIONS

## Remodeling

Brooks SL, Westesson PL, Eriksson L et al: Prevalence of osseous changes in the temporomandibular joint of asymptomatic persons without internal derangement, *Oral Surg Oral Med Oral Pathol* 73:118-122, 1992.

Moffett BC, Johnson LC, McCabe JB et al: Articular remodeling in the adult human temporomandibular joint, *Am J Anat* 115:119-141, 1964.

## Degenerative Joint Disease

de Leeuw R, Boering G, Stegenga B et al: Temporomandibular joint osteoarthrosis: clinical and radiographic characteristics 30 years after nonsurgical treatment—a preliminary report, *Cranio* 11:15-24, 1993.

Helenius LMJ, Tervahartiala P, Helenius I et al: Clinical, radiographic and MRI findings of the temporomandibular joint in patients with different rheumatic diseases, *Int J Oral Maxillofac Surg* 35:983-989, 2006.

Kurita H, Uehara S, Yokochi M et al: A long-term follow-up study of radiographically evident degenerative changes in the temporomandibular joint with different conditions of disk displacement, *Int J Oral Maxillfoacial Surg* 35:49-54, 2006.

Mayne JG, Hatch GS: Arthritis of the temporomandibular joint, *J Am Dent Assoc* 79:125-130, 1969.

Radin EL, Paul IL, Rose RM: Role of mechanical factors in pathogenesis of primary osteoarthritis, *Lancet* 1:519-522, 1972.

Sato H, Fujii T, Yamada N et al: Temporomandibular joint osteoarthritis: a comparative clinical and tomographic study pre- and post-treatment, *J Oral Rehabil* 21:383-395, 1994.

### Rheumatoid Arthritis

Gynther GW, Tronje G, Holmlund AB: Radiographic changes in the temporomandibular joint in patients with generalized osteoarthritis and rheumatoid arthritis, *Oral Surg Oral Med Oral Pathol Oral Radiol Endod* 81:613-618, 1996.

Larheim TA, Smith HJ, Aspestrand F: Rheumatic disease of the temporomandibular joint: MR imaging and tomographic manifestations, *Radiology* 175:527-531, 1990.

Syrjänen SM: The temporomandibular joint in rheumatoid arthritis, *Acta Radiol Diagn (Stockh)* 26:235-243, 1985.

### Juvenile Chronic Arthritis

Ganik R, Williams FA: Diagnosis and management of juvenile rheumatoid arthritis with TMJ involvement, *Cranio* 4:254-262, 1986.

Hu Y-S, Schneiderman ED: The temporomandibular joint in juvenile rheumatoid arthritis, I: computed tomographic findings, *Pediatr Dent* 17:46-53, 1995.

Hu Y-S, Schneiderman ED, Harper RP: The temporomandibular joint in juvenile rheumatoid arthritis, II: relationship between computed tomographic and clinical findings, *Pediatr Dent* 18:312-319, 1996.

Karhulahti T, Ylijoki H, Rönning O: Mandibular condyle lesions related to age at onset and subtypes of juvenile rheumatoid arthritis in 15-year-old children, *Scand J Dent Res* 101:332-338, 1993.

### Psoriatic Arthritis

Koorbusch GF, Zeitler DL, Fotos PG et al: Psoriatic arthritis of the temporomandibular joints with ankylosis, *Oral Surg Oral Med Oral Pathol* 71:267-274, 1991.

Wilson AW, Brown JS, Ord RA: Psoriatic arthropathy of the temporomandibular joint, *Oral Surg Oral Med Oral Pathol* 70:555-558, 1990.

### Ankylosing Spondylitis

Locher MC, Felder M, Sailer HF: Involvement of the temporomandibular joints in ankylosing spondylitis (Bechterew's disease), *J Craniomaxillofac Surg* 24:205-213, 1996.

Ramos-Remus C, Major P, Gomez-Vargas A et al: Temporomandibular joint osseous morphology in a consecutive sample of ankylosing spondylitis patients, *Ann Rheum Dis* 56:103-107, 1997.

### Septic Arthritis

Leighty SM, Spach DH, Myall RW et al: Septic arthritis of the temporomandibular joint: review of the literature and report of two cases in children, *Int J Oral Maxillofac Surg* 22:292-297, 1993.

Sembronio S, Albiero AM, Robiony M et al: Septic arthritis of the temporomandibular joint successfully treated with arthroscopic lysis and lavage: case report and review of the literature, *Oral Surg Oral Med Oral Pathol Oral Radiol Endod* 103:e1-6, 2007.

## ARTICULAR LOOSE BODIES

Ardekian L, Faquin W, Troulis MJ et al: Synovial chondromatosis of the temporomandibular joint: report and analysis of eleven cases, *J Oral Maxillofac Surg* 63:941-947, 2005.

Carls FR, von Hochstetter A, Engelke W et al: Loose bodies in the temporomandibular joint, *J Craniomaxillofac Surg* 23:215-221, 1995.

Chuong R, Piper MA: Bilateral pseudogout of the temporomandibular joint: report of a case and review of the literature, *J Oral Maxillofac Surg* 53:691-694, 1995.

Dijkgraaf LC, Liem RS, de Bont LG et al: Calcium pyrophosphate dihydrate crystal deposition disease: a review of the literature and a light and electron microscopic study of a case of the temporomandibular joint with numerous intracellular crystals in the chondrocytes, *Osteoarthritis Cartilage* 3:35-45, 1995.

Lustmann J, Zeltser R: Synovial chondromatosis of the temporomandibular joint: review of the literature and case report, *Int J Oral Maxillofac Surg* 18:90-94, 1989.

Orden A, Laskin DM, Lew D: Chronic preauricular swelling, *J Oral Maxillofac Surg* 47:390-397, 1989.

Pynn BR, Weinberg S, Irish J: Calcium pyrophosphate dihydrate deposition disease of the temporomandibular joint: a case report and review of the literature, *Oral Surg Oral Med Oral Pathol Oral Radiol Endod* 79:278-284, 1995.

Yu Q, Yang J, Wang P et al: CT features of synovial chondromatosis in the temporomandibular joint, *Oral Surg Oral Med Oral Pathol Oral Radiol Endod* 97:524-528, 2007.

## TRAUMA

### Effusion

Emshoff R, Brandimaier I, Bertram S et al: Magnetic resonance imaging findings of osteoarthrosis and effusion in patients with unilateral temporomandibular joint pain, *Int J Oral Maxillofac Surg* 31:598-602, 2002.

Schellhas KP, Wilkes CH: Temporomandibular joint inflammation: comparison of MR fast scanning with T1- and T2-weighted imaging techniques, *AJR Am J Roentgenol* 153:93-98, 1989.

Schellhas KP, Wilkes CH, Baker CC: Facial pain, headache, and temporomandibular joint inflammation, *Headache* 29:229-232, 1989.

Westesson P-L, Brooks SL: Temporomandibular joint: relationship between MR evidence of effusion and the presence of pain and disk displacement, *AJR Am J Roentgenol* 159:559, 1992.

### Dislocation

Kai S, Kai H, Nakayama E et al: Clinical symptoms of open lock position of the condyle: relation to anterior dislocation of the temporomandibular joint, *Oral Surg Oral Med Oral Pathol* 74:143-148, 1992.

Ohura N, Ichioka S, Sudo T et al: Dislocation of the bilateral mandibular condyle into the middle cranial fossa: review of the literature and clinical experience, *J Oral Maxillofac Surg* 64:1165-1172, 2006.

Wijmenga JP, Boering G, Blankestijn J: Protracted dislocation of the temporomandibular joint, *Int J Oral Maxillofac Surg* 15:380-388, 1986.

### Fracture

Choi J, Oh I-K: A follow-up study of condyle fracture in children, *Int J Oral Maxillofac Surg* 34:851-858, 2005.

Dahlström L, Kahnberg KE, Lindahl L: Fifteen years follow-up on condylar fractures, *Int J Oral Maxillofac Surg* 18:18-23, 1989.

Gerhard S, Ennemoser T, Rudisch A et al: Condylar injury: magnetic resonance imaging findings of the temporomandibular joint soft tissue changes, *Int J Oral Maxillofac Surg* 36: 214-218, 2007.

Horowitz I, Abrahami E, Mintz SS: Demonstration of condylar fractures of the mandible by computed tomography, *Oral Surg* 54:263-268, 1982.

Lindahl L, Hollender L: Condylar fractures of the mandible, II: a radiographic study of remodeling processes in the temporomandibular joint, *Int J Oral Surg* 6:153-165, 1977.

Pharoah MJ: Radiology of the temporomandibular joint. In Zarb GA, Carlsson BJ, Mohl ND, editors: Temporomandibular joint and masticatory muscle disorders, ed 2, Copenhagen, 1994, Munksgaard.

Raustia AM, Pyhtinen J, Oikarinen KS et al: Conventional radiographic and computed tomographic findings in cases of fracture of the mandibular condylar process, *J Oral Maxillofac Surg* 48:1258-1264, 1990.

Schellhas KP: Temporomandibular joint injuries, *Radiology* 173:211-216, 1989.

### Neonatal Fractures

Pharoah MJ: Radiology of the temporomandibular joint. In Zarb GA, Carlsson BJ, Mohl ND, editors: *Temporomandibular joint and masticatory muscle disorders,* ed 2, Copenhagen, 1994, Munksgaard.

Worth HM: Radiology of the temporomandibular joint. In Zarb GA, Carlsson GE, editors: *Temporomandibular joint function and dysfunction,* Copenhagen, 1979, Munksgaard.

### Ankylosis

Ferretti C, Bryant R, Becker P et al: Temporomandibular joint morphology following post-traumatic ankylosis in 26 patients, *Int J Oral Maxillofac Surg* 34:376-381, 2005.

Rowe NL: Ankylosis of the temporomandibular joint, *J R Coll Surg Edinb* 27:67-79, 1982.

Wood RE, Harris AM, Nortjé et al: The radiologic features of true ankylosis of the temporomandibular joint: an analysis of 25 cases, *Dentomaxillofac Radiol* 17:121-127, 1988.

## TUMORS

### Benign Tumors

James RB, Alexander RW, Traver JG Jr: Osteochondroma of the mandibular coronoid process: report of a case, *Oral Surg* 37:189-195, 1974.

Nwoku AL, Koch H: The temporomandibular joint: a rare localisation for bone tumors, *J Maxillofac Surg* 2:113-119, 1974.

Pharoah MJ: Radiology of the temporomandibular joint. In Zarb GA, Carlsson BJ, Mohl ND, editors: *Temporomandibular joint and masticatory muscle disorders,* ed 2, Copenhagen, 1994, Munksgaard.

Svensson B, Isacsson G: Benign osteoblastoma associated with an aneurysmal bone cyst of the mandibular ramus and condyle, *Oral Surg Oral Med Oral Pathol* 76:433-436, 1993.

Thoma KH: Tumors of the mandibular joint, *J Oral Surg Anesth Hosp Dent Serv* 22:157-167, 1964.

Worth HM: Radiology of the temporomandibular joint. In Zarb GA, Carlsson GE, editors: *Temporomandibular joint function and dysfunction,* Copenhagen, 1979, Munksgaard.

### Malignant Tumors

Morris MR, Clark SK, Porter BA et al: Chondrosarcoma of the temporomandibular joint: case report, *Head Neck Surg* 10:113-117, 1987.

Rubin MM, Jui V, Cozzi GM: Metastatic carcinoma of the mandibular condyle presenting as temporomandibular joint syndrome, *J Oral Maxillofac Surg* 47:507-510, 1989.

Takehana dos Santos D, Cavalcanti MGP: Osteosarcoma of the temporomandibular joint: report of 2 cases, *Oral Surg Oral Med Oral Pathol Oral Radiol Endod* 94:641-647, 2002.

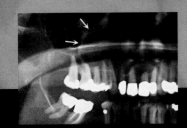

# CHAPTER 27

# Paranasal Sinuses

Axel Ruprecht • Ernest W.N. Lam

The paranasal sinuses are the four paired sets of air-filled cavities of the craniofacial complex composed of the maxillary, frontal, and sphenoid sinuses and the ethmoid air cells. The maxillary sinuses are of particular importance to the dentist because of their proximity to the teeth and their associated structures. Consequently, abnormalities arising from within the maxillary sinuses can cause symptoms that may mimic diseases of odontogenic origin, and conversely, abnormalities that arise in and around the teeth may affect the sinuses or mimic the symptoms of sinus disease.

Part or all of the paranasal sinuses may appear on radiographs made for dental purposes, including maxillary periapical, occlusal, and panoramic radiographs. All the paranasal sinuses can appear on skull radiographs made for orthodontic or orthognathic surgical purposes (see Chapter 12), although not necessarily in the most diagnostic fashion. Therefore, the dentist should have some familiarity with variations to the normal appearances of the sinuses and the more common diseases that may affect them.

## Normal Development and Variations

The paranasal sinuses develop as invaginations from the nasal fossae into their respective bones (maxillary, frontal, sphenoid, and ethmoid). Consequently, the mucosal lining of the paranasal sinuses is similar to that found in the nasal cavity, but with slightly fewer mucus glands. In the absence of disease the epithelial cilia move mucus toward their respective communications with the nasal fossae.

The maxillary sinuses (sometimes called the maxillary antra or antra of Highmore) are the first to develop in the second month of intrauterine life. An invagination develops in the lateral wall of the nasal fossa in the middle meatus, and the sinus enlarges laterally into the body of the maxilla. At birth, each sinus is a thin, small slit no more than 8 mm in length in its anteroposterior dimension. With time, the maxilla becomes progressively more pneumatized as the air cavity expands further into the bone both laterally under the orbits toward the zygomatic bone and inferiorly toward the alveolar process. Consequently, it may be very common to see the inferior or "dependent" portion of the air-filled maxillary sinus and floor near, or superimposed over, the roots of the premolar or molar teeth to some degree.

The floor of the maxillary sinus is a thin, radiopaque line on radiographs. Where the alveolar process of the maxilla is not well pneumatized, the floor of the maxillary sinus may not be visible on periapical radiographs (Fig. 27-1, *A*), or it may be seen superior to the roots of the maxillary premolar and/or molar teeth (Fig. 27-1, *B*).

With greater pneumatization of the alveolar process, the floor of the maxillary sinus may appear to undulate around the roots of the teeth or be superimposed over the roots of the adjacent teeth, giving the appearance that the tooth roots have penetrated the sinus floor (Fig. 27-1, *C* and *D*). The very close relationship between the tooth roots and the maxillary sinus is referred to as "draping." Closer examination of the periapical aspect of the teeth usually reveals intact laminae durae and periodontal ligament spaces around the tooth root apices. In some instances, the appearance of the maxillary sinus may be mistakenly confused with a benign space-occupying lesion (Fig. 27-2).

In patients with considerable pneumatization extending into the alveolar process of the maxilla, the lamina dura of a premolar or molar tooth may form a portion of the sinus floor. In addition to the alveolar process, the maxillary pneumatization may extend into the palatal, zygomatic, and frontal processes of the maxilla, which can be appreciated in plain films but are more notable in advanced imaging such as computed tomography (CT) or magnetic resonance imaging (MRI) (Fig. 27-3).

Hypoplasia of the maxillary sinuses occurs unilaterally in about 1.7% of patients and bilaterally in 7.2%. In these patients, the radiographic images of the affected sinus may appear more radiopaque than normal because of the relatively large amount of surrounding maxillary bone. The configuration of the maxillary sinus walls frequently helps to distinguish between a hypoplastic sinus and one that is pathologically radiopaque. A Waters view will show an inward bowing of the sinus wall resulting in a smaller than normal air cavity. In contrast, extensive enlargement of the maxillary and other paranasal sinuses is a well-known feature of acromegaly.

The development of the frontal sinuses does not usually begin until the fifth or sixth year. These sinuses develop either directly as extensions from the nasal fossae or from anterior ethmoid air cells (see Fig. 27-4, *B*). In about 4% of the population, the frontal sinuses fail to develop. As with the other paranasal sinuses, the right and left frontal sinus cavities develop separately, and as they expand, they approach each other in the midline. In most instances, a thin bony septum may separate the two cavities. In the adult, the frontal sinuses are often asymmetric cavities located above the supraorbital ridges and the nasion; however, in some patients the sinuses may also extend posteriorly over the orbits.

The sphenoid sinus begins growth in the fourth fetal month as invaginations from the sphenoethmoidal recesses of the nasal fossae. Located in the body of the sphenoid bone, the right and left sphenoid sinuses are separated by a bony septum and are usually asymmetric in size and shape. The overall size of the sinus is quite variable, and

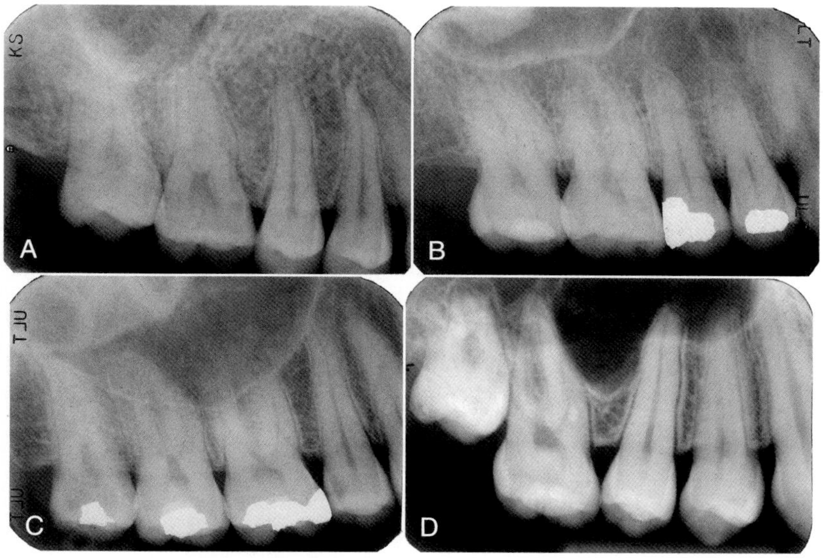

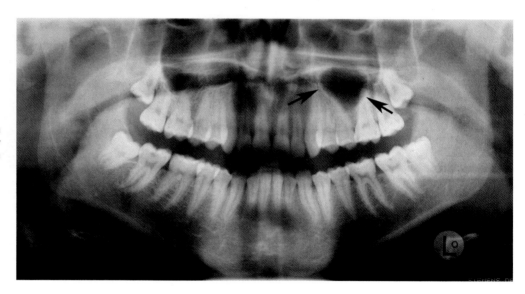

FIG. **27-1** The range of normal of the position of the maxillary sinus relative to the premolar and molar teeth are shown in periapical images **A** to **D**. There is no apparent floor in **A,** with progressively more pneumatization of the alveolar process in **B** and **C**; draping of the maxillary sinus border over the apices of the teeth is particularly evident in **D**.

FIG. **27-2** A panoramic image of a loculus *(arrows)* of the left maxillary sinus draping mimicking a benign space-occupying lesion.

like the maxillary sinuses, the sphenoid sinus may extend beyond the body of the sphenoid bone into the dorsum sella, the clinoid processes, the greater or lesser wings, and the pterygoid processes. The osteum of the sphenoid sinus is a relatively large-diameter opening, which may explain why blockages of the sphenoid sinus osteum are uncommon (see the section on mucoceles later in this chapter).

The ethmoid air cells extend into the ethmoid bones during the fifth fetal month and continue to enlarge until the end of puberty. They consist of multiple interconnected, or sometimes separate, small air-filled chambers that border the medial aspects of the orbital cavities (Fig. 27-4, *A* and *B*). The number of air cells varies considerably, with each ethmoid bone containing between 8 and 15 cells. In some cases, the ethmoid air cells may extend into the neighboring maxillary, lacrimal, frontal, sphenoid, and palatine bones.

The function of the paranasal sinuses is controversial. Some of the putative roles that have been ascribed to the sinuses include heating and humidification of inhaled air, helping to reduce cranial weight, and insulation or protection of deeper vital structures. Indeed, the paranasal sinuses may also have no function whatsoever and may be evolutionarily unwanted space.

## Diseases Associated with the Paranasal Sinuses

Because the maxillary sinus is of most concern to the dentist, the following text emphasizes diseases related to the maxillary sinus.

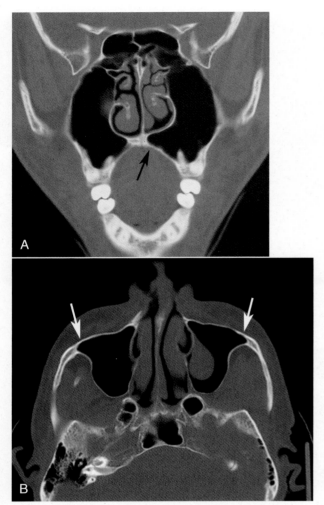

FIG. **27-3** An example of pneumatization of the maxillary sinus into the palatal process of the maxilla *(arrow)* in this coronal CT image **(A)** and examples of pneumatization of the zygomatic process of the maxilla in this axial CT image **(B)**; also note the retention pseudocyst in the left maxillary sinus.

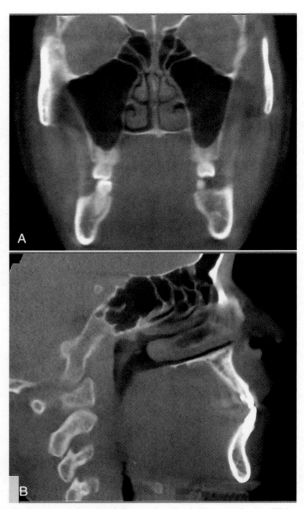

FIG. **27-4** Normal coronal **(A)** and sagittal **(B)** cone-beam CT images of the maxillary sinus and ethmoid air cells **(A)** and the frontal and sphenoid sinuses and ethmoid air cells **(B)**.

## DEFINITION

Diseases associated with the maxillary sinuses include both intrinsic diseases (originating primarily from tissues within the sinus) and those that originate outside the sinus (most commonly diseases arising from odontogenic tissues) that either impinge on or infiltrate the sinus. These types of diseases include inflammatory odontogenic disease, odontogenic cysts, benign and malignant odontogenic neoplasms, bone dysplasias, and trauma.

## CLINICAL FEATURES

The clinical signs and symptoms of maxillary sinus disease include a feeling of pressure, altered voice characteristics, pain on head movement, percussion sensitivity of the teeth or cheek region, regional dysesthesia, paresthesia or anesthesia, and swelling of the facial structures adjacent to the maxilla.

When the clinical signs indicate that maxillary sinus disease may be related to the alveolar process of the maxilla or teeth, it is reasonable for the dentist to proceed with the initial radiologic investigation. If there are positive findings, the patient should be referred to an oral and maxillofacial radiologist to complete the examination. The application of specific imaging modalities is reviewed in the following section.

## APPLIED DIAGNOSTIC IMAGING

A periapical radiograph provides a detailed, albeit limited, view of the alveolar recess and floor of the maxillary antrum. If during this examination the dentist suspects an abnormality, a maxillary lateral occlusal projection may be used for a more extensive view of the antrum. The panoramic radiograph depicts both maxillary sinuses, revealing greater internal structure and parts of the inferior, posterior, and anteromedial walls. It is difficult to compare the internal radiopacities of the right and left sinus in the panoramic image because of variations that result from overlapping phantom images of other structures.

Specialized skull views are the next step in the investigation. The standard series of plane radiographic views of the sinuses includes the Waters (occipitomental), lateral, submentovertex, and Caldwell (15-degree posteroanterior) skull views. The Waters projection is optimal for visualization of the maxillary sinuses, especially to compare internal radiopacities, and the frontal sinuses and ethmoid air cells. If the Waters view is made with the mouth open, parts of the sphenoid sinuses may also be visualized. The submentovertex view may be useful in evaluating the lateral and posterior borders of the maxillary sinuses and the ethmoid air cells. The Caldwell view is most useful in evaluating the frontal sinuses and ethmoid air cells. The lateral skull view allows examination of all four pairs of the paranasal sinuses, but with each member of a pair superimposed on the other.

CT and MRI have become increasingly important for evaluation of sinus disease and have virtually replaced plane radiography and conventional tomography for investigations of the paranasal sinuses. Because CT and MRI provide multiple sections through the sinuses in different planes, they may contribute significantly to delineating the extent of disease and the final diagnosis. High-resolution axial and coronal CT and MRI examinations are the most revealing imaging techniques for the paranasal sinuses and the adjacent structures and areas.

CT examination is appropriate to determine the extent of disease in patients who have chronic or recurrent sinusitis. Indeed, coronal CT provides superior visualization of the ostiomeatal complex (the region of the ostium of the maxillary sinus and the ethmoidal ostium) and nasal cavities and for demonstrating any reaction in the surrounding bone to sinus disease. MRI provides superior visualization of the soft tissues, especially the extension of infiltrating neoplasms into the sinuses or surrounding soft tissues, or the differentiation of retained fluid secretions from soft tissue masses in the sinuses.

## Intrinsic Diseases of the Paranasal Sinuses

The following are abnormalities that originate from tissues within the sinuses.

## INFLAMMATORY DISEASE

Inflammation may result from a variety of causes such as infection, chemical irritation, allergy, introduction of a foreign body, or facial trauma. The radiographic changes associated with inflammation include thickened sinus mucosa, air-fluid levels in the sinuses, polyps, empyema, and retention pseudocysts. Viral infections may, however, not cause any radiographic change in a sinus.

### Mucositis

#### Synonym
Thickened sinus mucosa

#### Definition
The mucosal lining of the paranasal sinuses is composed of respiratory epithelium and is normally about 1 mm thick. Normal sinus mucosa is not visualized on radiographs; however, when the mucosa becomes inflamed from either an infectious or allergic process, it may

increase in thickness 10 to 15 times, which may be seen radiographically. This inflammatory change is referred to as mucositis.

#### Clinical Features
The thickness of sinus mucosa in an asymptomatic individual may vary considerably over a relatively short period of time. Consequently, the discovery of thickened mucosa in an individual who is otherwise asymptomatic does not necessarily imply that further investigations are warranted or that treatment is required. Most of the inflammatory episodes that result in thickening of the mucosal lining of the sinuses are unrecognized by the patient and are discovered only incidentally on a radiograph.

#### Radiographic Features
The image of thickened mucosa is readily detectable in the radiograph as a noncorticated band noticeably more radiopaque than the air-filled sinus, paralleling the bony wall of the sinus (Fig. 27-5).

### Sinusitis

#### Definition
Sinusitis is a condition involving generalized inflammation of the paranasal sinus mucosa caused by an allergen, bacteria, or a virus. Sinusitis may cause blockage of drainage through the ostiomeatal complex. Inflammatory changes may lead to ciliary dysfunction and retention of sinus secretions. Perhaps 10% of inflammatory episodes of the maxillary sinuses are extensions of dental infections. The term *pansinusitis* describes sinusitis affecting all the paranasal sinuses. In children with pansinusitis, the possibility of cystic fibrosis should be considered.

#### Clinical Features
Acute maxillary sinusitis is often a complication of the common cold, which is accompanied by a clear nasal discharge or pharyngeal drainage. After a few days, the stuffiness and nasal discharge increase, and the patient may complain of pain and tenderness to pressure or swelling over the involved sinus. The pain may also be referred to the premolar and molar teeth on the affected side, and these teeth may also be sensitive to percussion, although this is more commonly seen in bacterial sinusitis. Under these conditions, a green or greenish yellow

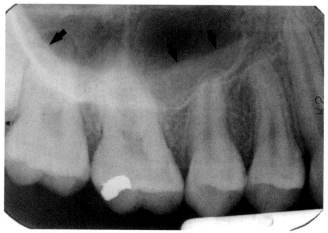

FIG. **27-5**  Thickened sinus mucosa is portrayed as a radiopaque band paralleling the contour of the maxillary antral floor.

nasal discharge may also be appreciated. This finding requires that the teeth be ruled out as a possible source of the pain or infection. However, the key signs and symptoms are those of sepsis: fever, chills, malaise, and an elevated leukocyte count. Acute sinusitis is the most common of the sinus conditions that cause pain.

Chronic maxillary sinusitis is typically a sequela of an acute infection that fails to resolve by 3 months. In general, no external signs occur, except during periods of acute exacerbations when increased pain and discomfort are apparent. Chronic sinusitis is often associated with anatomic derangements including deviation of the nasal septum and the presence of concha bullosa (pneumatization of the middle concha) that inhibit the outflow of mucus. Chronic sinusitis is also often associated with allergic rhinitis, asthma, cystic fibrosis, and dental infections.

### Radiographic Features

Thickening of sinus mucosa and the accumulation of secretions that accompany sinusitis reduce the air content of the sinus and cause it to become increasingly radiopaque. The most common radiopaque patterns that occur in the Waters view are localized mucosal thickening along the sinus floor, generalized thickening of the mucosal lining around the entire wall of the sinus, and near-complete or complete radiopacification of the sinus (Figs. 27-6 and 27-7). Such changes are best seen in the maxillary sinuses, but the frontal and sphenoid sinuses may be similarly affected. Scrutinizing the area around the maxillary ostium on any of the views from Waters projections to CT images may reveal the presence of thickened mucosal tissue, which may cause blockage of the ostium. Mucosal thickening in just the base of the sinus may not represent sinusitis. Rather, it may represent the more

localized thickening that can occur in association with rarefying osteitis from a tooth with a nonvital pulp. This may, however, progress to involve the entire sinus.

The image of thickened sinus mucosa on the radiograph may be uniform or polypoid. In the case of an allergic reaction, the mucosa tends to be more lobulated. In contrast, in cases of infection, the thickened mucosal outline tends to be smoother, with its contour following that of the sinus wall. The inability to perceive the delicate walls of the ethmoid air cells is a particularly sensitive sign of ethmoid sinusitis.

An air-fluid level resulting from the accumulation of secretions may also be present. Because the radiopacities of transudates, exudates, blood, and pathologically altered mucosa are similar, the differentiation among them relies on their shape and distribution. When present, fluid appears radiopaque and occupies the inferior aspect of the sinus. The border between the radiopaque fluid and the relatively radiolucent antrum is horizontal and straight, or with a meniscus (see

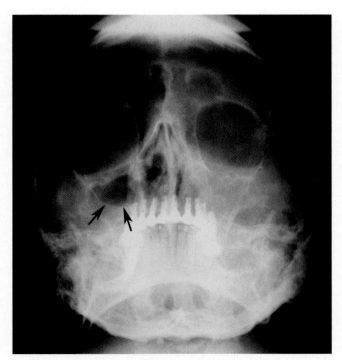

FIG. **27-6**  Waters view demonstrating complete radiopacification of the left maxillary and frontal sinuses, and ethmoid air cells. An air-fluid level is visible in the right maxillary sinus *(arrows)*.

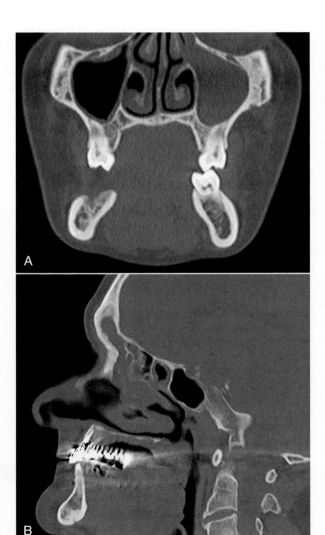

FIG. **27-7**  Coronal **(A)** view of the maxillary sinuses showing complete radiopacification of the left sinus and circumferential mucosal thickening of the right sinus, and sagittal **(B)** CT image of mucositis of the ethmoid air cells.

Fig. 27-6). It is possible to confirm that one is viewing an air-fluid interface by tilting the head and making another radiograph. This changes the orientation of the fluid level, which eliminates any doubt as to its fluid nature. However, when attempting to verify this, sufficient time should be allowed between the first and second exposures for the fluid level to change. If a significant proportion of the fluid is mucous, some minutes may be required before it attains its new level. To demonstrate an air-fluid level, the central ray of the x-ray beam must be horizontal and at the level of the air-fluid interface. Chronic sinusitis may result in persistent radiopacification of the sinus with sclerosis and thickening of the sinus wall (Fig. 27-8). Resorption of the bony border is unusual.

The resolution of acute sinusitis becomes apparent on the radiograph as a gradual increase in the radiolucency of the sinus. This can first be recognized when a small clear area appears in the interior of the sinus; the thickened mucous membrane gradually shrinks so that it begins to follow the outline of the bony wall. In time the mucous membrane again becomes radiographically invisible, and the sinus appears normal. In chronic sinusitis the inflammation may stimulate the sinus periosteum to produce bone, resulting in thick sclerotic borders of the maxillary antrum.

## Management

The goals of treatment of sinusitis are to control the infection, promote drainage, and relieve pain. Acute sinusitis is usually treated medically with decongestants to reduce mucosal swelling and with antibiotics in the case of a bacterial sinusitis. Chronic sinusitis is primarily a disease of obstruction of the ostia; thus the goal is ventilation and drainage. This is often accomplished through endoscopic surgery to enlarge obstructed ostia or by establishing an alternate path of drainage.

## Retention Pseudocyst

### Synonyms

Antral pseudocyst, benign mucous cyst, mucous retention cyst, mucous retention pseudocyst, mesothelial cyst, pseudocyst, interstitial cyst, lymphangiectatic cyst, false cyst, retention cyst of the maxillary sinus, benign cyst of the antrum, benign mucosal cyst of the sinus, serous nonsecretory retention pseudocyst, and mucosal antral cyst

### Definition

The term *retention pseudocyst* is used to describe several related conditions. The actual pathogenesis of these lesions is controversial; however, because their clinical and radiographic features are similar, no attempt is made here to distinguish them. One etiology suggests that blockage of the secretory ducts of seromucous glands in the sinus mucosa may result in a pathologic submucosal accumulation of secretions, resulting in swelling of the tissue. A second theory suggests that the serous nonsecretory retention cyst arises as a result of cystic degeneration within an inflamed, thickened sinus lining. Both types of lesions are called pseudocysts because they are not lined with epithelium.

### Clinical Features

Retention pseudocysts may be found in any of the sinuses at any time of the year but occur more often in the early spring or fall. This suggests that they might have to do with changes in seasonal temperatures or with heating or air conditioning in buildings. Most studies have found that the retention pseudocyst is more common in males.

The retention pseudocyst rarely causes any signs or symptoms, and thus the patient is usually unaware of the lesion. It often is noticed as an incidental finding on radiographs made for other purposes. However, when the pseudocyst completely fills the maxillary sinus cavity, it may prolapse (extrude) through the ostium and cause nasal obstruction and postnasal discharge. This may be the only clinical evidence of the presence of the pseudocyst. Because either type of retention pseudocyst may enlarge and fill a sinus cavity, it frequently ruptures as a result of abrupt pressure changes caused by sneezing or blowing of the nose. If this does not happen, the expanding pseudocyst may herniate through the ostium into the nasal cavity, where it subsequently ruptures. The pseudocyst may be present on radiographic examination of the maxillary sinus, perhaps absent only a few days later, only to reappear on subsequent examinations.

The maxillary sinus is the most common site of retention pseudocysts, although they are occasionally found in the frontal or sphenoid

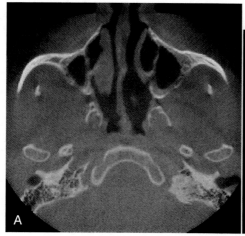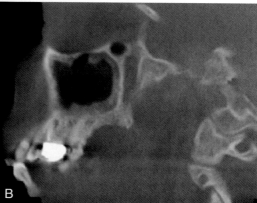

FIG. 27-8 Axial **(A)** and sagittal **(B)** cone-beam CT images show peripheral bony thickening of the left maxillary sinus from chronic sinusitis.

sinuses. Antral retention pseudocysts are not related to extractions or associated with periapical disease.

### Radiographic Features

*Location.* Partial images of retention pseudocysts of the maxillary antrum may appear on maxillary posterior periapical radiographs (Fig. 27-9, *A*), but they are best demonstrated in extraoral radiographs (Fig. 27-9, *B*). Although pseudocysts may occur bilaterally, usually only a single pseudocyst develops. Occasionally more than one pseudocyst may form in a single sinus. These pseudocysts usually form on the floor of the sinus (Fig. 27-9, *D*), although some may form on the lateral walls or the roof (Fig. 27-9, *C*). Retention pseudocysts may vary in size from that of a fingertip to completely filling the sinus and making it radiopaque.

*Periphery and Shape.* Retention pseudocysts usually appear as well-defined, noncorticated, smooth, dome-shaped radiopaque masses. Because the lesion originates within the sinus, no osseous border surrounds it. The base of the lesions may be narrow or more commonly broad.

*Internal Structure.* The internal aspect is homogeneous and more radiopaque than the surrounding air of the sinus cavity (see Fig. 27-9, *B*). The radiopacity of the lesion is caused by the accumulation of fluid and, as such, normal osseous landmarks may often be seen through its image.

*Effects on Surrounding Structures.* There are no effects on the surrounding structures, and thus it is of note that the sinus floor is intact. When a pseudocyst occurs adjacent to the root of a tooth, the lamina dura surrounding the root is intact and there is a normal width of the periodontal ligament space.

### Differential Diagnosis

It is important to distinguish retention pseudocysts from odontogenic cysts (for example, radicular or dentigerous cysts, or keratocysts), antral polyps, or any rounded neoplastic mass. This can usually be

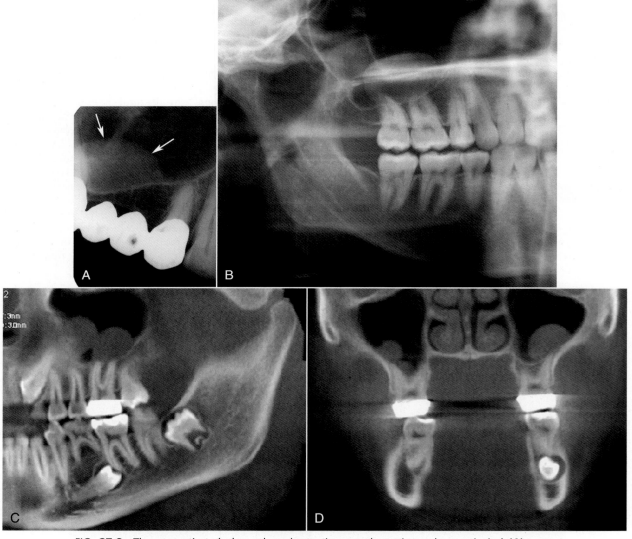

FIG. **27-9** The noncorticated, dome-shaped retention pseudocyst imaged on periapical **(A)**, panoramic **(B)** and reconstructed panoramic **(C)**, and coronal **(D)** cone-beam CT images. Retention pseudocysts have noncorticated borders, indicating that they arise from within the sinus.

done radiographically and by the patient's history. Commonly, the floor of the antrum is displaced by the odontogenic cyst, and the border of the cyst becomes coincident with the bony sinus floor. In some instances, periodic fenestrations can be seen through the bony sinus floor or cyst border. The retention pseudocyst is dome shaped but lacks the thin marginal radiopaque line representing the corticated border characteristic of the odontogenic cyst or tumor. The odontogenic cyst is also more rounded or tear drop shaped, and in the case of a radicular cyst, the lamina dura of the involved tooth or teeth is not intact in the apical area.

Antral polyps of infectious or allergic origin may be distinguished radiographically from a retention pseudocyst in that they are more often multiple. They are also commonly associated with a thickened mucous membrane, which is less frequently observed with retention pseudocysts.

Neoplasms may also mimic a retention pseudocyst. If they are benign and originating from outside the sinus, they are separated from the cavity of the sinus by a radiopaque border, similar to the odontogenic cysts. Malignant neoplasms may destroy the osseous border of the sinus, whether they arise from within the sinus or from the alveolar process. The neoplasm is, however, less likely to be as dome shaped as the retention pseudocyst.

### Management
Retention pseudocysts in the maxillary sinus usually require no treatment because they customarily resolve spontaneously without any residual effect on the antral mucosa.

### Polyps

### Definition
The thickened mucous membrane of a chronically inflamed sinus frequently forms into irregular folds called polyps. Polyposis of the sinus mucosa may develop in an isolated area or in a number of areas throughout the sinus.

### Clinical Features
Polyps may cause displacement or destruction of bone. In the ethmoid air cells, polyps may cause destruction of the medial wall of the orbit (lamina papyracea of the ethmoid bone) and a unilateral proptosis.

### Radiographic Features
A polyp may be differentiated from a retention pseudocyst on a radiograph by noting that a polyp usually occurs with a thickened mucous membrane lining because the polypoid mass is no more than an accentuation of the mucosal thickening. In the case of a retention pseudocyst, however, the adjacent mucous membrane lining is not usually apparent. If multiple retention pseudocysts are seen within a sinus, the possibility of sinus polyposis should be entertained.

The radiographic image of the bone displacement or destruction associated with polyps may mimic a benign or malignant neoplasm. Because many sinus neoplasms are asymptomatic, examination of a paranasal sinus that reveals bone destruction associated with radiopacification is an indication for biopsy and should not be delayed by initial conservative treatment.

### Antrolith

### Definition
Antroliths occur within the maxillary sinuses and are the result of deposition of mineral salts such as calcium phosphate, calcium carbonate, and magnesium around a nidus, which may be introduced into the sinus (extrinsic) or could be intrinsic such as masses of stagnant or inspissated mucous or cellular debris in sites of previous inflammation.

### Clinical Features
The smaller antroliths are usually asymptomatic and usually are discovered as incidental findings on radiographic examination. If they continue to grow, the patient may have associated sinusitis, blood-stained nasal discharge, nasal obstruction, or facial pain.

### Radiographic Features
*Location.* Antroliths occur within the maxillary sinus and thus are positioned above the floor of the maxillary antrum in either periapical or panoramic radiographs (Fig. 27-10).

*Periphery and Shape.* Antroliths have a well-defined periphery and may have a smooth or irregular shape.

*Internal Structure.* The internal aspect may vary in density from a barely perceptible radiopacity to an extremely radiopaque structure. The internal density may be homogenous or heterogeneous, and in

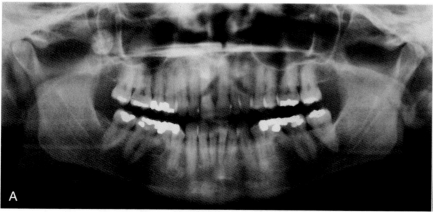
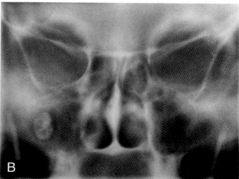

FIG. **27-10** The alternating circular radiopaque and radiolucent pattern of an antrolith is seen on a panoramic image **(A)** superimposed over the posterior wall of the right maxillary sinus. The coronal multidirectional tomographic image **(B)** confirms the location of the antrolith within the sinus and, furthermore, shows the antrolith not to be attached to the adjacent sinus wall.

some instances alternating layers of radiolucency and radiopacity in the form of laminations may be seen.

## Differential Diagnosis

Antroliths may be distinguished from root fragments in the sinus by inspection of the mass for the usual root anatomy such as the presence of a root canal. A displaced root fragment in the sinus may move when radiography is performed with the head in different positions, unless it is lodged between the bone and the sinus lining. Rhinoliths are similar calcifications but are found within the nasal fossae. Postero-anterior and lateral skull views help identify the location of a rhinolith.

## Management

An otolaryngologist may need to remove symptomatic antroliths.

## Mucocele

### Synonyms
Pyocele and mucopyocele

### Definition

A mucocele is an expanding, destructive lesion that results from a blocked sinus ostium. The blockage may result from intra-antral or intranasal inflammation, polyp, or neoplasm. The entire sinus thus becomes the pathologic cavity. As mucous secretions accumulate and the sinus cavity fills, the increase in intra-antral pressure results in thinning, displacement, and, in some cases, destruction of the sinus walls. When the cavity is filled with pus, it is termed an *empyema, pyocele,* or *mucopyocele.*

### Clinical Features

A mucocele in the maxillary sinus may exert pressure on the superior alveolar nerves and thus cause radiating pain. The patient may first complain of a sensation of fullness in the cheek, and the area may swell. This swelling may first become apparent over the anteroinferior aspect of the antrum, the area where the wall is thin, or destroyed. If the lesion expands inferiorly, it may cause loosening of the posterior teeth in the area. If the medial wall of the sinus is expanded, the lateral wall of the nasal cavity will deform and the nasal airway may be obstructed. Should it expand into the orbit, it may cause diplopia (double vision) or proptosis (protrusion of the globe of the eye).

## Radiographic Features

*Location.* About 90% of mucoceles occur in the ethmoid air cells and frontal sinuses and rarely in the maxillary and sphenoid sinuses.

*Periphery and Shape.* The normal shape of the sinus is changed into a more circular, "hydraulic" shape as the mucocele enlarges.

*Internal Structure.* The internal aspect of the sinus cavity is uniformly radiopaque (Fig. 27-11, *A*).

*Effects on Surrounding Structures.* The shape of the sinus changes as its margins are displaced outward and the bone expands. Septa and the bony walls may be severely thinned. When the mucocele is associated with the maxillary antrum, teeth may be displaced or roots resorbed. In the frontal sinus the usually scalloped border is smoothed by expansion, and the intersinus septum may be displaced (Fig. 27-11, *B*). The supramedial border of the orbit may be displaced or destroyed. In the ethmoid air cells, displacement of the lamina papyracea may occur, displacing the contents of the orbit. In the sphenoid sinus the expansion may be in a superior direction, suggesting a pituitary neoplasm.

## Differential Diagnosis

Although it may not be possible to distinguish between a mucocele in the maxillary antrum and a cyst or neoplasm, any suggestion that the lesion is associated with an occluded ostium should strengthen the likelihood of a mucocele. Blockage of the ostium is usually the result of a previous surgical procedure, although a deviated nasal septum or polyps may be a factor. A large odontogenic cyst displacing the maxillary antral floor may mimic a mucocele. Look for any remnants of the internal aspect of the antrum between the wall of the cyst and the wall of the antrum. CT is the imaging method of choice for making these distinctions.

## Management

Treatment of the mucocele is usually surgical, with a Caldwell-Luc operation to allow excision of the lesion. The prognosis is excellent.

## Neoplasms

Benign neoplasms of the paranasal sinuses other than inflammatory polyps are rare. The radiographic images of such benign neoplasms are nonspecific. Usually the involved portion of the sinus appears

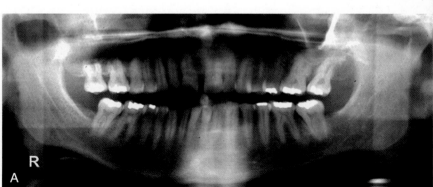
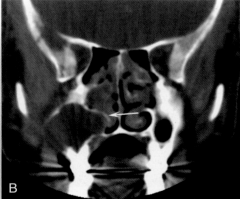

FIG. **27-11** A mucocele has caused the radiopacification of the right maxillary sinus. Note the lack of a distinct border to the sinus on the panoramic image **(A).** A coronal CT image **(B)** through the mucocele shows expansion into the nasal fossa *(arrow)* and the infratemporal fossa.

radiopaque because of the presence of a mass, and there may be displacement of adjacent sinus borders.

The most common malignant neoplasms of the paranasal sinuses are squamous cell carcinomas and, to a lesser extent, malignant salivary gland neoplasms. Of carcinomas of the paranasal sinuses, 74% originate in the maxillary sinus. Although radiopacification is a feature of both the inflammatory conditions and neoplasms, bone destruction is more common with malignant neoplasms.

## BENIGN NEOPLASMS OF THE PARANASAL SINUSES

### Papilloma

#### Definition
The epithelial papilloma is a rare neoplasm of respiratory epithelium that occurs in the nasal cavity and paranasal sinuses. It occurs predominantly in men.

#### Clinical Features
Unilateral nasal obstruction, nasal discharge, pain, and epistaxis may occur. The patient may have complained of recurring sinusitis for years and a subsequent nasal obstruction on the same side as the sinusitis. The epithelial papilloma, although benign, has a 10% incidence of associated carcinoma.

#### Radiographic Features
The features may not be specific, and the diagnosis can be made only by histopathologic examination of the tissue.
*Location.* The epithelial papilloma is usually in the ethmoidal or maxillary sinus. It may also appear as an isolated polyp in the nose or sinus.
*Internal Structure.* This neoplasm appears as a homogeneous radiopaque mass of soft tissue density.
*Effects on Surrounding Structures.* If bone destruction is apparent, it is the result of pressure erosion.

### Osteoma

#### Definition
The osteoma is the most common of the mesenchymal neoplasms in the paranasal sinuses. For a detailed description, see Chapter 22.

#### Clinical Features
Osteomas are almost twice as common in males as females and are most common in the second, third, and fourth decades. Most are usually slow growing and asymptomatic and thus are usually detected as an incidental finding in an examination made for another purpose. When symptoms do occur, they are the result of obstruction of the sinus ostium or infundibulum or are the result of erosion or deformity, orbital involvement, or intracranial extension. Those growing in the maxillary sinus may extend into the nose and cause nasal obstruction or a swelling of the side of the nose. They may expand the sinus and produce swelling of the cheek or hard palate. In cases extending to the orbit, the patient may have proptosis. In some cases, external fistulae have occurred. Osteomas of the maxillary sinus have been described after Caldwell-Luc operations.

#### Radiographic Features
*Location.* Although osteomas occasionally develop in the maxillary sinus, they more often occur in the frontal and ethmoidal sinuses.

The incidence in the maxillary antrum varies between 3.9% and 28.5% of the incidence in all paranasal sinuses.
*Periphery and Shape.* The osteoma is usually lobulated or rounded and has a sharply defined margin (Fig. 27-12).
*Internal Structure.* The internal aspect is homogeneous and extremely radiopaque.

#### Differential Diagnosis
The differential diagnosis includes antrolith, mycolith, teeth, odontomas, or odontogenic neoplasms, although these are all usually not as homogeneous in appearance as the osteoma.

## MALIGNANT NEOPLASMS OF THE PARANASAL SINUSES

Malignant neoplasms of the paranasal sinuses are rare, accounting for less than 1% of all malignancies in the body. Squamous cell carcinoma, comprising 80% to 90% of the cancers in this site, is by far the most common primary malignant neoplasm of the paranasal sinuses. Other primary neoplasms include adenocarcinoma, carcinomas of salivary gland origin, soft and hard tissue sarcomas, melanoma, and malignant lymphoma. Factors that contribute to a poor prognosis for cancer of the paranasal sinuses include the advanced stage of the disease when it is finally diagnosed and the close proximity of vital anatomic structures. The clinical signs and symptoms may masquerade as an inflammatory sinusitis. The early primary lesions may only appear as a soft tissue mass in the sinus before they cause bone destruction. The lesion may become extensive, involving the entire sinus, with radiographic evidence of bone destruction before symptoms become apparent. Therefore any unexplained radiopacity in the maxillary sinus of an individual older than 40 years should be investigated thoroughly.

### Squamous Cell Carcinoma

#### Definition
Squamous cell carcinoma likely originates from metaplastic epithelium of the sinus mucosal lining.

#### Clinical Features
The most common symptoms of cancer in the maxillary sinus are facial pain or swelling, nasal obstruction, and a lesion in the oral cavity. The mean age of the patient is 60 years (range, 25 to 89 years). Twice as many men as women are affected. Lymph nodes are involved in about 10% of cases, and the symptoms are present for about 5 months before diagnosis.

The symptoms produced by malignant neoplasms in the maxillary sinus depend on which wall(s) of the sinus is/are involved. The medial wall is usually the first to become eroded, leading to such nasal signs and symptoms as obstruction, discharge, bleeding, and pain. These symptoms may appear trivial, and their significance may not be appreciated. Lesions that arise on the floor of the sinus may first produce dental signs and symptoms, including expansion of the alveolar process, unexplained pain and altered sensation of the teeth, loose teeth, swelling of the palate or alveolar ridge, and ill-fitting dentures. The neoplasm may erode the sinus floor and penetrate into the oral cavity. Such oral manifestations appear in 25% to 35% of patients with cancer in the maxillary sinus. When the lesion penetrates the lateral wall, facial and vestibular swelling becomes apparent and the patient may complain of pain and hyperesthesia of the maxillary teeth. Involvement of the sinus roof and the floor of the orbit cause

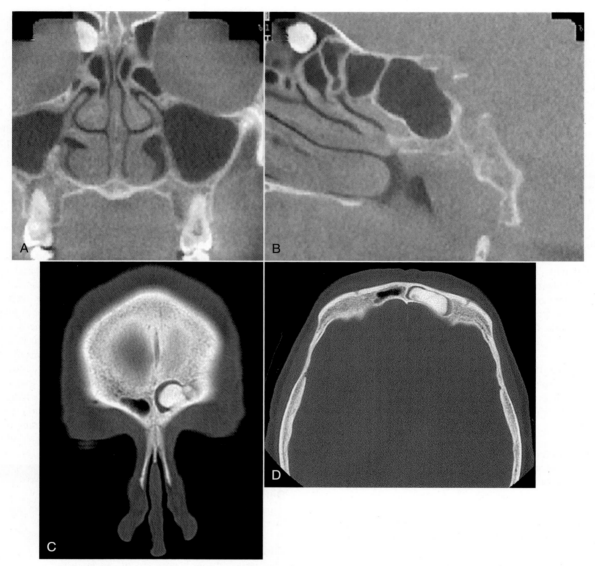

FIG. **27-12** Coronal **(A)** and sagittal **(B)** cone-beam CT images show an osteoma attached to the lateral wall of an anterior ethmoid air cell and coronal **(C)** and axial **(D)** CT images of an osteoma in the frontal sinus. (Courtesy Dr. Eugene Yu, Princess Margaret Hospital.)

signs and symptoms related to the eye: diplopia, proptosis, pain, and hyperesthesia or anesthesia and pain over the cheek and upper teeth. Invasion and penetration of the posterior wall lead to invasion of the muscles of mastication, causing painful trismus, obstruction of the eustachian tube causing a stuffy ear, and referred pain and hyperesthesia over the distribution of the second and third divisions of the fifth nerve.

### Radiographic Features

Sometimes the radiographic findings, especially in early malignant disease of the paranasal sinuses, are nonspecific. It may not be possible to differentiate the early manifestations in radiographs of the maxillary sinus from the radiopacity of the sinus that develops in sinusitis and polyp formation. Evidence relies on changes seen in the surrounding bone, the sinus walls, and the maxillary alveolar process.

*Location.* Most carcinomas occur in the maxillary sinuses, but involvement of the frontal and sphenoid sinuses is also comparatively common.

*Internal Structure.* The internal aspect of the maxillary sinus has a soft tissue radiopaque appearance.

*Effects on Surrounding Structures.* As the lesion enlarges, it may destroy sinus walls and in general, cause irregular radiolucent areas in the surrounding bone. A detailed examination of the adjacent alveolar process may reveal bone destruction around the teeth or irregular widening of the periodontal ligament space. Frequently the medial wall of the maxillary sinus is thinned or destroyed, although there may also be destruction of the floor and anterior or posterior walls that may be detected in the panoramic film. The medial wall of the maxillary sinus is best seen on the Caldwell and Waters projections. In addition to loss of the medial wall, it may extend into the nasal cavity.

### Additional Imaging

If a conventional radiograph of any radiopacified sinus reveals the slightest suggestion of bone destruction, advanced imaging is imperative (Fig. 27-13). On CT, the most characteristic sign of malignancy is invasion into the soft tissue facial planes beyond the sinus walls (Fig. 27-14). Consequently, CT is useful in revealing the extent of paranasal sinus neoplasms, especially when extension into the orbit, infratemporal fossa, or cranial cavity has occurred. MRI examinations are excellent for revealing the extent of soft tissue penetration into adjacent structures and in differentiating mucus accumulation from the soft tissue mass of the neoplasm.

### Differential Diagnosis

The differential diagnosis includes all the conditions that may cause radiopacity of the antrum, such as sinusitis, large retention pseudocysts, and odontogenic cysts. It is important to note that bone destruction may also occur in infectious and some benign conditions. Neoplasms should be suspected in any older patient in whom chronic sinusitis develops for the first time without an obvious cause.

### Management

Treatment of squamous cell carcinoma in the paranasal sinuses generally combines surgery and radiation therapy. Malignant neoplasms in the paranasal sinuses usually have a poor prognosis because they are usually well advanced by the time of diagnosis. Other factors contributing to the poor prognosis include frequently inaccurate preoperative staging and the complex anatomy of the region.

## Pseudotumor

### Synonyms

Invasive fungal sinusitis, inflammatory pseudotumor, fibroinflammatory pseudotumor, plasma cell granuloma, sinonasal fungal disease, mucormycosis, aspergillosis, zygomycosis of the paranasal sinuses, and *Rhizopus* sinusitis

### Definition

Pseudotumor is a descriptive name for a group of apparently related diseases of fungal origin that occur in the paranasal sinuses and in other parts of the head and neck.

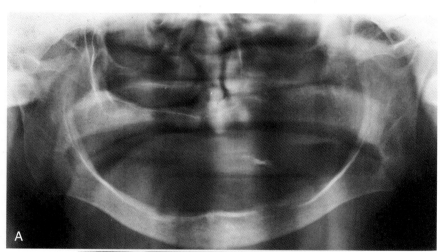

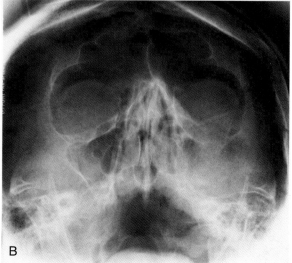

FIG. **27-13   A,** This panoramic image of a squamous cell carcinoma shows a loss of definition of the cortex of the left maxillary sinus, nasal floor, and alveolar crest. **B,** The Waters view of the same patient shows a similar loss of cortical integrity to the lateral wall of the left maxilla and radiopacification of the left maxillary sinus. (Courtesy Dr. K. Dolan.)

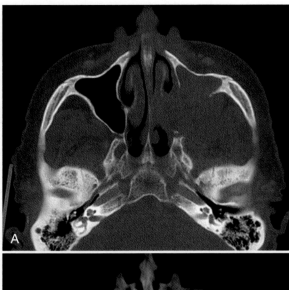

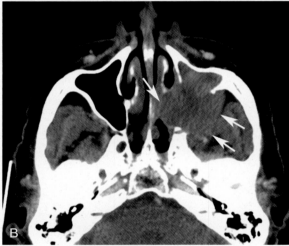

FIG. **27-14** **A,** This axial bone algorithm CT image of a squamous cell carcinoma of the left maxillary sinus shows destruction of the posterolateral wall and the medial wall of the sinus. **B,** The same axial image slice with soft tissue algorithm demonstrates extension of the malignant tumor into the surrounding soft tissues *(arrows)*.

### Clinical Features

Pseudotumor often occurs after a series of recurrent infections. The symptoms may not be very specific. There may be recurring pain and a mass simulating a neoplasm. The latter may cause erosion of the walls of the involved sinus and proptosis if the orbit is involved. Altered nerve function resulting from involvement of the nerve or occlusion of blood vessels by the mass has also been reported. Although cases have been reported in otherwise healthy individuals, many cases appear in patients who are immunocompromised or who have systemic diseases such as diabetes mellitus, von Willebrand disease, or myelodysplasia.

### Radiographic Features

The radiographic findings in pseudotumor include masses simulating malignant neoplasms that cause erosion of bony walls of the involved sinuses.

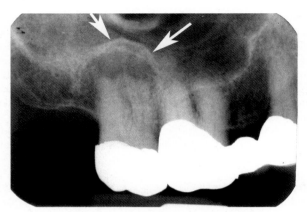

FIG. **27-15** The halolike appearance of bone surrounding the roots of a maxillary second molar is the result of periosteal new bone formation and displacement of the adjacent maxillary sinus floor *(arrows)*.

### Differential Diagnosis

The differential diagnosis includes benign and malignant neoplasms.

### Management

The treatment of pseudotumor, which can include debridement of the sinuses and administration of antifungal medication, a Caldwell-Luc surgical approach, and therapy, reflects the differences in the specific lesions included under the term pseudotumor of the sinuses, the exact location of the disease, the organism involved, and the medical status of the patient.

## Extrinsic Diseases Involving the Paranasal Sinuses

### INFLAMMATORY DISEASES

Dental inflammatory lesions such as periodontal disease or rarefying or sclerosing osteitis may cause a localized mucositis in the adjacent floor of the maxillary antrum. This is a result of the diffusion of inflammatory exudate (mediators) beyond the cortical floor of the antrum and into the periosteum and the mucosal lining of the sinus. The localized type of mucositis related to dental inflammatory disease usually resolves in days or weeks after successful treatment of the underlying cause.

### Radiographic Features

The involved mucosa presents as a homogeneous radiopaque, ribbon-shaped shadow that follows the contour of the floor of the maxillary sinus (see Fig. 27-5). The thickened mucosa is usually centered directly above the inflammatory lesion.

## Periostitis

### Definition

As previously described, the exudate from dental inflammatory lesions can diffuse through the cortical boundary of the antral floor. These products can strip and elevate the periosteal lining of the cortical bone of the floor of the maxillary antrum, stimulating the periosteum to produce an elevated thin layer of new bone adjacent to the root apex of the involved tooth (Fig. 27-15). The presence of one or more halolike layer(s) of new bone indicates inflammation of the periosteum.

### Radiographic Features

Although the periosteal tissue is not visible on the radiograph per se, this is referred to as periosteal new bone formation. This new bone may take the form of one or more thin radiopaque lines, or the line may be very thick. This new bone should be centered directly above the inflammatory lesion.

## BENIGN ODONTOGENIC CYSTS AND TUMORS

### Odontogenic Cysts

Odontogenic cysts are the most common group of extrinsic lesions that encroach on the maxillary sinuses. The most common are radicular cysts, followed by dentigerous cysts and odontogenic keratocysts (see Chapter 21 for detailed descriptions). As the odontogenic cyst grows, its border becomes indistinguishable from the sinus border. With continued growth, the cyst encroaches on the space of the sinus, displaces its borders, and the air-filled space decreases in volume (Fig. 27-16). A thin radiopaque line divides the contents of the cyst from the sinus cavity. This appearance is in contrast to a retention pseudocyst, which, being inside the sinus, does not have a cortex around its periphery.

### Radiographic Features

*Periphery and Shape.* The invaginating cyst has a curved or oval shape defined by a corticated border.

*Internal Structure.* The internal structure of the cyst is homogeneous and radiopaque relative to the air-filled sinus cavity. The degree of radiopacity may appear to be that of bone resulting from the extreme contrast to the radiolucent air within the sinus.

*Effects on Surrounding Structures.* The cyst may displace the floor of the maxillary antrum. Large dentigerous or odontogenic keratocysts can displace third molars as far as the floor of the orbit. In some cases the cyst may enlarge to the point that it has encroached on almost the entire sinus, and the residual sinus space may appear as a thin crescent of air adjacent to the cyst (see Fig. 27-16, *B*).

### Differential Diagnosis

Odontogenic cysts must be differentiated from the relatively common retention pseudocyst. Although both lesions may have similar shapes, only odontogenic cysts have a cortex at the periphery (Fig. 27-17). If the odontogenic cyst were to become infected, the cortex may be thickened or lost in some areas. In the latter instance, it may become difficult to determine whether the lesion has arisen from outside or from within the sinus. However, in most cases careful scrutiny of the lesion will reveal some remaining cyst cortex. Also, the relationship to neighboring teeth may help to make this decision. This is true for all odontogenic cysts, including radicular cysts, dentigerous cysts, and keratocysts (Fig. 27-18). It is not usually possible to differentiate a dentigerous cyst from an odontogenic keratocyst that has a pericoronal relationship to the third molar. Very large cysts may completely efface the sinus cavity. When this occurs, no radiographic evidence may exist of the air space left, and it may appear as if the cyst is within the sinus. In this case, because of the radiopacity of the cyst, the appearance may resemble sinusitis with radiopacification of the sinus. Evaluation of such conditions is aided by noting that the wall of the cyst is often thicker and more regular than that of a sinus. In addition, the normal vascular markings on the wall of the maxillary sinus are not present on the walls of a cyst. A cyst that occupies the entire sinus usually causes expansion of the medial wall (middle meatus) of the sinus and will alter the sigmoid contour of the posterolateral wall of the sinus as viewed in axial CT images.

An antral loculation may occasionally have a round shape and sometimes appear to have a cortex. However, because the loculation contains air, which is more radiolucent than the fluid within a cyst, the loculation appears more radiolucent than the surrounding antrum.

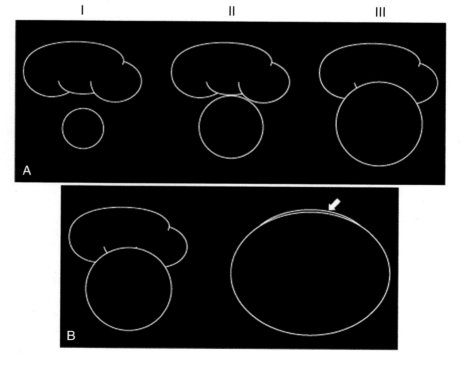

FIG. **27-16 A,** An odontogenic cyst or tumor develops adjacent to the floor of a sinus (*I*). As the lesion enlarges, it abuts the maxillary sinus floor (*II*) and ultimately displaces the floor superiorly as it enlarges (*III*). The border of the cyst and the border of the sinus are now the same line of bone. **B,** The lesion, as it continues to enlarge, may encroach on almost all the space of the sinus, leaving a small saddlelike sinus over it (*arrow*). The appearance may mimic sinusitis.

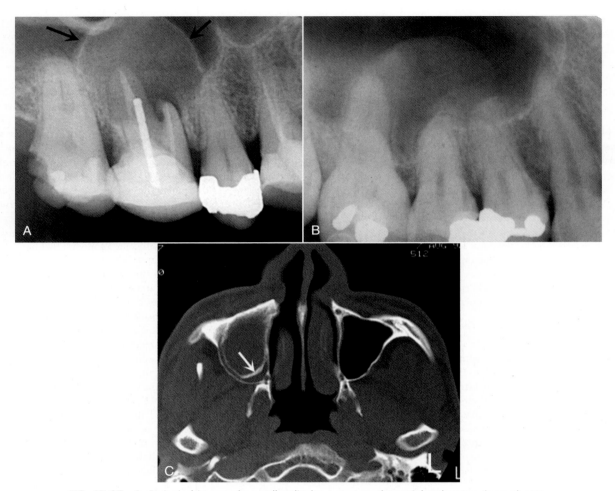

FIG. **27-17   A,** Periapical image of a small radicular cyst; note the peripheral cortex *(arrows)* compared with **B,** a periapical image of a pseudocyst; note the lack of a peripheral cortex. **C,** Axial CT image of a large radicular cyst; note the peripheral cortex *(arrow)* inside the outer cortex of the sinus.

After the successful treatment of an odontogenic lesion in the maxilla, healing will ensue in the affected area. This may include "collapse" of the bony cavity and remodeling of the sinus floor. The end result is the appearance of an irregularly shaped bone formation along the floor of the sinus.

### Odontogenic Tumors

Generally, benign odontogenic tumors can cause facial deformity, nasal obstruction, and displacement or loosening of teeth. For detailed descriptions of specific tumors, see Chapter 22. The nature of bony barriers in this region of the face, and the relatively good blood supply, are probably also responsible for efficient local spread. Some odontogenic tumors, particularly the ameloblastoma and the myxoma, show a more aggressive pattern of growth in the maxilla and have a close proximity to vital structures in the skull base. Therefore management of such tumors in the maxillae is often more aggressive than in cases involving the mandible.

#### Radiographic Features
***Periphery and Shape.*** The enlarging tumor may have a curved, oval, or multilocular shape that may be defined by a thin cortical border as it encroaches on the sinus. More aggressively growing tumors may even lack a portion of the border.

***Internal Structure.*** The internal structure of the tumor may have coarse or fine septae or regions of dystrophic calcification, depending on the histopathologic nature of the tumor.

***Effects on Surrounding Structures.*** The tumor may displace the floor of the maxillary antrum and cause thinning of the peripheral cortex. As with odontogenic cysts, in some cases the tumor may enlarge to the point where it has almost completely encroached on the sinus air space, and this residual space may appear as a thin saddle over the tumor.

The bony walls of the sinus may be thinned or eroded, and adjacent structures may be displaced. A tooth or part of a tooth may be embedded in the neoplasm.

## FIBROUS DYSPLASIA

Fibrous dysplasia may arise adjacent to any of the paranasal sinuses, cause displacement of sinus borders, and result in a smaller sinus on the affected side. For a detailed description of fibrous dysplasia, see Chapter 24.

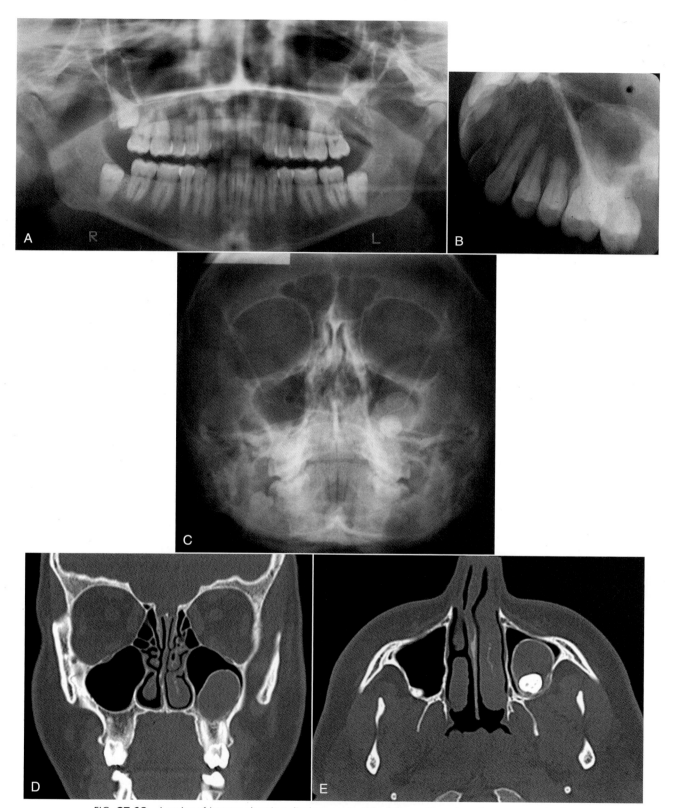

FIG. **27-18**   A series of images showing displacement of the left maxillary sinus floor as a result of a developing dentigerous cyst associated with the maxillary left third molar. The corticated periphery of the cyst is well seen in the panoramic, occlusal, and Waters images (**A, B,** and **C**). The coronal CT image (**D**) shows the displaced floor of the left maxillary sinus, and the axial image (**E**) shows the bowing of the posterior sinus wall and the impacted tooth adjacent to it.

## Clinical Features

The involvement of the facial skeleton with fibrous dysplasia can result in facial asymmetry, nasal obstruction, proptosis, pituitary gland compression, impingement on cranial nerves, or sinus obliteration. Sinus obliteration results when the expanding dysplastic bone encroaches on it. The lesion may displace the roots of teeth and cause teeth to separate or migrate, but it usually does not cause root resorption. Fibrous dysplasia is more common in children and young adults, and growth of the dysplastic bone usually ceases at the age of skeletal maturity.

## Radiographic Features

*Location.* The posterior maxilla is the most common location for fibrous dysplasia.

*Periphery.* The lesion itself is usually not well defined, tending to blend into the surrounding bone. The external cortex of the bone as well as the sinus floor is intact but displaced.

*Internal Structure.* The normal radiolucent maxillary antrum may be partially or totally replaced by the increased radiopacity of this lesion. The degree of radiopacity depends on its stage of development and the relative amounts of bone and fibrous tissue present. Usually the radiopaque areas have the characteristic "ground-glass" appearance on extraoral radiographs or an "orange-peel" appearance on intraoral views (Fig. 27-19).

*Effects on Surrounding Structures.* Fibrous dysplasia may replace most of the sinus by encroaching on and displacing the antral walls, elevating the orbital floor, or obstructing the nasal fossa.

## Differential Diagnosis

The diagnosis of fibrous dysplasia in a relatively young person is usually not difficult. In contrast, Paget's disease of bone does not usually obliterate the sinus. Ossifying fibroma, which may have an appearance that is similar to that of fibrous dysplasia, may also have a soft tissue capsule and may be more expansile. In some cases, however, the differential diagnosis of ossifying fibroma involving the antrum and fibrous dysplasia can be extremely difficult. The shape of the new bone encroaching on the internal aspect of the antrum often parallels the original shape of the external walls of the antrum in fibrous dysplasia.

## DENTAL STRUCTURES DISPLACED INTO THE SINUSES

### Definition

Tooth roots may be fractured from various forms of trauma, including iatrogenic causes. They may be displaced into the sinus during extraction or subsequent attempts to retrieve them.

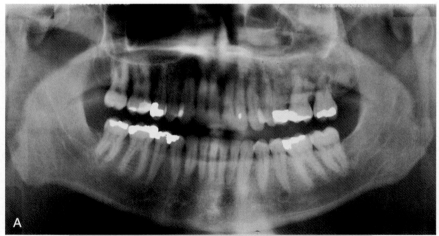

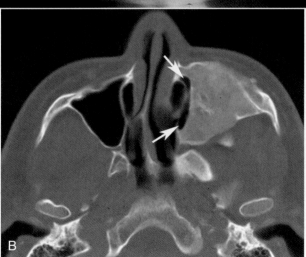

FIG. **27-19** **A,** Panoramic image of involvement of the left maxillary sinus with fibrous dysplasia; note the radiopacification of the left maxillary sinus compared with the right sinus. **B,** Axial CT image of the same case revealing almost complete filling of the sinus; a small medial segment remains *(arrows)*. Note the very fine homogeneous bone pattern of the fibrous dysplasia.

## Clinical Features

No specific features may be visible if the root was displaced into the sinus recently. However, the dentist may note the absence of the root fragment on examining the extracted tooth and may be unable to locate it anywhere else. Sometimes asking the patient to hold his or her nose while attempting to breathe out through it, similar to a Valsalva maneuver, will cause bubbles to appear within the blood contained within the fresh extraction socket.

If the patient has had the root or tooth in the sinus for a number of days, the presenting symptom may be sinusitis (see the previous discussion on sinusitis).

## Radiographic Features

*Location.* Premolar or molar teeth or root fragments may be displaced into the sinus because of their proximity. These may be found anywhere within the sinus, but more often they are located near the floor of the sinus because of gravity. Sometimes they may be submucosal, between the osseous wall of the sinus and the periosteum.

Lateral maxillary occlusal views are useful for examining the maxillary sinus for displaced teeth or root fragments. Other radiographs made along a different projection axis, such as a Waters view, may help in the three-dimensional localization.

*Periphery and Shape.* No immediate evidence of change may be appreciated in the sinus, even when an oroantral fistula has been created. The disruption of the sinus wall may be difficult or impossible to see on radiographs if it is not in the mesial, distal, or superior (apical) part of the alveolar process.

*Internal Structure.* In the early stages, no internal structural changes are present, except that the dental fragment may appear as a radiopaque mass of a size corresponding to the missing tooth or tooth root fragment.

*Effects on Surrounding Structures.* The dental fragment usually has no effect on surrounding structures; however, a sinusitis may result (see changes described earlier in this chapter under sinusitis). A break in the floor of the maxillary sinus caused by the displacement of the tooth or fragment into the sinus may be present but difficult to appreciate.

## Differential Diagnosis

Bony masses that are exostoses of the sinus wall or floor or septae within the sinus may mimic dental root fragments or even whole teeth. Antroliths may also have a similar appearance. The shape of the radiopacity or the presence of a pulp canal or layer of enamel may help in the differential diagnosis. It may also be possible to displace the tooth fragment by having the patient move the head abruptly between views. If the root tip remains in its socket, it may be superimposed radiographically over the maxillary sinus, but the presence of a lamina dura and periodontal ligament space indicate a position within the alveolar process.

The displaced tooth or root fragment may be subperiosteal, and thus interior to the osseous wall of the sinus, but not within the antral lumen. Alternatively, the root may have been forced out of the socket into the surrounding bone, into the submucosal space, or surrounding anatomic space such as the infratemporal space. Another possibility is for the fragment to be displaced into a cyst that was preoperatively mistaken for a loculus of the sinus cavity. Use of radiographs at different angles should help localize the dental structure.

## Management

Management ranges from following up the patient to see whether a small root tip will be removed from the sinus through the ostium by ciliary action to surgically entering the sinus by a Caldwell-Luc procedure to remove the dental structure. Sinusitis may develop and should be managed with the appropriate treatment.

For other trauma involving the paranasal sinuses, see Chapter 29.

# SUGGESTED READINGS

## NORMAL DEVELOPMENT AND VARIATIONS

Dodd GD, Jing BS: *Radiology of the nose, paranasal sinus and nasopharynx,* Baltimore, 1977, Williams & Wilkins.

DuBrul EL: *Sicher's oral anatomy,* ed 7, St. Louis, 1980, Mosby.

Grant JCB: *A method of anatomy,* Baltimore, 1958, Williams & Wilkins.

Hengerer AS: Embryonic development of the sinuses, *Ear Nose Throat J* 63:134-136, 1984.

Karmody CS, Carter B, Vincent ME: Developmental anomalies of the maxillary sinus, *Trans Sect Otolaryngol Am Acad Ophthalmol Otolaryngol* 84:723-728, 1977.

Lusted LB, Keats TE: *Atlas of roentgenographic measurement,* ed 3, Chicago, 1972, Year Book Medical Publishers.

Ritter FN: *The paranasal sinuses: anatomy and surgical technique,* St. Louis, 1973, Mosby.

Scuderi AJ, Harnsberger HR, Boyer RS: Pneumatization of the paranasal sinuses: normal features of importance to the accurate interpretation of CT scans and MR images, *AJR Am J Roentgenol* 160:1101-1104, 1993.

Shapiro R: *Radiology of the normal skull,* Chicago, 1981, Year Book Medical Publishers.

Som PM: The paranasal sinuses. In Bergeron RT, Osborn AG, Som PM, editors: *Head and neck imaging: excluding the brain,* St. Louis, 1984, Mosby.

Takahashi R: The formation of the human paranasal sinuses, *Acta Otolaryngol Suppl (Stockh)* 408:1-28, 1984.

## APPLIED DIAGNOSTIC IMAGING

Lloyd GA: Diagnostic imaging of the nose and paranasal sinuses, *J Laryngol Otol* 103:453-460, 1989.

Zinreich SJ: Imaging of chronic sinusitis in adults: x-ray, computed tomography, and magnetic resonance imaging, *J Allergy Clin Immunol* 90:445-451, 1992.

## INFLAMMATORY CHANGES

Robinson K: Roentgenographic manifestations of benign paranasal disease, *Ear Nose Throat J* 63:144, 1984.

## THICKENED MUCOUS MEMBRANE

### Mucositis

Dolan K, Smoker W: Paranasal sinus radiology, Part 4A: maxillary sinuses, *Head Neck Surg* 5:345-362, 1983.

Killey HC, Kay LA: *The maxillary sinus and its dental implications,* Bristol, 1975, John Wright.

## PERIOSTITIS

### Sinusitis

Druce HM: Diagnosis and medical management of recurrent and chronic sinusitis in adults. In Gershwin ME, Incaudo GA, editors: *Diseases of the sinuses,* Ottawa, Canada, 1996, Humana Press.

Fireman P: Diagnosis of sinusitis in children: emphasis on the history and physical examination, *J Allergy Clin Immunol* 90:433-436, 1992.

Incaudo G, Gershwin ME, Nagy SM: The pathophysiology and treatment of sinusitis, *Allergol Immunopathol (Madr)* 14:423-434, 1986.

Kennedy DW: First-line management of sinusitis: a national problem? Surgical update, *Otolaryngol Head Neck Surg* 103:884-886, 1990.

Killey HC, Kay LA: *The maxillary sinus and its dental implications,* Bristol, 1975, John Wright.

Palacios E, Valvassori G: Computed axial tomography in otorhinolaryngology, *Adv Otorhinolaryngol* 24:1-8, 1978.

Paparella MM: Mucosal cyst of the maxillary sinus, *Arch Otolaryngol* 77: 650-670, 1963.

Poyton HG: Maxillary sinuses and the oral radiologist, *Dent Radiogr Photogr* 45:43-50, 1972.

Reilly JS: The sinusitis cycle, *Otolaryngol Head Neck Surg* 103:856-861, 1990.

Shapiro GG, Rachelefsky GS: Introduction and definition of sinusitis, *J Allergy Clin Immunol* 90:417-418, 1992.

Zinreich SJ: Imaging of chronic sinusitis in adults: x-ray, computed tomography, and magnetic resonance imaging, *J Allergy Clin Immunol* 90:445-451, 1992.

### EMPYEMA

Ash JE, Raum M: *An atlas of otolaryngic pathology,* New York, 1956, American Registry of Pathology.

Groves J, Gray RF: *A synopsis of otolaryngology,* Bristol, 1985, John Wright.

### POLYPS

Potter GD: Inflammatory disease of the paranasal sinuses. In Valvassori GE, Potter GD, Hanefee WN, editors: *Radiology of the ear, nose and throat,* Philadelphia, 1982, WB Saunders.

### RETENTION PSEUDOCYSTS

Allard RH, van der Kwast WA, van der Waal JI: Mucosal antral cysts: review of the literature and report of a radiographic survey, *Oral Surg Oral Med Oral Pathol* 51:2-9, 1981.

Dolan K, Smoker W: Paranasal sinus radiology, Part 4A: maxillary sinuses, *Head Neck Surg* 5:345-362, 1983.

Gothberg K, Little JW, King DR et al: A clinical study of cysts arising from mucosa of the maxillary sinus, *Oral Surg* 41:52-58, 1976.

Hardy G: Benign cysts of the antrum, *Ann Otol Rhinol Laryngol* 48:649, 1939.

Kadymova MI: Lymphangiectatic (false) cysts of the maxillary sinuses and their relation with allergy, *Vestn Otorhinolaringol* 28:58, 1966.

Kaffe I, Littner MM, Moskona D: Mucosal-antral cysts: radiographic appearance and differential diagnosis, *Clin Prev Dent* 10:3-6, 1988.

McGregor GW: Formation and histologic structure of cysts of the maxillary sinus, *Arch Otolaryngol* 8:505, 1928.

Mills CP: Secretory cysts of the maxillary antrum and their relationship to the development of antrochoanal polypi, *J Laryngol Otol* 73:324-334, 1959.

Poyton HG: *Oral radiology,* Baltimore, 1982, Williams & Wilkins.

Ruprecht A, Batniji S, el-Neweihi E: Mucous retention cyst of the maxillary sinus, *Oral Surg Oral Med Oral Pathol* 62:728-731, 1986.

Shafer WG, Hine MK, Levy BM: *A textbook of oral pathology,* ed 4, Philadelphia, 1983, WB Saunders.

van Norstrand AWP, Goodman WS: Pathologic aspects of mucosal lesions of the maxillary sinus, *Otolaryngol Clin North Am* 9:21-34, 1976.

### MUCOCELE

Atherino C, Atherino T: Maxillary sinus mucopyoceles, *Arch Otolaryngol* 110:200, 1984.

Jones JL, Kaufman PW: Mucopyocele of the maxillary sinus, *J Oral Surg* 39:948, 1981.

Zizmor JK, Noyek AM: The radiologic diagnosis of maxillary sinus disease, *Otolaryngol Clin North Am* 9:93, 1976.

### ODONTOGENIC CYSTS

Killey HC, Kay LA: The maxillary sinus and its dental implications, Bristol, 1975, John Wright.

Poyton H: Maxillary sinuses and the oral radiologist, *Dent Radiogr Photogr* 45:43-50, 1972.

Van Alyea OE: *Nasal sinuses,* Baltimore, 1951, Williams & Wilkins.

### Odontogenic Keratocysts

MacDonald-Jankowski DS: The involvement of the maxillary antrum by odontogenic keratocysts, *Clin Radiol* 45:31-33, 1992.

### NEOPLASMS

Goepfert H, Luna MA, Lindberg RD et al: Malignant salivary gland tumors of the paranasal sinuses and nasal cavity, *Arch Otolaryngol* 109:662-668, 1983.

St-Pierre S, Baker SR: Squamous cell carcinoma of the maxillary sinus: analysis of 66 cases, *Head Neck Surg* 5:508-513, 1983.

### Epithelial Papilloma

Rogers JH, Fredrickson JM, Noyek AM: Management of cysts, benign tumors, and bony dysplasia of the maxillary sinus, *Otolaryngol Clin North Am* 9:233-247, 1976.

### Osteoma

Dolan K, Smoker W: Paranasal sinus radiology, Part 4B: maxillary sinuses, *Head Neck Surg* 5:428-446, 1983.

Goodnight J, Dulguerov P, Abemayor E: Calcified mucor fungus ball of the maxillary sinus, *Am J Otolaryngol* 14:209-210, 1993.

Reuben BM: Odontoma of the maxillary sinus: a case report, *Quintessence Int Dent Dig* 14:287-290, 1983.

Samy LL, Mostofa H: Osteoma of the nose and paranasal sinuses with a report of twenty-one cases, *J Laryngol Otol* 85:449-469, 1971.

### Ameloblastoma

Hames RS, Rakoff SJ: Diseases of the maxillary sinus, *J Oral Med* 27:90-95, 1972.

Reaume C, Wesley RK, Jung B et al: Ameloblastoma of the maxillary sinus, *J Oral Surg* 38:520-521, 1980.

### Malignant Neoplasms of the Paranasal Sinuses

Batsakis JG: *Tumors of the head and neck,* ed 2, Baltimore, 1979, Williams & Wilkins.

St-Pierre S, Baker S: Squamous cell carcinoma of the maxillary sinus: analysis of 66 cases, *Head Neck Surg* 5:508-513, 1983.

Zizmor J, Noyek AM: Cysts, benign tumors and malignant tumors of the paranasal sinuses, *Otolaryngol Clin North Am* 6:487-508, 1973.

### Squamous Cell Carcinoma

Batsakis JG, Rice DH, Solomon AR: The pathology of head and neck tumors: squamous and mucous-gland carcinomas of the nasal cavity, paranasal sinuses and larynx: part 6, *Head Neck Surg* 2:497-508, 1980.

Bridger M, Beale F, Bryce D: Carcinoma of the paranasal sinuses: a review of 158 cases, *J Otolaryngol* 7:379-388, 1978.

Eddleston B, Johnson R: A comparison of conventional radiographic imaging and computed tomography in malignant disease of the paranasal sinuses and the post-nasal space, *Clin Radiol* 34:161-172, 1983.

Haso AN: CT of tumors and tumor-like conditions of the paranasal sinuses, *Radiol Clin North Am* 22:119-130, 1984.

Larheim TA, Kolbenstvedt A, Lien H: Carcinoma of maxillary sinus, palate and maxillary gingiva, occurrence of jaw destruction, *Scand J Dent Res* 92:235-240, 1984.

Lund VJ, Howard DJ, Lloyd GA: CT evaluation of paranasal sinus tumors for cranio-facial resection, *Br J Radiol* 56:439-446, 1983.

Mancuso A, Hanafee WN, Winter J et al: Extensions of paranasal sinus tumors and inflammatory disease: an evaluation by CT and pluridirectional tomography, *Neuroradiology* 16:449-453, 1978.

St-Pierre S, Baker SR: Squamous cell carcinoma of the maxillary sinus: analysis of 66 cases, *Head Neck Surg* 5:508-513, 1983.

Thomas GK, Kasper KA: Ossifying fibroma of the frontal bone, *Arch Otolaryngol* 83:43-46, 1966.

Tsaknis PJ, Nelson JF: The maxillary ameloblastoma: an analysis of 24 cases, *J Oral Surg* 38:336-342, 1980.

Weber A, Tadmore R, Davis R et al: Malignant tumors of the sinuses: radiologic evaluation, including CT scanning, with clinical and pathologic correlation, *Neuroradiology* 16:443-448, 1978.

*Pseudotumor*

Butugan O, Sanchez TG, Gonçalez F et al: Rhinocerebral mucormycosis: predisposing factors, diagnosis, therapy, complications and survival, *Rev Laryngol Otol Rhinol (Bord)* 117:53, 1996.

Del Valle Zapico A, Rubio Suárez A, Mellado Encinas A et al: Mucormycosis of the sphenoid sinus in an otherwise healthy patient: case report and literature review, *J Laryngol Otol* 110:471-473, 1996.

Ishida M, Taya N, Noiri T et al: Five cases of mucormycosis in paranasal sinuses, *Acta Otolaryngol* 501(Suppl):92-96, 1993.

Lee BL, Holland GN, Glasgow BJ: Chiasmal infarction and sudden blindness caused by mucormycosis in AIDS and diabetes mellitus, *Am J Ophthalmol* 122:895-896, 1996.

Muzaffar M, Hussain SI, Chughtai A: Plasma cell granuloma: maxillary sinuses, *J Laryngol Otol* 108:357-358, 1994.

Ng TT, Campbell CK, Rothera M et al: Successful treatment of sinusitis caused by Cunninghamella bertholetiae, *Clin Infect Dis* 19:313-316, 1994.

Ozhan S, Araç M, Isik S et al: Pseudotumor of the maxillary sinus in a patient with von Willebrand's disease, *AJR Am J Roentgenol* 166:950-951, 1996.

Perolada Valmana JM, Morera Perez C, Blanes Julia M et al: Mucormycosis of the paranasal sinuses, *Rev Laryngol Otol Rhinol (Bord)* 117:51-52, 1996.

Som PM, Brandwein MS, Maldjian C et al: Inflammatory pseudotumor of the maxillary sinus: CT and MR findings in six cases, *AJR Am J Roentgenol* 163:689-692, 1994.

Tkatch LS, Kusne S, Eibling D: Successful treatment of zygomycosis of the paranasal sinuses with surgical debridement and amphotericin B colloidal dispersion, *Am J Otolaryngol* 14:249-253, 1993.

Utas C, Unlühizarci K, Okten T et al: Acute renal failure associated with rhinosinuso-orbital mucormycosis infection in a patient with diabetic nephropathy [letter], *Nephron* 71:235, 1995.

Zapater E, Armengot M, Campos A et al: Invasive fungal sinusitis in immunosuppressed patients: report of three cases, *Acta Otorhinolaryngol Belg* 50:137-142, 1996.

*FIBROUS DYSPLASIA*

Malcolmson KG: Ossifying fibroma of the sphenoid, *J Laryngol Otol* 81:87-92, 1967.

Thomas GK, Kasper KA: Ossifying fibroma of the frontal bone, *Arch Otolaryngol* 83:43-46, 1966.

Wong A, Vaughan CW, Strong MS: Fibrous dysplasia of temporal bone, *Arch Otolaryngol* 81:131-133, 1965.

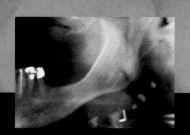

# CHAPTER 28

# Soft Tissue Calcification and Ossification

Laurie C. Carter

The deposition of calcium salts, primarily calcium phosphate, usually occurs in the skeleton. When it occurs in an unorganized fashion in soft tissue, it is referred to as heterotopic calcification. This soft tissue mineralization may develop in a wide variety of unrelated disorders and degenerative processes. Heterotopic calcifications may be divided into three categories:

- Dystrophic calcification
- Idiopathic calcification
- Metastatic calcification

Dystrophic calcification refers to calcification that forms in degenerating, diseased, and dead tissue despite normal serum calcium and phosphate levels. The soft tissue may be damaged by blunt trauma, inflammation, injections, the presence of parasites, soft tissue changes arising from disease, and many other causes. This calcification usually is localized to the site of injury. Idiopathic calcification (or calcinosis) results from deposition of calcium in normal tissue despite normal serum calcium and phosphate levels. Examples include chondrocalcinosis and phleboliths. Metastatic calcification results when minerals precipitate into normal tissue as a result of higher than normal serum levels of calcium (e.g., hyperparathyroidism, hypercalcemia, of malignancy) or phosphate (e.g., chronic renal failure). Metastatic calcification usually occurs bilaterally and symmetrically.

When the mineral is deposited in soft tissue as organized, well-formed bone, the process is known as heterotopic ossification. The term *heterotopic* indicates that bone has formed in an abnormal (extraskeletal) location. The heterotopic bone may be all compact bone, or it may show some trabeculae and fatty marrow. The deposits may range from 1 mm to several centimeters in diameter, and one or more may be present. The causes range from posttraumatic ossification, bone produced by tumors, and ossification caused by diseases such as progressive myositis ossificans and ankylosing spondylitis.

## Clinical Features

Sites of heterotopic calcification or ossification may not cause significant signs or symptoms; they most often are detected as incidental findings during radiographic examination.

## Radiographic Features

Soft tissue opacities are fairly common, present on about 4% of panoramic radiographs. In most cases the goal is to identify the calcification correctly to determine whether treatment or further investigation is required. Some soft tissue calcifications require no intervention or long-term surveillance, whereas others may be life threatening and the

underlying cause requires treatment. When the soft tissue calcification is adjacent to bone, it sometimes is difficult to determine whether the calcification is within bone or soft tissue. Another radiographic view at right angles is useful. The important criteria to consider in arriving at the correct interpretation are the anatomic location, number, distribution, and shape of the calcifications. Analysis of the location requires knowledge of soft tissue anatomy, such as the position of lymph nodes, stylohyoid ligaments, blood vessels, laryngeal cartilages, and the major ducts of the salivary glands.

## Dystrophic Calcification

### GENERAL DYSTROPHIC CALCIFICATION OF THE ORAL REGIONS

#### Definition

Dystrophic calcification is the precipitation of calcium salts into primary sites of chronic inflammation or dead and dying tissue. This process is usually associated with a high local concentration of phosphatase, as in normal bone calcification, an increase in local alkalinity, and anoxic conditions within the inactive or devitalized tissue. A long-standing chronically inflamed cyst is a common location of dystrophic calcification.

#### Clinical Features

Common soft tissue sites include the gingiva, tongue, lymph nodes, and cheek. Dystrophic calcifications may produce no signs or symptoms, although occasionally enlargement and ulceration of overlying soft tissues may occur, and a solid mass of calcium salts sometimes can be palpated.

#### Radiographic Features

The radiographic appearance of dystrophic calcification varies from barely perceptible, fine grains of radiopacities to larger, irregular radiopaque particles that rarely exceed 0.5 cm in diameter. One or more of these radiopacities may be seen, and the calcification may be homogeneous or may contain punctate areas. The outline of the calcified area usually is irregular or indistinct. Common sites are long-standing chronically inflamed cysts (Fig. 28-1) and polyps (Fig. 28-2).

### CALCIFIED LYMPH NODES

#### Definition

Dystrophic calcification occurs in lymph nodes that have been chronically inflamed because of various diseases, frequently granulomatous disorders. The lymphoid tissue becomes replaced by hydroxyapatite-

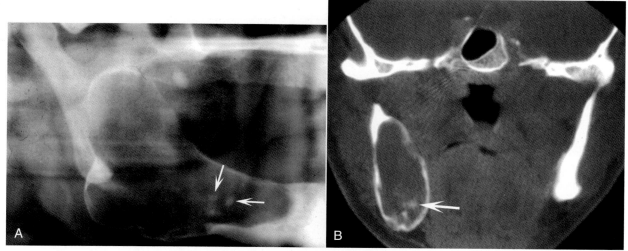

FIG. **28-1**   **A,** A large residual cyst with ill-defined calcifications seen in a panoramic image *(arrows).* **B,** A coronal computed tomographic image with bone algorithm of the same case, which demonstrates the dystrophic calcification within the cyst *(arrow).*

like calcium salts, nearly effacing all of nodal architecture. The presence of calcifications in lymph nodes implies disease, either active or the result of previously treated pathosis. In the past, tuberculosis was the most common disease causing calcified lymph nodes (scrofula or cervical tuberculous adenitis). Other well-known causes of lymph node calcification include bacille Calmette-Guérin vaccination, sarcoidosis, cat-scratch disease, rheumatoid arthritis and systemic sclerosis, lymphoma previously treated with radiation therapy, fungal infections, and metastases from distant calcifying neoplasms, most notably metastatic thyroid carcinoma.

## Clinical Features

Calcified lymph nodes are generally asymptomatic, and these nodes are first discovered as an incidental finding on a panoramic radiograph. The most commonly involved nodes are the submandibular and superficial and deep cervical nodes and, less commonly, the pre-auricular and submental nodes. When these nodes can be palpated, they are hard, lumpy, round to oblong masses.

## Radiographic Features

*Location.* The most common location is the submandibular region, either at or below the inferior border of the mandible near the angle, or between the posterior border of the ramus and cervical spine. The image of the calcified node sometimes overlaps the inferior aspect of the ramus. Lymph node calcifications may affect a single node or a linear series of nodes in a phenomenon known as lymph node "chaining" (Fig. 28-3).

*Periphery.* The periphery is well defined and usually irregular, occasionally having a lobulated appearance similar to the outer shape of cauliflower. This irregularity of shape is of great significance in distinguishing node calcifications from other potential soft tissue calcifications in the area.

*Internal Structure.* The internal aspect is without pattern but may vary in the degree of radiopacity, giving the impression of a collection of spherical or irregular masses. Occasionally the lesion has a laminated appearance, or the radiopacity may appear only on the surface of the node (eggshell calcification).The pattern of nodal cal-

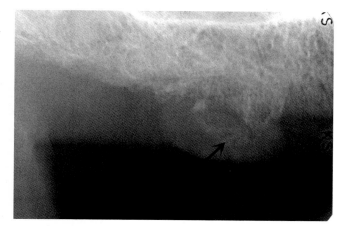

FIG. **28-2**   A periapical film showing the soft tissue mass, inflammatory fibrous hyperplasia, emanating from the edentulous ridge. This soft tissue mass contains a dystrophic calcification *(arrow).*

cification does not reliably distinguish between benign and malignant disease.

## Differential Diagnosis

Differentiation between a single calcified lymph node and a sialolith in the hilar region of the submandibular gland may be difficult because both may appear near or adjacent to the inferior cortex of the mandible just anterior to the angle. Usually a sialolith has a smooth outline, whereas a calcified lymph node is usually irregular and sometimes lobulated. The differentiation can be made if the patient has symptoms related to the submandibular salivary gland (see Chapter 31). Occasionally sialography may be necessary to make the differentiation. Another calcification that may have a similar appearance in this region is a phlebolith; however, phleboliths are usually smaller and multiple, with concentric radiopaque and radiolucent rings, and their shape may mimic a portion of a blood vessel.

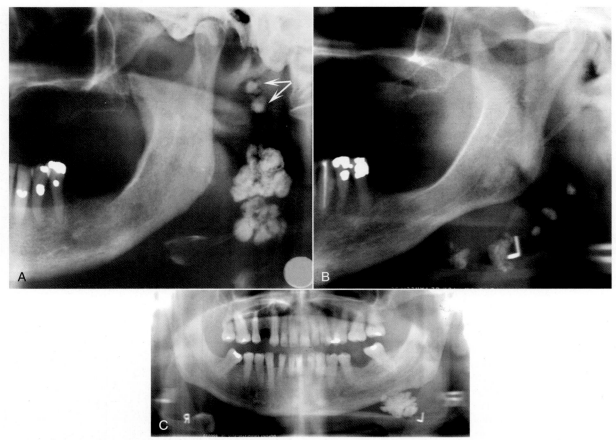

FIG. **28-3** Examples of dystrophic calcification in the lymph nodes. **A,** Two large examples positioned behind the ramus with a cauliflower-like shape and two smaller examples in a more superior position *(arrows).* **B,** Several smaller examples positioned below the lower border of the mandible. **C,** A larger example.

## Management

Calcified lymph nodes usually do not require treatment; however, the underlying cause should be established in case treatment is required, such as in the case of active disease.

### Dystrophic Calcification in the Tonsils

## Synonyms

Tonsillar calculi, tonsil concretions, and tonsilloliths

## Definition

Tonsillar calculi are formed when repeated bouts of inflammation enlarge the tonsillar crypts. Incomplete resolution of organic debris (dead bacteria and pus, epithelial cells, and food) can serve as the nidus for dystrophic calcification.

## Clinical Features

Tonsilloliths usually present as hard, round, white or yellow objects projecting from the tonsillar crypts, usually of the palatine tonsil. Small calcifications usually produce no clinical signs or symptoms. However, pain, swelling, fetor oris, dysphagia, or a foreign body sensation on swallowing has been reported with larger calcifications. Giant tonsilloliths stretching lymphoid tissue resulting in ulceration and extrusion are much less common. These calcifications have been

reported to occur between 20 and 68 years of age; they are found more often in older age groups.

## Radiographic Features

*Location.* In the panoramic film, tonsilloliths appear as single or multiple radiopacities that overlap the mid portion of the mandibular ramus in the region where the image of the dorsal surface of the tongue crosses the ramus in the oropharyngeal air spaces. Tonsilloliths frequently appear on the panoramic radiograph immediately inferior to the mandibular canal (Fig. 28-4).

*Periphery.* The most common appearance of tonsilloliths is a cluster of multiple small, ill-defined radiopacities. Rarely this calcification may attain a large size.

*Internal Structure.* These calcifications appear slightly more radiopaque than cancellous bone and approximately the same as cortical bone.

## Differential Diagnosis

The clinical differential diagnosis includes calcified granulomatous disease, syphilis, mycosis, or lymphoma, which may produce a firm tonsillar mass. The essential radiographic differential diagnosis is a radiopaque lesion within the mandibular ramus, such as a dense bone island. When in doubt, a right-angle view such as a posteroanterior skull view or an open Towne's view may show that the calcification

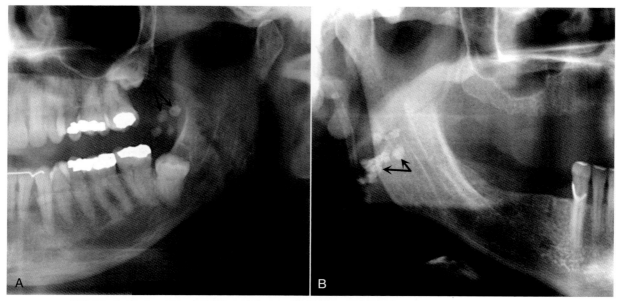

FIG. **28-4**   Dystrophic calcification of the tonsils. These two examples show positions anterior to the ramus **(A)** and overlapping the posterior aspect of the ramus **(B)** *(arrows)*. Note the calcified stylohyoid ligament.

lies to the medial aspect of the ramus. Three-dimensional imaging such as computed tomography (CT) or cone beam CT may be necessary for precise localization.

### Treatment

No treatment is required for most tonsillar calcifications. In symptomatic patients, tonsilloliths may be expressed manually, possibly with the patient under sedation to suppress the gag reflex. However, large calcifications with associated symptoms are removed surgically. Treatment of asymptomatic tonsilloliths may be considered in elderly patients with mechanical deglutition disorders and the immunocompromised because of the risk for aspiration pneumonia.

## CYSTICERCOSIS

### Definition

When humans ingest eggs or gravid proglottids from the parasite *Taenia solium* (pork tapeworm), the covering of the eggs is digested in the stomach and the larval form (*Cysticercus cellulosae*) of the parasite is hatched. The larvae penetrate the mucosa, enter the blood vessels and lymphatics, and are distributed in the tissues all over the body but preferentially locate to brain, muscle, skin, liver, lungs, and heart. They are also found in the oral and perioral tissues, especially the muscles of mastication. In tissues other than the intestinal mucosa, the larvae eventually die and are treated as foreign bodies, causing granuloma formation, scarring, and calcification approximately 3 months later. These areas in the tissues are called cysticerci. There is currently an increased incidence of cysticercosis in the American Southwest and urban Northeast, especially among Koreans and Hispanics. The problem is much worse in developing countries of Central and South America, Asia, and Africa, where there is fecal contamination of agricultural soil and pork is a valued food.

### Clinical Features

Mild cases of cysticercosis are completely asymptomatic. More severe cases have symptoms that range from mild to severe gastrointestinal upset with epigastric pain and severe nausea and vomiting. Invasion of the brain may result in seizures, headache, visual disturbances, acute obstructive hydrocephalus, irritability, loss of consciousness, and death. Examination of the oral mucosa may disclose palpable, well-circumscribed soft fluctuant swellings, which resemble a mucocele or benign mesenchymal neoplasm. Multiple small nodules may be felt in the region of the masseter and suprahyoid muscles and in the tongue, buccal mucosa, or lip.

### Radiographic Features

While alive, larvae are not visible radiographically. Death of the parasites and development of calcifications in subcutaneous and muscular sites occurs approximately 5 years after the initial infection.

*Location.*   The locations of calcified cysticerci include the muscles of mastication and facial expression, the suprahyoid muscle, and the postcervical musculature, as well as in the tongue, buccal mucosa, or lip.

*Periphery and Shape.*   Multiple well-defined elliptic radiopacities are viewed, resembling grains of rice.

*Internal Structure.*   The internal aspect is homogeneous and radiopaque.

### Differential Diagnosis

Cysticercus may appear similar to a sialolith. However, the small size of the calcified nodules of cysticerci and their widespread dissemination, particularly in brain and muscles, are highly suggestive of the diagnosis.

### Management

Although basic sanitation (proper preparation of pork and avoiding fecal contamination of water supplies and vegetables) is needed to extinguish this source of infection, the symptoms that accompany the initial infestation are best treated by a physician using an antihelminthic such as praziquantel. After the larvae have settled and calcified in the oral tissues, however, they are harmless. However, it is important to carry out a detailed investigation in each patient to rule out the presence of the parasite in other locations.

## Arterial Calcifications

Two distinct patterns of arterial calcification can be identified both radiographically and histologically, Monckeberg's medial calcinosis and calcified atherosclerotic plaque.

### MONCKEBERG'S MEDIAL CALCINOSIS (ARTERIOSCLEROSIS)

#### Definition
The hallmark of arteriosclerosis is the fragmentation, degeneration, and eventual loss of elastic fibers followed by the deposition of calcium within the medial coat of the vessel.

#### Clinical Features
Most patients are asymptomatic initially, although late in the course of the disease may have clinical pathosis such as cutaneous gangrene, peripheral vascular disease, and myositis as a result of vascular insufficiency. Patients with Sturge-Weber syndrome also develop intracranial arterial calcifications.

#### Radiographic Features
*Location.* Medial calcinosis involving the facial artery or, less commonly, the carotid artery, may be viewed on panoramic radiographs.

*Periphery and Shape.* The calcific deposits in the wall of the artery outline an image of the artery. From the side, the calcified vessel appears as a parallel pair of thin, radiopaque lines (Fig. 28-5) that may have a straight course or a tortuous path and is described as a "pipe stem" or "tram-track" appearance. In cross-section, involved vessels will display a circular or ringlike pattern.

*Internal Structure.* There is no internal structure because the diffuse, finely divided calcium deposits occur solely in the medial wall of the vessels.

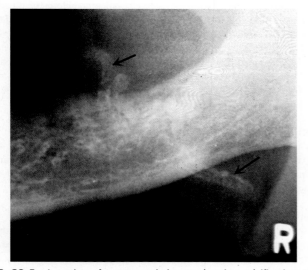

FIG. **28-5**  A section of a panoramic image showing calcification of a blood vessel, probably the facial vein *(arrows)*.

#### Differential Diagnosis
The radiographic appearance of arteriosclerosis is so distinctive as to be pathognomonic of the condition.

#### Management
Evaluation of the patient for occlusive arterial disease and peripheral vascular disease may be appropriate. In addition, hyperparathyroidism may be considered because medial calcinosis frequently develops as a metastatic calcification in patients with this condition.

### CALCIFIED ATHEROSCLEROTIC PLAQUE

#### Definition
Atheromatous plaque in the extracranial carotid vasculature is the major contributing source of cerebrovascular embolic and occlusive disease. Dystrophic calcification can occur in the evolution of plaque within the intima of the involved vessel.

#### Radiographic Findings
*Location.* Atherosclerosis first develops at arterial bifurcations as a result of increased endothelial damage from shear forces at these sites. When calcification has occurred, these lesions may be visible in the panoramic radiograph in the soft tissues of the neck either superior or inferior to the greater cornu of the hyoid bone (where the common carotid artery splits into the external and internal carotid arteries) and adjacent to the cervical vertebrae C3, C4, or the intervertebral space between them (Fig. 28-6).

*Periphery and Shape.* These soft tissue calcifications are usually multiple and irregular in shape and sharply defined from the surrounding soft tissues and they have a vertical linear distribution.

*Internal Structure.* The internal aspect is composed of a heterogeneous radiopacity with radiolucent voids.

#### Differential Diagnosis
Calcified triticeous cartilage may be mistaken for atheromatous plaque, although the uniform size, shape, and location of calcified triticeous cartilage in the laryngeal cartilage skeleton identify this innocuous condition.

#### Management
Many published case reports and case series report individual instances of patients with calcified carotid atheromata on panoramic radiographs who were found to have clinically significant stenoses with a heightened risk for a cerebrovascular accident. However, further research needs to be conducted with case-control or cohort studies with a control group to determine whether calcified carotid atheromas represent an independent risk factor for stroke. In the meantime, patients with calcified carotid atheromata, especially those with established risk factors for cerebrovascular and cardiovascular disease, should be referred to their physicians for further investigation.

## Idiopathic Calcification

### SIALOLITH

#### Definition
Sialoliths are stones found within the ducts of salivary glands (also see Chapter 31). Mechanical conditions contributing to a slow flow rate and physiochemical characteristics of the gland secretion both contribute to the formation of a nidus and subsequent precipitation of calcium and phosphate salts.

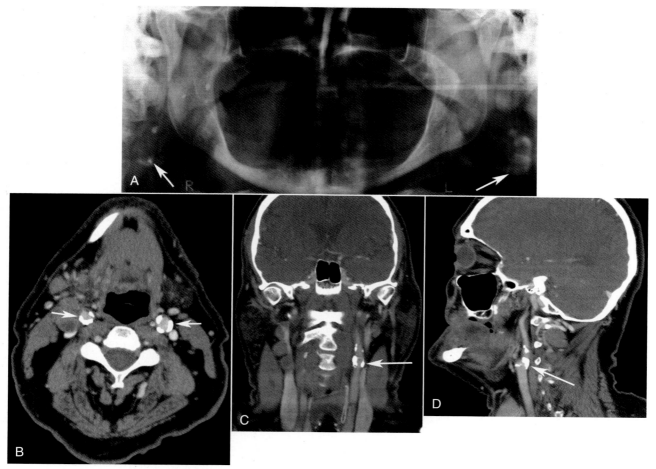

FIG. **28-6** **A,** Panoramic image with bilateral examples of calcifications associated with the carotid arteries *(arrows).* **B,** Axial CT image of the same case with soft tissue algorithm showing bilateral calcification with the walls of the carotid arteries *(arrows).* **C** and **D,** Coronal and sagittal CT images of the same case demonstrating the carotid calcifications *(arrows).*

## Clinical Features

Sialoliths are most common in the submandibular glands of men in their middle and later years. They usually occur singly (70% to 80%) but may be multiple, especially in the parotid gland. Patients with salivary stones may be asymptomatic, but they usually have a history of pain and swelling in the floor of the mouth and in the involved submandibular gland or in the cheek in the case of parotid sialoliths. This discomfort may intensify at mealtimes, when salivary flow is stimulated. Because the stone usually does not block the flow of saliva completely, the pain and swelling gradually subside. As many as 9% of patients have recurrent sialolithiasis, and about 10% of patients with sialolithiasis also have nephrolithiasis.

## Radiographic Features

*Location.* The submandibular gland is involved more often (83% to 94% of cases) than the parotid gland (4% to 10%) or the sublingual gland (1% to 7%), probably because the submandibular gland has a longer and more tortuous duct, an uphill flow in the proximal portion, and more viscous saliva with a higher mineral content. About half of submandibular stones lie in the distal portion of Wharton's duct, 20% in the proximal portion, and 30% in the gland itself.

*Periphery and Shape.* Sialoliths located in the duct of the submandibular gland usually are cylindric and very smooth in their outlines. Stones that form in the hilus of a submandibular gland tend to be larger and more irregularly shaped (Fig. 28-7).

*Internal Structure.* Some stones are homogeneously radiopaque, and others show evidence of multiple layers of calcification (Fig. 28-8, *A*). Less than 20% of submandibular gland sialoliths and 40% of those in the parotid gland are radiolucent because of the low mineral content of the parotid secretions.

## Applied Radiology

Salivary stones occasionally are seen on periapical views superimposed over the mandibular premolar and molar apices (Fig. 28-8, *C*). The best view for visualizing stones in the distal portion of Wharton's duct is a standard mandibular occlusal view using half the usual exposure time, which displays the floor of the mouth without overlap from the mandible. Stones in a more posterior location are best visualized on lateral oblique views of the mandible or on a panoramic film. To demonstrate stones in the parotid gland duct, the clinician places a periapical film in the buccal vestibule, reduces the exposure time, and orients x-ray beam through the cheek. Also, stones in the parotid duct

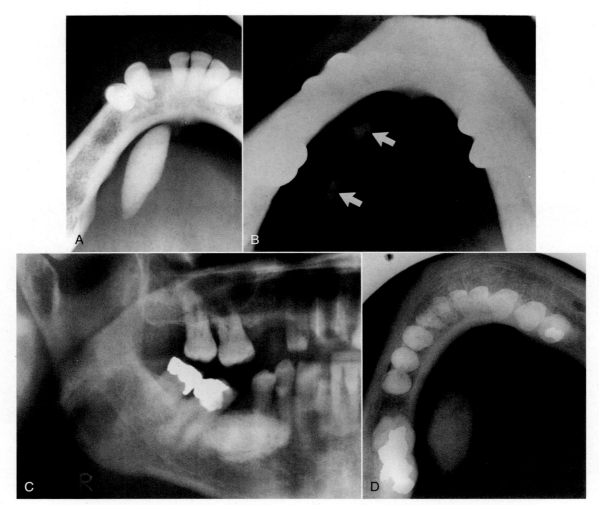

FIG. **28-7**   **A** and **B,** Standard occlusal projections of single and multiple examples of calcified sialo-liths *(arrows)* in the duct of a submandibular gland. Exposure times have been reduced to better demonstrate these calcifications, which are less calcified than the mandible. In another example **(C),** the image of the sialolith is superimposed over the mandibular alveolar process in this cropped pan-oramic image. **D,** Occlusal view of the same case.

can be seen if the patient "blows out" the cheek as an anteroposterior skull view is exposed. An open-mouth lateral skull projection can be used or sometimes visible in a panoramic view (Fig. 28-8, *B*). When radiographs to detect sialoliths are produced, the exposure time should be reduced to about half of normal. This helps in detecting stones that are lightly calcified. If a noncalcified stone is suspected, sialography is used (see Chapter 31).

### Differential Diagnosis

Sialoliths can be distinguished from other soft tissue calcifications because they usually are associated with pain or swelling of the involved salivary gland. Other calcifications (e.g., lymph nodes) are asymptomatic. If the diagnosis is unclear, the clinician can prescribe a sialogram.

### Management

Small stones often may be "milked out" through the duct orifice by bimanual palpation. If the stone is too large or located in the proximal duct, nonsurgical or minimally invasive sialolithotomy using intra-

corporeal lithotriptors is becoming a popular treatment modality. In cases of exceedingly large sialoliths, surgical removal of the stone or gland may be required.

## PHLEBOLITHS

### Definition

Intravascular thrombi, which arise from venous stagnation, some-times become organized or even mineralized. Such mineralization begins in the core of the thrombus and consists of crystals of apatite with calcium phosphate and calcium carbonate. Phleboliths are calci-fied thrombi found in veins, venulae, or the sinusoidal vessels of hemangiomas (especially the cavernous type).

### Clinical Features

In the head and neck, phleboliths nearly always signal the presence of a hemangioma. In an adult, phleboliths may be the sole residua of a childhood hemangioma that has long since regressed. The involved soft tissue may be swollen, throbbing, or discolored by the presence

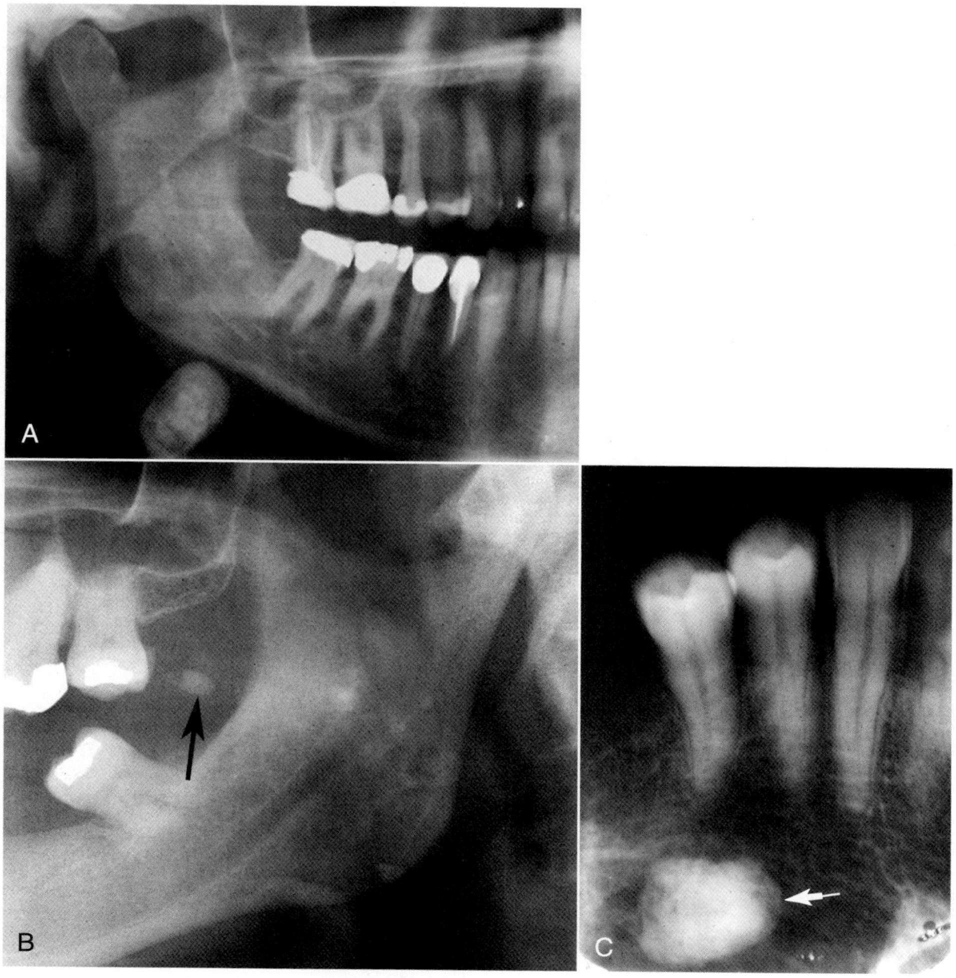

FIG. **28-8** **A,** Cropped panoramic image of a submandibular gland sialolith; note the position and also the hint at a laminated internal pattern. **B,** Cropped panoramic image of a sialolith *(arrow)* involving the parotid gland. **C,** Intraoral periapical image of superimposed sub-mandibular sialolith that could be difficult to differentiate from a dense bone island without an occlusal film. (**B** courtesy Drs. John Lovas and Nick Hogg, Dalhousie University.)

of veins or a soft tissue hemangioma. Hemangiomas often fluctuate in size, associated with changes in body position or during a Valsalva maneuver. Applying pressure to the involved tissue should cause a blanching or change in color if the lesion is vascular in nature. Auscultation may reveal a bruit in cases of cavernous hemangioma but not in the capillary type.

### Radiographic Features

*Location.* Phleboliths most commonly are found in hemangiomas (see Chapter 22).

*Periphery and Shape.* In cross-section the shape is round or oval, up to 6 mm in diameter with a smooth periphery. If the involved blood vessel is viewed from the side, the phlebolith may resemble a straight or slightly curved sausage.

*Internal Structure.* The internal aspect may be homogeneously radiopaque but more commonly has the appearance of laminations, giving phleboliths a bull's-eye or "target" appearance. A radiolucent center may be seen, which may represent the remaining patent portion of the vessel (Fig. 28-9).

### Differential Diagnosis

A phlebolith may have a shape similar to that of a sialolith. Sialoliths usually occur singly; if more than one is present, they usually are oriented in a single line, whereas phleboliths are usually multiple and

have a more random, clustered distribution. The importance of correctly identifying phleboliths lies in the identification of a possible vascular lesion such as a hemangioma. This is critical if surgical procedures are contemplated.

## LARYNGEAL CARTILAGE CALCIFICATIONS

### Definition

The small, paired triticeous cartilages are found within the lateral thyrohyoid ligaments. Both the thyroid and triticeous cartilages consist of hyaline cartilage, which has a tendency to calcify or ossify with advancing age.

### Clinical Features

Calcification of tracheal cartilages is an incidental radiographic finding with no clinical features.

### Radiographic Features

*Location.* The calcified triticeous cartilage is located on a lateral skull or panoramic radiograph within the soft tissues of the pharynx inferior to the greater cornu of the hyoid bone and adjacent to the superior border of C4. The superior cornu of a calcified thyroid cartilage appears medial to C4 and is superimposed on the prevertebral soft tissue (Fig. 28-10).

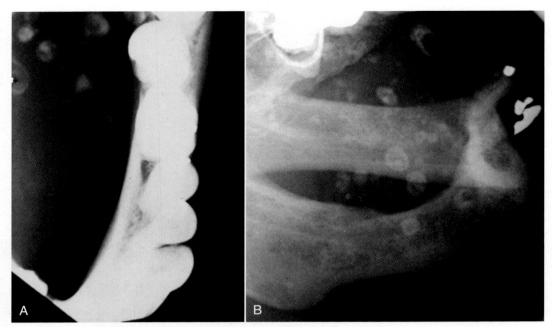

FIG. **28-9**   Phleboliths are soft tissue dystrophic calcifications found in veins. They are usually associated with hemangiomas.

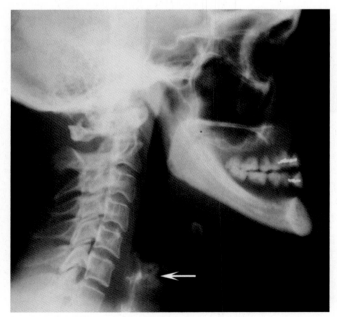

FIG. **28-10**   A lateral cephalometric film revealing calcification of the thyroid cartilage *(arrow)*.

*Periphery and Shape.* The word *triticeous* means "grain of wheat," and the cartilage measures 7 to 9 mm in length and 2 to 4 mm in width. The periphery of the calcified triticeous cartilage is well defined and smooth, and the geometry is exceedingly regular. Usually only the top 2 to 3 mm of a calcified thyroid cartilage will be visible at the lower edge of a panoramic radiograph with 6-inch systems.

*Internal Structure.* Calcified tracheal cartilages generally present a homogeneous radiopacity but may occasionally demonstrate an outer cortex.

### Differential Diagnosis
Calcified triticeous cartilage may be confused with calcified atheromatous plaque in the carotid bifurcation, but the solitary nature and extremely uniform size and shape of the former should be discriminatory.

### Management
No treatment is needed for calcified tracheal cartilages, but careful attention to the differences in morphology and location enable the clinician to distinguish between calcified triticeous cartilage and calcified carotid atheromata.

## RHINOLITH/ANTROLITH

### Definition
Calcareous concretions that occur in the nose (rhinoliths) or the antrum of the maxillary sinus (antroliths) arise from the deposition of nasal, lacrimal, and inflammatory mineral salts such as calcium phosphate, calcium carbonate, and magnesium by accretion around a nidus. In cases of rhinolith, the nidus is usually an exogenous foreign body (coins, beads, etc.), especially in the pediatric population. The route of entry is usually anterior, but some may enter the choana posteriorly during sneezing, coughing, or emesis. The nidus for an antrolith is usually endogenous (root tip, bone fragment, blood clot, inspissated mucus, etc.), especially in the adult population.

### Clinical Features
The patient may be asymptomatic for extended periods of time, but the expanding mass may impinge on the mucosa, producing pain,

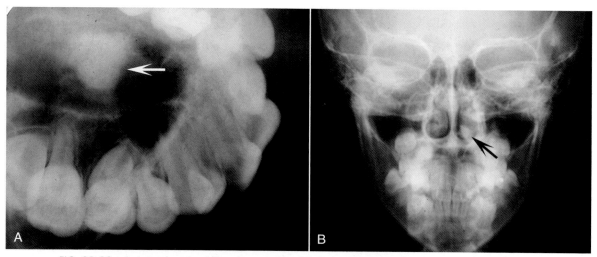

FIG. 28-11  **A,** Lateral occlusal film shows a rhinolith *(arrow)* positioned above the floor of the nose.
**B,** Posteroanterior skull film of the same case demonstrating that the rhinolith is positioned within the nasal fossa *(arrow).*

congestion, and ulceration. The patient may have a unilateral purulent rhinorrhea, sinusitis, headache, epistaxis, anosmia, fetor, and fever.

### Radiographic Features

*Location.* Rhinoliths develop in the nose (Fig. 28-11), whereas antroliths develop in the antrum of the maxillary sinus (see Fig. 27-10).

*Periphery and Shape.* These stones have a variety of shapes and sizes, depending on the nature of the nidus.

*Internal Structure.* They may present as homogeneous or heterogeneous radiopacities, depending on the nature of the nidus, and may sometimes have laminations. Occasionally the density will exceed the surrounding bone.

### Differential Diagnosis

The differential diagnosis includes osteoma, odontoma, surgical ciliated cyst, and mycolith.

### Management

Patients should be referred to an otorhinolaryngologist for endonasal surgical removal of the mass. In some cases, lithotripsy has been used to debulk large rhinoliths.

## Metastatic Calcification

Calcification of the soft tissues in the oral region caused by conditions involving elevated serum calcium and phosphate levels, such as hyperparathyroidism (see Chapter 25) or hypercalcemia of malignancy, are extremely rare.

## Heterotopic Bone

### OSSIFICATION OF THE STYLOHYOID LIGAMENT

#### Definition

Embryologically, the styloid process arises from the second branchial arch (Reichert cartilage), which consists of four sections that give rise to the stylohyoid complex. Ossification of the stylohyoid ligament usually extends downward from the base of the skull and commonly occurs bilaterally. However, in rare cases the ossification begins at the lesser horn of the hyoid and in fewer still in a central area of the ligament.

### Clinical Features

The ossified ligament usually can be detected by palpation over the tonsil as a hard, pointed structure. Only a minority of patients have symptoms and there is very little correlation between the extent of ossification and the intensity of the accompanying symptoms. Symptoms related to this ossified ligament are termed Eagle syndrome, which is expressed as one of two subtypes: classic Eagle syndrome resulting from cranial nerve impingement, and the carotid artery syndrome, resulting from impingement on the carotid vessels. When this entity is associated with discomfort and the patient has a recent history of neck trauma (typically tonsillectomy), the condition is called classic Eagle syndrome. The ossified stylohyoid complex and local scar tissue are thought to cause symptoms by impinging on cranial nerves V, VII, IX, X, or XII, all of which pass in close proximity to the styloid process. Symptoms may include vague, nagging to intense pain in the pharynx on swallowing, turning the head, or opening the mouth, especially on yawning, and tinnitus or otalgia. Clinical findings without a history of neck trauma constitute carotid artery syndrome. The patient may describe referred pain along the distribution of the external (ECA) or internal carotid artery (ICA). This is the result of mechanical impingement of the involved artery and stimulation of its sympathetic nerve plexus. When the ECA is impinged and stimulated, the patient may feel suborbital facial pain. Symptoms when the ICA is affected may include eye pain, temporal or parietal headache, aphasia, visual symptoms, weakness, and transient hemispheric ischemia with vertigo or syncope, notably on turning the head to the ipsilateral side. In these patients, pain is produced by mechanical irritation of sympathetic nerve tissue in the arterial wall, producing regional carotidynia. This may occur even in the absence of ossification of the stylohyoid complex. Only deviation of the styloid process, usually medially, is required for the tip of

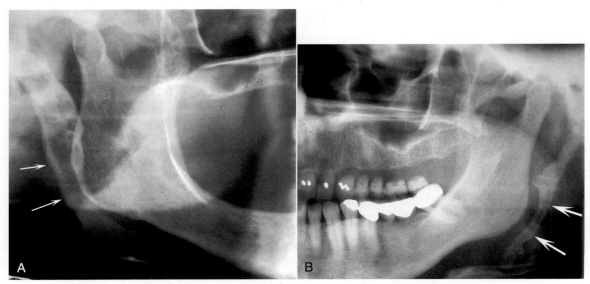

FIG. **28-12** **A** and **B,** Examples of prominent ossification of the stylohyoid ligament *(arrows);* these individuals did not have any symptoms.

the process to impinge an artery. These individuals usually are older than 40 years. This condition is more prevalent than classic Eagle syndrome.

### Radiographic Features

Ossification of the stylohyoid ligament is detected fairly commonly as an incidental feature on panoramic radiographs. In one study, approximately 18% of a population examined showed ossification of more than 30 mm of the stylohyoid ligament. The ligament may have at least some calcification in individuals of any age.

*Location.* In a panoramic image the linear ossification extends forward from the region of the mastoid process and crosses the posteroinferior aspect of the ramus toward the hyoid bone. The hyoid bone is positioned roughly parallel to or superimposed on the posterior aspect of the inferior cortex of the mandible.

*Shape.* The styloid process appears as a long, tapering, thin, radiopaque process that is thicker at its base and projects downward and forward (Fig. 28-12). It normally varies from about 0.5 to 2.5 cm in length. The ossified ligament has roughly a straight outline, but in some cases some irregularity may be seen in the outer surface. The farther the radiopaque ossified ligament extends toward the hyoid bone, the more likely it is that it will be interrupted by radiolucent, jointlike junctions (pseudoarticulations).

*Internal Structure.* Small ossifications of the stylohyoid ligament appear homogeneously radiopaque. As the ossification increases in length and girth, the outer cortex of this bone becomes evident as a radiopaque band at the periphery.

### Differential Diagnosis

The symptoms accompanying stylohyoid ligament ossification and Eagle syndrome or stylohyoid syndrome generally are vague; however, when they occur with the distinctive radiographic evidence of ligament ossification, little chance exists that the complaint will be confused with another entity. Occasionally, though, the symptoms may be similar to those seen in temporomandibular joint dysfunction.

### Management

Most patients with ossification of the stylohyoid ligament are asymptomatic, and no treatment is required. For patients with vague symptoms, a conservative approach of reassurance and steroid or lidocaine injections into the tonsillar fossa would be recommended initially. However, for patients with persistent or intense symptoms, the recommended treatment is amputation of the stylohyoid process (stylohyoidectomy).

## OSTEOMA CUTIS

### Definition

Osteoma cutis is a rare soft tissue ossification in the skin. Approximately 85% of cases occur as a result of acne of long duration, developing in a scar or chronic inflammatory dermatosis. Histologically these lesions are areas of dense viable bone in the dermis or subcutaneous tissue. They occasionally are found in diffuse scleroderma, replacing the altered collagen in the dermis and subcutaneous septa.

### Clinical Features

Osteoma cutis can occur anywhere, but the face is the most common site. The tongue is the most common intraoral site (osteoma mucosae or osseous choristoma). Osteoma cutis does not cause any visible change in the overlying skin other than an occasional color change that may appear yellowish white. If the lesion is large, the individual osteoma may be palpated. A needle inserted into one of the papules is met with stonelike resistance. Some patients have numerous (dozens to hundreds) of lesions, usually on the face in females and on the scalp or chest in males. This form is known as multiple miliary osteoma cutis.

### Radiographic Features

*Location.* Radiographically, osteoma cutis most commonly appears in the cheek and lip regions (Fig. 28-13). In this location the image can be superimposed over a tooth root or alveolar process, giving the appearance of an area of dense bone. Accurate localization can be achieved by placing an intraoral film between the cheek and alveolar process to image the cheek alone. As an alternative, a postero-anterior skull view with the cheek blown outward by use of a soft tissue technique of 60 peak kilovolts helps localize osteomas in the skin.

*Periphery and Shape.* Osteoma cutis appears as smoothly outlined, radiopaque, washer-shaped images. These single or multiple radiopacities usually are very small, although the size can range from 0.1 to 5 cm.

*Internal Structure.* The internal aspect may be homogeneously radiopaque but usually has a radiolucent center that represents normal fatty marrow, giving the lesion a donut appearance radiographically. Trabeculae occasionally develop in the marrow cavity of larger osteomas. Individual lesions of calcified cystic acne resemble a snowflake-like radiopacity, which corresponds to the clinical location of the scar.

### Differential Diagnosis

The differential diagnosis should include myositis ossificans, calcinosis cutis, and osteoma mucosae. If the blown-out cheek technique is used, the lesions of osteoma cutis appear much more superficial than mucosal lesions. Myositis ossificans is of greater proportions, in some cases causing noticeable deformity of the facial contour.

### Management

No treatment is required, but these osteomas occasionally are removed for cosmetic reasons. Resurfacing of the skin with the erbium:yttrium-aluminum-garnet laser with tretinoin cream has been successful in treating multiple miliary osteoma cutis. More recently, good cosmetic results have been reported with a needle microincision-extirpation technique in patients with multiple miliary osteoma cutis.

## MYOSITIS OSSIFICANS

### Definition

In myositis ossificans; fibrous tissue and heterotopic bone form within the interstitial tissue of muscle and associated tendons and ligaments. Secondary destruction and atrophy of the muscle occur as this fibrous tissue and bone interdigitate and separate the muscle fibers. There are two principal forms: localized and progressive.

### Localized (Traumatic) Myositis Ossificans

#### Synonyms

Posttraumatic myositis ossificans and solitary myositis

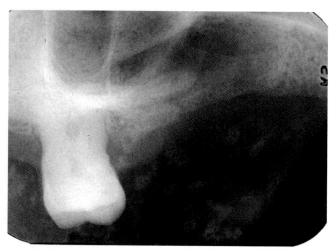

FIG. **28-13**  Osteoma cutis is seen here as faint radiopaque calcifications in the cheek.

### Definition

Localized myositis ossificans results from acute or chronic trauma or from heavy muscular strain caused by certain occupations and sports. Muscle injury from multiple injections (occasionally from dental anesthetic) also may be a cause. Skeletal muscle has limited capacity for regeneration after significant physical trauma. The injury leads to considerable hemorrhage into the muscle or associated tendons/fascia. It has been proposed that exuberant proliferation of vascular granulation tissue subsequently undergoes metaplasia to cartilage and bone during the healing process. The term *myositis* is misleading because no inflammation is involved. The fibrous tissue and bone form within the interstitial tissue of the muscle; no actual ossification of the muscle fibers occurs.

### Clinical Features

Localized myositis ossificans can develop at any age in either sex, but it occurs most often in young men who engage in vigorous activity. The site of the precipitating trauma remains swollen, tender, and painful much longer than expected. The overlying skin may be red and inflamed, and when the lesion involves a muscle of mastication, opening the jaws may be difficult. After about 2 or 3 weeks, the area of ossification becomes apparent in the tissues; a firm intramuscular mass can be palpated. The localized lesion may enlarge slowly, but eventually it stops growing. The lesion may appear fixed, or it may be freely movable on palpation.

### Radiographic Features

*Location.* The most commonly involved muscles of the head and neck are the masseter and sternocleidomastoid. However, other muscles of mastication may be involved, such as the medial and lateral pterygoid and the temporalis muscles. The anterior attachments of the temporalis as well as the medial pterygoid muscles are at risk of injury on administration of mandibular block anesthesia. Usually a radiolucent band can be seen between the area of ossification and

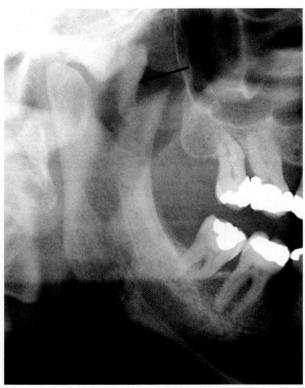

FIG. **28-14** Soft tissue ossification extending from the coronoid process in a superior direction, following the anatomy of the temporalis muscle *(arrow)*. This condition arose after several attempts were made to provide a submandibular nerve block, leaving the patient unable to open the mandible.

adjacent bone, and the heterotopic bone may lie along the long axis of the muscle (Fig. 28-14).

*Periphery and Shape.* The periphery commonly is more radiopaque than the internal structure. There is a variation in shape from irregular oval to linear streaks (pseudotrabeculae) running in the same direction as the normal muscle fibers. These pseudotrabeculae are characteristic of myositis ossificans and strongly imply a diagnosis.

*Internal Structure.* The internal structure varies with time. Within the third or fourth week after injury, the radiographic appearance is a faintly homogeneous radiopacity. This organizes further, and by 2 months a delicate lacy or feathery radiopaque internal structure develops. These changes indicate the formation of bone; however, this bone does not have a normal-appearing trabecular pattern. Gradually the image becomes denser and better defined, maturing fully in about 5 to 6 months. After this period the lesion may shrink.

## Differential Diagnosis
The differential diagnosis of localized myositis ossificans includes ossification of the stylohyoid ligament and other soft tissue calcifications. However, both the form and location of myositis ossificans often are enough to make the differential diagnosis. Other lesions to consider are bone-forming tumors. Although tumors such as osteo-

genic sarcoma can form a linear bone pattern (see Chapter 23), the tumor is contiguous with the adjacent bone, and signs of bone destruction often are present.

## Management
Rest and limitation of use are recommended to diminish the extent of the calcific deposit. Surgical excision of the entire calcified mass with intensive physiotherapy to minimize postsurgical scarring is the recommended treatment.

### Progressive Myositis Ossificans

## Definition
Progressive myositis ossificans is a rare hereditary disease with autosomal dominant transmission, but less commonly it arises as a result of spontaneous mutation. It is more common in males and causes symptoms from early infancy. Progressive formation of heterotopic bone occurs within the interstitial tissue of muscles, tendons, ligaments, and fascia, and the involved muscles atrophy.

## Clinical Features
In most cases the heterotopic ossification starts in the muscles of the neck and upper back and moves to the extremities. The disease commences with soft tissue swelling that is tender and painful and may show redness and heat, indicating the presence of inflammation. The acute symptoms subside, and a firm mass remains in the tissues. This condition may affect any of the striated muscles, including the heart and diaphragm. In some cases the spread of ossification is limited; in others it becomes extensive, affecting almost all the large muscles of the body. Stiffness and limitation of motion of the neck, chest, back, and extremities (especially the shoulders) gradually increase. Functional deficits are progressive and handicapping. Advanced stages of the disease result in the "petrified man" condition. During the third decade the process may spontaneously arrest; however, most patients die during the third or fourth decades. Premature death usually results from respiratory embarrassment or from inanition through the involvement of the muscles of mastication.

## Radiographic Features
The radiographic appearance of progressive myositis ossificans is similar to that described for the limited form. The heterotopic bone more commonly is oriented along the long axis of the involved muscle (Fig. 28-15). Osseous malformation of the regions of muscle attachment, such as the mandibular condyles, also may be seen.

## Differential Diagnosis
In the initial stages of the disease, distinguishing between progressive myositis ossificans and rheumatoid arthritis may be difficult. However, the presence of specific anomalies suggests the diagnosis. In the case of calcinosis, the deposits of amorphous calcium salts frequently resorb, but in progressive myositis ossificans, the bone never disappears.

## Management
No effective treatment exists for progressive myositis ossificans. Nodules that are traumatized and that ulcerate frequently should be excised. If interference with respiration or respiratory infection occurs in the later stages of the disease, supportive therapy may be required.

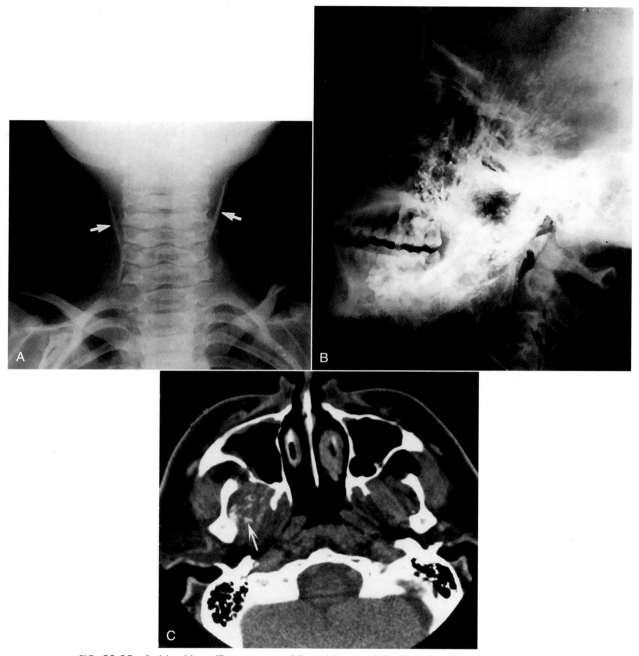

FIG. **28-15** **A,** Myositis ossificans, seen as bilateral linear calcifications *(arrows)* of the sternohyoid muscle. **B,** Extensive ossification of the masseter and temporalis muscles. **C,** An axial CT scan with soft tissue algorithm demonstrating calcifications in the lateral pterygoid muscle *(arrow).* (**A** courtesy Dr. H. Worth, Vancouver, British Columbia; **B** from Shawkat AH: Myositis ossificans: report of a case, *Oral Surg* 23:751-754, 1967.)

## SUGGESTED READINGS

Banks K, Bui-Mansfield L, Chew F et al: A compartmental approach to the radiographic evaluation of soft-tissue calcifications, *Semin Roentgenol* 40:391-407, 2005.

Carter L: Clinical indications as a basis for ordering extraoral imaging studies, *Compendium* 25:95-102, 2004.

Keberle M, Robinson S: Physiologic and pathologic calcifications and ossifications in the face and neck, *Eur Radiol* 17:2103-2111, 2007.

Monsour PA, Romaniuk K, Hutchings RD: Soft tissue calcifications in the differential diagnosis of opacities superimposed over the mandible by dental panoramic radiography, *Aust Dent J* 36:94-101, 1991.

Worth HM: *Principles and practice of oral radiologic interpretation*, St. Louis, 1963, Mosby.

### CALCIFIED LYMPH NODES

Eisenkraft B, Som P: The spectrum of benign and malignant etiologies of cervical node calcification, *AJR Am J Roentgenol* 172:1433-1437, 1999.

Paquette M, Terezhalmy G, Moore W: Calcified lymph nodes, *Quint Int* 34:562-563, 2003.

## DYSTROPHIC CALCIFICATION IN THE TONSILS

Ansai T, Takehara T: Tonsillolith as a halitosis-inducing factor, *Br Dent J* 198:263-264, 2005.

Dal Rio A, Franchi-Teixeira A, Nicola E: Relationship between the presence of tonsilloliths and halitosis in patients with chronic caseous tonsillitis, *Br Dent J Published on-line November 23*, 2007.

Mandel L: Multiple bilateral tonsilloliths: case report, *J Oral Maxillofac Surg* 66:148-150, 2008.

## CYSTICERCOSIS

Delgado-Azañero WA, Mosqueda-Taylor A, Carlos-Bregni R et al: Oral cysticercosis: a collaborative study of 16 cases, *Oral Surg Oral Med Oral Pathol Oral Radiol Endod* 103:528-533, 2007.

Ribeiro A, Luvizotto M, Soubhia A et al: Oral cysticercosis: case report, *Oral Surg Oral Med Oral Pathol Oral Radiol Endod* 104:e56-e58, 2007.

## CALCIFIED BLOOD VESSEL

Almog DM, Horev T, Illig K et al: Correlating carotid artery stenosis detected by panoramic radiography with clinically relevant carotid artery stenosis determined by duplex ultrasound, *Oral Surg Oral Med Oral Pathol Oral Radiol Endod* 94:768-773, 2002.

Carter LC, Tsimidis K, Fabiano J: Carotid calcifications on panoramic radiography identify an asymptomatic male patient at risk for stroke: a case report, *Oral Surg Oral Med Oral Pathol Oral Radiol Endod* 85:119-122, 1998.

Friedlander AH, Altman L: Carotid artery atheromas in postmenopausal women: their prevalence on panoramic radiographs and their relationship to atherogenic risk, *J Am Dent Assoc* 132:1130-1136, 2001.

Mupparapu M, Kim I: Calcified carotid artery atheroma and stroke, *J Am Dent Assoc* 138:483-492, 2007.

## RHINOLITH/ANTROLITH

Güneri P, Kaya A, Caliskan M: Antroliths: survey of the literature and report of a case, *Oral Surg Oral Med Oral Pathol Oral Radiol Endod* 99:517-521, 2005.

Kaushik V, Bhalla R, Pahade A: Rhinolithiasis, *ENT Ear Nose Throat J* 83:512, 514, 2004.

Munoz A, Pedrosa I, Villafruela M: "Eraseroma" as a cause of rhinolith: CT and MRI in a child, *Neuroradiology* 39:824-826, 1997.

Orhan K, Kocyigit D, Kisnisci R et al: Rhinolithiasis: an uncommon entity of the nasal cavity, *Oral Surg Oral Med Oral Pathol Oral Radiol Endod* 101:e28-e32, 2007.

Pinto LS, Campagnoli EB, de Souza Azevedo R et al: Rhinoliths causing palatal perforation: case report and literature review, *Oral Surg Oral Med Oral Pathol Oral Radiol Endod* 104:e42-e46, 2007.

## SIALOLITH

Ho V, Currie WJ, Walker A: Sialolithiasis of minor salivary glands, *Br J Oral Maxillofac Surg* 30:273-275, 1992.

McGurk M, Escudier M, Thomas B et al: A revolution in the management of obstructive salivary gland disease, *Dent Update* 33:28-30, 2006; erratum: *Dent Update* 33:83, 2006.

Nahlieli O, Nakar L, Nazarian Y et al: Sialoendoscopy: a new approach to salivary gland obstructive pathology, *J Am Dent Assoc* 137:1394-1400, 2006.

Nakayama E, Okamura K, Mitsuyasu T et al: A newly developed interventional sialendoscope for a completely nonsurgical sialolithectomy using intracorporeal electrohydraulic lithotripsy, *J Oral Maxillofac Surg* 65:1402-1405, 2007.

Williams MF: Sialolithiasis, *Otolaryngol Clin North Am* 32:819-834, 1999.

## PHLEBOLITHS

Altug H, Büyüksoy V, Okçu K, Dogan N: Hemangiomas of the head and neck with pheboliths: clinical features, diagnostic imaging, and treatment of 3 cases, *Oral Surg Oral Med Oral Pathol Oral Radiol Endod* 103:e60-e64, 2007.

Chuang C-C, Lin H-C, Huang C-W: Submandibular cavernous hemangiomas with multiple phleboliths masquerading as sialolithiasis, *J Chin Med Assoc* 68:441-443, 2005.

Kakimoto N, Tanimoto K, Nishiyama H et al: CT and MR imaging features of oral and maxillofacial hemangioma and vascular malformation, *Eur J Radiol* 55:108-112, 2005.

## CALCIFIED TRACHEAL CARTILAGES

Ahmad M, Madden R, Perez L: Triticeous cartilage: prevalence on panoramic radiographs and diagnostic criteria, *Oral Surg Oral Med Oral Pathol Oral Radiol Endod* 99:225-230, 2005.

Carter L: Discrimination between calcified triticeous cartilage and calcified carotid atheroma on panoramic radiography, *Oral Surg Oral Med Oral Pathol Oral Radiol Endod* 90:108-110, 2000.

Mupparrapu M, Vuppalapati A: Ossification of laryngeal cartilages on lateral cephalometric radiographs, *Angle Orthod* 75:196-201, 2005.

## OSSIFIED STYLOHYOID LIGAMENT

Bafaqeeh SA: Eagle syndrome: classic and carotid artery types, *J Otolaryngol* 29:88-94, 2000.

Balbuena L, Hayes D, Ramirez SG et al: Eagle's syndrome (elongated styloid process), *South Med J* 90:331-334, 1997.

Chuang WC, Short JH, McKinney AM et al: Reversible left hemispheric ischemia secondary to carotid compression in Eagle syndrome: surgical and CT angiographic correlation, *AJNR Am J Neuroradiol* 28:143-145, 2007.

Eagle WW: Elongated styloid process, symptoms and treatment, *AMA Arch Otolaryngol* 67:172-176, 1958.

## OSTEOMA CUTIS

Baskan EB, Turan H, Tunali S et al: Miliary osteoma cutis of the face: treatment with the needle microincision-extirpation method, *J Dermatol Treat* 18:252-254, 2007.

Farhood V, Steed DL, Krolls SO: Osteoma cutis: cutaneous ossification with oral manifestations, *Oral Surg* 45:98-103, 1978.

Hughes PS: Multiple miliary osteomas of the face ablated with the erbium: YAG laser, *Arch Dermatol* 135:378-380, 1999.

Shigehara H, Honda Y, Kishi K et al: Radiographic and morphologic studies of multiple miliary osteomas of cadaver skin, *Oral Surg Oral Med Oral Pathol Oral Radiol Endod* 86:121-125, 1998.

Thielen AM, Stucki L, Braun RP et al: Multiple cutaneous osteomas of the face associated with chronic inflammatory acne, *J Eur Acad Dermatol Venereol* 20:321-326, 2006.

## MYOSITIS OSSIFICANS

Kaplan FS, McCluskey W, Hahn G et al: Genetic transmission of fibrodysplasia ossificans progressive: report of a family, *J Bone Joint Surg Am* 75:1214-1220, 1993.

Sarac S, Sennaroglu L, Hosal AS et al: Myositis ossificans in the neck, *Eur Arch Otorhinolaryngol* 256:199-201, 1999.

Spinazze R, Heffez L, Bays R: Chronic progressive limitation of mouth opening, *J Oral Maxillofac Surg* 56:1178-1186, 1998.

St.-Hilaire H, Weber W, Ramer M et al: Clinicopatholgic conference: trismus following dental treatment, *Oral Surg Oral Med Oral Pathol Oral Radiol Endod* 98:261-266, 2004.

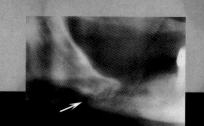

# CHAPTER 29

# Trauma to Teeth and Facial Structures

Ernest W.N. Lam

Radiologic examination is essential for evaluating trauma to the teeth and jaws. The presence, location, and orientation of fracture planes and fragments can be determined, and the involvement of nearby vital anatomic structures can be assessed. Furthermore, foreign objects that have become embedded within the soft tissues as a result of trauma can be detected. Follow-up images are useful in evaluating the extent of healing after an injury and long-term changes resulting from the trauma.

## Applied Radiology

The ideal imaging study may be difficult to perform after trauma because of the nature of the injury and patient discomfort. Although the prescription of the appropriate images should be ordered only after a careful clinical examination, in some cases this is not always possible. If plane radiography is to be used, multiple images should be made at differing angles, including at least two views made at right angles to each other. These views will typically consist of intraoral, panoramic, and lateral oblique projections of the mandible for dentoalveolar and mandibular injuries, and posteroanterior, Waters, submentovertex, Towne, and lateral projections for midface and skull injuries. In many centers, computed tomographic imaging (CT) has replaced plane radiography as the standard imaging modality whether for isolated trauma or more widespread complex injuries.

Although a panoramic image may be useful for localizing the area of an injury, it may not have the image resolution to reveal injuries involving the anterior mandible or maxillae or the teeth. Dentoalveolar trauma always requires intraoral images to obtain adequate anatomic detail. A minimum of two intraoral periapical images should be made at different horizontal x-ray beam angulations to identify fractures, and it is important to image not only the involved teeth but also the teeth of the opposing arch. Occlusal views may be particularly useful depending on the severity of the trauma and the ability of the patient to open the mouth.

If a tooth or a large fragment of a tooth is missing, a chest or abdominal image may be considered to locate the tooth. If there are lacerations in the lips or cheek, a soft tissue image of the area may be obtained by placing an intraoral film or receptor in the mouth adjacent to the traumatized soft tissue and then exposing it. If the laceration is in the tongue, a standard mandibular occlusal image may be exposed or the tongue can be protruded and then imaged.

## MANDIBULAR FRACTURES

Although the panoramic image may be a good initial image to make for assessing mandibular fractures, the intraoral cross-sectional occlusal view of the mandible may provide important information about body or alveolar process fractures in the tooth-supporting areas. If a panoramic image is not available, lateral oblique views of the mandible should be made.

The open mouth Towne view may be particularly useful in cases of suspected trauma to the mandibular condylar head and neck areas. These views are important to supplement lateral views of the temporomandibular joint, especially in cases of nondisplaced greenstick fractures of the condylar neck. For suspected multiple and complex fractures of the mandible, CT is the imaging modality of choice. Magnetic resonance imaging may be useful to assess soft tissue injury to the temporomandibular joint capsule or articular disk.

## MAXILLOFACIAL FRACTURES

Although some centers continue to rely on plane radiography for suspected localized trauma to the maxillofacial skeleton, CT is the imaging method of choice for more widespread complex fractures.

### RADIOGRAPHIC SIGNS OF FRACTURE

Fractures are often erroneously referred to as "lines" in spite of their three-dimensional nature. Fractures represent planes of cleavage through a tooth or bone, and these planes extend deep into the tissues. Therefore, a fracture may be missed if the plane of the fracture is not aligned with the direction of the incident x-ray beam on a single-plane image.

The following are general signs that may indicate the presence of a fracture of a tooth or bone:

1. The presence of one or two usually sharply defined radiolucent lines within the anatomic boundaries of a structure. If the line or lines extend beyond the boundaries of the mandible, more than likely they represent an overlapping structure. If a line extends beyond the boundaries of a tooth root, the line may represent a superimposed neurovascular canal.
2. A change in the normal anatomic outline or shape of the structure. A mandible that is noticeably asymmetric between the left and right sides may be fractured. A fracture of the mandible may also

manifest as a change in the contour of the occlusal plane at the location of the fracture site.

3. A loss of continuity of an outer border. This may appear as a gap in the continuity of the otherwise smooth tooth or cortical border. Such a gap may also produce a steptype defect where the two fragments have become displaced relative to one-another.

4. An increase in the radiopacity of a structure. This can be caused by the overlapping of two fragments of tooth or bone such that a particular area appears "doubly" radiopaque.

## Traumatic Injuries of the Teeth

### Concussion

#### Definition

The term *concussion* refers to a crush injury to the vascular structures at the tooth apex and the periodontal ligament resulting in inflammatory edema. No displacement and only minimal loosening of the tooth occurs. The injury may result in mild avulsion of the tooth from its socket, causing its occlusal surface to make premature contact with an opposing tooth during mandibular closing.

#### Clinical Features

The patient usually complains that the traumatized tooth is tender to touch, which can be confirmed by gentle horizontal or vertical percussion of the tooth. The tooth may also be sensitive to biting forces, although patients will usually try to modify their occlusion to avoid contacting the traumatized tooth.

#### Radiographic Features

The radiographic appearance of a dental concussion may be subtle. No radiographic changes may be found or localized widening of the apical periodontal ligament space may be seen (Fig. 29-1).

Reduction in the size of the pulp chamber and root canals may develop in the months and years after traumatic injury to the teeth (Fig. 29-2). This may be particularly evident in teeth that are still developing. If the pulp becomes necrotic, there may be no further deposition of (secondary) dentin as the odontoblasts and the pulpal stem cell populations die. The development of rarefying osteitis may ensue, and in rare cases, internal root resorption (Fig. 29-2).

#### Management

Because significant displacement of the tooth or teeth does not occur, the appropriate treatment is conservative and may include slight adjustment of the opposing teeth (if necessary) or the application of a flexible splint. Periodic monitoring in the first year with repeated vitality testing and radiographs are indicated.

### Luxation

#### Definition

Luxation is a dislocation of the tooth from its socket after severing of the periodontal attachment. Such teeth are both abnormally mobile and displaced. Subluxation of the tooth denotes an injury to the supporting structures of the tooth that results in abnormal loosening of the tooth without frank dislocation.

Depending on their magnitude and direction, traumatic forces can cause intrusive luxation (displacement of a tooth into the alveolar process), extrusive luxation (partial displacement of a tooth out of its socket), or lateral luxation (movement of a tooth in a direction other than intrusive or extrusive displacement). In intrusive and lateral luxation, comminution or crushing of the alveolar process may accompany tooth dislocation.

The movement of the apex and disruption of the circulation to the traumatized tooth that accompanies luxation can produce either temporary or permanent changes to the dental pulp, and these changes may result in pulpal necrosis. If the pulp survives the traumatic incident, the rate of dentin formation may accelerate and continue until it obliterates the pulp chamber and root canal. This may take place in permanent and deciduous teeth.

#### Clinical Features

An adequate clinical history is helpful in identifying luxation and ordering the appropriate radiographs. Subluxated teeth are in their normal location but are abnormally mobile. There may be extrava-

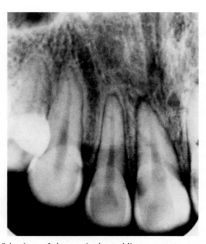

FIG. **29-1** Widening of the periodontal ligament spaces of the incisors after dental concussion.

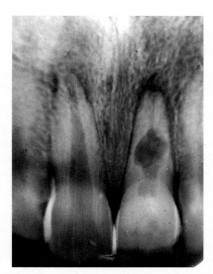

FIG. **29-2** Obliteration of the pulp chamber but not the root canal, internal root resorption, and an incisal fracture of the maxillary left central incisor after dental concussion. As well, note the area of rarefying osteitis involving the maxillary right central incisor and the widened pulp chamber and canal.

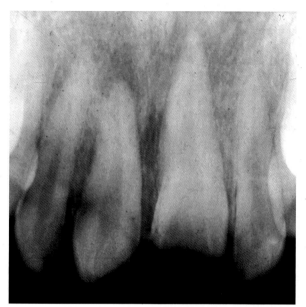

FIG. **29-3**  Intruded maxillary central incisor after trauma. Note the fractured incisal edges of both central incisors.

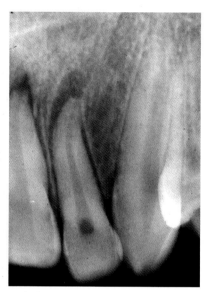

FIG. **29-4**  Extruded maxillary lateral incisor after trauma. Note the localized increase to the width of the apical periodontal ligament space.

sated blood emanating from the gingival crevice, indicating periodontal ligament damage, and they may be extremely sensitive to percussion and masticatory forces.

The clinical crowns of intruded teeth may appear reduced in height. Maxillary incisors may be intruded so deeply into the alveolar process that they appear to be completely avulsed or lost. The displaced tooth may cause some damage to adjacent teeth, particularly if any developing permanent teeth are present in the underlying bone.

Depending on the orientation and magnitude of the force and the shape of the root, it may be pushed through the buccal or, less commonly, the lingual cortex of the alveolar process where it may be seen and palpated. On repeated vitality testing, the sensitivity of a luxated tooth may be temporarily decreased or undetectable, especially shortly after the injury. Vitality may return, however, after weeks or even several months.

Usually two or more teeth are involved in luxation injuries, and the teeth most frequently affected are the deciduous and permanent maxillary incisors. The mandibular teeth are seldom affected. The type of luxation appears to vary with age and this may reflect changes to the nature of maturing bone. Intrusions and extrusions are often found in the deciduous dentition. In the permanent dentition, the intrusive type of luxation is seen less frequently.

### Radiographic Features

Radiographic examinations of luxated teeth may demonstrate the extent of injury to the root, periodontal ligament, and alveolar process. A radiograph made at the time of injury serves as a valuable reference point for comparison with subsequent radiographs. As with dental concussion, the minor damage associated with subluxation may be subtle and limited to elevation of the tooth from its socket. The sole radiographic finding may be a widening of the apical portion of the periodontal ligament space. Elevation of the tooth may not be radiographically apparent.

The depressed position of the crown of an intruded tooth is often apparent on a radiograph (Fig. 29-3), although a minimally intruded tooth may be difficult to demonstrate radiographically. Intrusion may result in partial or total obliteration of the apical periodontal ligament space. Multiple radiographic projections, including occlusal views, may be necessary to show the direction of tooth displacement and the relationship of the displaced tooth to adjacent teeth and the outer cortex of bone.

A tooth that has been extruded may demonstrate varying degrees of apical widening of the periodontal ligament space, depending on the magnitude of the extrusive force (Fig. 29-4). A laterally luxated tooth with some degree of extrusion may show a widened periodontal ligament space, with greater width on the side of impact.

### Management

A subluxated permanent tooth may be restored to its normal position by digital pressure shortly after the accident. If inflammation precludes repositioning, minimal reduction of opposing teeth may be necessary to minimize any discomfort. The use of a flexible splint may provide additional stability and prevent further damage to the pulp and periodontal ligament. A subluxed deciduous tooth may potentially damage its underlying successor. Consequently, extraction may be considered. If the alveolar bone over the root of a luxated tooth has been fragmented and displaced, the fragments should be repositioned by digital pressure. A subluxated primary tooth should be periodically examined after the injury. If it causes some discomfort as the result of extrusion, it can be removed without undue concern for occlusal problems. Subluxed permanent teeth should be monitored in the same manner as those teeth that have been concussed.

### Avulsion

#### Definition

*Avulsion* is the term used to describe the complete displacement of a tooth from the alveolar process. Teeth may be avulsed by direct trauma when the force is applied directly to the tooth or by indirect trauma (i.e., when indirect force is applied to teeth as a result of the jaws striking together). Avulsion occurs in about 15% of traumatic injuries

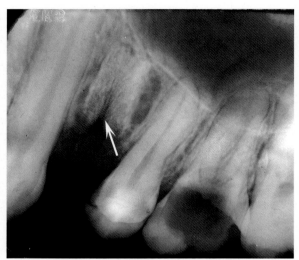

FIG. **29-5**   Bone formation during healing of a first premolar tooth socket. Note how the bone is developing from the lateral walls of the socket. The central radiolucent line *(arrow)* may have a similar appearance to that of a pulp canal, falsely giving the impression of a retained tooth fragment.

to the teeth, with fights being responsible for the avulsion of most permanent teeth and accidental falls accounting for the traumatic loss of most deciduous teeth.

### Clinical Features

Maxillary central incisors are the most commonly avulsed teeth from both dentitions. Most often only a single tooth is lost. Typically this injury occurs in a relatively young age group when the permanent central incisors are just erupting. Fractures of the alveolar process and lip lacerations may be seen with an avulsed tooth.

### Radiographic Features

In a recent avulsion, the lamina dura of the empty socket is apparent and usually persists for several months. The missing tooth may be displaced into the adjacent soft tissue, and its image may project over the alveolar process on an image, giving the false impression that it lies within the bone. Therefore, to differentiate between an intruded tooth and an avulsed tooth lying within the adjacent soft tissues, a soft tissue image of the lacerated lip or tongue should be made. In some instances new bone within the healing socket may be very dense and simulate a retained root tip (Fig. 29-5).

### Management

If the avulsed tooth is not found by clinical or radiographic examination, a chest or abdominal radiograph may be considered to locate it within the airway or gastrointestinal tract. Reimplanting permanent teeth after avulsion is possible; however, the prognosis of the reimplantation is dependent on the condition of the tooth while it is outside the mouth, the time it is out of its socket, and the viability of the residual periodontal ligament fibers. Endodontic therapy may be necessary after reimplantation and there may be external root resorption in the months and years after reimplantation. Reimplanting an avulsed deciduous tooth carries the danger of interfering with the underlying developing permanent tooth.

## FRACTURES OF THE TEETH

### Dental Crown Fractures

#### Definition

Fractures of the dental crown account for about 25% of traumatic injuries to the permanent teeth and 40% of injuries to the deciduous teeth. The most common event responsible for the fracture of permanent teeth is a fall, followed by accidents involving vehicles (e.g., bicycles, automobiles) and blows from foreign objects striking the teeth. Fractures involving only the crown normally fall into three categories:

1. Fractures that involve only the enamel without the loss of enamel substance (infraction of the crown or crack)
2. Fractures that involve enamel or enamel and dentin with loss of tooth substance but without pulpal involvement (uncomplicated fracture)
3. Fractures that pass through enamel, dentin, and pulp with loss of tooth substance and exposure of the pulp (complicated fracture)

#### Clinical Features

Fractures of the dental crowns most frequently involve anterior teeth. Infractions or cracks in the enamel are quite common but frequently are not readily detectable. Illuminating crowns with indirect light (directing the beam along the long axis of the tooth) causes cracks to appear distinctly in the enamel. Histologic studies show that they pass through the enamel but not into the dentin. The pattern and distribution of these cracks are unpredictable and apparently relate to the trauma.

Uncomplicated crown fractures that do not involve dentin usually occur at the mesioincisal or distoincisal corners of the maxillary central incisor. Loss of the central portion of the incisal edge may also occur. Fractures that involve dentin can be recognized by the contrast in color between dentin and the peripheral layer of enamel. The exposed dentin is usually sensitive to chemical, thermal, and mechanical stimulation. In deep fractures, the pink blush of the pulp may be appreciated through the thin remaining dentin wall.

Uncomplicated fractures that involve both the enamel and the dentin of permanent teeth are more common than complicated fractures are. In contrast, the incidence of complicated and uncomplicated fractures is about equal in the deciduous teeth.

Complicated crown fractures are distinguishable by bleeding from the exposed pulp or by droplets of blood forming from pinpoint exposures. The pulp is visible and may extrude from the open pulp chamber if the fracture is old. The exposed pulp is sensitive to most forms of stimulation.

#### Radiographic Features

Radiographs provide information regarding the location and extent of the fracture and the relationship of the fracture plane and fragment to the pulp chamber. As well, the stage of root development of the involved tooth can be assessed with radiography (Fig. 29-6). This initial image also provides a means of comparison for follow-up examinations of the involved teeth.

#### Management

Although crown infractions do not require treatment, the vitality of the tooth should be evaluated. The sharp edges of enamel that result from an uncomplicated fracture should be smoothed and may require restoration for cosmetic reasons. It is reasonable to delay this procedure for a number of weeks until the pulp has recovered and secondary dentin is laid down. The prognosis for teeth with fractures limited to the enamel is quite good, and pulpal necrosis develops in fewer than 2% of such cases. If a fracture involves both dentin and enamel, the frequency of pulpal necrosis is about 3%. Oblique fractures have a worse prognosis than horizontal fractures because potentially a greater amount of dentin is exposed. The frequency of pulpal necrosis increases greatly with concussion and mobility of the tooth.

Treatment of complicated crown fractures of permanent teeth may involve pulp capping, pulpotomy, or pulpectomy, depending on the stage of root formation. If a coronal fracture of a deciduous tooth involves the pulp, it is usually best treated by extraction.

## Dental Root Fractures

### Definition
Fractures of tooth roots are uncommon and account for fewer than 7% of traumatic injuries to permanent teeth and about half that many in deciduous teeth. This difference probably results from the fact that the deciduous teeth are less firmly anchored in the alveolar process.

### Clinical Features
Most root fractures occur in maxillary central incisors. The coronal fragments are usually displaced lingually and slightly extruded. The degree of mobility of the crown relates to the level of the fracture. That is, the closer the fracture plane is located to the apex, the more stable the tooth is. When testing the mobility of a traumatized tooth, place a finger over the alveolar process. If movement of only the crown is detected, a root fracture is likely. Fractures of the root may occur with fractures of the alveolar process, which are commonly not detected. This is most often observed in the anterior region of the mandible where root fractures are infrequent. Although root fracture is usually associated with temporary loss of sensitivity (by all usual criteria), the sensitivity of most teeth returns to normal within about 6 months.

### Radiographic Features
Fractures of the dental root may occur at any level and involve one (Fig. 29-7) or all the roots of multirooted teeth. Most of the fractures confined to the root occur in the middle third of the root.

The ability of an image to reveal the presence of a root fracture depends on the relative angulation of the incident x-ray beam to the fracture plane and the degree of distraction of the fragments. If the x-ray beam is well aligned with the fracture plane, a single sharply defined radiolucent line confined to the anatomic limits of the root may be seen. If, however, the orientation of the x-ray beam is not well aligned and meets the fracture plane in a more oblique manner, the fracture plane may appear as a more poorly defined single line or as two lines that converge at the mesial and distal surfaces of the root. The appearance of a comminuted root fracture may also appear less well defined. Most nondisplaced root fractures are usually difficult to demonstrate radiographically, and several views at differing angles may be necessary. In some instances when the fracture line is not visible, the only evidence of a fracture may be a localized increase in the width of the periodontal ligament space adjacent to the fracture site (Fig. 29-8).

Longitudinal root fractures are relatively uncommon but are most likely in teeth with posts that have been subjected to trauma. The width of the fracture plane tends to increase with time, probably because of resorption of the fractured surfaces. Over time,

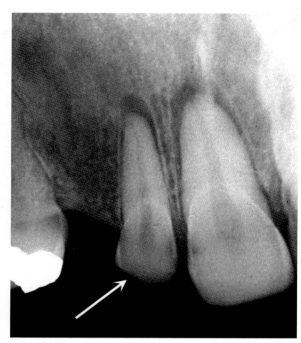

FIG. **29-6**    An incisal edge fracture involving the right maxillary lateral incisor *(arrow)* and subluxation of both the central and lateral incisors. Note the increases to the widths of the apical periodontal ligament spaces.

calcification and obliteration of the pulp chamber and canal may be seen.

### Differential Diagnosis
The superimposition of soft tissue structures such as the lip, ala of the nose, or nasolabial fold over the image of a root may suggest a root fracture. To avoid this diagnostic error, it should be noted that the soft tissue image of the lip line usually extends beyond the tooth margins. Fractures of the alveolar process may also overlap the root and suggest a root fracture.

### Management
Fractures in the middle or apical third of the root of permanent teeth can be manually reduced to the proper position and immobilized. Prognosis is generally favorable because the incidence of pulpal necrosis is about 20% to 24%. The more apical the fracture is, the better the prognosis. Endodontic therapy is performed when evidence of pulpal necrosis exists. It is common for bone resorption to occur at the site of the fracture rather than at the apex. When the fracture occurs in the coronal third of the root, the prognosis is poor and extraction is indicated unless the apical portion of the root fragment can be extruded orthodontically and restored. The roots of fractured deciduous teeth that are not badly dislocated may be retained with the expectation that they will be normally resorbed. Attempts at removal may result in damage to the developing succedaneous tooth.

## Vertical Root Fractures

### Definition
Vertical root fractures represent fracture planes that run lengthwise from the crown toward the apex of the tooth. Usually both sides of a root are involved. The crack is usually oriented in the facial-

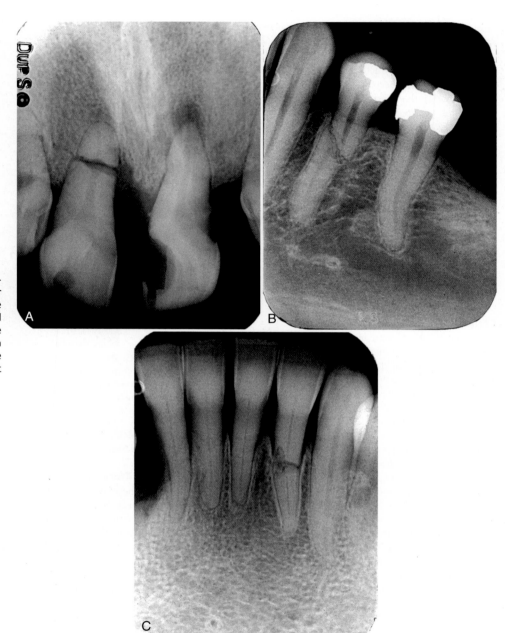

FIG. **29-7**  **A,** A recent horizontal fracture of the right maxillary central incisor and apical rarefying osteitis involving the adjacent left central incisor. **B,** A healed fracture with slight displacement of the fragments. **C,** A healed fracture with an increase in the distance between the fracture segments as a result of root resorption.

lingual plane in both anterior and posterior teeth. These fractures usually occur in the posterior teeth in adults, especially in mandibular molars. They are usually iatrogenic, after insertion of retention screws or pins into teeth. Uncrowned posterior teeth that have been treated endodontically are most at risk. Large occlusal forces are another etiology for vertical root fracture, particularly in restored teeth.

### Clinical Features
Patients with vertical root fractures complain of persistent low-level dull pain, often of long duration, the so-called cracked tooth syndrome. This pain is elicited by applying pressure to the involved tooth.

The patient may have rarefying osteitis or a history of repeated failed endodontic therapy. Occasionally, definitive diagnosis can be made only by inspection after surgical exposure.

### Radiographic Features
If the central ray of the x-ray beam lies along the plane of the fracture, the fracture may be visible as a radiolucent line on the image. Usually, however, radiography is not useful in identifying vertical root fractures in their early stages. Later, if rarefying osteitis develops, there will be evidence of bone loss (Fig. 29-9). The widening of the periodontal ligament space and this bone loss may not be centered at the apex but often positioned more coronally toward the alveolar crest.

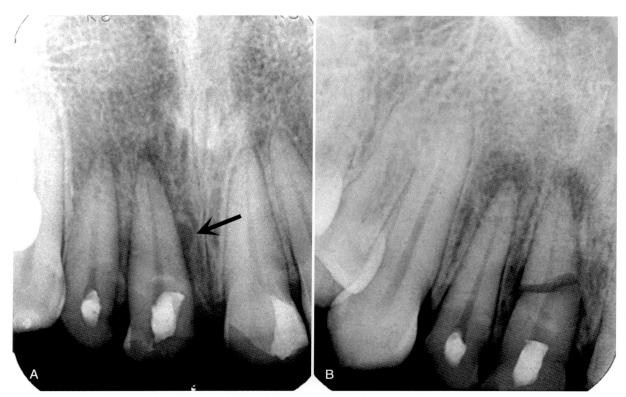

FIG. **29-8    A,** Subtle evidence of a root fracture involving the root of the maxillary right central incisor. Although a fracture plane is not apparent on the mesial aspect of the root because of malalignment of the x-ray beam, there is widening of the periodontal membrane space on the mesial surface *(arrow)* at the site of the fracture. **B,** Later dislocation of the root fragments.

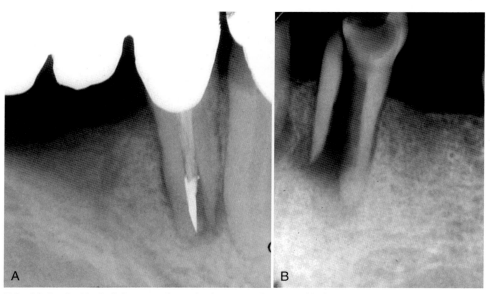

FIG. **29-9    A,** Vertical fracture through the root of a mandibular first premolar that has been endodontically treated. The fracture plane extends through the root canal and there is more displacement between the root fragments at the apex of the root. **B,** A vertical root fracture through the root of a mandibular canine with significant displacement of the fragments.

Inflammatory lesions may also extend apically from the alveolar crest and may resemble periodontal lesions.

### Management

Single-rooted teeth with vertical root fractures must be extracted. Multirooted teeth may be hemisected and the intact remaining half of the tooth restored with endodontic therapy and a crown.

### Combination Crown and Root Fractures

#### Definition

Crown/root fractures involve both the crown and root(s). Although uncomplicated fractures may occur, crown/root fractures usually involve the pulp. About twice as many affect the permanent as the deciduous teeth. Most crown/root fractures of the anterior teeth are the result of direct trauma. Many posterior teeth are predisposed to such fractures by large restorations or extensive caries.

#### Clinical Features

The fracture plane of a typical crown/root fracture of an anterior tooth extends obliquely from the labial surface near the gingival third of the crown to a position apical to the gingival attachment on the lingual surface. Displacement of the fragments is usually minimal. Crown/root fractures occasionally present with bleeding from the pulp. Because these teeth are sensitive to occlusal forces that may cause separation of the fragments, a patient with a crown/root fracture usually complains of pain during mastication.

#### Radiographic Features

These fractures are often not visible on the radiographic image because the x-ray beam is rarely aligned with the plane of the fracture. Also, distraction of the fragments is usually not present. Vertical crown/root fractures that are oriented in a mainly tangential orientation relative to the direction of the x-ray beam are readily apparent on the image. Unfortunately, this is not common.

#### Management

Removal of the coronal fragment permits the evaluation of the extent of the fracture. If the coronal fragment includes as much as 3 to 4 mm of clinical root, successful restoration of the tooth is doubtful and removal of the residual root is recommended. If the crown/root fracture is vertically oriented, prognosis is poor regardless of treatment.

If the pulp is not exposed and the fracture does not extend more than 3 to 4 mm below the epithelial attachment, conservative treatment is likely to be successful. Uncomplicated crown/root fractures are frequently encountered in posterior teeth, and with crown lengthening procedures the tooth is likely to be restorable. If only a small amount of root is lost with the coronal fragment but the pulp has been compromised, it is likely that the tooth can be restored after endodontic treatment.

## Traumatic Injuries to the Facial Bones

Facial fractures most frequently affect the zygomatic bones or mandible and, to a lesser extent, the maxillae. Radiography plays a crucial role in the diagnosis and management of traumatic injuries to these and the other facial bones.

Superficial signs of injury such as soft tissue swelling, hematoma formation, or hemorrhage from a laceration or abrasion may focus the radiologic examination. Localized injuries may be investigated with plane radiography. In this instance, it is important to make at least two views of the injured site at right angles to one another to assess the presence, location, extent, and displacement of a fracture. Some fractures may not be readily apparent if the x-ray beam is not oriented parallel to the plane of the fracture. More and more commonly, plane radiography is being replaced by CT, even for localized injuries. For more widespread trauma, CT is the imaging modality of choice.

## MANDIBULAR FRACTURES

The most common mandibular fracture sites are the condyle, body, and angle, followed less frequently by the parasymphyseal region, ramus, coronoid process, and alveolar process. Trauma to the mandible is often associated with other injuries, most commonly concussion (loss of consciousness) and other fractures, usually of the maxillae, zygomatic bones, and cranial vault.

The most common causes of mandibular fractures are assault, falls, and sports injuries. About half of all mandibular fractures occur in individuals between 16 and 35 years old, and injuries in males are reportedly three times more common than in females. Moreover, fractures are more likely to occur on weekend days than on other days of the week.

### Mandibular Body Fractures

#### Definition

The mandible is the most commonly fractured facial bone. It is important to realize that a fracture of the mandibular body on one side is frequently accompanied by a fracture of the condylar neck on the opposite side. Trauma to the anterior mandible may result in unilateral or bilateral fractures of the condylar necks. When a localized heavy force is directed posteriorly to the mandible, there may be fractures of the angle, ramus, or even the coronoid process. In children, fractures of the mandibular body usually occur in the anterior region.

Mandibular fractures are classified as being either favorable or unfavorable, depending on the orientation of the fracture plane. Unfavorable fractures are those in which the action of muscles attached to the mandibular fragments displace the fragments away from one another. For example, if a fracture plane in the body of the mandible slants obliquely posteriorly and inferiorly from the base of the anterior border of the ramus, the masseter and medial pterygoid muscles may displace the ramal fragment superiorly and away from the body of the mandible. In favorable fractures, the muscle action tends to reduce the fracture.

#### Clinical Features

A history of injury is typical, substantiated by some evidence of the trauma that caused the fracture, such as injury to the overlying skin. Frequently the patient has swelling and a deformity that is accentuated when the patient opens the mouth. A discrepancy is often present in the occlusal plane, and manipulation may produce crepitus or abnormal mobility. Intraoral examination may reveal ecchymosis in the floor of the mouth. In the case of bilateral fractures to the mandible, a risk exists that the digastric, mylohyoid, and omohyoid muscles will displace the anterior mandibular fragment posteriorly and inferiorly, causing impingement on the airway.

#### Radiographic Features

The radiographic examination of a suspected mandibular fracture may include intraoral or occlusal views, a panoramic view, postero-

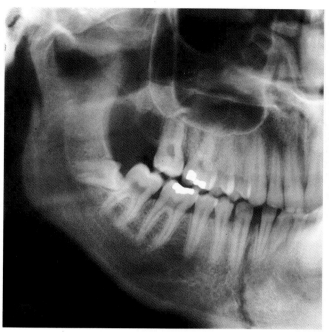

FIG. **29-10**  Cropped panoramic image shows a fracture through the right parasymphyseal region and a condylar neck fracture on the same side. Note the step defect on the posterior surface of the mandibular ramus.

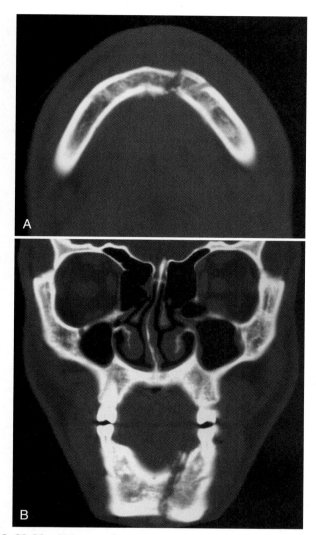

FIG. **29-11**  CT images show a minimally displaced mandibular para-symphyseal fracture in the axial **(A)** and coronal **(B)** planes.

anterior or submentovertex plain radiographic views, or CT. Intraoral images may, given their higher resolution, reveal fractures that extra-oral plane images may fail to reveal.

The margins of fracture planes usually appear as sharply defined radiolucent lines of separation that are confined to the structure of the mandible (Fig. 29-10). They are best visualized when the x-ray beam is oriented along the plane of the fracture. Displacement of the fragments results in a cortical discontinuity or "step" (Fig. 29-11) or an irregularity in the occlusal plane. Occasionally, the margins of the fracture overlap each other, resulting in an area of increased radiopacity at the fracture site.

Nondisplaced mandibular fractures may involve one or both buccal and lingual cortical plates. An incomplete fracture involving only one cortical plate is often called a greenstick fracture; these usually occur in children. An oblique fracture that involves both corti-cal plates may cause some diagnostic difficulties if the fracture lines in the buccal and lingual plates are not superimposed (Fig. 29-12). In this case, two lines are seen that converge at the periphery, suggesting two distinct fractures when in reality only one exists. A right-angle view such as an occlusal view may be useful.

### Differential Diagnosis

The superimposition of soft tissue images on the image of the man-dible may simulate fractures. A narrow air space between the dorsal surface of the tongue and the soft palate superimposed across the angle of the mandible in a panoramic image may simulate a fracture. The air space between the dorsal surface of the tongue and the poste-rior pharyngeal wall can appear similar to a fracture on lateral views of the mandible. Similar appearances can occur in the region of soft palate where it superimposes over the ramus.

### Management

The management of a fracture of the mandible presents a variety of surgical problems that involve the proper reduction, fixation, and immobilization of the fractured bone fragments. Minimally displaced fractures are managed by closed reduction and intermaxillary fixa-tion, whereas fractures with more severely displaced fragments may require open reduction. Treatment for fractures of the body often includes antibiotic therapy because a tooth root may be in the line of the fracture. When the fracture line involves third molars, severely mobile teeth, or teeth with at least half their roots exposed in the fracture line, the involved teeth are often extracted to reduce the risk of infection and problems with fixation.

### Mandibular Condyle Fractures

#### Definition

Fractures involving the mandibular condyle can be divided into con-dylar neck fractures and condylar head fractures. Condylar neck frac-tures are more common and are located below the condylar head. When a condylar neck fracture occurs, the head is usually displaced

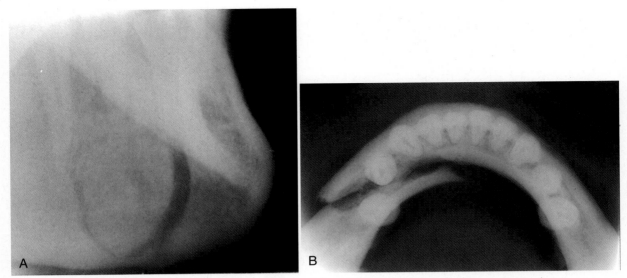

FIG. **29-12    A,** A lateral oblique image of the right mandible in the premolar region shows what appears to be two fracture lines that converge at the inferior cortex. **B,** The true occlusal image of the mandible of the same case demonstrates only a single fracture plane. Therefore the two lines seen in **A** reflect the obliquity of the fracture plane relative to the x-ray beam.

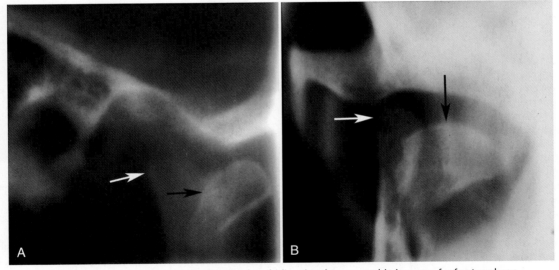

FIG. **29-13**    Corrected sagittal and coronal multidirectional tomographic images of a fractured condylar head. The condylar head has been displaced anteriorly *(black arrow)* in the sagittal view **(A)** and medially *(black arrow)* in the coronal view **(B)** as a result of contraction of the lateral ptyergoid muscle. The residual condylar neck *(white arrow in both images)* can be seen.

medially, inferiorly, and anteriorly as a result of contraction of the lateral pterygoid muscle (Figs. 29-13 and 29-14). Fractures of the condylar head may result in a vertical cleft dividing the condylar head fragments or may produce multiple fragments in a compression-like injury. Almost half the patients with condylar fractures also have fractures in the mandibular body.

## Clinical Features

The clinical symptoms of a fractured condylar head are not always apparent, so the preauricular area must be carefully examined and

palpated. The patient may have pain on opening or closing the mouth or trismus from local swelling. An anterior open bite may be present with only distal molar contacts and there may be deviation of the mandible on opening. A significant feature may be the inability of the patient to protrude the mandible because the lateral pterygoid muscle is attached to the condyle.

## Radiographic Features

Nondisplaced fractures of the condylar process may be difficult to detect on plain radiographic or panoramic images. CT is the imaging modality of choice because it will enable the clinician to visualize the three-dimensional relationship of the displaced condylar head to the glenoid fossa and to adjacent anatomical structures in the skull base and infratemporal fossa (Figs. 29-15 and 29-16).

Studies of remodeled previously fractured condyles show that young persons have much greater remodeling potential than do adults. In children younger than 12 years, most fractured condyles show a radiographic return to normal morphology after healing, whereas in teenagers the remodeling is less complete. In adults, only minor remodeling is observed. The extent of remodeling is also greater with fractures of the condylar head than with condylar neck fractures with displacement of the condylar head. The most common deformities are medial inclination of the condyle, abnormal shape of the condyle, shortening of the neck, erosion, and flattening. Early condylar fractures commonly result in hypoplasia of the ipsilateral side of the mandible.

## Management

The technical details of treating condylar fractures vary according to whether one or both condyles are involved, the extent of displacement, and the occurrence and severity of concomitant fractures. The treatment is directed to relieve acute symptoms, restore proper anatomic relationships, and prevent bony ankylosis. If a malocclusion develops, intermaxillary fixation may be provided in an attempt to restore proper occlusion. Often condylar head and neck fractures are not reduced because of the morbidity of the procedure and the size and position of the fracture fragments.

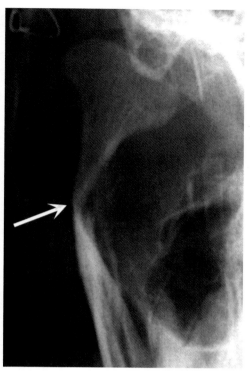

FIG. **29-14**  A periorbital view of the mandibular condyle showing a greenstick fracture of the condylar neck.

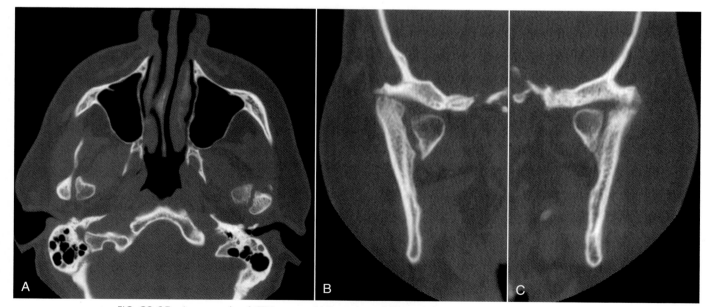

FIG. **29-15**  An example of CT images of bilateral condylar neck fractures showing medial displacement of the condylar heads in line with the lateral pterygoid muscles in the axial image **(A)** and medial displacement in the coronal images **(B** and **C)**; also in **C** there is osseous ankylosis between the residual condylar neck and the temporal bone.

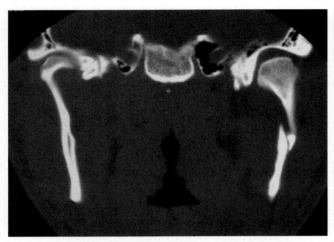

FIG. **29-16** Coronal CT image shows medial displacement and rotation of a condylar neck fracture.

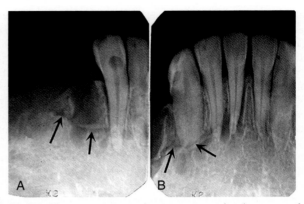

FIG. **29-17** These two images demonstrate an alveolar process fracture extending from the distal aspect of the mandibular right cuspid in an anterior direction (arrows) and through the tooth socket of the right central incisor.

## Fractures of the Alveolar Processes

### Definition
Simple fractures of the alveolar process may involve the buccal or lingual cortical plates of the alveolar processes of the maxillae or mandible. Commonly these fractures are associated with traumatic injuries to teeth that are luxated with or without dislocation. Several teeth are usually affected, and the fracture plane is most often horizontally oriented. Some fractures extend through the entire alveolar process (in contrast to the simple fracture that involves only one cortical plate), and the fracture plane may be located apical to the teeth or involve the tooth socket. These are also commonly associated with dental injuries and extrusive luxations with or without root fractures.

### Clinical Features
A common location of alveolar fractures is the anterior maxilla. Simple alveolar fractures are relatively rare in the posterior segments of the arches. In this location, fracture of the buccal plate usually occurs during removal of a maxillary posterior tooth. Fractures of the entire alveolar process occur in the anterior and premolar regions and in an older age group.

A characteristic feature of an alveolar process fracture is marked malocclusion with displacement and mobility of the fragment, and when the practitioner tests the mobility of a single tooth, the entire fragment of bone moves. The teeth in the fragment will have a recognizable dull sound when percussed and the attached gingiva may have lacerations. The detached bone may include the floor of the maxillary sinus, in which case bleeding from the nose on the involved side may occur as well as ecchymosis of the buccal vestibule.

### Radiographic Features
Periapical radiographs, if they can be made, will often not reveal fractures of a single cortical wall of the alveolar process, although evidence exists that the teeth have been luxated. However, a fracture of the anterior labial cortical plate may be apparent on an occlusal radiograph or on a lateral extraoral image of the mandible if bone displacement has occurred and the x-ray beam is oriented at near right angles to the direction of bone displacement. Fractures of both cortical plates of the alveolar process are usually apparent (Fig. 29-17).

The closer the fracture is to the alveolar crest, the greater the possibility that root fractures are present. It may be difficult to differentiate a root fracture from an overlapping fracture line of the alveolar bone. Several images produced with different projection angles may help with this differentiation. If the fracture plane is truly associated with the tooth, the line should not shift relative to the tooth. Fractures of the posterior alveolar process may involve the floor of the maxillary sinus and result in abnormal thickening of the sinus mucosa or the accumulation of blood and sinus secretions, in which case an air-fluid level may be appreciated.

### Management
Fractures of the alveolar process are treated by repositioning the displaced teeth and associated bone fragments with digital pressure. Gingival lacerations are sutured. If the luxated permanent teeth are splinted and stable, intermaxillary fixation may not be necessary. Teeth that have lost their vascular supply may eventually require endodontic treatment.

A soft diet for 10 to 14 days is recommended. Antibiotic coverage is provided because of communication with tooth sockets.

## MIDFACIAL FRACTURES INCLUDING MAXILLARY FRACTURES

### Definition
Fractures of the midfacial region one or multiple bones in the skull are discussed in this section.

## Orbital Blow-Out Fractures

### Definition
The blow-out fracture is generated as a result of a direct blow to the orbit by an object that is too large to enter the orbital cavity, such as a fist or a baseball. In this fracture, one or more of the walls of the orbit are damaged, but the orbital rim remains intact. The most common fractures involve the medial wall of the orbit formed by the lamina papyracea of the ethmoid bone and the floor of the orbit that separates this space from the maxillary sinus.

### Clinical Features
Periorbital edema is a common feature of the orbital blow-out fracture, as is enophthalmos. Eye movements may be restricted if one or

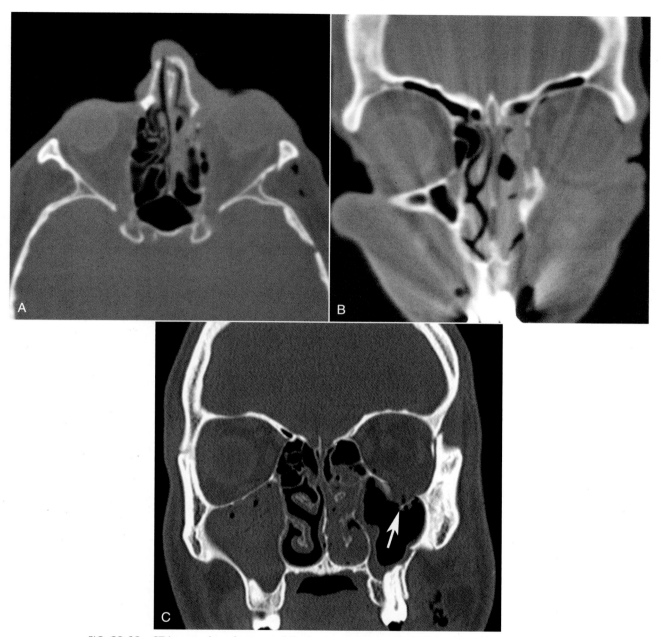

FIG. **29-18**   CT images show fractures of the lamina papyracea of the left ethmoid bone in the axial **(A)** and coronal **(B)** planes. Note the fluid/soft tissue densities in the adjacent ethmoid air cells. **C,** This coronal CT image demonstrates a blow-out fracture of the orbit; note the discontinuity in the floor of the orbit and herniation of soft tissue into the maxillary sinus *(arrow).*

more of the periorbital muscles becomes entrapped in the bony defect created by the fracture. If the ethmoid air cells are involved, there may be epistaxis.

### Radiographic Features
The Waters view or CT (Fig. 29-18) may demonstrate a discontinuity of the lamina papyracea in a medial wall blow-out fracture or the accumulation of soft tissue in the roof of the maxillary sinus in an orbital floor blow-out. Coronal CT may show the classic "trap door" appearance of the displaced orbital floor to best advantage. Soft tissue

CT images will show soft tissue densities or air-fluid levels in the adjacent ethmoid air cells (Fig. 29-18) or maxillary sinus or herniation of periorbital fat and entrapment of periorbital muscle through the bony defect in the orbital floor.

### Management
Surgical repair may be attempted for patients who have severely affected eye movements as a result of muscle entrapment or unacceptable enopthalmos.

## Zygomatic Fractures

### Definition

Unilateral fractures involving the zygomatic bone may include tripod fractures, in which the zygomatic bone and adjacent areas of the maxillary, frontal, sphenoid, and temporal bones may be involved, or zygomatic arch fractures, in which the zygomatic process of the temporal bone is fractured. Bilateral zygomatic fractures can occur in association with Le Fort type II and III fractures (described in the following section).

Injuries to the zygomatic bone or arch usually result from a forceful blow to the cheek or side of the face. Although zygomatic bone injuries may displace the fragment(s) medially, support by the adjacent temporalis and masseter muscles may limit displacement.

### Clinical Features

Flattening of the upper cheek with tenderness and dimpling of the skin over the side of the face may occur, although some of the clinical characteristics of zygomatic fractures may not be apparent much longer than an hour after trauma because they may be masked by edema. In most cases, periorbital ecchymosis and hemorrhage into the sclera (near the outer canthus) occur. Additional symptoms may include unilateral epistaxis (for a short time after the accident), anesthesia or paresthesia of the cheek, and compromised eye movements. The presence of diplopia suggests a significant injury to the floor of the orbit. Mandibular movement may be limited if the displaced zygomatic bone impinges on the coronoid process.

### Radiographic Features

Because of edema obscuring the clinical features, the radiographic examination may provide the only means of determining the pres-

ence and extent of the injury. The occipitomental (Waters) view provides a good image of the zygomatic bone and midface that will show the displaced fracture fragment (Fig. 29-19). An underexposed submentovertex projection (the so-called jug-handle view) provides a good view of the zygomatic arch and can often show the V-shaped deformity of the zygomatic process of the temporal bone. CT is, however, the imaging modality of choice for these fractures (Fig. 29-20).

The zygomatic arch may fracture at its weakest point, about 1 cm posterior to the zygomaticotemporal suture. Separation or fracture of the frontozygomatic suture may also occur. Fractures do not usually occur through the zygomaticomaxillary suture; however, in some cases, a fracture plane may extend obliquely involving the inferior rim of the orbit and the lateral wall of the maxilla. If the fracture plane involves the maxillary sinus, the sinus may exhibit increased radiopac-

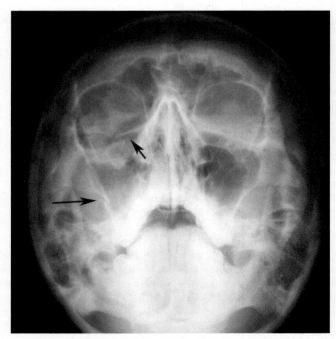

FIG. **29-19** Waters view shows a tripod fracture involving the right zygomatic bone. Note the fracture through the right orbital rim and lateral wall of the maxillary sinus. As well, there is radiopacification of the right maxillary sinus.

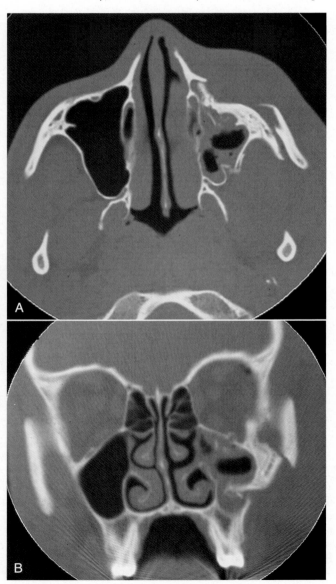

FIG. **29-20** Axial **(A)** and coronal **(B)** CT images show depression and rotation of a left tripod fracture. An air-fluid level is also visible in the left maxillary sinus.

ity as a result of the accumulation of blood and mucus secretions, an air-fluid level.

Panoramic images of the zygomatic arch often reveal the zygomaticotemporal suture as a radiolucent line that may even have the appearance of a discontinuity in the inferior border. This is a variation of normal anatomy and should not be misinterpreted as a fracture.

### Management

When symptoms include minimal displacement of the zygomatic arch and no cosmetic deformity or impairment of eye movement, no treatment may be required. Otherwise, reduction is usually indicated. Fractures of the zygomatic bone and arch may be reduced through an intraoral or extraoral approach.

## LE FORT FRACTURES

Complex fractures involving multiple facial bones may be quite variable but often follow general patterns classified by the French surgeon Rene Le Fort. By definition, all Le Fort fractures include fractures of one of the pterygoid plates of the sphenoid bone, and although Le Fort fractures may be bilateral, they are most often unilateral.

The radiographic interpretation of fractures of the midface is difficult because of the complex anatomy in this region and the multiple superimpositions of structures. CT is the diagnostic imaging method of choice for complex facial fractures. CT imaging provides multiple image slices in orthogonal planes through the face, allowing for the display of osseous structures without the complication of overlapping anatomy that is problematic with plane radiography. CT also provides suitable image detail to detect secondary changes associated with trauma, including herniation of orbital fat and extraocular muscle, soft tissue swelling or emphysema, and blood/fluid accumulation. As an aid in determining the spatial orientation of fractures or bone fragments, the CT images may be reformatted so that three-dimensional images may be evaluated.

### Le Fort I (Horizontal Fracture)

#### Definition

The Le Fort I fracture is a relatively horizontal fracture in the body of the maxilla that results in detachment of the alveolar process and adjacent bone of the maxilla from the middle face. This fracture is the result of a horizontally directed traumatic force directed posteriorly at the base of the nose. The fracture plane passes superior to the roots of the teeth and nasal floor and posteriorly through the base of the maxillary sinus and the tuberosity to the pterygoid processes (Fig. 29-21). In the unilateral fracture, an auxiliary fracture exists in the midline of the palate. The unilateral fracture must be distinguished from a fracture within the alveolar process (discussed previously) that does not extend to the midline or involve the ptyergoid plates posteriorly. Fractures of the mandible (54%) and zygomatic bone (23%) may also be found in these patients.

#### Clinical Features

If the fragment is not distally impacted, it can be manipulated by holding onto the teeth. If the fracture line is at a high level, the fragment may include the pterygoid muscle attachments, which pull the fragment posteriorly and inferiorly. As a result, the posterior maxillary teeth contact the mandibular teeth first, resulting in an anterior open bite, retruded chin, and long face. If the fracture is at a low level, no displacement may occur. Other symptoms may include associated swelling and bruising about the eyes, pain over the nose and face, deformity of the nose, and flattening of the middle of the face. Epistaxis is inevitable, and occasionally double vision and varying degrees of paresthesia over the distribution of the infraorbital nerve may occur. Manipulation may reveal a mobile maxilla and crepitation.

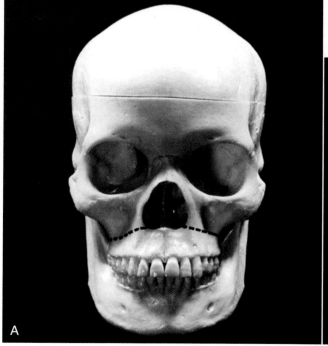 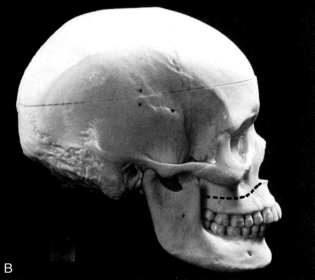

FIG. **29-21**   Usual position of a Le Fort I fracture on frontal (**A**) and lateral (**B**) views.

## Radiographic Features

CT imaging will reveal an air-fluid level or radiopacification in the maxillary sinus (Fig. 29-22, *A*). Coronal images may reveal the plane of the fracture extending posteriorly through the maxilla, whereas coronal or axial images together may reveal involvement of the pterygoid plates posteriorly. Three-dimensional reconstructions of the CT data set may show the plane of the fracture to greatest advantage (Fig. 29-22, *B*).

## Management

If the fracture is not displaced and is at a relatively low level in the maxilla, it can be treated by intermaxillary fixation. Those that are high, with the fragment displaced posteriorly or with pronounced separation, require craniomaxillary fixation in addition to intermaxillary fixation.

## Le Fort II (Pyramidal Fracture)

### Definition

The Le Fort II fracture has a pyramidal shape on posteroanterior skull images, hence the name. It results from a violent force applied posteriorly and superiorly through the base of the nose. This force separates the maxilla from the base of the skull. The fracture plane extends from the bridge of the nose inferiorly, laterally, and posteriorly through the nasal and lacrimal bones, the orbital floor and inferior rim obliquely, and inferiorly across the maxilla and posteriorly to the pterygoid processes (Figs. 29-23 and 29-24). The frontal and ethmoid sinuses are involved in about 10% of cases, especially in severe comminuted fractures.

## Clinical Features

In contrast to the Le Fort I fracture, which may be characterized by only slight swelling about the upper lips, the Le Fort II injury results in massive edema and marked swelling of the middle third of the face. Typically, ecchymosis develops around the eyes within minutes of the injury. The edema is likely to be so severe that it is impossible to see the globes. The conjunctivas over the inner quadrants of the eyes are bloodshot, and if the zygomatic bones are involved, this ecchymosis extends to the outer quadrant.

The broken nose is displaced because the face has fallen, and the nose and face are lengthened. An anterior open bite occurs. Epistaxis is inevitable, and cerebrospinal fluid rhinorrhea may also result. Palpation reveals the discontinuity of the lower borders of the orbits. By applying pressure between the bridge of the nose and the palate, the "pyramid" of bone can be moved. Other common symptoms include double vision and variable degrees of paresthesia over the distribution of the infraorbital nerve.

## Radiographic Features

The radiographic examination reveals fractures of the nasal bone, frontal process of the maxilla, infraorbital rim, and orbital floor. More inferiorly and posteriorly, there would be involvement of the zygomatic bone or zygomatic process of the maxilla, separation of the zygomaticomaxillary suture, and fracture of the lateral wall of the maxillary sinus and the pterygoid plates. Involvement of the ethmoid air cells, and frontal and maxillary sinuses, would result in thickening of the sinus

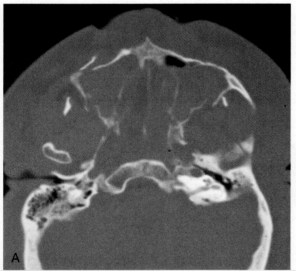

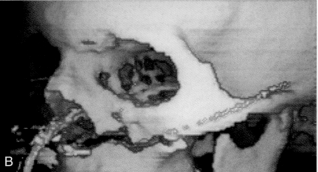

FIG. **29-22** **A,** Axial image of Le Fort I fractures involving the anterior and posterolateral walls of the right and left maxilla and the pterygoid plates. Radiopacification of the maxillary sinuses is also seen with a small retained collection of air in the left maxillary sinus. **B,** Three-dimensional reconstruction of the image data shows extension of the fracture plane from above the base of the nose posteriorly through the maxillary tuberosity.

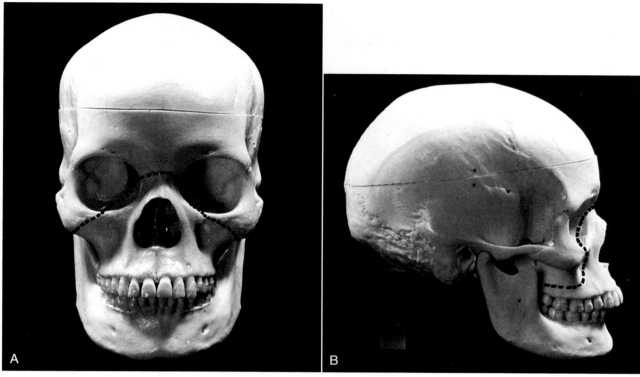

FIG. **29-23**    Usual position of the Le Fort II fracture on frontal **(A)** and lateral **(B)** views.

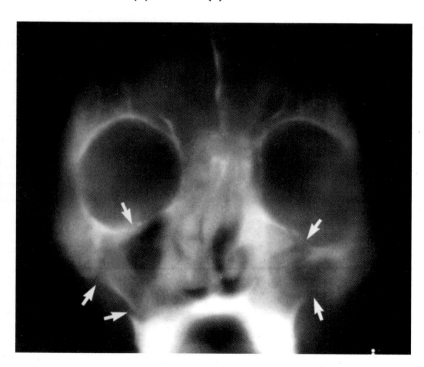

FIG. **29-24**    Coronal tomographic view of a Le Fort II fracture. Note the fractures through the orbital rims bilaterally. As well, there are fractures through the ethmoid bones and the lateral walls of the maxillae *(arrows)*. (Courtesy Dr. C. Schow, Galveston, Tex.)

mucosa or the accumulation of blood-fluid levels in the air spaces. CT is the imaging modality of choice for such complex fractures.

## Management

The treatment of this fracture is accomplished by reduction of the displaced maxilla by intermaxillary fixation, open reduction, and interosseous wiring of the infraorbital rims and plating of the accompanying fractures of the nose, nasal septum, and orbital floor. Repair of the detached medial canthal ligaments may also be required. Leakage of cerebrospinal fluid requires the attention of a neurosurgeon if the posterior or superior walls of the frontal sinuses are involved.

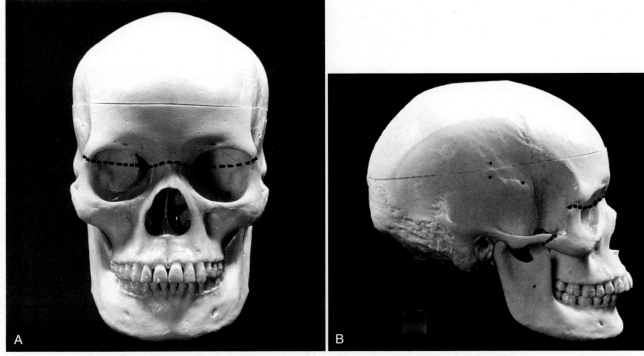

FIG. **29-25**    Usual position of the Le Fort III fracture on frontal **(A)** and lateral **(B)** views.

## Le Fort III (Craniofacial Disjunction)

### Definition

A Le Fort III midface fracture results when the traumatic force is of sufficient magnitude to completely separate the middle third of the facial skeleton from the cranium. The fracture plane usually extends from the nasal bone and frontal process of the maxilla or nasofrontal and maxillofrontal sutures, across the orbital floor, through the ethmoid air cells and sphenoid sinus to the zygomaticofrontal sutures (Fig. 29-25). More posteriorly and inferiorly, the fracture plane passes across the pterygomaxillary fissure and separates the bases of the pterygoid plates from the sphenoid bone. If the maxilla is displaced and freely movable, a fracture must also have occurred in the area of the zygomaticotemporal suture. Because the zygomatic bone or zygomatic arch is involved, these injuries are, as a rule, associated with multiple other maxillary fractures. Mandibular fractures are also observed in half the cases.

### Clinical Features

Craniofacial disjunction produces a clinical appearance similar to that of a pyramidal fracture. However, this injury is considerably more extensive. The soft tissue injuries are severe, with massive edema. The nose may be blocked with blood or blood clot, or cerebrospinal fluid rhinorrhea may be present. Bleeding may occur into the periorbital tissues and the conjunctiva, and a number of eye signs of neurologic importance are likely to be present. A "dished-in" or concave deformity of the face is characteristic of this fracture pattern, as is an anterior open bite because of the retroclined positions of the maxillary incisors with only the posterior teeth in occlusion. Even on mandibular opening, the patient is unable to separate the molars. Intraoral and extraoral palpation reveals irregular contours and step deformities, and crepitation is also apparent when the fragments are moved.

### Radiographic Features

It is virtually impossible to document these multiple fractures with plain films. Therefore CT images in concert with the clinical information are required. The main radiographic findings are distractions of the frontonasal, frontomaxillary, zygomaticofrontal, and zygomaticotemporal sutures and fractures through the nasal bone, frontal process of the maxilla, orbital floor, and pterygoid plates (Fig. 29-26). Associated fractures involving the walls of all the paranasal sinuses will result in radiopaque air-fluid levels with mucosal thickening. Three-dimensional reconstructions show the fracture planes and the large bone fragments (Fig. 29-26, *D* and *E*).

### Management

The associated severe soft tissue injury necessitates airway management, initial hemorrhage control, and repair of lacerations. Surgery may be delayed until the edema has sufficiently resolved. The treatment of transverse fractures is complicated because fixation of the loose middle third of the facial skeleton is difficult because of the fact that fractures of the zygomatic arch occur. The only possibilities are external immobilization or immobilization within the tissues. In the former, the loose maxilla is suspended by wires through the cheeks from a metal head frame (halo) or fixed by external pins anchored in bone. The other possibility is immobilization within the tissues by using internal wiring to the closest solid bone superior to the fracture. A number of complications may develop during or after this treatment.

## Monitoring the Healing of Fractures

Radiographic examination of the facial bones after trauma is usually necessary to measure the degree of reduction from treatment and to monitor the continued immobilization of the fracture site during repair. Typically, monitoring of this type is accomplished by use of

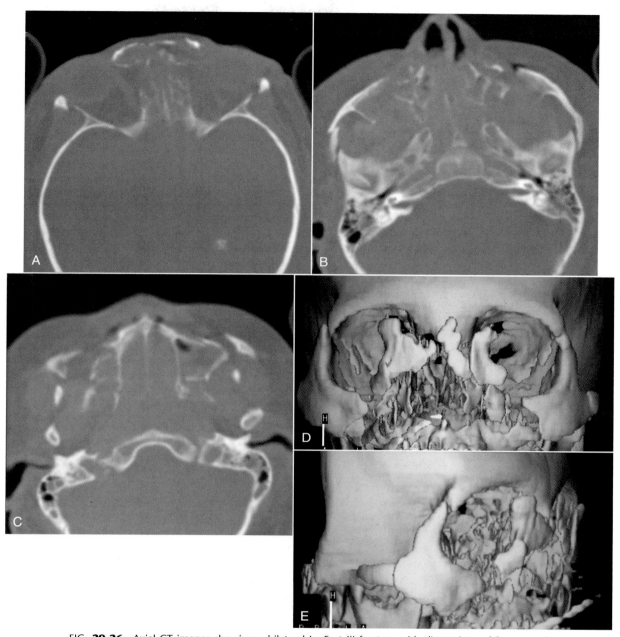

FIG. **29-26**  Axial CT images showing a bilateral Le Fort III fracture with distractions of frontonasal **(A)**, frontomaxillary, zygomaticofrontal, and zygomaticotemporal sutures **(B)** and fractures of nasal bone, frontal process of the maxilla, orbital floor, and pterygoid plates **(C).** Note the near-total radiopacification of the maxillary sinuses. Three-dimensional reconstructions, frontal view **(D)** and lateral view **(E),** of the axial CT images reveal substantial fragmentation of the periorbital bones, zygomatic bone, and arch, posteriorly.

plain radiography. The monitoring of fracture repair should include examination of both the alignment of the cortical plates of the involved bone and remodeling and remineralization of the fracture site. During normal healing the fracture line increases in width about 2 weeks after reduction of the fracture. This results from the resorption of the fractured ends and small sequestered fragments of bone. Evidence of remineralization usually occurs 5 to 6 weeks after treatment. Unlike the long bones of the skeleton, rarely is a callus formed in healing jaw fractures. The complete remodeling of the fracture site

with obliteration of the fracture line may take several months. On rare occasions, fracture lines may persist for years, even when the patient has made a clinically complete recovery. Possible complications of healing include malalignment of the fracture segments and inflammatory lesions related to nonvital teeth near or in the line of the fracture. Other complications include nonunion of the fractured segments seen as increased width of fracture line, cortication of the fractured surfaces, and rounding of the sharp edges of the segments. The development of osteomyelitis of the fracture site will appear as an increase in sclerosis of the surrounding bone, inflammatory periosteal new bone, and development of sequestra.

## SUGGESTED READINGS

Brook IW, Wood N: Aetiology and incidence of facial fractures in adults, *Int J Oral Surg* 12:293-298, 1983.

Daffner RH: Imaging of facial trauma, *Curr Probl Diagn Radiol* 26:153-184, 1997.

Dingman TM, Natvig AC: *Surgery of facial fractures*, Philadelphia, 1967, WB Saunders.

Gerlock AJ Jr, Sinn DP, McBride KL: *Clinical and radiographic interpretation of facial fractures*, Boston, 1981, Little, Brown.

Hunter JG: Pediatric maxillofacial trauma, *Pediatr Clin North Am* 39: 1127-1143, 1992.

Kaban LB: Diagnosis and treatment of fractures of the facial bones in children 1943-1993, *J Oral Maxillofac Surg* 51:722-729, 1993.

Koltai PJ, Rabkin D: Management of facial trauma in children, *Pediatr Clin North Am* 43:1253-1275, 1996.

Laine FJ, Conway WF, Laskin DM: Radiology of maxillofacial trauma, *Curr Probl Diagn Radiol* 22:145-188, 1993.

Matteson SR, Deahl ST, Alder ME et al: Advanced imaging methods, *Crit Rev Oral Biol Med* 7:346-395, 1996.

Matteson SR, Tyndall DA: Pantomographic radiology. Part II. Pantomography of trauma and inflammation of the jaws, *Dent Radiogr Photogr* 56:21-48, 1983.

Newman J: Medical imaging of facial and mandibular fractures, *Radiol Technol* 69:417-435, 1998.

Shumrick KA: Recent advances and trends in the management of maxillofacial and frontal trauma, *Facial Plast Surg* 9:16-28, 1993.

### TRAUMA TO TEETH

Andreasen JO: *Traumatic injuries of the teeth*, Philadelphia, 1981, WB Saunders.

Andreasen JO, Andreasen FM, Skeie A et al: Effect of treatment delay upon pulp and periodontal healing of traumatic dental injuries—a review article, *Dent Traumatol* 18:116-128, 2002

Josell SD, Abrams RG: Traumatic injuries to the dentition and its supporting structures, *Pediatr Clin North Am* 29:717-741, 1982.

### LUXATION

Andreasen JO: Luxation of permanent teeth due to trauma: a clinical and radiographic follow-up study of 189 injured teeth, *Scand J Dent Res* 78:273-286, 1970.

### AVULSION

Donaldson M, Kinirons MJ: Factors affecting the time of onset of resorption in avulsed and replanted incisor teeth in children, *Dent Traumatol* 17:205-209, 2001

### TOOTH CROWN FRACTURE

Ravn JJ: Follow-up study of permanent incisors with enamel fractures as a result of acute trauma, *Scand J Dent Res* 89:213-217, 1981.

Ravn JJ: Follow-up study of permanent incisors with enamel-dentin fracture after acute trauma, *Scand J Dent Res* 89:355-365, 1981.

Stockton LW, Suzuki M: Management of accidental and iatrogenic injuries to the dentition, *J Can Dent Assoc* 64:378-382, 1998.

### CRACKED TOOTH SYNDROME

Fox K, Youngson CC: Diagnosis and treatment of the cracked tooth, *Prim Dent Care* 4:109-113, 1997.

Turp JC, Gobetti JP: The cracked tooth syndrome: an elusive diagnosis, *J Am Dent Assoc* 127:1502-1507, 1996.

### TOOTH ROOT FRACTURE

Cvek M, Mejare I, Andreason JO: Healing and prognosis of teeth with intraalveolar fractures involving the cervical part of the root, *Dent Traumatol* 18:57-65, 2002

Hovland EJ: Horizontal root fractures: treatment and repair, *Dent Clin North Am* 36:509-525, 1992.

Luebke RG: Vertical crown-root fractures in posterior teeth, *Dent Clin North Am* 28:883-894, 1984.

Majorana A, Pasini S, Bardellini E et al: Clinical and epidemiological study of traumatic root fractures, *Dent Traumatol* 18:77-80, 2002

Schetritt A, Steffensen B: Diagnosis and management of vertical root fractures, *J Can Dent Assoc* 61:607-613, 1995.

Schmidt BL, Stern M: Diagnosis and management of root fractures and periodontal ligament injury, *J Calif Dent Assoc* 24:51-55, 1996.

Walton RE, Michelich RJ, Smith GN: The histopathogenesis of vertical root fractures, *J Endodont* 10:48-56, 1984.

Wright EF: Diagnosis, treatment, and prevention of incomplete tooth fractures, *Gen Dent* 40:390-399, 1992.

### COMPUTED TOMOGRAPHY OF JAW FRACTURES

Creasman CN, Markowitz BL, Kawamoto HK Jr et al: Computed tomography versus standard radiography in the assessment of fractures of the mandible, *Ann Plast Surg* 29:109-113, 1992.

Johnson DH: CT of maxillofacial trauma, *Radiol Clin North Am* 22:131-144, 1984.

Kassel EE, Noyek AM, Cooper PW: CT in facial trauma, *J Otolaryngol* 12:2-15, 1983.

Marsh JL, Vannier MW, Gado M et al: In vivo delineation of facial fractures: the application of advanced medical imaging technology, *Ann Plast Surg* 17:364-376, 1986.

Raustia AM, Pyhtinen J, Oikarinen KS et al: Conventional radiographic and computed tomographic findings in cases of fracture of the mandibular condylar process, *J Oral Maxillofac Surg* 48:1258-1264, 1990.

### TRAUMA TO THE MANDIBLE

Bailey BJ, Clark WD: Management of mandibular fractures, *Ear Nose Throat J* 62:371-378, 1983.

Chayra GA, Meador LR, Laskin DM: Comparison of panoramic and standard radiographs for the diagnosis of mandibular fractures, *J Oral Maxillofac Surg* 44:677-679, 1986.

Clark WD: Management of mandibular fractures, *Am J Otolaryngol* 13: 125-132, 1992.

Ellis E III, Moos KF, El-Attar A: Ten years of mandibular fractures: an analysis of 2,137 cases, *Oral Surg* 59:120-129, 1985.

Olson RA, Fonseca RJ, Zeitler DL et al: Fractures of the mandible: a review of 580 cases, *J Oral Maxillofac Surg* 40:23-28, 1982.

Reiner SA, Schwartz DL, Clark KF et al: Accurate radiographic evaluation of mandibular fractures, *Arch Otolaryngol Head Neck Surg* 115:1083-1085, 1989.

Winstanley RP: The management of fractures of the mandible, *Br J Oral Maxillofac Surg* 22:170-177, 1984.

### CONDYLAR FRACTURES

Consensus Conference on Open or Closed Management of Condylar Fractures, 12th ICOMS, Budapest, 1995, *Int J Oral Maxillofac Surg* 27:243-267, 1998.

Dahlström L, Kahnberg KE, Lindahl L: 15 year follow-up on condylar fractures, *Int J Oral Maxillofac Surg* 18:18-23, 1989.

Dimitroulis G: Condylar injuries in growing patients, *Aust Dent J* 42: 367-371, 1997.

Hall MB: Condylar fractures: surgical management, *J Oral Maxillofac Surg* 52:1189-1192, 1994.

Hayward JR, Scott RF: Fractures of the mandibular condyle, *J Oral Maxillofac Surg* 51:57-61, 1993.

Sahm G, Witt E: Long-term results after childhood condylar fractures: a computer-tomographic study, *Eur J Orthod* 11:154-160, 1989.

Silvennoinen U, Iizuka T, Lindqvist C et al: Different patterns of condylar fractures: an analysis of 382 patients in a 3-year period, *J Oral Maxillofac Surg* 50:1032-1037, 1992.

Walker RV: Condylar fractures: nonsurgical management, *J Oral Maxillofac Surg* 52:1185-1188, 1994.

## FRACTURES OF THE ALVEOLAR PROCESS

Andreasen JO: Fractures of the alveolar process of the jaw: a clinical and radiographic follow-up study, *Scand J Dent Res* 78:263-272, 1970.

Giovannini UM, Goudot P: Radiologic evaluation of mandibular and dentoalveolar fractures, *Plast Reconstr Surg* 109:2165-2166, 2002.

## TRAUMA TO THE MAXILLA

Banks P: *Kiley's fractures of the middle third of the facial skeleton,* Bristol, UK, 1981, Wright.

Close LG: Fractures of the maxilla, *Ear Nose Throat J* 62:365-370, 1983.

Luce EA: Developing concepts and treatment of complex maxillary fractures, *Clin Plast Surg* 19:125-131, 1992.

Marciani RD: Management of midface fractures: fifty years later, *J Oral Maxillofac Surg* 51:960-968, 1993.

Teichgraeber JF, Rappaport NJ, Harris JH Jr: The radiology of upper airway obstruction in maxillofacial trauma, *Ann Plast Surg* 27:103-109, 1991.

Tung TC, Chen YR, Santamaria E et al: Dislocation of anatomic structures into the maxillary sinus after craniofacial trauma, *Plast Reconstr Surg* 101:1904-1908, 1998.

## ZYGOMATIC COMPLEX FRACTURES

Fujii N, Yamashiro M: Classification of malar complex fractures using computed tomography, *J Oral Maxillofac Surg* 41:562-567, 1983.

McLoughlin P, Gilhooly M, Wood G: The management of zygomatic complex fractures—results of a survey, *Br J Oral Maxillofac Surg* 32:284-288, 1994.

Prendergast ML, Wildes TO: Evaluation of the orbital floor in zygoma fractures, *Arch Otolaryngol Head Neck Surg* 114:446-450, 1988.

Sands T, Symington O, Katsikeris N et al: Fractures of the zygomatic complex: a case report and review, *J Can Dent Assoc* 59:749-755, 1993.

Winstanley RP: The management of fractures of the zygoma, *Int J Oral Surg* 10(1 Suppl):235-240, 1981.

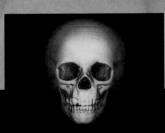

# CHAPTER 30

# Developmental Disturbances
# of the Face and Jaws

Carol Anne Murdoch-Kinch

D evelopmental disturbances affect the normal growth and differentiation of craniofacial structures. As a consequence, they are usually first discovered in infancy or childhood. Many of the conditions discussed in this chapter have an unknown etiology. Some are caused by known and recently discovered genetic mutations, whereas others result from environmental factors. These conditions result in a variety of abnormalities of the face and jaws including abnormalities of structure, shape, organization, and function of hard and soft tissues.

## Common Developmental Abnormalities

There are a multitude of conditions that affect the morphogenesis of the face and jaws, many of which are rare syndromes. This chapter briefly reviews the more common developmental abnormalities that may be encountered in dental practice.

## CLEFT LIP AND PALATE

### Definition

A failure of fusion of the developmental processes of the face during fetal development may result in a variety of facial clefts. Cleft lip/palate (CL/P) and cleft palate (CP) are the most common developmental craniofacial anomalies. Their incidence varies with geographic location, ethnicity, and socioeconomic status. In Caucasian populations the incidence of cleft lip is 1 : 800 to 1 : 1000 live births, and the incidence of cleft palate is approximately 1 : 1000. Cleft lip with or without cleft palate and cleft palate are two different conditions with different etiologies. CL/P results from a failure of fusion of the medial nasal process with the maxillary process. This condition can range in severity from a unilateral cleft lip to bilateral complete clefting through the lip, alveolus, and hard and soft palate in the most severe cases. CP develops from a failure of fusion of the lateral palatal shelves. The minimal manifestation of cleft palate is a submucous cleft. Here, the palate appears to be intact except for notching of the uvula (bifid uvula) or notching in the posterior border of the hard palate detectable by palpation. The most severe presentation is complete clefting of the hard and soft palate. The precise etiology of orofacial clefting is not completely understood. However, most cases of CL/P and CP are considered to be multifactorial with a strong genetic component. CL/P and CP can each be associated with other abnormalities, as part of a genetic malformation syndrome such as 22q.11 deletion syndrome (velocardiofacial syndrome—cleft palate and facial and cardiac abnormalities) or van der Woude syndrome (cleft lip and/or cleft palate and lip pits). Other factors that are implicated in the development of orofacial clefts include nutritional disturbances (prenatal folate deficiency); environmental teratogenic agents (maternal smoking, in utero exposure to anticonvulsants); stress, which results in increased secretion of hydrocortisone; defects of vascular supply to the involved region; and mechanical interference with the fusion of the embryonic processes (cleft palate in Pierre Robin sequence). Clefts involving the lower lip and mandible are extremely rare.

### Clinical Features

The frequency of CL/P and CP varies with sex and race but in general CL/P is most common in males and CP is more common in females. Both conditions are more common in Asians and Hispanics than blacks or Caucasians. The severity of CL/P varies from a notch in the upper lip to a cleft involving only the lip to extension into the nostril, resulting in deformity of the ala of the nose. As CL/P increases in severity, the cleft will include the alveolar process and palate. Bilateral cleft lip is more frequently associated with CP. CP also varies in severity, ranging from involvement of only the uvula or soft palate to extension all the way through the palate to include the alveolar process in the region of the lateral incisor on one or both sides. With involvement of the alveolar process there is an increase in frequency of dental anomalies in the region of the cleft, including missing, hypoplastic, and supernumerary teeth and enamel hypoplasia. Dental anomalies are also more prevalent in the mandible in these patients. In both CL/P and CP the palatal defects interfere with speech and swallowing. Affected individuals with palatal clefts are also at increased risk for recurrent middle ear infections because of the abnormal anatomy and function of the eustachian tube.

### Radiographic Features

The typical appearance is a well-defined vertical radiolucent defect in the alveolar bone, including numerous associated dental anomalies (Figs. 30-1 and 30-2). These may include the absence of the maxillary lateral incisor and the presence of supernumerary teeth in this region. Often the involved teeth are malformed and poorly positioned. In patients with CL/P, there may be a mild delay in the development of maxillary and mandibular teeth and an increased incidence of hypodontia in both arches. The osseous defect may extend to include the floor of the nasal cavity. In patients with a repaired cleft, a well-defined osseous defect may not be apparent but only a vertically short alveolar process at the cleft site.

## Management

Management of CL/P and CP is complex, requiring the coordinated efforts of a multidisciplinary team known as a cleft palate team. This team usually includes a plastic and reconstructive surgeon, an oral and maxillofacial surgeon, an ear, nose, and throat surgeon, an orthodontist, a dentist, a speech therapist, a psychologist, a nutritionist, and a social worker. Clefts of the palate are usually surgically repaired within the first year of life, whereas clefts of the lip are usually repaired within the first 3 months to aid in feeding and maternal-infant bonding. The bone in the cleft site is often augmented with bone grafting before replacement of missing teeth with either fixed or removable prosthodontics or dental implants. Orthodontic treatment is usually necessary to recreate a normal arch form and functional occlusion.

## CROUZON SYNDROME

### Synonyms

Craniofacial dysostosis, syndromic craniosynostosis, and premature craniosynostosis

### Definition

Crouzon syndrome (CS) is an autosomal dominant skeletal dysplasia characterized by variable expressivity and almost complete penetrance. It is one of many diseases characterized by premature craniosynostosis (closure of cranial sutures). Its incidence is estimated at 1:25,000 births. Of these cases, 33% to 56% may arise as a consequence of spontaneous mutations, with the remaining being familial. CS is caused by a mutation in fibroblast growth factor receptor II on

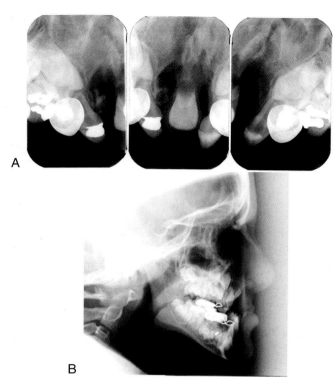

FIG. **30-1**  Cleft lip/palate results in defects in the alveolar ridge and abnormalities of the dentition. **A,** Bilateral clefts of the maxilla in the lateral incisor regions and defects of the dentition. **B,** Lateral cephalometric view showing underdevelopment of the maxilla.

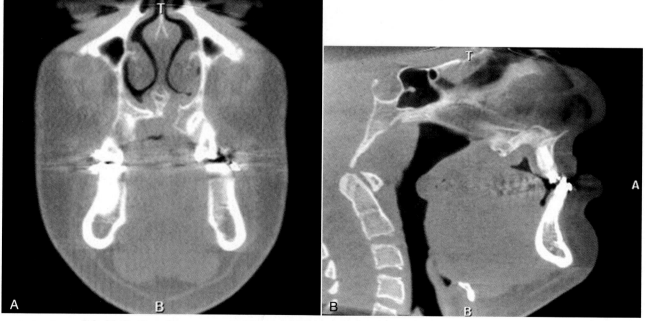

FIG. **30-2**  Cone-beam computed tomographic images of patient with left unilateral cleft lip/palate. **A,** Coronal view. Note the discontinuity in the nasal floor visible on the patient's left side. **B,** Sagittal view of same patient, showing the maxillary hypoplasia and deficient palatal anatomy. (Images courtesy Dr. Sean Edwards, Department of Oral and Maxillofacial Surgery, University of Michigan, Ann Arbor, Mich.)

chromosome 10. Mutations at this site are also responsible for other craniosynostosis syndromes with similar facial features but clinically visible limb abnormalities. In patients with CS the coronal suture usually closes first and eventually all cranial sutures close early. There is also premature fusion of the synchondroses of the cranial base. The subsequent lack of bone growth perpendicular to the synchondroses and cranial coronal sutures produces the characteristic cranial shape and facial features.

### Clinical Features

Patients characteristically have brachycephaly (short skull front to back), hypertelorism (increased distance between eyes), and orbital proptosis (protruding eyes) (Fig. 30-3, *A* and *B*). In familial cases, the minimal criteria for diagnosis are hypertelorism and orbital proptosis. Patients may become blind as a result of early suture closure and increased intracranial pressure. The nose often appears prominent and pointed because the maxilla is narrow, and short in a vertical and an anteroposterior dimension. The anterior nasal spine is hypoplastic and retruded, failing to provide adequate support to the soft tissue of the nose. The palatal vault is high and the maxillary arch narrow and retruded, resulting in crowding of the dentition.

### Radiographic Features

*General Radiographic Features.* The earliest radiographic signs of cranial suture synostosis are sclerosis and overlapping edges. Sutures that normally should look radiolucent on the skull film will not be detectable or will show sclerotic changes. Interestingly, on rare occasions the facial features may present before radiographic evidence of sutural synostosis. Premature fusion of the cranial base leads to diminished facial growth. In some cases, prominent cranial markings are noted, which are also seen in normally growing patients, but are more prominent because of an increase in intracranial pressure from the growing brain. These markings may be seen as multiple radiolucencies appearing as depressions (so-called digital impressions) of the inner surface of the cranial vault, which results in a beaten metal appearance (see Fig. 30-3, *C* to *E*).

*Radiographic Features of the Jaws.* The lack of growth in an anteroposterior direction at the cranial base results in maxillary hypoplasia, creating a Class III malocclusion in some patients. The maxillary hypoplasia contributes to the characteristic orbital proptosis because the maxilla forms part of the inferior orbital rim and if severely hypoplastic fails to adequately support the orbital contents. The mandible is typically smaller than normal but appears prognathic in relation to the severely hypoplastic maxilla.

### Differential Diagnosis

Premature craniosynostosis, either isolated or part of a genetic syndrome, is a fairly common disorder.

The incidence of CS is reported to range from 1:2100 to 1:2500 births. Other causes of craniosynostosis must be differentiated from CS, including other syndromic forms of craniosynostosis and nonsyndromic coronal craniosynostosis. The characteristic facial features must be present to suggest CS.

### Management

The craniofacial features of CS worsen over time because of the abnormal craniofacial growth. Early diagnosis permits surgical and orthodontic treatment from infancy through adolescence, coordinated by a craniofacial team. The objectives of these treatments are to allow normal brain growth and development by preventing increased intracranial pressure, protect the eyes by providing adequate bony support, and improve facial esthetics and occlusal function. Because of early diagnosis and improvements in medical and dental care, most patients have normal intelligence and can expect a normal life span.

## HEMIFACIAL MICROSOMIA

### Synonyms

Hemifacial hypoplasia, craniofacial microsomia, lateral facial dysplasia, Goldenhar syndrome, and oculoauriculovertebral dysplasia

### Definition

Hemifacial microsomia (HFM) is the second most common developmental craniofacial anomaly after cleft lip and palate, affecting approximately 1:56,000 live births. Patients with HFM typically display reduced growth and development of half of the face as a result of abnormal development of the first and second branchial arches. This malformation sequence is usually unilateral but occasionally may involve both sides (craniofacial microsomia). When the whole side of the face is involved, the mandible, maxilla, zygoma, external and middle ear, hyoid bone, parotid gland, vertebrae, fifth and seventh cranial nerves, musculature, and other soft tissues are diminished in size and sometimes fail to develop. Delayed dental eruption and hypodontia on the affected side have also been reported. Most cases occur spontaneously, but familial cases demonstrating autosomal dominant inheritance have been reported. There is a male predominance of 3:2 and a right side predominance of 3:2. Cases with vertebral abnormalities and epibulbar dermoids have been considered to form a separate category within this condition, known as Goldenhar syndrome or oculoauriculovertebral dysplasia.

### Clinical Features

HFM is usually apparent at birth. Patients with this condition have a striking appearance caused by progressive failure of the affected side to grow, which gives the involved side of the face a reduced dimension. In addition, aplasia or hypoplasia of the external ear (microtia) is common, and the ear canal is often missing. In some patients the skull is diminished in size. In about 90% of cases, there is malocclusion on the affected side. The midsagittal plane of the patient's face is curved toward the affected side. The occlusal plane will often be canted up to the affected side.

### Radiographic Features

The primary radiographic finding is a reduction in the size of the bones on the affected side. This change is clearest in the mandible, which may show a reduction in the size of or, in severe cases, lack of any development of the condyle, coronoid process, or ramus. The body is reduced in size, and a portion of the distal aspect may be missing (Fig. 30-4). The dentition on the affected side may show a reduction in the number or size of the teeth. Computed tomographic (CT) examination shows a reduction in the size of the muscles of mastication and muscles of facial expression and hypoplasia or atresia of the auditory canal and ossicles of the middle ear. The course of the facial nerve is often shown to be abnormal on CT examination of the temporal bone.

### Differential Diagnosis

The features of hemifacial microsomia are characteristic. Condylar hypoplasia, especially that caused by a fracture at birth or by juve-

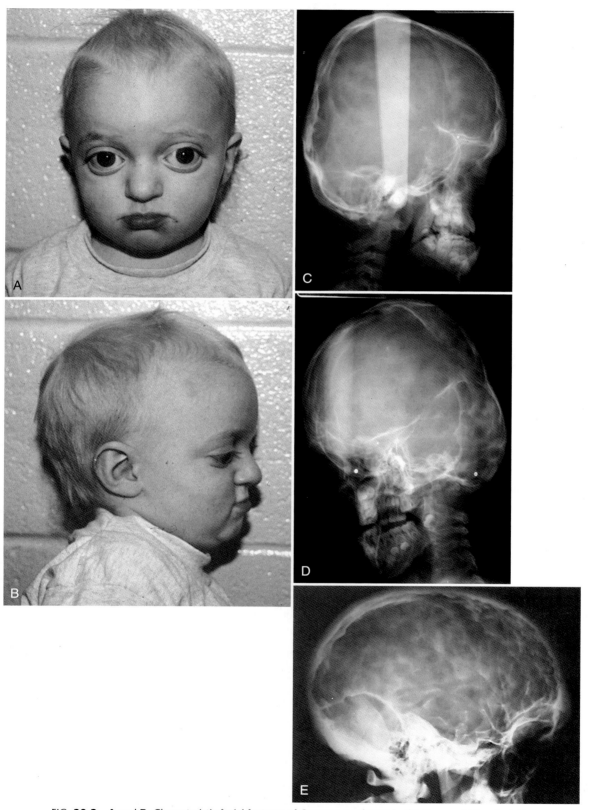

FIG. **30-3**  **A** and **B,** Characteristic facial features of Crouzon syndrome in this 2-year-old boy include orbital proptosis, hypertelorism, and midfacial hypoplasia. Rarely, they may precede the radiographic features of sutural synostosis. **C,** Lateral and, **D,** 45-degree skull views demonstrating the short anterior-posterior dimension of the skull, digital impressions, and hypoplastic maxilla. **E,** Lateral skull of another patient demonstrating prominent digital markings. (Courtesy Department of Radiology, Baylor University Hospital, Dallas, Tex.)

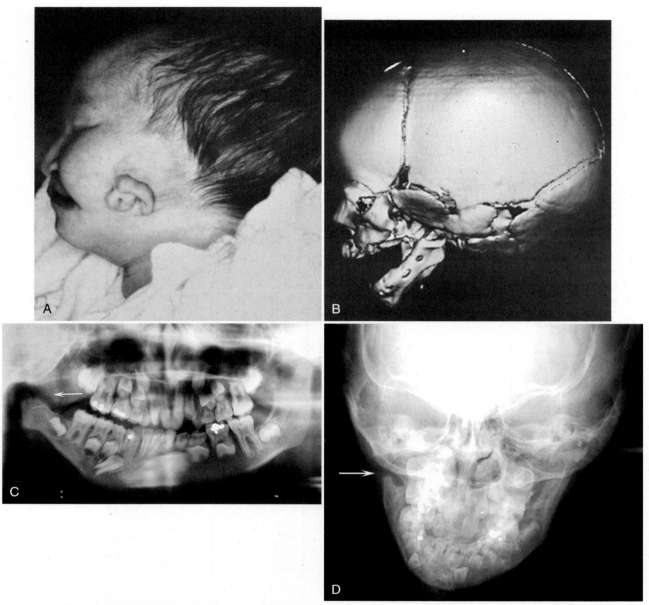

FIG. **30-4** **A** and **B,** Hemifacial microsomia, showing reduced size and malformation of the left ear and left side of the mandible. **A,** Clinical photograph of infant with hemifacial microsomia. **B,** Three-dimensional CT image of the affected side shows the extent of the bony malformation. Note the complete absence of the temporomandibular joint and coronoid process as well as auditory canal atresia. **C** and **D,** A panoramic image and a posteroanterior skull view of other cases showing lack of development of ramus, coronoid process, and condyle *(arrows).* (**A** and **B,** courtesy Dr. Arlene Rozzelle, Children's Hospital of Michigan, Detroit, Mich.)

nile arthrosis (Boering's arthrosis), may be similar, but it does not produce the ear changes (see Chapter 26). Exposure of the face of a child to radiation therapy during growth also may result in under-development of the irradiated tissues. In progressive hemifacial atrophy (Parry-Romberg syndrome), the changes will become more severe over time but are generally not present at birth, and the ears are normal.

## Management

The mandibular abnormalities may be corrected by conventional orthognathic surgery or distraction osteogenesis to lengthen the ramus on the affected side. Orthodontic intervention may correct or prevent malocclusion. The ear abnormalities may be repaired by plastic surgery or corrected with maxillofacial prosthetics, and the hearing loss may be partly corrected by hearing aids. In bilateral cases with profound hearing loss (Goldenhar syndrome), cochlear implants may be used to correct severe hearing loss.

## TREACHER COLLINS SYNDROME

### Synonym
Mandibulofacial dysostosis

### Definition
Treacher Collins syndrome (TCS) is an autosomal dominant disorder of craniofacial development. It is the most common type of mandibulofacial dysostosis, with an incidence of 1:50,000. TCS has variable expressivity and complete penetrance. Approximately half of cases arise as the result of sporadic mutation; the rest are familial. TCS is caused by a mutation in the *TCOF1* gene on chromosome 5.

### Clinical Features
Individuals with TCS have a wide range of anomalies, depending on the severity of the condition. The most common clinical findings are relative underdevelopment or absence of the zygomatic bones, resulting in a small narrow face; a downward inclination of the palpebral fissures; underdevelopment of the mandible, resulting in a down-turned, wide mouth; malformation of the external ears; absence of the external auditory canal; and occasional facial clefts (Fig. 30-5, *A* and *B*). The palate develops with a high arch or cleft in 30% of cases. Hypoplasia of the mandible and a steep mandibular angle results in an Angle Class II anterior open-bite malocclusion. Hypoplasia or atresia of the external ear, auditory canal, and ossicles of the middle ear may result in partial or complete deafness.

### Radiographic Features
A striking finding is the hypoplastic or missing zygomatic bones and hypoplasia of the lateral aspects of the orbits. The auditory canal, mastoid air cells, and articular eminence often are smaller than normal or are absent. The maxilla and especially the mandible are hypoplastic, showing accentuation of the antegonial notch and a steep mandibular angle, which gives the impression that the body of the mandible is bending in an inferior and posterior direction (see Fig. 30-5, *C* to *E*). The ramus is especially short. The condyles are positioned posteriorly and inferiorly. The maxillary sinuses may be underdeveloped or absent.

### Differential Diagnosis
Other disorders that may result in severe hypoplasia of the entire mandible include condylar agenesis, Hallermann-Streiff syndrome, Nager syndrome, and Pierre Robin sequence, which can be a part of several other genetic syndromes.

### Management
Comprehensive treatment of TCS is optimally provided by a multidisciplinary craniofacial team. Growth of the facial bones during adolescence results in some cosmetic improvement. Surgical intervention, including bilateral distraction osteogenesis of the mandible, may be used to improve the osseous defects. Treatment of the external ear defects may involve plastic and reconstructive surgery or maxillofacial prosthetics. Hearing aids or cochlear implants may be used to treat the hearing loss, depending on the severity. Coordinated orthodontics and orthognathic surgery are often used to treat the malocclusion and improve function and esthetics.

## CLEIDOCRANIAL DYSPLASIA

### Synonym
Cleidocranial dysostosis

### Definition
Cleidocranial dysplasia (CCD) is an autosomal dominant malformation syndrome affecting bones and teeth; it affects both sexes equally. Its prevalence is estimated at 1:1,000,000. It can be inherited or arise as a result of sporadic mutation. CCD is caused by a mutation in the *Runx2* gene on chromosome 6. This gene codes for anoasteoblast-specific transcription factor. It has variable expressivity and almost complete penetrance.

### Clinical Features
Although the disease affects the entire skeleton, CCD primarily affects the skull, clavicles, and dentition. Affected individuals have been shown to be of shorter stature than unaffected relatives, but not short enough for this to be considered a form of dwarfism. The face appears small in contrast to the cranium as a result of hypoplasia of the maxilla and a brachycephalic skull (reduced anteroposterior dimension with increased skull width), and the presence of frontal and parietal bossing. The paranasal sinuses may be underdeveloped. There is delayed closure of the cranial sutures and the fontanels may remain patent years beyond the normal time of closure. The bridge of the nose may be broad and depressed, with hypertelorism (excessive distance between the eyes). The complete absence (aplasia) or reduced size (hypoplasia) of the clavicles allows excessive mobility of the shoulder girdle (Fig. 30-6, *A* and *B*).

The dental abnormalities produce most of the morbidity associated with CCD and are often the reason for diagnosis in mildly affected individuals. Characteristically, patients with this disease show prolonged retention of the primary dentition and delayed eruption of the permanent dentition. Extraction of primary teeth does not adequately stimulate eruption of underlying permanent teeth. A study of teeth from patients with CCD revealed a paucity or a complete absence of cellular cementum on both erupted and unerupted teeth. Often unerupted supernumerary teeth are present, and considerable crowding and disorganization of the developing permanent dentition may occur. Recently the number of supernumerary teeth has been correlated with a reduction in skeletal height in these patients.

### Radiographic Features
*General Radiographic Features.* The characteristic skull findings are brachycephaly, delayed or failed closure of the fontanels, open skull sutures, and multiple wormian bones (small, irregular bones in the sutures of the skull that are formed by secondary centers of ossification in the suture lines) (see Fig. 30-6, *C* to *G*). In the most severe cases, very little formation of the parietal and frontal bones may occur. Typically the clavicles are underdeveloped to varying degrees and, in approximately 10% of cases, they are completely absent. Other bones also may be affected, including the long bones, vertebral column, pelvis, and bones of the hands and feet.

*Radiographic Features of the Jaws.* In CCD the maxilla and paranasal sinuses characteristically are underdeveloped, resulting in maxillary micrognathia. The mandible is usually normal size. A patent (open) mandibular symphysis has been reported in 3% of adults and 64% of children. Several investigators have described the alveolar bone overlying unerupted teeth as being denser than usual, with a

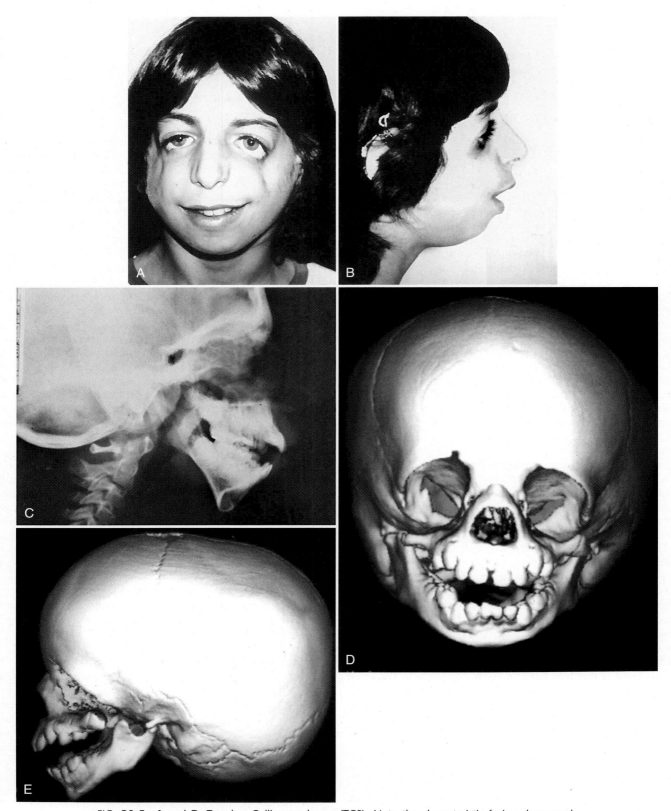

FIG. **30-5  A** and **B**, Treacher Collins syndrome (TCS). Note the characteristic facies: downward-sloping palpebral fissures, colobomas of the outer third of the lower lids, depressed cheekbones, receding chin, little if any nasofrontal angle, and a nose that appears relatively large. **C**, Lateral skull image demonstrating short mandibular rami, steep mandibular angle, and an anterior open bite. The zygomas are poorly formed. **D** and **E**, Three-dimensional CT images of young child with TCS show the extent of the bony abnormalities, including the bilateral auditory canal atresia, aplasia of the zygomatic arch, and hypoplasia of the mandibular ramus with characteristic "curved" shape of the mandibular body and pronounced antegonial notching.

coarse trabecular pattern in the mandible. This correlates with the histologic findings of decreased resorption and multiple reversal lines. It may account for the delayed eruption in teeth not mechanically obstructed by supernumerary and other unerupted teeth.

***Radiographic Features Associated with the Teeth.*** Characteristic features include prolonged retention of the primary dentition

and multiple unerupted permanent and supernumerary teeth (Fig. 30-7). The number of supernumerary teeth varies; as many as 63 in one individual have been reported. The unerupted teeth develop most commonly in the anterior maxilla and premolar regions of the jaws. Many resemble premolars and these unerupted teeth may develop dentigerous cysts. The supernumerary teeth develop, on average,

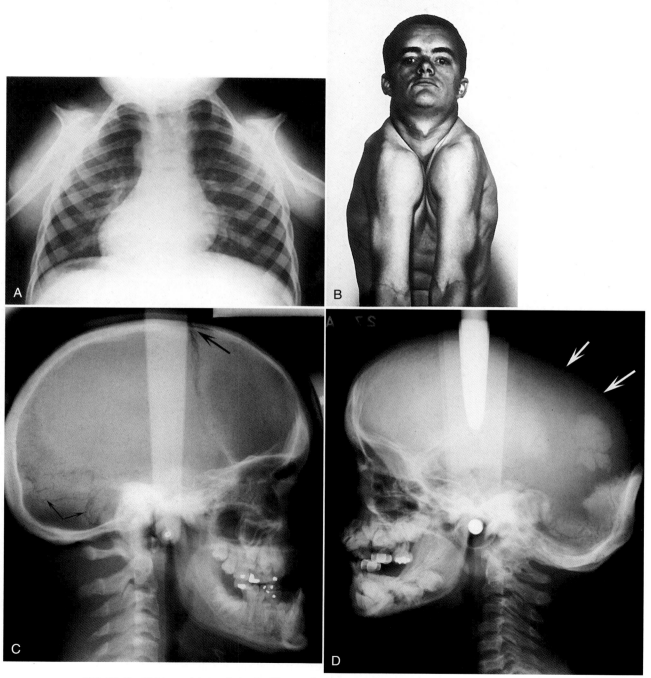

FIG. **30-6**  Cleidocranial dysplasia. **A,** Chest radiograph; note the absence of clavicles. **B,** The result is excessive mobility of the shoulders. Note also the frontal bossing and underdeveloped maxilla. **C,** On a lateral radiograph, note the wormian (sutural) bones in the occipital region *(arrows)* and the open fontanel *(large arrow).* **D,** A lateral skull film showing a lack of development of the parietal bones *(arrows).*

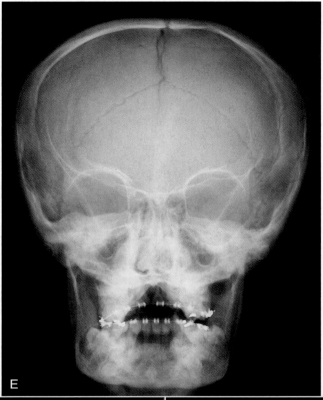

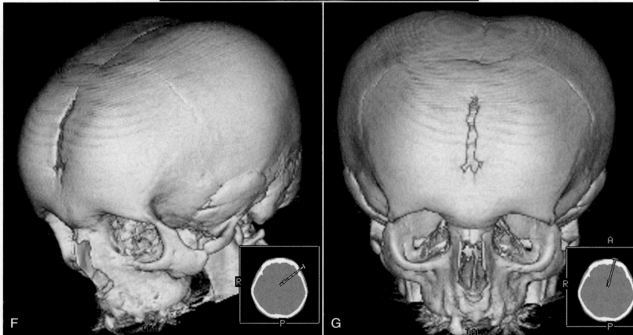

FIG. **30-6, cont'd    E,** A posteroanterior skull film. The brachycephaly results in a light bulb–like shape to the silhouette of the skull and mandible. **F,** Three-dimensional CT reconstruction with oblique orientation shows the typical skull shape; note the parietal and frontal bossing and open metopic suture in this 18-year-old man. **G** shows the light-bulb shape of the skull and the open metopic suture. (**A** courtesy Department of Radiology, Baylor University Hospital, Dallas, Tex., **F** and **G** courtesy Dr. Sean Edwards, Department of Oral and Maxillofacial Surgery, University of Michigan, Ann Arbor, Mich.)

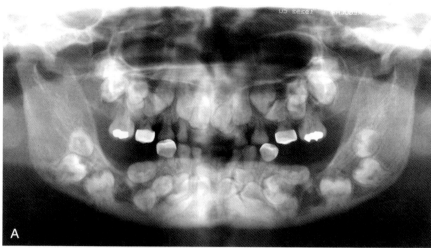

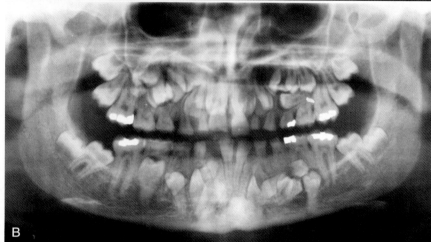

FIG. **30-7** **A** and **B**, Panoramic images of cleido-cranial dysplasia; note the prolonged retention of the primary dentition and multiple unerupted supernumerary teeth and the lack of normal coronoid notches. **C,** Axial CT view revealing multiple unerupted teeth, useful in identification and localization of the unerupted teeth. (**C** courtesy Dr. Sean Edwards, Department of Oral and Maxillofacial Surgery, University of Michigan, Ann Arbor, Mich.)

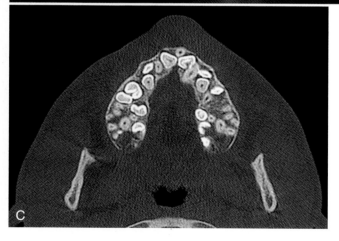

4 years later than the corresponding normal teeth. Because of this, it has been proposed that the supernumerary teeth represent a third dentition.

### Differential Diagnosis

CCD may be identified by the family history, excessive mobility of the shoulders, clinical examination of the skull, and pathognomonic radiographic findings of prolonged retention of the primary teeth with multiple unerupted supernumerary teeth. Other conditions associated with multiple unerupted and supernumerary teeth, such as Gardner's syndrome and pycnodysostosis must be considered in the differential diagnosis.

### Management

In CCD dental care should include the removal of primary and supernumerary teeth to improve the possibility of spontaneous eruption of the permanent teeth. The bone overlying the normal permanent teeth should be removed to expose the crown when half of the root is formed to aid their eruption. Autotransplantation of teeth has been shown to be a successful strategy to treat older patients. Ideally patients should be identified early, before the age of 5 years, to take advantage of combined orthodontic/surgical treatment. Prosthodontic rehabilitation with dental implants has been used in some cases. Patients should be monitored for development of distal molars and cysts until late adolescence. Surgical treatment of the bony defects of the skull is often done to address esthetic concerns. In those cases, three-dimensional CT imaging is used to visualize the size and thickness of such defects and plan for harvesting of bone graft material from other parts of the skull (see Fig. 30-6, *A* to *C*).

## HEMIFACIAL HYPERPLASIA

### Synonyms
Hemifacial hypertrophy and hemihyperplasia

### Definition
Hemifacial hyperplasia is a condition in which half of the face, including the maxilla alone or with the mandible, or in concert with other parts of the body, grows to unusual proportions. The cause of this condition is unknown. Some cases are associated with genetic diseases such as Beckwith-Weidemann syndrome.

### Clinical Features
Hemifacial hyperplasia begins at birth and usually continues throughout the growing years. In some cases it may not be recognized at birth, but it becomes more apparent with growth. It often occurs with other abnormalities, including mental deficiency, skin abnormalities, compensatory scoliosis, genitourinary tract anomalies, and various neoplasms, including Wilms' tumor of the kidney, adrenocortical tumor, and hepatoblastoma (Beckwith-Weidemann syndrome). Females and males are affected with approximately equal frequency. The dentition of affected individuals may show unilateral enlargement, accelerated development, and premature loss of primary teeth. The tongue and alveolar bone enlarge on the involved side.

### Radiographic Features
Radiographic examination of the skulls of these patients reveals, on the affected side, enlargement of the bones, including the mandible (Fig. 30-8), maxilla, zygoma, and frontal and temporal bones. There have been a few cases reported involving only one side of the maxilla or one side of the mandible.

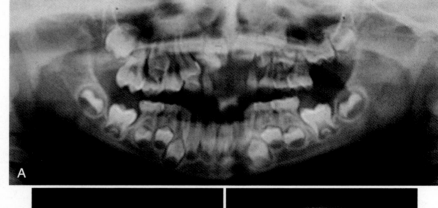

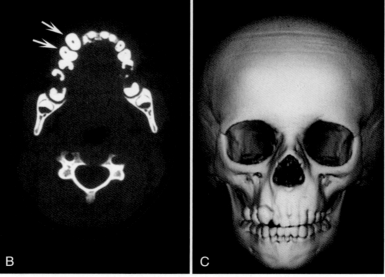

FIG. **30-8** Hemifacial hyperplasia, revealing enlargement of the right maxilla only. **A,** Panoramic radiograph shows accelerated dental development limited to the right maxilla in a 5-year-old boy. **B,** A CT axial image with bone algorithm of the same patient demonstrating enlargement of the maxillary cuspid and first bicuspid *(arrows)* compared with the contralateral side. **C,** Three-dimensional CT scan shows the subtle bony enlargement of the right maxilla and the right cuspid.

## Differential Diagnosis

The differential diagnosis should consider hemifacial hypoplasia of the opposite side, arteriovenous aneurysms, hemangioma, and congenital lymphedema. Also, severe condylar hyperplasia that may involve half of the mandible should be considered (see Chapter 26). The presence of enlarged teeth together with rapid eruption of the dentition suggests hemifacial hyperplasia. Cases limited to one side of the maxilla must be differentiated from monostotic fibrous dysplasia and segmental odontomaxillary dysplasia, both of which have characteristic changes in the radiographic appearance of the alveolar bone not present in hemifacial hyperplasia.

## Management

There have not been a significant number of cases of hemifacial hyperplasia reported with long-term follow-up to make definitive recommendations for treatment. Although most cases are isolated, a child with suspected hemifacial hyperplasia should be referred to a medical geneticist for diagnosis and early detection of one of several genetic syndromes that can be associated with this condition.

## SEGMENTAL ODONTOMAXILLARY DYSPLASIA

### Synonym

Hemimaxillofacial dysplasia

## Definition

Segmental odontomaxillary dysplasia (SOD) is a developmental abnormality of unknown etiology that affects the posterior alveolar process of one side of one maxilla, including the teeth and attached gingiva.

## Clinical Features

The abnormality is always unilateral and results in enlargement of the alveolar process, gingiva, and teeth. Frequently teeth are missing (most commonly the premolars), and some of the teeth that remain are unerupted. Unilateral hypertrichosis and mild facial enlargement have been reported in a few cases. Most cases are detected in childhood because a parent notices the lack of tooth eruption or mild facial asymmetry or the dentist notices missing premolars radiographically.

## Radiographic Features

The density of the maxillary alveolar process is increased, with a greater number of thick trabeculae that appear to be aligned in a vertical orientation, having an appearance similar to that of some intraosseous hemangiomas (Fig. 30-9). The roots of the deciduous teeth are larger than on the unaffected side and usually are splayed in shape. The crowns of the deciduous teeth and sometimes the permanent teeth are enlarged. Enlargement of pulp chambers and irregular resorption of the roots of deciduous teeth also may be seen. The maxillary sinus does not pneumatize the alveolar process and thus

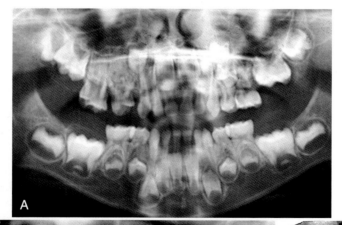

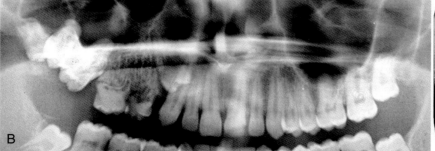
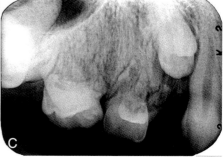

FIG. 30-9   **A,** A panoramic view of segmental odontomaxillary dysplasia. Note the large left maxillary deciduous molars compared with the right side and the lack of formation of the bicuspids, delayed eruption of the first molar, and the dense bone pattern of the left maxillary alveolar process. **B** and **C,** A second case demonstrating the coarse trabecular pattern of the right maxillary alveolar process and delayed eruption of the maxillary right first bicuspid and molars.

appears smaller than on the contralateral side. There is often delayed eruption of the first and second permanent molars.

### Differential Diagnosis

Other conditions that must be differentiated from SOD include segmental hemifacial hyperplasia, monostotic fibrous dysplasia, and regional odontodysplasia. Hemifacial hyperplasia is not associated with coarse vertically oriented trabeculae in the bone; monostotic fibrous dysplasia is not typically associated with missing teeth and, unlike SOD, will continue to show disproportionate growth of the affected side; and regional odontodysplasia typically is associated with ghost teeth and is not associated with expansion and alteration in trabecular pattern in the alveolar bone.

## LINGUAL SALIVARY GLAND DEPRESSION

### Synonyms

Lingual mandibular bone depression, developmental salivary gland defect, Stafne defect, Stafne bone cyst, static bone cavity, and latent bone cyst

### Definition

Lingual mandibular bone depressions represent a group of concavities in the lingual surface of the mandible where the depression is lined with an intact outer cortex. Historically, they were referred to as pseudocysts because they resemble cysts radiographically, but they are not true cysts because no epithelial lining is present. The most common location is within the submandibular gland fossa and often close to the inferior border of the mandible. This lingual posterior variant (LP) of these depressions was first described by Stafne in 1942. This well-defined deep depression is thought to result from or be associated with growth of the salivary gland adjacent to the lingual surface of the mandible. Similar defects have also been described in the anterior region near the apical region of the bicuspids, associated with the sublingual glands (lingual anterior variant or LA) and very rarely on the medial surface of the ascending ramus, associated with the parotid gland (medial ramus variant or MR). In LP developmental bone defects investigated surgically, an aberrant lobe of the submandibular gland has been described to extend into the bony depression; however, CT imaging of some of these defects reveals fat tissue and no evidence of gland. The etiology remains unknown, but the condition is a developmental anomaly that has been documented to develop in patients as old as 30 years and as young as 11 years. These defects may continue to slowly grow in size.

### Clinical Features

Although lingual mandibular bone depressions appear to be relatively rare, with an incidence of LP of about 0.10% to 0.48%, it is likely that many go unreported. LA incidence is even less at 0.009%. They are asymptomatic and next to impossible to palpate and, generally discovered only incidentally during radiographic examination of the area. In a recent review of a large number of cases, males predominated females at 6.1:1, with a peak incidence in the fifth and sixth decades.

### Radiographic Features

A lingual mandibular bone depression is a well-defined round, ovoid, or, occasionally, lobulated radiolucency that ranges in diameter from 1 to 3 cm (Fig. 30-10). The LP defect is located below the inferior alveolar nerve canal and anterior to the angle of mandible, in the region of the antegonial notch and submandibular gland fossa. Rare LA examples are located in the apical region of the mandibular premolars or cuspids and are related to the sublingual gland fossa, above the mylohyoid muscle. The margins of the radiolucent defect are well defined by a dense sclerotic radiopaque margin of variable width, which is usually thicker on the superior aspect. This appearance is the result of the x rays passing tangentially through the relatively thick walls of the depression. This cortical outline is often less distinct in the LA variant. The LP defect may involve the inferior border of the mandible. CT images reportedly reveal tissue of fat density within the defect (Fig. 30-11), or in some cases there is continuity of the tissue within the defect with the adjacent salivary gland.

### Differential Diagnosis

The appearance and location of the radiographic image of this developmental bone defect are characteristic and easily identified. Lingual mandibular bone depressions can be readily differentiated from odontogenic lesions such as cysts because the epicenter of odontogenic lesions is located above the inferior alveolar canal. However, when the defect is related to the sublingual gland and appears above the canal, odontogenic lesions should be considered in the differential diagnosis.

### Management

Recognition of the lesion should preclude any treatment or surgical exploration or the need for advanced imaging such as CT. The defect may increase in size with time. There are rare reports of salivary gland neoplasms developing in the soft tissue within the defect. Destruction of the well-defined cortex of the defect may indicate the presence of a neoplasm.

## FOCAL OSTEOPOROTIC BONE MARROW

### Synonym

Marrow space

### Definition

*Focal osteoporotic bone marrow* is a radiologic term indicating the presence of radiolucent defects within the cancellous portion of the jaws. Histologic examination reveals normal areas of hematopoietic or fatty marrow. The etiology is unknown but has been postulated to be (1) bone marrow hyperplasia, (2) persistent embryologic marrow remnants, or (3) sites of abnormal healing after extraction, trauma, or local inflammation. This entity is a variation of normal anatomy.

### Clinical Features

Focal osteoporotic bone marrow defects are usually clinically asymptomatic and are commonly an incidental radiographic finding. These marrow spaces are more common in middle-aged women.

### Radiographic Features

A common site for focal osteoporotic bone marrow is the mandibular molar-premolar region. Other sites include the maxillary tuberosity region, mandibular retromolar area, edentulous locations, occasionally the furcation region of mandibular molars, and rarely near the apex of teeth. The radiographic appearance of focal osteoporotic bone marrow space is quite variable. The internal aspect is radiolucent because of the presence of fewer trabeculae in comparison with the surrounding bone. The periphery may be ill defined and blending or may appear to be corticated. The immediate surrounding bone is normal without any sign of a bone reaction (Fig. 30-12).

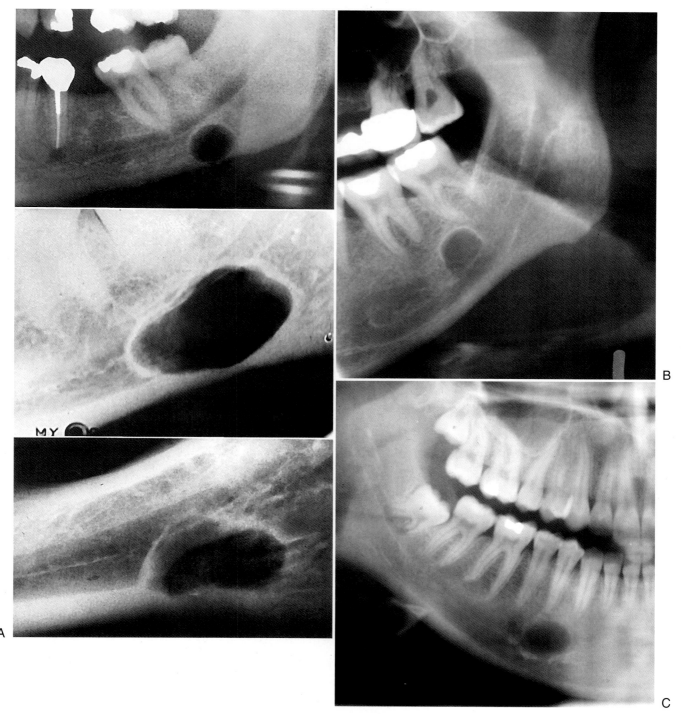

FIG. **30-10   A,** Lingual mandibular bone depressions of the posterior variant usually are seen as sharply defined radiolucencies beneath the mandibular canal in the region of the submandibular gland fossa. These defects can erode the inferior border of the mandible. **B,** An unusual variant with a superior position above the inferior alveolar canal. **C,** An anterior variant within the sublingual gland fossa.

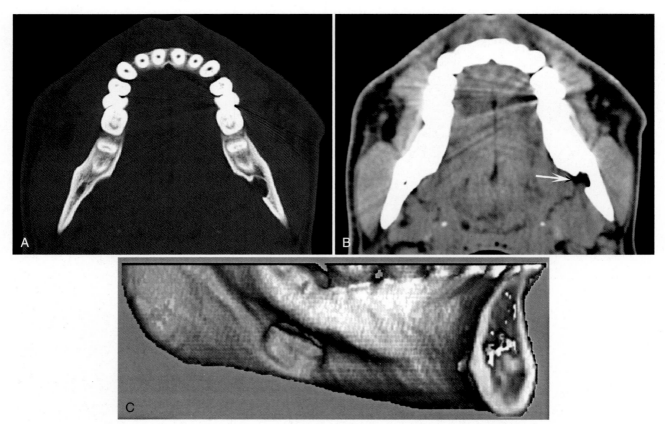

FIG. **30-11** CT scans of lingual mandibular bone depressions, posterior variant. **A** and **B,** Axial bone and soft tissue windows of the same case. Note the well-defined defect extending from the medial surface of the mandible and the corresponding soft tissue image, which shows radiolucent tissue within the defect that has the density equivalent of fat tissue *(arrow).* **C,** A three-dimensional, reformatted CT image revealing a defect extending from the medial surface of the mandible.

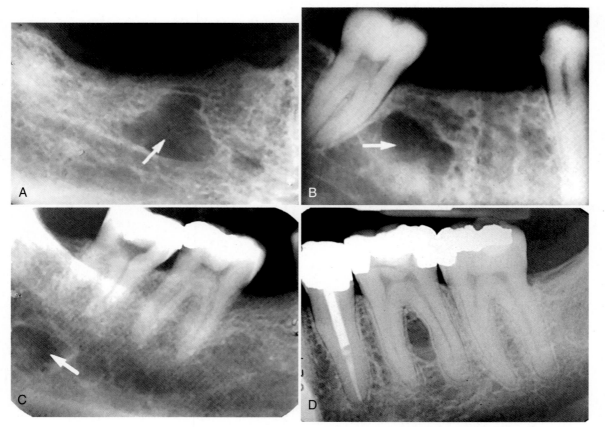

FIG. **30-12** **A** through **C,** Focal osteoporotic bone marrow defect, seen as a radiolucency *(arrow).* A few internal trabeculae may be present, and the periphery varies from well defined to ill defined. **D,** An example located in the furcation of a mandibular first molar. The periodontal ligament space and lamina dura are intact.

## Differential Diagnosis

A small simple bone cyst may have a similar appearance because there is usually no bone reaction at the periphery of a simple bone cyst. When osteoporotic bone marrow occurs in the furcation region or at the apex of a tooth, the differential diagnosis includes the presence of an inflammatory lesion. If the area is normal bone marrow, the lamina dura should be intact. Very early inflammatory lesions that have not yet stimulated a visible osteoblastic response may appear similar.

## Management

No treatment is required for the osteoporotic bone marrow space. Prior radiographs of the region should always be obtained if available. When doubt exists about the true nature of the radiolucency, a longitudinal study with films at 3-month intervals may be prescribed. The marrow space should not increase in size.

# BIBLIOGRAPHY

Cohen MM Jr, McLean RE: *Craniosynostosis: diagnosis, evaluation, and management,* ed 2. New York, 2000, Oxford University Press.

Gorlin RJ, Cohen MM Jr, Hennekam RCM: *Syndromes of the head and neck,* ed 4, New York, 2001, Oxford University Press.

Neville BW, Damm DD, Allen CM et al: *Oral and maxillofacial pathology,* ed 2, Philadelphia, 2002, WB Saunders.

Worth HM: *Principles and practice of oral radiologic interpretation,* Chicago, 1963, Year Book.

## CLEFT LIP AND CLEFT PALATE

Habel A, Sell D, Mars M: Management of cleft lip and palate, *Arch Dis Child* 74:360-366, 1996.

Harris EF, Hullings JG: Delayed dental development in children with isolated cleft lip and palate, *Arch Oral Biol* 35:469-473, 1990.

Hibbert SA, Field JK: Molecular basis of familial cleft lip and palate, *Oral Dis* 2:238-241, 1996.

Honein MA, Rasmussen SA, Reefhuis J et al: Maternal and environmental tobacco smoke exposure and the risk of orofacial clefts, *Epidemiology* 18:226-233, 2007.

Shapira Y, Lubit E, Kuftinec MM: Hypodontia in children with various types of clefts, *Angle Orthod* 70:16-21, 2000.

Wyszynski DF, Beaty TH, Maestri NE: Genetics of nonsyndromic oral clefts revisited, *Cleft Palate Craniofac J* 33:406-417, 1996.

## CROUZON SYNDROME

Murdoch-Kinch CA, Bixler D, Ward RE: Cephalometric analysis of families with dominantly inherited Crouzon syndrome: an aid to diagnosis in family studies, *Am J Med Genet* 77:405-411, 1998.

Tuite GF, Evanson J, Chong WK et al: The beaten copper cranium: a correlation between intracranial pressure, cranial radiographs, and computed tomographic scans in children with craniosynostosis, *Neurosurgery* 39:691-699, 1996.

## HEMIFACIAL MICROSOMIA

Maruko E, Hayes C, Evans CA et al: Hypodontia in hemifacial microsomia, *Cleft Palate Craniofac J* 38:15-19, 2001

Monahan R, Seder K, Patel P et al: Hemifacial microsomia: etiology, diagnosis and treatment, *J Am Dent Assoc* 132:1402-1408, 2001.

Sze RW, Paladin AM, Lee S et al: Hemifacial microsomia in pediatric patients: asymmetric abnormal development of the first and second branchial arches. *AJR Am J Roentgenol* 178:1523-1530, 2002.

## TREACHER COLLINS SYNDROME

Herman TE, Siegel MJ: Special imaging casebook: Treacher Collins syndrome, *J Perinatol* 16:413-415, 1996.

Posnick JC: Treacher Collins syndrome: perspectives in evaluation and treatment, *J Oral Maxillofac Surg* 55:1120-1133, 1997.

## CLEIDOCRANIAL DYSPLASIA

Golan I, Baumert U, Hrala BP et al: Dentomaxillofacial variability of cleidocranial dysplasia: clinicoradiological presentation and systematic review, *Dentomaxillofacial Radiol* 32:347-354, 2003

McGuire TP, Gomes PP, Lam DK et al: Cranioplasty for midline metopic suture defects in adults with cleidocranial dysplasia, *Oral Surg Oral Med, Oral Pathol Oral Radiol Endod* 103:175-179, 2007

Seow WK, Hertzberg J: Dental development and molar root length in children with cleidocranial dysplasia, *Pediatr Dent* 17:101-105, 1995.

Yoshida T, Kanegane H, Osata M et al: Functional analysis of RUNX2 mutations in Japanese patients with cleidocranial dysplasia demonstrates novel genotype-phenotype correlations, *Am J Hum Genet* 71:724-738, 2002.

## HEMIFACIAL HYPERPLASIA

Fraumeni JF Jr, Geiser CF, Manning MD et al: Wilms' tumor and congenital hemihypertrophy: report of five new cases and review of the literature, *Pediatrics* 40:886-899, 1967.

Hoyme HE, Seaver LH, Procopio F et al: Isolated hemihyperplasia (hemihypertrophy): report of a prospective multicenter study of the incidence of neoplasia and review, *Am J Med Genet* 79:274-278, 1998.

Kogon SL, Jarvis AM, Daley TD et al: Hemifacial hypertrophy affecting the maxillary dentition: report of a case, *Oral Surg Oral Med Oral Pathol* 58:549-553, 1984.

## SEGMENTAL ODONTOMAXILLARY DYSPLASIA

Danforth RA, Melrose RJ, Abrams AM et al: Segmental odontomaxillary dysplasia: report of eight cases and comparison with hemimaxillofacial dysplasia, *Oral Surg Oral Med Oral Pathol* 70:81-85, 1990.

Miles DA, Lovas JL, Cohen MM Jr: Hemimaxillofacial dysplasia: a newly recognized disorder of facial asymmetry, hypertrichosis of the facial skin, unilateral enlargement of the maxilla, and hypoplastic teeth in two patients, *Oral Surg Oral Med Oral Pathol* 64:445-448, 1987.

Packota GV, Pharoah MJ, Petrikowski CG: Radiographic features of segmental odontomaxillary dysplasia: a study of 12 cases, *Oral Surg Oral Med Oral Pathol Oral Radiol Endod* 82:577-588, 1996.

## LINGUAL MANDIBULAR BONE DEPRESSION

Parvizi F, Rout PG: An ossifying fibroma presenting as Stafne's idiopathic bone cavity, *Dentomaxillofac Radiol* 26:361-363, 1997.

Philipsen HP, Takata T, Reichart PA et al: Lingual and buccal mandibular bone depressions: a review based on 583 cases from a world-wide literature survey, including 69 new cases from Japan, *Dentomaxillofac Radiol* 31:281-290, 2002.

## FOCAL OSTEOPOROTIC BONE MARROW

Schneider LC, Mesa ML, Fraenkel D: Osteoporotic bone marrow defect: radiographic features and pathogenic factors, *Oral Surg* 65:127-129, 1988.

Standish SM, Shafer WG: Focal osteoporotic bone marrow defects of the jaws, *J Oral Surg Anesth Hosp Dent Serv* 20:123-128, 1962.

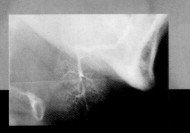

# CHAPTER 31

# Salivary Gland Radiology

Byron W. Benson

## Definition of Salivary Gland Disease

Dental diagnosticians have responsibility for detecting disorders of the salivary glands. A familiarity with salivary gland disorders and applicable current imaging techniques is an essential element of the clinician's armamentarium. Both major and minor salivary glands may be involved pathologically; however, this chapter deals only with the major glands. Salivary gland disease processes may be divided into the following clinical categories: inflammatory disorders, noninflammatory disorders, and space-occupying masses. Inflammatory disorders are acute or chronic and may be secondary to ductal obstruction by sialoliths, trauma, infection, or space-occupying lesions such as neoplasia. Noninflammatory disorders are metabolic and secretory abnormalities associated with diseases of nearly all the endocrine glands, malnutrition, and neurologic disorders. Space-occupying masses are cystic or neoplastic; the neoplasms are benign or malignant.

## Clinical Signs and Symptoms

Diseases of the major salivary glands may have single or multiple clinical features. Swellings in the areas of the parotid and submandibular glands should create a clinical suspicion of salivary gland disease. Pain and altered salivary flow may be present. Because the periodicity and longevity of these symptoms are important in the differential diagnosis, a review of the medical history and physical condition of the patient may provide important information. A history of skin, endocrine, or swallowing abnormalities may suggest a systemic collagen disease or metabolic disorder.

## Differential Diagnosis of Salivary Enlargements

### ENLARGEMENTS OF THE PAROTID AREA

Unilateral enlargements of the parotid area are categorized by the presence of a discrete, palpable mass or a diffuse swelling. If no mass is apparent, sialadenitis should be considered. Sialadenitis may be primary or secondary to ductal obstruction (retrograde). A mass superficial to the gland may represent lymphadenitis, infected preauricular cyst, infected sebaceous cyst, benign lymphoid hyperplasia, or extraparotid tumor. A mass intrinsic to the gland suggests a neoplasm (benign or malignant), intraglandular lymph node, or hamartoma.

Rapid growth, facial nerve paralysis, rock-hard texture, pain, and older age of occurrence are clinically suggestive of malignant neoplasms.

The differential diagnosis of asymptomatic bilateral enlargements of the parotid area may include benign lymphoepithelial lesion, Sjögren syndrome, alcoholism, medication (iodine and certain heavy metals), and Warthin tumor. Painful bilateral enlargement may occur after radiation treatment or as a result of bacterial or viral sialadenitis (including mumps) when accompanied by systemic symptoms.

A differential diagnosis of diffuse facial swelling in the parotid region, but not related to abnormalities of the gland, includes hypertrophy of the masseter muscle, accessory parotid gland, lesions related to the temporomandibular joint, and osteomyelitis of the ramus of the mandible. A palpable mass superficial to the gland suggests lymphadenitis, an infected preauricular or sebaceous cyst, benign lymphoid hyperplasia, or extraparotid tumor (Box 31-1).

## ENLARGEMENTS OF THE SUBMANDIBULAR AREA

Unilateral enlargement of the submandibular area associated with tender lymph nodes is suggestive of sialadenitis, which may be primary or secondary to ductal obstruction or decreased salivary flow (retrograde). Unilateral enlargement without tender lymph nodes suggests a neoplasm, cyst, lymphoepithelial lesion, or fibrosis. An intraglandular mass may be neoplastic or cystic. Neoplasms of the submandibular gland have a greater chance of being malignant than do those of the parotid gland. In turn, sublingual gland neoplasms have a still greater chance of being malignant than do those of the submandibular glands. Rapid growth, rock-hard texture, pain, and older age of occurrence are clinically suggestive of malignancy. Masses superficial or adjacent to the submandibular gland may be lymph nodes or extraglandular neoplasms.

Bilateral enlargement of the submandibular gland area suggests bacterial or viral sialadenitis. Although mumps is primarily a viral infection of the parotid glands, it may also occur in the submandibular glands. Other causes of swelling in the submandibular region include Sjögren syndrome, enlarged lymph nodes, submandibular space infection, and branchial cleft cyst (see Box 31-1).

## Applied Diagnostic Imaging of the Salivary Glands

Diagnostic imaging of salivary gland disease may be undertaken to differentiate inflammatory processes from neoplastic disease, distin-

## Differential Diagnosis of Enlargements in the Salivary Gland Areas

### Parotid Gland Area
**UNILATERAL**
- Bacterial sialadenitis
- Sialodochitis
- Cyst
- Benign neoplasm
- Malignant neoplasm
- Intraglandular lymph node
- Masseter muscle hypertrophy
- Lesions of adjacent osseous structures

**BILATERAL**
- Bacterial sialadenitis
- Viral sialadenitis (mumps)
- Sjögren syndrome
- Alcoholic hypertrophy
- Medication-induced hypertrophy (iodine, heavy metals)
- Human immunodeficiency virus–associated multicentric cysts
- Masseter muscle hypertrophy
- Accessory salivary glands
- Temporomandibular joint–related lesions

### Submandibular Gland Area
**UNILATERAL**
- Bacterial sialadenitis
- Sialodochitis
- Fibrosis
- Cyst
- Benign neoplasm
- Malignant neoplasm

**BILATERAL**
- Bacterial sialadenitis
- Sjögren syndrome
- Lymphadenitis
- Branchial cleft cyst
- Submandibular space infection

conditions are the most common disorders and primarily involve the ductal system, conventional sialography is commonly the most appropriate next imaging modality. If the patient is allergic to the iodine contrast agent used in sialography, magnetic resonance imaging (MRI), computed tomography (CT), or ultrasonography (US) may be selected as alternative imaging modalities. Recent studies comparing the diagnostic yield of MRI with that of sialography suggest that MRI might replace sialography in the future as the imaging modality of choice for ductal pathosis. Sialography or CT is the best imaging modality for the detection of sialoliths (sialolithiasis). If sialography eliminates inflammatory disorders or suggests the presence of a space-occupying mass (either cystic or solid), then contrast-enhanced CT or MRI is appropriate for evaluation. US is an alternative technique to differentiate cystic lesions from solid masses and to identify advanced autoimmune lesions. Functional disorders such as xerostomia are appropriately imaged with sialography or scintigraphy. Scintigraphy can provide important physiologic information that may be helpful in forming the differential diagnosis.

## PLAIN FILM RADIOGRAPHY

Plain film radiography is a fundamental part of the examination of the salivary glands and may provide sufficient information to preclude the use of more sophisticated and expensive imaging techniques. It has the potential to identify unrelated pathoses in the areas of the salivary glands that may be mistakenly identified as salivary gland disease, such as resorptive or osteoblastic changes in adjacent bone causing periauricular swelling mimicking a parotid tumor. Panoramic and conventional posteroanterior (PA) skull radiographs may demonstrate bony lesions, thus eliminating salivary pathosis from the differential diagnosis. Unilateral or bilateral functional or congenital hypertrophy of the masseter muscle may clinically mimic a salivary tumor. A plain film extraoral radiograph may demonstrate a deep antegonial notch, overdeveloped mandibular angle, and exostosis on the outer surface of the angle in cases of masseter hypertrophy.

Plain film radiographs are useful when the clinical impression, supported by a compatible history, suggests the presence of sialoliths (stones or calculi). Such an examination should include both intraoral and extraoral images to demonstrate the entire region of the gland. Sialoliths may be multiple at different locations. It is expedient to decrease the usual exposure by about half to avoid overexposure of the sialoliths. However, this technique is limited by the fact that 20% of the sialoliths of the submandibular gland and 40% of those of the parotid gland are not well calcified, rendering them radiolucent and not visible in plain films. Radiolucent sialoliths are rarely found in the sublingual glands.

## INTRAORAL RADIOGRAPHY

Sialoliths in the anterior two thirds of the submandibular duct are typically imaged with a cross-sectional mandibular occlusal projection as described in Chapter 8 (Fig. 31-1). The posterior part of the duct is demonstrated with an over-the-shoulder occlusal projection view, where the directing cone is placed on the shoulder and central ray directed in an anterior direction through the angle of the mandible, with the patient's head tilted to the unaffected side and rotated back (Fig. 31-2).

Parotid sialoliths are more difficult to demonstrate than the submandibular variety as a result of the tortuous course of Stensen duct around the anterior border of the masseter and through the buccina-

guish diffuse disease from focal suppurative disease, identify and localize sialoliths, and demonstrate ductal morphology. In addition, diagnostic imaging attempts to determine the anatomic location of a tumor, differentiate benign from malignant disease, demonstrate the relationship between a mass and adjacent anatomic structures, and aid in the selection of biopsy sites.

## ALGORITHM FOR DIAGNOSTIC IMAGING

Plain film radiography is an appropriate starting point for imaging the major salivary glands from a cost-benefit point of view. It can demonstrate sialoliths and the possible involvement of adjacent osseous structures. Because obstructive and associated inflammatory

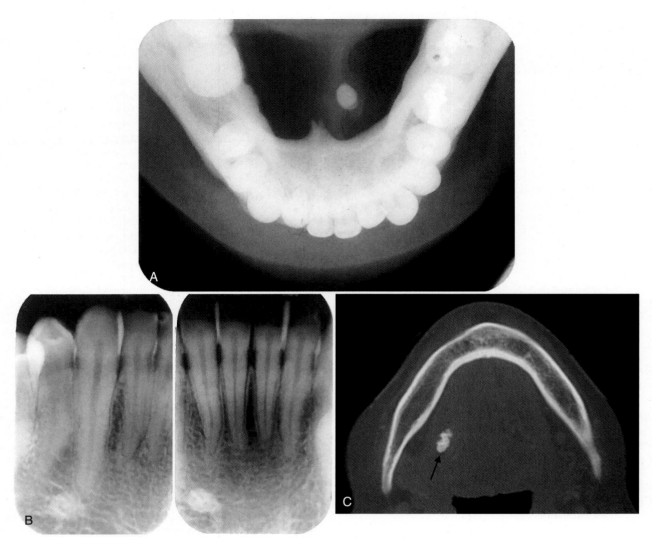

FIG. **31-1 A,** Underexposed mandibular occlusal radiograph demonstrating radiopaque sialolith in Wharton duct. Note the classic laminated appearance. **B,** Periapical radiographs of the same case. The radiopaque calculus can be localized lingual to the teeth by applying appropriate object localization rules. **C,** An axial bone algorithm CT image showing a sialolith in the submandibular duct *(arrow).*

tor muscle. As a rule, only sialoliths anterior to the masseter muscle can be imaged on an intraoral film. To demonstrate sialoliths in the anterior part of the duct, an intraoral film packet is held with a hemostat inside the cheek, as high as possible in the buccal sulcus and over the parotid papilla. The central ray is directed perpendicular to the center of the film.

## EXTRAORAL RADIOGRAPHY

A panoramic projection frequently demonstrates sialoliths in the posterior duct or reveals intraglandular sialoliths in the submandibular gland if they are within the image layer (see Fig. 31-2). The image of most parotid sialoliths is superimposed over the ramus and body of the mandible, making oblique lateral radiographs of the mandible of limited value. To demonstrate sialoliths in the submandibular gland, the lateral projection is modified by opening the mouth, extending the chin, and depressing the tongue with the index finger.

This improves the image of the sialolith by moving it inferior to the mandibular border.

Sialoliths in the distal portion of Stensen duct or in the parotid gland are difficult to demonstrate by intraoral or lateral extraoral views. However, a PA skull projection with the cheeks puffed out may move the image of the sialolith free of the bone, rendering it visible on the projected image (see Fig. 31-2). This technique may also demonstrate interglandular sialoliths that may be obscured during sialography.

## CONVENTIONAL SIALOGRAPHY

First performed in 1902, sialography is a radiographic technique where a radiopaque contrast agent is infused into the ductal system of a salivary gland before imaging with plain films, fluoroscopy, panoramic radiography, conventional tomography, or CT. Sialography remains the most detailed way to image the ductal system (Fig. 31-3).

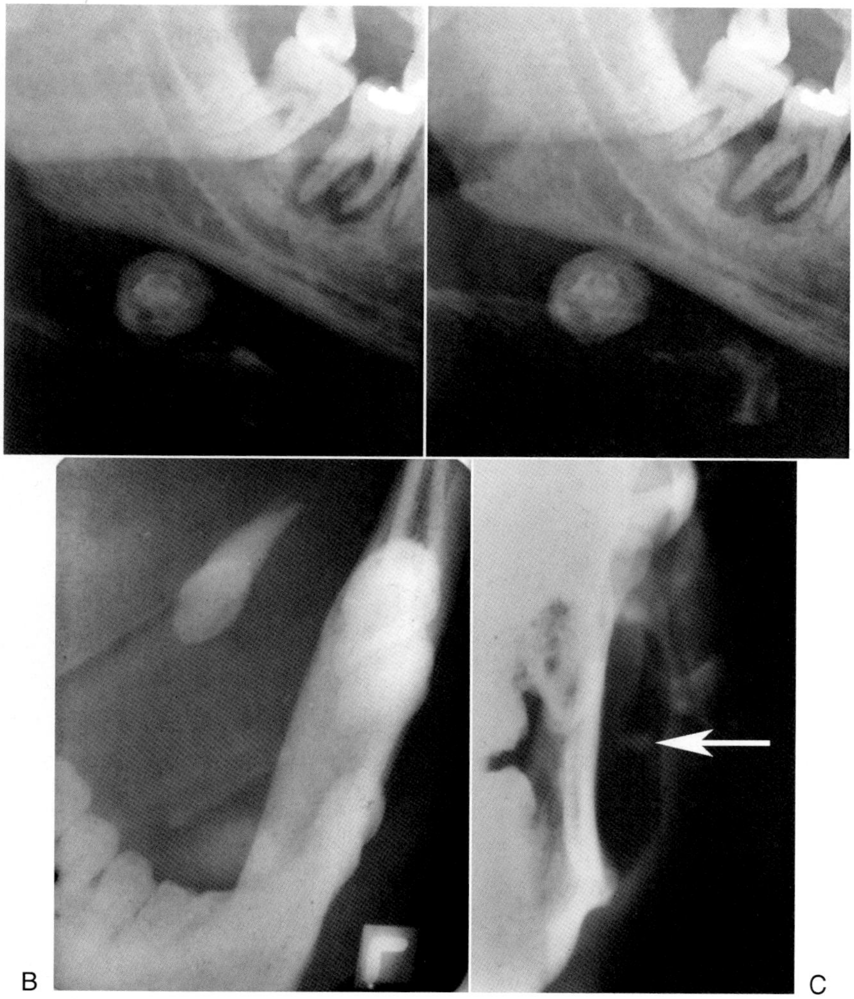

FIG. **31-2  A,** Stereoscopic panoramic plain film projection. Note the laminated appearance of this sialolith in the submandibular gland. The image of the sialolith is magnified because of its relatively lingual placement in the image layer. Taken from slightly different horizontal angles, a three-dimensional appearance can be obtained when viewed with stereobinoculars. **B,** Over-the-shoulder occlusal projection revealing a sialolith. **C,** Anteroposterior skull view with cheek blown out to provide air contrast to reveal a parotid sialolith *(arrow).*

The parotid and submandibular glands are more readily studied with this technique. Although the sublingual gland is difficult to infuse intentionally, it may be fortuitously opacified while the Wharton duct is infused to image the submandibular gland.

A survey or "scout" film is usually made before the infusion of the contrast solution into the ductal system as an aid in verifying the optimal exposure factors and patient positioning parameters and for the detection of radiopaque sialoliths or extraglandular pathosis.

With this technique, a lacrimal or periodontal probe is used to dilate the sphincter at the ductal orifice before the passage of a cannula (blunt needle or catheter) connected by extension tubing to a syringe containing contrast agent. Lipid-soluble (e.g., Ethiodol) or non–lipid-soluble (e.g., Sinografin) contrast solution is then slowly infused until the patient feels discomfort (usually between 0.2 and 1.5 ml, depending on the gland being studied). These iodine-containing agents render the ductal system radiopaque. The filling phase can be monitored by fluoroscopy or with static films. The intent is to opacify the ductal system all the way to the acini. The image of the ductal system appears as "tree limbs," with no area of the gland devoid of ducts. With acinar filling, the "tree" comes into "bloom," which is the typical appearance of the parenchymal opacification phase (Fig. 31-4). The gland is allowed to empty for 5 minutes without stimulation.

If postevacuation images suggest contrast retention, a sialogog such as lemon juice or 2% citric acid may be administered to augment evacuation by stimulating secretion. Non–lipid-soluble contrast agents are preferred because of reports of inflammatory reactions subsequent to inadvertent extravasation of lipid-soluble agents.

Sialography is indicated for the evaluation of chronic inflammatory diseases and ductal pathoses. Contraindications include acute infection, known sensitivity to iodine-containing compounds, and immediately anticipated thyroid function tests.

## COMPUTED TOMOGRAPHY

CT is useful in evaluating structures in and adjacent to salivary glands; it displays both soft and hard tissues and minute differences in soft tissue densities. Thin axial and coronal images with soft tissue algorithm commonly after intravenous administration of a contrast agent are typically acquired (Fig. 31-5). (See Chapter 14 for a description of the CT process.) Glandular tissues are usually easily discernible from surrounding fat and muscle. The parotid glands are more radiopaque than the surrounding fat but less opaque than adjacent muscles. Although the submandibular and sublingual glands are similar in density to adjacent muscles, they are readily identified on the basis of

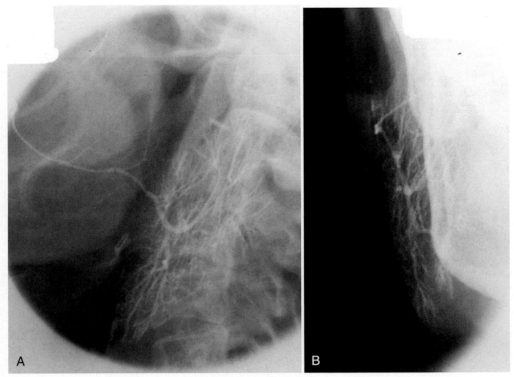

FIG. **31-3    Sialography. A,** Lateral projection of the parotid demonstrating opacification all the way to the terminal ducts and acini. **B,** Anteroposterior projection of the same gland demonstrating "parenchymal blushing" from acinar opacification. (Courtesy Oral and Maxillofacial Imaging Center, Baylor College of Dentistry, Dallas, Tex.)

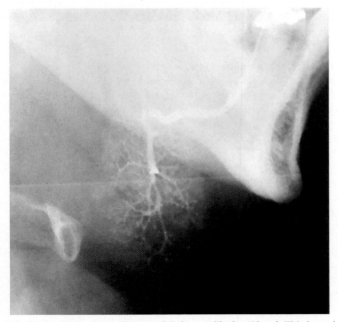

FIG. **31-4    Sialogram of Normal Submandibular Gland.** This lateral view demonstrates parenchymal blushing. Normal fine branching is visible. Lack of parenchymal blushing at the anteroinferior margin is caused by radiographic burnout.

shape and location. The submandibular and sublingual glands are most easily identified on directly acquired contrast-enhanced coronal CT scans. CT is useful in assessing acute inflammatory processes and abscesses as well as cysts, mucoceles, and neoplasia. Calcifications such as sialoliths are also well depicted with CT.

## MAGNETIC RESONANCE IMAGING

MRI typically provides a different and better soft tissue contrast resolution than does CT; it also results in fewer problems with streak artifacts from metallic dental restorative materials (Fig. 31-6). (See Chapter 14 for a description of the basic concepts and principles of MRI.) Axial views are acquired for all sequences, with coronal and sagittal views as needed. Noncontrast T1- and T2-weighted sequences are obtained, followed by T1-weighted postcontrast, fat-suppressed images. Fast-spin echo T2-weighted images may also require fat suppression.

Although indications for CT and MRI occasionally overlap, MRI is usually the imaging method of choice because of superior display of salivary gland masses, internal structures, and regional extension of the lesions into adjacent tissues or spaces, especially in examining the submandibular glands. The use of intravenous contrast (most commonly gadolinium) is helpful in distinguishing between cystic and solid masses and in the evaluation of perineural spread of malignant tumors. Studies have shown MRI with evoked salivation as a natural contrast medium to accurately reveal ductal morphology and to identify sialoliths.

## SCINTIGRAPHY (NUCLEAR MEDICINE, POSITRON EMISSION COMPUTED TOMOGRAPHY)

Nuclear medicine, or scintigraphy, provides a functional study of the salivary glands, taking advantage of the selective concentration of specific radiopharmaceuticals in the glands. (See Chapter 14 for a description of the nuclear medicine procedures used to acquire images.) When $^{99m}$Tc-pertechnetate is injected intravenously, it is concentrated in and excreted by glandular structures, including the salivary, thyroid, and mammary glands. The radionuclide appears in the ducts of the salivary glands within minutes and reaches maximal concentration within 30 to 45 minutes. A sialogog is then administered to evaluate secretory capacity. All major salivary glands can be studied at once.

Although this technique has high diagnostic sensitivity, it lacks specificity and demonstrates little morphology. Pathosis may be demonstrated by an increased, decreased, or absent radionuclide uptake (Fig. 31-7). Lesions that concentrate $^{99m}$Tc-pertechnetate are Warthin tumors and oncocytomas. The diagnosis of salivary gland tumors from nuclear medicine scans is not completely reliable. Because of relatively low image resolution, CT and MRI are preferred for the evaluation of salivary masses. A recent advance in nuclear medicine is positron emission computed tomography (PET). In spite of a much greater resolution than scintigraphy, PET has not been useful classifying salivary tumors as benign or malignant.

## ULTRASONOGRAPHY

Compared with CT and MRI, US has the advantages of being relatively inexpensive, widely available, painless, easy to perform, and noninvasive. (For a full description of US, see Chapter 14.) The primary application of US is the differentiation of solid masses from cystic ones (Fig. 31-8). Recent studies suggest that this technique may

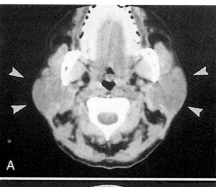
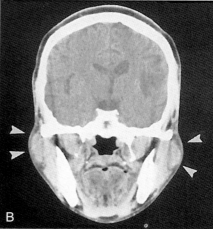

FIG. **31-5  CT Images with Soft Tissue Algorithm. A,** Axial view demonstrating bilateral enlargement of the parotid glands *(arrowheads).* **B,** Coronal view of the same patient. The clinical/histopathologic diagnosis was autoimmune parotitis. (Courtesy Department of Radiology, Baylor University Medical Center, Dallas, Tex.)

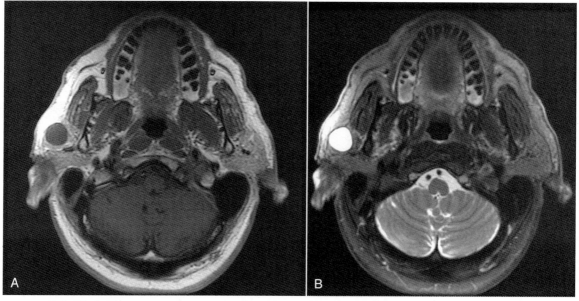

FIG. **31-6**  These magnetic resonance images reveal a lymphoepithelial cyst involving the right parotid gland. **A,** This axial T1-weighted image reveals a well-defined circular lesion involving the right parotid gland with an internal signal isointense to muscle, and the matching T2-weighted image **(B)** reveals that the lesion has a high internal signal because of the fluid content.

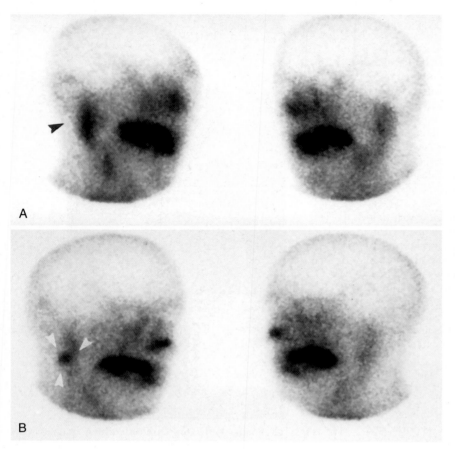

FIG. **31-7  Scintigraphy. A,** $^{99m}$Tc-pertechnetate scan of the salivary glands (right and left anterior oblique views) demonstrates increased uptake of radioisotope in the right parotid gland *(black arrowhead).* **B,** Scintigram taken after administration of a sialogog (lemon juice) demonstrates retention of isotope in right parotid gland *(white arrowheads).* This is a typical presentation of salivary stasis, Warthin tumor, or oncocytoma.

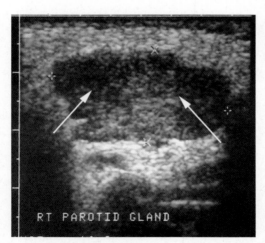

FIG. **31-8**  **Ultrasonography (US) Image of Right Parotid Gland.** A well-delineated solid mass is suggested by echo returns within the lesion *(arrows).* US appearance is typical of a benign salivary tumor. (Courtesy Department of Radiology, Baylor University Medical Center, Dallas, Tex.)

also be helpful in detecting sialoliths and diagnosing advanced autoimmune lesions (Sjögren syndrome).

## Image Interpretation of Salivary Gland Disorders

### OBSTRUCTIVE AND INFLAMMATORY DISORDERS

#### Sialolithiasis

**Synonyms**
Calculus and salivary stones

**Definition**
Sialolithiasis is the formation of a calcified obstruction within the salivary duct.

**Clinical Features**
Sialoliths can obstruct the secretory ducts, resulting in chronic retrograde infections because of a decrease in salivary flow. Clinical symptoms include intermittent swelling and pain with eating and signs of infection. Sialoliths may form in any of the major or minor salivary glands or their ducts, but usually only one gland is involved. The submandibular gland and Wharton duct are by far the most frequently involved (83% of cases). If one stone is found, at least a one in four chance exists that others are present.

## Radiographic Features

Depending on their degree of calcification, sialoliths may appear either radiopaque or radiolucent on radiographic examinations (20% to 40% of cases may not be calcified enough to be radiopaque and are sometimes referred to as "mucous plugs") (see Fig. 31-1). Sialoliths vary in shape from long cigar shapes to oval or round shapes. When visible, they usually have a homogeneous radiopaque internal structure. Sialography is helpful in locating obstructions that are undetectable with plain radiography, especially if the sialoliths are radiolucent. The contrast agent usually flows around the sialolith, filling the duct proximal to the obstruction (Fig. 31-9 and 31-10). The ductal system is frequently dilated proximal to the obstruction and implies the presence of an obstruction even when it is not visible. The contrast agent that flows around the sialolith is more radiopaque and may obscure small sialoliths. Radiolucent sialoliths appear as ductal filling defects (see Figs. 31-9 and 31-12). Sialography should not be performed if a radiopaque stone has been shown by plain radiography to be in the distal portion of the duct because the procedure may displace it proximally into the ductal system, complicating subsequent removal. CT may also detect minimally calcified sialoliths not visible on plain films.

US is of limited value in the diagnosis of inflammatory and obstructive diseases, but recent studies indicate it is fairly reliable in demonstrating sialoliths. More than 90% of stones larger than 2 mm are detected as echo-dense spots with a characteristic acoustic shadow.

Sialoliths must be differentiated from phleboliths and dystrophic calcification of lymph nodes. Phleboliths typically demonstrate a radiolucent center. Calcified lymph nodes usually appear to be "cauliflower" shaped. In the panoramic image palatine tonsilliths have a similar location as parotid sialoliths, superimposed over the ramus, but can be differentiated in that they are typically multiple and punctate.

## Treatment

Treatment of sialolithiasis may consist of encouragement of spontaneous discharge through the use of sialogogs to stimulate secretion. Sialography may also stimulate discharge, especially if an oil-based contrast agent is used. If discharge does not occur, the sialolith may be removed by surgery or by more conservative retrieval methods, and as a last resort the involved salivary gland may be removed.

## Bacterial Sialadenitis

### Synonyms

Parotitis and submandibulitis

### Definition

Bacterial sialadenitis is an acute or chronic bacterial infection of the terminal acini or parenchyma of the salivary glands.

### Clinical Features

Acute bacterial infections most commonly affect the parotid gland, but the submandibular gland may also be involved. Most cases are unilateral and may occur at any age. The typical clinical presentation is swelling, redness, tenderness, and malaise. Enlarged regional lymph nodes and suppuration may also be noted. Those most commonly afflicted are elderly persons, postoperative patients, and debilitated patients who have poor hygiene as a result of reduced salivary secretion and retrograde infection by the oral flora (usually *Staphylococcus aureus* and *Streptococcus viridans*). Reduced salivary secretion may also be drug related or the result of occlusion of a major duct. Untreated acute suppurative infections typically form abscesses. Diagnosis is based on clinical observation, systemic symptoms, and the expression of pus from the duct.

Chronic inflammation may affect any of the major salivary glands, causing extensive swelling and culminating in fibrosis. This may be a consequence of an untreated acute sialadenitis or associated with some type of obstruction resulting from sialolithiasis, noncalcified organic debris, or stricture (scar or fibrosis) formation in the excretory ducts. Bacteria or viruses may not be detected in the gland or saliva. The parotid is most often involved. During periods of painful swelling, pus may be expressed from the ductal orifice and salivary stimulation may cause pain. Episodic in nature, signs of generalized sepsis are seldom present. The obstruction may be congenital or

FIG. **31-9  A,** This partial image of a standard mandibular occlusal film reveals the presence of a sialolith *(arrow)*. **B,** Sialograph of the same patient demonstrating flow of contrast past the stone *(short arrows)* and a negative filling defect *(long arrow)* from a smaller radiolucent sialolith. The proximal secondary ducts within the gland show abnormal irregular widening indicating sialodochitis.

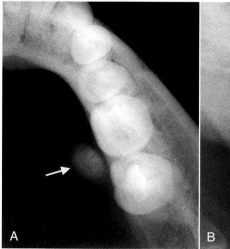
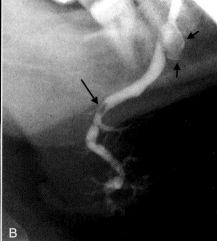

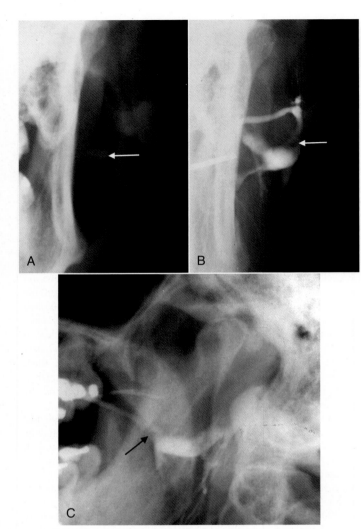

FIG. **31-10** **A,** Cropped view of a posteroanterior skull view as part of a parotid investigation; the cheek has been puffed out, providing air contrast and revealing a poorly calcified sialolith *(arrow).* **B,** Cropped view of a posteroanterior skull view of the sialograph of the same patient with the negative filling defect representing the sialolith *(arrow)* seen in **A. C,** Lateral view of the same patient revealing the filling defect *(arrow)* and abnormal dilation of the proximal ducts.

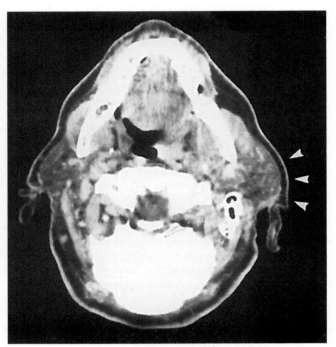

FIG. **31-11** **Contrast-Enhanced CT Image.** The left parotid gland *(arrows)* is larger than the right, with no suggestion of abscess formation. This appearance is consistent with diffuse parotitis and cellulitis. (Courtesy Department of Radiology, Baylor University Medical Center, Dallas, Tex.)

caused by sialolithiasis, trauma, infection, or neoplasia. Typical clinical symptoms are intermittent swelling, pain when eating, and superimposed infection resulting from salivary stasis.

## Radiographic Features

Sialography is contraindicated in acute infections because disrupted ductal epithelium may allow extravasation of contrast agent, resulting in a foreign body reaction and severe pain. This technique is appropriate for use in cases of suspected chronic infections. Epithelial flattening may lead to mildly dilated terminal ducts and saclike acini, which is demonstrable with sialography. The saclike acinar areas are referred to as sialectasia. An even distribution throughout the gland is seen in recurrent parotitis and autoimmune disorders. If connected to the ductal system, abscess cavities may fill with contrast media during sialography. Abscess cavities appear on CT as walled-off areas of lower attenuation within an enlarged gland. US may distinguish between diffuse inflammation (echo-free, light image) and suppuration (less echo-free, darker image) and detect sialoliths greater than 2 mm in diameter. US examination may also demonstrate abscess cavities, if present and may be the study of choice for recurrent parotitis, especially in children. Contrast-enhanced CT may demonstrate glandular enlargement (Fig. 31-11). However, MRI is an appropriate alternative examination in cases in which sialography is contraindicated or not technically possible. On MRI, inflamed glands are usually enlarged and demonstrate a lower tissue signal on T1-weighted images and a higher signal on T2-weighted images than that of the surrounding muscle. Advanced sialadenitis may present in combination with sialolithiasis, sialodochitis, abscess formation, and fistulas.

## Treatment

Treatment of bacterial sialadenitis typically begins conservatively with attention to oral hygiene, local massage, increased fluid intake, and the use of oral sialogogs (sour citrus fruit wedges or salivary stimulants). An appropriate antibiotic regimen may also be indicated. If symptoms continue, surgical remedies ranging from partial to total excision of the gland may be considered.

## Sialodochitis

### Synonym
Ductal sialadenitis

### Definition
Sialodochitis is an inflammation of the ductal system of the salivary glands.

## Clinical Features

Sialectasia or dilation of the ductal system is a prominent sialographic presentation of sialodochitis. It is common in both the submandibular (Fig. 31-12) and parotid glands. If interstitial fibrosis develops, it is apparent in sialograms as a sausage-string appearance of the main duct and its major branches produced by alternate strictures and dilations. Recently these changes have been seen with the use of thin-section MRI. Scintigraphy and CT are not typically indicated in the diagnosis of inflammatory ductal diseases of the salivary glands. They are costly and nonspecific and typically do not provide any more useful information than sialography does.

## Treatment

The management of sialodochitis is similar to that described for sialadenitis.

### Autoimmune Sialadenitis

## Synonyms

Myoepithelial sialadenitis, Sjögren syndrome, benign lymphoepithelial lesion, Mikulicz disease, sicca syndrome, dacryosialoadenopathia atrophicans, and autoimmune sialosis

## Definition

Autoimmune sialadenitis represents a group of disorders that affect the salivary glands and share an autosensitivity. The range of clinical and histopathologic manifestations suggests that these disorders represent different developmental stages of the same immunologic mechanisms, differing only in the extent and intensity of tissue reaction. Different forms may share a common etiology.

## Clinical Features

The clinical manifestations range from recurrent painless swelling of the salivary glands (usually the parotid gland) to a stage that includes enlargement of the lacrimal glands. Glandular swelling may be accompanied by xerostomia and xerophthalmia (primary Sjögren syndrome), and subsequently by a connective tissue disease such as rheumatoid arthritis, progressive systemic sclerosis, systemic lupus erythematosus, or polymyositis (secondary Sjögren syndrome). The

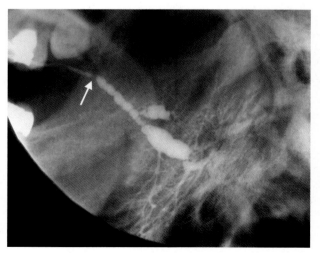

FIG. **31-12**  Lateral view of a sialogram of a parotid gland demonstrating a negative fill defect *(arrow)* representing a noncalcified sialolith and prominent intermittent stricture and dilation of the main and secondary ducts, which is typical of advanced sialodochitis.

process may progress to benign lymphoepithelial lesions that can assume the proportions of a tumor. A presumptive diagnosis can be made on the basis of any two of the following three features: dry mouth, dry eyes, and rheumatoid disease. The disease is most common in adults, primarily in the 40- to 60-year-old age group with a 90% to 95% female prevalence. The childhood form is only one-tenth as common as the adult form and there is much less chance of advanced parotid disease. Studies have shown a 44 times greater risk for development of non-Hodgkin lymphoma than in control subjects. Mikulicz disease has been included within the diagnosis of primary Sjögren syndrome but represents a unique condition consisting of enlargement of the lacrimal and salivary glands and characterized by few autoimmune reactions.

## Radiographic Features

Sialography is helpful in the diagnosis and staging of autoimmune disorders. The early stages of disease are witness to the initiation of punctate (less than 1 mm) and globular (1 to 2 mm) spheric collections of contrast agent evenly distributed throughout the glands. These collections are referred to as sialectases (Fig. 31-13). At this stage, the main duct may appear normal, but the intraglandular ducts may be narrowed or not even evident. Sialectasia typically remains after the administration of a sialogog, which is an indication that contrast agent is pooled extraductally.

As the disease progresses, the collections of contrast agent increase in size (greater than 2 mm in diameter) and are irregular in shape. These pools of contrast agent are termed *cavitary sialectases*. These larger sialectases are fewer in number and less uniformly distributed throughout the glands than are punctate or globular sialectases (Fig. 31-14). Progressively larger cavities of contrast agent and dilation of the main ductal system may also be present. At the end point of this disorder, complete destruction of the gland occurs. Cavitation and glandular fibrosis are the result of recurrent inflammation. The differential diagnosis of this appearance would include chronic bacterial or granulomatous infections and multiple parotid cysts associated with human immunodeficiency virus (HIV) infection. However, diffuse cervical lymphadenopathy is common in HIV disease and uncommon in Sjögren syndrome. Thin-section MRI has been shown to be reliable in depicting sialodochitis and sialectasia, especially when globular changes are present.

## Treatment

The management of autoimmune disorders of the salivary glands is directed toward relief of symptoms. Underlying systemic rheumatoid conditions are typically treated with anti-inflammatory agents, corticosteroids, and immunosuppressive therapeutic agents. Salivary stimulants, increased fluid intake, and artificial saliva and tears are symptomatic treatment regimens for the eyes and mouth. More advanced inflammatory changes may be treated surgically by local or total excision of the symptomatic gland.

# NONINFLAMMATORY DISORDERS

### Sialadenosis

## Synonym

Sialosis

## Definition

Sialadenosis is a nonneoplastic, noninflammatory enlargement of primarily the parotid salivary glands. It is usually related to metabolic

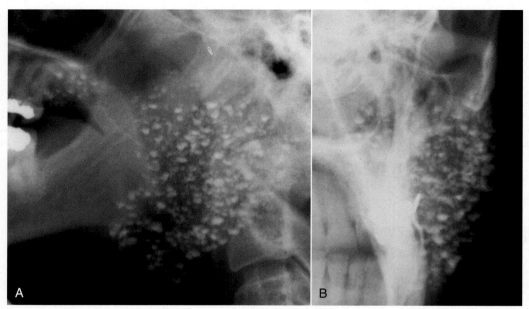

FIG. **31-13** **Conventional Sialography of Left Parotid. A,** Lateral projection demonstrates punctate sialectases distributed throughout the gland, which is suggestive of autoimmune sialadenitis. Clinical/histopathologic diagnosis was Sjögren syndrome. **B,** Anteroposterior projection of the same gland.

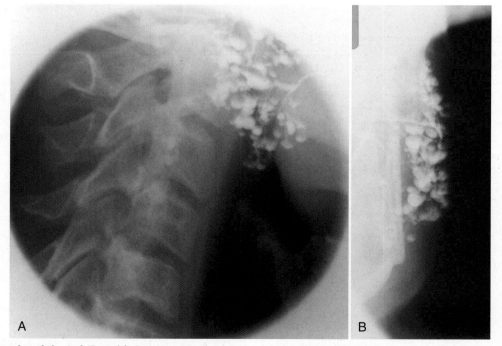

FIG. **31-14** **Sialography of the Left Parotid.** Punctate (small spheric), globular (larger spheric), and cavitary (larger, irregular) sialectases with some dilation of the main duct are suggestive of advanced autoimmune disease with parenchymal destruction with retrograde infection in lateral **(A)** and anteroposterior **(B)** projections. Clinical/histopathologic diagnosis was Sjögren syndrome. (Courtesy Oral and Maxillofacial Imaging Center, Baylor College of Dentistry, Dallas, Tex.)

and secretory disorders of the parenchyma associated with diseases of nearly all the endocrine glands (hormonal sialadenoses), protein deficiencies, malnutrition in alcoholics (dystrophic-metabolic sialadenoses), vitamin deficiencies, and neurologic disorders (neurogenic sialadenoses).

## Clinical Features
Affected glands are typically enlarged.

## Radiographic Features
Sialography may demonstrate enlargement of the affected glands or a normal appearance. In enlarged glands, the ducts will be splayed. CT and MRI provide a more straightforward depiction of the glands but are nonspecific and require correlation with the clinical findings and history.

## Treatment
The management of sialadenosis hinges on identifying the cause of the metabolic or secretory disorder. Conservative treatment, including local massage, increased fluid intake, and the use of oral sialogogs (sour citrus fruit wedges or salivary stimulants), is appropriate.

## Cystic Lesions

### Definition
Cysts of the salivary glands are rare (less than 5% of all salivary gland masses) and most commonly occur unilaterally in the parotid gland (see Fig. 31-6). They may be congenital (branchial), lympho-epithelial, dermoid, or acquired, including mucous retention cysts (obstructions from any etiology). Cystic salivary lesions may be intraglandular or extraglandular in nature and may progress to such proportions that they are clinically palpable and must be distinguished from neoplasia. Cystic neoplasms do occur, but they are discussed separately in this chapter. Mucous extravasation pseudocysts lack an epithelial lining and result from ductal rupture. Ranulas are retention cysts that usually occur as a result of obstruction of the sublingual duct. Benign lymphoepithelial cysts are thought to be sequelae of cystic degeneration of salivary inclusions within lymph nodes. Multicentric parotid cysts associated with HIV have been reported and are termed benign lymphoepithelial lesions of human immunodeficiency syndrome. These lesions are accompanied by cervical lymphadenopathy, occur bilaterally, and are usually in the superficial portion of the parotid gland (Fig. 31-15). Secondary parotitis may develop.

### Radiographic Features
On sialographic examination, cystic masses may be indirectly visualized only by the displacement of the ducts arching around them. Cystic lesions typically appear as well-circumscribed, nonenhancing (with contrast), low-density areas when examined on CT. Cysts appear as well-circumscribed, high-signal areas on T2-weighted MRI, but they do not enhance after gadolinium contrast, as do benign mixed tumors. When imaged with US, cysts are sharply marginated and echo free (represented as a dark area) (Fig. 31-16).

### Treatment
Management of cystic lesions is typically surgical, involving local or total excision of the gland.

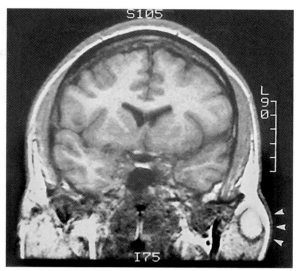

FIG. **31-15  Coronal Section MRI.** The high-signal mass *(arrows)* in the left parotid gland was diagnosed as a cyst. This patient was found to be HIV positive. (Courtesy Department of Radiology, Baylor University Medical Center, Dallas, Tex.)

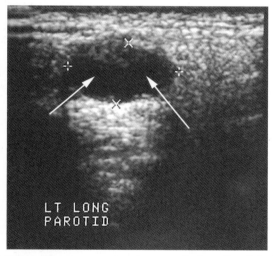

FIG. **31-16  Ultrasonography Image of the Parotid Gland.** Echo-free mass with well-defined margins presents a typical cystic appearance *(arrows)*. (Courtesy Department of Radiology, Baylor University Medical Center, Dallas, Tex.)

## BENIGN TUMORS

Salivary gland tumors are relatively uncommon and occur in less than 0.003% of the population. They account for about 3% of all tumors. Some 80% of the salivary tumors arise in the parotid, 5% in the submandibular, 1% in the sublingual, and 10% to 15% in the minor salivary glands. The majority (70% to 80%) of these tumors occur in the superficial lobe of the parotid gland. Most are benign or low-grade malignancies. High-grade malignancies are uncommon. The chance of neoplasms of major salivary glands being benign varies directly with the size of the gland.

## Radiographic Features

Benign tumors and low-grade malignancies may have a similar appearance, with well-defined margins, which are most apparent on CT or MRI examinations. Because of the higher density of the submandibular gland, which can equal that of the neoplasm and obscure the tumor, intravenous contrast enhancement is required during the CT examination. This causes the tumor to appear more radiopaque because the vascularity of the tumor is greater than that of the adjacent salivary gland tissue. MRI is a preferential modality for salivary gland neoplasia, especially for the submandibular gland, because of its superior soft tissue contrast resolution. On US examination, benign masses are typically less echogenic than parenchyma, sharply defined, and of essentially homogeneous echo strength and density. Benign tumors may present as low-intensity (dark) or high-intensity (light) tissue signals on MRI, although the relative intensity of the signal may indicate the presence of lipid, vascular, or fibrous tissues. Sialography may suggest a space-occupying mass when the ducts are compressed or smoothly displaced around the lesion (the "ball-in-hand" appearance) (Fig. 31-17).

## Treatment

The management of benign tumors of the major salivary glands is typically surgical. Benign tumors of the parotid gland may be either partially or totally excised. Submandibular and sublingual glands are invariably totally excised.

## Benign Mixed Tumor

### Synonym

Pleomorphic adenoma

### Definition

The benign mixed tumor is a neoplasm arising from the ductal epithelium of major and minor salivary glands exhibiting epithelial and mesenchymal components.

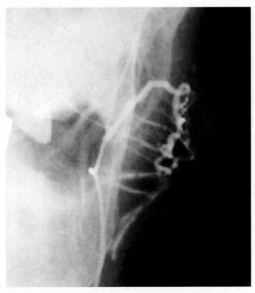

FIG. **31-17 Sialogram of Left Parotid (Anteroposterior View).** A mass within the gland is inferred by the appearance of the ducts displaced around the lesion. This is referred to as the "ball-in-hand" appearance, which is suggestive of a space-occupying mass. (Courtesy Department of Radiology, Baylor University Medical Center, Dallas, Tex.)

## Clinical Features

The benign mixed tumor accounts for 75% of all salivary gland tumors; 80% are found in the parotid gland, 4% in the submandibular gland, 1% in the sublingual gland, and 10% in the minor salivary glands. This tumor typically occurs in the fifth decade of life as a slow-growing, unilateral, encapsulated, asymptomatic mass. A slight female predilection exists. Recurrence occurs in 50% of cases after excision. Malignant transformation is reported in up to 15% of untreated cases.

## Radiographic Features

The CT presentation of the benign mixed tumor is a sharply circumscribed infrequently lobulated and essentially round homogeneous lesion that has a higher density than the adjacent glandular tissue (Fig. 31-18, A). Calcifications within the tumor are commonly seen and are well depicted on CT. This tumor has various tissue signals in different MRI techniques such as relatively low (dark) in T1-weighted, intermediate on proton density-weighted, and homogeneous high-intensity (bright) on T2-weighted images (Fig. 31-18). Foci of low signal intensity (dark areas) usually represent areas of fibrosis or dystrophic calcifications. If a calcification is present (signal void) the diagnosis favors a benign mixed tumor; otherwise, it is difficult to differentiate this tumor from other parotid masses.

Benign mixed tumor does not usually concentrate $^{99m}$Tc-pertechnetate. Therefore the tumor appears as a cold spot when examined by scintigraphy. Solid tumors larger than 5 mm are usually well visualized.

## Warthin Tumor

### Synonym

Papillary cystadenoma lymphomatosum, adenolymphoma, and lymphomatous adenoma

### Definition

Warthin tumor is a benign tumor arising from proliferating salivary ducts trapped in lymph nodes during embryogenesis of the salivary glands.

### Clinical Features

Warthin tumor is the second most common benign neoplasm of the salivary glands, accounting for 2% to 6% of the parotid tumors. In the parotid, it is usually found in the inferior lobe of the gland. This unusual type of tumor is a slow-growing, painless, round-to-ovoid mass. In 20% of cases the tumors are multiple. Warthin tumor typically afflicts males older than 40 years and may be unilateral or bilateral (Fig. 31-19).

### Radiographic Features

CT and MRI are the preferred techniques for imaging Warthin tumor. The CT and MRI appearance of this tumor is not specific and is typical of benign salivary tumors as described for the benign mixed tumor. On CT, this tumor may be of either soft tissue or cystic density. On MRI, it is heterogeneous and may demonstrate hemorrhagic foci. Warthin tumor is characteristically intensely hot on $^{99m}$Tc-pertechnetate scans. Oncocytoma (oxyphilic adenoma) may also accumulate the $^{99m}$Tc-pertechnetate but is uncommon and more likely to be bilateral (see Fig. 31-7). Oncocytoma has been reported to be present in essentially everyone older than 70 years. The US presentation of Warthin tumor is that of a solid mass (anechoic), if the mass is not cystic, as some are (see Fig. 31-8).

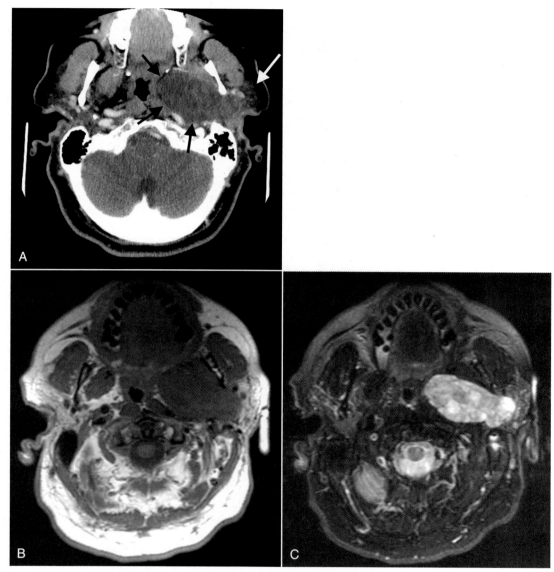

FIG. **31-18** **CT and MRI Images of a Pleomorphic Adenoma. A,** In the axial CT soft tissue algorithm image, note the well-defined periphery *(black arrows)* and the internal density that is less than surrounding muscles. The remaining parotid gland *(white arrow)* is displaced laterally. **B,** In the axial MRI T1-weighted image, the tissue signal of the tumor is isointense with muscle. **C,** In the T2-weighted image, note the increased signal of the tumor, which is now hyperintense to muscle.

## Hemangioma

### Synonym
Vascular nevus

### Definition
Hemangioma is a benign neoplasm of proliferating endothelial cells (congenital hemangioma) and vascular malformations, including lesions resulting from abnormal vessel morphogenesis.

### Clinical Features
Hemangioma is the most frequently occurring nonepithelial salivary neoplasm, accounting for 50% of the cases. As many as 85% arise in the parotid gland. It is the most common salivary gland tumor during infancy and childhood. The average age at diagnosis is 10 years, with 65% occurring in the first two decades of life. They are frequently unilateral and asymptomatic. A 2:1 female-to-male predilection exists. Treatment is by local excision for those who do not undergo spontaneous remission.

### Radiographic Features
Phleboliths are common in this tumor. They appear as discrete soft tissue calcifications with a radiolucent center and are best identified on plain films and CT. Displaced ducts curving about the mass may also be apparent on sialography. The CT presentation of hemangioma is a soft tissue mass that is well distinguished from surrounding tissue, especially when intravenous contrast enhancement is used. On MRI, the tumor has a signal similar to that of adjacent muscle on

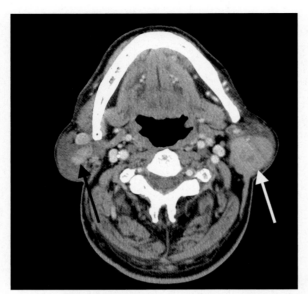

FIG. **31-19** An axial soft tissue algorithm CT image of a case of bilateral Warthin tumor, a large tumor involving the left parotid *(white arrow)* and a much smaller tumor on the right side *(black arrow)*.

T1-weighted images and a very high signal on T2-weighted images. Although US usually demonstrates well-defined margins in the hemangioma, ill-defined margins may also be noted. Strongly hypoechoic hemangioma may have a complex US appearance resulting from the multiple interfaces in the lesion. Phleboliths image as multiple hyperechoic areas within the body of the gland itself.

## MALIGNANT TUMORS

About 20% of tumors in the parotid are malignant compared with 50% to 60% of submandibular tumors, 90% of sublingual tumors, and 60% to 75% of minor salivary gland tumors.

### Radiographic Features

The radiographic presentation of malignant tumors is variable and is related to the grade, aggressiveness, location, and type of tumor. In many cases it is not possible to determine whether a tumor is malignant or benign (Fig. 31-20). However, features such as ill-defined margins (Fig. 31-21), invasion of adjacent soft tissues (such as fat spaces), and destruction of adjacent osseous structures are considered to be typical indicators of malignancy.

### Treatment

The management of malignant tumors of the major salivary glands is typically surgical. Low-grade malignant tumors of the parotid gland may be either partially or totally excised. Submandibular and sublingual glands are invariably totally excised. High-grade tumors may require radical neck dissection. Combinations of surgery, therapeutic radiation, and chemotherapy may also be used.

### Mucoepidermoid Carcinoma

#### Definition

Mucoepidermoid carcinoma is a malignant tumor composed of a variable admixture of epidermoid and mucous cells arising from the ductal epithelium of the salivary glands.

### Clinical Features

This is the most common malignant salivary gland tumor (35%). Just over half occur in the major salivary glands, most commonly the parotid gland; the rest are found in the minor glands, with the palate being the most frequent location. The aggressiveness of the lesion varies with its histologic grade. A wide age range exists, with the highest prevalence in the fifth decade of life. A slight predilection for females exists. The low-grade variety rarely metastasizes. Clinically, this tumor appears as a movable, slowly growing, painless nodule not unlike a benign mixed tumor. It is usually only 1 to 4 cm in diameter. The prognosis is good; the 5-year survival rate is greater than 95%.

In contrast to low-grade mucoepidermoid carcinomas, high-grade tumors often cause facial pain and paralysis, have ill-defined margins, and are relatively immobile. Metastasis by blood and lymph are common, with recurrence in half the patients after excision. The prognosis is poor and varies with the histologic grade; the 5-year survival rate may be as low as 25%.

### Radiographic Features

Low-grade mucoepidermoid carcinomas are typically not apparent on plain films unless destructive changes to adjacent osseous structures have occurred. The sialographic, CT, MRI, US, and scintigraphic presentations of this tumor are similar to those previously described for benign salivary tumors. However, low-grade mucoepidermoid carcinoma may present a lobulated or irregularly sharply circumscribed appearance on contrast enhanced CT or MRI (Fig. 31-22). Cystic area may present and, rarely, calcifications may be seen.

The radiographic diagnosis of high-grade mucoepidermoid carcinoma typically relies on the appearance of irregular margins and ill-defined form when the mass is examined with CT or MRI. In CT images, the tumor as an irregular homogeneous mass, slightly denser than the gland parenchyma. If intravenous contrast is added to the CT study, the result is a sharply defined homogeneous mass that is considerably more opaque. CT is also a reliable technique for the detection of invasion of adjacent osseous structures.

In contrast to low-grade malignancies and benign neoplasms, high-grade mucoepidermoid carcinoma, like most high-grade malignancies, has homogeneous low signal intensity (dark) on T1-weighted images, but T2-weighted images are more heterogeneous and intense (brighter) than T1-weighted images but still slightly darker (low signal) relative to the surrounding tissues. Regardless of clinical presentation and margins, low signal intensity is suggestive of a high-grade malignancy. Cavitary sialectasia and ductal displacement may be noted on sialographic images of this tumor.

### Malignant Mixed Tumor

#### Synonyms

Carcinoma ex mixed tumor, carcinoma ex pleomorphic adenoma, and malignant pleomorphic adenoma

#### Definition

The malignant mixed tumor is composed of three distinct types of tumors. The most common is carcinoma ex mixed tumor, which arises from the epithelial components of a preexisting benign mixed tumor. The other two, which are extremely rare, are a true malignant mixed tumor (from both epithelial and mesenchymal components of a mixed tumor) and the metastasizing mixed tumor, which appears histologically benign but behaves in a malignant fashion.

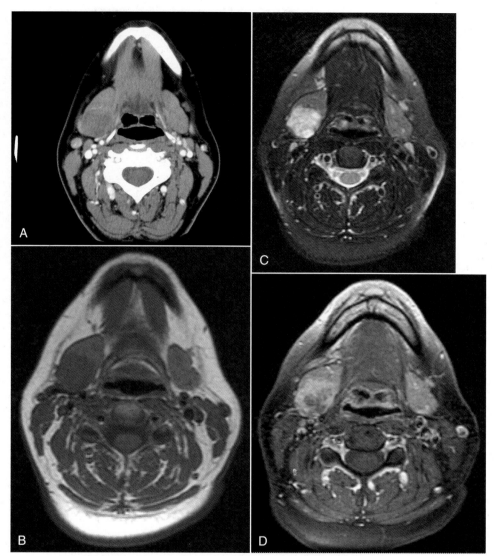

FIG. **31-20** These four axial CT and magnetic resonance images depict an adenoid cystic carcinoma of the right submandibular gland. Note the well-defined periphery, making it difficult to differentiate from a benign tumor. **A,** The internal density of the tumor in this soft tissue algorithm CT image is almost equal to the remaining gland. **B,** The tissue signal in this T1-weighted magnetic resonance image is very slightly less than the remaining gland. However, in **C,** a T2-weighted magnetic resonance image, the high signal of the tumor contrasts with the remaining gland. Similarly, in **D,** a T1-weighted postgadolinium, fat-saturation image, the tumor has a higher signal than in the remaining gland.

## Clinical Features

The malignant mixed tumor typically begins as a slowly growing mass that suddenly undergoes rapid proliferation, often accompanied by pain and facial paralysis. Metastasis is early and the prognosis is unfavorable.

## Radiographic Features

The presentation of this tumor is similar to that of the high-grade mucoepidermoid carcinoma previously described. MRI is usually superior to CT for tumor definition.

## OTHER MALIGNANT AND METASTATIC TUMORS

Although the incidence of other malignant tumors of the major salivary glands is low, a significant variety exists in their histogenesis. Of

all malignant salivary gland tumors, 23% are adenoid cystic carcinomas; however, the majority of these neoplasms develop in the minor salivary glands.

Adenocarcinoma accounts for 6.4% of all salivary gland malignancies, with acinic cell carcinoma, primary lymphoma, and squamous cell carcinoma occurring with even less frequency. Pain, paresthesia, and even paralysis may be present, especially in high-grade tumors. Interestingly, the pain associated with acinic cell carcinoma is not considered to be as grave a sign as in other malignant salivary tumors. Tumor spread may be by direct invasion or metastasis. Adenoid cystic carcinoma also spreads along nerve sheaths and is best demonstrated on postcontrast MRI where nerve enhancement and enlargement is present. Metastasis of tumors of the salivary glands is not unusual. Metastatic lesions in the parotid gland are more common than in the other salivary glands because of the extensive lymphatic and

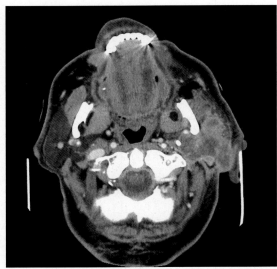

FIG. **31-21** This axial soft tissue algorithm CT image reveals an adenocarcinoma of the left parotid gland. Almost all the gland has been replaced by this ill-defined tumor that has some peripheral enhancement and lower density internal structure, likely representing necrotic regions.

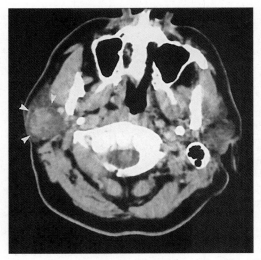

FIG. **31-22** Contrast-enhanced axial soft tissue algorithm CT image demonstrating a mass in right parotid gland with a poorly marginated, heterogeneous, slightly lobulated appearance *(white arrows)*. Poorly defined margins suggest a low-grade malignancy rather than a benign tumor, although the CT appearance of both is similar. Histopathologic diagnosis was low-grade mucoepidermoid carcinoma. (Courtesy Department of Radiology, Baylor University Medical Center, Dallas, Tex.)

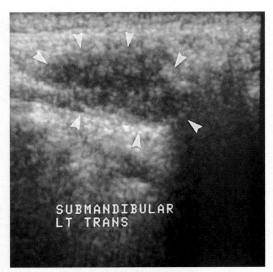

FIG. **31-23** **Ultrasonography.** The mass in the submandibular gland *(arrows)* demonstrates a heterogeneous hypoechoic pattern compared with the adjacent tissue. The histopathologic diagnosis was adenoid cystic carcinoma. (Courtesy Department of Radiology, Baylor University Medical Center, Dallas, Tex.)

### Radiographic Features

The presentation of these tumors is nonspecific and similar to that of the high-grade mucoepidermoid carcinoma previously described. US may demonstrate echo-free cystic areas in adenoid cystic carcinomas (Fig. 31-23).

## SUGGESTED READINGS

Del Balso AM, Ellis GE, Hartman KS et al: Diagnostic imaging of the salivary glands and periglandular regions. In Del Balso AM, editor: *Maxillofacial imaging,* Philadelphia, 1990, WB Saunders.

Freling NJM: Imaging of salivary gland disease, *Semin Roentgenol* 35:12-20, 2000.

Harnsberger HR, Hudgins PA, Wiggins RW III et al: *Pocket radiologist, head and neck 100 top diagnoses,* Salt Lake City, 2002, Amirsys.

Harnsberger HR, Hudgins R, Wiggins P et al: *Diagnostic imaging head and neck,* Salt Lake City, 2004, Amirsys.

Lufkin RB, Hanafee WN: *MRI of the head and neck,* New York, 1992, Raven Press.

Rabinov K, Weber AL: *Radiology of the salivary glands,* Boston, 1985, GK Hall Medical Publishers.

Rankow RM, Polayes IM: *Diseases of the salivary glands,* Philadelphia, 1976, WB Saunders.

Rice DH, Becker TS: The salivary glands. In Hanafee WN, Ward PH, editors: *Clinical correlations in the head and neck,* vol 2, New York, 1994, Thieme Medical Publishers.

Seifert G, Miehlke A, Hanbrich J et al: *Diseases of the salivary glands,* Stuttgart, Germany, 1986, George Thieme Verlag.

Van den Akker HP: Diagnostic imaging in salivary gland disease, *Oral Surg* 66:625-637, 1988.

Watson MG: Investigation of salivary gland disease, *Ear Nose Throat J* 68:84, 87-93, 1989.

### PLAIN FILM RADIOGRAPHY

Ollerenshaw R, Ross SS: Radiological diagnosis of salivary gland disease, *Br J Radiol* 24:538-548, 1951.

Silvers AR, Som PM: Salivary glands, *Radiol Clin North Am* 36:941-966, 1998.

circulatory components of the parotid gland. Most metastatic lesions of the parotid gland occur through the lymphatic system and include squamous cell carcinoma, lymphoma, and melanoma. Although considerably fewer lesions are the result of hematogenous dissemination, metastasis from the lung, breast, kidney, and gastrointestinal tract has been reported.

Weissman JL: Imaging of the salivary glands, *Semin Ultrasound CT MR* 16:546-568, 1995.

Yousem DM, Kraut MA, Chalian AA: Major salivary gland imaging, *Radiology* 216:19-29, 2000.

## CONVENTIONAL SIALOGRAPHY

Drag NA, Brown JE, Wilson RF: Pain and swelling after sialography: is it a significant problem? *Oral Surg Oral Med Oral Pathol Oral Radiol Endod* 90:385-388, 2000.

Eisenbud L, Cranin N: The role of sialography in the diagnosis and therapy of chronic obstructive sialadenitis, *Oral Surg Oral Med Oral Pathol* 16:1181-1199, 1963.

Kalk WW, Vissink A, Spijkervet HK et al: Parotid sialography for diagnosing Sjögren syndrome, *Oral Surg Oral Med Oral Pathol Oral Radiol Endod* 94:131-137, 2002.

Manashil GB: *Clinical sialography*, Springfield, 1978, Charles C Thomas.

Whaley K, Blair S, Low PS et al: Sialographic abnormalities in Sjögren's syndrome, rheumatoid arthritis, and other arthritides and connective tissue diseases: a clinical and radiological investigation using hydrostatic sialography, *Clin Radiol* 23:474-482, 1972.

Varghese JC, Thornton F, Lucey BC et al: A prospective comparative study of MR sialography and conventional sialography of salivary duct disease, *AJR Am J Roentgenol* 173:1497-1503, 1999.

Yune HY, Klatte EC: Current status of sialography, *Am J Roentgenol Radiumt Ther Nucl Med* 115:420-428, 1972.

## COMPUTED TOMOGRAPHY OF THE MAJOR SALIVARY GLANDS

Bryan RN, Miller RH, Ferreyro RI et al: Computed tomography of the major salivary glands, *AJR Am J Roentgenol* 139:547-554, 1982.

Casselman JW, Mancuso AA: Major salivary gland masses: comparison of MR imaging and CT, *Radiology* 165:183-189, 1987.

Kosaka M, Kamiishi H: New strategy for the diagnosis of parotid gland lesions utilizing three-dimensional sialography, *Comput Aided Surg* 5:42-45, 2000.

Lloyd RE, Ho KH: Combined CT scanning and sialography in the management of parotid tumors, *Oral Surg Oral Med Oral Pathol* 65:142-144, 1988.

## MAGNETIC RESONANCE IMAGING OF THE MAJOR SALIVARY GLANDS

Browne RFJ, Golding SJ, Watt-Smith SR: The role of MRI in facial swelling due to presumed salivary gland disease, *Br J Radiol* 74:127-133, 2001.

Jäger L, Menauer F, Holzknecht N et al: MR sialography of the submandibular duct—an alternative to conventional sialography and US? *Radiology* 216:665-671, 2000.

Jungehulsing M, Fischbach R, Schroder U et al: Magnetic resonance sialography, *Otolaryngol Head Neck Surg* 121:488-494, 1999.

Kaneda T, Minami M, Ozawa K et al: MR of the submandibular gland: normal and pathologic states, *AJNR Am J Neuroradiol* 17:1575-1581, 1996.

Mandelblatt S, Braun IF, Davis PC et al: Parotid masses: MR imaging, *Radiology* 163:411-414, 1987.

Som PM, Biller HF: High-grade malignancies of the parotid gland; identification with MR imaging, *Radiology* 173:823-826, 1989.

Swartz JD, Rothman MI, Marlowe FI et al: MR imaging of parotid mass lesions: attempts at histopathologic differentiation, *J Comput Assist Tomogr* 13:789-796, 1989.

## NUCLEAR MEDICINE (SCINTIGRAPHY) OF THE MAJOR SALIVARY GLANDS

Chaudhuri TK, Stadalnik RC: Salivary gland imaging, *Semin Nucl Med* 10:400-401, 1980.

Garcia RR: Differential diagnosis of tumors of the salivary glands with radioactive isotopes, *Int J Oral Surg* 3:330-334, 1974.

Greyson ND, Noyek AM: Radionuclide salivary scanning, *J Otolaryngol Suppl* 10:1-47, 1982.

Keyes JW Jr, Harkness BA, Greven KM et al: Salivary gland tumors: pretherapy evaluation with PET, *Radiology* 192:99-102, 1994.

Mishkin FS: Radionuclide salivary gland imaging, *Semin Nucl Med* 11:258-265, 1981.

Van den Akker HP, Busemann-Sokole E: Absolute indications for salivary gland scintigraphy with $^{99m}$Tc-pertechnetate, *Oral Surg* 60:440-447, 1985.

## ULTRASONOGRAPHY OF THE MAJOR SALIVARY GLANDS

Gooding GAW: Gray scale ultrasound of the parotid gland, *AJR Am J Roentgenol* 134:469-472, 1980.

Gritzmann G: Sonography of the salivary glands, *AJR Am J Roentgenol* 153:161-166, 1989.

Mandel LK. Ultrasound findings in HIV-positive patients with parotid swellings, *J Oral Maxillofac Surg* 59:283-286, 2001.

Martinoli C, Derchi LE, Solbiati L et al: Color doppler sonography of salivary glands, *AJR Am J Roentgenol* 163:933-941, 1994.

Rothberg R, Noyek AM, Goldfinger M et al: Diagnostic ultrasound imaging of parotid disease-a contemporary clinical perspective, *J Otolaryngol* 13:232-240, 1984.

Shimizu M, Ussmüller J, Donath K et al: Sonographic analysis of recurrent parotitis in children: a comparative study with sialographic findings, *Oral Surg Oral Med Oral Pathol Oral Radiol Endod* 86:606-615, 1998.

## OBSTRUCTIVE AND INFLAMMATORY DISORDERS

Aung W, Yamada I, Umehara I et al: Sjögren's syndrome: comparison of assessments with quantitative salivary gland scintigraphy and contrast sialography, *J Nucl Med* 41:257-262, 2000.

Brook I: Acute bacterial suppurative parotitis: microbiology and management, *J Craniofac Surg* 14:37-40, 2003.

Gonzales L, Mackenzie AH, Tarar RA: Parotid sialography in Sjögren's syndrome, *Radiology* 97:91-93, 1970.

Hughes M, Carson K, Hill J: Scintigraphic evaluation of sialadenitis, *Br J Radiol* 67:328-331, 1994.

Kassan SS, Moutsopoulos HM: Clinical manifestations and early diagnosis of Sjögren syndrome, *Arch Intern Med* 164:1275-1284, 2004.

Langlais RP, Kasle MJ: Sialolithiasis: the radiolucent stones, *Oral Surg Oral Med Oral Pathol* 40:686-690, 1975.

Lemon SI, Imbesi SG, Shikhman AR: Salivary gland imaging in Sjögren syndrome , *Future Rheumatol* 2:83-92, 2007.

Scully C: Sjögren's syndrome: clinical and laboratory features, immunopathogenesis, and management, *Oral Surg Oral Med Oral Pathol* 62:510-523, 1986.

Som PM, Shugar JM, Train JS et al: Manifestations of parotid gland enlargement: radiographic, pathologic, and clinical correlation—part 1, the autoimmune pseudosialectasias, *Radiology* 141:415-419, 1981.

Yamamoto Y, Harada S, Ohara, M et al: Clinical and pathological differences between Mikulicz's disease and Sjögren's syndrome, *Rheumatology (Oxford)* 44:227-234, 2005.

## NONINFLAMMATORY DISORDERS

Chilla R: Sialadenosis of the salivary glands of the head. Studies on the physiology and pathophysiology of parotid secretion, *Adv Otorhinolaryngol* 26:1-38, 1981.

## CYSTS AND NEOPLASMS

Boahene DKO, Olsen KD, Lewis JE et al: Mucoepidermoid carcinoma of the parotid gland—the Mayo Clinic experience, *Arch Otolaryngol Head Neck Surg* 130:849-856, 2004.

Boles R, Raines J, Lebovits M et al: Malignant tumors of salivary glands: a university experience, *Laryngoscope* 90:729-736, 1980.

Byrne MN, Spector JG, Garvin CF et al: Preoperative assessment of parotid masses: a comparative evaluation of radiographic techniques to histologic diagnosis, *Laryngoscope* 99:284-292, 1989.

Day TA, Deveikis J, Gillespie MB et al: Salivary gland neoplasms, *Curr Treat Options Oncol* 5:11-26, 2004.

Del Balso AM, Williams E, Tane TT: Parotid masses: current modes of diagnostic imaging, *Oral Surg* 54:360-364, 1982.

Eneroth CM: Salivary gland tumors in the parotid gland and the palate region, *Cancer* 27:1415-1418, 1971.

Gottesman RI, Som PM, Mester J et al: Observations on two cases of apparent submandibular gland cysts in HIV positive patients: MR and CT findings, *J Comput Assist Tomogr* 20:444-447, 1996.

Mirich DR, McArdle CB, Kulkarni MV: Benign pleomorphic adenomas of the salivary glands: surface coil MR imaging versus CT, *J Comput Assist Tomogr* 11:620-623, 1987.

Thawley SE, Panbje WR: *Comprehensive management of head and neck tumors*, Philadelphia, 1987, WB Saunders.

Tsai SC, Hsu HT: Parotid neoplasms: diagnosis, treatment, and intraparotid facial nerve anatomy, *J Laryngol Otol* 116:359-362, 2002.

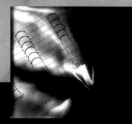

# Dental Implants

Byron W. Benson • Vivek Shetty

Few advances in dentistry have been as remarkable as the use of dental implants (Fig. 32-1) to restore orofacial form and function. Implant technology has enabled the dentist to help affected patients regain the ability to chew normally and function without embarrassment. With the application of precise surgical and prosthodontic techniques, implant-facilitated restorations allow for a very predictable prosthodontic successful rehabilitation of a broad spectrum of patients with very challenging needs. The predictable results of contemporary implant systems derive, in part, from increasingly sophisticated imaging techniques used in all phases of implant treatment. These imaging modalities contribute information for every stage of the treatment, extending from presurgical diagnosis and treatment planning through surgical placement and postoperative assessment of the implant, to the prosthetic restoration and long-term surveillance phase.

Acceptance of dental implantology as an integral part of conventional practice makes it necessary for the general dentist to be knowledgeable of implant imaging techniques and their clinical application. With the exception of the occasional subperiosteal, blade, and transosteal implant systems (Figs. 32-2 and 32-3), dental implants used today are almost exclusively root-form devices (see Fig. 32-1) embedded within the jaw bone (endosseous implants). The focus of this chapter is not only to provide information regarding the various imaging technologies available but also their specific application and the potential information that each can provide to facilitate the placement of endosseous implant restorations.

## Diagnostic Imaging for Dental Implants

Basic imaging, such as panoramic and periapical radiographs, are generally useful and cost-effective but do not provide the cross-sectional visualization or interactive image analysis that can be obtained with more sophisticated imaging techniques. The various imaging techniques can be applied to various phases of the surgical and restorative procedures (Table 32-1). The selection of a specific imaging technique should be based on the technique best suited to provide the information required by the implant team—the restorative dentist, surgeon, and radiologist (Table 32-2).

## Imaging Techniques

The ideal imaging technique for dental implant care should have several essential characteristics, including the ability to visualize the implant site in the mesiodistal, facial-lingual, and superoinferior dimensions; the ability to allow reliable, accurate measurements; a capacity to evaluate trabecular bone density and cortical thickness; a capacity to correlate the imaged site with the clinical site; reasonable access and cost to the patient; and minimal radiation risk. Usually a combination of radiographic techniques is used. Available radiographic techniques include intraoral radiography (film and digital), cephalometric radiography, panoramic radiography, and conventional tomography, as well as cone-beam and multidetector computed tomography (CBCT, MDCT). The following is a review of these imaging techniques as applied to dental implant case management.

## INTRAORAL RADIOGRAPHY

Intraoral images may be acquired on analog film or as digital images. Periapical and occlusal radiographic films provide images with superior resolution and sharpness. Periapical radiographs commonly are used to evaluate the status of adjoining teeth and remaining alveolar bone in the mesiodistal dimension. They also have been used for determining vertical height, architecture, and bone quality (bone density, amount of cortical bone, and amount of trabecular bone). Although readily available and relatively inexpensive, periapical radiography has geometric and anatomic limitations. Periapical radiographs, made on a dentate arch, typically are made with the paralleling technique, creating an image with minimal foreshortening and elongation (Fig. 32-4). Because of variations in the morphology of the residual edentulous alveolar ridge (Fig 32-5), the ridge may not have the same "long axis" as a tooth. Thus the position of the image receptor may not result in an accurate display of the height of the alveolar ridge as a result of image foreshortening and elongation. Also, it frequently is not possible to place the image receptor either superior or inferior enough to capture an image of the entire maxillary or mandibular ridge. It is reported that 25% of mandibular periapical radiographs do not demonstrate the mandibular canal. In cases when the canal was identifiable, only 53% of measurements from the alveolar crest to the superior wall of the mandibular canal were accurate within 1 mm.

Because periapical radiographs are unable to provide any cross-sectional information, occlusal radiographs are used on occasion to determine the facial-lingual dimensions of the mandibular alveolar ridge. Although somewhat useful, the occlusal image records only the widest portion of the mandible, which typically is located inferior to the alveolar ridge. This may give the clinician the impression that more bone is available in the cross-sectional (facial-lingual)

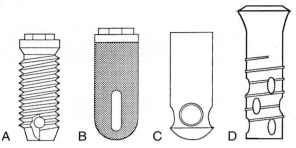

FIG. **32-1** Four common types of root-form implant fixtures. **A,** Brånemark. **B,** IMZ. **C,** Integral. **D,** ITI.

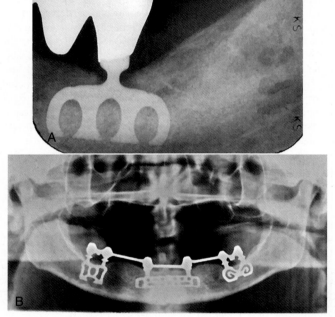

FIG. **32-2** **A,** Blade implant integrated with bone to support a fixed bridge (periapical radiograph of a mandibular molar). **B,** Three blade implants integrated with bone using common abutments to support a mandibular denture region. (**A** courtesy Krishan Kapur, DDS, Los Angeles, Calif.)

dimension than actually exists. The occlusal technique is not useful in imaging the maxillary arch because of anatomic limitations.

## LATERAL AND LATERAL-OBLIQUE CEPHALOMETRIC RADIOGRAPHY

Lateral cephalometric radiography provides an image of known magnification (usually 7% to 12%) that documents axial tooth inclinations and the dentoalveolar ridge relationships in the midline of the jaws. The soft tissue profile also is apparent on this film and can be used to evaluate profile alterations after prosthodontic rehabilitation. This projection can provide a cross-sectional view of only the maxillary and mandibular midline. Images of nonmidline structures are superimposed on the contralateral side, complicating the evaluation of other implant sites. Occasionally, lateral-oblique cephalometric radiography is used with one side of the mandibular body positioned parallel to the film cassette. Image magnification on these views is not predictable because the body of the mandible is not the same distance from the film as is the rotation center of the cephalostat (used to calculate object-film distance for image magnification values). Thus measurements made from these radiographs are not reliable. In general, cephalometric radiographs have significant limitations but may be useful in placement of some implants near the midline for overdentures.

## PANORAMIC RADIOGRAPHY

Although the resolution and sharpness of panoramic radiographs are less than those of intraoral radiographs, panoramic projections certainly provide a broader visualization of the jaws and adjoining ana-

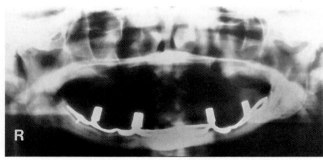

FIG. **32-3** Subperiosteal implant used for aiding denture support.

| TABLE **32-1** *Stage of Treatment* | | |
| --- | --- | --- |
| STAGE OF TREATMENT | TIME (mo) | RADIOGRAPHIC PROCEDURES |
| Treatment planning | −1 | PA, pan, tomo, CBCT/MDCT, ceph |
| Surgery (placement) | 0 | PA, pan, tomo, CBCT/MDCT, ceph for correction of problems |
| Healing | 0-3 | PA, pan, tomo, CBCT/MDCT, ceph for correction of problems |
| Remodelling | 4-12 | PA, pan |
| Maintenance (without problems) | 13+ | PA, pan, (following approximately every 3 years) |
| Complications | Anytime | PA, pan, CBCT/MDCT (as indicated) |

*PA,* Periapical; *pan,* panoramic radiography; *tomo,* conventional tomography; *CBCT,* cone-beam computed tomography; *MDCT,* multidetector computed tomography; *ceph,* lateral/lateral-oblique cephalometric radiography.

TABLE **32-2**
*Imaging Technique*

| IMAGING TECHNIQUE | APPLICATIONS | ADVANTAGES | DISADVANTAGES |
|---|---|---|---|
| Intraoral periapical radiography | S, M, E, A | Readily available<br>High image definition<br>Minimal distortion<br>Least cost and radiation exposure | Limited imaging area<br>No facial-lingual dimension<br>Limited reproducibility<br>Image elongation and foreshortening |
| Panoramic radiography | S, M, E, A | Readily available<br>Large imaging area<br>Minimal cost and radiation exposure | No facial-lingual dimension<br>Image distortion<br>Technique errors common<br>Inconsistent magnification<br>Geometric distortion |
| Conventional tomography | S, M, E, A | Minimal superimposition<br>Facial-lingual dimension<br>Uniform magnification<br>Measurements accurate within about 1 mm<br>Moderate cost<br>Simulates placement with software | Less image definition than plain films<br>Somewhat limited availability<br>Special training for interpretation<br>Sensitive to technique errors<br>Greater radiation exposure for multiple sites |
| Reformatted cone-beam computed tomography | M, E, A | Allows evaluation of all possible sites<br>No superimposition<br>Uniform magnification<br>Measurements accurate within about 1 mm<br>Estimates internal bone density<br>Simulates placement with software | Limited availability<br>Sensitive to technique errors<br>Some metallic image artifacts<br>Special training for interpretation<br>Moderate cost and radiation exposure<br>Volume averaging contributes to measurement error |
| Reformatted multidetector computed tomography | M, E, A | Allows evaluation of all possible sites<br>No superimposition<br>Uniform magnification<br>Measurements accurate within about 1 mm<br>Estimates internal bone density<br>Simulates placement with software | Limited availability<br>Sensitive to technique errors<br>Metallic image artifacts<br>Special training for interpretation<br>Higher cost and radiation exposure<br>Volume averaging contributes to measurement error |

*S,* Single implant: *M,* multiple implants (two to five); *E,* edentulous (6+); *A,* augmentation.

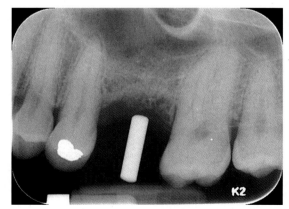

FIG. **32-4** An intraoral periapical radiograph of a potential implant site. The imaging stent indicates the desired axis of insertion.

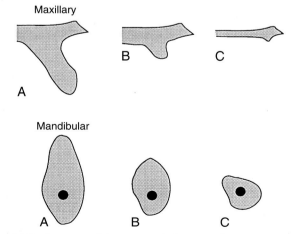

FIG. **32-5** Patterns of bone morphology in the anterior maxilla *(above)* and posterior mandible *(below)* in potential implant therapy patients. Minimal resorption **(A)**, moderate resorption **(B)**, and severe resorption **(C)** of alveolar bone. (Modified from Brånemark P-I, Zarb GA, Albrektsson T: *Tissue-integrated prostheses: osseointegration in clinical dentistry,* Chicago, 1985, Quintessence.)

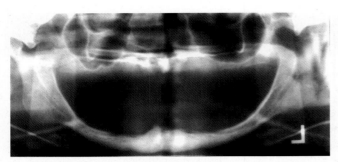

FIG. **32-6** Evaluation of potential implant sites by panoramic radiograph; note the severe atrophy of the maxillary and mandibular alveolar process.

tomic structures. Panoramic radiography units are widely available, making this imaging technique very useful and popular as a screening and assessment instrument. This technique is useful in making preliminary estimations of crestal alveolar bone and cortical boundaries of the mandibular canal, maxillary sinus, and nasal fossa (Fig. 32-6).

Information acquired from panoramic radiographs must be applied judiciously because this technique has significant limitations as a definitive presurgical planning tool. Angular measurements on panoramic radiographs tend to be accurate, but linear measurements are not. Image size distortion (magnification) varies significantly between films from different panoramic units and even within different areas of the same film. Vertical measurements are unreliable because of foreshortening and elongation of the anatomic structures because the x-ray beam is not perpendicular to the long axis of the anatomic structures or to the plane of the image receptor. The negative vertical angulation of the x-ray beam also causes lingually positioned objects such as mandibular tori to be projected superiorly on the film, resulting in an overestimation of vertical bone height. Furthermore, the anatomic vertical axis varies within the image, particularly in nonmidline areas. Compared with contact radiographs of dissected anatomic specimens, only 17% of panoramic measurements between the alveolar crest and superior wall of the mandibular canal were found to be accurate within 1 mm.

Similarly, dimensional accuracy in the horizontal plane of panoramic radiographs is highly dependent on the position of the structures of interest relative to the central plane of the image layer. The horizontal dimension of images of structures located facial or lingual to the central plane but still within the image layer tends to be minified or magnified. The degree of horizontal size distortion is difficult to ascertain on panoramic radiographs because the shape of the image layer is configured to a population average and the anatomic morphology of only a few individuals conforms totally to that image layer. In summary, horizontal image magnification with panoramic radiographs varies from 0.70 to 2.2 times the actual size, which some manufacturers report as a 1.25 average magnification (at the central plane of the image layer). Errors in patient positioning can further exacerbate measurement error in the horizontal dimension. The deficient dimensional accuracy of the two-dimensional panoramic image is further limited by the lack of any cross-sectional information.

## CONVENTIONAL TOMOGRAPHY

Used as an adjunct to screening radiographs, cross-sectional tomograms enhance visualization of the available bone by providing reli-

able dimensional measurements at proposed implant sites, especially the cross-sectional (facial-lingual) dimension. Tomographic machines were readily available but now are being replaced with CBCT machines. This technique produces a cross-sectional, flat-plane image layer that is perpendicular to the x-ray beam. Images of anatomic structures of interest are relatively sharp, and images of structures outside the image layer are blurred beyond recognition by the motion of the x-ray tube and image receptor. The thickness, orientation, and anatomic location of the image layer can be predetermined and manipulated. To obtain reliable measurements, it is critical that the image layer be a true cross-section of the curve of the alveolar process, rather than oblique. Scout images (usually a submentovertex, occlusal, or panoramic projection) or wax bite registrations or dental models are commonly used to determine the appropriate cross-sectional angulation. The complex (multidirectional) tube motion of current conventional tomographic units minimizes image superimposition and provides fixed, uniform image magnification, thus allowing for accurate measurements. Complex tube motion also permits use of a thicker image layer while retaining diagnostic quality. A thicker image layer is desirable to maximize image contrast, making the identification of structures such as the mandibular canal more predictable. Conventional tomographic images may be acquired as analog films or digital images.

The dimensional accuracy of cross-sectional tomograms is particularly useful in measuring the distance between the alveolar crest and adjacent structures, such as the floor of the nasal fossa, maxillary sinus floor, mandibular canal, mental canal, and inferior mandibular cortex. The appropriate buccal-lingual axis of insertion of the implant may also be assessed preoperatively. Measurements are directly acquired from the images and subsequently corrected by the magnification factor used. As an alternative, acetate overlays with appropriately magnified 1-mm grids may be used with film-based images or on digital monitors when the display is life sized (Fig. 32-7). Published research suggests a measurement error of less than 1 mm in optimal images. Typically, two to three cross-sectional tomographic slices are required to adequately image each intended implant site. Conventional tomography is especially convenient in the planning of single implants or multiple implants within a quadrant (Fig. 32-8).

## REFORMATTED CONE-BEAM AND MULTIDETECTOR COMPUTED TOMOGRAPHY

Patients who are edentulous or who are being considered for multiple implants and augmentation procedures may be best imaged with either CBCT or MDCT to investigate all possible implant sites. For traditional MDCT, a lateral scout image of the selected jaw with the necessary alignment corrections for the mandible or maxilla is typically an essential initial step for the MDCT study. The jaws are aligned so that the acquired axial computed tomographic image slices are parallel to the occlusal plane. These axial images are thin (1-2 mm) and overlapping, resulting in approximately 30 axial image slices per jaw. The image information of these sequential axial images can be postprocessed to produce multiple two-dimensional images in various planes, using a computer-based process called multiplanar reformatting (MPR).

CBCT images are acquired with an initial scout image followed by a single revolution imaging sequence. The vertical height of the imaging sequence can be adjusted to include only one jaw, both, or a larger area, especially if the temporomandibular joint needs to be

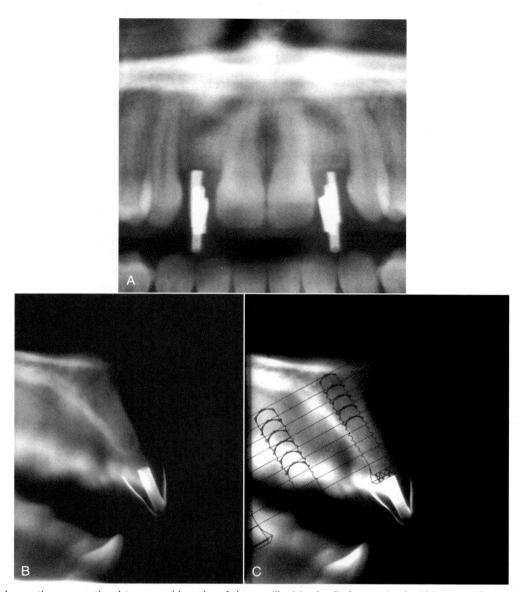

FIG. **32-7**   Complex-motion conventional tomographic series of the maxilla. Metal cylinders retained within an acrylic imaging stent are used to indicate the planned implant sites. Foil strips have been placed on the stent to indicate desired buccal and lingual contours of the restoration. **A,** A scout panoramic radiograph used to orient subsequent tomograms. **B,** Cross-sectional tomograms appropriate for measuring the height and width of the alveolar ridge, as well as the axial orientation of the proposed implant. **C,** A clear plastic overlay is placed over the tomogram to visualize implant placement and determine desired length. The overlay is the same magnification as the tomographic image. (Courtesy Oral and Maxillofacial Imaging Center, Baylor College of Dentistry, Dallas, Tex.)

included in the imaged area. MPR processing is also accomplished with the CBCT data.

The reformatted images of both types of computed tomographic data result in three basic image types: axial images with a computer-generated superimposed curve of the alveolar process and the associated reformatted alveolar cross-sectional images and panoramic-like images. An axial image that includes the full contour of the mandible (or maxilla) at a level corresponding to the dental roots is typically selected as a reference for the reformatting process. With use of a computer program, a series of sequential dots on the selected axial scan are connected to develop a customized arch or curve unique for each jaw. The computer program then generates a series of lines per-

pendicular to the curve of the individual arch. These lines are made at constant intervals (usually 1 to 2 mm) and numbered sequentially on the axial and panoramic (curved linear) images to indicate the position at which each cross-sectional slice will be reconstructed (Figs. 32-9 and Fig. 32-10). Cross-sectional alveolar reconstructions are made perpendicular to the curve, and panoramic (curved linear) reconstructions are made parallel with the curve. Three-dimensional representations may also be constructed in various orientations.

Such reformatted images provide the clinician with accurate two-dimensional diagnostic information in all three dimensions. Typical computed tomographic studies provide information on the continu-

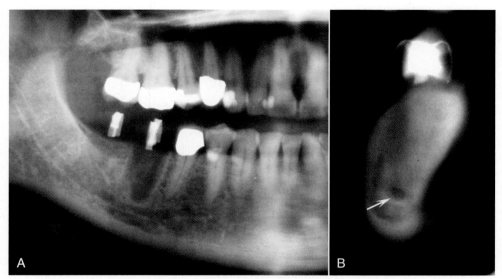

FIG. **32-8**    Complex-motion conventional tomographic series of the mandible. Metal cylinders retained within an acrylic imaging stent have been used to indicate the planned implant sites. **A,** Scout panoramic radiograph used to orient the subsequent tomograms. **B,** Cross-sectional tomogram appropriate for measuring the height and width of the alveolar ridge and the axial orientation of the proposed implant. Note the mandibular canal *(arrow)*. (Courtesy Oral and Maxillofacial Imaging Center, Baylor College of Dentistry, Dallas, Tex.)

ity of the cortical bone plates, residual bone in the mandible and maxilla, the relative location of adjoining vital structures, and the contour of soft tissues covering the osseous structures. Studies have reported that 94% of computed tomographic measurements between the alveolar crest and wall of the mandibular canal were accurate within 1 mm. Reformatted images from CBCT data have been shown to be of equivalent measurement accuracy as MDCT data. These reformations are also useful in the planning augmentation procedures such as a sinus lift and can provide an estimate of the internal density. A three-dimensional image can provide a visualization of the overall morphology of the intended implant site.

Reformatted CBCT/MDCT images may be printed as life size on photographic prints or radiographic film. If the study is to be viewed electronically as individual static images on a monitor, a measurement scale is typically incorporated into the image for calibration. Alternatively, the reformatted study may also be viewed with interactive software. The panoramic (curved linear) images are helpful in identifying mesial-distal relationships and noncorticated mandibular canals. However, the quality of the reformatted computed tomographic study depends on the ability of the patient to remain still during image acquisition because movement may produce geometric image distortion. Because of the shorter acquisition times, this is less of an issue with CBCT. Metallic restorations can cause streak image artifacts, but this can be avoided by aligning the jaws so that the acquired axial scans are parallel to the occlusal plane, which sometimes keeps the artifact from obscuring the alveolar crest. Metallic artifacts are less prominent on CBCT by nature of the image acquisition physics. All the images in computed tomographic studies for dental implant studies should be adequately interpreted by an oral and maxillofacial radiologist or other appropriately trained dentist or physician. This is especially important because a rather large anatomic area outside the region of interest is included in the primary images and must be reviewed.

## Preoperative Planning

Radiographic visualization of potential implant sites is an important extension of clinical examination and assessment. Radiographs help the clinician visualize the alveolar ridges and adjacent structures in all three dimensions and guide the choice of site, number, size, and axial orientation of the implants. Site selection includes consideration of adjacent anatomic structures such as the incisive and mental foramina, inferior alveolar canal, existing teeth, nasal fossae, and maxillary sinuses. Conditions, including retained root fragments, impacted teeth, and any osseous pathoses that could compromise the outcome, must be identified and located relative to the site of the proposed implant.

Diagnostic images of potential implant sites can provide information about the quality and quantity of bone that would be adequate to support the implant fixture. The quality of bone includes assessment of the cortical bone because it is best suited to withstand the functional loading forces of dental implants. There is a greater likelihood of successful osseous integration when there is a thicker cortical bone. A greater number of internal trabeculae per unit area is also advantageous.

Bone quantity is assessed by documenting the height and width of available alveolar bone and the morphology of the ridge. The chances of a successful outcome will increase with a greater amount of bone available for anchorage. A cross-sectional image to document the facial-lingual width and height of the ridge, along with the inclination of the bone contours, is especially useful in the preoperative planning phase. Alveolar ridge width measurements aid in selecting the implant diameter and implant placement to maximally engage cortical bone. Ridge height measurements help select the largest appropriate fixture to maximize anchorage and distribution of masticatory forces. Frequently, morphologic features such as osseous undercuts and ridge concavities that are not immediately apparent on clinical examination become evident with cross-sectional imaging.

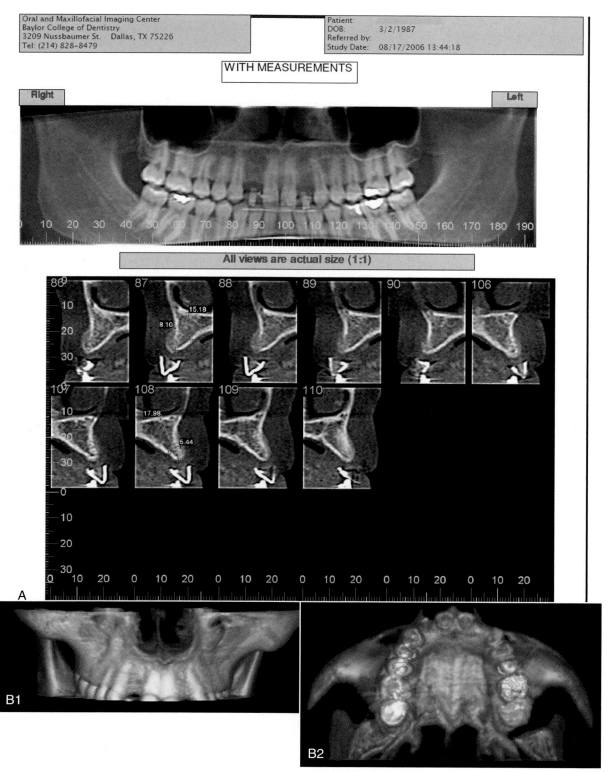

FIG. **32-9**  Reformatted cone-beam CT study of the maxilla. **A,** Panoramic-like curved linear and alveolar cross-sectional reconstructed images using an imaging stent incorporating radiopaque strips to define the buccal and palatal contours of the planned prosthesis. Note the measurements on the cross-section images. **B,** Three-dimensional reformatted images to visualize the morphology of the intended implant sites. (Courtesy Oral and Maxillofacial Imaging Center, Baylor College of Dentistry, Dallas, Tex.)

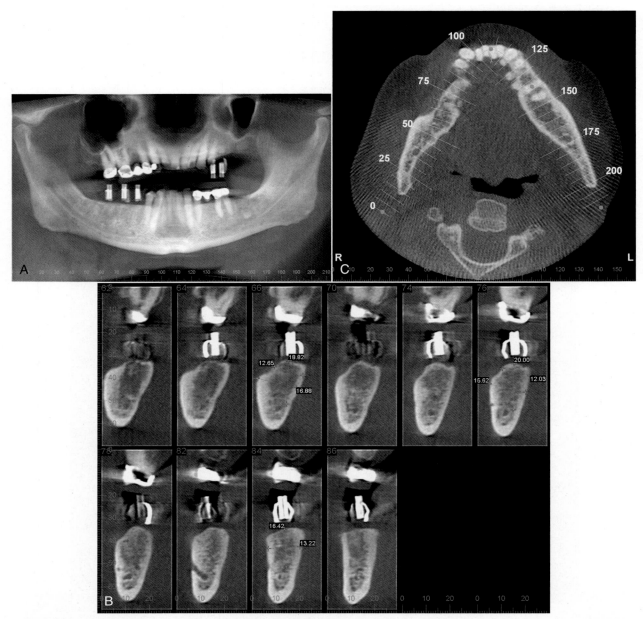

FIG. **32-10**   Reformatted cone-beam CT study of the mandible. **A,** Panoramic-like curved linear reconstructed image. The imaging stent incorporates copper cylinders for the path of insertion and radiopaque strips defining the buccal and lingual contours of the proposed prosthesis. The copper cylinders will allow the imaging stent to be used as a surgical guide when the implants are placed. **B,** Correlating cross-sectional images. **C,** Reformatted axial image through the alveolar ridge depicting the panoramic arc and correlated cross-sectional images. (Courtesy Oral and Maxillofacial Imaging Center, Baylor College of Dentistry, Dallas, Tex.)

Accurate bone measurements are essential for determining the optimal size and length and orientation of the proposed implants. When measurements are made on any image, the fact that the magnification factor of the image might vary with the imaging technique used must be considered. Except for specialized interactive reformatted computed tomography implant programs; all other radiographic images have a magnification factor, which must be taken into account when the dimensions of the bone are calculated. The measurements obtained from the images (usually in millimeters) are divided by the magnification factor for that particular imaging technique. As described earlier, the magnification factor of some techniques may be variable (periapical, panoramic), and thus a constant magnification factor cannot be applied. With dental implant computed tomographic reformatting software, the image is reproduced in the actual size of the jaw without magnification. If the magnification factor is constant, clear plastic overlays with 1-mm grids or diagrams of available implant sizes already corrected for the specific magnification factor can be used directly on printed images or on the viewing monitor with the image displayed at 1:1. The magnification of electronic images can also be calibrated with the measurement tool.

## IMAGING STENTS

The clinical utility of presurgical imaging can be enhanced by the use of an imaging stent that helps relate the radiographic image and its information to a precise anatomic location or a potential surgical site. In the case of conventional and computed tomography, an imaging stent also facilitates correlation of the individual image slices to an anatomic location in the scout films. The intended implant sites are identified by markers made of radiopaque spheres or rods (metal, composite resin, or gutta-percha) retained within an acrylic stent (Fig. 32-11; see Fig. 32-7), which the patient wears during the imaging procedure so that images of the markers will be created in the diagnostic images. The imaging stent subsequently may be used as a surgical guide to orient the insertion angle of the guide bur and hence the angle of the implant. For optimal visualization, the width of the markers should be less than the thickness of the conventional tomographic image layer. Diagnostic dentures coated with barium paste may be used during imaging for localization and can also establish the spatial relationships between the anticipated prosthesis and the implant fixtures. Generally, nonmetallic radiopaque markers (gutta-percha, composite resin) are used in computed tomographic imaging because of the image artifacts that would be produced by metal markers. However, some metals scatter less than others. The metallic scatter artifact of some CBCT units appears to be less than that of MDCT units. Existing rootform implants do not produce a significant computed tomographic scatter artifact.

## INTERACTIVE DIAGNOSTIC SOFTWARE

Several different interactive software packages that can simulate implant orientation and placement on a computer screen before surgery have been developed. They are designed for use on personal computers, typically requiring a Windows (Microsoft, Redmond, Wash.) operating system. Diagnostic software is available for both conventional tomography and reformatted computed tomography. These programs provide an interactive analysis of potential implant sites for bone quantity, quality, and morphology and can simulate the surgical placement of the implant. Visualization of anatomic structures, volumetric analysis for bone grafts, and mechanical analysis of structural forces during restoration are also within the capability of the software packages (Fig. 32-12).

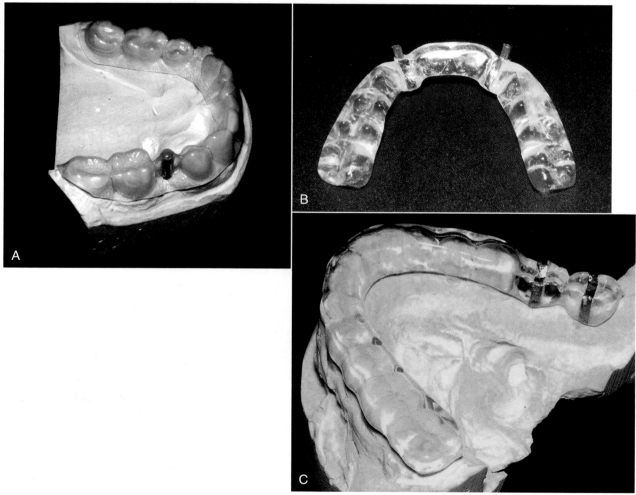

FIG. **32-11**   Three examples of imaging stents. **A,** A vacuum-formed imaging stent with a metal rod to indicate desired axis of insertion. **B,** A processed stent with metal cylinders marking the implant sites. This can also be used as a surgical stent by inserting the guide bur through the cylinders. **C,** A processed stent with insertion axis markers, along with a radiopaque strip outlining the buccal and lingual contours of the planned restoration. The stent provides an image of the emergence profile of the restored implant and can also be used as a surgical guide.

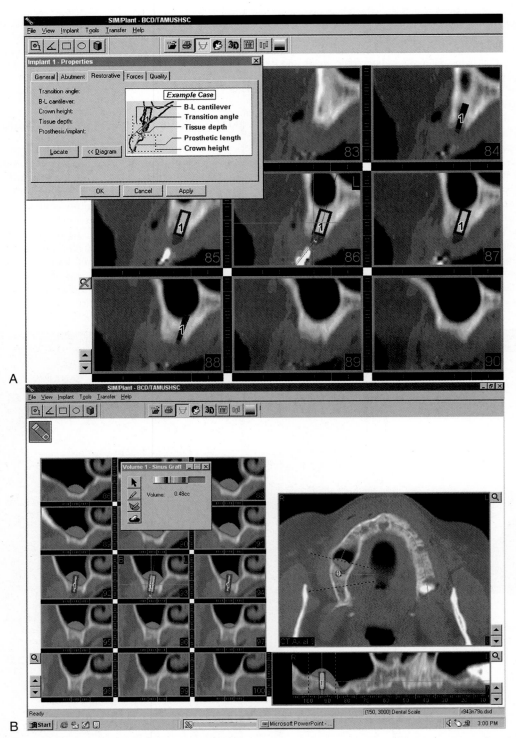

FIG. **32-12**   SIMPlant (Materialise, New Berne, Md.) interactive software. **A,** Simulation of implant placement and predicted restorative dimensions are displayed on cross-sectional images. **B,** The volume of bone grafting material for a sinus lift procedure is predicted in a case with inadequate alveolar ridge height.

## SELECTING DIAGNOSTIC IMAGING FOR PREOPERATIVE PLANNING

A good starting point would be to proceed with a panoramic image and possibly intraoral radiographs if greater image detail is required of any particular region of interest. These survey radiographs would help determine whether the patient is a good candidate for implant procedures. For instance, if there is a pathologic lesion in the planned implant site or if there is obviously inadequate vertical dimension from severe atrophy of the alveolar ridges, there is no sense in proceeding with more expensive imaging procedures such as conventional or computed tomography. If the initial scout films reveal reasonable potential implant sites, then either conventional or computed tomography can be used to obtain cross-sectional image slices of these sites (see Table 32-2 and Fig. 32-13). Generally, if images are required of all of the maxilla and mandible to evaluate possible implant sites, then computed tomography would be the best modality. If potential sites are restricted to a few selected regions, then conventional tomography would be a suitable choice. However, the ease of acquisition and relatively low radiation risk of CBCT makes this technique a very viable alternative study even for single implants.

## Intraoperative and Postoperative Assessments

Intraoral and panoramic radiographs usually are adequate for both intraoperative and postoperative assessments (Fig. 32-14). Intraoperative imaging may be required to confirm correct placement of the implant or to locate a lost implant (Fig. 32-15). The two aspects that are usually assessed with time after implant placement are the alveolar bone height around the implant and the appearance of the bone immediately adjacent to and surrounding the implant. If threaded rootform fixtures have been placed, the optimal radiographic image must separate the threads for best visualization. This may not always be a predictable procedure because the exact angulation of the implant is not known. The angulation of the x-ray beam must be within 9 degrees of the long axis of the fixture to open the threads on the image on most threaded fixtures (Fig. 32-16). Angular deviations of 13 degrees or more result in complete overlap of the threads. In general, periapical radiographs are appropriate for longitudinal assessments. However, in evaluating the bone height around an implant, an effort should be made to reproduce the vertical angulation of the central ray of the x-ray beam as closely as possible between

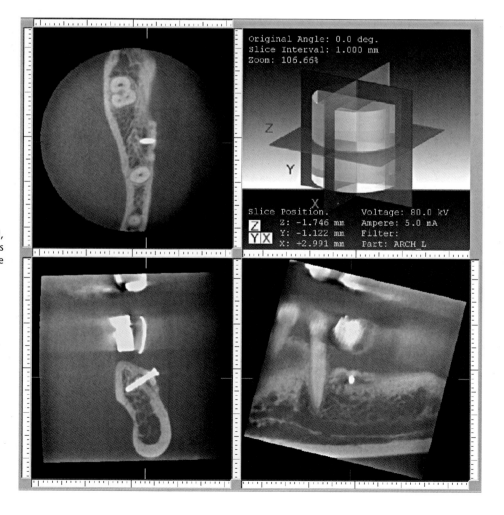

FIG. **32-13** Reformatted axial, coronal, and sagittal cone-beam CT images to assess the viability of an osseous graft before implant placement.

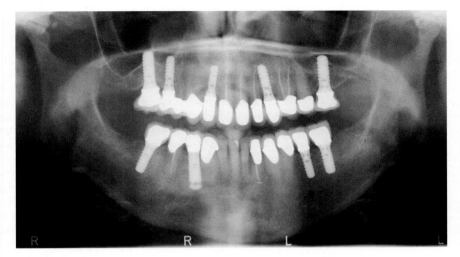

FIG. **32-14** A panoramic radiograph used for postoperative assessment of multiple successfully restored rootform implants. The threads are visualized on all of the implants except for the mandibular right premolar, which is a smooth cylinder.

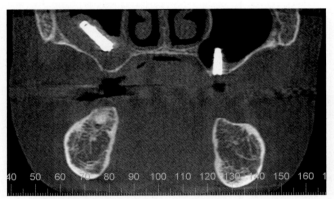

FIG. **32-15** Reformatted cone-beam CT study for postoperative assessment of an implant cylinder displaced into the right maxillary sinus, associated with mucositis in the right antrum. The implant on the left alveolus is not well supported by bone and extends well into the antrum. (Courtesy Oral and Maxillofacial Imaging Center, Baylor College of Dentistry, Dallas, Tex.)

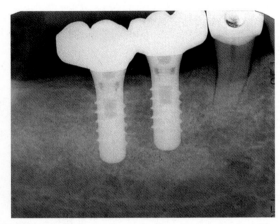

FIG. **32-16** A periapical radiograph of two successful dental implants. Note the close apposition of the bone to the surface of each implant. A minor amount of saucerization is present at the alveolar crest adjacent to the distal fixture.

radiographs to closely duplicate the image geometry. Mesial and distal marginal bone height is measured from a standard landmark at the collar of the implant or, in the case of threaded implants, by use of known interthread measurements and compared with bone levels in previous periapical radiographs. The presence of relatively distinct bone margins with a constant height relative to the implant suggests successful osseous integration. Any resorptive changes, if present, are evidenced by apical migration of the alveolar bone or indistinct osseous margins. These adverse changes are progressive and should be differentiated from the initial circumscribed resorptive osseous changes around the cervical area of the fixture occurring during the first 6 months that are induced by the surgical procedure itself (Fig. 32-17). Studies suggest that the rate of marginal bone loss after successful implantation is approximately 1.2 mm in the first year, subsequently tapering off to about 0.1 mm in succeeding years. Subtle areas of bone resorption adjacent to the fixture may be made more evident with intraoral digital images by evaluating a density

profile graph of radiographic density values, a feature available on most digital imaging units. If intraoral digital images are acquired at surgery, they may be compared with subsequent digital images either by subjective visualization or digital subtraction. Digital subtraction of sequential radiographs is a computerized process that may reveal areas of bone resorption not apparent visually but requires that the image geometry be reproduced between radiographic examinations. Occasionally, areas of marginal bone gain also may be noted.

The success of an implant can also be evaluated by the appearance of normal bone surrounding it and its apposition to the surface of the implant body. The development of a thin radiolucent area that closely follows the outline of the implant usually correlates to clinically detectable implant mobility; it is an important indicator of failed osseointegration (Fig. 32-18). Changes in the periodontal ligament space of associated teeth (natural abutment) are also useful in monitoring the functional competence of the implant-prostheses compos-

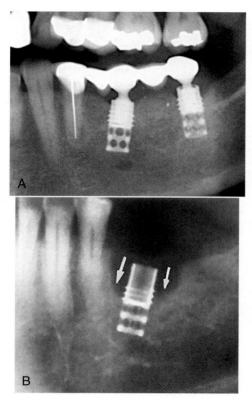

FIG. **32-17** **A,** Marginal bone loss around the cervical region of a rootform dental implant (portion of a panoramic radiograph). **B,** Periapical radiograph of moderate bone loss ("saucerization" type) around the cervical region of a rootform dental implant *(arrows).*

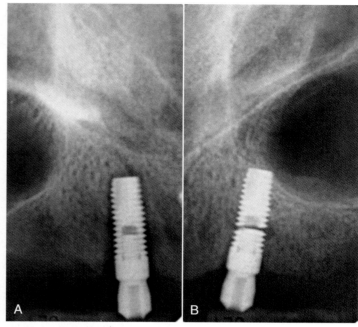

FIG. **32-18** **A,** Periapical radiograph of bone loss around a root-form dental implant (thin radiolucent band surrounding the implant), indicating failure of osseous integration. **B,** Periapical view of a fractured endosseous implant.

---

TABLE **32-3**
## *Radiographic Signs Associated with Failing Endosseous Implants*

| RADIOGRAPHIC APPEARANCE | CLIINICAL IMPLICATIONS |
| --- | --- |
| Thin radiolucent area that closely follows the entire outline of the implant | Failure of the implant to integrate with the adjoining bone |
| Crestal bone loss around the coronal portion of the implant | Osteitis resulting from poor plaque control, adverse loading, or both |
| Apical migration of alveolar bone on one side of the implant | Nonaxial loading resulting from improper angulation of the implant |
| Widening of the periodontal ligament space of the nearest natural (tooth) abutment | Poor stress distribution resulting from biomechanically inadequate prosthesis-implant system |
| Fracture of the implant fixture | Unfavorable stress distribution during function |

---

ite. Any widening of the periodontal ligament space compared with baseline radiographs indicates poor stress distribution and forecasts implant failure (Table 32-3). After successful implantation, radiographs may be made at regular intervals to assess the success or failure of the implant fixture. Advanced imaging studies may be necessary for adequate assessment in some cases (Figs. 32-19 and 32-20).

In summary, diagnostic imaging is an integral part of dental implant therapy for presurgical planning, intraoperative assessment, and postoperative assessment by use of a variety of imaging techniques. Cross-sectional imaging is increasingly considered essential for optimal implant placement, especially in the case of complex reconstructions.

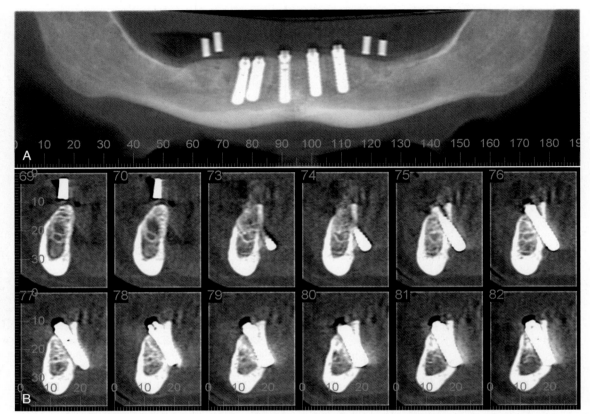

FIG. **32-19**  **A,** Panoramic-like curved linear reformatted cone-beam CT (CBCT) image initially made for implant planning. In this image, the existing implants appear reasonably normal in orientation. **B,** The cross-sectional reformatted CBCT images reveal nonrestorable ectopic placement of the existing implants with lingual cortical perforation and extension into the lingual tissues. (Courtesy Oral and Maxillofacial Imaging Center, Baylor College of Dentistry, Dallas, Tex.)

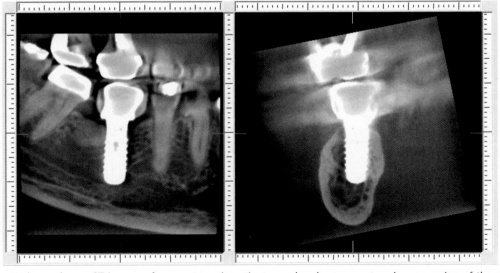

FIG. **32-20**  Reformatted cone-beam CT images of a symptomatic patient reveal embarrassment and compression of the mandibular canal by the implant.

# BIBLIOGRAPHY

## COMPARATIVE DOSIMETRY

Avendanio B, Frederiksen NL, Benson BW et al: Estimate of radiation detriment: scanography and intraoral radiology, *Oral Surg Oral Med Oral Pathol Oral Radiol Endod* 82:713-719, 1996.

Cohnen M, Kemper J, Möbes O et al: Radiation dose in dental radiology, *Eur Radiol* 12:634-637, 2002.

Frederiksen NL, Benson BW, Sokolowski TW: Risk assessment from film tomography used for dental implant diagnostics, *Dentomaxillofac Radiol* 23:123-127, 1994.

Frederiksen NL, Benson BW, Sokolowski TW: Effective dose and risk assessment from computed tomography of the maxillofacial complex, *Dentomaxillofac Radiol* 24:55-58, 1995.

Lecomber AR, Yoneyama Y, Lovelock DJ et al: Comparison of patient dose from imaging protocols for dental implant planning suing conventional radiography and computed tomography, *Dentomaxillofac Radiol* 30:255-259, 2001.

Ludlow JB, Davies-Ludlow LE, Brooks SL et al: Dosimetry of 3 CBCT devices for oral and maxillofacial radiology: CB Mercuray, NewTom 3G and i-CAT, *Dentomaxillofac Radiol* 35:219-226, 2006; erratum *Dentomaxillofac Radiol* 35:392.

Scaf G, Lurie AG, Mosier KM et al: Dosimetry and cost of imaging for osseointegrated implants with film-based and computed tomography, *Oral Surg Oral Med Oral Pathol Oral Radiol Endod* 83:41-48, 1997.

Schulze D, Heiland M, Thurmann H et al: Radiation exposure during midfacial imaging using 4- and 16-slice computed tomography, cone beam computed tomography systems and conventional tomography, *Dentomaxillofac Radiol* 33:83-86, 2004.

## COMPUTED TOMOGRAPHY (CBCT AND MDCT)

Hashimoto K, Kawashima S, Araki M et al: Comparison of image performance between cone-beam computed tomography for dental use and four-row multidetector helical CT, *J Oral Sci* 48:27-34, 2006.

Hatcher DC, Dial C, Mayorga C: Cone beam CT for presurgical assessment of implant sites, *J Calif Dent Assoc* 31:825-833, 2003.

Lascala CA, Panella J, Marques MM: Analysis of the accuracy of linear measurements obtained by cone beam computed tomography (CBCT–NewTom), *Dentomaxillofac Radiol* 33:291-294, 2004.

McGivney GP, Haughton V, Strandt JA et al: A comparison of computer-assisted tomography and data-gathering modalities in prosthodontics, *Int J Oral Maxillofac Implants* 1:55-68, 1986.

Rothman SLG: *Dental applications of computed tomography—surgical planning for implant placement*, Chicago, 1998, Quintessence.

Scarfe WC, Farman AG, Sukovic P: Clinical applications of cone-beam computed tomography in dental practice, *J Can Dent Assoc* 72:75-80, 2006.

Schwarz MS, Rothman SL, Rhodes ML et al: Computed tomography, I: preoperative assessment of the mandible for endosseous implant surgery, *Int J Oral Maxillofac Implants* 2:137-141, 1987.

Schwarz MS, Rothman SL, Rhodes ML et al: Computed tomography, II: preoperative assessment of the maxilla for endosseous implant surgery, *Int J Oral Maxillofac Implants* 2:143-148, 1987.

Sukovic P: Cone beam computed tomography in craniofacial imaging, *Orthod Craniofacial Res* 6(1 Suppl):31-36, 2003.

Wishan MS, Bahat O, Krane M: Computed tomography as an adjunct in dental implant surgery, *Int J Periodontics Restorative Dent* 8:30-47, 1988.

Zhang L, Zhu XR, Lee AK et al: Reducing metal artifacts in cone-beam CT images by preprocessing projection data, *Int J Radiat Oncol Biol Phys* 67:924-932, 2007.

## CONVENTIONAL TOMOGRAPHY

Ekestubbe A, Gröndahl K, Gröndahl HG: The use of tomography for dental implant planning, *Dentomaxillofac Radiol* 26:206-213, 1997.

Gröndahl K, Ekestubbe A, Gröndahl HG et al: Reliability of hypocycloidal tomography for the evaluation of the distance from the alveolar crest to the mandibular canal, *Dentomaxillofac Radiol* 20:200-204, 1991.

Stella JP, Tharanon W: A precise radiographic method to determine the location of the inferior alveolar canal in the posterior edentulous mandible: implications for dental implants, I: technique, *Int J Oral Maxillofac Implants* 5:15-22, 1990.

Stella JP, Tharanon W: A precise radiographic method to determine the location of the inferior alveolar canal in the posterior edentulous mandible: implications for dental implants, II: clinical application, *Int J Oral Maxillofac Implants* 5:23-29, 1990.

## GENERAL IMAGING TECHNIQUES

Benson BW: Diagnostic imaging for dental implant assessment, *Tex Dent J* 112:37-41, 1995.

Benson BW: Presurgical radiographic planning for dental implants, *Oral Maxillofac Surg Clin North Am* 13:751-761, 2001.

DeSmet E, Jacobs R, Gijbels F et al: The accuracy and reliability of radiographic methods for the assessment of marginal bone level around oral implants, *Dentomaxillofac Radiol* 31:176-181, 2002.

Holmes SM: iCAT scanning in the dental office, *Fortress Guardian* 9:2, 2007.

Milgrom P, Getz T: Implants: growing concern, *Dental Claims and Insurance News* 8:1, 1994 [newsletter].

Reddy MS, Wang IC: Radiographic determinants of implant performance, *Adv Dent Res* 13:136-145, 1999.

Sahiwal IG, Woody RD, Benson BW et al: Radiographic identification of nonthreaded endosseous dental implants, *J Prosthet Dent* 87:552-562, 2002.

Sahiwal IG, Woody RD, Benson BW et al: Radiographic identification of threaded endosseous dental implants, *J Prosthet Dent* 87:563-577, 2002.

Tyndall DA, Brooks SL: Selection criteria for dental implant site imaging: a position paper of the American Academy of Oral and Maxillofacial Radiology, *Oral Surg Oral Med Oral Pathol Oral Radiol Endod* 89:630-637, 2000.

## GENERAL IMPLANTOLOGY

Misch CE: *Dental implant prosthodontics*, St. Louis, 2005, Elsevier Mosby.

Miyamoto I, Tsuboi Y, Suwa H et al: Influence of cortical bone thickness and implant length on implant stability at the time of surgery—clinical, prospective, biomechianical, and imaging study, *Bone* 37:776-780, 2005.

Palmer RM, Smith BJ, Howe LC et al: *Implants in clinical dentistry*, Chicago, 1998, Quintessence.

Sahiwal I, Woody RD, Benson BW et al: Macro design morphology of endosseous dental implants, *J Prosthet Dent* 87:543-551, 2002.

## IMAGING STENTS

Cehreli MC, Aslan Y, Sahin S: Bilaminar dual-purpose stent for placement of dental implants, *J Prosthet Dent* 84:55-58, 2000.

Kopp KC, Koslow AH, Abdo OS: Predictable implant placement with a diagnostic/surgical template and advanced radiographic imaging, *J Prosthet Dent* 89:611-615, 2003.

Ku YC, Shen YF: Fabrication of a radiographic and surgical stent for implants with a vacuum former, *J Prosthet Dent* 83:252-253, 2000.

## INTERACTIVE COMPUTER SOFTWARE

Fortin T, Bosson JL, Coudert JL et al: Reliability of preoperative planning of an image-guiding system for oral implant placement based on 3-dimensional images: an in vivo study, *Int J Oral Maxillofac Implants* 18:886-893, 2003.

Guerrero ME, Jacobs R, Loubele M et al: State-of-the-art cone beam CT imaging for preoperative planning of implant placement, *Clin Oral Investig* 10:1, 2006.

Rosenfeld AL, Mandelaris GA, Tardieu PB: Prosthetically directed implant placement using computer software to ensure precise placement and predictable prosthetic outcomes, 1: diagnostics, imaging, and collaborative accountability, *Int J Periodontics Restorative Dent* 26:215-221, 2006.

## PANORAMIC RADIOGRAPHY

Tal H, Moses O: A comparison of panoramic radiography with computed tomography in the planning of implant surgery, *Dentomaxillofac Radiol* 20:40-42, 1991.

Truhlar RS, Morris HF, Ochi S: A review of panoramic radiography and its potential use in implant dentistry, *Implant Dent* 2:122-130, 1993.

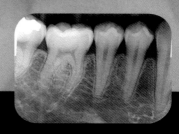

# Index

Page numbers followed by f indicate figures;
t, tables; b, boxes.